AF333643

Biomaterials Fabrication and Processing

HANDBOOK

Biomaterials Fabrication and Processing

HANDBOOK

Edited by

Paul K. Chu
Xuanyong Liu

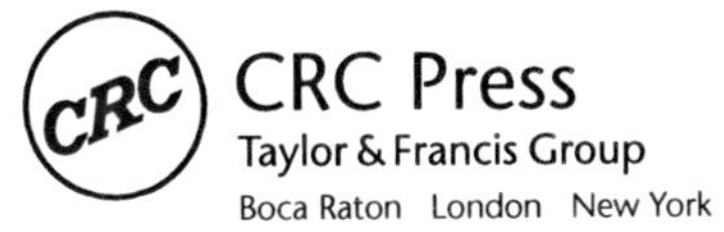

CRC Press
Taylor & Francis Group
Boca Raton   London   New York

CRC Press is an imprint of the
Taylor & Francis Group, an **informa** business

CRC Press
Taylor & Francis Group
6000 Broken Sound Parkway NW, Suite 300
Boca Raton, FL 33487-2742

© 2008 by Taylor & Francis Group, LLC
CRC Press is an imprint of Taylor & Francis Group, an Informa business

No claim to original U.S. Government works
Printed in the United States of America on acid-free paper
10 9 8 7 6 5 4 3 2 1

International Standard Book Number-13: 978-0-8493-7973-4 (Hardcover)

Library of Congress Cataloging-in-Publication Data

Biomaterials fabrication and processing handbook / [edited by] Paul K. Chu and Xuanyong Liu.
     p. ; cm.
   "A CRC title."
   Includes bibliographical references and index.
   ISBN 978-0-8493-7973-4 (alk. paper)
    1. Biomedical materials. 2. Biomedical engineering. I. Chu, Paul K. II. Liu, Xuanyong. III. Title.
   [DNLM: 1. Biocompatible Materials. 2. Biosensing Techniques. 3. Nanotechnology--methods. 4. Tissue Engineering--methods. QT 37 B61413 2008]

   R857.M3B5696 2008
   610.284--dc22   2007042613

**Visit the Taylor & Francis Web site at
http://www.taylorandfrancis.com**

**and the CRC Press Web site at
http://www.crcpress.com**

Contents

PART I   Tissue Engineering Scaffold Materials

PART II   Drug Delivery Systems

PART III Nano Biomaterials and Biosensors

PART IV Other Biomaterials

Contents vii

Preface

Biomaterials are used in the biomedical industry to replace or repair injured and nonfunctional tissues. The worldwide biomaterials market was worth over \$300 billion in 2005. This market is projected to grow at a rate of 20% per year, and a growing number of scientists and engineers are engaged in fabrication and research of biomaterials. Recognizing the ever increasing importance of biomaterials, a number of books on biomaterials were published in the past 20 years. The *Biomaterials Fabrication and Processing Handbook* is different from these published books in that it brings together the various aspects of fabrication and processing of the latest biomaterials, including tissue engineering scaffold materials, drug delivery systems, and nanobiomaterials and biosensors. Some common implant materials including hard tissue materials, blood-contacting materials, and soft tissue materials are also described in this book.

Tissue engineering involves the development of new materials or devices capable of interacting specifically with biological tissues. The key to tissue engineering is the preparation of scaffolds using materials with the appropriate composition and structure. In the drug industry, advances in drug delivery systems are very important. Controlled release can be obtained by selecting the appropriate materials to produce the drug delivery system. Attempts have been made to incorporate drug reservoirs into implantable devices for sustained and preferably controlled release. Nanotechnology also plays an important role in the biomedical and biotechnology industries and has been used in the preparation of drugs for protein delivery, tissue engineering, bones, cardiovascular biomaterials, hard tissue replacements, biosensors, and biological microelectromechanical systems (Bio-MEMS). This book covers the latest information pertaining to tissue engineering scaffold materials, drug delivery systems, and nanobiomaterials and biosensors.

The book has 21 chapters describing different types of biomaterials, and is divided into four sections, namely tissue engineering scaffold materials, drug delivery systems, nanobiomaterials and biosensors, and other biomaterials. The section on tissue engineering describes inorganic and composite bioactive scaffolds for bone tissue engineering, design, fabrication, and characterization of scaffolds via solid free-form fabrication techniques, control and monitoring of scaffold architecture for tissue engineering, rapid prototyping methods for tissue engineering applications, as well as design and fabrication principles of electrospinning of scaffolds. The section on drug delivery systems discusses nanoparticles in cancer drug delivery systems, polymeric nano/microparticles for oral delivery of proteins and peptides, nanostructured porous biomaterials for controlled drug release systems, and inorganic nanostructures for drug delivery. The section on nanobiomaterials and biosensors includes self-assembly of nanostructures as biomaterials, electrohydrodynamic processing of micro- and nanometer biological materials, fabrication and functions of biohybrid nanomaterials prepared via supramolecular approaches, polypyrrole nano- and microsensors and actuators for biomedical applications, as well as processing of biosensing materials and biosensors. The last section, which deals with other biomaterials, includes synthetic and natural degradable polymeric biomaterials, electroactive polymers as smart materials with intrinsic actuation properties such as new functionalities for biomaterials, blood-contacting surfaces, improvement of blood compatibility of biomaterials using a novel antithrombin–heparin covalent complex, surface modification of biomaterials using plasma immersion ion implantation and deposition, biomaterials for gastrointestinal medicine, repair, and reconstruction, and biomaterials for cartilage reconstruction and repair.

These chapters have been written by renowned experts in their respective fields, and this book is valuable to the biomaterials and biomedical engineering community. It is intended for a broad and diverse readership including bioengineers, materials scientists, physicians, surgeons, research students, practitioners, and researchers in materials science, bioengineering, and medicine.

Readers will be able to familiarize themselves with the latest techniques in biomaterials and processing. In addition, each chapter is accompanied by an extensive list of references for readers interested in pursuing further research.

The outstanding cooperation from contributing authors who devoted their valuable time and effort to write excellent chapters for this handbook is highly appreciated. We are also indebted to all our colleagues who have made this book a reality.

Paul K. Chu
Xuanyong Liu

Editors

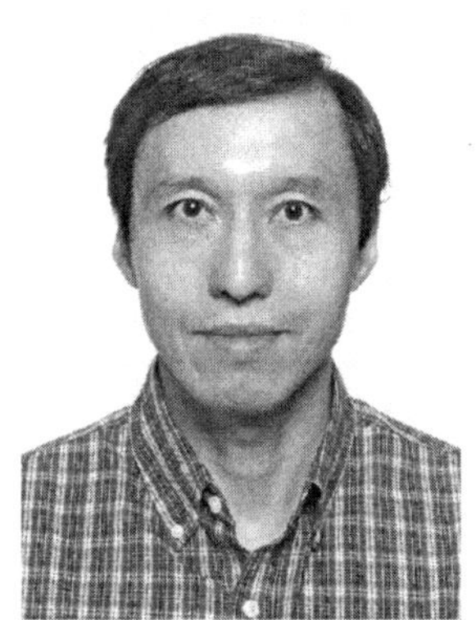

Paul K. Chu is a professor (chair) of materials engineering at the City University of Hong Kong. He received a BS in mathematics from The Ohio State University in 1977 and an MS and a PhD in chemistry from Cornell University in 1979 and 1982, respectively. Professor Chu's research activities are quite diverse, encompassing plasma surface engineering and various types of materials and nanotechnology. He has published over 550 journal papers and has been granted eight U.S. and three Chinese patents. He is a fellow of the IEEE, AVS, and HKIE, senior editor of *IEEE Transactions on Plasma Science*, associate editor of *International Journal of Plasma Science and Engineering*, and a member of the editorial board of *Materials Science & Engineering: Reports, Surface and Interface Engineering, and Biomolecular Engineering*. He is a member of the Plasma-Based Ion Implantation and Deposition International Committee, Ion Implantation Technology International Committee, and IEEE Plasma Science and Application Executive Committee.

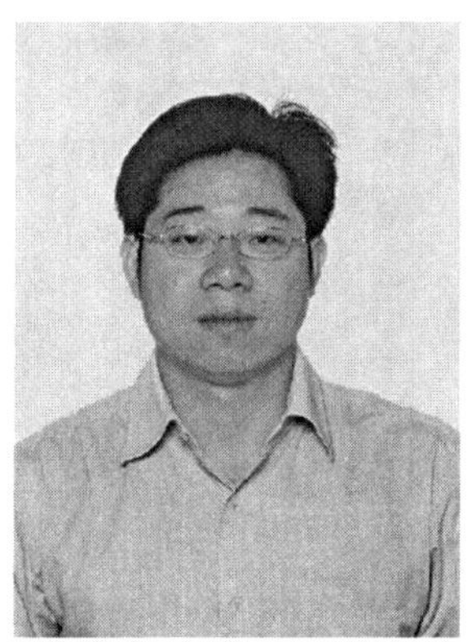

Xuanyong Liu is an associate professor of materials engineering at the Shanghai Institute of Ceramics, Chinese Academy of Sciences (SICCAS), and a professor at Hunan University. He received a BS and an MS in materials science and engineering from Hunan University in 1996 and 1999, respectively, and a PhD in materials science and engineering from SICCAS in 2002. His doctoral dissertation was awarded the National Excellent Doctoral Dissertation of People's Republic of China in 2004. Professor Liu's primary research focus is on surface modification of biomaterials. He has founded the Surface Engineering of Biomaterials Group in SICCAS and has published over 70 journal papers, including 14 papers on biomaterials.

Contributors

Arti Ahluwalia
Interdepartmental Research Center
  "E. Piaggio" and Department
  of Chemical Engineering
University of Pisa
Pisa, Italy

Hua Ai
National Engineering Research Center
  for Biomaterials
Sichuan University
Chengdu, China

Katsuhiko Ariga
WPI Center for Materials Nanoarchitectonics
National Institute for Materials Science
Tsukuba, Japan

Halil Murat Aydin
Institute for Science and Technology
  in Medicine
Keele University
Staffordshire, U.K.

Pierre Olivier Bagnaninchi
Institute for Science and Technology
  in Medicine
Keele University
Staffordshire, U.K.

Yevgeny Berdichevsky
Electrical and Computer Engineering
  Department
University of California
San Diego, California, U.S.A.

Leslie Roy Berry
Henderson Research Centre
Hamilton, Ontario, Canada

Aldo R. Boccaccini
Department of Materials
Imperial College
London, U.K.

Oana Bretcanu
Department of Materials
Imperial College
London, U.K.

Federico Carpi
Interdepartmental Research Centre
  "E. Piaggio"
University of Pisa
Pisa, Italy

Anthony Kam Chuen Chan
Henderson Research Centre
Hamilton, Ontario, Canada

Qi-Zhi Chen
Department of Materials
Imperial College
London, U.K.

Paul K. Chu
Department of Physics and Materials
  Science
City University of Hong Kong
Hong Kong, China

Robert Lewis Clark
Center for Biologically Inspired Materials
  and Material Systems
Pratt School of Engineering
Duke University
Durham, North Carolina, U.S.A.

Cassilda Cunha-Reis
Institute for Science and Technology
  in Medicine
Keele University
Staffordshire, U.K.

Richard M. Day
Department of Medicine
University College
London, U.K.

Danilo De Rossi
Interdepartmental Research Centre "E. Piaggio"
University of Pisa
Pisa, Italy

Sanjukta Deb
Department of Biomaterials
Dental Institute, King's College
London, U.K.

Andrew K. Ekaputra
Graduate Program in Bioengineering
National University of Singapore
Singapore

Miroslawa El Fray
Division of Biomaterials and Microbiological
  Technologies
Szczecin University of Technology Polymer
  Institute
Szczecin, Poland

Yujiang Fan
National Engineering Research Center
  for Biomaterials
Sichuan University
Chengdu, China

Ricky K.Y. Fu
Department of Physics and Materials Science
City University of Hong Kong
Hong Kong, China

Zhongwei Gu
National Engineering Research Center
  for Biomaterials
Sichuan University
Chengdu, China

Dietmar W. Hutmacher
Division of Regenerative Medicine
Institute of Health and Biomedical
  Innovation
Queensland University of Technology
Brisbane, Australia

So Yeon Kim
Division of Engineering Education
College of Engineering
Chungnam National University
Daejeon, South Korea

Menno L.W. Knetsch
Centre for Biomaterials Research
University of Maastricht
Maastricht, The Netherlands

Krzysztof J. Kurzydlowski
Division of Materials Design
Faculty of Materials Science and Engineering
Warsaw University of Technology
Warsaw, Poland

Young Moo Lee
School of Chemical Engineering
Hanyang University
Seoul, South Korea

Jifan Li
Hitachi Chemical Research Center
Irvine, California, U.S.A.

Yang Yang Li
Hitachi Chemical Research Center
Irvine, California, U.S.A.
and
Department of Physics and Materials Science
City University of Hong Kong
Hong Kong, China

Xuanyong Liu
Shanghai Institute of Ceramics
Chinese Academy of Sciences
Shanghai, China
and
Department of Physics and Materials Science
City University of Hong Kong
Hong Kong, China

Yanyan Liu
Shanghai Institute of Ceramics
Chinese Academy of Sciences
Shanghai, China
and
Laboratory of Special Functional Materials
Henan University
Kaifeng, China

Yu-Hwa Lo
Electrical and Computer Engineering
  Department
University of California
San Diego, California, U.S.A.

Bunichiro Nakajima
Hitachi Chemical Research Center
Irvine, California, U.S.A.

S. Sajeesh
Division of Biosurface Technology
Sree Chitra Tirunal Institute for Medical
 Sciences and Technology
Thiruvananthapuram, India

Chandra P. Sharma
Division of Biosurface Technology
Sree Chitra Tirunal Institute for Medical
 Sciences and Technology
Thiruvananthapuram, India

Wojciech Swieszkowski
Division of Materials Design
Faculty of Materials Science and Engineering
Warsaw University of Technology
Warsaw, Poland

Giovanni Vozzi
Interdepartmental Research Center "E. Piaggio"
 and Department of Chemical Engineering
University of Pisa
Pisa, Italy

Maria Ann Woodruff
Division of Regenerative Medicine
Institute of Health and Biomedical Innovation
Queensland University of Technology
Brisbane, Australia

Yiquan Wu
Center for Biologically Inspired Materials
 and Material Systems
Pratt School of Engineering
Duke University
Durham, North Carolina, U.S.A.

Ying Yang
Institute for Science and Technology
 in Medicine
School of Medicine
Keele University
Staffordshire, U.K.

Yu Yang
Shanghai Institute of Ceramics
Chinese Academy of Sciences
Shanghai, China

Yingchun Zhu
Shanghai Institute of Ceramics
Chinese Academy of Sciences
Shanghai, China

Ying-Jie Zhu
State Key Laboratory of High
 Performance Ceramics
 and Superfine Microstructures
Shanghai Institute of Ceramics
Chinese Academy of Sciences
Shanghai, China

Part I

Tissue Engineering Scaffold Materials

1 Inorganic and Composite Bioactive Scaffolds for Bone Tissue Engineering

Qi-Zhi Chen, Oana Bretcanu, and Aldo R. Boccaccini

CONTENTS

1.1   INTRODUCTION

Being a modern discipline, tissue engineering encounters various challenges, such as the development of suitable scaffolds that temporarily provide mechanical support to cells at an early stage of implantation until the cells are able to produce their own extracellular matrix (ECM) [1]. Numerous biomaterials and techniques to produce three-dimensional (3-D) tissue-engineering scaffolds have been considered; biomaterials include polymers, ceramics, and their composites, as discussed in the literature [1–3]. In this chapter, we present an up-to-date summary of the fabrication technologies for tissue-engineering scaffolds, including the choice of suitable materials and related fabrication techniques, with a focus on the development of synthetic scaffolds based on bioceramics, glasses, and their composites combined with biopolymers for bone regeneration. Being one of the most promising technologies, the replication method for the production of highly porous, biodegradable, and mechanically competent Bioglass®-derived glass-ceramic scaffolds is highlighted. The enhancement of scaffold properties and functions by surface modification is also discussed, and examples of novel approaches are given.

1.2   DESIGN OF 3-D SCAFFOLDS

In an organ, cells and their ECM are organized into 3-D tissues. Therefore, in tissue engineering a highly porous 3-D matrix (i.e., scaffold) is necessary to accommodate cells and to guide their growth and tissue regeneration in 3-D structures. This is particularly relevant in the field of bone tissue engineering and regeneration, bone being a highly hierarchical 3-D composite structure. Moreover, the structure of bone tissue varies with its location in the body. So the selection of configurations as well as appropriate biomaterials depends on the anatomic site for regeneration, the mechanical loads present at the site, and the desired rate of incorporation. Ideally, the scaffold should be porous enough to support cell penetration, tissue ingrowth, rapid vascular invasion, and nutrient delivery. Moreover, the matrix should be designed to guide the formation of new bones in anatomically relevant shapes, and its degradation kinetics should be such that the biodegradable scaffold retains its physical (e.g., mechanical) properties for at least 6 months (for *in vitro* and *in vivo* tissue regeneration) [1,3]. Important scaffold design parameters are summarized in Table 1.1.

The design of highly porous scaffolds involves a critical issue related to their mechanical properties and structural integrity, which are time dependent. For example, it has been reported that the compressive strength of hydroxyapatite scaffolds increases from ~10 to ~30 MPa because of tissue ingrowth *in vivo* [5]. This finding leads to a conclusion that it might not be necessary to have a starting scaffold with a mechanical strength equal to that of a bone, because cultured cells on the scaffold *in vitro* will create a biocomposite and increase the strength of the scaffold significantly.

Another factor that affects scaffold design is the need for vascularization and angiogenesis in the constructs [6]. *In vitro* engineering approaches face the problem of critical thickness while regenerating tissue in the absence of true vascularization: mass transportation into tissue is difficult beyond a thin peripheral layer of a tissue construct even if artificial means are used to supply nutrients and oxygen [7]. Diffusion barriers that are present *in vitro* are most likely to become more

TABLE 1.1

Scaffold Design Parameters for Bone Tissue Engineering [4]

Parameters	Requirements
Porosity	Maximum possible without compromising mechanical properties
Pore size	200–400 μm
Pore structure	Interconnected
Mechanical properties of the cancellous bone	
Tension and compression	Strength: 5–10 MPa
	Modulus: 50–100 MPa
Mechanical properties of the cortical bone	
Tension	Strength: 80–150 MPa
	Modulus: 17–20 GPa
Compression	Strength: 130–220 MPa
	Modulus: 17–20 GPa
	Fracture toughness: 6–8 MPa$\sqrt{m}$
Degradation properties	
Degradation time	Must be tailored to match the application in patients
Degradation mechanism	Bulk dissolution in medium
Biocompatibility	No chronic inflammation
Sterilizability	Sterilizable without altering material properties

deleterious *in vivo* due to lack of vascularization. Once the engineered tissue construct is placed in the body, vascularization becomes a key issue for further remodeling in the *in vivo* environment. Thus, angiogenesis is an essential step in the colonization of macroporous biomaterials during osteointegration. Capillaries bring osteoprogenitor cells and the nutriments that are required for their growth. They transport especially numerous angiogenic growth factors [8].

The main critical factors affecting bone formation are the pore size and pore interconnection of the scaffold. Pore size is related to the *in vivo* bone tissue ingrowth, allowing migration and proliferation of osteoblasts and mesenchymal cells, and matrix deposition in the empty spaces [9]. Pore interconnection provides the channel for cell distribution and migration allowing efficient *in vivo* blood vessel formation. An incomplete pore interconnection could limit blood vessels invasion. Small pore size could obstruct cell adhesion and bone ingrowth. Bone vascularization, besides providing nutrients essential for tissue survival, plays also a crucial role in coordinating the activity of bone cells and their migration for new bone formation [10].

Several studies have investigated the minimum pore size required to regenerate mineralized bone. The minimum requirement for pore size is considered to be around 100 μm due to cell size, migration requirements, and transport. However, pore sizes >300 μm are recommended due to enhanced growth rate of a new bone and the formation of capillaries [3,4,11]. Pore size in the range of 300–500 μm would promote vascularization and mass transportation of nutrients and waste products, while the scaffold would maintain good mechanical integrity during *in vitro* culture and *in vivo* transplantation [12].

It is equally important to notice that tissue-engineering scaffolds should have enhanced biological functions. Therefore, the incorporation of growth factors, such as bone growth factors (BGF) and vascularization growth factors (VGF), or specific peptide sequences into the scaffolds or on their surface is being considered as part of the integral design of scaffolds. Moreover, to improve cell attachment and growth, the surface of scaffolds' struts needs to be pretreated (a process called surface functionalization) [13–15]. The design of the surface properties of scaffolds is an important step to achieve their successful *in vitro* and *in vivo* applications. A few approaches to surface modification of scaffolds are discussed below.

1.3 SCAFFOLD MATERIALS FOR BONE TISSUE ENGINEERING

The first step in achieving a successful scaffold is to choose a suitable biomaterial. Natural bone matrix is a composite of biological ceramic (a natural apatite) and biological polymer. Carbonated hydroxyapatite $Ca_{10}(PO_4)_6(OH)_2$ accounts for nearly two-thirds of the weight of a bone. The inorganic component provides compressive strength to the bone. Roughly one-third of the weight of a bone is from collagen fibers. Collagen fibers are tough and flexible, and thus tolerate stretching, twisting, and bending. It is not surprising that polymers, ceramics, or their composites have been chosen for bone repair [16]. They can be either synthetic or naturally occurring ones. Table 1.2 lists synthetic and natural scaffold biomaterials that have been most widely investigated for bone regeneration, some of which are well-established and clinically applicable. In this section, the biocompatibility, biodegradability, and mechanical properties of these scaffold materials, which are the most essential factors to be considered in the fabrication of bone regeneration scaffold, are reviewed concisely. Particular attention is paid to a key issue that remains with almost all existing scaffold biomaterials, that is, mechanically strong materials (in crystalline structure) tend to be bioinert, and biodegradable materials (in amorphous structure) are, in general, mechanically weak. An exception, 45S5 Bioglass-derived glass-ceramic, is considered in more detail because the issue associated with the two apparently irreconcilable properties (mechanical strength and biodegradability) have been successfully addressed in this material [17].

1.3.1 BIOCERAMICS: CALCIUM PHOSPHATES

1.3.1.1 Biocompatibility

Since almost two-thirds of the weight of a bone is hydroxyapatite $Ca_{10}(PO_4)_6(OH)_2$, it seems logical to use this ceramic as a major component of scaffold materials for bone tissue engineering. Actually, hydroxyapatite and related calcium phosphates (e.g., β-tricalcium phosphate [β-TCP]) have been intensively investigated [16,18,21]. As expected, calcium phosphates have an excellent biocompatibility due to their close chemical and crystal resemblance to bone mineral [19,20]. Although they have not shown osteoinductive ability, they certainly possess osteoconductive properties as well as a remarkable ability to bind directly to bone [32–35]. A high number of *in vivo* and *in vitro* assessments have concluded that calcium phosphates, no matter which forms (bulk, coating, powder, or porous) and which phases (crystalline or amorphous) they are in, always support the attachment, differentiation, and proliferation of cells (such as osteoblasts and mesenchymal cells), with hydroxyapatite being the best among these scaffold materials [36]. Although the excellent biological performance of hydroxyapatite and related calcium phosphates has been well-documented, the slow biodegradation of their crystalline phases and the weak mechanical strength of their amorphous states limit their application in engineering of new bone tissue, especially at load-bearing sites.

1.3.1.2 Degradability

Typically, crystalline calcium phosphates have a long degradation time *in vivo*, often of the order of years [37]. The dissolution rate of synthetic hydroxyapatite depends on the type and concentration of the buffered or unbuffered solutions, pH of the solution, degree of the saturation of the solution, solid and solution ratio, length of suspension in the solution, as well as composition and crystallinity of the hydroxyapatite. In the case of crystalline hydroxyapatite, the degree of micro and macroporosities, defect in the structure, and amount and type of other phases present also have significant influence [39]. Crystalline hydroxyapatite exhibits the slowest degradation rate, compared with other calcium phosphates. The dissolution rate decreases in the following order [38]:

Amorphous hydroxyapatite $>$ all other calcium phosphates (e.g., TCP) $\gg$ crystalline hydroxyapatite.

TABLE 1.2

List of Promising Scaffold Biomaterials for Bone Regeneration

Biomaterials	Abbreviation	Application
Ceramics [16,18]		
Calcium phosphates [19–21]	CaP	
Hydroxyapatite	HA	Dental
Tricalcium phosphate	TCP	Drug delivery
Biphasic calcium phosphate: HA and TCP	BCP	Scaffolds
Bioactive glasses [22–25]		Dental
Bioglass		Drug delivery
Phosphate glasses		Scaffolds
Bioactive Glass-Ceramics [26,27]	A/W	Dental
Apatite-Wollastonite		Drug delivery
Ceravital		Scaffolds
Polymers [28–31]		
Synthetic degradable polymers		
Bulk biodegradable polymers		Sutures
Aliphatic polyester		Dental
Poly(lactic acid)	PLA	Orthopedic
Poly(D-lactic acid)	PDLA	Drug delivery
Poly(L-lactic acid)	PLLA	Scaffolds
Poly(D,L-lactic acid)	PDLLA	
Poly(glycolic acid)	PGA	
Poly(lactic-*co*-glycolic acid)	PLGA	
Poly(ε-caprolactone)	PCL	
Poly(hydroxyalkanoate)	PHA	
Poly(3- or 4-hydroxybutyrate)	PHB	
Poly(3-hydroxyoctanoate)	PHO	
Poly(3-hydroxyvalerate)	PHV	
Polydioxanone		
Poly(propylene fumarate)	PPF	
Surface bioerodible polymers		Drug delivery
Poly(ortho esters)	POE	
Poly(anhydrides)		
Poly(phosphazene)	PPHOS	
Natural degradable polymers		
Polysaccharides		
Hyaluronan	HyA	
Alginate		
Chitosan		
Proteins		
Collagen		
Fibrin		
Composites [12]		
Composed of the above-mentioned ceramics and polymers		

1.3.1.3 Mechanical Properties

The properties of synthetic calcium phosphates vary significantly with their crystallinity, grain size, porosity, and composition (e.g., calcium deficiency). In general, the mechanical properties of synthetic calcium phosphates decrease significantly with increasing content of amorphous phase, microporosity, and grain size. High crystallinity, low porosity, and small grain size tend to give

TABLE 1.3

Comparison of Mechanical Properties of Calcium Phosphates and Human Bone

Ceramics	Compressive Strength (MPa)	Tensile Strength (MPa)	Elastic Modulus (GPa)	Fracture Toughness (MPa√m)	References
Calcium phosphates	20–900	30–200	30–103	<1.0	39,42
Hydroxyapatite	>400	~40	~100	~1.0	39,42
Cortical bone	130–180	50–151	12–18	6–8	28,43–46

higher stiffness, higher compressive and tensile strength, and greater fracture toughness [39,40]. It has been reported that the flexural strength and fracture toughness of dense hydroxyapatite are much lower in a dry condition than in a wet condition [41]. The mechanical properties of hydroxyapatite and related calcium phosphates, as well as those of bone, are given in Table 1.3.

In brief, hydroxyapatite and related calcium phosphates exhibit excellent biocompatibility and osteoconductivity. However, these materials are poorly degradable in case of crystalline structures, and their amorphous counterparts are mechanically too fragile to be used for fabrication of highly porous tissue-engineering scaffolds.

1.3.2 BIOCERAMICS: BIOACTIVE SILICATE GLASSES

1.3.2.1 Biocompatibility

As early as in 1969, Hench and colleagues discovered that certain silicate glass compositions had excellent biocompatibility as well as the ability of bone bonding [23–25]. Through interfacial and cell-mediated reactions, bioactive glass develops a calcium-deficient, carbonated calcium phosphate surface layer that allows it to chemically bond to the host bone. This bone-bonding behavior is referred to as "bioactivity" and has been associated with the formation of a carbonated hydroxyapatite layer on the glass surface when implanted or when in contact with biological fluids [47–50]. Bioactivity is not an exclusive property of bioactive silicate glasses. Hydroxyapatite and related calcium phosphates also show an excellent bone-bonding ability, as discussed above. The capability of a material to form a biological interface with the surrounding tissue is critical in avoiding scaffold loosening *in vivo*.

Bioactive glasses have also been found to support enzyme activity [51–54], vascularization [55,56], as well as foster osteoblast adhesion, growth, and differentiation. Bioactive glasses were also shown to induce the differentiation of mesenchymal cells into osteoblasts [57–59] and to provide osteoconductivity [60].

A significant finding for the development of bone engineering is that the dissolution products from bioactive glasses exert a genetic control over osteoblast cycle and rapid expression of genes that regulate osteogenesis and the production of growth factors [61,62]. Silicon has been found to play a key role in the bone mineralization and gene activation, which has led to the substitution of silicon for calcium into synthetic hydroxyapatite. Investigations *in vivo* have shown that bone ingrowth into silicon-substituted hydroxyapatite granules was remarkably greater than that into pure hydroxyapatite [62,63].

The above-mentioned advantages make 45S5 Bioglass a very successful material in clinical applications, for example, for the treatment of periodontal disease (PerioGlas) and as a bone-filler material (NovaBone) [63,64]. Bioglass implants have also been used to replace damaged middle ear bones, restoring auditory capabilities of patients [64]. Recently bioactive glasses have gained attention as promising scaffold materials for bone tissue engineering [64–69]. Similar to calcium phosphates, the application of this material, particularly in tissue engineering, has encountered a hurdle caused by the conflict between the properties of biodegradability and mechanical reliability, which is discussed in Sections 1.3.2.3 and 1.3.3.4.

1.3.2.2 Biodegradability

The basic constituents of most bioactive glasses are SiO_2, Na_2O, CaO, and P_2O_5. The well-known 45S5 Bioglass contains 45% SiO_2, 24.5% Na_2O, 24.4% CaO, and 6% P_2O_5, in weight percent. The bioreactivity of the material is composition-dependent. Hench and coworkers [22] have systematically studied a series of glasses in the four-component systems with a constant 6 wt.% P_2O_5 content. This work is summarized in the ternary SiO_2–Na_2O–CaO diagram shown in Figure 1.1. In region A, the glasses are bioactive and bond to bone. In region B, glasses are nearly inert when implanted. Compositions in region C are resorbed within 10–30 days in tissue. In region D, the compositions are not technically practical.

The key advantage of bioactive glasses that makes them promising scaffold materials is the possibility of controlling a range of chemical properties and thereby the rate of bioresorption. The structure and chemistry of glasses, in particular sol–gel derived glasses [47,48], can be tailored at a molecular level by varying either composition, or thermal or environmental processing history. It is possible to design glasses with degradation properties specific to a particular application of bone tissue engineering.

1.3.2.3 Mechanical Properties

A primary disadvantage of bioactive glasses is their low fracture toughness (Table 1.4) because of their amorphous structure. Hence, many researchers sintered bioactive glasses at their crystallization temperatures in order to improve the mechanical performance of these materials. However, it was reported that crystallization of bioactive glasses could decrease the level of bioactivity [70]

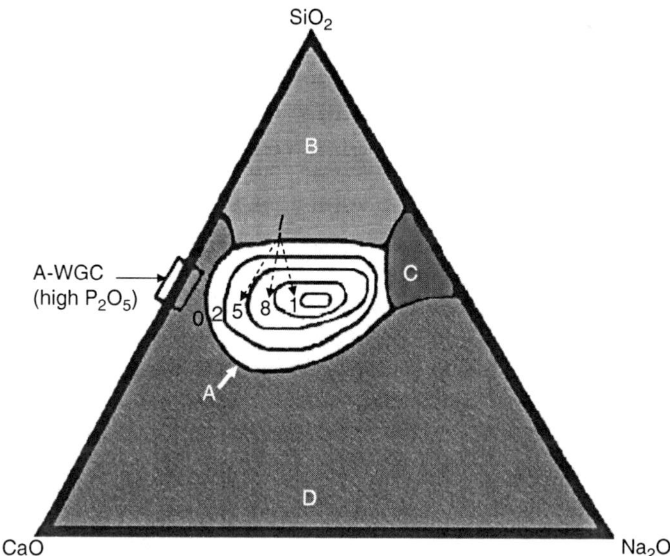

FIGURE 1.1 Compositional dependence (in wt.%) of bone bonding and soft tissue bonding of bioactive glasses and glass-ceramics. Bioactivity index I_B is defined as $I_B = 100/t_{0.5}$, where $t_{0.5}$ is the time taken for 50% of the interface to bond to bone. All compositions have a constant 6 wt.% of P_2O_5. In region A, the glasses are bioactive and bond to bone. In region B, glasses are nearly inert when implanted. Compositions in region C are resorbed within 10–30 days in tissue. In region D, the compositions are not technically practical. In the region where $I_B > 8$ (called region E), soft tissue bonding occurs. Apatite-wollastonite glass-ceramic (A-WGC) has higher P_2O_5 content [22].

TABLE 1.4

Mechanical Properties of Hydroxyapatite, 45S5 Bioglass, Glass-Ceramics, and Human Cortical Bone

Ceramics	Compression Strength (MPa)	Tensile Strength (MPa)	Elastic Modulus (GPa)	Fracture Toughness (MPa$\sqrt{m}$)	References
45S5 Bioglass	500	42	35	0.5–1	42,73
A-W	1080	215 (bend)	118	2.0	26
Parent glass of A-W	NA	72 (bend)	NA	0.8	26
Bioverit I	500	140–180 (bend)	70–90	1.2–2.1	74
Cortical bone	130–180	50–151	12–18	6–8	28,43–46

and even turn a bioactive glass into an inert material [71]. This is one of the disadvantages that limit the application of bioactive glasses as scaffold materials, as full crystallization occurs prior to significant densification upon heat treatment (i.e., sintering) [72]. Extensive sintering is necessary to densify the struts of a scaffold, which would otherwise be made up of loosely packed particles and thus the structure would be too fragile to handle. Most recently, Boccaccini's group at Imperial College London [17] reported on a phase transformation from a mechanically competent crystalline phase to a biodegradable amorphous calcium phosphate in 45S5 Bioglass-derived scaffolds. This phase transition, which takes place in a biological environment at body temperature, couples the two required properties (mechanical strength and biodegradability) in a single scaffold. A detailed characterization of this material is given in Section 1.3.3.4.

In summary, like hydroxyapatite and related calcium phosphates, bioactive glasses exhibit good biocompatibility and osteoconductivity. At the same time, all these materials, except 45S5 Bioglass-derived glass-ceramics, encounter a similar disadvantage, that is, a mechanically strong scaffold has to be achieved through crystallization, which unfortunately hampers the biodegradability of these materials.

1.3.3 BIOCERAMICS: GLASS-CERAMICS

Glasses can be strengthened by the formation of crystalline particles in the glass matrix upon heat treatment in the relevant glass-crystal region of its phase diagram. The resultant glass-ceramics usually exhibit better mechanical properties than both the parent glass and sintered crystalline ceramics (e.g., sintered hydroxyapatite) (Table 1.4). There are many biomedical glass-ceramics available for the repair of damaged bones. Among them, apatite-wollastonite (A-W), Ceravital, and Bioverit glass-ceramics have been intensively investigated [16,18]. Recently, a 45S5 Bioglass-derived glass-ceramic showed a great potential as a tissue-engineering scaffold material, as mentioned above (Section 1.3.2.3).

1.3.3.1 A-W Glass-Ceramics

In A-W glass-ceramic, the glass matrix is reinforced by β-wollastonite (CaSiO$_3$) crystals and a small amount of apatite phase, which precipitate successively at 870°C and 900°C, respectively [75]. Some mechanical properties of this glass-ceramic have been listed in Table 1.4. The high bending strength (215 MPa) of A-W glass-ceramic is due to the precipitation of wollastonite as well as apatite. These two precipitates also give the glass-ceramic a higher fracture toughness than that of both the glass and ceramic phases. It is believed that wollastonite effectively prevents straight propagation of cracks, causing them to deflect or branch out [26,75–77].

A-W glass-ceramic is capable of binding tightly to a living bone in a few weeks after implantation, and the implants do not deteriorate *in vivo* [78]. The excellent bone-bonding ability of A-W glass-ceramic is attributed to the glass matrix and apatite precipitates, whereas the *in vivo* stability as a whole is due to the inertness of β-wollastonite. Although the long-term integrity *in vivo* is desirable in the application of nonresorbable prosthesis, the material does not match the goal of tissue engineering, which demands biodegradable scaffolds.

1.3.3.2　Ceravital Glass-Ceramics [79]

"Ceravital" was coined to mean a number of different compositions of glasses and glass-ceramics and not only one product. Their basic network components include SiO_2, $Ca(PO_2)_2$, CaO, Na_2O, MgO, and K_2O, with ceramic additions being Al_2O_3, Ta_2O_5, TiO_2, B_2O_3, $Al(PO_3)_3$, SrO, La_2O_3, or Gd_2O_3. This material system was developed as solid fillers in the load-bearing conditions for the replacement of bone and teeth. It turned out, however, that their mechanical properties do not serve the purpose, and there has been virtually no research on the application of this material in tissue-engineering scaffolds.

1.3.3.3　Bioverit Glass-Ceramics [74]

Bioverit products are mica-apatite glass-ceramics. Mica crystals (aluminum silicate minerals) give the materials good machinability, and apatite crystals ensure the bioactivity of the implants. The mechanical properties of Bioverit materials (Table 1.4) allow them to be used as fillers in dental application. As regards bioreactivity, Bioverit implants show a hydrolytic stability *in vivo*. As for Ceravital glass-ceramics, no significant research has been carried out regarding the use of this glass-ceramic in tissue engineering.

1.3.3.4　45S5 Bioglass-Derived Glass-Ceramics

In 2005, Chen et al. [80] fabricated a 3-D, highly porous, mechanically competent, bioactive and biodegradable scaffold for the first time by the replication technique using 45S5 Bioglass powder. Under an optimum sintering condition (1000°C/h), nearly full densification of the foam struts occurred and fine crystals of $Na_2Ca_2Si_3O_9$ are formed, which conferred the scaffolds the highest possible compressive and flexural strength for this foam structure. Important findings in this work are that the mechanically strong crystalline phase $Na_2Ca_2Si_3O_9$ can transform into an amorphous calcium phosphate phase after immersion in simulated body fluid (SBF) for 28 days and that the transformation kinetics can be tailored by controlling the crystallinity of the sintered 45S5 Bioglass. As such, it was demonstrated that the goal of an ideal scaffold that provides good mechanical support temporarily while maintaining bioactivity and that can biodegrade at later stages at a tailorable rate can be achieved with these Bioglass-based scaffolds [17].

1.3.4　Naturally Occurring Biopolymers

Much research effort has been focused on naturally occurring polymers such as demineralized bone ECM [81], purified collagen [82,83], and chitosan [84] for tissue engineering applications. Theoretically, naturally occurring polymers should not cause response of foreign materials when implanted. They provide a natural substrate for cellular attachment, proliferation, and differentiation in their native state. For these reasons, naturally occurring polymers could be a favorite substrate for tissue engineering [28]. Table 1.5 provides a list of some of the naturally occurring polymers, their sources, and applications. Among them, collagen and chitosan are most widely investigated for bone engineering and are briefly discussed here.

1.3.4.1　Collagen and ECM-Based Materials

The most commonly used naturally occurring polymer is the structural protein collagen. Biomaterials derived from ECM include collagen and other naturally occurring structural and functional

TABLE 1.5
List of Naturally Occurring Polymers, Their Sources, and Applications [85]

Polymers	Source	Application
Collagen	Tendons and ligament	Multiapplications, including bone tissue engineering
Collagen-Glycosaminoglycan (GAG) (alginate) copolymers		Artificial skin grafts for skin replacement
Albumin	In blood	Transporting protein used as coating to form a thromboresistant surface
Hyaluronic acid	In the ECM of all higher animals	An important starting material for preparation of new biocompatible and biodegradable polymers that have applications in drug delivery, tissue engineering, and viscosupplementation
Fibrinogen–Fibrin	Purified from plasma in blood	Multiapplications, including bone tissue engineering
Chitosan	Shells of shrimps and crabs	Multiapplications, including bone tissue engineering

proteins. Natural polymers must be modified and sterilized before clinical use. All methods of stabilization and sterilization can moderately or severely alter the rate of *in vivo* degradation and change the mechanical and physical properties of the native polymers. Each method has certain advantages and disadvantages, and thus should be selectively utilized for scaffolds of specifically sited bone tissue engineering [86].

1.3.4.2 Chitosan

The use of chitosan for bone tissue engineering has been widely investigated [84,87]. This is in part due to the apparent osteoconductive properties of chitosan. Mesenchymal stem cells cultured in the presence of chitosan have demonstrated an increased differentiation to osteoblasts compared with cells cultured in the absence of chitosan [88]. It is also speculated that chitosan may enhance osteoconduction *in vivo* by entrapping growth factors at the wound site [89].

1.3.5 SYNTHETIC POLYMERS

Although naturally occurring polymers possess the above-mentioned advantages, their poor mechanical properties and variable physical properties with different sources of protein matrices have hampered their progress in broad applications in tissue engineering. Concerns have also been expressed regarding immunogenic problems associated with the introduction of foreign collagen [37].

Following the developmental efforts regarding the use of naturally occurring polymers as scaffolds, much attention has been paid to synthetic polymers. Synthetic polymers have high potential in tissue engineering not only because of their excellent processing characteristics, which can ensure their off-the-shelf availability, but also because of their advantage of being biocompatible and biodegradable [37,90]. Synthetic polymers have predictable and reproducible mechanical and physical properties (e.g., tensile strength, elastic modulus, and degradation rate) and can be manufactured with great precision. Although they are unfamiliar to cells and many have some shortcomings, such as eliciting persistent inflammatory reactions, being eroded, not being compliant or able to integrate with the host tissues, they may be replaced *in vivo* in a timely fashion by native constructs built by the cells seeded into them. It has been widely accepted that an ideal tissue-engineered bone substitute should be a synthetic scaffold, which is biocompatible and provides for cell attachment, proliferation and maturation, has mechanical properties to match those of the tissues at the site of implantation, and degrades at rates to match tissue replacement. Table 1.6 lists selected properties of synthetic, biocompatible, and biodegradable polymers that have been intensively investigated as scaffold materials for tissue engineering, type I collagen fibers being included for comparison.

1.3.5.1 Bulk Degradable Polymers

1.3.5.1.1 *Saturated Poly-α-Hydroxyesters (PLA, PGA, and PCL)*
The biodegradable synthetic polymers most often utilized for 3-D scaffolds in tissue engineering are the poly(α-hydroxyacids), including poly(lactic acid) (PLA) and poly(glycolic acid) (PGA), as well as poly(lactic-*co*-glycolide) (PLGA) copolymers [91]. PLA exists in three forms: L-PLA (PLLA), D-PLA (PDLA), and racemic mixture of D,L-PLA (PDLLA).

These polymers are popular for various reasons, among which biocompatibility and biodegradability stand out. These materials have chemical properties that allow hydrolytic degradation through de-esterification. After the process of degradation is over, the monomeric components of each polymer are removed through natural pathways: PGA can be converted to other metabolites or eliminated by other mechanisms, and PLA can be cleared through tricarboxylic acid cycle. The body already contains highly regulated mechanisms for completely removing monomeric components of lactic and glycolic acids. Due to these properties, PLA and PGA have been used in products such as degradable sutures and have been approved by the U.S. Food and Drug Administration (FDA) [28]. Other significant properties of these polymers are their very good processability, and their ability to exhibit a wide range of degradation rates, physical, mechanical, and other properties, which can be achieved by PLA and PGA of various molecular weights and their copolymers. However, these polymers undergo a bulk erosion process in contact with body fluids such that they can cause scaffolds to fail prematurely. In addition, abrupt release of these acidic degradation products can cause a strong inflammatory response [92,93].

In general, PGA degrades faster than PLA, as listed in Table 1.6. Their degradation rates decrease in the following order.

$$PGA > PDLLA > PLLA$$

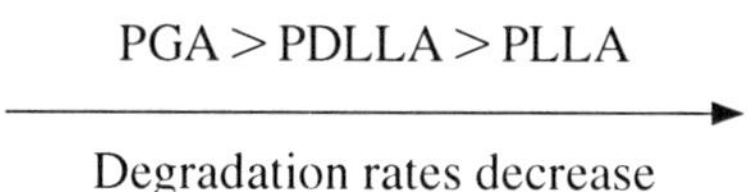

Degradation rates decrease

Table 1.6 also lists the mechanical properties of type I collagen, which is the major organic component of ECM in bone. The strength and ductility (e.g., ultimate elongation) of PLA and PGA are comparable to those of type I collagen fibers.

PDLLA has been extensively investigated as a biomedical coating material because of its excellent features with respect to implant surface [28,104]. In addition to its high mechanical stability [105], PDLLA also shows excellent biocompatibility *in vivo* and good osteoinductive potential [106]. PDLLA of low molecular weight can be combined with drugs like growth factors [106], antibiotics [107], or thrombin inhibitors [108] to establish a locally acting drug-delivery system. It is due to these desirable features that much more attention has recently been paid to PDLLA for applying it as a scaffold material for tissue engineering.

Highly porous 3-D scaffolds made of Bioglass-filled PDLLA and PLGA were fabricated by Boccaccini et al. [59]. Since then an increasing number of publications have emerged on this subject, as reviewed recently [12]. Porous PDLLA foams and Bioglass-filled PDLLA composite foams have both been fabricated, using thermally induced–phase separation (TIPS) technique [109,110]. Bioglass-filled PDLLA composite foams exhibit high bioactivity, assessed by the formation of hydroxyapatite

TABLE 1.6

Physical Properties of Synthetic, Biocompatible, and Biodegradable Polymers Investigated as Scaffold Materials

Polymers	Melting Point, T_m (°C)	Glass Transition Point, T_g (°C)	Degradation Time (months)	Tensile or Compressive* Strength (MPa)	Modulus (GPa)	Ultimate Elongation (%)	References
Bulk degradable polymers							
PDLLA	Amorphous	55–60	12–16	Pellet: 35–150* Film or disk: 29–35	Film or disk: 1.9–2.4	Pellet: 0.5–8.0 Film or disk: 5.0–6.0	90,94,95
PLLA	173–178	60–65	>24	Pellet: 40–120 Film or disk: 28–50 Fiber: 870–2300	Film or disk: 1.2–3.0 Fiber: 10–16	Pellet: 2.0–10.0 Film or disk: 2.0–6.0 Fiber: 12–26	90,94
PGA	225–230	35–40	6–12	Fiber: 340–920	Fiber: 7–14	Fiber: 15–25	90,96,97
PLGA	Amorphous	45–55	Adjustable	41.4–55.2	1.4–2.8	3–10	28
PPF			Bulk	2–30*			28,30
PCL	58	−72	Bulk			700	98
Surface erosive polymers							
Poly(anhydrides)	150–200		Surface	25–27 30–40*	0.14–1.4		28,30,99
Poly(ortho-esters)	30–100		Surface	4–16*	2.5–4.4		28,100
Polyphosphazene	−66–50	242	Surface				101,102
Type I collagen			Bulk	Uncross-linked fiber: 0.91–7.2 Cross-linked fiber: 46.8–68.8	Uncross-linked fiber: 1.8–46×10^{-3} Cross-linked fiber: 0.383–0.766	Uncross-linked fiber: 24.1–68.0 Cross-linked fiber: 11.6–15.6	103

on the strut surfaces upon immersion in SBF [111]. It has also been shown that the foams support the migration, adhesion, spreading, and viability of MG-63 cells (osteosarcoma cell line) [112].

Poly(ε-caprolactone) (PCL) is also an important member of the aliphatic polyester family. It has been used to effectively entrap antibiotic drugs and thus a construct made with PCL can be considered as a drug-delivery system, being used to enhance bone ingrowth and regeneration in the treatment of bone defects [113]. The degradation of PCL and its copolymers involves similar mechanisms to PLA, proceeding in two stages: random hydrolytic ester cleavage and weight loss through the diffusion of oligometric species from the bulk. It has been found that the degradation of PCL system with a high molecular weight ($\overline{M}_n$ of 50,000) is remarkably slow, requiring 3 years for complete removal from the host body [114].

1.3.5.1.2 Polyhydroxyalkanoates (PHB, PHBV, P4HB, PHBHHx, PHO)

Recently, polyhydroxyalkanoates (PHAs), another type of polyesters, have been suggested for tissue engineering because of their controllable biodegradation and high biocompatibility [115]. They are aliphatic polyesters as well, but produced by microorganisms under unbalanced growth conditions [116,117]. They are generally biodegradable (via hydrolysis) and thermoprocessable, making them attractive as biomaterials for application in medical devices and tissue engineering. Over the past years, PHA, particularly poly-3-hydroxybutyrate (PHB), copolymers of 3-hydroxybutyrate and 3-hydroxyvalerate (PHBV); poly 4-hydroxybutyrate (P4HB), copolymers of 3-hydroxybutyrate and 3-hydroxyhexanoate (PHBHHx); and poly 3-hydroxyoctanoate (PHO) were demonstrated to be suitable for tissue engineering and are reviewed in detail in Refs. 115,116.

Depending on the property requirement of different applications, PHA polymers can be either blended, surface modified, or composed with other polymers, enzymes, or inorganic materials to further adjust their mechanical properties or biocompatibility. The blending among the several PHA themselves can dramatically change their material properties and biocompatibility [115,116].

PHB is of particular interest for bone tissue application as it was demonstrated to produce a consistent favorable bone tissue adaptation response with no evidence of an undesirable chronic inflammatory response after an implantation period of up to 12 months [116]. The bone is formed close to the material and subsequently becomes highly organized, with up to 80% of the implant surface lying in direct apposition to the new bone. The materials showed no evidence of extensive structural breakdown *in vivo* during the implantation period of the study [118].

However, a drawback of some PHA polymers is their limited availability and the time-consuming extraction procedure from bacterial cultures that is required for obtaining sufficient processing amounts as described in the literature [115,119]. Therefore, the extraction process might be a challenge to a cost-effective industrial upscale production for large amounts of some PHA polymers.

1.3.5.1.3 Polypropylene Fumarate

Poly(propylene fumarate) (PPF) is an unsaturated linear polyester. Similar to PLA and PGA, the degradation products of PPF through hydrolysis (i.e., propylene glycol and fumaric acid) are biocompatible and readily removed from the body. The double bond along the backbone of the polymer permits cross-linking *in situ*, which causes a moldable composite to harden within 10–15 min. Mechanical properties and degradation time of the composite may be controlled by varying the PPF molecular weight. Therefore, preservation of the double bonds and control of molecular weight during PPF synthesis are critical issues [120]. PPF has been suggested for use as scaffold for guided tissue regeneration, often as part of an injectable bone replacement composite [121], and has been used as a substrate for osteoblast culture [122].

1.3.5.2 Surface Bioeroding Polymers

There is a family of hydrophobic polymers that undergo a heterogeneous hydrolysis process, which is predominantly confined to the polymer–water interface. This property is referred to as surface eroding as opposed to bulk degrading behavior. These surface bioeroding polymers have been intensively investigated as drug-delivery vehicles. The surface-eroding characteristic offers three key advantages over bulk degradation when used as scaffold materials: (1) retention of mechanical integrity over the degradative lifetime of the device, owing to the maintenance of mass to volume ratio; (2) minimal toxic effects (i.e., local acidity), owing to lower solubility and concentration of degradation products; and (3) significantly enhanced bone ingrowth into the porous scaffolds, owing to the increment in pore size as the erosion proceeds [123].

1.3.5.2.1 Poly(anhydrides)

Poly(1,3-*bis-p*-carboxyphenoxypropane anhydride) [124] and poly(erucic acid dimer anhydride) [125] are biodegradable polymers for controlled drug delivery in a form of implant or injectable microspheres. Studies in rabbits have shown that the osteocompatibility of poly(anhydrides) that undergo photocuring are comparable to PLA and that the implants of poly(anhydrides) show enhanced integration with the surrounding bones in comparison to PLA controls [126].

1.3.5.2.2 Poly(ortho-esters)

Poly(ortho-esters) (POE) scaffolds were coated with cross-linked acidic gelatine to improve surface properties for cell attachment. Preliminary *in vitro* and *in vivo* results revealed that POE did not show any inflammation and had little or no effect on bone formation while PLA provoked a chronic inflammatory response and inhibited bone formation [127,128].

1.3.5.2.3 Polyphosphazenes

These polymers seem to be potential bioerodible materials capable of controlled degradation and sustained drug delivery for therapeutic use [101,129] and bone regeneration [130]. Their tailored side groups enable a wide variety of hydrolytic properties to be designed into selected polymers for application in biological environments without the release of harmful degradation products at physiological concentration.

1.3.6 BIOCOMPOSITES

From a biological perspective, it is a natural strategy to combine polymers and ceramics to fabricate scaffolds for bone tissue engineering because native bone is the combination of a naturally occurring polymer and a biological apatite. From the point of view of materials science, a single material type does not always provide the necessary mechanical and chemical properties desired for a particular application. In these instances, composite materials designed to combine the advantages of both components may be most appropriate. Polymers and ceramics that degrade *in vivo* should be chosen for designing biocomposites for tissue-engineering scaffolds. While massive release of acidic degradation from polymers can cause inflammatory reactions [4,92,131], the basic degradation of calcium phosphate or bioactive glasses would buffer the acidic by-products of polymers and may thereby help to avoid the formation of an unfavorable environment for cells due to a decreased pH level. Mechanically, bioceramics are much stronger than polymers and play a critical role in providing mechanical stability to constructs prior to the synthesis of a new bone matrix by cells. However, ceramics and glasses are very fragile because of their intrinsic brittleness and flaw sensitivity. To capitalize on their advantages and minimize their shortcomings, ceramic and glass materials have been combined with various biopolymers to form composite biomaterials for osseous regeneration. Table 1.7 lists selected ceramic/glass–polymer composites, which were designed as biomedical devices or scaffold materials for bone tissue engineering, and their mechanical properties.

In general, all these synthetic composites have good biocompatibility. Kikuchi et al. [132], for instance, combined TCP with PLA to form a polymer–ceramic composite, which was found to possess the osteoconductivity of β-TCP and the degradability of PLA [132].

The research team led by Laurencin [147] synthesized porous scaffolds containing PLGA and hydroxyapatite, which were reported to combine the degradability of PLGA with the bioactivity of hydroxyapatite, fostering cell proliferation and differentiation as well as mineral formation

TABLE 1.7

Biocomposites Designed for Bone Tissue Engineering

Biocomposites					Compressive (C), Tensile(T), Flexural				
Ceramic	Polymer	Percentage of Ceramic (%)	Porosity (%)	Pore Size (μm)	Strength (F) (MPa)	Modulus (MPa)	Ultimate Strain (%)	Toughness (kJ/m^2)	References
Dense composites									
HA fiber	PDLLA	2–10.5 (vol.)	Not applicable		45 (F)	$1.75–2.47\times10^3$			133
	PLLA	10–70 (wt.)			50–60 (F)	$6.4–12.8\times10^3$	0.7–2.3		134
HA	PLGA	40–85 (vol.)			22 (F)	1.1×10^3		5.29	135,136
	Chitosan	40–85 (vol.)			12 (F)	2.15×10^3		0.092	136
	Chitosan+PLGA	40–85 (vol.)			43 (F)	2.6×10^3		9.77	136
	PPhos	85–95 (wt.)							137
	Collagen	50–72 (wt.)							138
β-TCP	PLLA-*co*-PEH	75 (wt.)			51 (F)	5.18×10^3			132
	PPF	25 (wt.)			7.5–7.7 (C)	191–134			139
A/W	PE	10–50 (vol.)			18–28 (F)	$0.9–5.7\times10^3$			140
Ca$_3$(CO$_3$)$_2$	PLLA	30 (wt.)			50 (C)	$3.5–6\times10^3$			141
Human cortical bone					50–150 (T) 130–180 (C)	$12–18\times10^3$			28,43–46
Porous composites									
Amorphous CaP	PLGA	28–75 (wt.)	75	>100		65			142,143
β-TCP	Chitosan–Gelatin	10–70 (wt.)		322–355	0.32–0.88 (C)	3.94–10.88			144
HA	PLLA	50 (wt.)	85–96	100×300	0.39 (C)	10–14			145
	PLGA	60–75 (wt.)	81–91	800–1800	0.07–0.22 (C)	2–7.5			146
	PLGA		30–40	110–150		337–1459			147
Bioglass	PLGA	75 (wt.)	43	89	0.42 (C)	51			64,148,149
	PLLA	20–50 (wt.)	77–80	~100 ~10	1.5–3.9 (T)	137–260	1.1–13.7		150
	PLGA	0.1–1 (wt.)		50–300					151
	PDLLA	5–29 (wt.)	94	~100 10–50	0.07–0.08 (C)	0.65–1.2	7.21–13.3		111,112,152
Phosphate glass A/W	PLA–PDLLA	40 (wt.)	93–97		0.017–0.020 (C)	0.075–0.12			153
	PDLLA	20–40 (wt.)	85.5–95.2	98–154					154
Human cancellous bone					4–12 (C)	100–500	1.65–2.11		155,156

[147,157,158]. Similarly, composites of bioactive glass and PLA were observed to form calcium phosphate layers on their surfaces and support rapid and abundant growth of human osteoblasts and osteoblast-like cells when cultured *in vitro* [109–112,148–154].

A comparison between the dense composites and cortical bone indicates that the most promising synthetic composite seems to be hydroxyapatite fiber–reinforced PLA composite [134], which, however, exhibit mechanical property values close to the lower values of the cortical bone. Other promising composite scaffolds reported in literature are those from Bioglass and PLLA or PDLLA [149–152]. They have a well-defined porous structure, for example obtained by thermally induced phase separation [151], at the same time their mechanical properties are close to (but lower than) those of cancellous bone.

1.3.7 SUMMARY

To design an ideal scaffold, which is bioresorbable, biocompatible, provides for cell attachment, proliferation, and maturation, and which disappears whenever a new bone forms allowing the new bone to undergo remodeling, it is necessary to weight up the *pros* and *cons* of the potential precursor materials, as summarized in Table 1.8.

Among the bioactive ceramics and glasses listed in Table 1.8, bioactive (silicate) glasses have remarkable advantages. The ability to enhance vascularization, the role of silicon in upregulating

TABLE 1.8

Advantages and Disadvantages of Synthetic Scaffold Biomaterials in Bone Tissue Engineering

Biomaterials	Positive	Negative
Calcium phosphates (e.g., HA, TCP, and BPCP)	1. Excellent biocompatibility 2. Supporting cell activity 3. Good osteoconductivity	1. Too fragile in amorphous structure 2. Nearly bioinert in crystalline phase
Bioactive glasses and glass-ceramics	1. Excellent biocompatibility 2. Supporting cell activity 3. Good osteconductivity 4. Vascularization 5. Upregulation of gene expression 6. Tailorable degradation rate	1. Mechanically brittle and weak in the glass state 2. Degrade slowly in crystalline structures, except for 45S5 Bioglass-derived glass-ceramics
Bulk biodegradable polymers (e.g., PLA, PGA, PLGA, PPF)	1. Good biocompatibility 2. Biodegradable with a wide range of degradation rates 3. Bioresorbable 4. Good processability 5. Good ductility	1. Inflammation caused by acid degradation products 2. Accelerated degradation rates cause collapse of scaffolds
Surface bioerodible polymers (e.g., POE, poly(anhydrides), poly(phosphazene))	1. Good biocompatibility 2. Retention of mechanical integrity over the degradative life of the device 3. Significantly enhanced bone ingrowth into the porous scaffolds, owing to the increment in pore size	1. They cannot be completely replaced by new bone tissue
Composites	1. Excellent biocompatibility 2. Supporting cell activity 3. Good osteoconductivity 4. Tailorable degradation rate 5. Improved mechanical properties	1. Fabrication techniques can be complex

gene expression, and the tailorable degradation rate make bioactive glasses promising scaffold materials over others, and so they could be the material of choice as the inorganic component of composite scaffolds. Although bioactive glasses are brittle with low fracture toughness (Table 1.4), they can be used in combination with polymers to form composite materials. The ability to couple mechanical strength with tailorable biodegradability makes 45S5 Bioglass-derived glass-ceramics advantageous over calcium phosphates (including hydroxyapatite), as well as other bioactive glasses and related glass-ceramics.

Between the two types of polymers, the bulk degradable type is more promising than the surface-erosive group, considering that being replaced by new bone tissue is one of the important criteria of an ideal scaffold material (Table 1.1). Finally, it is obvious that composites can be considered ideal scaffolding materials for bone tissue engineering if fabrication processes suitable for the production of 3-D structures of the required size and shape and amenable to commercialization are further developed and optimised.

1.4 FABRICATION OF TISSUE-ENGINEERING SCAFFOLDS

1.4.1 Fabrication of Inorganic Scaffolds

Porous ceramics can be produced by a variety of different processes [2,159], which may be classified into two main categories: (1) manual-based processing techniques and (2) computer-controlled fabrication processes, such as solid free-form (SFF) technology, which is also commonly known as rapid prototyping (RP) [160]. Most manual-based processing techniques can further be divided into two groups: conventional powder-forming processes and sol–gel techniques [161].

1.4.1.1 Powder-Forming Processes

A flowchart that is common to all powder-forming processes is shown in Figure 1.2, and the different steps involved in these processes are discussed in this section.

1.4.1.1.1 Preparation of Slurries
Slurry is a suspension of ceramic particles in a suitable liquid (e.g., water or ethanol) used to prepare green bodies. The inherent mechanism of pore formation in a powder compact is illustrated in Figure 1.3. Attractive forces that consist of hydrogen bonds, van der Waals forces, Coulomb's forces, and physical friction between particles cause agglomeration of particles. Addition of fillers to the

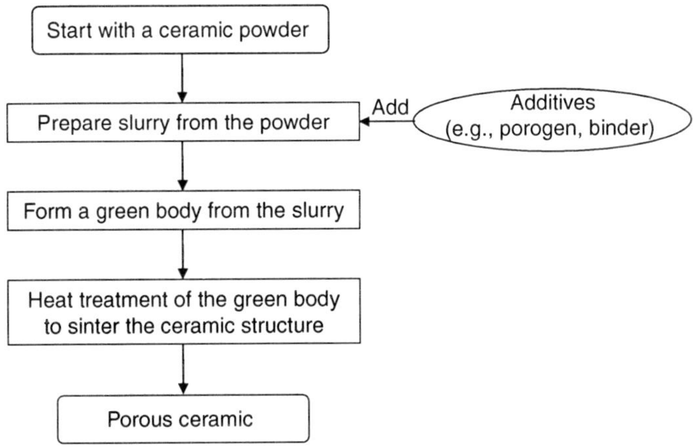

FIGURE 1.2 Flowchart of the powder-sintering method to produce porous ceramic scaffolds.

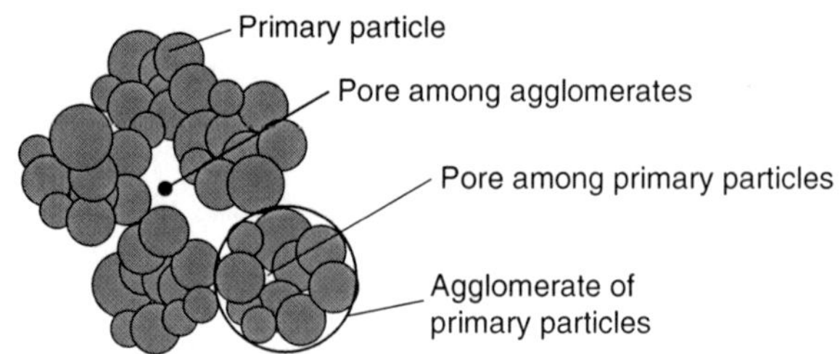

FIGURE 1.3 Schematic illustration of pores among agglomerates and particles [159].

TABLE 1.9
Methods for Obtaining Ceramic Bodies for 3-D Porous Ceramics [159]

Dry processes
Loose packing
Compaction
    Uniaxial pressing
    Cold isostatic pressing (CIPing)
Wet processes
Slip casting
Injection molding
Phase separation/freeze-drying
Polymer replication
Gelcasting

---

slurry, such as sucrose, gelatine, and PMMA microbeads, and a wetting agent (i.e., a surfactant) can increase porosity. These chemicals, which are called porogens, are evaporated or burned out during sintering, and as a result pores are formed [2,159]. One successful formulation has been the use of hydroxyapatite powder slurries (dispersed with vegetable oil) added with gelatine solution [162], which has led to porous scaffolds with interconnected pore structure with pore diameters of ~100 μm. A similar process has been used to prepare melt-derived Bioglass scaffolds using camphor ($C_{10}H_{16}O$) as the porogen [163].

Binders are also added to slurries. The most important function of a binder is to improve the strength of the green body in order to provide structural integrity for handling (green strength) before the product is sintered [164]. Polysaccharides [165], polyvinyl alcohol (PVA) [166], and polyvinyl butyl (PVB) [167] are the frequently added binders in bioceramic slurries.

1.4.1.1.2 Formation of Green Bodies

In ceramic production, a green body is always porous, and its structure largely determines that of the sintered product. Table 1.9 lists different methods of obtaining green bodies for 3-D porous ceramics. These methods can be classified into two categories: dry and wet processes [159]. They lead to different porous structures and pore volume fractions. Certain techniques, such as tape casting, extrusion, slurry dipping, and spraying, are not included here; because they aim at achieving a predetermined geometric shape of ceramic parts (such as rods, tubes, sheets, and coating on films), instead of a given porous structure. Except injection molding, all conventional processes listed in Table 1.9 have been applied to synthesize ceramic scaffolds for tissue engineering as discussed below.

Dry methods. The simplest way to prepare ceramic green bodies is the dry powder method where powders are directly compressed by pressing (uniaxially or isostatically) into molds, thereby forming green bodies. Pore diameters decrease and mechanical properties increase as the packing density of the particles in the green bodies increases. A densification step by sintering at high temperature is required (see Section 1.4.1.1.3). Mechanical properties can be increased further by hot-isostatic pressing (HIP) [168] or by uniaxial hot pressing. These pressure-assisted methods decrease the pore diameter as well. The addition of porogens, such as sucrose and camphor, enhances the formation of pores [159].

Slip casting. Slip is a creamy (relatively thick) slurry. In this method, the slurry is cast into a porous mold. The liquid of the slurry is absorbed into the porous mold, and as a result the particles in the slurry are filtered, which adhere to the mold surface. After this process, a porous green body is obtained through further drying [161,169].

Phase separation/freeze-drying. In this method, a ceramic slurry is poured into a container, which is immersed in a freezing bath. Thus, ice is stimulated to grow and ceramic particles are piled up between the columns of the growing ice. After the slurry is completely frozen, the container is dried in a drying vessel, usually under vacuum [170]. The pores are created by the ice crystals that sublimate at a reduced pressure. Freeze-drying removal of ice crystals creates 3-D interconnected pore channels with complex structures. The porous structure can be customized by the variation of the slurry concentration, freezing temperature, and pressure.

Replication technique. This method, which is also called the polymer-sponge method, was patented for the manufacturing of ceramic foams [171]. In the polymer-replication process, the green bodies of ceramic foams are prepared by coating a polymer (e.g., polyurethane) foam with a ceramic slurry. The polymer foam, which already has the desired macrostructure, simply serves as a sacrificial template for the ceramic coating. The polymer template is immersed in the slurry, which subsequently infiltrates the structure, and so the ceramic particles adhere to the surface of the polymer substrate. Excess slurry is squeezed out leaving a ceramic coating on the foam struts. After it is dried, the polymer is slowly burned out in order to minimize damage to the porous ceramic coating. After the removal of the polymer, the ceramic is sintered to the desired density. The process replicates the macroporous structure of the polymer foam and results in a rather distinctive microstructure within the struts. A flowchart of the process is given in Figure 1.4 [172]. This method has been applied for the preparation of foam-like scaffolds for tissue engineering, including porous calcium phosphates [173], Bioglass [80], and other inert bioceramics [172,174].

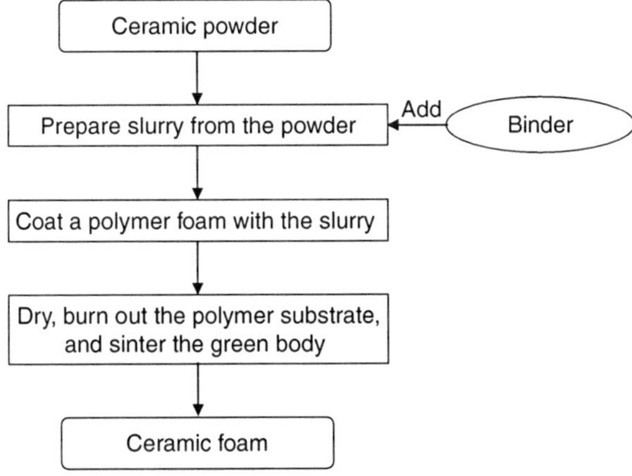

FIGURE 1.4   Flowchart of the replication process to produce a ceramic foam.

Apart from the slurry-immersion coating, electrospray coating techniques have also been applied together with the polymer-sponge process to produce ceramic foams, for example, Al_2O_3 [175] and ZrO_2 foams [176]. Unlike the foams produced by the slurry-immersion method, the struts of the ceramic foams produced by the process of electrospray coating contain fewer holes and cracks. This microstructure can lead to improved mechanical properties of the foams [176].

Another possibility investigated to improve the mechanical properties of foams made by the replication method is to apply a thin polymer coating on the porous structure. For example, to improve the mechanical stability of highly porous Bioglass-derived scaffolds produced by the replication technique [80], a polymer coating, such as poly(D,L-lactic acid) (PDLLA), was applied [177]. The coating thickness was approximately 3 µm on an average. Although the thin coating layer did not increase the mechanical strength of the foams considerably, it significantly improved the mechanical stability of the structure. The fracture energy of the coated foams was ~20 times higher than that of uncoated foams. More importantly, upon immersion in SBF, nanofibers of hydroxyapatite deposited within the PDLLA coating layer, eventually a nanocomposite layer, formed biomimetically on the strut surfaces. This method has remarkably improved the mechanical performance of the scaffolds in a biological environment [177].

Gelcasting. This method adopts one of the direct-foaming techniques mentioned in Table 1.10 to achieve highly porous green bodies. The foamed suspension is set through a direct-consolidation technique, listed in Table 1.10, that is, polymerization of organic monomers (i.e., gelation), in which the particles of the slurry are consolidated through polymerization reaction. A green body is formed after the gel is cast in a mold [178–180]. Figure 1.5 gives the flowchart of the gelcasting process.

Two factors are critical in the gelcasting process: (1) the gelation speed must be fast enough to prevent foam collapse, and (2) the gel rheology is important because the process involves casting. Systems of high fluidity are required in order to enable easy filling of small details in molds to allow production of high-complexity shapes. Gelcasting techniques have been applied to produce hydroxyapatite foams [181–183]. Gelcasting has also been combined with the replication process (described above in this section) to produce hydroxyapatite scaffolds with interconnected pores [184].

1.4.1.1.3 Sintering

The final step in the production of a ceramic foam is the densification of the green bodies by conducting a high temperature sintering process. Foams are normally dried at room temperature for at least 24 h prior to sintering. In this step, controlled heating is important to prevent collapse of the ceramic network. The heating rate, sintering temperature, and holding time depend on the ceramic starting materials. For example, values are in the range of 0.5–2°C/min, 1200–1350°C, and 2–5 h,

---

TABLE 1.10

Techniques of Direct Foaming and Direct Consolidation

Techniques	References
Direct foaming	20
1. Injection of gases through the fluid medium	
2. Mechanically agitating particulate suspension	
3. Blowing agents	
4. Evaporation of compounds	
5. Evaporation of gas by *in situ* chemical reaction	
Direct consolidation	178
1. Gelcasting	
2. Direct coagulation consolidation (DCC)	
3. Hydrolysis-assisted solidification (HAS)	
4. Freezing (quick set)	

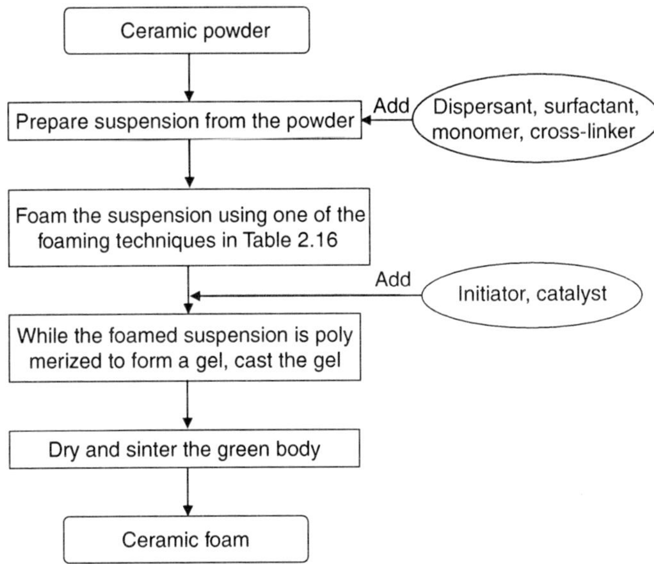

FIGURE 1.5 Flowchart of the gelcasting method to produce a ceramic foam.

respectively, in the case of porous hydroxyapatite [173,181,183,185]. It is worthwhile noticing that there is a narrow time–temperature window for densification of foams made from bioactive glasses, which are prone to crystallize while sintering by viscous flow. Hence the production of bioactive glass foams by powder-based methods presents difficulties [80].

1.4.1.2 Sol–Gel Techniques

1.4.1.2.1 Sol–Gel Process and Synthesis of Aerogel Ceramics

The sol–gel process is a well-developed, robust, and versatile "wet" technique for the synthesis of ceramics and glasses. By applying the sol–gel process, it is possible to fabricate inorganic materials in various forms: ultrafine or spherical shaped powders, thin film coatings, ceramic fibers, microporous inorganic membranes, monolithic ceramics and glasses, and extremely porous aerogel materials [186].

The processing path of aerogel ceramics starts with an alkoxide precursor. Alkoxide precursors, such as tetraethyl orthosilicate (TEOS) and triethoxyl orthophosphate (TEP), undergo hydrolysis and condensation reactions to form a sol. In case of silicate precursors, polymerization of —Si—OH groups continues after hydrolysis is complete, beginning the formation of the silicate (—Si—O—Si—) network. The network connectivity increases until it spans throughout the solvent medium. Eventually a wet gel forms. The wet gel is then subjected to controlled thermal processes of aging to strengthen the gel, drying to remove the liquid by-product of the polycondensation reaction, and thermal stabilization (or sintering) to remove organic species from the surface of the material; and as a result, a porous aerogel forms [2,187].

1.4.1.2.2 Production of Highly Porous Glasses

Highly porous glasses (or glass foams) have been developed by a slightly modified sol–gel process [188]. The sol–gel process is based on the polymerization reactions of metal alkoxide precursors (usually TEOS and TEP). These precursors are dissolved in a solvent, and a gel is formed by hydrolysis and condensation reactions. The gel is then subjected to controlled thermal processes of aging to strengthen the gel, drying to remove the liquid by-product of the polycondensation reaction, and thermal stabilization/sintering to remove organic species from the surface of the material (500–800°C). Sol–gel derived glass scaffolds are obtained by directly foaming the sol with the use

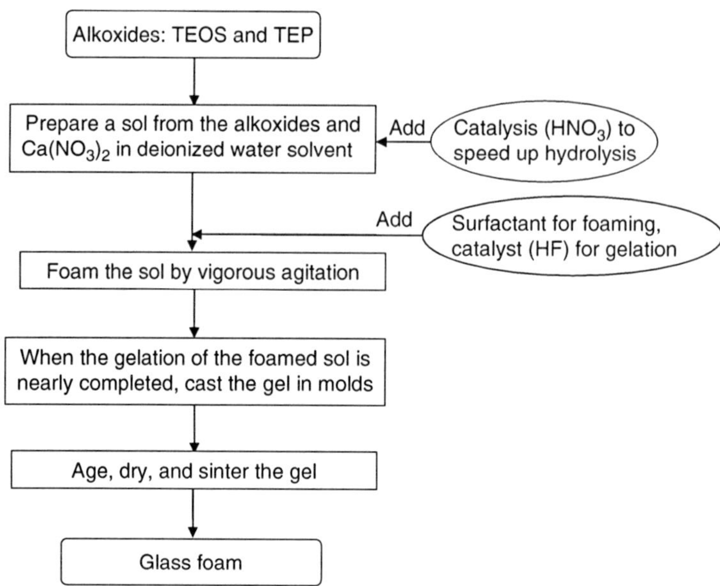

FIGURE 1.6 Flowchart of the production of bioactive glass foams using sol–gel technology.

of a surfactant and catalysts [188–190]. Therefore, after sol hydrolysis, the surfactant (e.g., Teepol, a detergent containing a low-concentration mixture of anionic and nonionic surfactants), water (improves foamability of surfactant), and the catalyst for polycondensation (e.g., HF) are added by vigorous agitation. A flowchart of the process is given in Figure 1.6. Porosity of the foam scaffolds is influenced by the foaming temperature, water content, and catalyst content. Sol–gel derived bioactive glass foams [191,192] and gelcast hydroxyapatite scaffolds [181,183] have shown favorable results in both *in vitro* and *in vivo* tests for bone regeneration.

1.4.1.3 Solid Free-Form Techniques

SFF techniques, also known as RP, are computer-controlled fabrication processes. They can rapidly produce highly complex 3-D objects using data generated by computer-aided design (CAD) systems. In a typical case, an image of a bone defect in a patient can be taken, which is used to develop a 3-D CAD model. The computer can then reduce the model to slices or layers. The 3-D objects are constructed layer-by-layer using RP techniques such as fused deposition modeling (FDM), selective laser sintering (SLS), 3-D printing (3-DP), or stereolithography [160]. Calcium phosphate scaffolds have been produced using the FDM process [193,194], SLS, 3-DP processes [160], stereolithography [195,196], and RP combined with replication technique [197]. The typical process chain for all SFF techniques is presented in Figure 1.7.

To date, only a small number of SFF techniques, such as 3-DP, FDM, and SLS, have been adopted for tissue-engineering scaffolds. The following paragraphs give brief descriptions of the principles on which these three techniques are based. Comprehensive technical details can be found in previous detailed reviews [160,198–201].

1.4.1.3.1 Three-Dimensional Printing

Three-dimensional printing employs ink-jet printing technology for processing materials from powders. Therefore, this technique is a combination of SFF and powder sintering. During fabrication, a printer head is used to print a liquid binder onto thin layers of powder following the object's profile being generated by the system computer. The subsequent stacking and printing layer recreates the full structure of the desired object.

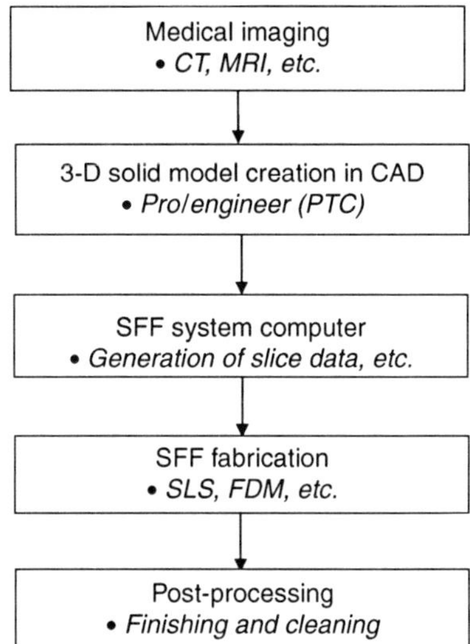

FIGURE 1.7 Flowchart of the typical rapid prototyping (RP) process [160].

1.4.1.3.2 Fused Deposition Modeling

FDM employs the concept of melt extrusion to deposit a parallel series of material rods that forms a material layer. In FDM, filament material stock (generally thermoplastic) is fed and melted inside a heated liquefier head before being extruded through a nozzle with a small orifice.

Indirect fabrication methods involving FDM have been applied for producing porous bioceramic implants. In this method, FDM was employed to fabricate wax molds containing the negative profiles of the desired scaffold microstructure. Ceramic scaffolds were then cast from the mold through a lost mold technique [193,194].

1.4.1.3.3 Selective Laser Sintering

SLS employs a CO_2 laser beam to selectively sinter polymer, ceramic, or polymer-ceramic composite powders to form material layers. The laser beam is directed onto the powder bed by a high precision laser scanning system. The fusion of material layers that are stacked on top of one another replicates the object's height [202,203].

1.4.1.4 Comparison of Fabrication Techniques for Ceramic or Glass Scaffolds

Table 1.11 lists the porosity, pore size, and mechanical properties of several porous ceramics produced by different techniques. Figure 1.8 shows typical pore structures produced by different techniques. Comparing the pore structures of ceramic scaffolds shown in Figure 1.8 with the structure of cancellous bone, it is evident that the pore morphology produced by the replication technique is the most similar one, containing completely interconnecting pores and solid material forming only the struts. The ceramic foams synthesized by gelcasting and sol–gel techniques come next in terms of structural similarity to cancellous bone, however, it is expected that these foams exhibit lower pore interconnectivity than foams made by the replication method.

The advantages of replication method over other ceramic foaming techniques are summarized in Table 1.12. In brief, the replication technique meets all criteria posed on the fabrication process of tissue-engineering scaffolds: suitable for commercialization, reproducible, cost-effective, safe, and capable of producing irregular or complex shapes. Contemporary authors consider the replication technique as the optimal technique for production of novel bioactive glass-ceramic scaffolds for bone tissue engineering [204].

TABLE 1.11

Porous Structures and Mechanical Properties of Porous Bioceramics Produced by Different Techniques

Technique	Materials	Porosity (%)	Pore Size (μm)	Closed (C) or Open (O)	Compressive/Flexural Strength (MPa)	References
Powder forming–sintering						
Dry process with porogens	Hydroxyapatite	NA	Varying between 40 and 100	C	NA	166
	Hydroxyapatite	67	250–400	O		205
	45S5 Bioglass	21	200–300	C		163
		42	80	C		206
						69
Phase separation/ freeze-drying	Al_2O_3	30–60	~50 in width, 300–500 in length	O	NA	170
Replication technique/coated by						
Slurry-immersion	Al_2O_3	87	Up to 800	O	NA	169
	TiO_2	74	385–700	O		165
	Glass-reinforced HA	85–97.5	Average size 420–560	O	0.01–0.175	185
	Hydroxyapatite	69–86	490–1130	O	0.03–0.29	173
	HA coated by PLGA	69–86	490–1130	O	0.31–4.03	173
	Bioglass	>90	400–800	O	0.4–0.5	80
Electrospray	Al_2O_3	96	~800	O		175
Gelcasting/foamed by						
Starch	Al_2O_3	23–70	10–80	C	NA	178

Vigorous stirring	Al_2O_3	70–92	Average size: 260–700 Range in 50–2000 NA 20–1000	Partly O/C NA	2–26	179
	Al_2O_3	NA	50–300	Partly O/C	3–20	180
	Hydroxyapatite	76.7–80.2	Cell: 100–500	Partly O/C		
	Hydroxyapatite	48	Window: 30–120	Partly O/C		
	Hydroxyapatite	NA				
Replication technique	Hydroxyapatite	70–77	200–400	O	4.4–7.4	181
	β-TCP+HA	73	NA	O	8	183
					1.6–5.8	182
					0.55–5	184
					9.8	207
Sol–gel/foamed by						
Burning PMMA beads	$CaO–SiO_2$ glass	70–95	~0.5	Partially O/C		208
Decomposition of H_2O_2	$(CH_3O)_4Si$		<0.7	Partially O/C		209
Burning EO-PO-EO blocks	SiO_2 glass		1–10	Partially O/C		210
Vigorous stirring	Bioactive glasses		Up to 600, size of cell windows mostly in 80–120	Partially O/C		189
Solid free-form (SFF)						
FDM	Al_2O_3	29–44	305–480	O	62–128	211
	β-TCP	29–44	305–480	O	0.25–1.45	211
	$CaO-Al_2O_3$	29–44	300	O	2–24	212
	PP-TCP composite	36–52	160	O	12.7–10	213
SLS	Calcium phosphates	30	200	O	13.8	214

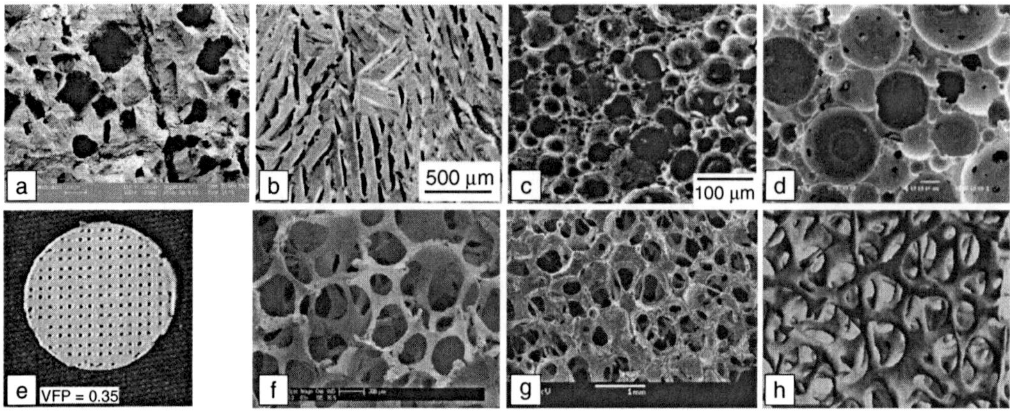

FIGURE 1.8 Typical structures of porous ceramics produced by different techniques: (a) porous hydroxyapatite produced by the powder method combined with PVA as a porogen additive [205], (b) porous alumina by freeze-drying method [170], (c) porous hydroxyapatite by gelcasting method [181], (d) bioactive glass foams by sol–gel technique [188], (e) porous β-TCP by solid free-form technique [211], (f) β-TCP+hydroxyapatite foam produced by the replication technique [207], (g) porous bioglass-based glass-ceramic foam by the replication technique [80], and (h) porous structure of cancellous bone [215].

TABLE 1.12
Advantages of the Replication Technique over Other Methods

1. Cancellous bone-like macroporous structure

   The porous structure produced by the replication technique is very similar to cancellous bone: highly porous network with open and highly interconnected porosity, compared with the rest of the techniques (see Figures 1.8 (f, g, h)).

2. High commercialization potential

   This technique is the simplest and most cost-effective method, and thus most suitable for commercialization, for example, compared with SFF. SFF-RP, which are expensive processes, it may be a method for producing specific and complex scaffold architectures.

3. Safety

   It does not involve any toxic chemicals, compared with sol–gel and gelcasting techniques, which use HF to accelerate polymerization.

4. Irregular or complex shape production ability

   It can produce scaffolds of irregular or complex shapes, compared with standard dry powder processing or sol–gel-based methods.

1.4.2 FABRICATION OF COMPOSITE SCAFFOLDS

The fabrication of polymer–ceramic composite scaffolds is based on conventional processes used for neat polymeric scaffolds. Numerous techniques have been developed to process porous polymer scaffolds for use in tissue engineering. Table 1.13 lists currently applied 3-D polymer scaffold fabrication technologies, based on Ref. 1. Excellent reviews can be found in the literature [1,216–219].

While intensive efforts have been made to develop the processing technologies of polymer scaffolds, relatively less attention has been paid to the fabrication of porous composite scaffolds. Among the technologies in Table 1.13, solvent casting with or without particle leaching [146,150,153,154] and TIPS combined with freeze-drying [109–112,144,145] seem to be the most applied method to the fabrication of polymer–ceramic composite scaffolds. In addition to these methods, there are

TABLE 1.13

3-D Fabrication Technologies of Polymer Scaffolds [1]

Fabrication Technology	Required Properties of Materials	Reproducibility	Available Pore Size (µm)	Porosity (%)	Architecture
Solvent casting/particle leaching	Soluble	User, material and technique sensitive	30–300	20–50	Spherical pores
Membrane lamination	Soluble	User, material and technique sensitive	30–300	<85	Irregular pores
Textile technology	Fibers	Machine controlled	20–100	<95	
Melt molding	Thermoplastic	Machine controlled	50–500	<80	
Extrusion/particle leaching	Thermoplastic	Machine controlled	<100	<84	Spherical pores
Emulsion freeze-drying	Soluble	User, material and technique sensitive	<200	<97	High volume of interconnected micropores
Thermally induced phase separation	Soluble	User, material and technique sensitive	<200	<97	High volume of interconnected micropores
Gas foaming	Amorphous	Material and technique sensitive	<100	10–30	High volume of noninterconnected micropores
Gas foaming/particle leaching	Amorphous	Material and technique sensitive	Micropores <50 Macropores <400	<97	Low volume of noninterconnected micropores combined with high volume of interconnected macropores
Three-dimensional printing	Soluble	Machine and computer controlled	45–150	<60	100% interconnected macrospores
Fused deposition modeling	Thermoplastic	Machine and computer controlled	>150	<80	100% interconnected macrospores

TABLE 1.14

Fabrication Methods of Three-Dimensonal Porous Composite Scaffolds

Fabrication Technique	Biocomposites		Percentage of Ceramic (%)	Porosity (%)	Pore Size (μm)	References
	Ceramic	Polymer				
Solvent casting/particle leaching	HA	PLGA	60–75 (wt.)	81–91	800–1800	146
	Bioglass	PLLA	20–50 (wt.)	77–80	~100 (macro) ~10 (micro)	150
	Phosphate glass	PLA–PDLLA	40 (wt.)	93–97		153
	A/W	PDLLA	20–40 (wt.)	85.5–95.2	98–154	154
Thermally induced phase separation/freeze-drying	β-TCP	Chitosan–gelatin	10–70 (wt.)		322–355	144
	HA	PLLA	50 (wt.)	85–95	100×300	145
	Bioglass	PDLLA	5–29 (wt.)	94	~100 (macro) 10–50 (micro)	109–112, 152, 221
Microsphere/sintering	Amorphous CaP	PLGA	28–75 (wt.)	75	>100	142, 143
	Bioglass	PLGA	75 (wt.)	43	89	149
Polymer foam/ceramic coating	HA	PLGA	40–85 (vol.)			135, 136
	Bioglass	PDLLA				109, 110, 222, 223
Ceramic foam/polymer coating	HA foam	PDLLA				173, 221–223

two other methods: microsphere sintering and foam coating, which have been considered extensively for the combination of ceramic and polymeric materials, as listed in Table 1.14 and shown in Figure 1.9. This section will briefly introduce the processing techniques for polymer-ceramic composite scaffolds.

1.4.2.1 Solvent Casting

Solvent casting of biocomposite scaffolds involves the dissolution of the polymer in an organic solvent, mixing it with ceramic granules, and casting the solution into a predefined 3-D mold. The solvent is subsequently allowed to evaporate. The main advantage of this processing technique is the ease of fabrication without the need of specialized equipment. The primary disadvantages of solvent casting are (1) the limitation in the shapes (typically flat sheets and tubes are the only shapes that can be formed), (2) the possible retention of toxic solvent within the polymer, and (3) the denaturation of the proteins and other molecules incorporated into the polymer by the use of solvents. The use of organic solvents to cast the polymer may decrease the activity of bioinductive molecules (e.g., protein). The detailed processing steps can be found in Ref. 65.

1.4.2.2 Solvent Casting or Particle Leaching and Microsphere Packing

Polymer-ceramic constructs can be fabricated by the solvent aggregation method. The polymer microspheres are first formed from traditional water oil/water emulsions. Solvent-aggregated polymer-ceramic scaffolds can then be constructed by mixing solvent, salt or sugar particles, ceramic granules, and prehardened microspheres [220]. A 3-D structure of controlled porosity

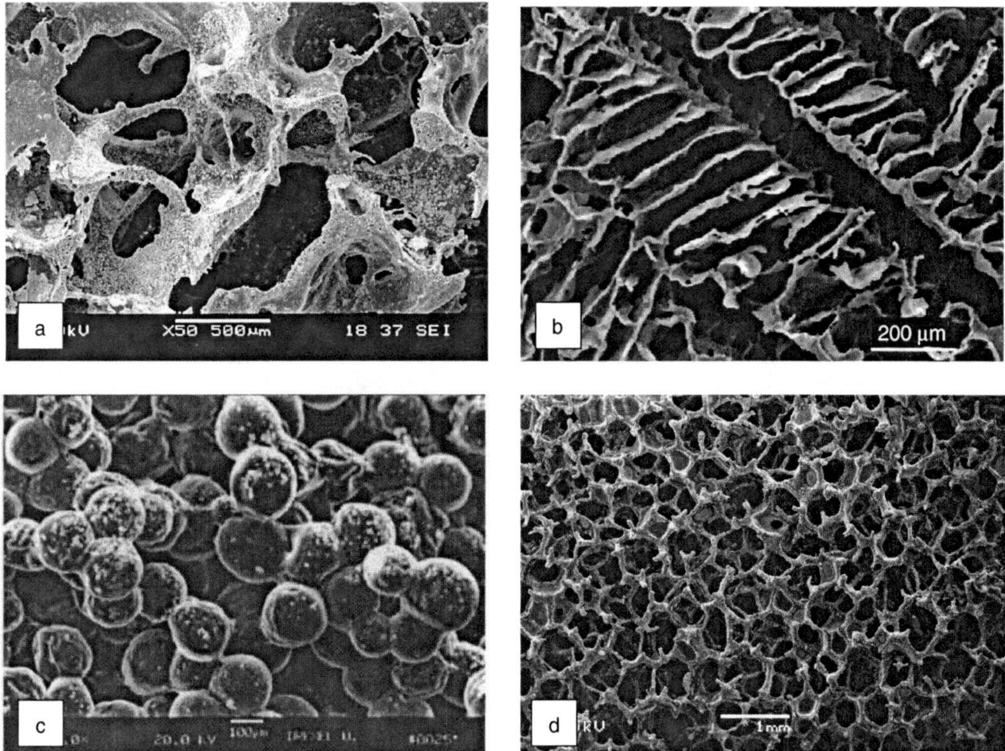

FIGURE 1.9 Typical structures of porous biocomposites by various techniques: (a) solvent casting or particle leaching [146,150], (b) phase separation or freeze-drying [145], (c) microsphere sintering [143], (d) polymer coating of Bioglass foam [177].

is formed based on this method combined with particle leaching and microsphere packing. This method shares similar advantages and disadvantages with the solvent casting technique. Details of the method are presented in Ref. 65.

1.4.2.3 Thermally Induced Phase Separation or Freeze-Drying

Three-dimensional porous structures can also be achieved through phase separation and evaporation. An approach to induce phase separation is to lower the temperature of the suspension of polymer and ceramic materials. The solvent is solidified first, forcing the polymer and ceramic mixture into the interstitial spaces. The frozen mixture is then lyophilized using a freeze dryer in which the ice solvent evaporates [109,144,145].

1.4.2.4 Microsphere Sintering

In this process, microspheres of a ceramic and polymer composite are synthesized first, using emulsion or solvent evaporation technique. Sintering the composite microspheres yields a 3-D porous scaffold [142,143].

1.4.2.5 Foam Coating

An alternative approach to address the combination of polymeric and ceramic materials is to coat bioactive ceramics onto polymeric foams [220–222]. The inverse method, known as polymer-coated ceramic scaffolds, has also been investigated [173,177,223], as discussed in Section 1.4.1.1.2.

1.5 SURFACE FUNCTIONALIZATION

The biocompatibility of biomaterials is related to cell behavior in contact with the biomaterial surface and particularly to cell adhesion to the surface. Surface characteristics of materials, such as topography (roughness), chemistry, or surface energy, play a key role in the cell adhesion behavior on biomaterials. The first stage in cell or material interactions involves cell attachment, adhesion, and spreading. The quality of this first phase will influence the cell's capacity to proliferate and to differentiate (second stage) in contact with the scaffold [224–228].

The process of bone tissue regeneration involves expression of genes and synthesis of proteins known to be important in the mineralization process. To ensure the *in vivo* biocompatibility of an implant, it is often necessary to modify the material surface, either physically by surface roughening, for example, or chemically, such as by attachment of chemically active species [228,229].

To improve the cell–substrate interaction, different strategies including surface modification have been developed. The functionalized surfaces can control not only the initial protein adsorption and production, but also the differentiation potential of different cells (such as human stem cells) [229]. The main strategies developed for surface modification are presented in Sections 1.5.1 through 1.5.4.

1.5.1 Protein Adsorption

This first phase of cell–implant interaction depends on protein adhesion. The proteins currently used for chemical surface modification of biomaterials are growth factors (or related proteins) and adhesion proteins (or related peptides). Members of the transforming growth factor-β family are widely studied: TGF-β1, bone morphogenetic proteins BMP-2, BMP-7, or osteogenic protein OP-1 [230–233]. Among adhesion proteins, RGD-peptides (contain a sequence of the amino acids: arginine R, glycine G, and aspartic acid D) have a high efficacy in promoting osteoblast adhesion [226,234,235].

All these proteins can be adsorbed *in vitro* from the serum containing media or *in vivo* from biological fluids. The pH, ionic composition of biological solution, temperature, and the functional group of proteins are the main factors determining protein adsorption on a specific substrate [226]. Another important factor that influences the protein adsorption is the surface energy. Positively and negatively charged substrates adsorb different proteins [226]. In general, proteins that have a number of positively charged residues are expected to show a high affinity for the anionic surfaces, due to electrostatic attractions. By an appropriate pretreatment of the ceramic substrate (e.g., in phosphate solution), the ionic charges from the surface can be modified, providing an increasing affinity of the proteins or other biomolecules [236].

1.5.2 Silane-Modified Surfaces (Silanization Technique)

The ability of organosilanes to bond to surfaces arises from the fact that the ethoxy groups ($-Si-(OCH_2CH_3)_3$) of aminosilanes, such as aminopropyltriethoxysilane (APTES), form silanols ($-Si-(OH)_3$) in aqueous solution. These silanol groups can then bond covalently to a suitable substrate, usually inorganic solids displaying appropriate surface chemical groups (such as –OH), thus leaving terminal (nonbonded) amino groups free to serve as attachment sites for biological modifiers like peptides and proteins. Attachment of biological modifiers to the terminal amino groups can be accomplished by either of the two processes: physisorption or chemisorption [226,227].

The functional groups such as methyl (–CH3), hydroxyl (–OH), carboxyl (–COOH), and amino (–NH2) groups are present in many biological molecules and have specific physical and chemical properties that influence the cellular process. By silanization, the substrate surface can be modified in order to immobilize specific biomolecules. The inclusion of all these functional groups, using silane modification techniques, especially on glass surfaces, provides a method that

TABLE 1.15

Functional Group Abbreviations, Chemical Formulae, and Silane Precursors for Silane-Modified Surfaces [235]

Functional Group	Formula	Precursor
NH_2	$-(CH_2)_3NH_3^+$	3-Aminopropyltrimethoxysilane
COOH	$-COO^-$	Trichlorovinylsilane[a]
OH	$-CH_2CH_2OH$	Trichlorovinylsilane[a]
C_6H_5	$-C_6H_5$	Phenyltrichlorosilane
CH_3	$-CH_3$	Dimethyldichlorosilane

[a] The COOH and OH surfaces were produced by a postsilanization modification of the vinyl surfaces.

produces well-defined and organized substrates with different surface chemistries and energies [225–228,235,236]. Table 1.15 presents the typical silane precursors for silane-modified surfaces.

1.5.3 TOPOGRAPHY (ROUGHNESS) MODIFICATION

The cell adhesion on ceramic substrates can be enhanced by modifying the surface roughness (e.g., by sandblasting, heat treatment, acid etching, etc.). Increased surface wettability or hydrophilicity has been associated with enhanced protein adsorption and, consequently, cell adhesion on biomaterials [237]. There has been, however, only limited work on developing techniques to modify the surface topography of 3-D ceramic or composite scaffolds [238–240], these techniques being developed especially for metallic implant for orthopedics.

Another strategy consists of immersing the ceramic substrate in an SBF to mimic the first stage of bone tissue integration on the *in vivo* implants. The integration of bone tissue on the bioactive ceramic or composite surfaces takes place by biomineralization of a thin layer of calcium phosphate at the interface between the implant and the bone tissue. Therefore, by soaking the bioactive biomaterial in SBF, a uniform thick-film composed of nanocrystallites of biologically active calcium phosphate is produced [241]. During this biomimetic process, the topography of the ceramic implant is modified by the precipitation of nanocrystals of calcium phosphate on its surface. The new nanoscaled texture of the bioactive ceramic implant can improve the cellular adhesion.

1.5.4 POLYMER COATINGS

Another strategy to improve the cell–scaffold interaction is coating the substrate with an organic phase, usually a biodegradable polymer [177]. Moreover, the strong interfacial adhesion between the ceramic biomaterial and the organic polymer is a key parameter in generating composites with good mechanical properties. A wide variety of polymers have been investigated for this application, including PLA, PGA, PLGA, PDLLA, PHA, and PCL [173,177,223,242–244]. It has been anticipated that the combination of ceramic scaffolds and appropriate biodegradable polymer coatings can enhance the interfacial adhesion of proteins.

1.6 CONCLUSIONS

Significant developments have been achieved in the design and fabrication of a variety of bioceramic and composite scaffolds, which have demonstrated outstanding properties for applications in bone tissue engineering. However, there are several challenges ahead for material scientists and tissue engineers, associated with, in particular, the improvement of biological functions and mechanical integrity of synthetic scaffolds. Vascularization is the single most important issue to be addressed prior to clinical applications of bioceramic and composite scaffolds. The effect of dissolution products of bio-active glasses on angiogenesis demonstrated recently both *in vivo* and *in vitro* offers another alternative to the development of 3-D scaffolds with improved vascularization potential [55]. As such, prevascularization by using VGF is a highly recommended strategy in the design of synthetic tissue scaffolds. Other relevant issues include the optimization of surface functionalization and surface topography of scaffolds, as well as the development of advanced scaffolds with the capability to release other biomolecules, such as antibiotics, vitamins, or BGF during their degradation *in vivo*.

REFERENCES

1. Hutmacher DW. Scaffolds in tissue engineering bone and cartilage. *Biomaterials* 2000; 21: 2529–2543.
2. Jones JR, Boccaccini AR. Cellular ceramics in biomedical applications: Tissue engineering. In: *Cellular Ceramics: Structure, Manufacturing, Processing and Applications*, Scheffler M, Colombo P (eds.), Wiley-VCH Verlag GmbH & Co. KGaA, Weinheim, 2005, pp. 550–573.
3. Karageorgiou V, Kaplan D. Porosity of 3D Biomaterial Scaffolds and Osteogenesis. *Biomaterials* 2005; 26: 5474–5491.
4. Temenoff JS, Lu L, Mikos AG. Bone tissue engineering using synthetic biodegradable polymer scaffolds. In: *Bone Engineering*, Davies JE (ed.), EM Squared, Toronto, 2000, pp. 455–462.
5. Tamai N, Myoui A, Tomita T, Nakase T, Tanaka J, Ochi T. Novel hydroxyapatite ceramics with an interconnective porous structure inhibit superior osteoconduction *in vivo*. *J Biomed Mater Res* 2002; 59: 110–117.
6. Sedrakyan S, Zhou ZY, Perin L, Leach K, Mooney D, Kim TH. Tissue engineering of a small hand phalanx with a porously casted polylactic acid-polyglycolic acid copolymer. *Tissue Eng* 2006; 12: 2675–2683.
7. Radisic M, Vunjak-Novakovic G. Cardiac tissue engineering. *J Serb Chem Soc* 2005; 70(3): 541–556.
8. Henno S, Lambotte JC, et al. Characterisation and quantification of angiogenesis in β-tricalcium phosphate implants by immunohistochemistry and transmission electron microscopy. *Biomaterials* 2003; 24: 3173–3181.
9. Mastrogiacomo M, Scaglionec S, et al. Role of scaffold internal structure on *in vivo* bone formation in macroporous calcium phosphate bioceramics. *Biomaterials* 2006; 27: 3230–3237.
10. Oudadesse H, Derrien AC, Lucas-Girot A. Statistical experimental design for studies of porosity and compressive strength in composite materials applied as biomaterials. *Eur Phys J Appl Phys* 2005; 31: 217–223.
11. Gittings JP, Turner IG, Miles AW. Calcium phosphate open porous scaffold bioceramics. *Key Eng Mater (Bioceramics 17)* 2005; 284–286: 349–352.
12. Rezwan K, Chen QZ, Blaker JJ, Boccaccini AR. Biodegradable and bioactive porous polymer/inorganic composite scaffolds for bone tissue engineering. *Biomaterials* 2006; 27(18): 3413–3431.
13. Koening AL, Grainger DW. Cell-synthetic surface interaction: Targeted cell adhesion (Chap: 66). In: *Methods of Tissue Engineering*, Atala A, Lanza RP (eds.), Academic Press, San Diego, CA, 2002, pp. 751–770.
14. Hermanson GT. *Bioconjugate Techniques*; Academic Press, San Diego, London, 1996.
15. Chen QZ, Rezwan K, Armitage D, Nazhat SN, Boccaccini AR. Surface functionalisation of 45S5 Bioglass-based scaffolds and its impact on bioactivity. *J Mater Sci Mater Med* 2006; 7: 979–987.
16. Hench LL, Wilson J. *An Introduction to Bioceramics*, 2nd Edition, World Scientific, London, 1999.
17. Chen QZ, Boccaccini AR. Coupling mechanical competence and bioresorbability in bioglass-derived tissue engineering scaffolds. *Adv Eng Mater* 2006; 8: 285–289.
18. *Handbook of Bioactive Ceramics*. Yamamuro T, Hench LL, Wilson J (eds.), CRC Press, Boca Raton, FL, 1990.
19. Jarcho M, Kay JF, Gumar KI, Doremus RH, Drobeck HP. Tissue, cellular and subcellular events at a bone-ceramic hydroxyapatite interface. *J Bioeng* 1977; 1: 79–92.
20. Jarcho M. Calcium phosphate ceramics as hard tissue prosthetics. *Clin Orthop Rel Res* 1981; 157: 259–278.
21. LeGeros RZ, LeGeros JP. Calcium phosphate ceramics: Past, present and future. *Bioceramics*, vol. 15, Proceedings of the 15th International Symposium on Ceramics in Medicine. Sydney, 4–8 December 2002, pp. 3–10.

22. Hench LL, Andersson O. Bioactive glasses. In: *An Introduction to Bioceramics*, 2nd Edition, Hench LL, Wilson J (eds.), World Scientific, London, 1999, pp. 41–62.

23. Hench LL, Splinter RJ, Allen WC. Bonding mechanisms at the interface of ceramic prosthetic materials. *J Biomed Mater Res Symp* 1971; 2(part 1): 117–141.

24. Hench LL, Paschall HA. Direct chemical bond of bioactive glass-ceramic materials to bone and muscle. *J Biomed Mater Res Symp* 1973; 4: 25–42.

25. Hench LL, Paschall HA. Histochemical response at a biomaterial's interface. *J Biomed Mater Res Symp* 1974; 5(part 1): 49–64.

26. Kokubo T. A/W glass-ceramic: Processing and properties. In: *An Introduction to Bioceramics*, Hench LL, Wilson J (eds.), World Scientific, Singapore, 1993, pp. 75–88.

27. Kokubo T, Ito S, Sakka S, Yamanuro T. Formation of a high-strength bioactive glass-ceramic in the system MgO-CaO-SiO_2-P_2O_5. *J Mater Sci* 1986; 21: 536–540.

28. Seal BL, Otero TC, Panitch A. Polymeric biomaterials for tissue and organ regeneration. *Mater Sci Eng R* 2001; 34R: 147–230.

29. Atala A, Lanza RP (eds.), *Methods of Tissue Engineering*, Academic Press, San Diego, CA, 2002.

30. Gunatillak PA, Adhikari R. Biodegradable synthetic polymers for tissue engineering. *Eur Cells Mater* 2003; 5: 1–16.

31. Garlotta D. A literature review of poly(lactic acid). *J Poly Environ* 2001; 9: 63–84.

32. Driskell TD, Hassler CR, McCoy LR. The significance of resorbable bioceramics in the repair of bone defects. *Proc 26th Ann Conf Med Bio* 1973; 15: 199–206.

33. Denissen HW, de Groot K, Kakkes P, van den Hooff A, Klopper PJ. Tissue response to dense apatite implants in rats. *J Biomed Mater Res* 1980; 14: 713–721.

34. Hollinger JO, Battistone GC. Biodegradable bone repair materials. *Clin Orthop Rel Res* 1986; 207: 290–305.

35. Hammerle CH, Olah AJ, Schid J, Fluckiger L, Gogolewski S, Winkler JR. The biological effect of natural bone mineral on bone neoformation on the rabbit skull. *Clin Oral Implants Res* 1997; 8: 198–207.

36. Brown S, Clarke I, Williams P (eds.), Bioceramics 14: Proceedings of the 14th International Symposium on Ceramics in Medicine, International symposium on ceramics in medicine, Nov 2001, Palm Springs, CA, pp. 213–269.

37. Vacanti CA, Bonassar LJ, Vacanti JP. Structure tissue engineering. In: *Principles of Tissue Engineering*, 2nd Edition, Lanza RP, Langer R, Vacanti J (eds.), Academic Press, San Diego, CA, 2000, pp. 671–682.

38. Oonishi H, Kushitani S, Iwaki H. Comparative bone formation in several kinds of bioceramic granules. In: *Bioceramics*, vol. 8, Proceedings of the 8th International Symposium on Ceramics in Medicine, Wilson J, Hench LL, Greenspan D (eds.), Elsevier Science Ltd., Tokyo, Japan, 1995, pp. 137–144.

39. LeGeros RZ, LeGeros JP. Dense hydroxyapatite. In: *An Introduction to Bioceramics*, 2nd Edition, Hench LL, Wilson J (eds.), World Scientific, London, 1999, pp. 139–180.

40. Kokubo T. Novel Biomedical materials based on glasses. In: *Bioceramics Applications of Ceramic and Glass Materials in Medicine*, Shackelford JF (ed.), Trans Tech Publications Ltd, Switzerland. *Mater Sci Forum*, vol. 293, 1999, pp. 65–82.

41. de Groot K, Lein CPAT, Wolke JGC, de Bliek-Hogervost JMA. Chemistry of calcium phosphate bioceramics. In: *Handbook of Bioactive Ceramics*, vol. 11, Yamamuro T, Hench LL, Wilson J (eds.), CRC Press, Boca Raton, FL, 1990, pp. 3–16.

42. Hench LL. Bioactive glasses and glasses-ceramics. In: *Bioceramics Applications of Ceramic and Glass Materials in Medicine*, Shackelford JF (ed.), Trans Tech Publication, Switzerland, 1999, pp. 37–64.

43. Nalla RK, Kinney JH, Ritchie RO. Mechanistic fracture criteria for the failure of human cortical bone. *Nature Mater* 2003; 2: 164–168.

44. Zioupos P, Currey JD. Changes in the stiffness, strength, and toughness of human cortical bone with age. *Bone* 1998; 22: 57–66.

45. Keaveny TM, Hayes WC. Mechanical properties of cortical and trabecular bone. In: *Bone. A Treatise, Volume 7: Bone Growth; B*, Hall BK (ed.), CRC Press, Boca Raton, FL, 1993, pp. 285–344.

46. Moore WR, Graves SE, Bain GI. Synthetic bone graft substitutes. *ANZ J Surg* 2001; 71: 354–361.

47. Clark AE, Hench LL. Calcium phosphate formation on sol-gel derived bioactive glasses. *J Biomed Mater Res* 1994; 28: 693–698.

48. Hench LL. Sol-gel materials for bioceramic applications. *Curr Opin Solid State Mater Sci* 1997; 2: 604–610.

49. Hench LL. Bioceramics. *J Am Ceram Soc* 1998; 81: 1705–1728.

50. Wilson J, Pigott GH, Schoen FJ, Hench LL. Toxicology and biocompatibility of Bioglass. *J Biomed Mater Res* 1981; 15: 805–811.

51. Lobel KD, Hench LL. *In-vitro* protein interactions with a bioactive gel-glass. *J Sol-Gel Sci Tech* 1996; 7: 69–76.

52. Lobel KD, Hench LL. *In vitro* adsorption and activity of enzymes on reaction layers of bioactive glass substrates. *J Biomed Mater Res* 1998; 39: 575–579.

53. Ohgushi H, Dohi Y, Yoshikawa T, Tamai S, Tabata S, Okunaga K, Shibuya T. Osteogenic differentiation of cultured marrow stromal stem cells on the surface of bioactive glass ceramics. *J Biomed Mater Res* 1996; 32: 341–348.

54. Aksay IA, Weiner S. Biomaterials—Is this really a field of research? *Curr Opin Solid State Mater Sci* 1998; 3: 219–220.

55. Day RM, Boccaccini AR, Sherey S, Roether JA, Forbes A, Hench LL, Gabe SM. Assessment of polyglycolic acid mesh and bioactive glass for soft-tissue engineering scaffolds. *Biomaterials* 2004; 25: 5857–5866.

56. Keshaw H, Forbes A, Day RM. Release of angiogenic growth factors from cells encapsulated in alginate beads with bioactive glass. *Biomaterials* 2005; 26: 4171–4179.

57. Schepers E, de Clercq M, Ducheyne P, Kempeneers R. Bioactive glass particulate material as filler for bone lesions. *J Oral Rehab* 1991; 18: 439–452.

58. Gatti AM, Valdre G, Andersson OH. Analysis of the *in vivo* reactions of a bioactive glass in soft and hard tissue. *Biomaterials* 1994; 15: 208–212.

59. Roether JA, Gough JE, Boccaccini AR, Hench LL, Maquet V, Jerome R. Novel bioresorbable and bioactive composites based on bioactive glass and polylactide foams for bone tissue engineering. *J Mater Sci Mater Med* 2002; 13: 1207–1214.

60. Oonishi H, Kushitani S, Yasukawa E, Iwaki H, Hench LL, Wilson J, Tsuji E, Sugihara T. Particulate bioglass compared with hydroxyapatite as a bone graft substitute. *Clin Orthop Relat Res* 1997; 334: 316–325.

61. Xynos ID, Edgar AJ, Buttery LDK, Hench LL, Polak JM. Ionic dissolution products of bioactive glass increase proliferation of human osteoblasts and induce insulin-like growth factor II mRNA expression and protein synthesis. *Biochem Biophys Res Commun* 2000; 276: 461–465.

62. Xynos ID, Hukkanen MVJ, Buttery LDK, Hench LL, Polak JM. Bioglass 45S5 stimulates osteoblast turnover and enhances bone formation *in vitro*: Implications and applications for bone tissue engineering. *Calcif Tissue Int* 2000; 67: 321–329.

63. Botelho CM, Brooks RA, Best SM, Lopes MA, Santos JD, Rushton N, Bonfield W, Human osteoblast response to silicon-substituted hydroxyapatite, *J. Biomed. Mater. Res.* A 2006; 79A: 723–730.

64. Hench LL. Bioceramics. *J Am Ceram Soc* 1998; 81: 1705–1728.

65. Laurencin CT, Lu HH, Khan Y. Processing of polymer scaffolds: Polymer-ceramic composite foams. In: *Methods of Tissue Engineering,* Atala A, Lanza RP (eds.), Academic Press, San Diego, CA, 2002, pp. 705–714.

66. Jones JR, Hench LL. Regeneration of trabecular bone using porous ceramics. *Curr Opin Solid State Mater Sci* 2003; 7: 301–307.

67. Livingston T, Ducheyne P, Garino J. *In vivo* evaluation of a bioactive scaffold for bone tissue engineering. *J Biomed Mater Res* 2002; 62: 1–13.

68. Kaufmann EABE, Ducheyne P, Shapiro IM. Evaluation of osteoblast response to porous bioactive glass (45S5) substrates by RT-PCR analysis. *Tissue Eng* 2004; 6: 19–28.

69. Yuan H, de Bruijn JD, Zhang X, van Blitterswijk CA, de Groot K. Bone induction by porous glass ceramic made from Bioglass (45S5). *J Biomed Mater Res Appl Biomater* 2001; 58: 270–276.

70. Peitl O, LaTorre GP, Hench LL. Effect of crystallization on apatite-layer formation of bioactive glass 45S5. *J Biomed Mater Res* 1996; 30: 509–514.

71. Li P, Zhang F, Kokubo T. The effect of residual glassy phase in a bioactive glass-ceramic on the formation of its surface apatite layer *in vitro*. *J Mater Sci Med* 1992; 3: 452–456.

72. Clupper DC, Hench LL. Crystallization kinetics of tape cast bioactive glass 45S5. *J Non-Crys Solid* 2003; 318: 43–48.

73. Hench LL, Kokubo T. Properties of Bioactive glasses and glass-ceramics. In: *Handbook of Biomaterial Properties*, Black J, Hastings G (eds.), Chapman & Hall, London, 1998, pp. 355–363.

74. Holand W, Vogel W. Mechinable and phosphate glass-ceramics. In: *An Introduction to Bioceramics,* Hench LL, Wilson J (eds.), World Scientific, Singapore, 1993, pp. 125–137.

75. Kokubo T. A/W glass-ceramic: Processing and properties. In: *An Introduction to Bioceramics*, 2nd Edition, Hench LL, Wilson J (eds.), World Scientific, London, 1999, pp. 75–88.

76. Rafferty A, Clifford A, Hill R, Wood D, Samuneva B, Dimitrova-Lukacs M. Influence of fluorine content in apatite mullite glass-ceramics. *J Am Ceram Soc* 2000; 83: 2833–2838.

77. Calver A, Hill RG, Stamboulis A. Influence of fluorine content on the crystallisation behaviour of apatite-wollastonite glass-ceramics. *J Mater Sci* 2004; 39: 2601–2603.

78. Yamamuro T. A/W glass-ceramic: Clinical applications. In: *An Introduction to Bioceramics*, Hench LL, Wilson J (eds.), World Scientific, Singapore, 1993, pp. 89–103.

79. Grodd UM, Muller-Mai C, Voigt C. Ceravital bioactive glass-ceramics. In: *An Introduction to Bioceramics*, Hench LL, Wilson J (eds.), World Scientific, Singapore, 1993, pp. 105–123.

80. Chen QZ, Thompson ID, Boccaccini AR. 45S5 Bioglass-derived glass-ceramic scaffolds for bone tissue engineering. *Biomaterials* 2006; 27: 2414–2425.

81. Russel JL, Block JE. Clinical utility of demineralised bone matrix for osseous defects, arthrodesis, and reconstruction: Impact of processing techniques and study methodology. *Orthopaedics* 1999; 22: 524–531.

82. Yaylaoglu MB, Yildiz C, Korkusuz F, Hasirci V. A novel osteochondral implant. *Biomaterials* 1999; 20: 1513–1520.

83. Du C, Cui FZ, Zhu XD, de Groot K. Three-dimensional nano Hap/collagen matrix loading with osteogenic cells in organ culture. *J Biomed Mater Res* 1999; 44: 407–415.

84. Brown CD, Hoffman AS. Modification of natural polymer: Chitosan. In: *Methods of Tissue Engineering*, Atala A, Lanza RP (eds.), Academic Press, San Diego, CA, 2002, pp. 565–574.

85. Atala A, Lanza RP. *Methods of Tissue Engineering*. Academic Press, San Diego, CA, 2002, pp. 505–574.

86. Badylak SE. Modification of natural polymers: Collagen. In: *Methods of Tissue Engineering*, Atala A, Lanza RP (eds.), Academic Press, San Diego, CA, 2002, pp. 505–514.

87. Wan ACA, Khor E, Hastings GW. Preparation of a chitin-apatite composites by *in situ* precipitation onto porous chitin scaffolds. *J Biomed Mater Res* 1998; 41: 541–548.

88. Klokkevold PR, Vandemark L, Kenney EB, Bernard GW. Osteogenesis enhanced by chitosan (poly-*n*-acetyl glucosaminoglycan) *in vitro, J Periodontol* 1996; 67: 1170–1175.

89. Muzzarelli RAA, Zucchini C, Ilari P, Pugnaloni A, Belmonte MM, Biagini G, Castaldini C. Osteoconductive properties of methyl-pyrrolidinone chitosan in an animal model. *Biomaterials* 1993; 14: 925–929.

90. Middleton JC, Tipton AJ. Synthetic biodegradable polymers as orthopaedic devices. *Biomaterials* 2000; 21: 2335–2346.

91. Langer R, Vacanti JP, Vacanti CA, Atala A, Freed LE, Vunjak-Novakovic G. Tissue engineering biomedical applications. *Tissue Eng* 1995; 1: 151–161.

92. Bergsma E, Rosema F, Bos R, de Bruijin W. Foreign body reaction to resorbable poly(L-lactic) bone plates and screws used for the fixation of unstable zygomatic fractures. *J Oral Maxillofacial Surg* 1993; 51: 666–670.

93. Martin C, Winet H, Bao J. Acidity near eroding polylactides-polyglycolide *in vitro* and *in vivo* in rabbit tibial bone chambers. *Biomaterials* 1996; 17: 2373–2380.

94. Lu LC, Mikos AG. Poly(lactic acid). In: *Polymer Data Handbook*. Mark JE (ed.), Oxford Press, Oxford, 1999, pp. 527–633.

95. Yang SF, Leong KF, Du ZH, Chua CK. The design of scaffolds for use in tissue engineering part I: Traditional factors. *Tissue Eng* 2001; 6: 679–689.

96. Lu LC, Mikos AG. Poly(glycolic acid). In: *Polymer Data Handbook*. Mark JE (ed.), Oxford Press, Oxford, 1999, pp. 566–569.

97. Ramakrishna S, Huang ZM, Kumar GV, Batchelor AW, Mayer J. *An Introduction to Biocomposites*. Imperial College Press, London, 2004, p. 36.

98. Iroh JO. Poly(ε-caprolactone). In: *Polymer Data Handbook*. Mark JE (ed.), Oxford Press, Oxford, 1999, pp. 361–362.

99. Yoda N. Synthesis of polyanhydrides II: New aromatic polyanhydrides with high melting points and fibre-forming properties. *Die Markromolekulare Chemie* 2003; 32: 1–12.

100. Kellomak M, Heller J, Tormala P. Processing and properties of two different poly(ortho esters). *J Mater Sci Mater Med* 2000; 11: 345–355.

101. Magill JH. Poly(phosphazenes), bioerodible. In: *Polymer Data Handbook*. Mark JE (ed.), Oxford Press, Oxford, 1999, pp. 746–749.

102. Laurencin CT, Lakshmi S. Polyphosphazene nanofibers for biomedical applications: Preliminary studies. In: *Proceedings of NATOASI Conference 2003*, September 1–12, 2003, Antalya, Turkey, pp. 281–300.

103. Kumudine C, Premachandra JK. In: *Polymer Data Handbook*. Mark JE (ed.), Oxford Press, Oxford, 1999, pp. 70–77.

104. Gollwitzer H, Ibrahim K, Meyer H, Mittelmeier W, Busch R, Stemberger A. Antibacterial poly(D,L-lactic acid) coating of medical implants using a biodegradable drug delivery technology. *J Antimicrob Chemother* 2003; 51: 585–591.

105. Schmidmaier G, Wildemann B, Stemberger A, Haas NP, Raschke M. Biodegradable poly(D,L-lactide) coating of implants for continuous release of growth factors. *J Biomed Mater Res Appl Biomater* 2001; 58: 449–455.

106. Schmidmaier G, Wildemann B, Bail H, Lucke M, Fuchs T, Stemberger A. Local application of growth factors (insulin-like growth factor-1 and transforming growth factor-beta 1) from a biodegradable poly(D,L-lactide) coating of osteosynthetic implants accelerates fracture healing in rats. *Bone* 2001; 28: 341–350.

107. Gollwitzer H, Ibrahim K, Meyer H, Mittelmeier W, Busch R, Stemberger A. Antibacterial poly(D,L-lactic acid) coating of medical implants using a biodegradable drug delivery technology. *J Antimicrob Chemother* 2003; 51: 585–591.

108. Herrmann R, Schmidmaier G, Markl B, Resch A, Hähnel I, Stemberger A. Antithrombogenic coatings of stents using a biodegradable drug delivery technology. *Thromb Haemostasis* 1999; 82: 51–57.

109. Maquet V, Boccaccini AR, Pravata L, Notingher I, Jerome R. Preparation, characterisation, and *in vitro* degradation of bioresorbable and bioactive composites based on Bioglass®-filled polylactide foams. *J Biomed Mater Res* 2003; 66: 335–346.

110. Maquet V, Boccaccini AR, Pravata L, Notingher I, Jerome R. Porous poly(α-hydroxyacid)/Bioglass® composite scaffolds for bone tissue engineering. I: Preparation and *in vitro* characterisation. *Biomaterials* 2004; 25: 4185–4194.

111. Blaker JJ, Gough JE, Maquet V, Notingher I, Boccaccini AR. *In vitro* evaluation of novel bioactive composites based on Bioglass®-filled polylactide foams for bone tissue engineering scaffolds. *J Biomed Mater Res A* 2003; 67A: 1401–1411.

112. Verrier S, Blaker JJ, Maquet V, Hench LL, Boccaccini AR. PDLLA/Bioglass® composites for soft-tissue and hard-tissue engineering: An *in vitro* cell biology assessment. *Biomaterials* 2004; 25: 3013–3021.

113. Pitt CG, Gratzel MM, Kimmel GL. Aliphatic polyesters. 2. The degradation of poly(D,L-lactide), poly(ϵ-caprolactone) and their copolymers *in vivo*. *Biomaterials* 1981; 2: 215–220.

114. Gabelnick HL. Biodegradable implants: Alternative approaches. In: *Advanced in Human Fertility and Reproductive Endocrinology*, Mishell DR (ed.), vol. 2, Long Acting Steroid Contraception, Raven Press, New York, 1983, pp. 149–173.

115. Chen GQ, Wu Q. The application of polyhydroxyalkanoates as tissue engineering materials. *Biomaterials* 2005; 26: 6565–6578.

116. Doi Y, Kitamura S, Abe H. Microbial synthesis and characterization of poly(3-hydroxybutyrate-*co*-3-hydroxyhexanoate). *Macromolecules* 1995; 28: 4822–4828.

117. Li HY, Du RL, Chang J. Fabrication, characterization, and *in vitro* degradation of composite scaffolds based on PHBV and bioactive glass. *J Biomater Appl* 2005; 20: 137–155.

118. Doyle C, Tanner ET, Bonfield W. *In vitro* and *in vivo* evaluation of polyhydroxybutyrate and of polyhydroxybutyrate reinforced with hydroxyapatite. *Biomaterials* 1991; 12: 841–847.

119. Verma S, Bhatia Y, Valappil S, Roy I. A possible role of poly-3-hydroxybutyric acid in antibiotic production in streptomyces. *Arch Microbiol* 2002; 179: 66–69.

120. Payne RG, Mikos AG. Synthesis of synthetic polymers: Poly(propylene fumarate). In: *Methods of Tissue Engineering*, Atala A, Lanza RP (eds.), Academic Press, San Diego, CA, 2002, pp. 649–652.

121. Yaszenski MJ, Payne RG, Hayes WC, Langer R, Aufdemorte TB, Mikos AG. The ingrowth of new bone tissue and initial mechanical properties of a degrading polymeric composite scaffold. *Tissue Eng* 1995; 1: 41–52.

122. Peter SJ, Lu L, Kim DJ, Stamatas GN, Miller MJ, Yaszemski MJ, Mikos AG. Effects of transforming growth factor β1 released from biodegradable polymer microparticles on marrow stromal osteoblasts cultured on poly(propylene fumarate) substrates. *J Biomed Mater Res* 2000; 50: 452–462.

123. Shastri VP, Zelikin A, Hildgen P. Synthesis of synthetic polymers: Poly(anhydrides). In: *Methods of Tissue Engineering*, Atala A, Lanza RP (eds.), Academic Press, San Diego, CA, 2002, pp. 609–617.

124. Domb AJ. Langer R. Poly(1,3-bis-p-carboxyphenoxypropane anhydride). In: *Polymer Data Handbook*, Mark JE (ed.), Oxford Press, Oxford, 1999, pp. 303–305.

125. Doma AJ, Langer R. Poly(erucic acid dimmer anhydride). In: *Polymer Data Handbook*, Mark JE (ed.), Oxford Press, Oxford, 1999, pp. 457–459.

126. Shastri V, Marini P, Padera R, Kirchain S, Tarcha P, Langer R. Osteocompatibility of photopolymerizable anhydride networks. *Mater Res Soc Symp Proc* 1999; 530: 93–98.

127. Solheim E, Sudmann B, Bang G, Sudmann E. Biocompatibility and effect on osteogenesis of poly(ortho ester) compared to poly(D,L-lactic acid). *J Biomed Mater Res* 2000; 49: 257–263.

128. Andriano KP, Gurny R, Heller J. Synthesis of synthetic polymers: Poly(ortho esters). In: *Methods of Tissue Engineering*, Atala A, Lanza RP (eds.), Academic Press, San Diego, CA, 2002, pp. 619–627.

129. Allcock HR. Syntheses of synthetic polymers: Polyphosphazenes. In: *Methods of Tissue Engineering*, Atala A, Lanza RP (eds.), Academic Press, San Diego, CA, 2002, pp. 597–608.

130. Laurencin CT, ElAmin SF, Ibim SE, Willougghby DA, Attawia M, Allcock HR, Ambrosio AA. A highly porous 3-dimensional polyphosphazene polymer matrix for skeletal tissue regeneration. *J Biomed Mater Res* 1996; 30: 133–138.

131. Bergsma EJ, Brujn W, Rozema FR, Bos RM, Boering G. Late tissue response to poly(L-lactide) bone plates and screws. *Biomaterials* 1995; 16: 25–31.

132. Kikuchi M, Tanaka J, Koyama Y, Takakuda K. Cell culture tests of TCP/CPLA composite. *J Biomed Mater Res* 1999; 48: 108–110.

133. Deng X, Hao J, Wang C. Preparation and mechanical properties of nanocomposites of poly(D,L-lactide) with Ca-deficient hydroxyapatite nanocrystals. *Biomaterials* 2001; 22: 2867–2873.

134. Kasaga T, Yoshio O, Masayuki N, Yoshihiro A. Preparation and mechanical properties of polylactide acid composites containing hydroxyapatite fibres. *Biomaterials* 2001; 22: 19–23.

135. Xu HHK, Simon Jr CG. Self-hardening calcium phosphate composite scaffold for bone tissue engineering. *J Orthopaedic Res* 2004; 22: 535–543.

136. Xu HHK, Quinn JB, Takagi S, Chow LC. Synergistic reinforcement of *in situ* hardening calcium phosphate composite scaffold for bone tissue engineering. *Biomaterials* 2004; 25: 1029–1037.

137. Greish YE, Bender JD, Lakshmi S, Brown PW, Allcock HR, Laurencin CT. Low temperature formation of hydroxyapatite-poly(alkloxybezoate)phosphatzene composites for biomedical applications. *Biomaterials* 2005; 26: 1–9.

138. Rodrigues CVM, Serricella P, Linhares ABR, Guerdes RM, Borojevic R, Rossi MA, Duarte MEL, Farina M. Characterization of a bovine collagen-hydroxyapatite composite scaffold for bone tissue engineering. *Biomaterials* 2003; 24: 4987–4997.

139. Peter SJ, Miller ST, Zhu G, Yasko AW, Mikos AG. *In vivo* degradation of poly(propylene fumarate)/β-tricalcium phosphate injectable composite scaffold. *J Biomed Mater Res* 1998; 41: 1–7.

140. Juhasz JA, Best SM, Brooks R, Kawashita M, Miyata N, Kokubo T, Nakamura T, Bonfield W. Mechanical properties of glass-ceramic A-W-polyethylene composites: Effect of filler content and particle size. *Biomaterials* 2004; 25: 949–955.

141. Kasuga T, Maeda H, Kato K, Nogami M, Hata K, Ueda M. Preparation of poly(lactide acid) composites coating calcium carbonate (vaterite). *Biomaterials* 2003; 24: 3247–3253.

142. Ambrosio AMA, Sahota JS, Khan Y, Laurencin CT. A novel amorphous calcium phosphate polymer ceramic for bone repair: I. Synthesis and characterization. *J Biomed Mater Res* 2001; 58: 295–301.

143. Khan YM, Katti DS, Laurencin CT. Novel polymer-synthesised ceramic composite-based system for bone repair: An *in vitro* evaluation. *J Biomed Mater Res* 2004; 69A: 728–737.

144. Yin Y, Ye F, Cui J, Zhang F, Li X, Yan K. Preparation and characterization of macroporous chitosan-gelatin/β-tricalcium phosphate composite scaffolds for bone tissue engineering. *J Biomed Mater Res* 2003; 67A: 844–855.

145. Zhang R, Ma PX. Poly(α-hydroxyl acids)/hydroxyapatite porous composites for bone-tissue engineering. I. Preparation and morphology. *J Biomed Mater Res* 1999; 44: 446–455.

146. Guan L, Davies JE. Preparation and characterisation of a highly macroporous biodegradable composite tissue engineering scaffold. *J Biomed Mater Res* 2004; 71A: 480–487.

147. Devin JE, Attawia MA, Laurencin CT. Three-dimensional degradable porous polymer-ceramic matrices for use in bone repair. *J Biomater Sci Poly Ed* 1996; 7: 661–669.

148. Stamboulis AG, Boccaccini AR, Hench LL. Novel biodegradable polymer/bioactive glass composites for tissue engineering applications. *Adv Eng Mater* 2002; 4: 105–109.

149. Lu HH, El-Amin AF, Scott KD, Laurencin CT. Three-dimensional, bioactive biodegradable, polymer-bioactive glass composite scaffolds with improved mechanical properties support collagen synthesis and mineralization of human osteoblast-like cells *in vitro*. *J Biomed Mater Res* 2003; 64A: 465–474.

150. Zhang K, Wang Y, Hillmayer MA, Francis LF. Processing and properties of porous poly(L-lactide)/ bioactive glass composites. *Biomaterials* 2004; 25: 2489–2500.

151. Blaker JJ, Day RM, Maquet V, Boccaccini AR. Novel bioresorbable poly(lactide-*co*-glycolide) (PLGA) and PLGA/Bioglass composite tubular foam scaffolds for tissue engineering applications. *Adv Mater Forum II Mater Sci Forum* 2004; 455–456: 415–419.

152. Blaker JJ, Maquet V, Jérôme R, Boccaccini AR, Nazhat SN. Mechanically anisotropic PDLLA/Bioglass® composite foams as scaffolds for bone tissue engineering. *Acta Biomaterialia* 2005; 1(6): 643–652.

153. Navarro M, Ginebra MP, Planell JA, Zeppetelli S, Ambrosio L. Development and cell response of a new biodegradable composite scaffold for guided bone regeneration. *J Mater Sci Mater Med* 2004; 15: 419–422.

154. Li H, Chang J. Preparation and characterisation of bioactive and biodegradable wollastonite/poly(D,L-lactic acid) composite scaffolds. *J Mater Sci Mater Med* 2004; 15: 1089–1095.

155. Giesen EBW, Ding M, Dalstra M, van Eijden TMGJ. Mechanical properties of cancellous bone in the human mandibular condyle are anisotropic. *J Biomech* 2001; 34: 799–803.

156. Yeni YN, Fyhrie DP. Finite element calculated uniaxial apparent stiffness is a consistent predictor of uniaxial apparent strength in human vertebral cancellous bone tested with different boundary conditions. *J Biomech* 2001; 34: 1649–1654.

157. Attawia MA, Herbert KM, Laurencin CT. Osteoblast-like cell adherence and migration through 3-dimensional porous polymer matrices. *Biochem Biophy Res Commun* 1995; 213: 639–644.

158. Laurencin CT, Attawia MA, Elgendy HE, Herbert KM. Tissue engineered bone-regeneration using degradable polymer: The formation of mineralized matrices. *Bone* 1996; 19: 93S–99S.

159. Ishizaki K, Komarneni S, Nanko M. *Porous Materials: Processing Technology and Applications*, Kluwer Academic Publisher, The Netherlands, 1998, pp. 12–66.

160. Leong KF, Cheah CM, Chua CK. Solid free-form fabrication of three-dimensional scaffolds for engineering replacement tissue and organs. *Biomaterials* 2003; 24: 2363–2378.

161. Reed JS. *Principles of Ceramic Synthesis*. 2nd edition, Wiley, Chichester, 1988.

162. Komlev VS, Barinov SM. Porous hydroxyapatite ceramics of bi-modal pore size distribution. *J Biomed Mater Res* 2002; 62: 30–36.

163. Livingston T, Ducheyne P, Garino J. *In vivo* evaluation of a bioactive scaffold for bone tissue engineering. *J Biomed Mater Res* 2002; 62: 1–13.

164. Reed JS. *Principles of Ceramic Synthesis*. 2nd edition, Wiley, Chichester, 1988, pp. 173–174.

165. Haugen H, Will J, Kohler A, Hopfner U. Ceramic TiO_2-foams: Characterisation of a potential scaffold, *J Eur Ceram Soc* 2004; 24: 661–668.

166. Andrade JCT, Camilli JA, Yawachi EY, Bertran CA. Behaviour of dense and porous hydroxyapatite implants and tissue response in rat femoral defects. *J Biomed Mater Res* 2002; 62: 30–36.

167. Kim HW, Lee SY, Bae CJ, Noh YJ, Kim HE, Kim HM, Ko JS. Porous ZrO_2 bone scaffold coated with hydroxyapatite with fluorapatite intermediate layer. *Biomaterials* 2003; 24: 3277–3284.

168. Zhao J, Xiao S, Lu X, Wang J, Weng J. A study on improving mechanical properties of porous HA tissue engineering scaffolds by hot isostatic pressing. *Biomed Mater* 2006; 1: 188–192.

169. Montanaro L, Jorand Y, Fantozzi G, Negro A. Ceramic foams by powder processing. *J Eur Ceram Soc* 1998; 18: 1339–1350.

170. Fukasawa T, Deng ZY, Ando M, Ohji T, Goto Y. Pore structure of porous ceramics synthesized from water based slurry by freeze-dry process. *J Mater Sci* 2001; 36: 2523–2527.

171. Schwartzalder K, Somers AV. Method of making a porous shape of sintered refractory ceramic articles. United States Patent No. 3090094, 1963.

172. Haugen H, Will J, Kohler A, Hopfner U. Ceramic TiO_2-foams: Characterisation of a potential scaffold. *J Eur Ceram Soc* 2004; 24: 661–668.

173. Miao X, Lim G, Loh KH, Boccaccini AR. Preparation and characterisation of calcium phosphate bone cement. *Mater Proc Prop Perf* (MP³) 2004; 3: 319–324.

174. Kim HW, Kin HE, Knowles JC. Hard-tissue-engineered zirconia porous scaffolds with hydroxyapatite sol-gel and slurry coatings. *J Biomed Mater Res B Appl Biomater* 2004; 70B: 270–277.

175. Jayasinghe SN, Edirisinghe MJ. A novel method of forming open cell ceramic foam. *J Porous Mater.* 2002; 9: 265–273.

176. Chen QZ, Zhang HB, Wang DZ, Edirisinghe MJ, Boccaccini AR. Improved mechanical reliability of bone tissue engineering (zirconia) scaffolds by electrospraying. *J Am Ceramic Soc* 2006; 89: 1534–1539.

177. Chen QZ, Boccaccini AR. Poly(D,L-lactic acid) coated 45S5 Bioglass-based scaffolds: Processing and characterisation. *J Biomed Mater Res A* 2006; 77A: 445–457.

178. Lyckfeldt O, Ferreira JMF. Processing of porous ceramics by 'starch consolidation.' *J Eur Ceram Soc* 1998; 18: 131–140.

179. Sepulveda P, Binner JGP. Processing of cellular ceramics by foaming and *in situ* polymerisation of organic monomers. *J Eur Ceram Soc* 1999; 20: 2059–2066.
180. Ortega FS, Valenzuela FAO, Pandolfelli VC. Gelcasting ceramic foams with alternative gelling agents. *Mater Sci* F 2003; 416: 512–518.
181. Sepulveda P, Binner JGP, Rogero SO, Higa OZ, Bressiani JC. Production of porous hydroxyapatite by the gel-casting of foams and cytoxic evaluation. *J Biomed Mater Res* 2000; 50: 27–34.
182. Sepulveda P, Bressiani AH, Bressiani JC, Meseguer L, Konig Jr B. *In vivo* evaluation of hydroxyapatite foams. *J Biomed Mater Res* 2002; 62: 587–592.
183. Tamai N, Myoui A, Tomita T, Nakase T, Tanaka J, Ochi T, Yoshikawa H. Novel hydroxyapatite ceramics with an interconnective porous structure exhibit superior osteoconduction *in vivo*. *J Biomed Mater Res* 2002; 59: 110–117.
184. Ramay HRR, Zhang M. Preparation of porous hydroxyapatite scaffolds by combination of the gel-casting and polymer sponge methods. *Biomaterials* 2003; 24: 3293–3302.
185. Callcut S, Knowles JC. Correlation between structure and compressive strength in a reticulate glass-reinforced hydroxyapatite foam. *J Mater Sci Mater Med* 2002; 13: 485–489.
186. Brinker CJ, Scherer GW. *Sol-Gel Science: The Physics and Chemistry of Sol-Gel Processing.* Academic Press, London, 1990.
187. Saravanapavan P, Hench LL. Mesoporous calcium silicate glasses. I. Synthesis. *J Non-Cryst Sol* 2003; 318: 1–13.
188. Sepulveda P, Jones JR, Hench LL. Bioactive sol-gel foams for tissue repair. *J Biomed Mater Res* 2002; 59: 340–348.
189. Jones JR, Hench LL. Factors affecting the structure and properties of bioactive foam scaffolds for tissue engineering. *J Biomed Mater Res B Appl Biomater* 2004; 68B: 36–44.
190. Jones JR, Ahir S, Hench LL. Large-scale production of 3D bioactive glass macroporous scaffolds for tissue engineering. *J Sol-Gel Sci Tech* 2004; 29: 179–188.
191. Lenza RFS, Jones JR, Vasconcelos WL, Hench LL. *In vitro* release kinetics of proteins from bioactive forms. *J Biomed Mater Res* 2003; 67A: 121–129.
192. Gough JE, Jones JR, Hench LL. Nodule formation and mineralization of human primary osteoblasts cultured on a porous bioactive glass scaffold. *Biomaterials* 2004; 25: 2039–2046.
193. Bose S, Avila M, Bandyopadhyay A. Processing of bioceramic implants via fused deposition process. *Proceedings of Solid Freeform Fabrication Symposium*, Austin, TX, 1998, pp. 629–636.
194. Hattiangadi A, Bandyopadhyay A. *Proceedings of Solid Freeform Fabrication Symposium*, Austin, TX, 1999, pp. 319–326.
195. Chu TMG, Orton DG, Hollister SJ, Feinberg SE, Halloran JW. Mechanical and *in vivo* performance of hydroxyapatite implants with controlled architectures. *Biomaterials* 2002; 23: 1283–1293.
196. Cornejo IA, McNulty TF, Lee S, Bianchi E, Danforth SC, Safari A. Development of bioceramics tissue scaffolds via fused deposition of ceramics. In: *Bioceramics: Materials and Applications*, George L (ed.) American Ceramic Society, Westeville, OH, 2000, pp. 183–195.
197. Jun IK, Koh YH, Kim HE. Fabrication of a highly porous bioactive glass-ceramic scaffold with a high surface area and strength. *J Am Ceram Soc* 2006; 89: 391–394.
198. Sachlos E, Czernuszka JT. Making tissue engineering scaffolds work. Review on the application of solid freeform fabrication technology to the production of tissue engineering scaffolds. *Euro Cells Mater* 2003; 5: 29–40.
199. Yang S, Leong AF, Du Z, Chua CK. The design of scaffolds for use in tissue engineering. Part II. Rapid prototyping techniques. *Tissue Eng* 2002; 8: 1–11.
200. Curodeau A, Sachs E, Caldarise S. Design and fabrication of casat orthopaedic implant with freeform surface textures from 3-D printed ceramic shell. *J Biomed Mater Res* 2000; 53: 525–535.
201. Das S, Hollister SJ. Tissue engineering scaffold. *Encyclopaedia of Materials: Science and Technology* 2003, pp. 1–7.
202. Lee GH, Barlow JW. Selective laser sintering of bioceramic materials for implants. *Proceedings of Solid Freeform Fabrication Symposium*, Austin, TX, 1993; pp. 376–380.
203. Lee GH, Barlow JW. Selective laser sintering of calcium phosphate powders. *Proceedings of Solid Freeform Fabrication Symposium*, Austin, TX, 1994, pp. 191–197.
204. Boccaccini AR, Chen QZ, Lefebvre L, Gremillard L, Chevalier J. Sintering, crystallisation and biodegradation behaviour of Bioglass®-derived glass–ceramics. *Faraday Discuss.*, 2007; 136: 27–44.
205. Tadic D, Beckmann F, Schwarz K, Epple M. A novel method to produce hydroxyapatite objects with interconnecting porosity that avoids sintering. *Biomaterials* 2004; 25: 3335–3340.

206. Kaufmann EABE, Ducheyne P, Shapiro IM. Evaluation of osteoblast response to porous bioactive glass (45S5) substrates by RT-PCR analysis. *Tissue Eng* 2004; 6: 19–28.

207. Ramay HRR, Zhang M. Biphasic calcium phosphate nanocomposite scaffolds for load bearing bone tissue engineering. *Biomaterials* 2004; 25: 5171–5180.

208. Yan H, Zhang K, Blanford CF, Fancis LF, Stein A. *In vitro* hydroxylcarbonate apatite mineralization of CaO-SiO$_2$ sol-gel glasses with three-dimensionally ordered macroporous structure. *Chem Mater* 2001; 13: 1374–1382.

209. Gun J, Lev O, Regev O, Pevzner S, Kucernak A. Sol-gel formation of reticular methyl-silicate materials by hydrogen peroxide decomposition. *J Sol-Gel Sci Tech* 1998; 13: 189–193.

210. Sato Y, Nakanish K, Hirao K, Jinnai H, Shibayama M, Melnichenko YB, Wignall GD. Formation of ordered macropore and templated nanopores in silica sol-gel system incorporated with EO-PO-EO tri-block copolymer. *Colloid Surface* 2001; 187–188: 117–122.

211. Bose S, Darsell J, Kintner M, Hosick H, Bandyopadhyay A. Pores size and pore volume effects on alumina and TCP ceramic scaffolds. *Mater Sci Eng* C 2003; 23C: 479–486.

212. Kalita SJ, Bose S, Hosick HL, Bandyopadhyay A. Porous calcium aluminate ceramics for bone-graft applications. *Mater Res Soc* 2002; 17: 3042–3049.

213. Kalita SJ, Bose S, Hosick HL, Bandyopadhyay A. Development of controlled porosity polymer-ceramic composite scaffolds via fused deposition modelling. *Mater Sci Eng C* 2003; 23C: 611–620.

214. Lee GH, Barlow JW, Fox WC, Aufdermorte TB. Biocompatibility of SLS-formed calcium phosphate implants. *Proceedings of Solid Freeform Fabrication Symposium*, Austin, TX, 1996, pp. 15–22.

215. Lu L, Mikos AG. The importance of new processing techniques in tissue engineering. *MRS Bull* 1996; 11: 28–32.

216. Thomas RC, Shung AK, Yaszemski MJ. Polymer scaffold processing. In: *Principles of Tissue Engineering*, 2nd Edition, Lanza RP, Langer R, Vacanti J (eds.), Academic Press, San Diego, CA, 2000, pp. 251–262.

217. Widmer MS, Mikos AG. Fabrication of biodegradable polymer scaffolds for tissue engineering. In: *Frontier in Tissue Engineering*, Patrick Jr CW, Mikos AG, Mcintire LV (eds.), Elsevier Science, New York, 1998, pp. 107–120.

218. Atala A, Lanza RP (ed.), *Methods of Tissue Engineering*, Academic Press, San Diego, CA, 2002, pp. 681–740.

219. Ma PX, Choi JW. Biodegradable polymer scaffolds with well-defined interconnected spherical pore network. *Tissue Eng* 2001; 7: 23–33.

220. Boccaccini AR, Blaker JJ. Bioactive composite materials for tissue engineering scaffolds. *Expert Rev Med Devices* 2005; 2: 303–317.

221. Gough JE, Arumugam M, Blaker J, Boccaccini AR. Bioglass coated poly(DL-lactide) foams for tissue engineering scaffolds. *Materialwissenschaft und Werkstofftechnik* 2003; 34: 654–661.

222. Roether JA, Boccaccini AR, Hench LL, Maquet V, Gautier S, Jerome R. Development and *in vitro* characterisation of novel bioresorbable and bioactive composite materials based on polylactide foams and Bioglass for tissue engineering applications. *Biomaterials* 2002; 23: 3871–3878.

223. Kim HW, Knowles JC, Kim HE. Hydroxyapatite porous scaffold engineered with biological polymer hybrid coating for antibiotic vancomycin release. *J Mater Sci Mater Med* 2005; 16: 189–195.

224. Anselme K. Osteoblast adhesion on biomaterials. *Biomaterials* 2000; 21: 667–681.

225. Siperko LM, Jacquet R, Landis WJ. Modified aminosilane substrates to evaluate osteoblast attachment, growth, and gene expression *in vitro*. *J Biomed Mater Res* 2006; 78A: 808–822.

226. Curran JM, Chen R, Hunt JA. Controlling the phenotype and function of mesenchymal stem cells *in vitro* by adhesion to silane-modified clean glass surfaces. *Biomaterials* 2005; 26: 7057–7067.

227. Glass-Brudzinski J, Perizzolo D, Brunette DM. Effects of substratum surface topography on the organization of cells and collagen fibers in collagen gel cultures. *J Biomed Mater Res* 2002; 61: 608–618.

228. Curran JM, Chen R, Hunt JA. The guidance of human mesenchymal stem cell differentiation *in vitro* by controlled modifications to the cell substrate. *Biomaterials* 2006; 27: 4783–4793.

229. Guo X, Zheng Q, et al. Bone regeneration with active angiogenesis by basic fibroblast growth factor gene transfected mesenchymal stem cells seeded on porous β-TCP ceramic scaffolds. *Biomed Mater* 2006; 1: 93–99.

230. Singhatanadgit W, Salih V, Olsen I. Up-regulation of bone morphogenetic protein receptor IB by growth factors enhances BMP-2-induced human bone cell functions. *J Cell Physiol* 2006; 209: 912–922.

231. Kuo AC, et al. Microfracture and bone morphogenetic protein 7 (BMP-7) synergistically stimulate articular cartilage repair. *Osteoarthr Cartilage* 2006; 14: 1126–1135.

232. Fricain JC, Pothuaud L, Durrieu MC, et al. Effects of cyclic RGD peptide functionalization on the quantitative bone ingrowth process in cellularized biphasic calcium phosphate ceramics. *Key Eng Mater* 2005; 284–286: 647–650.
233. Pallu S, Dard M, Jonczvk A, et al. Role of RGD-peptide in cbfa1/osf2 expression stimulation in human bone marrow stromal cells (HBMSC). *J Bone Miner Res* 2003, Suppl. 2; 18: S343.
234. Zhanga J, Jiang D. Increased cell response to zirconia ceramics by surface modification. *Appl Phys Lett* 2006; 89: 183–902.
235. Filippini P, Rainaldi G, et al. Modulation of osteosarcoma cell growth and differentiation by silane-modified surfaces. *J Biomed Mater Res* 2001; 55: 338–349.
236. Zurlinden K, Laub M, Jennissen HP. Chemical functionalization of a hydroxyapatite based bone replacement material for the immobilization of proteins. *Materialwissenschaft und Werkstofftechnik* 2005; 36: 820–827.
237. Webster TJ, et al. Specific proteins mediate enhanced osteoblast adhesion on nanophase ceramics. *J Biomed Mater Res* 2000; 51: 475–483.
238. Kruyt MC, Persson C, Johansson G, et al. Towards injectable cell-based tissue-engineered bone: The effect of different calcium phosphate microparticles and pre-culturing. *Tissue Eng* 2006; 12: 309–317.
239. Liu H, Slamovich EB, Webster TJ. Increased osteoblast functions among nanophase titania/poly(lactide-co-glycolide) composites of the highest nanometer surface roughness. *J Biomed Mater Res Part A* 2006; 78: 798–807.
240. Hildebrand HF, Blanchemain N, Mayer G, et al. Surface coatings for biological activation and functionalization of medical devices. *Surf Coating Tech* 2006; 200(22–23): 6318–6324.
241. Lee KY, et al. Ceramic bioactivity: Progresses, challenges and perspectives. *Biomed Mater* 2006; 1: R31–R37.
242. Lee HJ, Choi HW, Kim KJ, Lee SC. Modification of hydroxyapatite nanosurfaces for enhanced colloidal stability and improved interfacial adhesion in nanocomposites. *Chem Mater* 2006; 18: 5111–5118.
243. Misra SK, Valappil SP, Roy I, Boccaccini AR. Polyhydroxyalkanoate (PHA)/inorganic phase composites for tissue engineering applications. *Biomacromolecules* 2006; 7: 2249–2258.
244. Huang X, Mian X. Novel porous hydroxyapatite prepared by combining H_2O_2 foaming with PU sponge and modified with PLGA and bioactive glass. *J Biomater Appl* 2007; 21: 351–374.

2 Design, Fabrication, and Characterization of Scaffolds via Solid Free-Form Fabrication Techniques

Dietmar W. Hutmacher and Maria Ann Woodruff

CONTENTS

2.1 INTRODUCTION

The recently coined term "regenerative medicine" represents a shift in emphasis from current methods to replace tissues with medical devices and artificial organs toward more biological approaches, which focus on regeneration rather than replacement or repair. Regenerative medicine has many components, however, it can be argued that cell therapy and tissue engineering are currently the flagship areas. In addition, this technology has the potential to develop therapies for previously untreatable diseases and conditions. Examples of diseases that regenerative medicine might alleviate one day include diabetes, heart disease, renal failure, osteoporosis, and spinal cord injuries. The current generation of baby boomers would almost certainly rally behind the rationale to advance into regenerative medicine as it offers them the greatest hope for the most effective medical treatment and quality of life in their senior years. Beyond the obvious health benefits of regenerative medicine from a patient's point of view, this technology is desperately needed to challenge rising healthcare costs around the world.[1]

Unfortunately, to the disappointment of everyone involved, we must today reconcile the fact that cell-based therapies and tissue engineering have not lived up to the promises the pioneers of tissue engineering communicated two decades ago.[2] Although there have been some successes, it is widely recognized that tissue engineering is not yet showing significant progress in terms of clinical outcomes and commercialization. Part of the problem has been that we have failed to fully understand what regenerative medicine really means and to appreciate that regeneration here is synonymous with creation. More importantly, cell transplantation and the scaffold-based tissue engineering processes, for example, involve many different phases and substantially different scientific inputs, such that there has been insufficient integration of these phases within any holistic regenerative medicine technology platform.[1] Two major problems, within such a holistic technology platform, that tissue engineers need to overcome are (1) problems associated with "scale-up"[3,4] and (2) cell death of a significantly high number of cells after implantation.[4]

From an engineering point of view, large numbers of cells are needed to generate relatively small volumes of tissues. To ultimately be effective in patients, it is necessary to generate relatively large volumes of so-called neotissue, starting with very few cells. Differentiated cells, expanded *in vitro* under modern cell-culture protocols, more often than not lose efficacy. Cell implantation and its associated vascular disruption result in a relatively hypoxic host environment and subsequently lead to fast necrosis of a large number of the implanted cells. Hence, the potential for different cell types to be expanded *in vitro* and stay alive in a relatively hostile environment at the time of implantation is now being studied not only from a qualitative but also from a quantitative point of view. To be effective, cells should be easily procured, effectively expanded *in vitro*, survive the implantation, not be recognized as foreign, function normally, and not become malignant. In addition, it would also be quite convenient if no moral concerns or questions were generated as a result of the cell type used. There is a considerable debate concerning different cell sources. Mature cells have a relatively high oxygen requirement and a low potential for expansion (scale-up). Alternatively, there are several sources of "immature" cells. Immature cells commonly referred to as stem or progenitor cells may be classified as embryonic in origin or adult somatic stem cells. Despite being under great moral debate, the fact remains that embryonic and adult stem cells may have very similar potential to develop into the different cellular elements necessary for structural and functional tissue regeneration. Embryonic stem cells have been postulated to retain a greater ability to produce a healthier tissue. At this point in time, there is little evidence to support the goal that embryonic stem cells can be consistently driven to form only the cell type needed for the tissue to be engineered. Several excellent reviews[5–7] and books[8] have summarized the current knowledge on embryonic and adult somatic stem cells.

2.1.1 Scaffold-Based Tissue Engineering

It can be argued that the beginning of the "scaffold-based tissue engineering concept"—as we know it today—was in the mid-1980s when Dr. Joseph Vacanti of the Children's Hospital approached Dr. Robert Langer of Massachusetts Institute of Technology (MIT) with an idea to design scaffolds for cell delivery as opposed to seeding cells onto, or mixing cells into the currently available naturally occurring matrices, which possessed physical and chemical properties that were difficult to be manipulated, resulting in wide variations of the results produced *in vitro* and *in vivo*.[4,9]

Today, scaffold-based tissue engineering concepts involve the combination of viable cells, biomolecules, and a scaffold to promote the repair and regeneration of tissues as depicted schematically in Figure 2.1. The two *in vivo* images at the bottom show a medical grade polycaprolactone–tricalcium phosphate (mPCL–TCP) composite scaffold (14 mm × 12 mm × 5 mm) being inserted during pig surgery in a spinal fusion model and also an FDA-approved mPCL scaffold (50 mm × 50 mm × 2 mm) being utilized during human orbital floor fracture repair. The scaffold (Osteopore, Singapore) is intended to support cell migration, growth and differentiation, and guide tissue development and organization into a mature and healthy state. The science behind engineering tissue-engineered constructs (TECs) is still in its relative infancy, and various approaches and

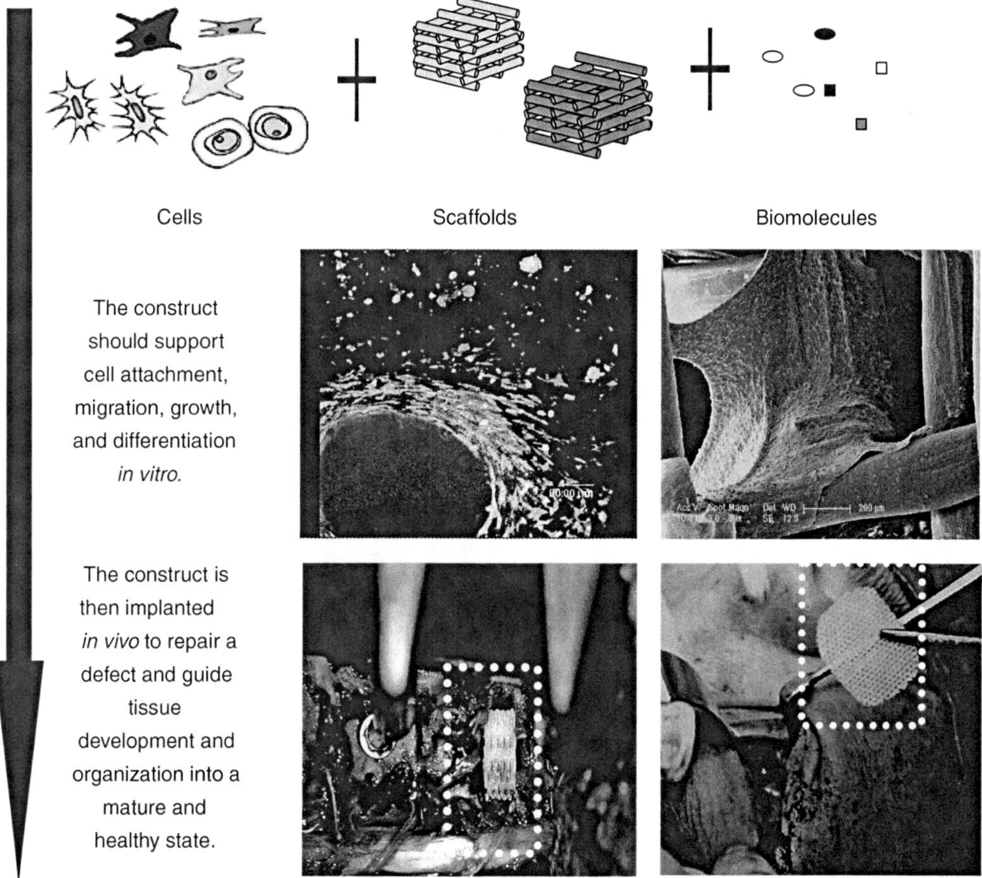

FIGURE 2.1 Scaffold-based tissue engineering aims to promote the repair and regeneration of tissues through the incorporation of cells and biomolecules within a 3-D scaffold system, which can be maintained *in vitro* culture conditions until implantation.

strategies are currently under experimental investigation. It is by no means clear what defines an ideal scaffold/cell or scaffold/neotissue construct, even for a specific tissue type. The considerations are complex and include architecture, structural mechanics, surface properties, degradation products, and composition of biological components. Furthermore one must consider the temporal and spatial variations in each of these factors both *in vitro* and *in vivo*.[10]

Scaffolds in TEC have certain minimum requirements for their biochemical, chemical, and physical properties. These properties include biocompatibility, angiogenesis, vascularization, and chemotaxis issues; the scaffold must not be an agent for allergic reaction and disease transmission, and it must possess suitable gross architectural qualities, which are possible to produce via a reproducible processing platform. There are also sterilization and administrative issues to contend with. Scaffolds must provide sufficient initial mechanical strength and stiffness to substitute for the mechanical function of the diseased or damaged tissue, which is aimed at repairing or regenerating. Scaffolds may not necessarily be required to provide complete mechanical equivalence to a healthy tissue, but stiffness and strength should be sufficient to at least support and transmit forces to the host tissue site in the context. For example, in skin tissue engineering, the construct should be able to withstand the wound contraction forces. In the case of bone engineering, external and internal fixation systems might be applied to take support and maintain the majority of load-bearing forces until the bone has matured.[11]

Cell and tissue remodeling is important for achieving stable biomechanical conditions and vascularization at the host site. Hence, the 3-D scaffold/tissue construct should maintain sufficient structural integrity during the *in vitro* and *in vivo* growth and remodeling process. The degree of remodeling depends on the tissue itself (e.g., skin 4–6 weeks, bone 4–6 months) and its host anatomy and physiology. Scaffold architecture has to allow for initial cell attachment and subsequent migration into and through the interconnecting pore volume, mass transfer of nutrients and metabolites, provision of sufficient space for development, and later remodeling of organized tissue. Figure 2.2 shows schematically the process of cell attachment till mineralization for a scaffold intended for bone engineering application.

The degradation and resorption kinetics of the scaffold need to be designed based on the relationships of mechanical properties, molecular weight (M_w/M_n), mass loss, and tissue development. A number of studies[12–15] have demonstrated the dependence of mechanical properties on scaffold porosity when designing and fabricating scaffolds via solid free-form fabrication (SFF). Logically, as porosity of the scaffold is increased (decline in material bulk) its mechanical properties would decrease correspondingly. This decline has been found to follow a power-law relationship (Figure 2.3).

In addition to these essentials of mechanics and geometry, a suitable construct will possess surface properties that are optimized for the attachment and migration of cell types of interest (depending on the targeted tissue). The external size and shape of the construct must also be considered, especially if the construct is to be customized for an individual patient.[2]

A number of fabrication technologies have been applied to process biodegradable and bioresorbable materials into 3-D polymeric scaffolds of high porosity and surface area.[16] From a scaffold

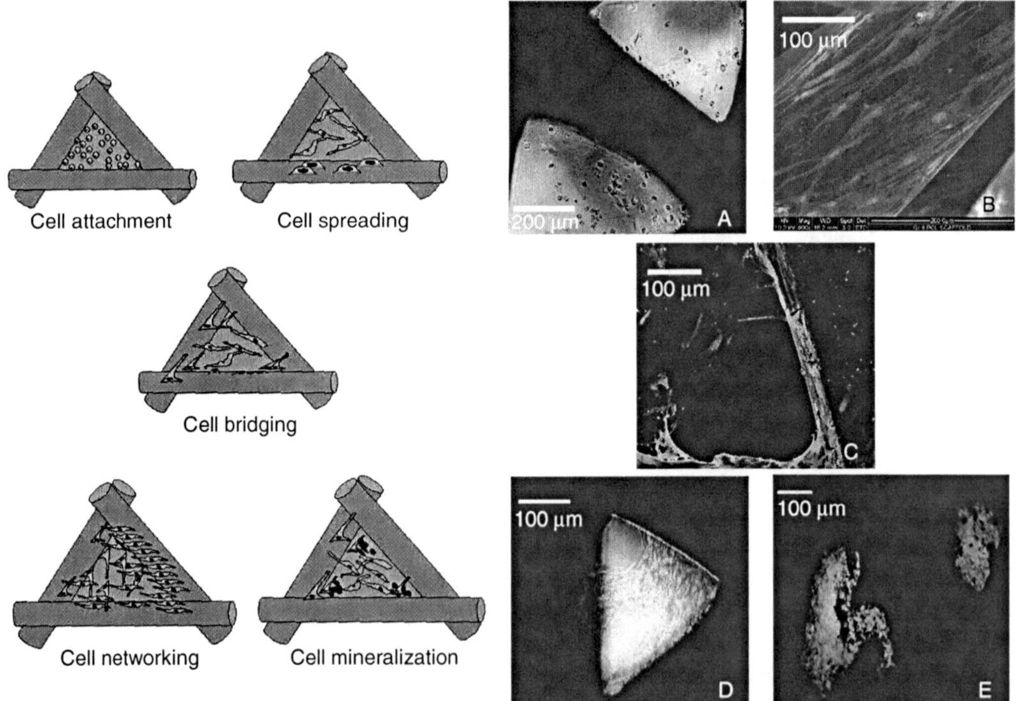

FIGURE 2.2 Sequences of scaffold neo-tissue formation, *in vitro*. Cells manually (pipetted) or dynamically (using a bioreactor) seeded and attach to the scaffold surface (A). Seeding efficiency is highly dependent upon the surface itself but also on the surface to volume ratio of the scaffold. Attachment is followed by cell spreading (B) and bridging across the scaffold pores (C), cell networking then follows (D) with subsequent cell mineralisation (E) providing a firm basis for successful transferral and implantation of the neo-tissue construct *in vivo*.

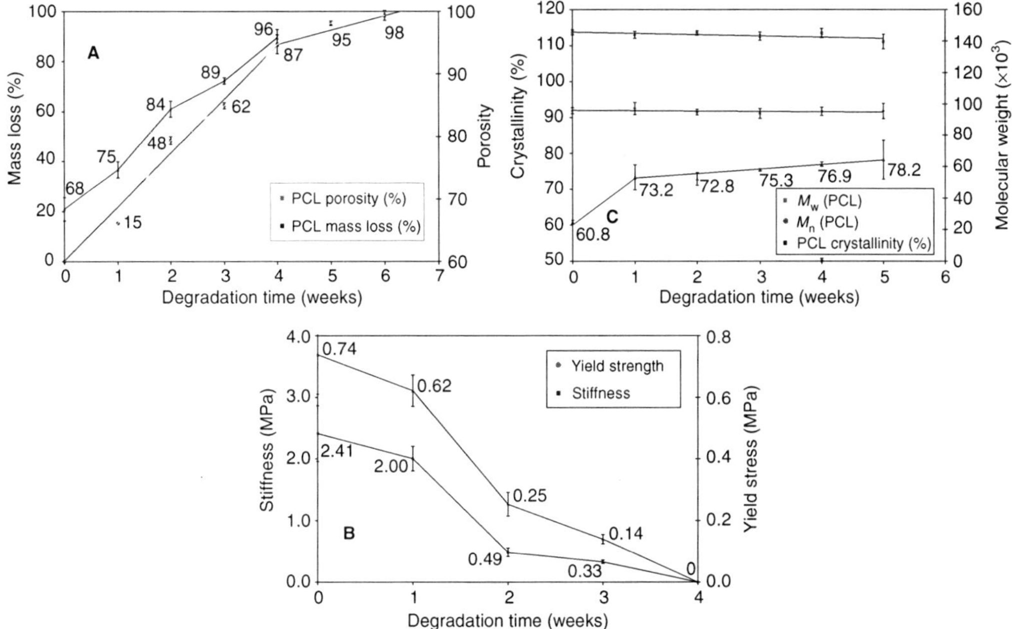

FIGURE 2.3 (A) Mean percentage mass loss of PCL scaffolds ($n = 6$) degraded over 6 weeks ($\pm$SD) and porosity ($n = 6$) degraded over 4 weeks ($\pm$SD). The mean porosity of the PCL scaffolds was $68 \pm 1.9\%$. The rate of porosity increment was observed to be uniform and linear throughout the 4 weeks. (B) The mean compressive mechanical properties, stiffness and yield stress, of the PCL scaffolds ($n = 6$) show the overall loss of compressive stiffness and yield stress, which was observed to advance in three phases. Stiffness initially declined from 2.4 to 2.0 MPa after the first week of degradation. From 1 to 2 weeks, the most drastic drop is found in stiffness falling to 0.5 MPa. Finally, from 2 to 4 weeks, there was a slow decrease in stiffness until it was undetectable after 4 weeks. Corresponding yield stresses reflected similar decreases over the three time periods. (C) Thermal analysis—differential scanning calorimetry (DSC): The mean crystallinity of the degraded PCL scaffolds ($n = 6$) was observed to progress in two stages; a sharp increase in crystallinity during the first week and a slower and more gradual increase thereafter. The final crystallinity measured at 5 weeks was $78.2 \pm 6.9\%$. In the meantime, the crystalline melting temperature was constant over the degradation period. The melting temperature was consistently measured to be 65°C. Mean percentage crystallinity and molecular weight (M_w and M_n, in g mol^{-1}) of PCL scaffolds degraded over 5 weeks ($\pm$SD). Crystallinity was observed to increase in two stages while both molecular weights remained constant over the period of 5 weeks. Polydispersity was constant at about 1.49. A second GPC peak was observed after 4 weeks. The average molecular weights (M_w and M_n) of the degraded PCL scaffolds were observed to remain relatively constant over the 5 weeks of degradation. The M_w averaged around 143,700 and M_n averaged around 95,500. A second peak appeared after 4 weeks and was about $M_w = 1720$ and $M_n = 1660$. (From Lam, C.X.F., Teoh, S.H., Hutmacher, D.W. Polymer International, 56, 718–728, 2007. With permission from Wiley and Elsevier.)

design and function view point, each processing methodology has its *pros* and *cons*. It is beyond the scope of this chapter to cover all scaffold fabrication techniques available. Hence, the authors aim to provide the reader with an overview of the methods that are currently most relevant for scaffold-based tissue engineering. The aim of this chapter is to compile information and to present this data in a comprehensive form. The key rationale, characteristics, and process parameters behind the currently used scaffold fabrication techniques are presented. The aim of this part of the book is to assist research teams with their choice for a specific 3-D scaffold processing technology, by providing the information for determining the critical issues. As discussed above, the current challenge in tissue engineering research is not only to design but also to fabricate reproducible, bioresorbable 3-D scaffolds, which are able to function correctly from both a mechanical and a biological perspective in a specific anatomical site.

2.2 SCAFFOLD DESIGN

2.2.1 INTRODUCTION

It is important to emphasize, at the outset, that the field of scaffold-based tissue engineering is still in its infancy, and many different approaches are under experimental investigation. Thus, it is by no means clear what defines an ideal scaffold/cell or scaffold/neotissue construct, even for a specific tissue type. Indeed, since some tissues perform multiple functional roles, it is unlikely that a single scaffold would serve as a universal foundation for the regeneration of even a single tissue. Hence, the considerations for scaffold design are complex. They include material composition, porous architecture, structural mechanics, surface properties, degradation properties and their products (degradation rate strongly depends on polymer type, impurities, manufacturing process, sterilization, device size, and the local environment), together with the composition of any biological component that may have been added to the scaffold to improve function. Furthermore one must also consider the behaviors and the consequences of how all the aforementioned factors may change with time.

Hollister[17] stated that approaches in scaffold design must be able to create hierarchical porous structures to attain desired mechanical function and mass-transport (permeability and diffusion) properties and to produce these structures within arbitrary and complex 3-D anatomical shapes. Hierarchical refers to the fact that features at scales from the nanometer to millimeter level will determine how well the scaffold meets conflicting mechanical function and mass-transport needs. Material chemistry together with processing determines the maximum functional properties that a scaffold can achieve, as well as how cells interact with the scaffold. However, mass-transport requirements for cell nutrition, pore interconnections for cell migration, and surface features for cell attachment necessitate a minimal requirement for scaffold morphology. The porous structure dictates that achievable scaffold properties fall between the theoretical maximum set by the material and the theoretical minimum of zero predicted by composite theories. The critical issue for design is then to compute the precise value of mechanical as well as mass-transport properties at a given scale based on more microscopic properties and structure.

Hence, for each envisioned application, successful TECs have certain minimum requirements from a biochemical, chemical, and physical perspective as described previously. Scaffolds are normally required to provide sufficient initial mechanical strength and stiffness to substitute for the mechanical function of the diseased or damaged tissue, which the TEC aims at repairing or regenerating. Scaffolds may not necessarily be required to provide a complete mechanical equivalence to a healthy tissue; indeed the variability in architecture for a single tissue type is so extensive that it is inconceivable that a single TEC would serve universal applications for even a single tissue. Nevertheless, stiffness and strength should be sufficient to at least either permit prerequisite cell seeding of the scaffold *in vitro* without compromising scaffold architecture or support and transmit forces in an *in vivo* healing site. Thus, in the context of skin tissue engineering the scaffold material should be sufficiently robust not only to resist change in shape as a result of the introduction of cells into the scaffold, each of which would be capable of exerting tractional forces, but also to withstand the wound contraction forces, which will be invoked during tissue healing *in vivo*. The same general rules would apply to bone engineering, although the external and internal fixation systems, or other supports or restrictions on patient activity during the early stage recovery, may lessen the importance of scaffold mechanical considerations during the *in vivo* phase.

Cell and tissue remodeling is important for achieving stable biomechanical conditions and vascularization at the host site. Hence, the 3-D scaffold/tissue construct should maintain sufficient structural integrity during the *in vitro* and/or *in vivo* growth and remodeling processes.

Scaffold architecture has to allow for initial cell attachment and subsequently migration into and throughout the matrix. It must enable mass transfer of nutrients and metabolites, provision of sufficient space for development, and later remodeling of organized tissue. The porosity and internal space within a degradable scaffold will increase with time, allowing increased space for tissue to develop or remodel.

2.2.2 Morphology/Architecture

Gibson and Ashby[18] classified porous solids into two general groups: foams and honeycombs. A honeycomb consisted of a regular two-dimensional array of polygonal pores each defined by a wall shared between adjacent pores (Figure 2.4). The pores were packed in planar arrays like the hexagonal cells of a honeycomb, as seen in Figure 2.4C.

The ASTM terminology[19] for porous materials is similar and classified into three groups: interconnecting (open pores), nonconnecting (closed pores), and a combination of both. When the pores are open, the foam material is usually drawn into struts forming the pore edges. A network of struts produces a low-density solid with pores connecting to each other through open faces. When the pores are closed, a network of interconnected plates produces a higher density solid. The closed pores are sealed off from adjacent neighbors.

Gibson and Ashby[18] describe that the mechanical properties of a porous solid depend mainly on its relative density, the properties of the material that make up the pore edges or walls, and the anisotropic nature, if any, of the solid. In general, the stiffness (E^*) and yield strength (σ^*), in compression, of porous solids were each related to the relative density by a power-law relationship. Given that most constructs require a high degree of porosity to accommodate mass transfer and tissue development, the volume fraction of the scaffold will necessarily be low. In all, especially in the most biomechanically challenging applications, it is likely that the test for the scaffold engineer is to

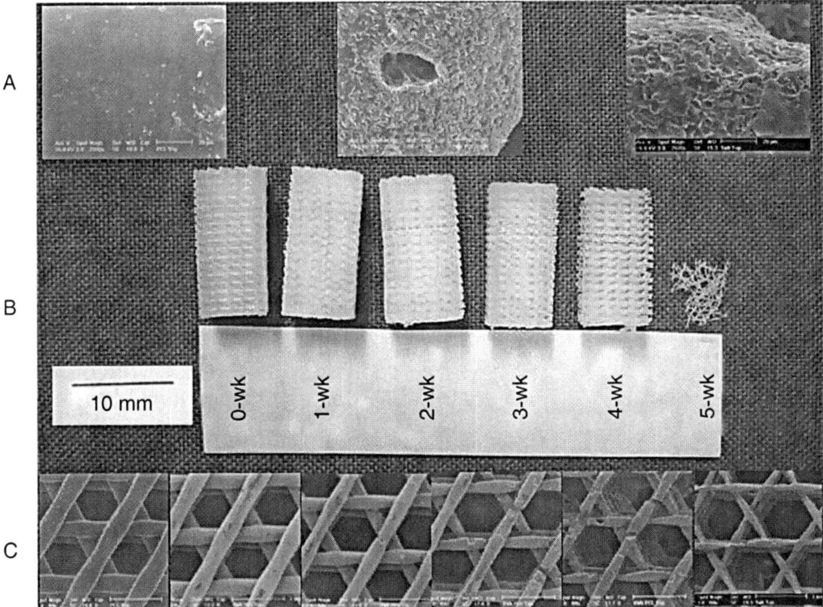

FIGURE 2.4 Microscopic and macroscopic views of NaOH-degraded PCL scaffolds from 0 to 5 weeks. Top inset (A) shows SEM micrographs (×2000 magnifications) of the surface texture of the scaffold filaments over time; 0-week, 1-week and 5-week (*left to right*). Middle inset (B) shows the macroscopic view of the degraded scaffolds. Bottom inset (C) shows SEM micrographs (×64) from 0 to 5 weeks. The scaffolds were observed to degrade via a surface erosion pathway homogenously throughout the scaffold structure, through the thinning of the filament diameters. (From Lam, C.X.F., Teoh, S.H., Hutmacher, D.W. Polymer International, 56, 718–728, 2007. With permission from Wiley and Elsevier.)

achieve sufficient stiffness and strength in a highly porous structure to provide adequate mechanical integrity. One of the most demanding applications is the repair and generation of musculoskeletal tissues, particularly bone, where scaffolds need to have a high elastic modulus to provide temporary mechanical support without showing symptoms of fatigue or failure, to be retained in the space they were designated for, and to provide the tissue with adequate space for growth. One of the fundamental challenges of scaffold design and material selection concerns the achievement of high enough initial strength and stiffness; the scaffold material must have both a sufficiently high interatomic and intermolecular bonding and a physical and chemical structure, which must in turn allow for hydrolytic attack and breakdown, *in vivo*, as the scaffold degrades over time.[20]

Porosity. A pore can be defined as a void space within a scaffold, whereas porosity can be considered as a collection of pores. Pore size and porosity are important scaffold parameters. Macropores (>50 μm) are of an appropriate scale to influence tissue function, for example, pores greater than 300 μm in size are typically recommended as optimal for bone in-growth in relation to vascularization of the construct. Micropores (<50 μm) are of a scale to influence cell function (e.g., cell attachment) given that mammalian cells typically are 10–20 μm in size. Nanoporosity refers to pore architectures or surface textures on a nanoscale (1–1000 nm).

There is often a compromise between porosity and scaffold mechanical properties. Increasing porosity may provide a greater pore volume for cell infiltration and extra cellular matrix (ECM) formation, but there is a concomitant decrease in mechanical properties in accordance with a power-law relationship.[11]

Pore interconnectivity. Pore interconnectivity is a critical factor and is often overlooked in scaffold design and characterization. A scaffold may be porous, but unless the pores are interconnecting (i.e., voids linking one pore to another), they serve no purpose and become superfluous within a scaffold intended for tissue engineering. The interconnecting pore size is more critical than pore size, and should be suitably large to support cell migration and proliferation in the initial stages and subsequent ECM infiltration of desired tissue. It is preferable that scaffolds for tissue engineering have 100% interconnecting pore volume, thereby maximizing the diffusion and exchange of nutrients (e.g., oxygen) and the eliminations of waste throughout the entire scaffold pore volume.

Pore characterization. As a measure of pore interconnectivity, the accessible pore volume, or permeability, of a scaffold can be measured. Accessible pore volume can be defined as the total volume of pores that can be infiltrated from all peripheral borders to the interior of the scaffold. Scaffold permeability can be measured by determining the flow rate of fluid flow through interconnecting pores. However, this technique is not suitable in scaffolds with large, 100% interconnected pore volumes as the scaffold provides no resistance to fluid flow. Alternatively, accessible pore volume as well as vol.% porosity, pore size distribution, and scaffold surface area to volume ratio (i.e., volume fraction) can be characterised using techniques such as mercury intrusion porosimetry, microcomputed tomography (μCT), or image analysis.[21] Mercury porosimetry is a popular technique based on the principle that the pressure required to force a nonwetting liquid such as mercury into pores, against the resistance of liquid surface tension, is indicative of the pore size, assuming that the pores are cylindrical in shape. However, the resolution of the technique is severely limited in scaffolds with large pore sizes (>500 μm) where low mercury intrusion pressures are necessary, and it has limitations when applied to materials that have irregular pore geometries. Alternative techniques such as μCT have been developed for analyzing bone architecture and more recently scaffold architecture to generate computer models of porous materials. Using 3-D μCT techniques, a much greater amount of information can be obtained to characterize pore architectures containing features ranging from 6 to >1500 μm, without the physical limitations associated with mercury porosimetry.[21] Scaffold fabrication is a critical step in the production of an appropriate scaffold and an increasingly popular technique for creating these tailor-made scaffolds in SFF.

2.3 SOLID FREE-FORM FABRICATION

2.3.1 Introduction

The tissue engineering fraternities are a long way off matching Nature in her ability to grow functioning tissues and organs. It is clear that much knowledge needs to be gained at all levels of tissue engineering, but from an engineering point of view the past decade has seen great advances in scaffold design. Starting with simple foams and fibers, it was quickly realized that connectivity between the pores, pore dimensions, and properties of the scaffold materials are of vital importance in facilitating cell seeding, migration, proliferation, and the production of extracellular matrix. Significant advances have also been made in incorporating bioactive molecules into scaffolds. As more is learned about the behavior of cells on micro and nanopatterned topographies, and plasma and chemically treated surfaces, future developments in scaffold fabrication technology are likely to be better tailored to produce designs and techniques that are targeted toward specific cell and tissue/ organ types, and even individual patients. Hybrid scaffold fabrication techniques have already been shown to be effective in pushing the limits of previously known techniques to meet the demands of more complex biological structures. One of the most pressing issues in current scaffold fabrication designs is the absence of vascularization; a strategy for addressing this issue is now of the utmost importance. Greater control of scaffold parameters is probably going to be just as important as vascularization in future scaffold designs. SFF has gained a lot of attention as it offers the ability to overcome some of the control problems that are already mentioned above.[2]

SFF and rapid prototyping (RP) are used to fabricate complex-shaped scaffolds by selectively adding materials, in a layer-by-layer, computer-generated process. Several SFF techniques are depicted in Figure 2.5.[17]

Lewis[22] coined the term "direct ink writing" and the term describes fabrication methods that employ a computer-controlled translation stage, which moves a pattern-generating device, that is, an ink-deposition nozzle, to create materials with controlled architecture and composition. Lewis divides them into filamentary-based approaches, such as robocasting (or robotic deposition) micropen writing and fused deposition, and droplet-based approaches, such as ink-jet printing and hot-melt printing. Ink designs that have been employed include highly shear thinning colloidal suspensions, colloidal gels, polymer melts, dilute colloidal fluids, waxes, and concentrated polyelectrolyte complexes. These inks solidify either through liquid evaporation, gelation, or a temperature- or solvent-induced phase change.

However, reviewing the current biomaterials and tissue engineering literature, it is concluded that the terms SFF and RP are mainly used to define the technologies described below namely, sterolithography, selective laser sintering, solid ground curing, three dimensional printing, extrusion and direct writing. Today, SFF provides a powerful instrument in the tissue engineer's toolbox for the generation of scaffold technology platforms.[17] One of the major benefits offered by SFF technology is the flexibility to create parts with highly reproducible architecture and compositional variation across the entire matrix due to the computer-controlled fabrication process. The application of SFF technologies in scaffold fabrication is wide and varied. Some of the more acknowledged techniques are described in the following sections. Figure 2.6 summarizes these technologies with regard to the dimensions of scaffolds, which can be fabricated using each respective technique.

2.3.1.1 Stereolithography

Stereolithography (SL) is one of the most commonly used rapid manufacturing and RP technologies. It is considered to provide high accuracy and good surface finish. SL is an additive fabrication process utilizing a vat of ultraviolet (UV)–sensitive photopolymer and a laser to build parts of a layer at a time. Each part is traced by the laser beam on the surface of the UV-sensitive photopolymer solidifying it. SL is based on the use of a focused UV laser, which is vector-scanned over the top of a liquid bath of a photopolymerizable material. The UV laser causes the bath to polymerize

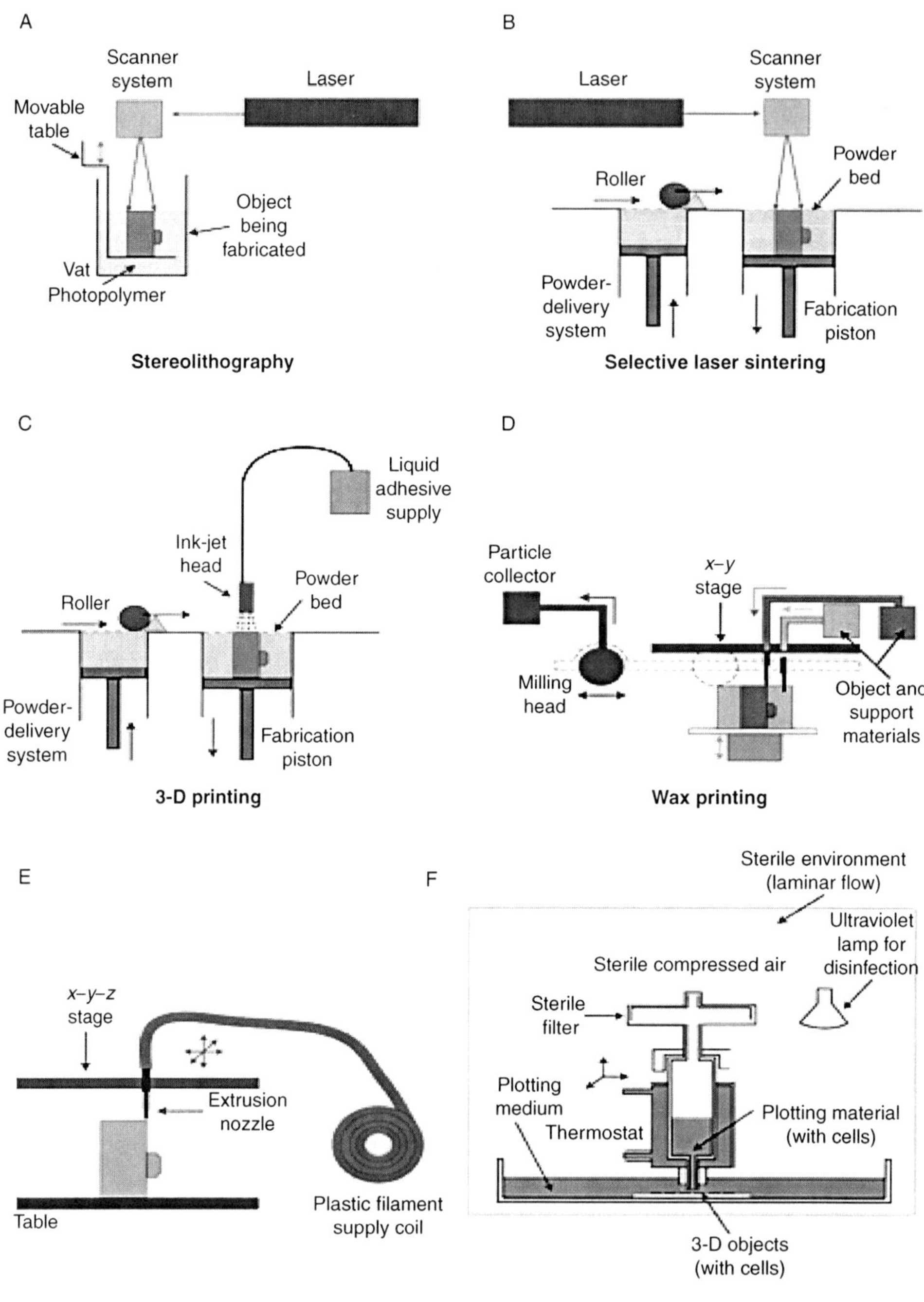

FIGURE 2.5 Schematics of SFF systems categorized by the processing technique. (A,B) Laser-based processing systems include the stereolithography system, which photopolymerizes a liquid (A) and the SLS systems, which sinter powdered material (B). In each system, material is swept over a build platform, which is lowered for each layer. (C,D) Printing-based systems, including 3-D printing (C) and a wax-printing machine (D). The 3-DP prints a chemical binder onto a powder bed. The wax-based system prints two types of wax material in sequence. (E,F) Nozzle-based systems. The fused deposition modeler prints a thin filament of material that is heated through a nozzle (E). The bioplotter prints material that is processed either thermally or chemically. (From Hollister, S.J., *Nat. Mater.* 4, 518–524, 2005. With permission from *Nature*.)

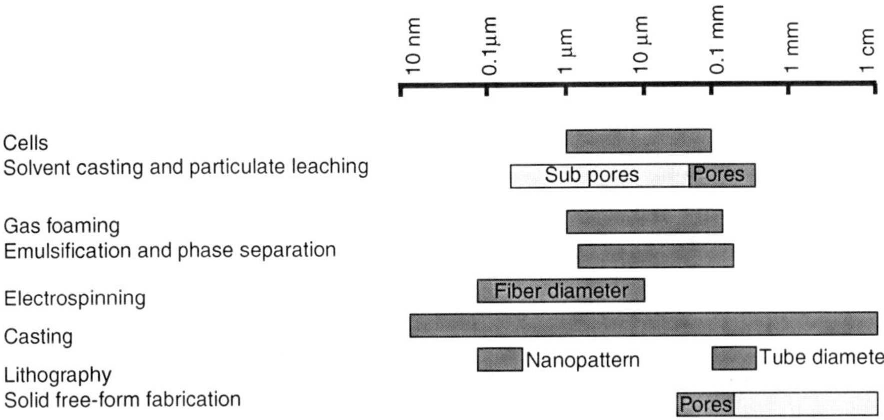

FIGURE 2.6 SFF fabrication techniques compared to other scaffold fabrication technologies and the dimensions of the generated scaffolds.

where the laser beam strikes the surface of the bath, resulting in the creation of a first solid plastic layer at and just below the surface. The solid layer is then lowered into the bath, and the laser-generated polymerization process is repeated for the generation of the next layer, and so on, until a plurality of superimposed layers forming the desired scaffold architecture is obtained. The most recently created layer in each case is always lowered to a position for the creation of the next layer slightly below the surface of the liquid bath. Once the scaffold is complete, the platform rises out of the vat and the excess resin is drained. The scaffold is then removed from the platform, washed of excess resin, and then placed in an UV oven for a final curing.

For industrial applications, the photopolymer resins are mixtures of simple low-molecular-weight monomers capable of forming solid long-chain polymers by chain reactions when activated by radiant energy within specific wavelength range. The commercial materials used by SL equipment are epoxy- or acrylate-based resins that offer strong, durable, and accurate parts or models. However, these materials cannot be used as scaffold materials due to the lack of biocompatibility and biodegradability. Hence, the limited availability of photopolymerizable biomaterials is a major constraint for the use of the SL technique in the design and fabrication of scaffolds for tissue engineering applications. However, biocompatible acrylic, anhydride, and polyethylene oxide (PEO)–based polymers may be explored in future research, as they are already typically at the clinical research stage as curable bioadhesives or injectable materials. A variation in laser intensity or traversal speed may be employed to alter the cross-link or polymer density within a layer so that the properties of the material can be varied from position to position within the scaffold. This variation enables the fabrication of so-called biphasic or triphasic matrix systems. Microstereolithography (MSL) in particular is thought to offer a great potential for the production of 3-D polymeric structures with micrometer resolution.

2.3.1.2 Selective Laser Sintering

Selective laser sintering (SLS) also uses a focused laser beam, but with the intention of sintering areas of a loosely compacted powder. In this method, a thin layer of powder is spread evenly onto a flat surface with a roller mechanism. The powder is then raster-scanned with a high-power laser beam. The powder material that is struck by the laser beam is fused, while the other areas of powder remain dissociated. Successive layers of powder are deposited and raster-scanned, one on top of one another, until an entire part is complete. Each layer is sintered deeply enough to bond it to the preceding layer. Wiria et al. have used SLS to produce biocompatible PCL/TCP scaffolds from starting powders; the scaffold demonstrated good osteoblast-like cell responses such as attachment levels and proliferation.[23] However, SLS has inherent material constraints for scaffold fabrication and is currently mainly used to make calcium phosphate–based scaffolds for bone engineering. The main drawback of SLS is that incorporation of sensitive biomolecules is difficult because of the need to locally heat the powder layer so as to sinter it. Antonov et al. produced 3-D bioactive, biodegradable scaffolds utilizing SLS using a different approach to conventional techniques. Instead of using infrared radiation ($\lambda = 10.6$ µm), which leads to polymer particles melting and fusing together, they used near-infrared ($\lambda = 0.97$ µm) laser radiation, which is not absorbed by particles. This meant the melting process was limited to just the polymer surface, which could render the polymer particles capable of encapsulating delicate bioactive species thus circumventing this important problem associated with traditional SLS.[24]

2.3.1.3 Solid Ground Curing

Besides the classical laser-based SL process, alternative processes using digital mask generators (e.g., liquid crystal displays or digital mirror devices [DMDs]) have been used successfully to build structures out of polymers and ceramics. In the RP literature this process is also termed solid ground curing (SGC) or digital light processing (DLP). In contrast to traditional UV-laser–based SL machines, DLP systems are significantly cheaper and therefore more versatile in respect to material modifications. At the same time DLP machines can expose a whole layer at once, whereas laser-based systems have to scan the contour of the object sequentially. DLP systems are based on a digital micromirror device. By projecting a bitmap onto the photosensitive resin, the liquid resin can be solidified selectively. Theoretically, DLP systems can be used to fabricate scaffolds with high resolution and geometric complexity. However, a prerequisite, and consequent limitation, is the availability of a light-curable biocompatible and bioresorbable polymer material. The wider application of SGC in designing scaffolds is mainly driven by developments of photochemically driven gelation technology of biomacromolecules that are chemically modified with photodimerizable groups.

2.3.2 Three-Dimensional Printing

The three-dimensional printing (3-DP) technology was developed at the MIT.[25] Three-dimensional printing is used to create a solid object by ink-jet printing a binder into selected areas of sequentially deposited layers of powder. Each layer is created by spreading a thin layer of powder over the surface of a powder bed. The powder bed is supported by a piston, which descends upon powder spreading and printing of each layer (or, conversely, the ink-jets and spreader are raised after printing of each layer, and the bed remains stationary). Instructions for each layer are derived directly from a computer-aided design (CAD) representation of the component. The area to be printed is obtained by computing the area of intersection between the desired plane and the CAD representation of the object. The individual sliced segments or layers are joined to form the 3-D structure. The unbound powder supports temporarily unconnected portions of the component as the scaffold is built but is removed after completion of the printing.

The solvent drying rate is an important variable in the production of scaffolds by 3-DP. Very rapid drying of the solvent tends to cause warping of the printed plotting of dots in 3-D with or without incorporation of cells. Much, if not all, of the warping can be eliminated by choosing a solvent with a low vapor pressure. It has been found that it is often an advantage to combine solvents to achieve minimal warping and adequate bonding between the biomaterial particles. Thus, an aggressive solvent can be mixed in small proportions with a solvent that has lower vapor pressure. After the binder has dried in the powder bed, the finished component can be retrieved, and the unbound powder is removed for postprocessing, if necessary.

The 3-DP process is capable of overcoming the limitations of some SFF techniques, such as those associated with manufacturing certain designs, for example, the overhanging structures. The solution lies in the layering of powders. As the layers are spread, there is always a supporting platform of powder for printing and binding to take place. Thus, as long as the parts are connected together, overhanging structures are of no difficulty. However, a drawback of the powder-supported and powder-filled structure is that the open pores must be able to allow the internal unbound powders to be removed, if the part is designed to be porous such as a scaffold for tissue engineering applications. The surface roughness and the aggregation of the powdered materials also affect the efficiency of removing the trapped materials. The resolution of the printer is limited by the specification of the nozzle size and position controller, which defines the print head movement. Another factor is the particle size of the powder, which simultaneously determines the layer thickness. A layer thickness between 100 and 400 µm can be achieved depending on the printer. The versatility of using a powdered material is advantageous, however, an obvious constraint of the 3-DP process is that most of the available biomaterials do not come in powder-form and need special processing conditions to get a powder that fulfils the requirements for 3-DP. Chen et al. used reverse SSF to create a negative mold (negative molds were first designed and then converted into SL data followed by 3-D printing of the mold) into which a poly-L-lactic acid (PLLA) solution could be poured and then phase-separated thermally to create 3-D nanofibrous scaffolds.[26] Taylor et al. used 3-D ink-jet printing in combination with CAD software to create sacrificial molds, bovine collagen was then cast into the mold, and the resulting scaffolds were shown to support the attachment and proliferation of human aortic valve interstitial cells.[27] More recently, tissue engineers were able to print cells in combination with hydrogels by simple modification of office ink-jet printers showing the proof of principle to one day create a tissue-engineered construct in a fully automated system.

2.3.3 Systems Based on Extrusion/Direct Writing

A number of groups have developed SFF machines, which can perform extrusion of strands/filaments and dots all employ extrusion of a material in a layered fashion to build a scaffold.[28] Depending on the type of machine, a variety of biomaterials can be used for scaffold fabrication. Schantz et al.[29] used FDM-fabricated polycaprolactone (PCL) scaffolds as burr hole plugs in a pilot study for cranioplasty. The clinical outcome after 12 months was positive, with all patients tolerating the implants with no adverse side effects reported, and good cosmetic and functionally stable cranioplasty observed in all cases. The second-generation scaffolds produced by FDM for bone engineering of Hutmacher's group are based on composites and have been evaluated *in vitro* and *in vivo*.[30]

The traditional definition of a composite material is a material with at least two phases, a continuous phase and a dispersed phase. The continuous phase is responsible for filling the volume and transferring loads to the dispersed phase. The dispersed phase is usually responsible for enhancing one or more properties of the composite. Most of the composites target an enhancement of mechanical properties such as stiffness and strength, but other properties may be of interest such as transport properties or density.

Matrix materials for composites can be metal, ceramic, polymeric, or biologic. It can be observed that metals and ceramics are always stiffer and can have larger strength than biologic hard tissue. Polymers are mostly more compliant (lower modulus) than hard tissue and can have strengths of the same order of magnitude than hard tissue. Biologic tissues show larger spectra of mechanical properties than the other materials. This picture clearly illustrates the great interest of compounding polymers and other materials to obtain composites that attain combinations of mechanical and biological properties similar to those of biologic hard tissue.

As in other areas of biomedical research, nature is seen as a guide to design new scaffold materials in the area of biocomposites. Mimicking the solutions found in natural materials is one of the most promising ways to reach the target set of properties needed for biomaterials. The development of materials for any replacement application should be based on the understanding of the structure to be substituted. This is true in many fields, but particularly exigent in scaffold-based tissue engineering. The demands upon the properties of the scaffold material largely depend on the site of implantation and the tissue function it has to restore. Ideally, a scaffold material should mimic the host tissue from a mechanical, chemical, biological, and functional points of view.

The main characteristics of the route by which the mineralized hard tissues are formed are that the organic matrix is laid down first, and the inorganic reinforcing phase grows within this organic matrix. Oyster shells, coral, ivory, pearls, sea urchin spines, and cuttlefish bone are just a few of the vast variety of biomineralized materials engineered by living creatures. Many of these biological structural materials consist of inorganic minerals combined with organic polymers. The study of these structures has generated a growing awareness that the adaptation of biological processes may lead to significant advances in the controlled fabrication of superior smart materials. However, to date, neither the elegance of the biomineral assembly mechanisms nor the intricate composite microarchitectures have been duplicated by nonbiological methods. But tissue engineers are trying very hard to implement the above-described principles of natural tissues to design and fabricate scaffolds.

Zhou et al.[20] studied so-called second-generation scaffolds made of medical grade polycaprolactone and 20% calcium phosphate *in vitro* and *in vivo*. Composite scaffolds were fabricated via FDM and were studied *in vivo* in conjunction with bone marrow stromal cell (BMSC) sheets for the engineering of structural and functional bone grafts. The constructs were fabricated and cultured *in vitro* before undergoing an 84-day *in vivo* trial using nude rats as shown in Figure 2.7.

The second-generation FDM scaffolds for bone engineering are now made of polymers and ceramics. Hutmacher's group at the University of Singapore has designed and built an RP machine as shown in Figure 2.8. The group has undertaken several studies (both *in vitro* and *in vivo*) utilizing FDM to produce scaffolds comprising medical grade polycaprolactone and 20% calcium phosphate, combined with collagen type I, which have been studied for up to 13 months in rat calvarial model. These scaffolds demonstrated superior bone regeneration compared with control (blank) defects as seen in Figure 2.9. Larger composite scaffolds have also been produced and placed as a bone graft in a high-load-bearing application in a pig spinal fusion model as seen in Figure 2.10. Collectively these methods demonstrate the versatility of FDM techniques in producing tailor-made scaffolds of different shapes, sizes, and compositions for specific anatomical applications.

A traditional FDM machine consists of a head-heated-liquefier attached to a carriage moving in the horizontal x–y plane. The function of the liquefier is to heat and pump the filament material through a nozzle to fabricate the scaffold following a programmed path, which is based on CAD model and the slice parameters. Once a layer is built, the platform moves down one step in the z-direction to deposit the next layer. Parts are made layer-by-layer with the layer thickness varying in proportion to the nozzle diameter chosen. FDM is restricted to the use of thermoplastic materials with good melt viscosity properties; cells or other theromosensitive biological agents cannot be encapsulated into the scaffold matrix during the fabrication process.

A variation of FDM process, the so-called precision extruding deposition (PED) system, was developed at Drexel University and tested.[31] The major difference between PED and conventional FDM is that the scaffolding material can be directly deposited without filament preparation. Pellet-formed PCL is fused by a liquefier temperature provided by two heating bands and respective thermal couples and is then extruded by the pressure created by a turning precision screw.

The pore openings facing the z-direction are formed in between the intercrossing of material struts/bars and are determined by user-defined parameter settings. However, the pore openings facing both the x- and y-directions are formed from voids created by the stacking of material layers, and hence, their sizes are restricted to the bar/strut thickness (diameter). As such, systems with a single extrusion head/liquefier do not allow variation in pore morphology in all three axes. A design method exists by extruding one strut/bar directly on top of each other to add design variability in the z-axis.[15]

Yang et al.[32] have prepared fine ceramic lattices (hydroxyapatite) using extrusion free forming utilizing a volatile solvent. The ceramic powder was compounded with binder and solvent, and after extrusion, the paste was solidified by evaporation, making it possible to form regular quasicrystal lattices; the filament spacing can be varied and the overall structure can be controlled by using a support structure, and all the organic contents can be removed on sintering at high temperatures, resulting in a pure ceramic lattice. Moroni et al.[33] have developed a technology to fabricate hollow

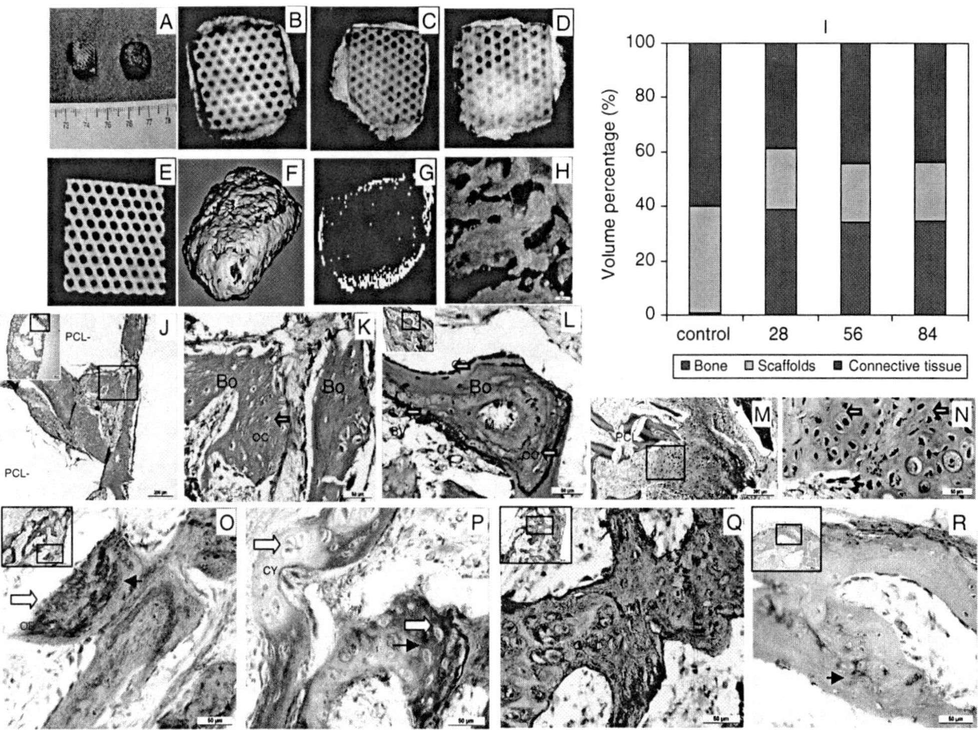

FIGURE 2.7 Constructs with BMSC sheet scaffolds (mPCL–TCP) were implanted into nude rat harvested after 28, 56, and 84 days. (A) Gross appearance of BMSC sheet scaffolds constructs with osteogenic induction (*right*) and noninduction (control) (*left*) after 4 weeks. (B) X-ray detected bone-like tissue formation in 28 days. (C) 56-day and (D) 84-day implants. (E) X-ray image of constructs without cell seeding (control). (F) Micro-CT demonstrated the overall highly mineralized tissue similar to cortical (golden) and cancellous (red) bone in implanted constructs after 28 days. (G) Micro-CT images disclosed the hard tissue formation within constructs. Mineralized tissue with similar density with cancellous bone was detected (darker areas) while the lighter color represented cortical bone. (H) Fluorescence was detected on the formed bone tissue after 28 days; the fluorescence came from the cFDA labeled BMSC. (I) Micro-CT quantification of implant tissue compositions depicted substantial bone formation in the induction group, accounting for 40% total volume for the 28, 56, and 84-day implantation, while the control group formed only connective tissue. (J) H&E staining shows lamellar bone-like tissue formed in both outer part and interior of constructs after 28 days. (K) High-magnification image shows well organized lamellar bone-like tissue (Bo) with distinct osteocytes located within bone tissue. (L) The typical osteoblasts (OB, black arrow) located on the surface of neomineralized tissue with marrow cavities and blood vessels in 56-day implants. (M) Safranin-O staining demonstrated that hypertrophic chondrocytes (white arrow) were observed in 56-day implants in very low numbers. High magnification shows the chondrocytes (white arrow) with weak safranin-O staining surrounded by the osteocyte (black arrow). (N) OCN staining. Strong signals (arrow head) were detected on neomineralized tissue while very weak to no signals were detected on chondrocyte like cells (O). (P) Collagen type I staining. Extensive staining was detected on the neomineralized tissue in constructs. (Q) Collagen type II staining. Limited signals (arrow head) were detected on chondrocyte-like cells while no staining for the mineralized tissues (R). BV, blood vessel+red blood cells; Ma, marrow; OB, osteoblast; Bo, bone; OC, osteocyte; CY, chondrocyte. Scale bar: (J) 200 μm; (H–Q) 50 μm. (Zhou, Y., Chen, F., Ho, S.T., Woodruff, M.A., Lim, T.M., Hutmacher, D.W. *Biomaterials.* 28, 814–824, 2007. With permission from Wiley and Elsevier.)

fibers with controllable hollow cavity diameter and shell thickness. They utilized viscous encapsulation to produce fibers with shell-core configuration via extrusion. The inner core polymer was then removed by selective dissolution. The extrudates were then organized into 3-D matrices, which can be customized into various shapes using RP.

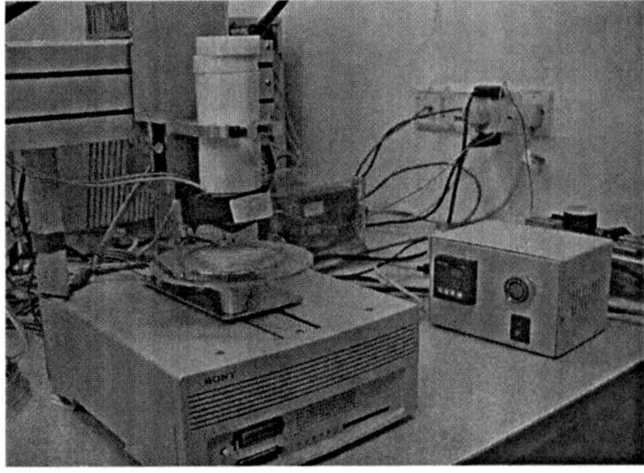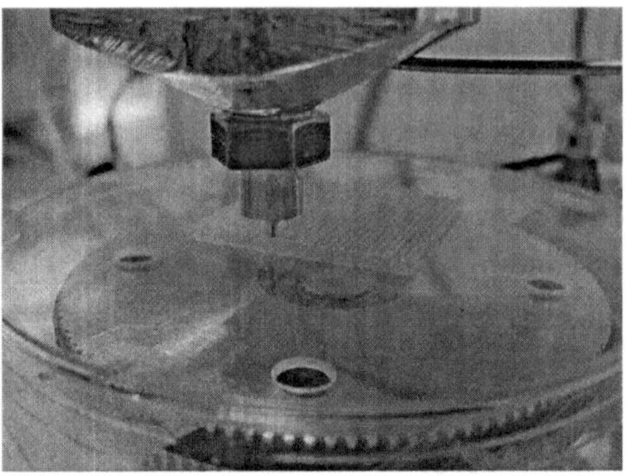

FIGURE 2.8 The group at the National University of Singapore designed and built a rapid prototyping (RP) machine and software, which is specifically dedicated to scaffold fabrication. The machine is based on an extrusion/dispenser head (multiple heads are also possible) by a three-axis robot (A). The process generates a scaffold from a computer file (STL, etc.) by building microstrands or dots. Depending on the machine setup, a tissue engineer can make use of a wide variety of polymer pastes/solutions (B, chitosan), and hot melts as well as dispersions and chemical reactive systems (e.g., fibrin glue).

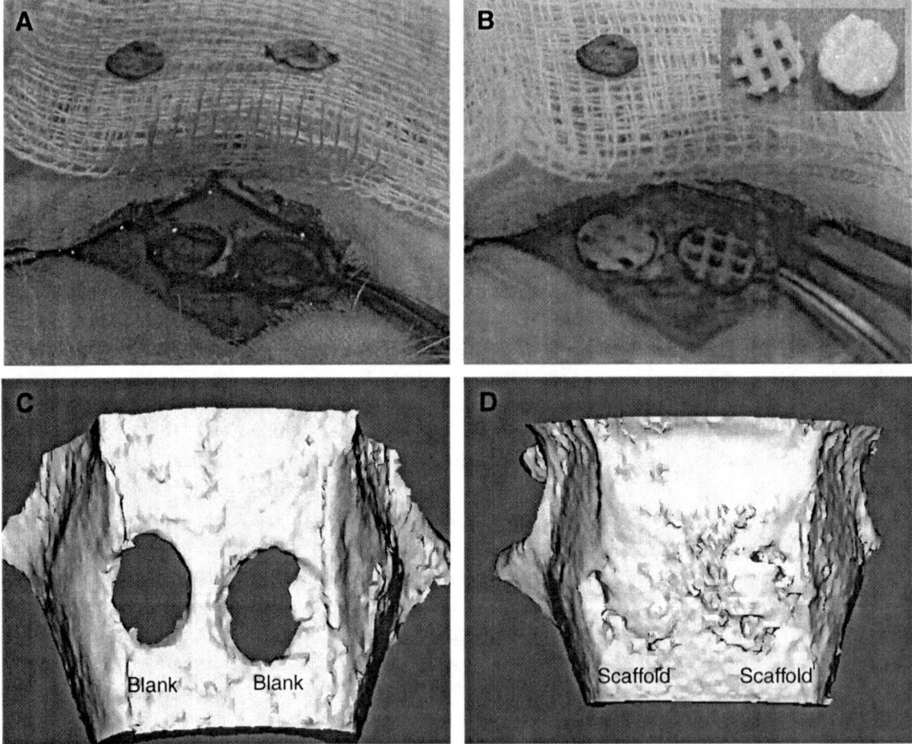

FIGURE 2.9 (A) Two full-thickness critical bone defects (5-mm diameter) were created in the rat parietal bone. Bone chips are shown. (B) Implantation of PCL/TCP-Col1 scaffolds into the defects (Inset: PCL–TCP scaffold (5-mm diameter and 1-mm thick, 0–900 lay-down pattern, 70% porosity) before treatment, *left*, and after lyophilization of 350 µg of rat tail collagen 1, *right*. (C,D) Micro-CT scanning of the skull defect showing the bone formation 13 months with and without scaffold implantation. It can be seen in (D) that there is formation of new bone, made possible by the implantation of the PCL/TCP/Col scaffold, which were produced via FDM.

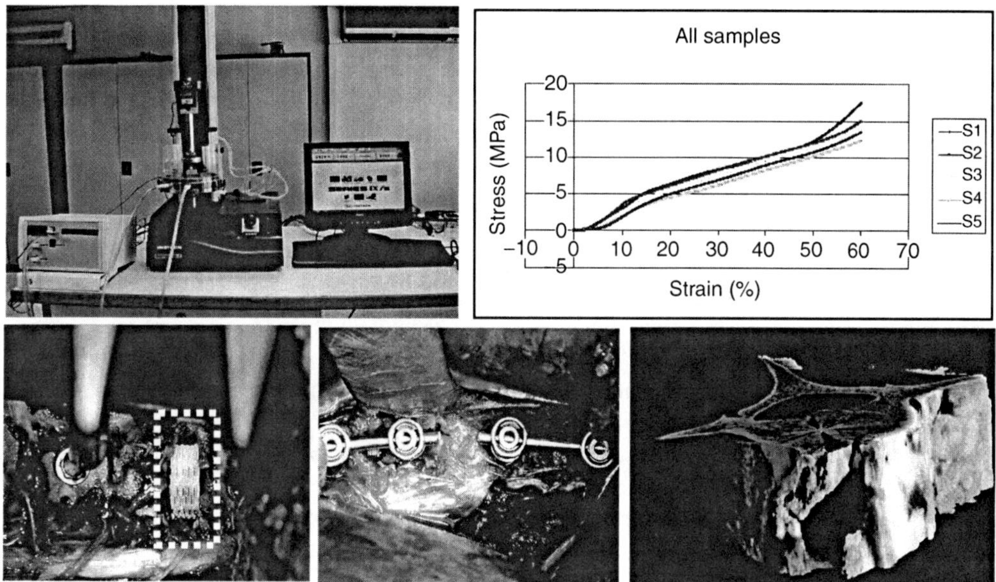

FIGURE 2.10 The second–generation FDM scaffolds for bone engineering are now made of polymers and ceramics.[11] Polymer/CaP composites confer favorable mechanical (pictures top row) and biochemical properties, including strength via the ceramic phase, toughness and plasticity via the polymer phase, more favorable degradation and resorption kinetics, and graded mechanical stiffness. Other advantages include improved cell seeding, and enhanced control and simplification of the incorporation and immobilization of biological factors PCL-TCP composite scaffolds (see white window left and middle picture lower row) placed as bone graft in a high load bearing application in a pig spinal fusion model. Three-month postoperative x-ray analysis shows no spinal bone fusion due to the scaffold becoming encapsulated with fibrous tissue (micro-CT, bottom right picture).

Mondrinos et al.[13] used indirect SFF by applying a drop on demand printing (DDP) fabrication process. A single universal porogen material was used to build a negative mold, which could then be injected with a wide range of biomaterials. Scaffolds comprising homogenous composites of PCL and calcium phosphate (10% or 20% w/w) were fabricated using injection molding of molten polymer–ceramic composites, followed by porogen dissolution with ethanol creating scaffold pore sizes as low as 200 µm. An inherent advantage of this technique is the ability to use multiple biomaterials for injection molding with a single ubiquitous porogen. Furthermore this technique circumvents the need to use cytotoxic solvents, which are common with many other polymer fabrication routes.

Yaszemski et al.[34] used poly(propylene fumarate) (PPF) as an injectable, biodegradable polymer, which has been used for fabricating preformed scaffolds in tissue engineering applications because of *in situ* crosslinking characteristics in combination with an SFF technique. To understand the effects of pore structure parameters on bone tissue in growth, 3-D PPF scaffolds with controlled pore architecture have been produced in this study from CAD models. The authors created original scaffold models with three pore sizes (300, 600, and 900 µm) and randomly closed 0%, 10%, 20%, or 30% of total pores from the original models in three planes. PPF scaffolds were fabricated by a series of steps involving 3-D printing of support/build constructs, dissolving build materials, injecting PPF, and dissolving support materials. To investigate the effects of pore size and interconnectivity on scaffolds, the authors compared the porosities between the models and PPF scaffolds fabricated thereby examined pore morphologies in surface and cross-section using scanning electron microscopy, and measured permeability using the falling head conductivity test.

PPF scaffolds with average pore sizes and pore shapes, that is, 600- and 900-μm pores, were similar to those of CAD models, but they depended on directions in those with 300-μm pores. Porosity and permeability of PPF scaffolds decreased as the number of closed pores in original models increased, particularly when the pore size was 300 μm, as the result of low porosity and pore occlusion. The authors conclude that their results show that 3-D printing in combination with injection molding can be applied to crosslinkable polymers to fabricate 3-D porous scaffolds with controlled pore structures, porosity, and permeability using their CAD models.

In the material science literature, another term for extrusion-based systems is used, namely, direct-write techniques, which rely on the formulation of colloidal inks for a given deposition scheme.[15] The techniques employed in direct writing are pertinent to many other fields besides scaffold fabrication such as the capability of controlling small volumes of liquid accurately. Direct-write techniques involving colloidal ink can be divided into two approaches: (1) droplet-based approach including direct ink-jet printing and hot-melt printing and (2) continuous (or filamentary) techniques.

The key to the versatile fabrication method of the SFF is its ability to literally build the model from its respective basic raw materials. However, the major limitations also lie in its methodology of building and bonding of raw materials together. For the SL technique the raw materials must be in a liquid form and must be photopolymerizable. The raw materials for the SLS must be able to melt and be severed cleanly, respectively; particles and layers must also be able to bond together based on the energy supplied. The 3-DP powder and binder combination must be compatible and must adhere the bulk material effectively. Finally, the FDM can only use a thermoplastic material. With these limitations on the building materials, SFF further restricts the list and availability of biomaterials that can be used for forming scaffolds or devices using this technology. Some researchers have begun to explore other options to exploit the macroscopic geometry and internal intrinsic architecture attainable by the SFF, along with its convenience and accuracy of duplication from medical imaging sources. An emerging method is to fabricate a negative mold based on the scaffold design and cast the scaffold using the desired materials, which may not be usable in an SFF setting. Indirect SFF routes rely on an additional molding step after fabricating the master pattern by RP.

In conclusion, indirect SFF adds further versatility and detail in scaffold design and fabrication. The previous restriction on casting was the inability of molds to produce complex geometry and internal architecture. But now with indirect SFF, traditional casting processes with these SFF molds can meet the specific tissue engineering requirements, including mechanical integrity and customized shapes. A highlighted advantage of indirect SFF is cost savings as the materials required for mold casting is substantially less and need not be processed into a dedicated form for any particular SFF process, such as processing into a powder for SLS and 3-DP. In addition, indirect SFF allows the usage of a wide range of materials or a combination of materials (composites or copolymers). However, some drawbacks still exist, including the resolution of the SFF method, as the cast model would inherit the errors and defects from the mold, such as cracks and dimensional changes. Also, a mold removal method must be developed to remove the mold while preserving the as-cast scaffold in an intact manner without disturbing its desired properties.

2.4　FUTURE DIRECTIONS

2.4.1　Introduction

The main challenge in preparing a useful TEC is to obtain a homogenous distribution of cells, and hence new tissue, throughout the entire 3-D scaffold volume. Furthermore, there exist two possibilities of incorporating cells into the scaffolds: (a) seeding of cells onto the surface of the scaffold subsequent to scaffold fabrication and (b) the incorporation of cells into the scaffold during the fabrication process. This second approach is of interest especially when incorporating cells into the scaffold material. Hence, the dream of tissue engineers is to build a structural and functional tissue *in vitro* by using SFF systems. The concept of organ printing by Mironov et al.[35,36] and robot-assisted construct fabrication aims at making this dream a reality.

2.4.2 Cell/Organ Printing

With the advantages of being inexpensive as well as high throughput, commercial thermal ink-jet printers have been modified to print biomolecules onto target substrates with little or no reduction of their bioactivities, resulting in the creation of DNA chips, protein arrays, and cell patterns. Most recently, by means of computer-assisted deposition, viable cells can be delivered to precise target positions within a matrix. Furthermore, using different cell types in combination with different hydrogels (bio-inks), which are then delivered to exact positions to mimic tissue structures of the original tissue, can be envisioned by using multiple nozzles. Thus, the printing of dissociated or aggregated cells based on specific patterns, and their subsequent fusion, may allow the development of replacement tissue or even whole organ substitutes.

Several groups have demonstrated the ability to extrude biopolymer solutions and living cells for 3-D tissue engineering applications. Sodium alginate solutions were deposited into calcium chloride solution using 3-D dispensing nozzles to produce a hydrogel TEC. Boland's group[37–39] proved the ability to print viable cells either by direct-writing or the ink-jet printing method. Since the physiological properties of mammalian cells strongly depend on the culture conditions and they are very sensitive to heat and mechanical stress, there was a major concern that the cells could be damaged or lysed by the conditions present during thermal printing. The temperature in the nozzle of the cartridge can be 300°C or higher. The study by Boland et al. indicates, however, that cells can be delivered successfully by using a modified ink-jet Hewlett-Packard (HP) printer, and most of these cells (>90%) were not lysed during printing. The HP ink-jet printer technology is based on vaporizing a micrometer-sized layer of liquid in contact with a thin-film resistor. As the timescales involved in the drop ejection process are small, there is not enough time for heat to diffuse into the bulk liquid. While the surface in contact with the liquid can peak at 250–350°C, the bulk liquid does not rise more than a couple (approximately 4–10°C) degrees above ambient. This situation could change, however, depending on the liquid and thermophysical properties of the ink. Although mammalian cells are more sensitive to high heat and strong mechanical stress than bacteria, their volume is also relatively small compared to the total volume of the printed droplet. The fact that these mammalian cells are viable, can proliferate, and differentiate indicates that damage from the heat and mechanical stress during the very short timescale of printing is avoided. Moreover, the $3 \times$ phosphate buffered saline (PBS) used for the cell print suspensions could have caused a further decrease in cell volume, because they are expected to shrink by osmosis in this hypertonic solution, effectively preventing clogging of the nozzle during printing. While these initial studies were mainly concerned with the survivability of cells, future studies will need to optimize the ink-jet technology along with the hydrogels to be successfully used in the field of tissue engineering.

Future studies will aim at modifying current ink-jet printers based on piezoelectric technology for possible use in cell printing.[40] However, there are some challenges in adapting commercial piezoprinters for organ printing. Commercial piezoprinters use a more viscous ink, and hence minimizing ink leakage and preventing formation of vapor is difficult. More viscous inks help to eliminate the need for complex fluid gates between the ink cartridge and print head to prevent the ink from backflow. However, this technique comes at the expense of requiring more power and higher vibration frequencies, both of which can break and damage the cell membranes. Typical commercial piezoprinters use frequencies up to 30 kHz and power sources ranging from 12 to 100 W. These frequencies create a problem because vibrating frequencies ranging from 15 to 25 kHz and power sources from 10 to 375 W are often used to disrupt cell membranes. Adapting piezoprinters for less viscous ink to lower the frequency and power would be challenging, since ink leakage and mist formation during printing could obscure the pattern. Future studies need to overcome these problems.[41]

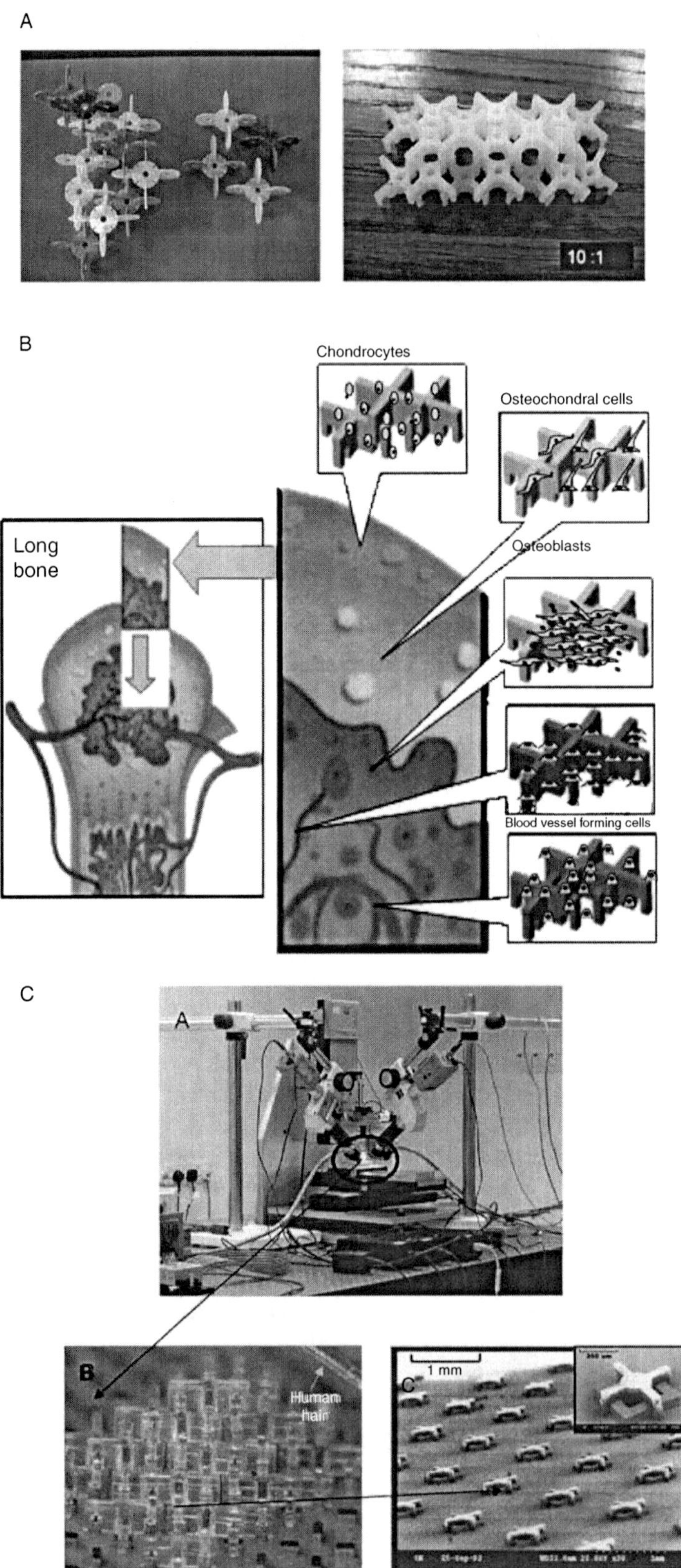
A
10 :1
B
Chondrocytes
Osteochondral cells
Osteoblasts
Blood vessel forming cells
Long
bone
C
A
B
Human
hair
1 mm
C

2.4.3 ROBOT-ASSISTED CONSTRUCT FABRICATION

A small number of groups work on this type of technology. This work was reviewed by Zhang et al.[42] The principle of microassembling a scaffold/cell construct is based on the same concept of assembling a structure using small building block units like Lego (Figure 2.11). Building blocks of different designs are first fabricated via lithography or microfabrication technologies and are then assembled by a dedicated precision-robot with four degrees of freedom microgripping capabilities, accomplishing a functional-sized scaffold with the required material, chemical, and physical properties. A monolithic shape memory alloy microgripper was used to manipulate and assemble the unit microparts into a scaffold structure. Even though preliminary data are promising, future studies need to show if this technique can be translated into clinically applicable concepts.

2.5 CONCLUSIONS

Scaffolds are of great importance for tissue engineering because they enable the fabrication of functional living implants utilizing cells directly obtained from cell culture. As the scaffolds for tissue engineering will be implanted in the human body, the scaffold materials should be nonantigenic, noncarcinogenic, nontoxic, nonteratogenic and possess high cell/tissue biocompatibility so that they will not trigger pathological reactions after implantation. Along with stringent material considerations, the macro and microstructural properties of the scaffold are also very important. In general, the scaffolds require specific individual external shapes and well-defined internal structure with interconnected porosity to host most cell types. From a biological point of view, the designed matrix should serve several functions, including (1) the ability to act as an immobilization site for transplanted cells, (2) the formation of a protective space to prevent unwanted tissue growth into the wound bed and allow healing with differentiated tissue, (3) directing the migration or growth of cells via surface properties of the scaffold, and (4) directing the migration or growth of cells via release of soluble molecules such as growth factors, hormones, and cytokines. Future work has to provide further compelling evidence that SFF offers the right balance of capability and practicality to be suitable for fabrication of materials in sufficient quantity and quality to move holistic tissue engineering technology platforms into a clinical application.

In addition to considerations of scaffold performance based on tissue engineering strategies, practical considerations of manufacture also arise. From a clinical point of view, it must be possible to manufacture scaffolds under good manufacturing practice (GMP) conditions in a reproducible and quality-controlled fashion at an economic cost and speed. To move the current tissue engineering practices to the next frontier, some manufacturing processes will be required to accommodate the incorporation of cells and growth factors during the scaffold fabrication process. To address this issue, novel manufacturing processes such as robotic assembly and machine- and computer-controlled

FIGURE 2.11   (A) Simple building blocks (*left*) were manually fabricated to illustrate the original concept for microassembly concept. The feasibility of designed parts was studied by using parts made 10× larger than the original parts (*right*). (B) A group at the National University of Singapore started developing a novel advanced manufacturing technique to fabricate scaffold/cell constructs for various tissue engineering applications in 2001. The idea was to assemble microscopic Lego-like building blocks into a scaffold. Based on this CAD-based and automated concept, the distribution of growth factors and living cells within the scaffold can be truly controlled in three dimensions so that scaffold/cell constructs with customized biological and physical properties can be realized. (C) The fabrication of these microparts is challenging due to their small size (0.5 μm × 0.5 μm × 0.2 μm overall, 60 μm thickness, ±5 μm tolerance) and complex 3-D shape. To facilitate the microassembly process, another challenge is the requirement that the parts need to be stably fixed on the wafer but at the same time are able to easily be removed by the microgripper. Currently, SU-8, a biocompatible material, is used to test the feasibility of the microassembly. (From Zhang, H., Hutmacher, D.W., Chollet, F., Poo, A.N., Burdet, E. Review Macromol. Biosci. 5, 477–489, 2005. With permission from Wiley.)

3-D cell encapsulation are under development. These approaches are working toward the enablement of the TEC to not only have a controlled spatial distribution of cells and growth factors, but also possess a versatility of scaffold material and microstructure within a specifically designed and fabricated construct for implantation in an intended anatomical site.

REFERENCES

1. Hutmacher DW. Regenerative medicine will impact, but not replace, the medical device industry (invited editorial). *Expet Rev Med Dev* 2006 Jul; 3(4): 409–412.
2. Lysaght MJ, Hazelhurst AL. Tissue engineering: the end of the beginning. *Engineering* 2004; 10: 309–320.
3. Archer R, Williams DJ. Why tissue engineering needs process engineering. *Nat Biotechnol* 2005; 23: 1353–1355.
4. Vacanti C. History of tissue engineering. *J Cell Mol Med* 2006; 10(3): 569–576.
5. Gadi P, Kuangshin T, Dima S, Yoram Z, Sangamesh K, Lakshmi SN, Cato TL, Dan G, Christine O. Structural and nanoindentation studies of stem cell-based tissue-engineered bone. *J Biomech* 2007; 40(2): 399–411.
6. Nicholas DE, Eileen G, Julia MP. Scaffolds for stem cells. *Mater Today* 2006; 9(12): 26–33.
7. Khalil P, Weiler V, Nelson P, Khalil M, Moosmann S, Mutschler W. Non-myeloablative stem cell therapy enhances microcirculation and tissue regeneration in murine inflammatory bowel disease. *Gastroenterology* 2006; 132(3): 944–954.
8. Bongso A, Lee EH. *Human Stem Cells: From Bench to Bedside*. World Scientific Press, Hackensack, NJ.
9. Vacanti JP. Beyond transplantation, the third annual Samuel Jason Mixter lecture. *Arch Surg* 1988; 123: 545–549.
10. Hutmacher DW. Scaffolds in tissue engineering bone and cartilage. *Biomaterials* 2000; 21(24): 2529–2543.
11. Hutmacher DW, Sittinger M, Risbud MV. Scaffold-based tissue engineering: rationale for computer-aided design and solid free-form fabrication systems. *Trends Biotechnol* 2004; 22(7): 354–362.
12. Moroni L, de Wijn JR, van Blitterswijk CA. 3D fiber-deposited scaffolds for tissue engineering: influence of pores geometry and architecture on dynamic mechanical properties. *Biomaterials* 2006; 27(7): 974–985.
13. Mondrinos MJ, Dembzynski R, Lu L, Byrapogu KC, Wootton DM, Lelkes PI, Zhou J. Porogen-based solid freeform fabrication of polycaprolactone-calcium phosphate scaffolds for tissue engineering. *Biomaterials* 2006; 27: 4399–4408.
14. Zein I, Hutmacher DW, Tan KC, Teoh SH. Fused deposition modeling of novel scaffold architectures for tissue engineering applications. *Biomaterials* 2002; 23(4): 1169–1185.
15. Lam CXF, Teoh SH, Hutmacher DW, *Comparison of Degradation of PCL & PCL-TCP Scaffolds in Alkaline Medium*. Polymer International 2007; 56: 718–728.
16. Woodfield TB, Bezemer JM, Pieper JS, van Blitterswijk CA, Riesle J. Scaffolds for tissue engineering of cartilage. *Crit Rev Eukaryot Gene Expr* 2002; 12(3): 209–236.
17. Hollister SJ. Porous scaffold design for tissue engineering. *Nat Mater* 2005; 4(7): 518–524.
18. Gibson LJ, Ashby MF. *Cellular Solids: Structure and Properties*. 2nd ed., Cambridge University Press, Cambridge, U.K., 1997.
19. American Standard for Testing and Methods ASTM D883-99, Standard Terminology Relating to Plastics, 1999.
20. Zhou Y, Chen F, Ho ST, Woodruff MA, Lim TM, Hutmacher DW. Combined marrow stromal cell sheet techniques and high strength biodegradable composite scaffolds for engineered functional bone grafts. *Biomaterials* 2007; 28(5): 814–824.
21. Ho ST, Hutmacher DW. A comparison of micro CT with other techniques used in the characterization of scaffolds. *Biomaterials* 2006; 27(8): 1362–1376.
22. Lewis JA, Gratson GM. *Mater Today* 2004; 7: 32.
23. Wiria FE, Leong KF, Chua CK, Liu Y. Polycaprolactone/hydroxyapatite for tissue engineering scaffold fabrication via selective lasr sintering. *Acta Biomaterialia* 2007; 3: 1–12.
24. Antonov EN, Bagratashvilli VN, Whittaker MJ, Barry JJA, Shakesheff KM, Konovalov AN, Popov VK, Howdle SM. Three dimensional bioactive and biodegradable scaffolds fabricated by surface selective laser sintering. *Adv Mater* 2005; 17(3): 327–329.

25. Cima M, Sachs E, Fan TL, Bredt JF, Michaels SP, Khanuja S, Lauder S, Lee SJ, Brancazio D, Curodeau A, Tuerck H. 1995 United States Patent 5387380.
26. Chen V, Smith LA, Ma PX. Bone regeneration on computer designed nano fibrous scaffolds. *Biomaterials* 2006; 27: 3973–3979.
27. Taylor PM, Sachlos E, Dreger SA, Chester AH, Czernuszka JT, Yacoub MH. Interaction of human valve interstitial cells with collagen matrices manufactured using rapid prototyping. *Biomaterials* 2006; 27: 2733–2737.
28. Hutmacher DW, Woodfield T, Dalton PD, Lewis JA. Scaffold design and fabrication. In: *Textbook on Tissue Engineering.* van Blitterswijk C, Thomsen P, Williams D, Hubbell J, Cancedda R, de Bruijn JD. (eds.) Elsevier 2008.
29. Schantz JT, Lim TC, Ning C, Teoh SH, Tan KC, Wang SC, Hutmacher DW. Cranioplasty after trephination using a novel biodegradable burr hole cover: technical case report. *Neurosurgery* 2006 Feb; 58(1 Suppl): ONS-E176; discussion ONS-E176.
30. Hutmacher DW (invited and key note lecture). Advances in the use of scaffold-based bone engineering. 28th Australasian Polymer Symposium & 16th annual meeting of the Australasian Society for Biomaterials. Rotorua, New Zealand, 5–9 February, 2006.
31. Sun W, Lal P. Recent development on computer aided tissue engineering: a review. *Comput Meth Programs Biomed* 2002; 67: 85–103.
32. Yang H, Yang S, Chi X, Evans RG. Fine ceramic lattices prepared by extrusion freeforming. *J Biomed Mater Res B Appl Biomater* 2006; 79B: 116–121.
33. Moroni L, Schotel R, Sohier J, de Wijn JR, van Blitterswijk CA. Polymer hollow fiber three-dimensional matrices with controllable cavity and shell thickness. *Biomaterials* 2006; 27: 5918–5926.
34. Esmaiel J, Bradford LC, Michael J, Yaszemski K-W, Lee MS, Shanfeng W, Lichun L. Fabrication and characterization of poly(propylene fumarate) scaffolds with controlled pore structures using 3-dimensional printing and injection molding. *Tissue Eng* 2006; 12: 10.
35. Mironov V, Boland T, Trusk T, Forgacs G, Markwald RR. Organ printing: computer-aided jet-based 3D tissue engineering. *Trends Biotechnol* 2003; 21(4): 157–161.
36. Jakab K, Neagu A, Mironov V, Forgacs G. Organ printing: fiction or science. *Biorheology* 2004; 41: 371–375.
37. Boland T, Mironov V, Gutowska A, Roth EA, Markwald RR. Cell and organ printing 2: fusion of cell aggregates in three-dimensional gels. *Anat Rec Part A* 2003; 272(2): 497–502.
38. Xu T, Jin J, Gregory C, Hickman JJ, Boland T. Inkjet printing of viable mammalian cells. *Biomaterials* 2005; 26: 93–99.
39. Boland T, Tao X, Damon BJ, Manley B, Kesari P, Jalota S, Bhaduri S. Drop on demand printing of cells and materials for designer tissue constructs. *Mater Sci Eng C* 2006.
40. Boland T, Xu T, Damon B, Cui X. Application of inkjet printing to tissue engineering. *Biotechnol J* 2006; 1(9): 910–917.
41. Mironov V, Reis N, Derby B. Review: bioprinting: a beginning. *Tissue Eng* 2006 Apr; 12(4): 631–634.
42. Zhang H, Hutmacher DW, Chollet F, Poo AN, Burdet E. Microrobotics and MEMS-based fabrication techniques for scaffold-based tissue engineering. Review *Macromol Biosci* 2005 Jun 24; 5(6): 477–489.

3 Control and Monitoring of Scaffold Architecture for Tissue Engineering

Ying Yang, Cassilda Cunha-Reis, Pierre Olivier Bagnaninchi, and Halil Murat Aydin

CONTENTS

3.1 INTRODUCTION

The loss or failure of an organ or tissue is one of the most frequent, devastating, and costly problems in healthcare.[1] With the increase in life expectancy, the aging-associated tissue loss or degeneration becomes more severe and frequent. The current therapeutic options to treat organ or tissue loss are based on transplanting the organ, performing surgical reconstruction, or using artificial implants.[2] Despite the advances in the medical field, all these therapeutic approaches display several limitations, and, in the majority of cases, they relieve the symptoms but do not cure the disease, since they are unable to provide tissue regeneration.[3]

The application of cells as therapeutic agents for disease as well as for repair and regeneration of tissues is one of the toughest challenges in modern therapeutics. Tissue engineering (TE) is an emerging multidisciplinary technique that offers great potential for developing new therapeutic strategies for the treatment of damaged tissues or organs.[4] TE combines engineering and life science approaches to guide specific cells to grow into the required tissue arrangement *in vitro*.[5] Synthetic or natural biodegradable macromolecules are used to produce temporary scaffolds, which provide a suitable environment for cells to eventually form the required functional tissue. Ideally, a small number of cells are collected from patients, then seeded in a temporary scaffold where they are expanded and cultured *in vitro*. During the *in vitro* culture period, biochemical and mechanical stimulations are applied to the cell–scaffold construct in order to direct cell proliferation and extracellular matrix (ECM) organization and to generate functional tissue-engineered constructs that meet the physiological requirements before being implanted into patients. After implantation, the tissue-engineered construct, integrated in the damaged area, would guide the formation of new functional tissue. Alongside the new tissue formation, the scaffold undergoes degradation releasing products that are readily incorporated in well-defined metabolic pathways, and more space is left available for further tissue growth.[6]

TE has demonstrated its great potential as a promising treatment for repair and regeneration of tissues and organs.[7,8] The success of TE will have great impact on general healthcare and quality of human life.

3.2 REQUISITES FOR ENGINEERING TISSUES

Cells, scaffolds, and culture environment are the three essential elements in engineering tissue constructs.[9] In an ideal situation, the patient himself is the cell source, eliminating all the problems regarding biocompatibility and transmission of pathogens. Nevertheless, the number of cells that can be obtained from certain tissues without causing donor site morbidity is generally very low. The use of adult stem cells (ASCs) is a very promising option to overcome this problem. ASCs are undifferentiated cells with a very high proliferation capacity found among differentiated cells in tissues or organs. These cells have the capacity of self-renewing and differentiating to yield the major specialized cell types of that tissue or organ. The presence of ASCs has been reported in several organs and tissues, such as the periosteum,[10] bone marrow,[11] muscle,[12] skin,[13,14] brain,[15] and fat tissue.[16,17] At the moment there is an increasing number of research focused on understanding the mechanisms that control the differentiation of ASCs into particular cell types and their potential use in tissue-engineering strategies. The state of the art for the research in this area has been reviewed elsewhere.[18,19]

The culture environment is another crucial element when developing an tissue-engineered construct. This environment must mimic the one found in the original tissue or organ as closely as possible. Ultimately, cell behavior is dictated by the complex coordination of a panoply of biochemical and biomechanical cues. In the field of bone TE, some studies have shown that applying perfusion systems to the constructs increases the expression of bone-related proteins by providing flow-mediated mechanical stimuli[20,21] and enhancing transport of nutrients and waste within the constructs. Other studies have shown that using bioreactors to apply cyclical load to the constructs increases the expression of bone-related proteins, compared with the nonloading ones.[22]

The authors' group has combined the application of mechanical and biochemical stimuli by developing a mechanoactive scaffold. This study has shown that in the presence of *in vitro* physiological loading regimes and release of calcium channel agonists incorporated in poly (L-lactic acid) (PLLA) scaffolds, the expression of collagen I and osteopontin and osteoid calcification were enhanced, when compared with controls.[23,24] These results indicate that agonist-encapsulated scaffolds can be used in the presence of load to enhance the production of load-bearing engineered tissue.

Scaffolds play a pivotal role in converting isolated cells to functional tissues because they initially endow cells with temporary shelter for anchoring, adhering, and settling down. The requirements of supporting the cell to grow into a functional tissue make it essential for the scaffold to have several unique features. The first one is obviously biocompatibility. High porosity is also a prerequisite, to provide space for the cells to settle down, generate ECM, and to guarantee an effective diffusion of nutrients, metabolites, biological cues, and gases across the scaffolds during the *in vitro* maturation. The porous structure also facilitates angiogenesis after implantation, thus blood vessels can grow and supply oxygen and nutrients to the center of the construct.[25] In addition to an appropriate porosity, the scaffold must display the required mechanical integrity to maintain the predesigned tissue structure and to guarantee a suitable performance when it is subjected to the local strain after implantation. The ability to degrade in the biological environment by either enzymatic or hydrolytic reaction is another feature of the scaffold. The degradation and elimination rate of the temporary template should correspond with the rate of tissue turnover.

When the final goal is to achieve a functional tissue construct, providing only the essential requisites for cell survival and proliferation is not enough. In their natural environment, the cells are integrated in tissues that display specific architectures usually optimized for specialized functions. Consequently, it is not surprising that several studies have shown that the cell behavior is highly influenced by the architecture of the scaffolds. These studies have shown that rather than just responding to the chemical composition of the scaffolds, the cells actually react to structural parameters, such as surface topography and the stiffness,[26,27] nanotopography,[28,29] fiber diameter,[30] and microgeometry.[31,32] Some authors have even shown that it is possible to direct cell migration to specific areas of scaffolds by using micropatterning techniques to create micropaths with specific architecture.[33,34] Nevertheless, one has to bear in mind that the possibility of extrapolating these studies to different contexts is fairly limited because they report the behavior of a particular cell type in a particular type of scaffold. The establishment of standard generalized cell behavior in a well-defined context is at the moment virtually impossible because of the high amount of variability stemming from the conditions used in different laboratories.

3.3 SCAFFOLDS FOR TISSUE ENGINEERING

3.3.1 MATERIALS

The materials used to fabricate scaffolds for TE are derived either from synthetic polymers, mainly from polyester family, or from natural materials, for example, collagen and chitosan. The mechanical properties and structural properties of these materials can be tailored by adjusting the molecular weight, crystallinity, and the ratio of comonomers in the copolymers.[35–38]

3.3.1.1 Synthetic Polymers

Poly(glycolic acid) (PGA), poly(lactic acid) (PLA), and their copolymers poly(lactic acid-*co*-glycolic acid) (PLGA) are a family of linear aliphatic polyesters, which are most frequently used in TE.[39] These polymers are among the few synthetic polymers approved by the U.S. Food and Drug Administration (FDA) for certain human-clinical applications.[40] They degrade through hydrolysis of the ester bonds,[41] and the ultimate products of their degradation are the monomers lactic and glycolic acids, which are further transformed into water and carbon dioxide in well-defined metabolic pathways.[42] Several studies have revealed that they are biocompatible and that their presence is well-tolerated *in vivo*.[43,44]

There are other linear aliphatic polyesters, such as poly(ε-caprolactone) (PCL), which are also used in TE research.[45–47] PCL degrades at a significantly slower rate than PLA, PGA, and PLGA. The slow degradation makes PCL less attractive for general TE applications but more attractive for long-term implants.[48] PCL-based copolymers have recently been synthesized to improve degradation properties.[49,50] Other important synthetic biodegradable polymers include poly(propylene fumarate) (PPF),[51] which degrades through hydrolysis of the ester bonds similar to glycolide and lactide polymers[52] and segmented polyurethanes whose structural variations enable the production of materials with a range of mechanical properties.[53] Synthetic polymers from the families of polyphosphoesters,[54] poly(ethylene oxide terephthalate)-poly(butylene terephthalate) (PEOT/PBT),[55] polyanhydrides[56] and poly(ortho esters)[57] are also under study for potential use in TE applications.

3.3.1.2 Natural Origin Polymers

Most of the interest in natural origin polymers stems from their biocompatibility, relative abundance, ease of processing, and possibility of mimicking the microenvironment found *in vivo*.

Collagen is present in most of the connective tissues of the body. Although there are 16 types of collagens, the most abundant one is collagen type I. The macromolecular fiber structure derived from a triple helix arrangement confers this polymer resistance to pressure. As a result, collagen acts as a structural matrix protein.[58,59] Collagen has been used in several TE applications, like human cornea reconstruction,[60] cardiac regeneration,[61] skin,[62] cartilage,[63] and bone regeneration.[64]

Alginate is composed of two repeating monosaccharides: L-guluronic acid and D-mannuronic acid. Repeated strands of these units form linear water-soluble polysaccharides. Once these polysaccharides are exposed to calcium ions, a three dimensional (3-D) gel quickly forms.[65] Therefore various drugs, growth factors, or cells can be encapsulated in the gel.[66] Alginate gels have been used in a wide range of TE, such as the regeneration of cardiac tissue,[61] liver,[67] pancreas,[68] cartilage,[69] and bone,[66,70] alone or as a blend.[71,72]

Among the wide range of available materials for TE applications, chitosan is considered to be very promising because of some of its properties like biocompatibility, biodegradability, and antibacterial activity.[73–78] Chitosan is a partially deacetylated derivative of chitin, found in arthropod exoskeletons. Structurally, chitosan is a linear polysaccharide consisting of β(1 → 4) linked D-glucosamine residues with a variable number of randomly located *N*-acetyl-glucosamine groups.[79] The presence of such chemical groups provides active sites for the grafting of relevant molecules for the improvement of cell–material interactions.[80,81] This polymer is degraded by the action of several enzymes,[82] but in an *in vivo* environment enzymatic degradation is mainly attributed to the action of lysozyme.[83,84] This polymer has been used in several studies as potential material for pancreas,[85] bone,[86,87] cartilage,[88,89] and skin[90,91] TE.

Other natural origin polymers with good potential in TE applications are starch,[83,92–96] polyhydroxybutyrate,[97,98] hyaluronic acid,[99,100] or silk.[101,102]

3.3.2 Processing Techniques to Control the Scaffolds' Architecture

Various techniques have been developed to produce scaffolds. The ultimate goal is to obtain highly interconnected porous scaffolds with required internal architectures suitable for different tissues.

3.3.2.1 Solvent-Based Techniques

Solvent-evaporation/particulate leaching is a technique that has been widely used to fabricate scaffolds for TE applications. In this technique, a polymer solution mixed with a porogen is cast into a mold filled with a porogen, usually a salt, such as sodium chloride. After the evaporation of the solvent, the salt crystals are leached away with water leaving empty spaces that form the pores of the scaffold.[103,104] Phase-separation techniques to produce porous scaffolds are based on the fact that under certain conditions, a homogeneous multicomponent system becomes thermodynamically unstable and tends to separate into more than one phase in order to lower the system free energy. For example, a polymer solution can separate into two phases: a polymer-rich phase and a polymer-lean phase. After the solvent is removed, the polymer-rich phase solidifies and the pores are formed.[105] Solid–liquid phase separation can be achieved by lowering the temperature to induce solvent crystallization from a polymer solution. After the removal of the solvent crystals (sublimation or solvent exchange), the space originally taken by the solvent crystals becomes pores.[106] Fabrication of scaffolds by freeze-drying and cryogel formation belongs to this category. The common shortcomings of the fabrication technologies discussed in this section are the lack of precise control of the 3-D pore architecture of the scaffolds and lack of with relative low pore interconnection. To tackle these problems, computer-assisted design and manufacture CAD/CAM is being adopted.[39]

3.3.2.2 Computer-Assisted Design and Manufacture

Lack of pore interconnection will result in a poor and nonefficient nutrients, gas, and waste exchange within the scaffolds. The internal architecture and topography of the scaffold not only affect cell attachment but also influence alignment, which can subsequently affect the organization of the generated ECM. Precise design and manufacture of scaffolds have stimulated a rapid development of solid free-form fabrication and rapid prototyping techniques for scaffold manufacture enabling formation of scaffolds with a controlled internal architecture. CAD/CAM techniques offer the advantage of producing well-controlled 3-D structure with regular micropattern for a range of biomaterials. Scaffolds produced by such means can be customized both in microstructure and overall size and shape for preparation of implants tailored to specific applications or even to individual patients. These techniques can be performed by applying the action of heat, light, or adhesives.[107,108] Selective laser sintering (SLS) and fused deposition modeling (FMS) are heat-based fabrication techniques.[109,110] These techniques involve the application of heat to fuse layers of material to each other by raising the biopolymer above its glass transition temperature and applying pressure.[110–112] In addition to heat-based fabrication, light can also be used to create polymer structures. Photopolymerization involves the use of light to initiate a chain reaction, resulting in the solidification of a liquid polymer solution. Stereolithography and photolithography are the photopolymerization techniques that have been used in the fabrication of TE scaffolds.[113–115]

Another approach to fabricate scaffolds is to bind polymers by using solvents or adhesives rather than heat or light, eliminating any biomaterial limitations such as heat compatibility or photoinitiator dependence. An example of this type of fabrication is 3-D printing (3-DP) in which a binder solution is deposited onto a biomaterial powder bed using an ink-jet printer. Three-dimensional structures of approximately 200–500 μm are fabricated, one layer at a time.[116,117] Like 3-DP, pressure-assisted microsyringe (PAM) fabrication also involves layer-by-layer deposition with the solvent acting as a binding agent.[118,119] Manjubala et al.[120] used a rapid prototyping technique (3-D printer) to produce scaffolds with chitosan and hydroxyapatites. The resulting scaffold has biomimetic mineral–organic composition and controlled macroporosity and reproducible microporous internal architecture. Results from *in vitro* cell culture experiments indicate that the architecture encourages cell growth from the periphery to the middle of the pores. Stevens et al.[34] have used a replica printing method to transfer stamps onto porous hydroxyapatite scaffolds. This replica printing is a simple and inexpensive method to control spatial distribution of cells, which promotes the hierarchical organization. Fukuda et al.[121] have developed a layer-by-layer deposition method to control micropatterned cell coculture. By the formation of electrostatic complexes, the surface can be switched from a cell–deterrent to a cell–adhesive surface.

3.4 MONITORING SCAFFOLDS' ARCHITECTURE

Quality control and adjustment of the scaffold manufacturing process are essential to achieve high-standard scaffolds. However, most scaffolds are made from highly crystalline polymers, which inevitably result in their opaque appearance. The 3-D opaque structure prevents the observation of internal uneven surface structures of the scaffold under normal optical instruments, such as the traditional light microscope. The inability to easily monitor the inner structure of scaffolds poses a major challenge for TE as it impedes the precise control and adjustment of the parameters affecting cell growth and ECM deposition in response to various mimicked culture conditions. In this section, rather than providing an extensive description of the principles of operation of the most commonly used imaging techniques, we outline their potential and limitations as monitoring tools for TE.

3.4.1 Microscopy

3.4.1.1 Scanning Electron Microscopy

A common way for assessing general structural features of the scaffolds is by scanning electron microscopy (SEM). In this technique, the samples are irradiated with a high-energy-focused electron beam. The excited molecules from the sample then emit secondary electrons that are detected in a scintillator photomultiplier, and the ensuing signal is turned into two-dimensional (2-D) intensity distribution, which can be viewed as a digital image. Because the brightness of the signal depends on the angle of the electron bean in relation to the surface, the obtained digital images reflect some features of 3-D structure. Most of the polymeric and biological samples are not good electron conductors. So, in order to achieve contrast, sample preparation involves coating with electronically dense molecules such as gold.

SEM can provide high-resolution images (up to 5 nm) evidencing general morphology, surface topography, pore geometry, cell distribution, and morphology. SEM is also useful for monitoring the morphological changes that occur along the *in vitro* culture. Nevertheless, this technique is limited to the surface of the scaffolds and is not suitable for assessing the 3-D structure of the scaffold, neither the cell distribution throughout the construct. The combination of SEM with physical methods such as mercury intrusion porosimetry, which determines porosity and pore interconnectivity, provides a more detailed description of the scaffolds' architecture.[122–124] However, besides the inability to provide 3-D information, SEM presents another severe limitation: the processing requirements. Not every sample can be easily processed for SEM analysis, and this is particularly verifiable for samples containing cells and ECM. Furthermore, this method is destructive and requires the sacrifice of the analyzed samples, which sometimes are so difficult to obtain.

3.4.1.2 Light and Fluorescence Microscopy

Light microscopy is a traditional but very powerful tool in the biological field. One of the most important areas relying on the use of microscopy is Histology. Histology is the study of animal and plant Tissue at a microscopic level. The use of conventional microscopy in combination with various biochemical stains that selectively enhance contrast, enables the distinction of individual components within a complex biological system. Traditional histological techniques have shown to be useful in the assessment of the evolution of engineered tissue constructs, since they have enabled the localization of cells, matrix proteins, and matrix calcification throughout the constructs, as well as the visualization of the morphological aspects of the scaffolds.[125,126] Figure 3.1 shows a light microscope image of the grown in a PLLA scaffold for 4 weeks. Another variant of histology is fluorescent immunohistochemistry. The principles are quite the same, but in this case the molecules of interest are marked with fluorescent dyes, usually linked to very specific antibodies[127], and the tissue sections are analysed in a fluorescent microscope. The high resolution and great contrast associated with a relatively low cost of operation make histology an essential technique in every biological laboratory. However, the penetration depth of visible and fluorescent light is very limited. Only thin and transparent samples can be visualized. Inevitably, all tissue or organ samples have to be cut into thin sections about 7 µm through conventional paraffin embedding and microtome sectioning before being examined by bright light or fluorescence microscopy. Alternatively cryo-sectioning can be used. These sample preparation methods and histological analysis are not only

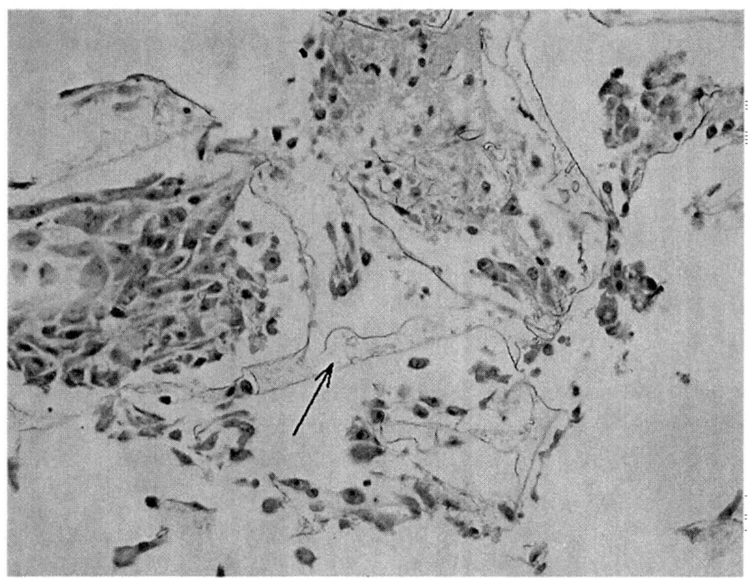

FIGURE 3.1 Light microscopy images of MG63 bone cells growth in a PLLA scaffold for 4 weeks (H&E staining) with 200× magnification. The arrow points to the porous wall of the PLLA scaffold.

time consuming, but may also introduce structural artifacts or lead to loss of some components because all biological specimens must be subjected to a dehydration and rehydration cycle. Changes in the hydration of the matrix may lead to the separation of the cells and matrix and the formation of lacunar spaces, thus impairing the factual examination of the constructs.[128] Most importantly, observation by microscopy is an end-point evaluation and a destructive analysis.

3.4.1.3   Confocal Microscopy

The emergence of confocal microscopy (CM) was a revolution in the field of microscopy. By labeling with fluorophores, optically nontransparent specimens can be visualized at high resolution in 3-D. CM enables the acquisition of sample images up to a few hundred micrometers thickness by using a focused laser beam and collecting the emitted fluorescent signal through a pinhole aperture that spatially rejects light from out of focus areas. Changing the plane of focus enables the rapid sample sectioning along the xz- or yz-plane to obtain sample cross-sections.[129] Optical sectioning eliminates the requirements of physical sectioning as in histological analysis, enabling the observation of viable cells in the scaffold and the online measurement of cell activities and tissue turnover. A confocal microscope image of a chitosan scaffold is presented in Figure 3.2.

The main drawbacks of CM are the limited penetration depth, the lack of temporal resolution, which renders it unsuitable to detect transient cell shape changes, and the requirement of fluorophores. Except for a few engineered tissues, for instance, skin and cornea, the engineered constructs are relatively thick, around a few millimeters to centimeter range. The penetration depth in CM limits the observation to few hundred micrometers from the surface of the constructs. Furthermore the fluorescent labeling may affect the long-term viability of cells in the constructs.

The use of CM in reflectance mode overcomes the requirement of fluorophores. In this case, the contrast is achieved by utilizing the inherent refractive index properties of the various cellular microstructures. The radiated laser beam is scattered irregularly by the heterogeneous tissue components. Backscattered in-focus signals are captured, transmitted to a spectrometer, and submitted for visualization. Usually, a laser light with near-infrared (near-IR) wavelengths is used for *in vivo* reflectance mode measurements. Even though this mode is more appropriate for *in vivo*

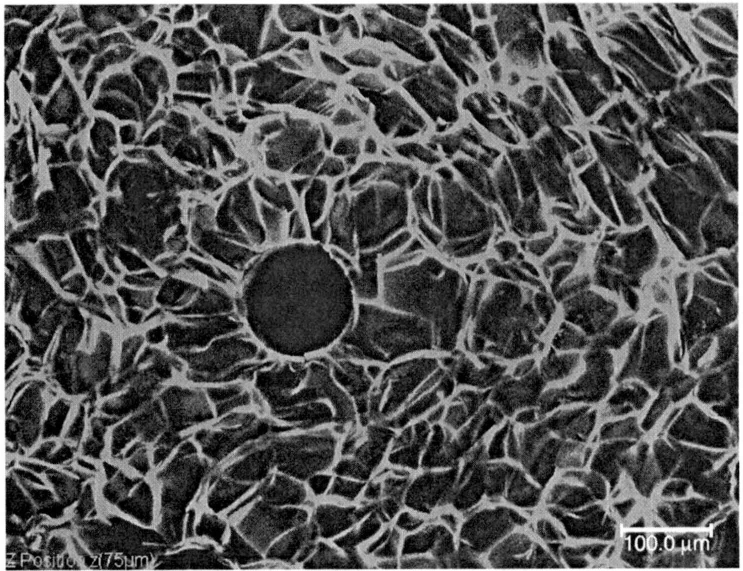

FIGURE 3.2   Confocal microscope image of a blank dual-mode chitosan scaffold.

tissue imaging because it dispenses with the use of fluorophores and allows the use of near-IR light, its resolution is lower than that achieved in traditional CM.[130]

A new imaging modality, multiphoton confocal microscopy (MCM) has been developed based on the fact that when photons of certain energy are fired almost simultaneously to a target molecule, they can cause an excitation similar to the one produced by the absorption of a single photon of higher energy. If the excited molecule is fluorescent, it can emit a single photon of fluorescence as if it were excited by a single higher energy photon. This characteristic makes the use of longer wavelength excitation lights possible (e.g., near-IR), leading to reduced light scattering in tissues and improved penetration depths, with reduced photobleaching and photodamage. This setup also simplifies multicolor imaging by allowing excitation of different fluorophores with the same laser, avoiding chromatic aberrations and providing a broad uninterrupted emission collection bandwidth. Furthermore, the use of near-IR light favors cell viability. The principles and applications of this technique are reviewed elsewhere.[131] Again, the limitation of MCM is its low specimen penetration depth.

3.4.2   Microcomputed Tomography

Microcomputed tomography (μ-CT) is an analog of x-ray CT scanner in the medical field. Its increasing popularity comes from its ability to provide precise quantitative and qualitative information on the 3-D morphology of specimens in great detail without resorting to physical sectioning. Moreover, due to the nondestructive character of the technique and the absence of processing requirements, the samples can be subjected to other tests eliminating the problem of sample scarcity. In this imaging technique, the source of contrast is the attenuation of x-rays by high-density materials. Consequently it has been used in the biological field preferentially for bone tissue analysis. In μ-CT scanning, the specimen is irradiated from the edges with x-rays in order to achieve a series of 2-D slices. As the radiation crosses each slice, the x-rays are attenuated, and the sprouting x-rays with reduced intensities are captured by a detector. The x-ray paths and the attenuation coefficients are derived from the detector measurements. Then, a 2-D pixel map is created from these computations, and each pixel is designated by a threshold value that corresponds to the attenuation coefficient measured at a similar location within the specimen. Because the attenuation coefficient correlates to the material density, the resultant 2-D maps reveal the material phases within the specimen, depending on the scanning resolution, which ranges from 1 to 50 μm. A 3-D reconstruction allows a close-up view of any specific location, thus the observation of pore shape, the measurement of pore size, and the thickness of strut or wall can be conducted in these close-ups.[132]

A scaffold made from polymeric materials has low x-ray attenuation, but the contrast between air and polymer is sufficiently high to differentiate them. Therefore, μ-CT has extra applications for the assessment of scaffolds' architecture, such as pore size, porosity, pore interconnectivity, quantification of microarchitectural parameters, and correlation with compressive mechanical properties of scaffolds.[133] In the context of TE, μ-CT scanning has mainly been used for monitoring mineralization within 3-D scaffolds *in vitro*, since bones have higher x-ray attenuation coefficient than soft tissue or polymeric materials. Numerous studies have reported the mineralization degree within the 3-D construct by μ-CT scanning method. A shortcoming of μ-CT scanning is that in most of the cases, the analysis has to be performed in a dry state since most scaffold materials have similar attenuation coefficient to water. This renders the online monitoring of tissue turnover fairly difficult to accomplish. Even though the online follow-up of scaffolds mineralization by μ-CT has been reported,[134] one should bear in mind that it was achieved by using low-voltage x-rays during short periods of time. Such conditions may not be sufficient to achieve the degree of detail required in some cases. Furthermore, the cellular response to such harsh conditions in long-term studies has not been reported so far.

3.4.3 Optical Coherence Tomography

Optical coherence tomography (OCT)[135] has recently emerged as a promising imaging technique, mainly for medical applications. The original development of OCT was for transparent tissues, such as cornea and retinal tissues.[136] The current OCT technology enables nontransparent soft and hard tissues to be examined *in vivo*,[137] for example, the skin,[138] gastrointestinal tract,[139] nervous systems,[140] cartilage,[141] and respiratory tract.[142] OCT is an imaging modality that can be used to study tissues or biological systems *in vivo* with near-histological, ultrahigh resolution. OCT is an interferometric technique. The light backscattered from the sample interferes with the light from the reference arm when the delay is within the coherence length of the source. The variation of the optical path in the reference arm allows in-depth scanning of the sample. Clearly, its features provide enormous potential to overcome a number of limitations currently experienced in TE for monitoring scaffold architecture and also tissue-engineered constructs.

In the last decade, the instrumentation of OCT has been continuously investigated and developed. The resolution, the penetration depth, and functionality of OCT have been improved dramatically. The image penetration depth of OCT determined by the scattering coefficient of the sample can be up to 2–3 mm in tissue. Depending on the light source, image resolutions of 1–15 μm have been achieved, which are at the same order of cell dimension, showing the potential to view cell morphology by this modality. Generally, a set of computer-controlled mirrors move the beam over the sample in *x*- and *y*-directions, allowing a 3-D reconstruction of the specimen. Most importantly, analysis with OCT can be realized in real time and in a nondestructive manner, without the need for excision and processing of specimens, providing a great amount of quantitative data regarding the tissue morphology.[143]

Some studies that focus the use of OCT in TE have been reported.[144] Yang et al.[145] have used this technique to image macrostructural morphology and delineate the morphology of cells and constructs in a developing *in vitro* engineered bone tissue. The authors have shown the potential for the use of OCT in noninvasive monitoring of cellular activities in 3-D developing engineered tissues. Since OCT provides both quantitative and qualitative data, it can further be adjusted to monitor scaffolds' degradation or erosion.

3.5 CONTROL AND MONITORING OF SCAFFOLD ARCHITECTURE FOR TISSUE ENGINEERING—A CASE STUDY

The clinical application of 3-D-engineered constructs with specific dimensions and architecture will most certainly rely on the development of computer-assisted techniques to manufacture the appropriate scaffolds for individual cases. Unfortunately, that achievement is still some steps ahead of what the actual state of the art in TE can provide. As it has been pointed out in this chapter, a great deal of research involving the response of cells to several stimuli in a 3-D dynamic environment needs to be done before that stage can be reached. Despite the array of highly controlled and reproducible morphological features that computer-assisted manufacturing techniques can offer, the implementation of these methods on the average TE laboratory is not realistic. In addition to a relatively high cost of operation, most of them are extremely time consuming and cannot generate the amount of scaffolds usually required for most biological studies in a practical timescale. In this section, we discuss the new manufacturing techniques developed by the authors' research group. These techniques enable alteration of scaffolds' architecture in terms of pore shapes and interconnectivity based on routine laboratory facilities. μ-CT and OCT have been explored to monitor the scaffolds' architecture in a nondestructive manner. In the case of OCT, this has been achieved under sterile conditions, which generates a new tool that sets in motion the online investigation of scaffold degradation and tissue turnover.

3.5.1 DEVELOPMENT OF NEW TECHNIQUES TO TAILOR SCAFFOLD ARCHITECTURE

The exploration of new scaffold manufacture techniques with high productivity, easy operation, and accurate control of scaffolds' architecture will be of great benefit for the TE research field since a large number of scaffolds are frequently required for comparison or optimization of the culture conditions in TE experiments. In the following sections, we present three techniques developed for the manufacture of scaffolds, with advantages over existing methods.

3.5.1.1 Controlling Pore Interconnectivity in Porous PLLA Scaffolds by Dual Porogen

Traditional solvent-evaporation and salt-leaching technique makes use of a single porogen, usually sodium chloride, to give rise to scaffolds with controllable porosity but poor pore interconnectivity.[24] This characteristic renders them improper to tissue culture because it reduces the diffusion of nutrients, gases, and metabolites across the scaffolds and impairs cell-to-cell contact. Based on this technique, we have developed a new approach to increase pore interconnectivity.[146] In this new approach, a dual porogen system is used: the water-soluble porogen, sodium chloride, creating macroporosity and the water-nonsoluble porogen, naphthalene, producing pore interconnections. The principle is illustrated in Figure 3.3.

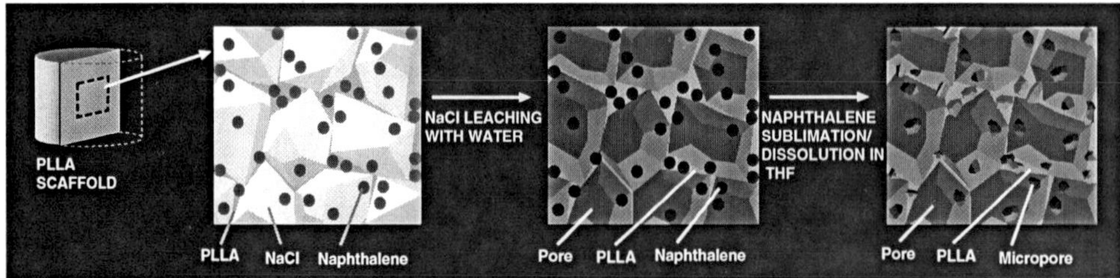

FIGURE 3.3 Schematic diagram showing the principle of solvent evaporation/particulate leaching with dual-porogen method. In this method, the NaCl crystals create the macroporosity, whereas the particles of naphthalene generate pore interconnections.

In brief, medical grade PLLA was dissolved in chloroform and mixed with 100–355 µm sodium chloride (NaCl) crystals and naphthalene with irregular shape and size around 5 µm to form a composite that was placed into a mold of 9 mm diameter. Following chloroform evaporation and polymer solidification, salt was leached from the polymer composite by placing scaffolds in double distilled water for 2–3 days, with gentle agitation, and then dried at room temperature. After NaCl salt was leached out by water, naphthalene was removed by tetrahydrofuran (THF), and this step was followed by the removal of THF by ethanol. Finally, the scaffolds were rinsed with distilled water and dried. Two different naphthalene/polymer ratios, 10% and 20%, were used to optimize the structural changes in the pore morphology.

3.5.1.2 Controlled Morphology and Degradation Rate in Fibrous Chitosan Scaffolds Produced by Wet Spinning

Fibers are very attractive structures for the production of scaffolds because they provide a large surface area as well as a considerably large porosity and interconnectivity, which can be optimized for specific applications. Our objective for choosing fibrous scaffolds was twofold: adjusting both the porosity and the degradation rate. In this study, based on a previously described wet-spinning technique,[75] a new method for tailoring the morphology of chitosan fiber-mesh scaffolds was developed. The starting material was chitosan powder with a deacetylation of 89% and a molecular weight of 366 kDa, purified by reprecipitation. To produce fibrous scaffolds, a 2% chitosan solution in 2% acetic acid was wet spun into a sodium hydroxide/sodium sulfate solution which, was acting as the precipitation agent. The diameter of the fiber and the porosity of the scaffolds were controlled by using different needles and changing the total volume of the chitosan solution used for spinning,[147] as described in Figure 3.4. Four types of cylindrical shape scaffolds (ϕ 5 mm $\times$ 4 mm) with fiber diameter of 65 and 105 µm and two different porosities ranging between 70% and 90% were produced. Two distinct degradation profiles were obtained from the four types of structures, which indicated the potential of this technique on adjusting several properties of these type of scaffolds.

3.5.1.3 Creation of Dual Pore Modes in Chitosan Scaffolds

Engineering specific organized tissue or organ demands equally specific scaffold architecture, which can guide cell and matrix growth in harmony with natural tissue organization. Chitosan scaffolds with dual pore modes have been fabricated aiming to generate engineered tendon. The dual pore mode chitosan scaffolds possess micropores and microchannels, which were fabricated based on a modification of a method described elsewhere.[148] A 2% chitosan solution was prepared by dissolving 95% deacetylated chitosan flakes in 1% v/v glacial acetic acid. The resulting solution was cast in a cylindrical plastic mold containing a needle array. Stainless steel needles of 250 µm diameter were used to produce 3 $\times$ 2 or 3 $\times$ 4 arrays. Constructs were frozen overnight at $-20°C$ and subsequently freeze-dried. The remaining acetic acid in the resulting scaffolds with microchannels was removed in a gradient of ethanol (i.e., 100%, 70%, and 50%) since the use of sodium hydroxide to neutralize acetic acid leads to the change of crystallinity, which results in deformation and shrinkage of the scaffolds.[149] Finally, the scaffolds were stored in phosphate-buffered saline (PBS).

3.5.2 MONITORING THE SCAFFOLDS' ARCHITECTURE

Development of nondestructive and online imaging technique to monitor the scaffolds' architecture provides dual benefit for TE. The monitoring enables controlling the fabrication process and adjusting processing parameter in a rapid mode. More importantly, the imaging system can investigate the degradation and tissue turnover processes within the scaffolds. µ-CT and OCT have been applied to assess the scaffolds described in section 3.5.1.1–3.5.1.3. The experimental work described in this section (3.5.2) sets a good example of how the new imaging modalities can be beneficial for TE.

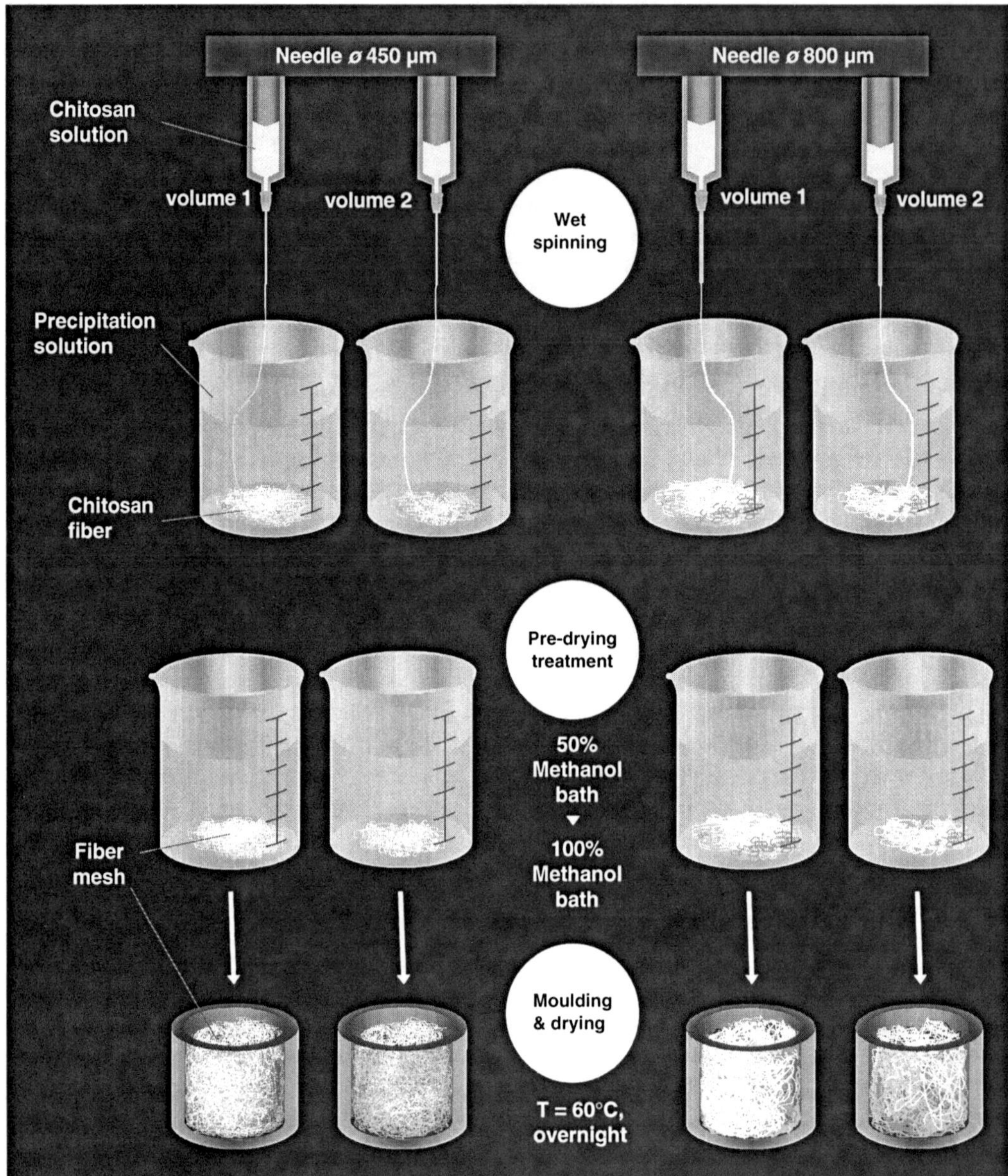

FIGURE 3.4 Schematic diagram demonstrating the method to tailor the morphology of fibrous chitosan scaffolds produced by wet spinning. By using various needle diameters and molding different volumes of fibers, it is possible to obtain a range of scaffolds with distinct morphologies.

3.5.2.1   Microcomputed Tomography

Selected porous PLLA scaffolds and fibrous chitosan scaffolds have been cross-examined by µ-CT (Scanco µ-CT40) using 55 kV energy and 144 µA intensity (Figure 3.5). The effective resolution of the reconstructions was 6 µm. A Gauss filter and threshold were applied to the reconstructions to segment the scaffold structure, which was initially analyzed for porosity, surface area, and filament thickness. The percentage of polymer here denominated bone volume (BV), the total volume (TV), and the ratio (BV:TV), which were obtained using the Scanco Medical µ-CT software. BV is used

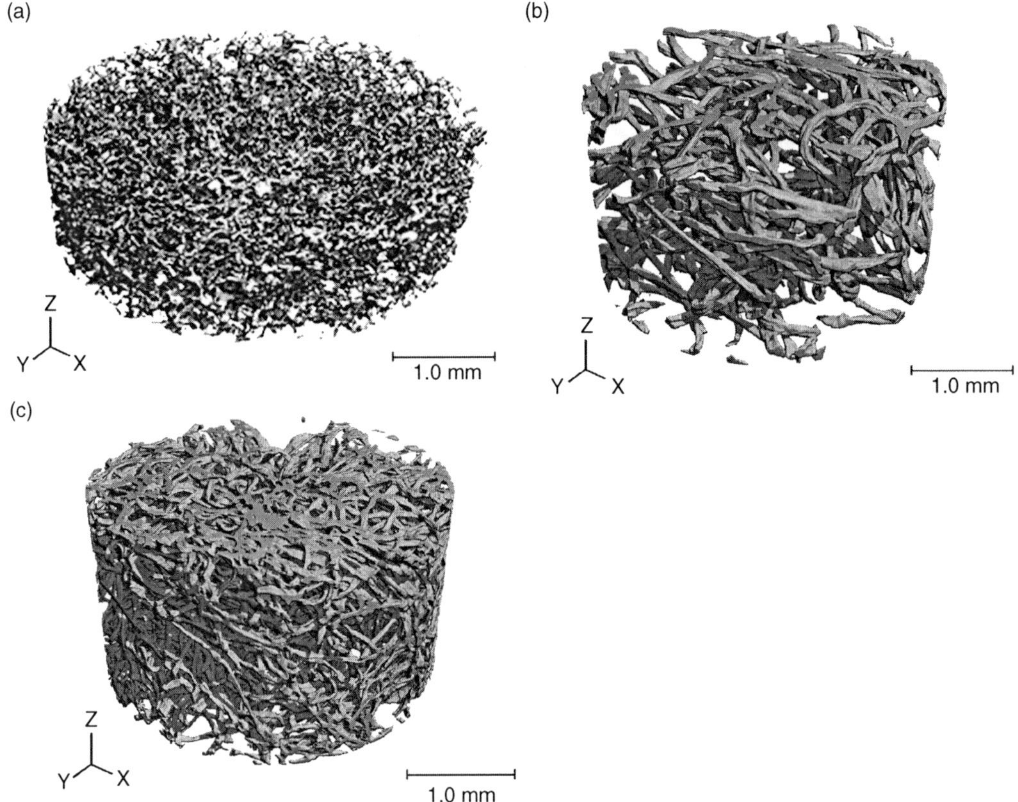

FIGURE 3.5 Micro-CT images of (a) PLLA scaffold with pore size of 255–350 µm, (b) fibrous chitosan scaffold with fiber diameter around 105 µm and porosity of 85%, and (c) fibrous chitosan scaffold with fiber diameter around 65 µm and porosity of 95%.

to indicate the densest material under investigation, in this instance, PLLA and chitosan. So pores occupy the remaining volume within the volume of interest (VOI). The porosity is calculated by subtracting the percentage of polymer out of the total volume. The clearly characterized morphology of the fibrous and porous scaffolds is shown in Figure 3.5. In addition, the quantitative data such as pore size and porosity can be easily derived from it.

3.5.2.2 Optical Coherence Tomography

An all-fiber time-domain OCT, based on a Michelson interferometer, was used for the study (Figure 3.6). The detailed description of the system can be found elsewhere.[150] Briefly, the system employed a 1300 nm superluminescent diode with a bandwidth of 52 nm, which was coupled into the port 1 of a circulator. A 50/50 fiber coupler splits the beam from port 2 to the reference and sample arms. Port 3 is connected to the balanced detector for heterodyne detection. The signal-to-noise ratio (SNR) of the system is measured at 90 dB with the use of a 4-OD neutral density filter with a scanning speed of 100 Hz. The depth-scan was performed by a double-pass grating-based scanning system to scan rapidly the optical delay in the reference arm. The measurement beam was scanned over the sample by a mirror controlled by the galvanometer. The system has a measured x–z resolution of 16 µm $\times$ 14 µm in free space. The scans presented in this study were scaled according to a mean refractive index of 1.4, commonly adopted for biological material. A linear x–y stage has been equipped to collect successive scans, allowing a 3-D reconstruction of the sample images. The step of successive scans was chosen as 25 µm.

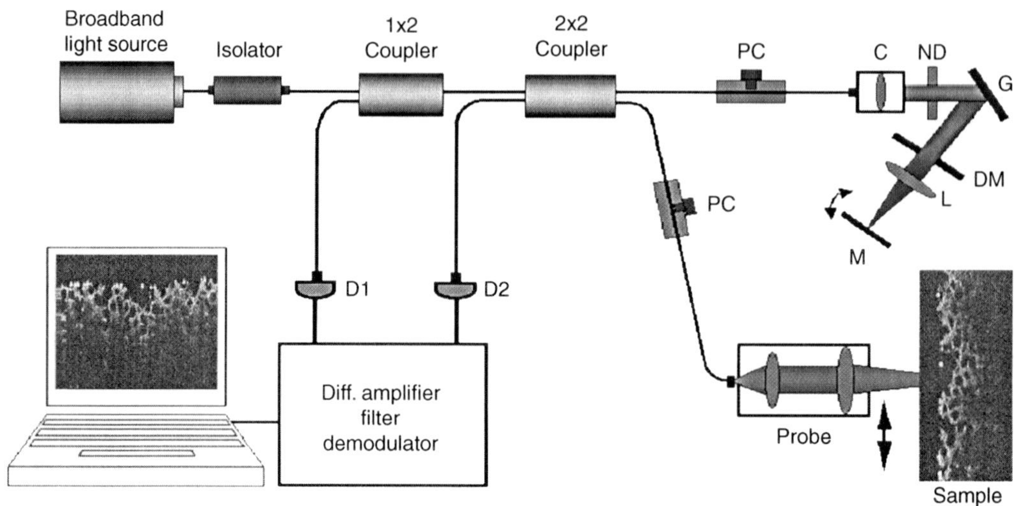

FIGURE 3.6 Schematic representation of OCT system setups used for the current investigations, where PC denotes the polarization controller, C the collimator, ND the neutral density filter, G the grating, DM the double pass mirror, L the optical lens, M the reflecting mirror and D the detector.[145]

The pore size in the PLLA scaffold made by single porogen was controlled between 255 and 350 μm, yielding a porosity of approximately 90% by the weight fraction of PLLA and salt in the scaffolds. When the salt crystal size is altered while maintaining the polymer/salt weight ratio, the resultant scaffolds have different pore sizes but a similar porosity. Figure 3.7a gives an example of the resulting OCT images from such scaffolds where an imaging depth of around 1 mm was achieved despite the highly scattering nature of the scaffold. The top view image of the same scaffold from reconstruction (Figure 3.7b) clearly presented the porous structure. The imaging contrast was primarily provided by the difference in scattering coefficient among the polymer, PLLA, and PBS in which the measurements were performed. The polymer backscattered the light, thereby appearing brighter, while the pores appear as a dark area in the OCT image. Such contrast gives us an opportunity to estimate the porosity from the OCT images. By using a commercial software, for example, Volocity, Improvision, the porosity has been derived as 70%, which was close to the value estimated by stoichiometry.

Figure 3.8a shows the scaffold produced by dual porogen, NaCl and naphthalene, in comparison with the same pore-size scaffold made by a single porogen, NaCl (Figure 3.8b). The corresponding cross-section images are presented in Figure 3.9. Striking morphological changes can be seen when compared with Figure 3.7a. First, the pore size in these scaffolds was smaller since 106–255 μm. NaCl porogen was used in these scaffolds, demonstrating that OCT image can clearly distinguish pore size variations in these scaffolds. Secondly, pore interconnection has been obviously increased in the dual porogen–produced scaffolds. Introducing naphthalene as the second porogen in solvent-casting and salt-leaching process resulted in the improvement of the pore interconnectivity. By using 20% naphthalene, highly interconnected pore structures were achieved. This interconnection feature has been further confirmed by SEM analysis.[146] SEM images of the scaffolds prepared with and without naphthalene are given in Figure 3.10. Extra-small pores presented in the pore wall were visualized in the scaffolds produced with naphthalene. Figure 3.11 is a typical OCT image of porous chitosan scaffolds with microchannels. The porous structure was clearly seen and the channels were well-delimitated. The interconnected micropores have diameters ranging from 50 to 150 μm, while the microchannels have a width of 250 μm. The typical image of the specimens shows a penetration depth of more than 1 mm. On the other hand, the fibrous chitosan scaffolds exhibited a characterized morphology in OCT image. The diameter of the fibers was very clearly delimitated, allowing the examination of the distribution of the fibers inside the scaffold (Figure 3.12).

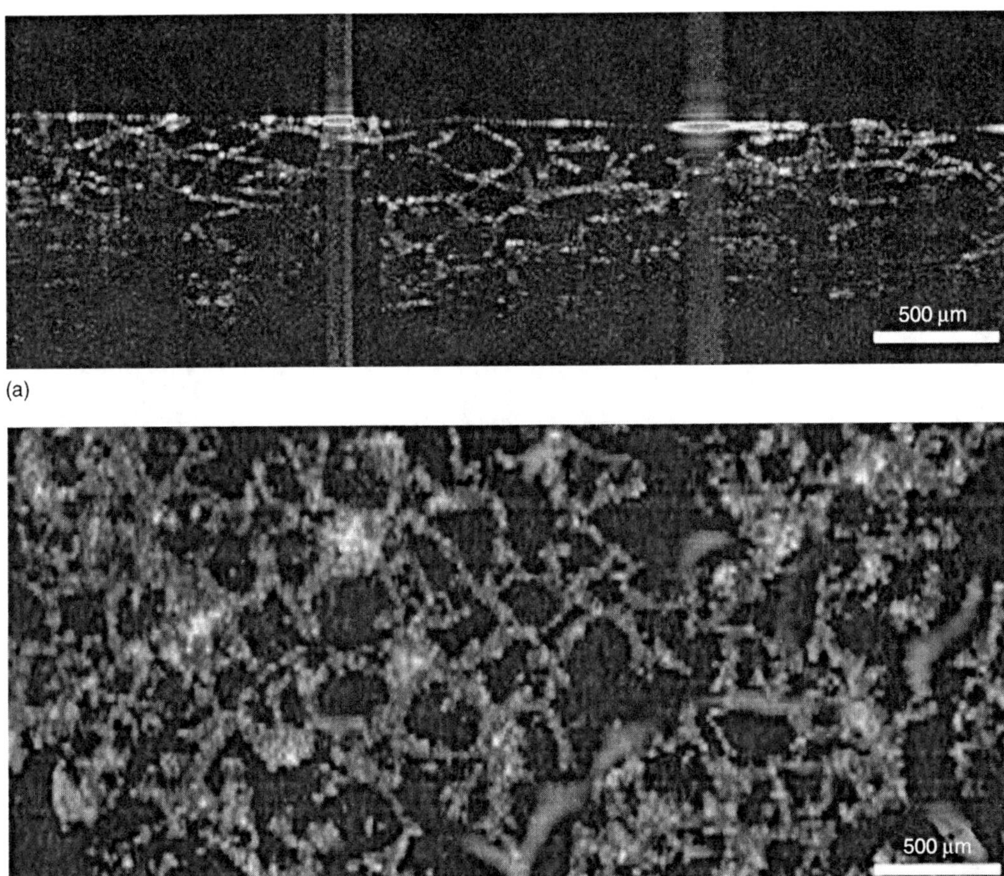

(a)

(b)

FIGURE 3.7 OCT image of a porous PLLA scaffold generated by single porogen technique: (a) cross-section and (b) top view from reconstruction. The pore size ranged from 255 to 350 μm.

3.5.3 DISCUSSION

Development of relatively simple, fast, and highly productive techniques to manufacture scaffolds with the required external and internal architecture is an interesting research area in biomaterials and TE field. Its success will greatly benefit and promote the study of engineered tissues. The main objective for achieving high-quality scaffolds is to increase pore interconnection at the same time maintaining the mechanical strength in order to overcome the poor diffusion efficiency of nutrients and gas within the center of scaffolds. Furthermore, the internal architecture should fit the requirement for specific tissues.

In the reported case study, we have developed a dual porogen system for solvent-evaporation and salt-leaching technique. OCT and SEM image have shown that the pore interconnection increased with this technique. It has been found that it can also tailor the interconnectivity by changing the percentage of the second porogen, that is, naphthalene. Sodium chloride and naphthalene have different mechanisms for pore formation within scaffolds. Macropores are created by dissolving the NaCl crystal in water, leaving an empty space within the polymer composites (see Figure 3.7), while naphthalene remains undissolved. Thus, during the removal of NaCl, naphthalene remained in the scaffolds until the macropores were formed (see Figure 3.3). In this study, either 255–350 μm or 106–255 μm pores were formed first. Uniquely, naphthalene volatilized and sublimed at room temperature. Thus, the

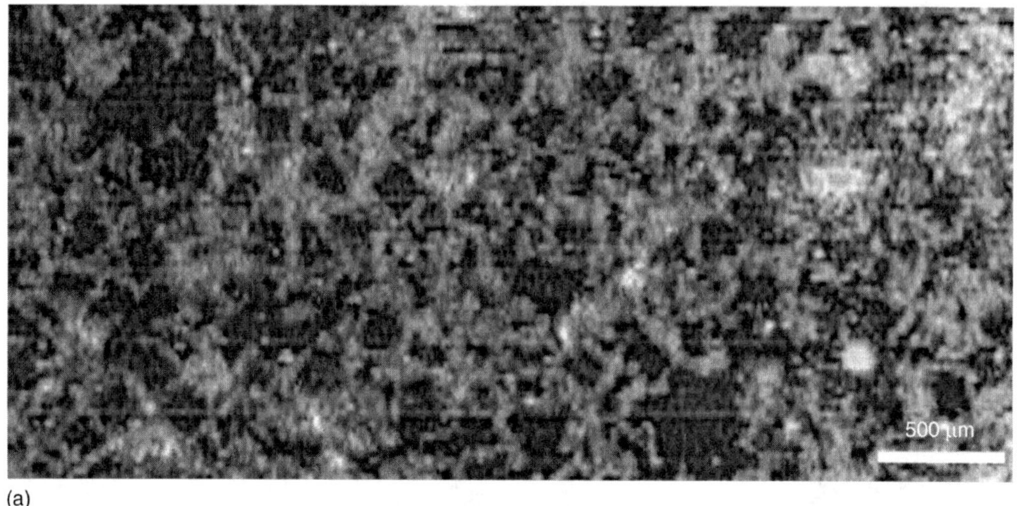

(a)

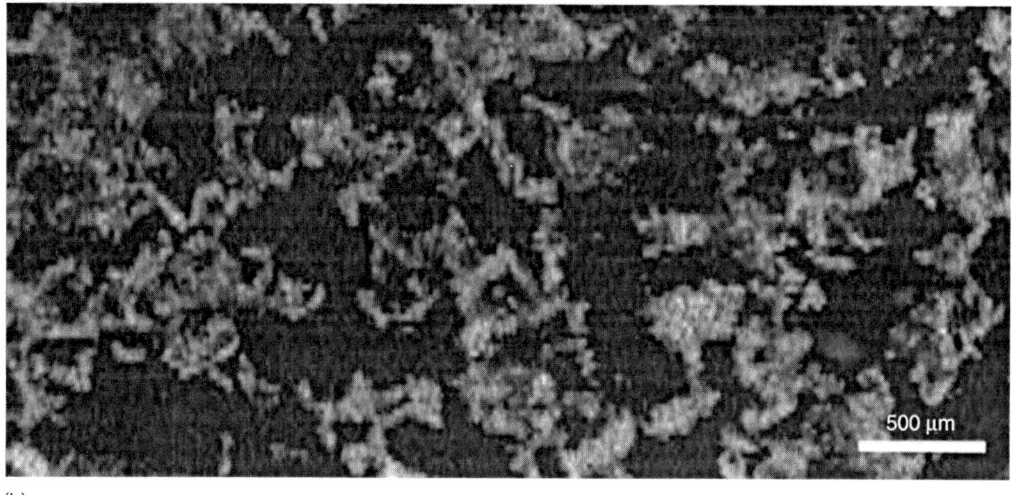

(b)

FIGURE 3.8 Top view OCT images of porous PLLA scaffolds generated by (a) single porogen and (b) dual porogen. The pore size ranged from 106 to 255 μm. The concentration of the second porogen, that is, naphthalene, was 20%.

trapped naphthalene can be removed either by slow sublimation or dissolution in organic solvent. We utilized THF as the solvent to remove naphthalene because THF has low influence on PLLA. With such sequential pore generation, we can control the pore interconnectivity. In fact, the pores generated by naphthalene were much smaller than those generated by NaCl because when naphthalene was mixed with the PLLA solution, it was a fine powder. It is the presence of these fine pores on the wall of the larger pores that enhances the scaffold pore interconnection, allowing a better exchange of nutrients and gas. The unique feature of this technique is that it neither requires complicated facilities nor comprehensive processing methods, and the process can maintain a high productivity.

The manufacturing of fibrous scaffolds is another efficient way to generate highly interconnected porous scaffolds. With proper precipitation solvent, wet-spinning method can produce scaffolds with different porosity and fiber diameter. Interestingly, it has been found that with the change of porosity or diameter of the fibrous chitosan scaffold, it is possible to tailor the degradation rate of

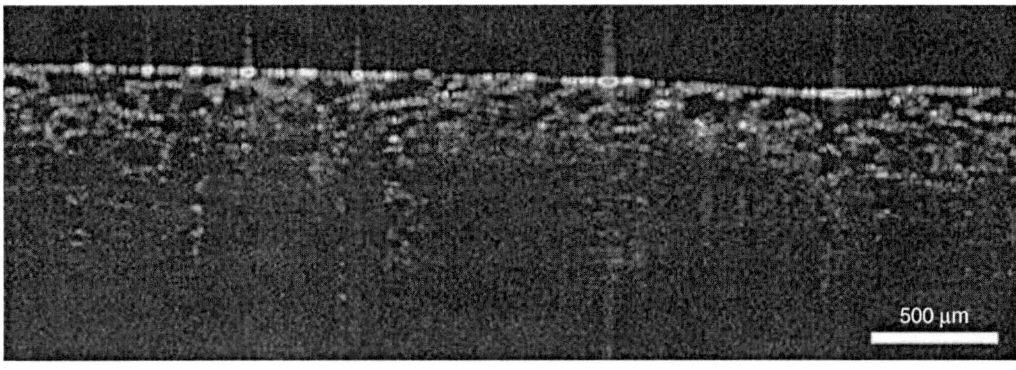

(a)

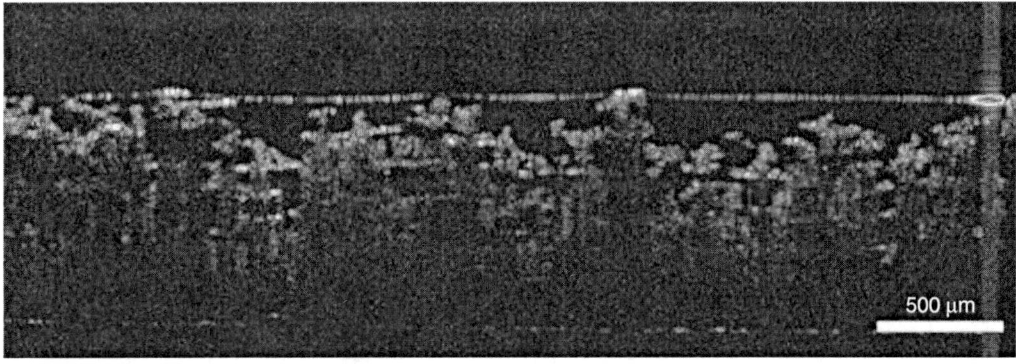

(b)

FIGURE 3.9 Cross-section of the OCT images for the same PLLA scaffolds in Figure 3.8 by (a) single porogen and (b) dual porogen.

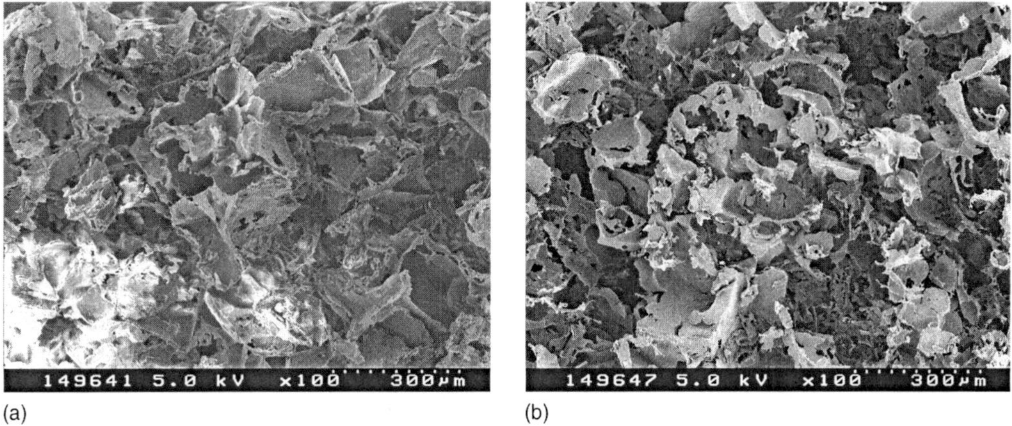

(a)   (b)

FIGURE 3.10 SEM images of porous PLLA scaffolds generated by (a) single porogen and (b) dual porogen. The pore size ranged from 106 to 255 µm. The concentration of the second porogen, that is, naphthalene, was 20%.

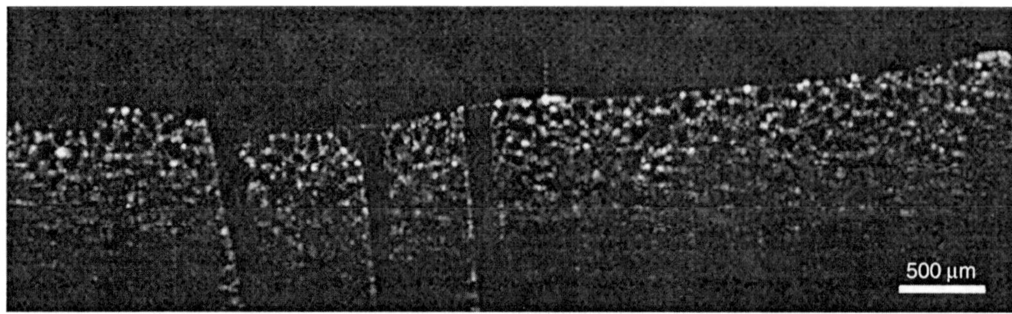

FIGURE 3.11 OCT image of porous chitosan scaffold with microchannels. The micropores ranged from 50 to 100 μm. The microchannel diameter was around 250 μm.

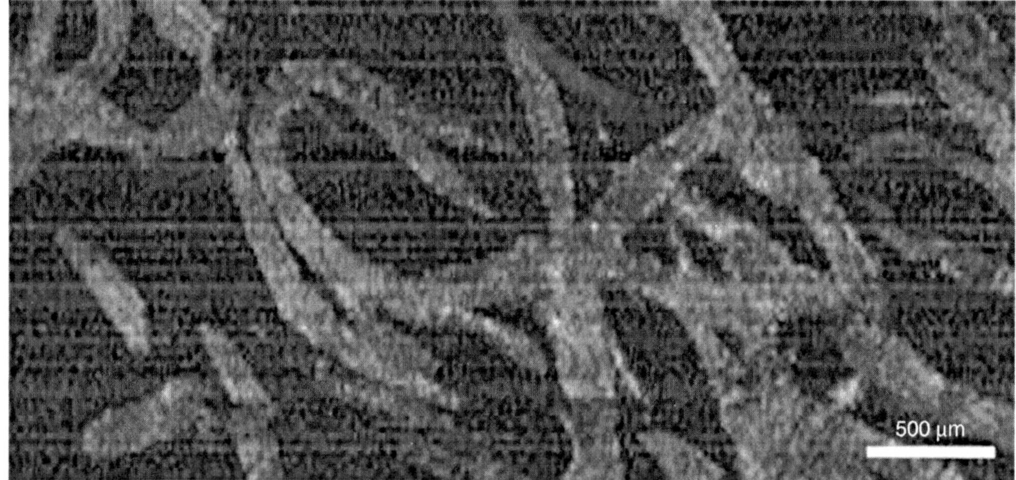

FIGURE 3.12 OCT image of a fibrous chitosan scaffold. The diameter of the fibers was around 105 μm and porosity of 95%.

chitosan scaffolds without interfering with the chemical composition of the polymer, which creates another technique to alter chitosan degradation profile by physical means in contrast to the usual chemical manipulation of the deacetylation degree.[148]

The microporous chitosan scaffold with microchannels is specifically designed for tendon TE. A tendon has a high degree of organization of the ECM. The ECM, mainly composed of collagen type I, is organized in a hierarchy of bundles of different sizes, which are uniaxially orientated[151] in a proteoglycans matrix. Such structure endows the tendon its biomechanical function, withstanding high tensile stress. So, to be functional, tendon TE has to create an environment for the formation of orientated ECM organization. Consequently, parameters affecting both production and organization of the ECM have to be considered during the generation of scaffolds for tendon TE. Our dual-mode chitosan scaffold fulfills such requirements. The micropores improve chemotransport while the microchannels are the main sites for the seeding and growth of the tenocytes. The longitudinal geometry of the channel induced or guided tenocytes to form bundle-like cell–ECM complex. We have been testing such hypothesis using specific internal architecture scaffold as a cue for better engineering. By culturing these microchannels scaffolds in a perfusion system, tendon cells are mechanically stimulated by fluid shear stress in the microchannel improving the rate of collagen production.[152]

From this study, it emerges that OCT can become a powerful tool to monitor scaffold architecture. The advantages of OCT over other modalities are based on several aspects. First, it is a nondestructive technique. Thus there is no sample preparation requirement. Similar to ultrasound, OCT scan will produce a clear internal cross-section image. However, OCT can obtain a much higher resolution compared with ultrasound without direct contact with the specimen, which eliminates the contamination of sample and provides a valuable feature for monitoring specimens under sterile conditions. Not requiring any labeling or contrast agent in OCT measurement is another remarkable feature. Unlike confocal microscopy, OCT image is based on the backscattering and not on fluorescence. There is no fluorescent labeling required. Due to the nondestructive, direct, and noncontact measurement features, the monitoring of scaffolds can be performed along the time under sterile conditions. In fact, we have applied OCT to monitor the scaffold degradation and cell growth within scaffolds in our laboratory,[153] which requires the quantification of pore size and porosity variation.

To establish a quantitative estimation of porosity, we have developed two methods. The first one is the local porosity. Variations of scaffold porosity, occurring as a result of the original polymer/salt ratio, and various culture conditions were quantified using Matlab software (Mathworks Inc.). A local porosity analysis, in which large and continuous defects (i.e., pore size > 500 μm) were excluded, was adopted to quantify the porosity of the construct. For each scan, a threshold was set to discriminate between true empty pores and the pore walls. After binarization, the local porosity was calculated by a block processing method,[154] and the results were displayed as a gradient color map as shown in Figure 3.13. Block size was chosen in order to take into account inside construct

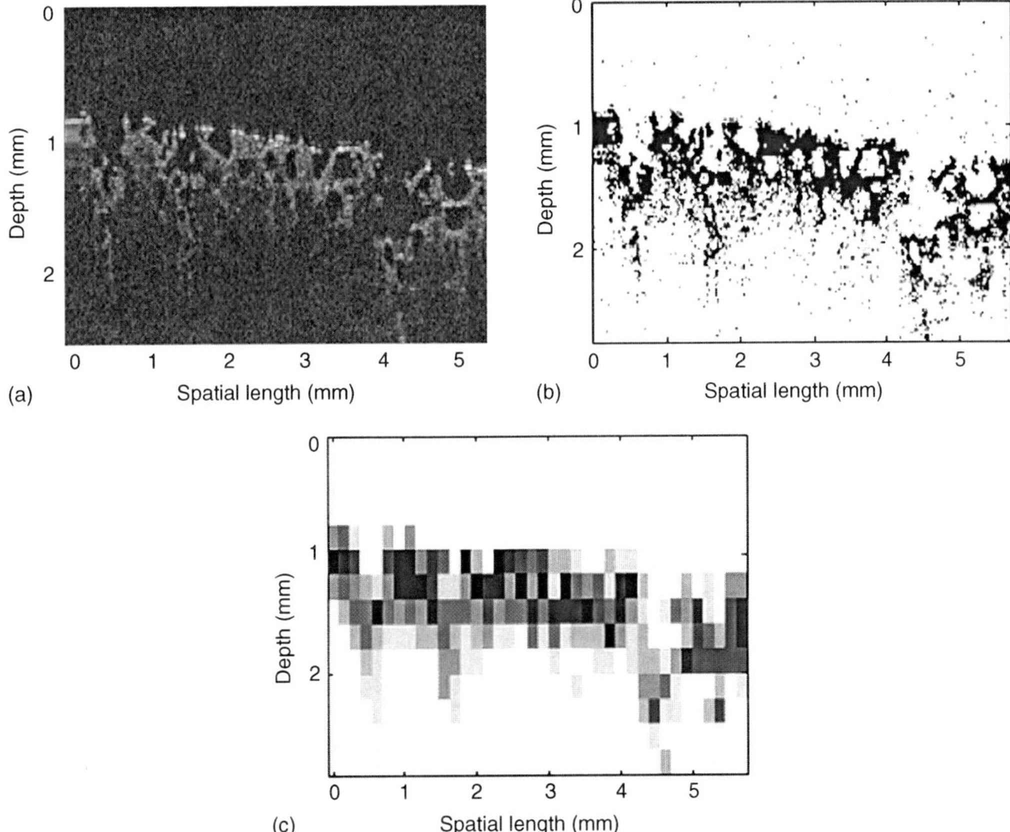

FIGURE 3.13 Demonstration of how to calculate local porosity based on an OCT image: (a) OCT image of a blank PLLA scaffold, (b) the threshold image by block processing, and (c) the local porosity map after binarization.

pores for the porosity calculation and to reject the void space in the picture and the degradation effects. As a result, the mean local porosity of the cultured scaffold can be assessed. Alternatively, when full 3-D reconstruction of the sample is available, a professional image processing software can be used to generate porosity data. Some calculations presented in this chapter were performed with the help of a commercial software, Volocity, Improvision. It has to be noted that some discrepancies exist in the calculation of porosity with different modalities such as μ-CT and OCT. Different imaging modalities yield slightly different results. Thus, monitoring the porosity variation due to degradation or tissue formation should be performed using the same modality.

3.6 FINAL REMARKS

In conclusion, to generate functional tissues by the TE principle, development of reliable and efficient techniques to control architecture of scaffolds is in high demand. In this chapter, we have shown that CAD/CAM techniques will be indispensable tools on providing scaffolds with the required architecture. Nevertheless these techniques are not accessible to every laboratory, and alternative ways to produce scaffolds with high productivity, easy operation, and accurate control of the architecture to perform biological studies are required. The presented case study demonstrates that it is possible to achieve this goal by using dual porogen technique and fabrication of fibrous scaffold. Formation of dual or multiple mode of internal architecture in scaffolds such as micropore along with microchannels can mimic specific tissue structure and promote organized tissue formation. OCT as a nondestructive, high resolution, and online measurement modality has demonstrated its high potential for monitoring scaffold architecture and the variations associated with cell growth and ECM deposition.

ACKNOWLEDGMENTS

This work was performed with partial financial support from the Biotechnology and Biology Sciences Research Council, U.K. (BBS/B/04277); the Engineering and Physical Sciences Research Council, U.K. (GR/S11510/01); and EXPERTISSUES Network of Excellence (NoE)–NMP3-CT-2004-500283. Cassilda Cunha-Reis would like to acknowledge Marie Curie Actions: Alea Jacta EST—MEST-CT-2004-008104 for funding her PhD. The authors would like to acknowledge António Pinto for preparing the illustrations for this chapter.

REFERENCES

1. Lalan, S., Pomerantseva, I. and Vacanti, J.P., Tissue engineering and its potential impact on surgery, *World J Surg*, 25, 1458, 2001.
2. Shieh, S.J. and Vacanti, J.P., State-of-the-art tissue engineering: from tissue engineering to organ building, *Surgery*, 137, 1, 2005.
3. Minas, T. and Nehrer, S., Current concepts in the treatment of articular cartilage defects, *Orthopedics*, 20, 525, 1997.
4. Ahsan, T. and Nerem, R.M., Bioengineered tissues: the science, the technology, and the industry, *Orthod Craniofac Res*, 8, 134, 2005.
5. Langer, R. and Vacanti, J.P., Tissue engineering, *Science*, 260, 920, 1993.
6. Stock, U.A. and Vacanti, J.P., Tissue engineering: current state and prospects, *Annu Rev Med*, 52, 443, 2001.
7. Eaglstein, W.H. and Falanga, V., Tissue Engineering and development of Apligraf, a human skin equivalent, *Clin Ther*, 19, 894, 1997.
8. Marston, W.A., Dermagraft, a bioengineered human dermal equivalent for the treatment of chronic nonhealing diabetic foot ulcer, *Expert Rev Med Devices*, 1, 21, 2004.
9. Risbud, M., Tissue engineering: implications in the treatment of organ and tissue defects, *Biogerontology*, 2, 117, 2001.

10. Breitbart, A.S., Grande, D.A., Kessler, R., Ryaby, J.T. et al., Tissue engineered bone repair of calvarial defects using cultured periosteal cells, *Plast Reconstr Surg*, 101, 567, 1998.
11. Caplan, A.I., Reuben, D. and Haynesworth, S.E., Cell-based tissue engineering therapies: the influence of whole body physiology, *Adv Drug Deliv Rev*, 33, 3, 1998.
12. Peng, H. and Huard, J., Muscle-derived stem cells for musculoskeletal tissue regeneration and repair, *Transpl Immunol*, 12, 311, 2004.
13. Jahoda, C.A. and Reynolds, A.J., Hair follicle dermal sheath cells: unsung participants in wound healing, *Lancet*, 358, 1445, 2001.
14. Fernandes, K.J., Mckenzie, I.A., Mill, P., Smith, K.M. et al., A dermal niche for multipotent adult skin-derived precursor cells, *Nat Cell Biol*, 6, 1082, 2004.
15. Mckay, R., Renfranz, P. and Cunningham, M., Immortalized stem cells from the central nervous system, *C R Acad Sci III*, 316, 1452, 1993.
16. Zuk, P.A., Zhu, M., Mizuno, H., Huang, J. et al., Multilineage cells from human adipose tissue: implications for cell-based therapies, *Tissue Eng*, 7, 211, 2001.
17. De Ugarte, D.A., Morizono, K., Elbarbary, A., Alfonso, Z. et al., Comparison of multi-lineage cells from human adipose tissue and bone marrow, *Cells Tissues Organs*, 174, 101, 2003.
18. Tuan, R.S., Boland, G. and Tuli, R., Adult mesenchymal stem cells and cell-based tissue engineering, *Arthritis Res Ther*, 5, 32, 2003.
19. Barrilleaux, B., Phinney, D.G., Prockop, D.J. and O'connor K.C., Review: ex vivo engineering of living tissues with adult stem cells, *Tissue Eng*, 12, 3007, 2006.
20. Gomes, M.E., Sikavitsas, V.I., Behravesh, E., Reis, R.L. et al., Effect of flow perfusion on the osteogenic differentiation of bone marrow stromal cells cultured on starch-based three-dimensional scaffolds, *J Biomed Mater Res A*, 67, 87, 2003.
21. Cartmell, S.H., Porter, B.D., Garcia, A.J. and Guldberg, R.E., Effects of medium perfusion rate on cell-seeded three-dimensional bone constructs in vitro, *Tissue Eng*, 9, 1197, 2003.
22. Ignatius, A., Blessing, H., Liedert, A., Schmidt, C. et al., Tissue engineering of bone: effects of mechanical strain on osteoblastic cells in type I collagen matrices, *Biomaterials*, 26, 311, 2005.
23. Yang, Y., Magnay, J.L., Cooling, L. and El, H.A., Development of a 'mechano-active' scaffold for tissue engineering, *Biomaterials*, 23, 2119, 2002.
24. Wood, M.A., Yang, Y., Thomas, P.B. and Haj, A.J., Using dihydropyridine-release strategies to enhance load effects in engineered human bone constructs, *Tissue Eng*, 12, 2489, 2006.
25. Perets, A., Baruch, Y., Weisbuch, F., Shoshany, G. et al., Enhancing the vascularization of three-dimensional porous alginate scaffolds by incorporating controlled release basic fibroblast growth factor microspheres, *J Biomed Mater Res A*, 65, 489, 2003.
26. Discher, D.E., Janmey, P. and Wang, Y.L., Tissue cells feel and respond to the stiffness of their substrate, *Science*, 310, 1139, 2005.
27. Huang, Y., Siewe, M. and Madihally, S.V., Effect of spatial architecture on cellular colonization, *Biotechnol Bioeng*, 93, 64, 2006.
28. Berry, C.C., Dalby, M.J., Mccloy, D. and Affrossman, S., The fibroblast response to tubes exhibiting internal nanotopography, *Biomaterials*, 26, 4985, 2005.
29. Chung, T.W., Wang, Y.Z., Huang, Y.Y., Pan, C.I. et al., Poly(epsilon-caprolactone) grafted with nano-structured chitosan enhances growth of human dermal fibroblasts, *Artif Organs*, 30, 35, 2006.
30. Badami, A.S., Kreke, M.R., Thompson, M.S., Riffle, J.S. et al., Effect of fibre diameter on spreading, proliferation, and differentiation of osteoblastic cells on electrospun poly(lactic acid) substrates, *Biomaterials*, 27, 596, 2006.
31. Berry, C.C., Campbell, G., Spadiccino, A., Robertson, M. et al., The influence of microscale topography on fibroblast attachment and motility, *Biomaterials*, 25, 5781, 2004.
32. Downing, B.R., Cornwell, K., Toner, M. and Pins, G.D., The influence of microtextured basal lamina analog topography on keratinocyte function and epidermal organization, *J Biomed Mater Res A*, 72, 47, 2005.
33. Recknor, J.B., Sakaguchi, D.S. and Mallapragada, S.K., Directed growth and selective differentiation of neural progenitor cells on micropatterned polymer substrates, *Biomaterials*, 27, 4098, 2006.
34. Stevens, M.M., Mayer, M., Anderson, D.G., Weibel, D.B. et al., Direct patterning of mammalian cells onto porous tissue engineering substrates using agarose stamps, *Biomaterials*, 26, 7636, 2005.
35. Timmins, M.R. and Lenz, R.W., Enzymatic biodegradation of polymers: The polymer chemists' perspective, *Trends Polym Sci*, 2, 15, 1994.

36. Tsuji, H., In vitro hydrolysis of blends from enantiomeric poly(lactide)s. Part 4: well-homo-crystallized blend and nonblended films, *Biomaterials*, 24, 537, 2003.
37. Tsuji, H., Ogiwara, M., Saha, S.K. and Sakaki, T., Enzymatic, alkaline, and autocatalytic degradation of poly(L-lactic acid): effects of biaxial orientation, *Biomacromolecules*, 7, 380, 2006.
38. Srivastava, R.K. and Albertsson, A.C., Porous scaffolds from high molecular weight polyesters synthesized via enzyme-catalyzed ring-opening polymerization, *Biomacromolecules*, 7, 2531, 2006.
39. Ma, X., Scaffolds for tissue fabrication, *Materials Today*, 7, 30, 2004.
40. Athanasiou, K.A., Niederauer, G.G. and Agrawal, C.M., Sterelization, toxicity, biocompatibility and clinical applications of polylactic acid polyglycolic acid copolymers, *Biomaterials*, 17, 93, 1996.
41. Li, S., Hydrolytic degradation characteristics of aliphatic polyesters derived from lactic and glycolic acids, *Journal of Biomedical Materials Research*, 48, 342, 1999.
42. Agrawal, C.M. and Athanasiou, K.A., Technique to control pH in vicinity of biodegrading PLA-PGA implants, *J Biomed Mater Res (Appl Biomater)*, 38, 105, 1997.
43. Burdick, J.A., Padera, R.F., Huang, J.V. and Anseth, K.S., An investigation of the cytotoxicity and histocompatibility of in situ forming lactic acid based orthopedic biomaterials, *J Biomed Mater Res*, 63, 484, 2002.
44. Shi, G., Cai, Q., Wang, C., Lu, N. et al., Fabrication and biocompatibility of cell scaffolds of poly(L-lactic acid) and poly(L-lactic-*co*-glycolic acid), *Polymers for Advanced Technologies*, 13, 2002.
45. Serrano, M.C., Pagani, R., Vallet-Regi, M., Pena, J. et al., In vitro biocompatibility assessment of poly(epsilon-caprolactone) films using L929 mouse fibroblasts, *Biomaterials*, 25, 5603, 2004.
46. Darling, A.L. and Sun, W., Free-form fabrication and micro-CT characterization of poly-epsilon-caprolactone tissue scaffolds, *IEEE Eng Med Biol Mag*, 24, 78, 2005.
47. Serrano, M.C., Portoles, M.T., Vallet-Regi, M., Izquierdo, I. et al., Vascular endothelial and smooth muscle cell culture on NaOH-treated poly(epsilon-caprolactone) films: a preliminary study for vascular graft development, *Macromol Biosci*, 5, 415, 2005.
48. Kweon, H., Yoo, M.K., Park, I.K., Kim, T.H. et al., A novel degradable polycaprolactone networks for tissue engineering, *Biomaterials*, 24, 801, 2003.
49. Zeng, J., Chen, X., Liang, Q., Xu, X. et al., Enzymatic degradation of poly(L-lactide) and poly(epsilon-caprolactone) electrospun fibres, *Macromol Biosci*, 4, 1118, 2004.
50. Cho, H. and An, J., The effect of epsilon-caproyl/D,L-lactyl unit composition on the hydrolytic degradation of poly(D,L-lactide-ran-epsilon-caprolactone)-poly(ethylene glycol)-poly(D,L-lactide-ran-epsilon-caprolactone), *Biomaterials*, 27, 544, 2006.
51. Wang, S., Lu, L. and Yaszemski, M.J., Bone-tissue-engineering material poly(propylene fumarate): correlation between molecular weight, chain dimensions, and physical properties, *Biomacromolecules*, 7, 1976, 2006.
52. Wolfe, M.S., Dean, D., Chen, J.E., Fisher, J.P. et al., In vitro degradation and fracture toughness of multilayered porous poly(propylene fumarate)/beta-tricalcium phosphate scaffolds, *J Biomed Mater Res*, 61, 159, 2002.
53. Guan, J., Fujimoto, K.L., Sacks, M.S. and Wagner, W.R., Preparation and characterization of highly porous, biodegradable polyurethane scaffolds for soft tissue applications, *Biomaterials*, 26, 3961, 2005.
54. Reddi, A.H., Symbiosis of biotechnology and biomaterials: applications in tissue engineering of bone and cartilage, *J Cell Biochem*, 56, 192, 1994.
55. Claase, M.B., Grijpma, D.W., Mendes, S.C., De Bruijn, J.D. et al., Porous PEOT/PBT scaffolds for bone tissue engineering: preparation, characterization, and in vitro bone marrow cell culturing, *J Biomed Mater Res A*, 64, 291, 2003.
56. Burkoth, A.K., Burdick, J. and Anseth, K.S., Surface and bulk modifications to photocrosslinked polyanhydrides to control degradation behavior, *J Biomed Mater Res*, 51, 352, 2000.
57. Kellomaki, M., Heller, J. and Tormala, P., Processing and properties of two different poly (ortho esters), *J Mater Sci Mater Med*, 11, 345, 2000.
58. Bhattacharjee, A. and Bansal, M., Collagen structure: the Madras triple helix and the current scenario, *IUBMB Life*, 57, 161, 2005.
59. Brodsky, B. and Persikov, A.V., Molecular structure of the collagen triple helix, *Adv Protein Chem*, 70, 301, 2005.
60. Doillon, C.J., Watsky, M.A., Hakim, M., Wang, J. et al., A collagen-based scaffold for a tissue engineered human cornea: physical and physiological properties, *Int J Artif Organs*, 26, 764, 2003.

61. Zimmermann, W.H. and Eschenhagen, T., Cardiac tissue engineering for replacement therapy, *Heart Failure Rev*, 8, 259, 2003.

62. Tremblay, P.L., Hudon, V., Berthod, F., Germain, L. et al., Inosculation of tissue-engineered capillaries with the host's vasculature in a reconstructed skin transplanted on mice, *Am J Transplant*, 5, 1002, 2005.

63. Bartlett, W., Gooding, C.R., Carrington, R.W., Skinner, J.A. et al., Autologous chondrocyte implantation at the knee using a bilayer collagen membrane with bone graft. A preliminary report, *J Bone Joint Surg Br*, 87, 330, 2005.

64. Wahl, D.A. and Czernuszka, J.T., Collagen-hydroxyapatite composites for hard tissue repair, *Eur Cell Mater*, 11, 43, 2006.

65. Gutowska, A., Jeong, B. and Jasionowski, M., Injectable gels for tissue engineering, *Anat Rec*, 263, 342, 2001.

66. Abbah, S.A., Lu, W.W., Chan, D., Cheung, K.M. et al., In vitro evaluation of alginate encapsulated adipose-tissue stromal cells for use as injectable bone graft substitute, *Biochem Biophys Res Commun*, 347, 185, 2006.

67. Selden, C. and Hodgson, H., Cellular therapies for liver replacement, *Transpl Immunol*, 12, 273, 2004.

68. Song, Y.C., Chen, Z.Z., Mukherjee, N., Lightfoot, F.G. et al., Vitrification of tissue engineered pancreatic substitute, *Transplant Proc*, 37, 253, 2005.

69. Yamaoka, H., Asato, H., Ogasawara, T., Nishizawa, S. et al., Cartilage tissue engineering using human auricular chondrocytes embedded in different hydrogel materials, *J Biomed Mater Res A*, 78, 1, 2006.

70. Stevens, M.M., Marini, R.P., Schaefer, D., Aronson, J. et al., In vivo engineering of organs: the bone bioreactor, *Proc Natl Acad Sci USA*, 102, 11450, 2005.

71. Li, Z. and Zhang, M., Chitosan-alginate as scaffolding material for cartilage tissue engineering, *J Biomed Mater Res A*, 75, 485, 2005.

72. Wayne, J.S., Mcdowell, C.L., Shields, K.J. and Tuan, R.S., In vivo response of polylactic acid-alginate scaffolds and bone marrow-derived cells for cartilage tissue engineering, *Tissue Eng*, 11, 953, 2005.

73. Vandevord, P.J., Matthew, H.W., Desilva, S.P., Mayton, L. et al., Evaluation of the biocompatibility of a chitosan scaffold in mice, *J Biomed Mater Res*, 59, 585, 2002.

74. Lahiji, A., Sohrabi, A., Hungerford, D.S. and Frondoza, C.G., Chitosan supports the expression of extracellular matrix proteins in human osteoblasts and chondrocytes, *J Biomed Mater Res*, 51, 586, 2000.

75. Tuzlakoglu, K., Alves, C.M., Mano, J.F. and Reis, R.L., Production and characterization of chitosan fibres and 3-D fibre mesh scaffolds for tissue engineering applications, *Macromol Biosci*, 4, 811, 2004.

76. Silva, R.M., Silva, G.A., Coutinho, O.P., Mano, J.F. et al., Preparation and characterisation in simulated body conditions of glutaraldehyde crosslinked chitosan membranes, *J Mater Sci Mater Med*, 15, 1105, 2004.

77. Malafaya, P.P.B., Pedro, A.J., Peterbauer, A., Gabriel, C. et al., Chitosan particles agglomerated scaffolds for cartilage and osteochondral tissue engineering approaches with adipose tissue derived stem cells, *J Mater Sci Mater Med*, 16, 1077, 2005.

78. Silva, S.S., Santos, M.I., Coutinho, O.P., Mano, J.F. et al., Physical properties and biocompatibility of chitosan/soy blended membranes, *J Mater Sci Mater Med*, 16, 575, 2005.

79. Suh, J.-K.F. and Matthew, H.W.T., Application of chitosan-based polysaccharide biomaterials in cartilage tissue engineering: a review, *Biomaterials*, 21, 2589, 2000.

80. Di Martino, A., Sittingerc, M. and Risbud, M.V., Chitosan: A versatile biopolymer for orthopaedic tissue-engineering, *Biomaterials*, 26, 5983–5990, 2005.

81. Ho, M.H., Wang, D.M., Hsieh, H.J., Liu, H.C. et al., Preparation and characterization of RGD-immobilized chitosan scaffolds, *Biomaterials*, 26, 3197, 2005.

82. Zhang, H. and Neau, S.H., In vitro degradation of chitosan by a commercial enzyme preparation: effect of molecular weight and degree of deacetylation, *biomaterials*, 22, 1653, 2001.

83. Marques, A.P., Reis, R.L. and Hunt, J.A., Evaluation of the potential of starch-based biodegradable polymers in the activation of human inflammatory cells, *J Mater Sci Mater Med*, 14, 167, 2003.

84. Varum, K.M., Myhr, M.M., Hjerde, R.J. and Smidsrod, O., In vitro degradation rates of partially N-acetylated chitosans in human serum, *Carbohydr Res*, 299, 99, 1997.

85. Cui, W., Kim, D.H., Imamura, M., Hyon, S.H. et al., Tissue-engineered pancreatic islets: culturing rat islets in the chitosan sponge, *Cell Transplant*, 10, 499, 2001.

86. Cho, B.C., Chung, H.Y., Lee, D.G., Yang, J.D. et al., The effect of chitosan bead encapsulating calcium sulfate as an injectable bone substitute on consolidation in the mandibular distraction osteogenesis of a dog model, *J Oral Maxillofac Surg*, 63, 1753, 2005.
87. Liu, H., Li, H., Cheng, W., Yang, Y. et al., Novel injectable calcium phosphate/chitosan composites for bone substitute materials, *Acta Biomater*, 2006.
88. Hoemann, C.D., Sun, J., Legare, A., Mckee, M.D. et al., Tissue engineering of cartilage using an injectable and adhesive chitosan-based cell-delivery vehicle, *Osteoarthritis Cartilage*, 13, 318, 2005.
89. Griffon, D.J., Sedighi, M.R., Schaeffer, D.V., Eurell, J.A. et al., Chitosan scaffolds: interconnective pore size and cartilage engineering, *Acta Biomater*, 2, 313, 2006.
90. Lin, S.J., Jee, S.H., Hsaio, W.C., Lee, S.J. et al., Formation of melanocyte spheroids on the chitosan-coated surface, *Biomaterials*, 26, 1413, 2005.
91. Adekogbe, I. and Ghanem, A., Fabrication and characterization of DTBP-crosslinked chitosan scaffolds for skin tissue engineering, *Biomaterials*, 26, 7241, 2005.
92. Gomes, M.E., Ribeiro, A.S., Malafaya, P.B., Reis, R.L. et al., A new approach based on injection moulding to produce biodegradable starch-based polymeric scaffolds: morphology, mechanical and degradation behaviour, *Biomaterials*, 22, 883, 2001.
93. Marques, A.P., Reis, R.L. and Hunt, J.A., The biocompatibility of novel starch-based polymers and composites: in vitro studies, *Biomaterials*, 23, 1471, 2002.
94. Costa, S.A. and Reis, R.L., Immobilisation of catalase on the surface of biodegradable starch-based polymers as a way to change its surface characteristics, *J Mater Sci Mater Med*, 15, 335, 2004.
95. Salgado, A.J., Figueiredo, J.E., Coutinho, O.P. and Reis, R.L., Biological response to pre-mineralized starch based scaffolds for bone tissue engineering, *J Mater Sci Mater Med*, 16, 267, 2005.
96. Gomes, M.E., Holtorf, H.L., Reis, R.L. and Mikos, A.G., Influence of the porosity of starch-based fibre mesh scaffolds on the proliferation and osteogenic differentiation of bone marrow stromal cells cultured in a flow perfusion bioreactor, *Tissue Eng*, 12, 801, 2006.
97. Williams, D., The proving of polyhydroxybutyrate and its potential in medical technology, *Med Device Technol*, 16, 9, 2005.
98. Shishatskaya, E.I. and Volova, T.G., A comparative investigation of biodegradable polyhydroxyalkanoate films as matrices for in vitro cell cultures, *J Mater Sci Mater Med*, 15, 915, 2004.
99. Price, R.D., Myers, S., Leigh, I.M. and Navsaria, H.A., The role of hyaluronic acid in wound healing: assessment of clinical evidence, *Am J Clin Dermatol*, 6, 393, 2005.
100. Nehrer, S., Domayer, S., Dorotka, R., Schatz, K. et al., Three-year clinical outcome after chondrocyte transplantation using a hyaluronan matrix for cartilage repair, *Eur J Radiol*, 57, 3, 2006.
101. Horan, R.L., Antle, K., Collette, A.L., Wang, Y. et al., In vitro degradation of silk fibroin, *Biomaterials*, 26, 3385, 2005.
102. Wang, Y., Blasioli, D.J., Kim, H.J., Kim, H.S. et al., Cartilage tissue engineering with silk scaffolds and human articular chondrocytes, *Biomaterials*, 27, 4434, 2006.
103. Moore, M.J., Jabbari, E., Ritman, E.L., Lu, L. et al., Quantitative analysis of interconnectivity of porous biodegradable scaffolds with micro-computed tomography, *J Biomed Mater Res A*, 71, 258, 2004.
104. Sander, E.A., Alb, A.M., Nauman, E.A., Reed, W.F. et al., Solvent effects on the microstructure and properties of 75/25 poly(D,L-lactide-*co*-glycolide) tissue scaffolds, *J Biomed Mater Res A*, 70, 506, 2004.
105. Lin, H.R. and Yeh, Y.J., Porous alginate/hydroxyapatite composite scaffolds for bone tissue engineering: preparation, characterization, and in vitro studies, *J Biomed Mater Res B Appl Biomater*, 71, 52, 2004.
106. Liu, L., Zhang, L., Ren, B., Wang, F. et al., Preparation and characterization of collagen-hydroxyapatite composite used for bone tissue engineering scaffold, *Artif Cells Blood Substit Immobil Biotechnol*, 31, 435, 2003.
107. Tsang, V.L. and Bathia, S.N., Three-dimensional tissue fabrication, *Adv Drug Deliv Rev*, 56, 1635, 2004.
108. Hutmacher, D.W., Sittinger, M. and Risbud, M.V., Scaffold-based tissue engineering: rationale for computer-aided design and solid free-form fabrication systems, *Trends Biotechnol*, 22, 354, 2004.
109. Tan, K.H., Chua, C.K., Leong, K.F., Cheah, C.M. et al., Selective laser sintering of biocompatible polymers for applications in tissue engineering, *Biomed Mater Eng*, 15, 113, 2005.
110. Chim, H., Hutmacher, D.W., Chou, A.M., Oliveira, A.L. et al., A comparative analysis of scaffold material modifications for load-bearing applications in bone tissue engineering, *Int J Oral Maxillofac Surg*, 35, 928, 2006.

111. Hao, L., Savalani, M.M., Zhang, Y., Tanner, K.E. et al., Selective laser sintering of hydroxyapatite reinforced polyethylene composites for bioactive implants and tissue scaffold development, *Proc Inst Mech Eng [H]*, 220, 521, 2006.

112. Cai, H., Azangwe, G. and Shepherd, D.E., Skin cell culture on an ear-shaped scaffold created by fused deposition modelling, *Biomed Mater Eng*, 15, 375, 2005.

113. Cooke, M.N., Fisher, J.P., Dean, D., Rimnac, C. et al., Use of stereolithography to manufacture critical-sized 3D biodegradable scaffolds for bone ingrowth, *J Biomed Mater Res B Appl Biomater*, 64B, 65, 2003.

114. Dhariwala, B., Hunt, E. and Boland, T., Rapid prototyping of tissue-engineering constructs, using photopolymerizable hydrogels and stereolithography, *Tissue Eng*, 10, 1316, 2004.

115. Sodian, R., Loebe, M., Hein, A., Martin, D.P. et al., Application of stereolithography for scaffold fabrication for tissue engineered heart valves, *Asaio J*, 48, 12, 2002.

116. Seitz, H., Rieder, W., Irsen, S., Leukers, B. et al., Three-dimensional printing of porous ceramic scaffolds for bone tissue engineering, *J Biomed Mater Res B Appl Biomater*, 74, 782, 2005.

117. Sherwood, J.K., Riley, S.L., Palazzolo, R., Brown, S.C. et al., A three-dimensional osteochondral composite scaffold for articular cartilage repair, *Biomaterials*, 23, 4739, 2002.

118. Vozzi, G., Flaim, C., Ahluwalia, A. and Bhatia, S., Fabrication of PLGA scaffolds using soft lithography and microsyringe deposition, *Biomaterials*, 24, 2533, 2003.

119. Bianchi, F., Vassalle, C., Simonetti, M., Vozzi, G. et al., Endothelial cell function on 2D and 3D micro-fabricated polymer scaffolds: applications in cardiovascular tissue engineering, *J Biomater Sci Polym Ed*, 17, 37, 2006.

120. Manjubala, I., Woesz, A., Pilz, C., Rumpler, M. et al., Biomimetic mineral-organic composite scaffolds with controlled internal architecture, *J Mater Sci Mater Med*, 16, 1111, 2005.

121. Fukuda, J., Khademhosseini, A., Yeh, J., Eng, G. et al., Micropatterned cell co-cultures using layer-by-layer deposition of extracellular matrix components, *Biomaterials*, 27, 1479, 2006.

122. Borden, M., El-Amin, S.F., Attawia, M. and Laurencin, C.T., Structural and human cellular assessment of a novel microsphere-based tissue engineered scaffold for bone repair, *Biomaterials*, 24, 597, 2003.

123. Min, B.M., Lee, G., Kim, S.H., Nam, Y.S. et al., Electrospinning of silk fibroin nanofibres and its effect on the adhesion and spreading of normal human keratinocytes and fibroblasts in vitro, *Biomaterials*, 25, 1289, 2004.

124. Sarazin, P., Roy, X. and Favis, B.D., Controlled preparation and properties of porous poly(L-lactide) obtained from a co-continuous blend of two biodegradable polymers, *Biomaterials*, 25, 5965, 2004.

125. Jager, M., Feser, T., Denck, H. and Krauspe, R., Proliferation and osteogenic differentiation of mesenchymal stem cells cultured onto three different polymers in vitro, *Ann Biomed Eng*, 33, 1319, 2005.

126. Stangenberg, L., Schaefer, D.J., Buettner, O., Ohnolz, J. et al., Differentiation of osteoblasts in three-dimensional culture in processed cancellous bone matrix: quantitative analysis of gene expression based on real-time reverse transcription-polymerase chain reaction, *Tissue Eng*, 11, 855, 2005.

127. Curran, J.M., Chen, R. and Hunt, J.A., The guidance of human mesenchymal stem cell differentiation in vitro by controlled modifications to the cell substrate, *Biomaterials*, 27, 4783, 2006.

128. Guilak, F., Volume and surface area measurement of viable chondrocytes in situ using geometric modelling of serial confocal sections, *J Microsc*, 173, 245, 1994.

129. Jones, C.W., Smolinski, D., Keogh, A., Kirk, T.B. et al., Confocal laser scanning microscopy in orthopaedic research, *Prog Histochem Cytochem*, 40, 1, 2005.

130. Meyer, L.E., Otberg, N., Sterry, W. and Lademann, J., In vivo confocal scanning laser microscopy: comparison of the reflectance and fluorescence mode by imaging human skin, *J Biomed Opt*, 11, 044012, 2006.

131. Zipfel, W.R., Williams, R.M. and Webb, W.W., Nonlinear magic: multiphoton microscopy in the biosciences, *Nat Biotechnol*, 21, 1369, 2003.

132. Ho, S.T. and Hutmacher, D.W., A comparison of micro CT with other techniques used in the characterization of scaffolds, *Biomaterials*, 27, 1362, 2006.

133. Lin, A.S., Barrows, T.H., Cartmell, S.H. and Guldberg, R.E., Microarchitectural and mechanical characterization of oriented porous polymer scaffolds, *Biomaterials*, 24, 481, 2003.

134. Cartmell, S., Huynh, K., Lin, A., Nagaraja, S. et al., Quantitative microcomputed tomography analysis of mineralization within three-dimensional scaffolds in vitro, *J Biomed Mater Res A*, 69, 97, 2004.

135. Huang, D., Swanson, E.A., Lin, C.P., Schuman, J.S. et al., Optical coherence tomography, *Science*, 254, 1178, 1991.

136. Hee, M.R., Izatt, J.A., Swanson, E.A., Huang, D. et al., Optical coherence tomography of the human retina, *Arch Ophthalmol*, 113, 325, 1995.
137. Tomlins, P.H. and Wang, R.K., Theory, developments and applications of optical coherence tomography, *J Phys D—Appl Phys*, 2519, 2005.
138. Gladkova, N.D., Petrova, G.A., Nikulin, N.K., Radenska-Lopovok, S.G. et al., In vivo optical coherence tomography imaging of human skin: norm and pathology, *Skin Res Technol*, 6, 6, 2000.
139. Fujimoto, J.G., Brezinski, M.E., Tearney, G.J., Boppart, S.A. et al., Optical biopsy and imaging using optical coherence tomography, *Nat Med*, 1, 970, 1995.
140. Boppart, S.A., Bouma, B.E., Pitris, C., Southern, J.F. et al., In vivo cellular optical coherence tomography imaging, *Nat Med*, 4, 861, 1998.
141. Drexler, W., Stamper, D., Jesser, C., Li, X. et al., Correlation of collagen organization with polarization sensitive imaging of in vitro cartilage: implications for osteoarthritis, *J Rheumatol*, 28, 1311, 2001.
142. Yang, Y., Whiteman, S., Gey Van Pittius, D., He, Y. et al., Use of optical coherence tomography in delineating airways microstructure: comparison of OCT images to histopathological sections, *Phys Med Biol*, 49, 1247, 2004.
143. Fujimoto, J.G., Optical coherence tomography for ultrahigh resolution in vivo imaging, *Nat Biotechnol*, 21, 1361, 2003.
144. Mason, C., Markusen, J.F., Town, M.A., Dunnill, P. et al., The potential of optical coherence tomography in the engineering of living tissue, *Phys Med Biol*, 49, 1097, 2004.
145. Yang, Y., Dubois, A., Qin, X.P., Li, J. et al., Investigation of optical coherence tomography as an imaging modality in tissue engineering, *Phys Med Biol*, 51, 1649, 2006.
146. Aydin, H.M., Yang, Y., Piskin, E. and El Haj, A., Optimizing Degradable Scaffolds for Cranium Tissue Repair, *Eur. Cell Mater.*, 11, 23, 2006.
147. Cunha-Reis, C., Tuzlakoglu, K., Baas, E., Yang, Y. et al., Influence of porosity and fibre diameter on the degradation of chitosan fibre-mesh scaffolds and cell adhesion, *J Mater Sci Mater Med*, 18, 195, 2007.
148. Bagnaninchi, P.O., Dikeakos, M., Veres, T. and Tabrizian, M., Towards on-line monitoring of cell growth in microporous scaffolds: Utilization and interpretation of complex permittivity measurements, *Biotechnol Bioeng*, 84, 343, 2003.
149. Madihally, S.V. and Matthew, H.W., Porous chitosan scaffolds for tissue engineering, *Biomaterials*, 20, 1133, 1999.
150. Wang, R.K., Xu, X.Q., Tuchin, V.V. and Elder, J.B., Concurrent enhancement of imaging depth and contrast for optical coherence tomography by hyperosmotic agents, *J Opt Soc Am B*, 18, 948, 2001.
151. Jozsa, L., Kannus, P., Balint, J.B. and Reffy, A., Three-dimensional ultrastructure of human tendons, *Acta Anat (Basel)*, 142, 306, 1991.
152. Bagnaninchi, P.O., Yang, Y., Zghoul, N., Maffulli, N. et al., Chitosan microchannels scaffolds for tendon tissue engineering characterized by optical coherence tomography, *Tissue Eng*, 13, 323, 2007.
153. Yang, Y., Bagnaninchi, P.O. and El Haj, A., Application of optical coherence tomography in tissue engineering, *Eur Cell Mater*, 11, 69, 2006.
154. Yang, Y., Bagnaninchi, P.O., Wood, M.A., El Haj, A. et al., Monitoring cell profile in tissue engineering by optical coherence tomography, *SPIE*, 51, 5695, 2005.

4 Rapid Prototyping Methods for Tissue Engineering Applications

Giovanni Vozzi and Arti Ahluwalia

CONTENTS

4.1 INTRODUCTION

Tissue engineering can be defined as the development of biological substitutes to restore, maintain, or improve tissue functions and is based on the application of principles and methods of engineering and life sciences toward a fundamental understanding of structure–function relationships in normal and pathological mammalian tissues. This is an emerging interdisciplinary area of research and technology that has the potential of revolutionizing our methods of health care treatment and dramatically improving the quality of life for millions of people throughout the world. Several approaches to tissue engineering have been established of which the most common approach is based on scaffold-guided tissue formation *in vitro*. A scaffold is a biodegradable and biocompatible three-dimensional (3-D) porous structure, which can support cell adhesion and growth. Typically cells are seeded onto biodegradable polymeric scaffolds, and the constructs in some way reform the intrinsic tissue structures [1]. The scaffold approach to tissue engineering first emerged in the early 1990s, and since then much of the work has focused on scaffolds in the form of sponges or foams, which possess a random microstructure. More recently as a result of a hypothesis that tissues must have a prearranged spatial architecture in order to function correctly, much attention has shifted to designer scaffolds. This hypothesis is based on the fact that a large number of organs possess a well-defined internal structure, which is essential to their function. Thus, in order to realize 3-D constructs for tissue repair and reconstruction, it is necessary to guide cell growth on structures with an established topology, which replicates that of natural tissue. As a result, several different microfabrication techniques for biomaterial scaffolds have been developed. Most of these techniques arise from preexisting manufacturing methodologies such as photolithography, silicon micromachining, and the realization of pseudomechanical microcomponents. We can distinguish two groups of methodologies: one based on the realization of two-dimensional (2-D) structures and the other on the fabrication of 3-D scaffolds. In this chapter, we focus exclusively on 3-D methods borrowed from the well-established field of computer-aided design/computer-aided manufacturing (CAD/CAM) and rapid prototyping (RP).

4.2 MICROFABRICATION OF THREE-DIMENSIONAL STRUCTURES: RAPID PROTOTYPING

RP, which is synonymous with solid free-from fabrication (SFF), refers to the fabrication of 2-D or 3-D structures using a preprogrammed computer graphics file containing layer-by-layer maps of the structures. Figure 4.1 schematizes this structure in terms of the liver, one of the most complex organs in the body. These maps are reconstructed through computer-aided fabrication (usually an x-, y-, z-positioning system), much as a 3-D printer would do. Each layer is about 0.01–1 mm thick (this depends very much on the manufacturing process as well as the resolution required), and a 3-D object is built-up through the assembly of successive 2-D layers, or what we call a pseudo-3-D (PS3D), sometimes also known as 2½ D. Nowadays RP is the chosen method of production for manufacturing complex objects, surpassing traditional techniques such as milling and turning. However, it should be noted that rapid is a relative term, and it usually takes several minutes to several hours to produce an object.

The RP process can be subdivided into three main units:

- Generation and conversion of the CAD model
- Realization of the prototype
- Postprocessing

In the first phase, a 3-D object is decomposed into a stratified structure using appropriate software, such as AutoCAD. The layers are then codified into step-by-step instructions for the control system, which drives the x-, y-, z-positioner. Currently, RP for tissue engineering scaffolds is associated with the use of CAD design files originating from computerized tomography (CT) data. Their most appropriate application is in the bone tissue engineering, where high-resolution micro-CT can reveal structural features of the order of 5 μm. In the case of soft tissues, architecture is not only harder to define, but also more difficult to image with high resolution, because information on structure is reconstructed largely from histological specimens. Conversion of histological images into a layer-by-layer and step-by-step scaffold is hindered by the lack of contrast and nonspecificity of stains (such as eosin and hematoxylin). It is very difficult to identify cell contours and separate them from the contents of the extracellular matrix (ECM). Soft-tissue scaffolds are therefore generally constructed with a repetitive grid consisting of squares, triangles, or hexagons. In fact, one of the most challenging aspects of scaffold design for nonbony biological tissues is the extraction of structural features, and the conversion of these into a repetitive algorithm describing an appropriate locus of points or lines in a given plane.

Once the architecture has been chosen, the three-axis positioners proceed to the actual fabrication of the structure, following the location maps provided by the controller. This process can be quite complicated, since binders, powders, and fillers are usually involved.

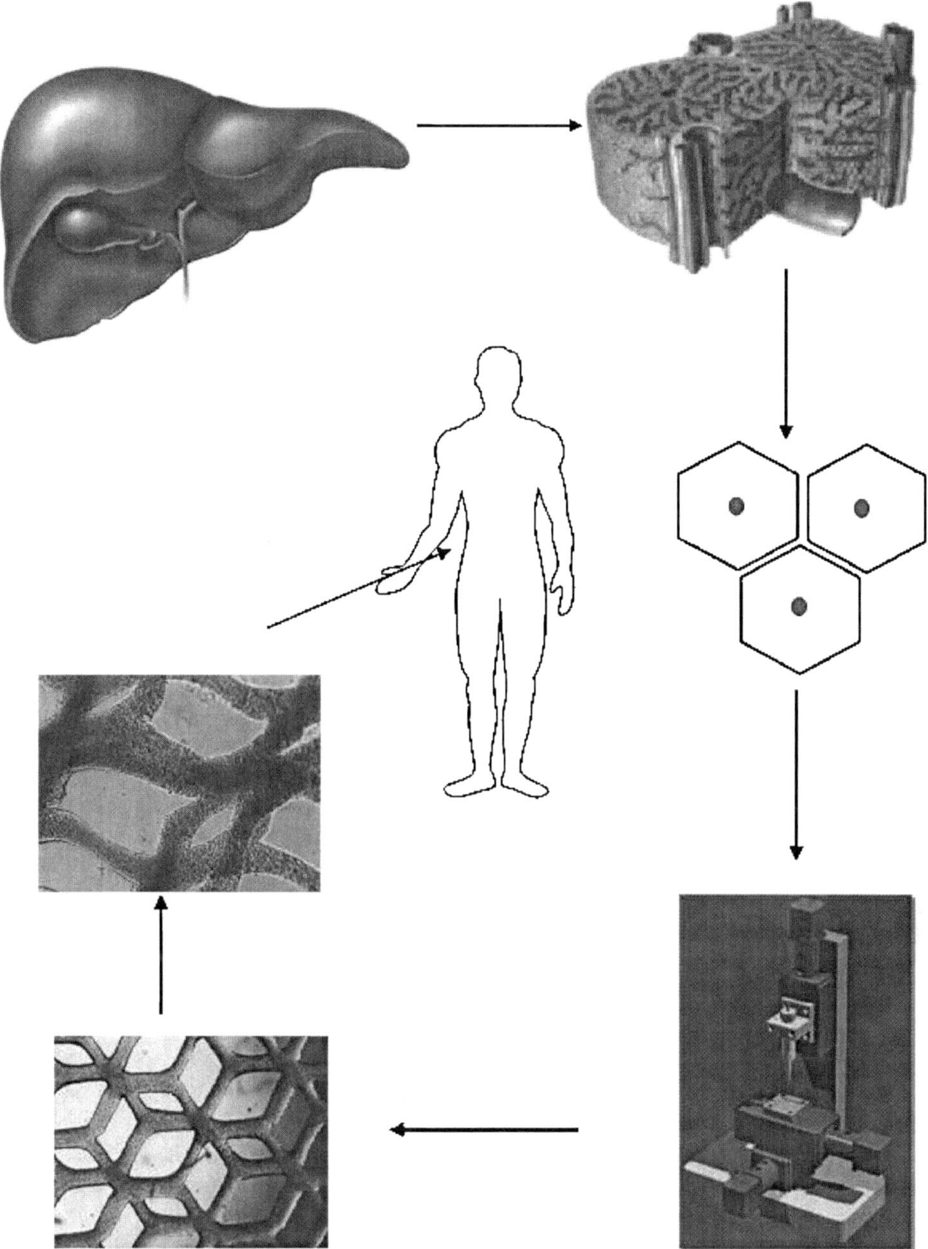

FIGURE 4.1 Rapid prototyping scheme: CAD/CAM SFF.

The final phase can be described as a cleaning and polishing phase, where the waxes or fillers are melted or dissolved away. These three steps usually vary for each method and will be illustrated individually for the description of the tissue engineering RP application.

As illustrated in Figure 4.2, several types of RP methods are available for tissue engineering, and all but one of them have been adapted from existing manufacturing technologies. Almost all RP methods are based on PS3D except those constructs that are poured into 3-D sacrificial molds, which are then destroyed during postprocessing. In this case, the sacrificial mold is inevitably manufactured through PS3D methods.

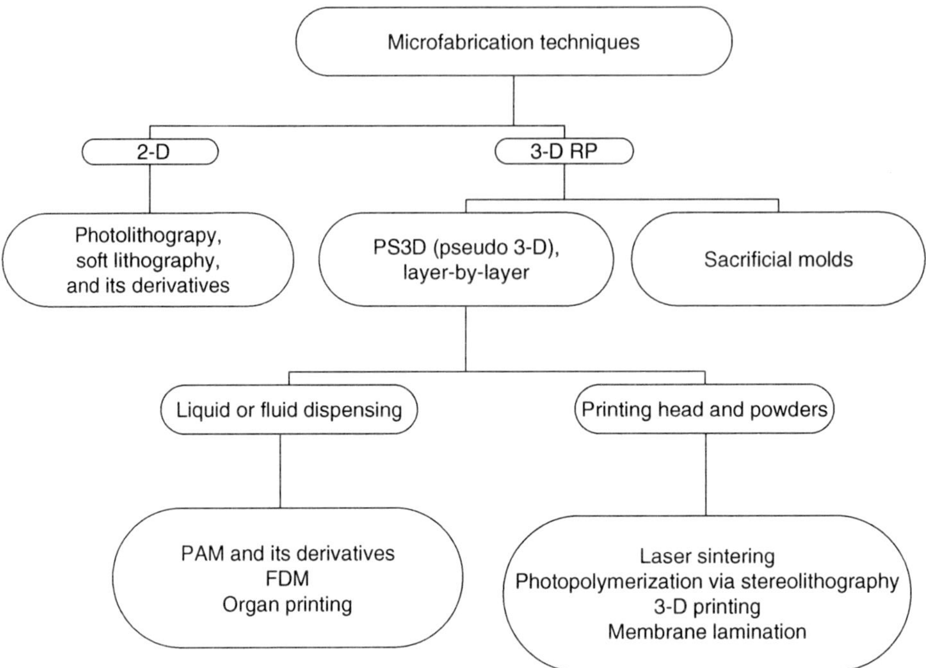

FIGURE 4.2 Classification of RP methods.

We will use the classification suggested by Yeong et al. [2], which subdivides RP methods into PS3D solution or fluid-based systems and printing head and powder-based fabrication, in addition a third class is added, which is based on the use of sacrificial molds. Pressure-assisted microsyringe (PAM), ink-jet organ printing, and fused deposition modeling (FDM) are some of the processes that use solutions. RP methods such as 3-D printing (3-DP) and laser sintering fall into the second class of fabrication, which relies on the use of a printing head emitting a binder such as light, heat, or a solvent.

4.3 MATERIALS USED FOR TISSUE ENGINEERING SCAFFOLDS

One of the most critical aspects of tissue engineering is the choice of biomaterial. Typically biomaterials fall into two main categories: biological polymers and synthetic polymers. Biological polymers are rarely used in RP because of their delicate nature; they denature easily, are difficult to sterilize, and often do not possess adequate mechanical properties to allow the creation of freestanding porous 3-D structures. However, some reports using collagen containing RP scaffolds have been published. In particular, Sachlos et al. [3] have used reconstituted collagen composites, which were poured in the rapid-prototyped sacrificial molds. Biological hydrogels such as gelatin and alginate have also been employed, despite the fact that their floppiness makes them difficult to manage and assemble, and in general the resolutions obtained are low [4,5]. Synthetic polymers are, however, the preferred material for most systems. The most commonly used synthetic polymers for the realization of 3-D scaffolds for tissue engineering are the polyesters—polylactide (PLA), lactide/glycolide co polymers (PLGA), and polycaprolactone (PCL). Often synthetic polymers are incapable of supporting an adequate degree of cell adhesion and must be surface treated or modified with appropriate ligands. These synthetic polymers, also perform poorly in mechanical terms, being too compliant for bone tissue but too rigid for soft tissue. It is therefore becoming increasingly common to use composites or blends, and hydroxyapatite is very often used to render synthetic polymers more rigid for bone engineering applications [6]. The positive trend toward the employment of

TABLE 4.1

A Comparison of Well-Known Microfabrication Methods, Their Resolution, and Limits (References Are Given in the Text)

Technique	Materials Used	RTM Ratio (cm^2/min)	Resolution (μm)	Cells Used	Limits
Membrane lamination	Bioerodable polymers (PLA, PLGA, etc.), bioceramics	Low (<1)	1000	Osteoblasts	Structures not really porous, low resolution
3-D printing	Bioerodable polymers (PLA, PLGA, etc.), hydroxyapatite	Medium (about 1)	300	Various types	Presence of polymeric grains and of excess solvent
Laser sintering	Calcium phosphates, polymers (PLA, PLGA, etc.)	Medium to high	<400	Osteoblasts	Presence of polymeric grains and of excess solvent
Photopolymerization	Photopolymeric resins	0.5 (medium)	250	Osteoblasts	Use of photo-sensitive polymers and initiators, which may be toxic
Fused deposition modeling	Bioerodable polymers (PLA, PLGA, etc.)	7 (very high)	200	Various types	Limited to nonthermolabile materials. Layered structure is very evident
Sacrificial molds—multiphase ink-jet printing	Bioerodable polymers (PLA, PLGA, etc.), collagen	0.1 (low)	300	Various types	Complex to realize, build materials limited, low fidelity
Pressure-assisted microsyringe	Bioerodable polymers (PLA, PLGA, etc.), gels (alginate)	1 (medium)	5–10	Neurons, endothelial cells, fibroblasts, hepatocytes, muscle	Highly water soluble materials cannot be used. Extrusion head is very small
Organ printing	Cells and thermoreversible gels	Medium (about 1)	100	Hepatocytes	Limited range of gels available
Bioplotter	Gels and polymers	Medium	50	Various types	Gels have low fidelity

hybrid materials with different chemical and mechanical properties should result in major improvements in this field.

These materials are either used in powder or solid form, as in the case of laser sintering, 3-DP, or FDM or as solutions as with the PAM or photopolymerization. Obviously different materials are suited to different methods, and some methods are limited to a very narrow range of polymers, particularly in the case of photopolymerization and ink-jet organ printing. Table 4.1 lists some of the different materials employed in RP for tissue engineering.

4.4 RESOLUTION AND RESOLUTION/TIME OF MANUFACTURE RATIO AND GEOMETRY

Table 4.1 clearly shows that RP methods have a wide range of resolutions ranging from 5 to 1000 μm. Prior to discussing the issue of cell response to spatial patterns or geometry and topography, it is necessary to define these terms in the context of this chapter. We define geometry as the 2-D or 3-D spatial organization of cells, referring to spatial dimensions over five times greater than that of the cell. Topography, on the other hand, can be defined as surface features and relief with dimensions of the order of cell size. Thus topography is local, whereas geometry is global. Geometry is easier to control and design using RP whereas topography is harder to define and is a dynamic feature in tissue engineering because cells will remodel a substrate.

It has been amply demonstrated that cells react to the topography of their substrate on which they are seeded [7]. Furthermore it is important to note that characteristic topographical dimensions may vary significantly from one cell type to another. In addition, the adhesion and motility of cells may be enhanced by their contact with a surface with topological features. It has also been shown that the dimensions and aspect ratios of structures can affect the reaction of cells to a marked extent, but despite several studies, we are still far from a full understanding of the events involved [8]. However, much effort is being directed toward the study of the phenomena that guide cell reaction to the geometry of the substrate on which they are seeded, and also the reason why some cell functions are either enhanced or suppressed according to the spatial patterns or geometry [9]. The scaffold-based tissue engineering is founded on the principle that the microstructural environment of a cell undoubtedly conditions its behavior. However, there are no hard-and-fast rules as to which type of geometry or topography is most suitable for this process, and as mentioned in Section 4.2, there are no algorithms or rules to define soft-tissue microarchitecture.

At present there is no RP method, which enables scaffolds with a precision of less than a few microns to be fabricated, and it is likely that smaller features would necessitate elimination of the term rapid, since time is sacrificed at the expense of resolution. We can define the resolution/time of manufacture ratio (RTM ratio) as the maximum resolution (expressed as the inverse of minimum feature length, d) divided by the time (t) required to realize a unit volume (V) of scaffold. The RTM ratio is then

$$\text{RTM} = \frac{1/d}{t/V}$$

and has been quantified where possible in Table 4.1. The higher this number is, the more efficient is the RP method, and the better it lends itself to a high throughput scaffold production. Here we have only used the manufacture time without considering solvent extraction, sterilization, cell seeding, and proliferation times since these times will vary greatly with the selected application.

RP methods can also be characterized in terms of their fidelity, that is, the match between structural features of the scaffolds and the actual CAD design. Obviously no technique has 100% fidelity; in particular, methods that involve melting, swelling, or the use of solvents will show deviations from the input design where usually the scaffold features are larger and less defined than the specified features.

In our experience, the optimum resolution for RP is the order of cell dimensions, or a few tens of microns [10]. In most tissues the functional element is only a few cell diameters [11], so any architectural dimensions greater than this diameter would probably comprise spatial control of cell organization, which is the underlying philosophy behind scaffold-based tissue engineering.

4.5   FLUID-BASED RP MICROFABRICATION

Fluid-based RP methods use a solution or melt of polymer, which is extruded through a syringe mounted on an arm or on the z-axis of a 3-D micropositioner. The material of the upper layer is bonded to that of the lower layer in order to obtain a 3-D scaffold. Often an intermediate supporting layer is required to avoid collapse of the structure during fabrication, which is then sacrificed in the postprocessing phase.

This group includes all the PAM-like methods, FDM and its variants, fiber spinning, and different types of ink-jet-based organ printing. The resolution is generally a function of the viscosity of the polymeric solution extruded as well as the diameter of the deposition head.

4.5.1 Pressure-Assisted Microsyringe System

The pressure-assisted microsyringe (PAM) technique, developed at the Interdepartmental Research Center "E. Piaggio" at the University of Pisa, is based on the use of a microsyringe that allows the deposition of a wide range of polymers, as well as hydrogels [12]. The system consists of a stainless-steel syringe with a 10–20 μm glass capillary needle, as shown in Figure 4.3. A solution of the polymer, in a volatile solvent, is placed inside the syringe and expelled from the tip by the application of filtered, compressed air. The syringe is mounted on the z-axis of a three-axis micropositioning system, which was designed and built in-house. A supporting substrate, usually glass, is placed on the two horizontal motors and is moved relative to the syringe. The control software is developed in C++ (a programming language) with a user-friendly graphical interface and allows a wide range of patterns with a well-defined geometry to be designed and deposited. Within horizontal plane, the resolution of PAM-fabricated parts is 5–600 μm. This resolution depends on the pressure applied to the syringe, the viscosity of the solution, the motor speed, and the dimensions of the syringe tip.

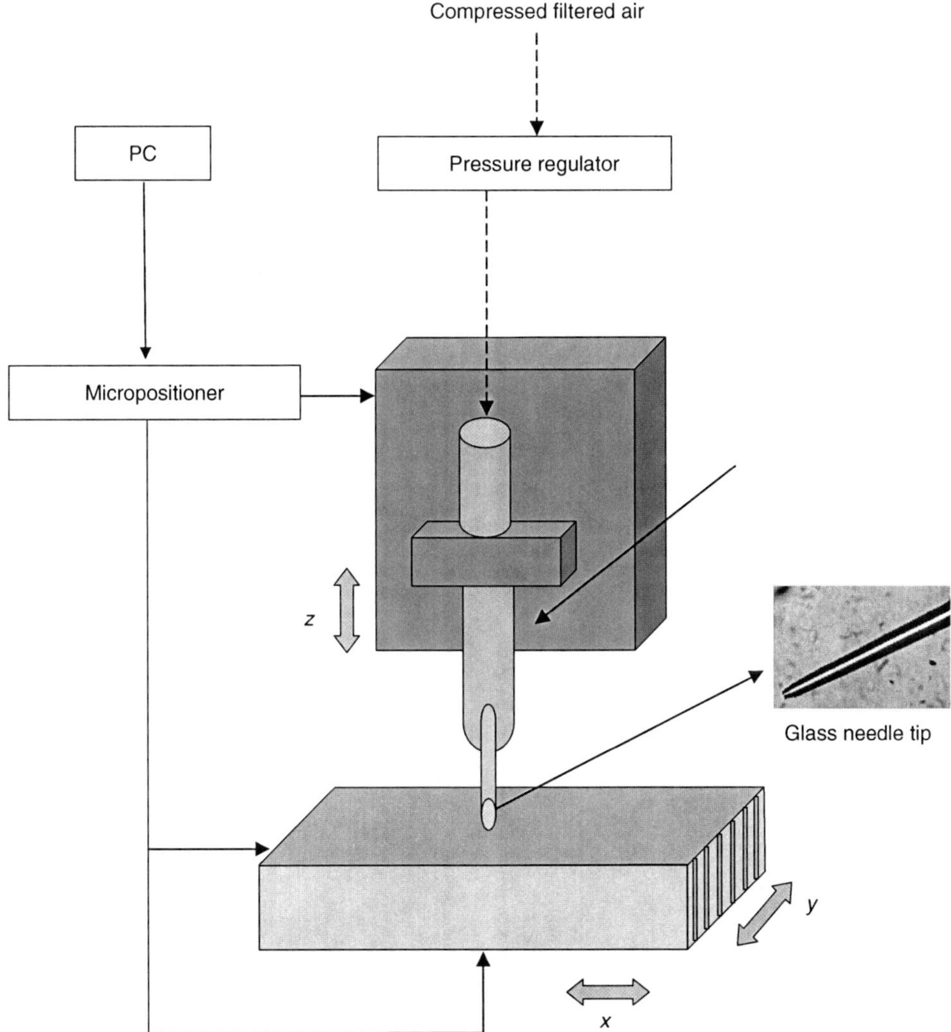

FIGURE 4.3 Block diagram of the pressure-assisted microfabrication (PAM) system. The inset illustrates the capillary needle with an inner diameter of 20 μm.

After the first layer has been deposited, subsequent layers are deposited by moving the syringe up along the z-axis by an amount corresponding to the height of each layer. To avoid collapse of over-hanging structures during the fabrication process, a water-soluble polymeric spacer of about 10–20 μm is deposited between layers. Different layers can be built from different polymers in different patterns, adding to the flexibility of the technique. Once the microfabrication steps are completed, the scaffolds are rinsed with water to remove the polymeric spacer for creating interspaces where the cells can penetrate and adhere to initiate the proliferation process. Typically it takes about 30 s to realize a 2-D layer of 1 cm × 1 cm. In the case of 3-D scaffolds, the postprocessing phase requires about 6–24 h of rinsing. Examples of the scaffolds realized with PAM are shown in Figure 4.4.

The PAM method has the highest resolution among the RP methods and has been adapted by several research groups [5]. Its main drawbacks are the low vertical dimensions (due to the high resolution) and as a result a fairly low RTM ratio, which implies that thick constructs take over an hour to fabricate. Furthermore, the incorporation of the small particles such as hydroxyapatite and nanotubes requires a capillary needle with a larger exit diameter to avoid clogging of the syringe, so precluding high resolutions.

4.5.2 FUSED DEPOSITION MODELING

FDM is an RP process that extrudes polymeric materials in molten form through the use of a heated deposition head developed at the National University of Singapore (NUS). The system is composed of a microcontrolled mechanical arm, which moves in the horizontal plane on which the extrusion head is positioned. A filament of polymer is drawn into the head through the use of rollers, where

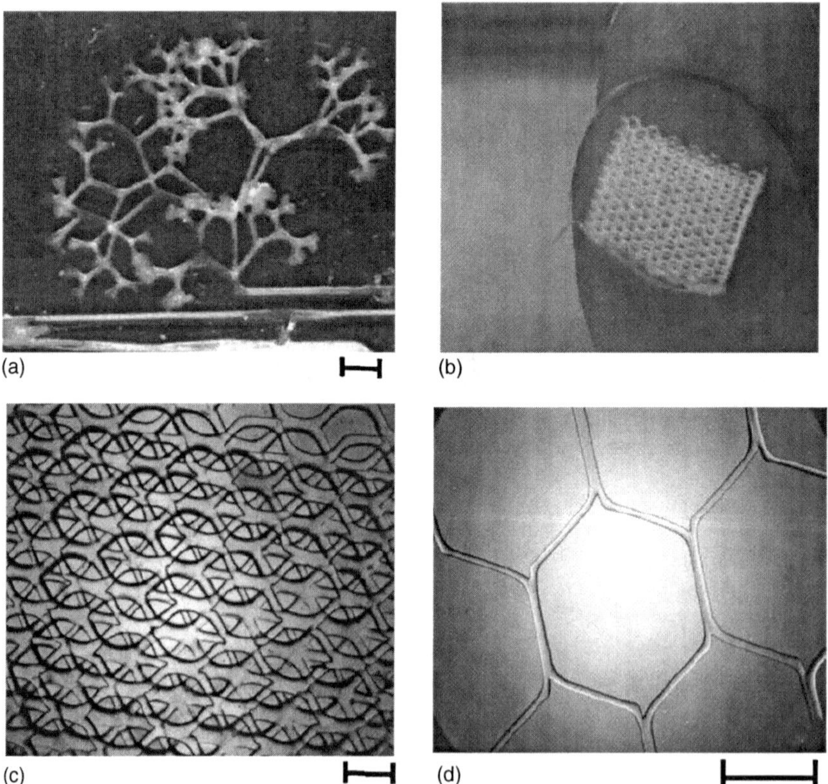

FIGURE 4.4 Typical (a) fractal (scale bar 1 mm), (b) 3-D hexagonal, (c) 3-D hexagonal detail (scale bar 500 μm), and (d) high-resolution 2-D hexagonal (scale bar 500 μm) scaffolds of PLGA obtained by PAM.

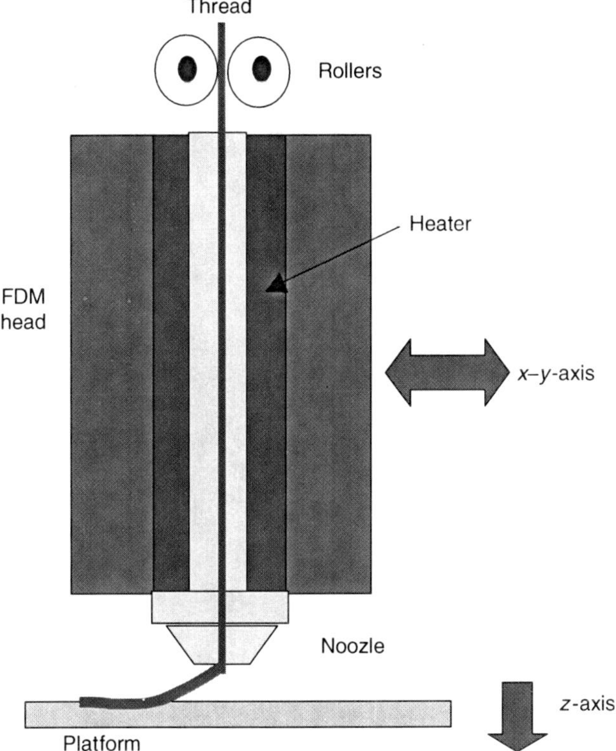

FIGURE 4.5 Schematic representation of fused deposition modeling.

it is heated to near fusion. The semimolten extrudate is driven through a needle having a diameter of 1.27 mm onto a substrate mounted on a platform, and solid objects are built string-by-string as the platform moves down (Figure 4.5). The FDM-fabricated structures have a lateral resolution of a few hundred microns [13]. Several improvements to the FDM system have been reported by the NUS group, in particular, the extrusion head has been modified to enable incorporation of particles or granules rather than filaments and hence renamed as precision extrusion deposition and precision extrusion manufacturing (PED and PEM) [2].

The main limitation of this technique is its resolution since many cell types are smaller than 50 μm. Small scaffolds are difficult to produce because previous layers may melt during heating, whereas larger structures tend to split or peel along layers due to insufficient bonding. Furthermore, because the extrusion is forced by a heating system, this method cannot be used with thermolabile materials. On the other hand, it has the highest RTM ratio of all RP methods because the postprocessing phase is practically nonexistent as there are no intervening layers or binders and solvents to remove as with most other techniques.

4.5.3 ORGAN PRINTING

Mironov et al. [14] developed an ink-jet printer that can print gels, single cells, and cell aggregates. This method, which is known as organ printing, relies on the use of a thermosensitive gel to generate sequential layers for cell printing. This nontoxic biodegradable gel is a liquid below 20°C and solidifies above 32°C. Living cells are sprayed onto the solidified thin layers of the thermoreversible gel, which also serves as printing paper. The printers used are old commercial printers adapted by washing out the ink cartridges and refilling them with cell suspensions. The software that controls

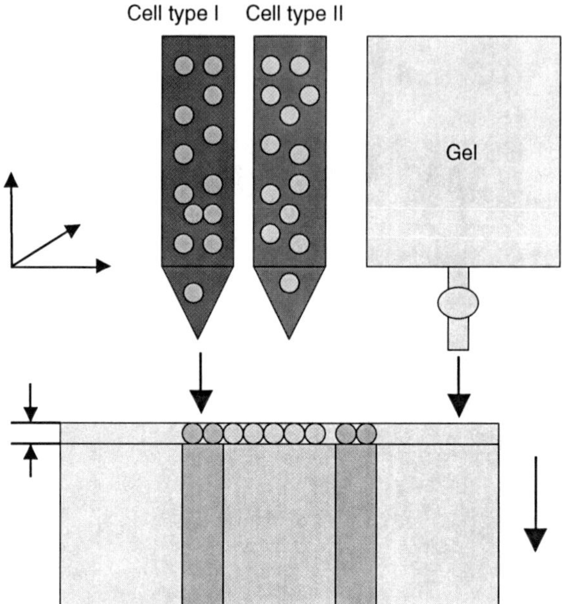

FIGURE 4.6￼A representation of the organ printing concept.

the viscosity, electrical resistances, and temperature of the printing fluids has been reprogrammed and the feed systems altered. As defined by Mironov et al. [14], organ printing includes the many different printer designs and components of the deposition process, for example, jet-based cell printers, cell dispensors or bioplotters, the different types of 3-D hydrogels, and varying cell types. The concept is schematized in Figure 4.6.

With this method the resolution is about 100 µm, and in fact several cell aggregates are formed within the drops. Due to the use of an ink-jet head, cells may be damaged during spraying due to the high shear stress by the piezoelectric actuator, and obviously the choice of materials is also restricted to a narrow range of biocompatible thermoreversible hydrogels.

4.6 PRINTING HEAD AND POWDER-BASED MICROFABRICATION

In this section, we include all the techniques where the polymeric powders or liquids are placed on the x–y plane of the system, and the working head (laser, ink-jet head, etc.) realizes microstructures in which the resolution is a function of the grain dimensions or of the printing head beam or drop size.

4.6.1 MEMBRANE LAMINATION

Membrane lamination consists of the realization of membranes having a thickness between 500 and 2000 µm. They are then cut by a laser beam or scissors in the form of predetermined, 2-D shapes. Once the basic elements are ready, the structure is assembled layer-by-layer using microcontrolled and microactuated system controlled by CAD/CAM software. Lamination is obtained by wetting an absorbent material such as paper, cloth, or a sponge with an organic solvent. Light pressure is applied to the exposed surface of each membrane for a sufficient amount of time to wet each surface. The resulting bilayer-laminated structure is gently compressed to ensure sufficient adhesion between the wet surfaces of the first and the second membranes. This procedure is repeated with the bilayer or resulting multilayer-laminated structure until the desired 3-D shape is obtained. The final laminated structure is dried to ensure complete solvent evaporation [15]. Since the resolution of this method is insufficient for most tissue engineering applications, it has been replaced by more precise techniques.

4.6.2 THREE-DIMENSIONAL PRINTING

Originally developed for rapid-prototyping ceramics and metal objects such as molds for investment casting, three-dimensional printing (3-DP) has since been applied to the fabrication of drug delivery devices and tissue scaffolds from biomedical polymers. It allows simultaneous fabrication and surface modification of 3-D devices. A schematic description of the 3-DP process is shown in Figure 4.7.

A thin layer of powder (0.05–0.20 mm) is first spread on the top of a piston. An ink-jet printhead then prints a liquid binder onto the layer wherever the particles are to be bonded together to form the solid part of the object. Colloidal silica is commonly used as a binder in ceramic systems, while organic solvents such as chloroform, which swell and partially dissolve individual powder particles, are suitable for polymer systems [16].

Each printed droplet is 50–80 μm in diameter, and a CAD/CAM program controls its position. After the first layer is printed, the piston is dropped, and the sequential steps of powder spreading and printing are repeated. Scaffolds possessing complex internal features can be created because during the building process, the powder bed allows the formation of channels and overhangs as supports for objects. Furthermore, multiple printheads containing different solutions can be readily employed to modify local surface chemistries and compositions. At the end of the process, the scaffold is lifted from the powder bed, and the loose powder is removed. The resulting product is a solid, continuous 3-D structure with well-defined internal microarchitectures. The resolution of features is approximately 300 μm. Interconnected pores can be generated in the walls of polymer

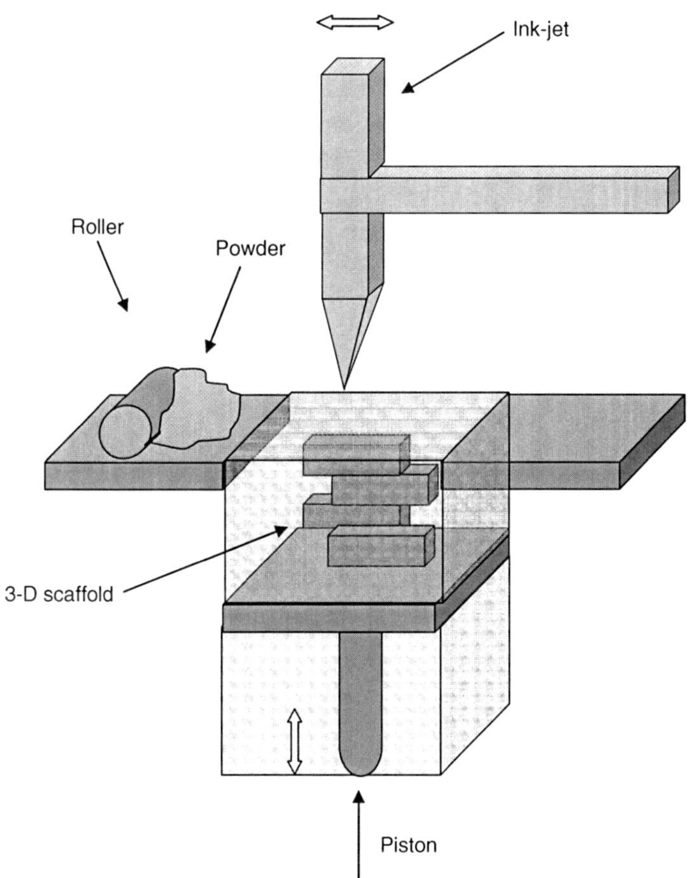

FIGURE 4.7 Basic scheme of the 3-D printing method.

devices by inclusion of a porogen in the powder [17]. Therics Inc. uses a 3-DP system to produce bone fillers composed of PLGA and tricalcium phosphate (TCP), the first example of an RP commercial product specifically for tissue engineering.

With 3-DP it is often difficult to remove excess polymer grains, and the residual amount of solvent is only reduced by 10–15% in weight. As mentioned, this system allows the realization of polymeric structures with a lateral resolution of approximately 0.3 mm, which is suboptimal if precise control of cell positioning is required. Its RTM ratio is about 1, thus placing it at the high end of manufacturing efficiency.

4.6.3 LASER SINTERING

This microfabrication system uses a laser beam in order to realize polymeric microstructures. A polymer powder layer is placed on the substrate, and an infrared laser beam locally raises a given spot to the temperature of glass transition, thereby fusing the polymeric grains. Once a layer has been appropriately patterned, the substrate is moved down, and a new polymer powder layer is applied. Excess polymer powder is left in loco during the fabrication process because it prevents collapse of overhangs, but then it can be rather difficult to remove during the postprocessing phase.

CAD/CAM software is employed for designing the structures layer-by-layer and for controlling the laser beam and the motion of the micropositioner where the laser beam and substrate for deposition are mounted, as schematized in Figure 4.8 [18].

This technique is typically used to realize bone implants with calcium phosphate powders or ceramics but has also been successfully employed for polymers and gels such as PCL and

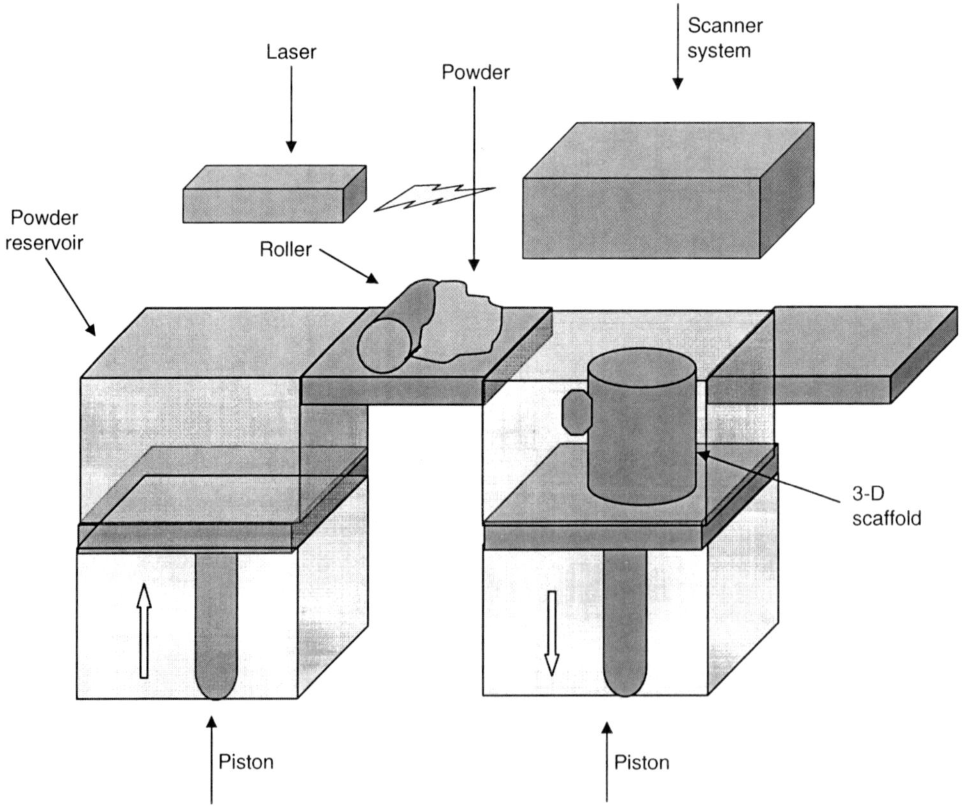

FIGURE 4.8   The laser-sintering process.

polysaccharides [19]. One of the main advantages of laser sintering is the ability to incorporate particles such as hydroxyapatite into the scaffold with minimum effort where the particles are simply added to the polymer, which fuses around them [6].

In laser sintering, the resolution of the system depends on laser spot size, thermal conductivity and absorption of the polymer, and the grain size. A commercial device, Sinter Station 2500 (DTM, USA), has a laser beam with a 400 μm spot. Heat conduction inevitably makes the precision of the system rather larger than the spot size. At present, new systems with better resolutions are being developed. Much effort is also being dedicated to resolve the problem of the presence of excess powder by using ultrasonic vibrations, compressed air, and particular solvents.

4.6.4 PHOTOPOLYMERIZATION

Photopolymerization is a method based on the polymerization of photopolymeric resins in a site-specific manner. The photopolymeric resins are mixtures of simple monomers with low molecular weight that form a long chain polymer when they are activated by light. An initiator or a catalyst is often required for polymerization to occur (these are toxic to cells) and the light source must have a high frequency (usually ultraviolet).

Site-specific polymerization takes place either by scanning a laser beam over the surface of the liquid prepolymer—a process known as stereolithography—or by irradiating a mask placed above the surface. In both methods, irradiated zones become solid whereas the other areas remain liquid. Once the layer has polymerized, a fresh layer of prepolymer is applied. In theory, the laser spot could also be focused at different heights, but the depth of action is limited by the absorption of the liquid. The second technique requires the fabrication of a different mask for each layer and cannot strictly be defined as RP. Using the data in Ref. 20, an RTM ratio of about 0.5 can be estimated, which places this method among the more efficient techniques.

The main limitation of RP by photopolymerization is the use of acrylic or epoxy photopolymeric materials, which are often not biocompatible. Currently attempts are being made to extend this methodology to bioerodable polymers and biological polymers. For example, Dhariwala et al. [20] have used a commercial stereolithography machine to polymerize poly(ethylene oxide) and poly(ethylene glycol) dimethacrylate hydrogel using a photoinitiator. In their setup, a 250 μm ultraviolet light spot was rastered over a layer of prepolymer containing living cells, as schematized in Figure 4.9. The results demonstrated that the cells were very sensitive to the initiator and remained viable only at very low initiator concentrations.

4.7 OTHER RP METHODS

Two further techniques that are worth mentioning are the sacrificial mold method and fiber spinning. The former uses rapid-prototyped molds to cast melts, solutions, or even powders, whereas the latter is not strictly RP at present but can be used to build nanoscale features on microfabricated scaffolds.

4.7.1 SACRIFICIAL MOLDS

A limited number of techniques using sacrificial molds have been reported, and this is likely due to the complexity of the fabrication process. Firstly, a plastic mold of the microstructure to be realized is constructed through one of the RP methods described above, usually ink-jet printing or 3-DP. Secondly, a deposition head then fills up the empty spaces present in the microstructure with a selected biopolymer thereby forming the scaffold. The polymer mold that simply constructs the support for the 3-D structure is then removed or sacrificed by bathing it in an appropriate solvent. In theory, using more heads, complex and multipolymeric structures can be rapidly realized.

Sachlos et al. [3] reported a two-phase ink-jet–based method to prepare molds of Protobuild (phase 1) and Protosupport (phase 2). The phase 2 material was dissolved away leaving a 3-D

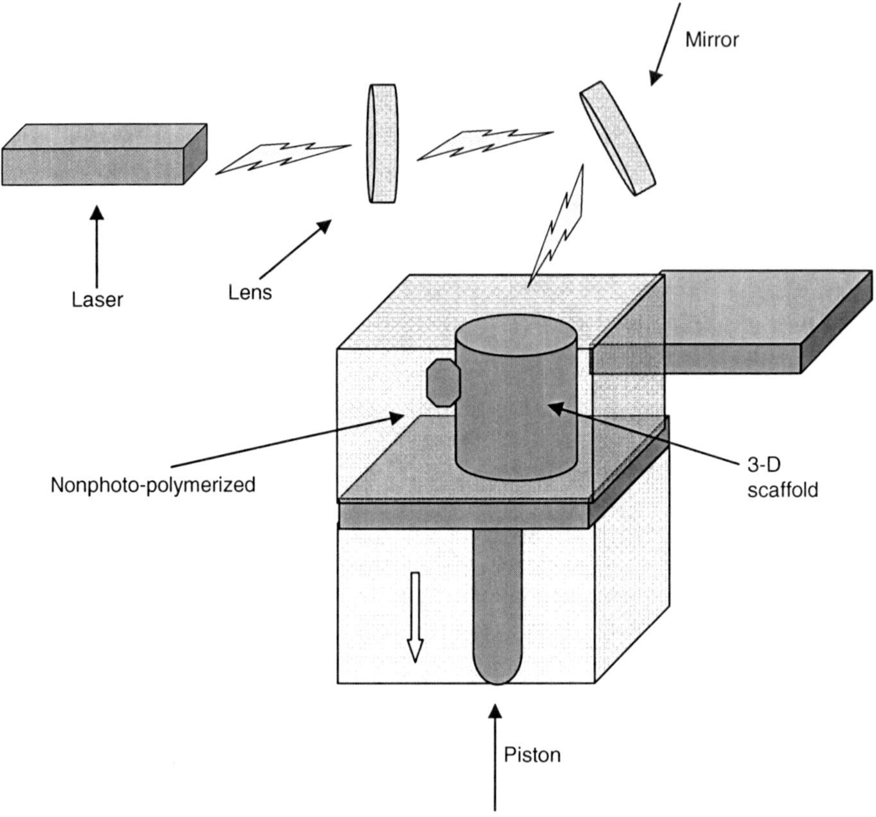

FIGURE 4.9 Scheme of photopolymerization using laser stereolithography.

structure with interconnected channels. Subsequently collagen dispersion was poured into the channels and solidified through freeze-drying. Finally the phase 1 build material was dissolved away, leaving a collagen containing 3-D scaffold with features of about 200 μm. A very similar method was recently reported in which polypropylene fumarate was injected into a mold fabricated using two-phase ink-jet printing. Phase 1 and phase 2 materials were wax (removed by heating and solvent) and polystyrene (dissolved with acetone), respectively. The final PPF scaffold has a resolution of a few hundred microns and is mainly delimited by the precision of the ink-jet printer [21]. The process is outlined in Figure 4.10.

The use of sacrificial molds adds to the complexity of the design, fabrication, and postprocessing of scaffolds but eliminates the pseudo-3-D layered effect, which gives rise to the characteristic steps that are observed in all other RP scaffolds. The final structure is a homogeneous monolith with channels, pores, and overhangs. However, this feature is obtained at the expense of extremely long manufacture times; the RTM ratio is the lowest of all the RP methods described in this chapter. Besides its complexity, a major disadvantage of this method is the inability to use different materials in different areas and the limitations on choice of biomaterials, which have to be insoluble in the solvent used to degrade the mold. Furthermore, owing to the multiple steps involved, the fidelity of the scaffold is quite low. On the other hand, it is one of the few RP methods that can be used to produce scaffolds composed of proteins such as collagen.

4.7.2 ELECTROSPINNING

Although not strictly an RP method at present, electro or fiberspinning has the potential to become an RP method by appropriate eletrostatic and mechanical control of the deposition plane.

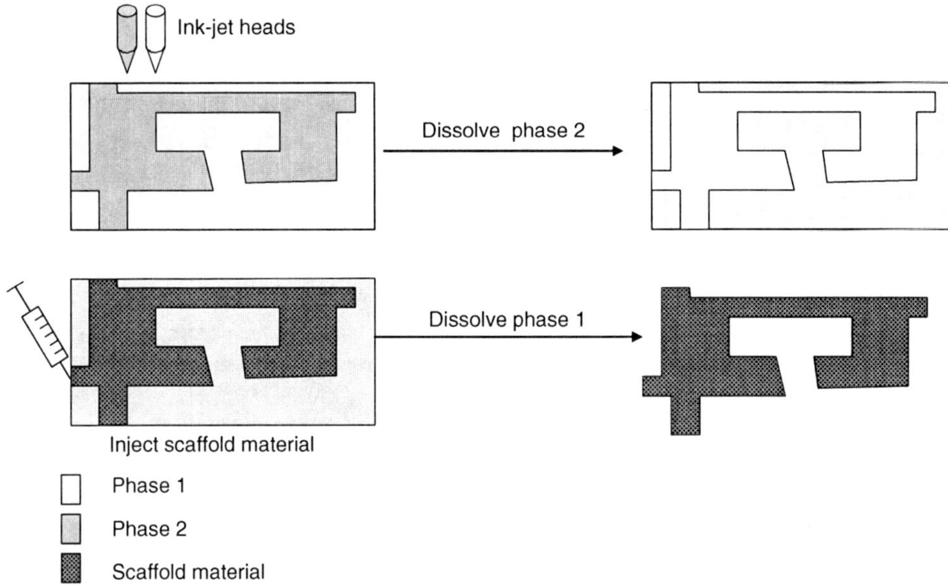

FIGURE 4.10 The process of obtaining an RP scaffold through the use of a sacrificial mold.

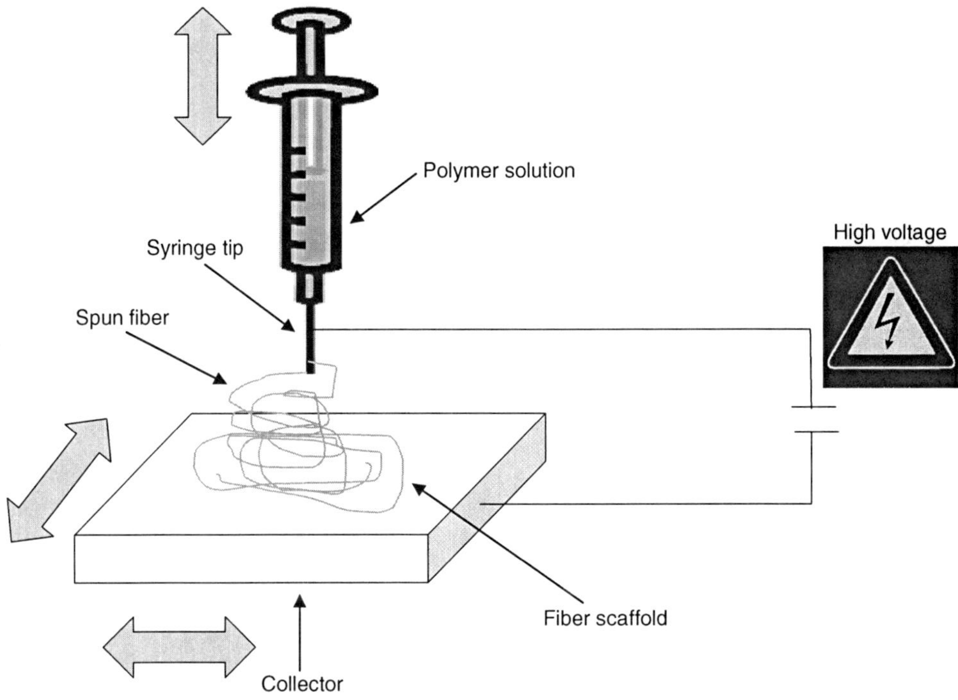

FIGURE 4.11 Schematic of the electrospinning technique.

In electrospinning, a syringe is loaded with a polymer solution, which is forced out by the application of a high voltage to the syringe tip. This action causes a high-speed jet of polymer to exit from the tip and land on an appropriate collector, usually a flat plate or a rotating cylinder, as illustrated in Figure 4.11. Polymer fibers with diameters ranging from a few nanometers to several microns can thus be produced. A wide range of materials can be spun using this method, including the classic biodegradable polyesters, gels such as gelatin and polyvinyl alcohol, and proteins (the range of possible polymers is much wider than any of the RP methods reported in Table 4.1). Furthermore, the method is also highly tunable, in the sense that fiber diameter and quality is dependent on several parameters, for example, viscosity, dipole moment, conductivity, and applied potential. Several designs and configurations of needle tips have been also proposed, such as multiple tips and coaxial tips, which allow the strands to be deposited as hollow fibers. Interested readers are encouraged to consult the excellent review by Pham et al. [22].

At present the collector system where fibers are laid is very simple, but we envisage more sophisticated and fast moving collection systems, which could enable site-specific fiber deposition and orientation and render the electrospinning method RP. We predict that its manufacturing efficiency in terms of RTM ratio is likely to be astonishingly high, possibly a degree of magnitude over that of FDM because of the high speed with which the polymer jet is ejected from the needle tip and the high surface to volume ratio produced by very thin fibers.

4.8   INTEGRATION OF RP METHODS

None of the techniques so far developed can meet the requirements of resolution, RTM ratio, or flexibility of materials for the realization of a multifunctional scaffold for tissue engineering. An emerging trend now is to use the combination of technologies to integrate features at different scales. In an earlier work, we integrated the PAM technique with site-specific surface modification [23]. Ideally this approach should also combine one or more RP methods. At present, electrospinning, although not strictly RP, is most commonly integrated with other processing methods to produce microscale networks with higher order networks. An example of this method is the integration of fiber bonding with electrospinning. The resulting 3-D scaffolds comprise a macro and a nanofibrillar network, which is able to support cell viability and differentiation into bone cells [24]. The electrospinning technique has also been combined with a wet-spun macrofibrillar network to create structure-mimicking vessels [25].

Zhang et al. [26] have recently proposed a technique to fabricate scaffold or cell constructs for tissue engineering by the assembly of microscopic building blocks, realized with different methods such as bioplotter and FDM techniques in order to mimic the original topology of tissues.

We are certain that this new trend will bring about improvements in design and production capacity of RP scaffolds.

4.9   COMMERCIAL RP SYSTEMS FOR TISSUE ENGINEERING SCAFFOLDS

RP systems appear to be fairly expensive and bulky, but this is not always the case particularly as far as fabrication of tissue engineering products is concerned. The maximum size of scaffold desired is usually no larger than a few centimetres squared, and the fabrication costs are actually only a small fraction of the total cost of a cell-based 3-D structure, not to mention that of future preclinical and clinical trails. Some of the RP systems and products described in this chapter are available commercially, but at present these devices and the scaffolds are still very much a niche product used more for research than for medical applications.

Therics Inc. is a company that produces a line of beta-TCP (β-TCP) products as bone fillers using a patented technology, Theriform (www.therics.com). Theriform technology is based on the 3-DP method, which was the first RP technology to be applied for tissue engineering. The company currently has eight products, two of which are FDA approved with positive clinical results.

PAM-fabricated scaffolds are marketed by Biodigit (www.biodigit.it) for use in cardiac tissue engineering and are mainly employed for research purposes. They are available in a variety of materials from biodegradable polyesters to polyurethanes as well as alginates.

Sciperio Inc. (www.sciperio.com) claims to be developing a new *in vivo* direct-deposition machine for the fabrication of *in vivo* tissue using advanced minimally invasive techniques, vision and diagnostic imaging systems, biological sensing systems, ultrashort-pulse-laser tissue ablation, and the fabrication and assembly of 3-D tissue constructs. The system described is essentially a dream tissue engineering factory, which has been envisaged by several researchers. According to Sciperio, the tool will be able to deposit a wide variety of cells (e.g., stem cells, endothelial cells, chondrocytes, T-cells, dendritic cells), growth factors, nutrients, ECM proteins, and biocompatible structural materials with exquisite precision.

Envisiontec (www.envisiontec.de) has developed the bioplotter technology, invented at the Freiburg Materials Research Centre in 1999. The system is based on a 3-D dispenser and allows processing a magnitude of materials including various biochemical systems and even living cells. CAD data handling and machine/process control are done through a system-specific pseudo-3-D CAD/CAM software. The bioplotter principle is based on dispensing a plotting material into a plotting medium to cause solidification of the material and to compensate gravity force through buoyancy. In the presence of a temperature-controlled plotting medium, the solidification of the material during plotting into the medium can be modulated by precipitation reactions, phase transitions, or chemical reactions. The bioplotter is the only commercial RP system available at fairly reasonable cost.

Neatco and Dimarix (www.dimatix.com) have created a cartridge-style printhead that allows users to fill their own fluids and print immediately with different materials. For the moment the systems are still used for liquid printing DNA arrays or sensors, but they can potentially be employed for organ printing. Each single-use cartridge has 16 nozzles linearly spaced at 254 μm with a typical drop size of 10 pL and can be replaced to facilitate printing of a series of fluids.

There is no doubt that in future the number of scaffolds available on the market will increase steadily. It should, however, be kept in mind that the road ahead to the real medical applications of RP scaffolds is still long and arduous. An emerging critical factor that should be considered in all design and processing phases is the application of good manufacturing practice (GMP) principles and standards to RP methods and products for biomedical use. Scaffolds should be considered as biomedical devices for advanced therapeutics, and RP technologies are therefore a key part of the manufacturing and validation processes.

4.10 DISCUSSION: LIMITATIONS AND CRITIQUES

In this review, we have given a general description of the state of the art of RP methods for the realization of scaffolds for tissue engineering applications. There is no doubt that the microstructural environment of a cell conditions its behavior, and scaffold-based tissue engineering is founded on this very principle. However, as yet we do not have any rules or guidelines on just what this microstructure should be and in general very little effort has been made toward defining structural design parameters. Until we establish architectural canons for biological tissue, the main advantage of RP technologies over other material processing methods is their ability to generate reproducible and repetitive structures with controlled porosity, which do not vary from batch to batch and at present adhering to an industrial rather than biological requirement.

As summarized in Table 4.1, it is clear that a large variety of RP techniques exist, and the choice of one method with respect to another depends on manufacturing efficiency and the desired resolution as well as on the polymer chosen for fabrication; there is no optimal or unique RP method. Each RP technique must be matched with a particular organ considering cell density, cell size, organizational and nutritional requirements, as well as mechanical matching between scaffold and tissue.

It can also be argued that RP fits the tissue engineering paradigm better than the classical subtractive fabrication methods such as milling or turning. In RP the object or prototype is created through an additive process not dissimilar to the process of biological development in which cells

TABLE 4.2

Differences between Biological Tissue Development and Tissue Engineering Using Scaffolds

Tissue Development	RP Scaffold Approach
Not scaffold dependent	A porous biodegradable scaffold is necessary
Cells create their matrix and extend in three dimensions from a "point source"	Takes place through pseudo-3-D fabrication: through layer-by-layer assembly of 2-D
Environment and structure modulated in real time	Preprogrammed architecture
Complex multicomponent materials	Usually one material
Soft and wet	Often hard and dry

assemble and organize through a process of accumulation and accretion rather than degradation and attrition. However, the differences between tissue development and scaffold-based tissue engineering, some of which are listed in Table 4.2, should be kept in mind. Cell assembly and organization is an immensely complicated process and depends on the correct orchestration of biochemical signals with spatial and other physical stimuli. Simply seeding cells on a porous scaffold with the same shape as the end organ and hoping for a functional tissue to form has already been shown to be insufficient. Indeed, despite the enormous economic resources injected into tissue engineering, very few products are actually viable from a commercial [27] or even medical point of view [28].

In this sense, scaffold fabrication techniques through RP are not stand-alone tissue engineering tools but, taking into account the intricate complexity of living systems, must be integrated with other micro and macroscale techniques. For instance, that scaffolds must be accompanied by pre- or postsurface modification usually thorough the immobilization of adhesion proteins, which is already well established. Other supporting elements such as soluble growth factors, incubators, or bioreactors are also mandatory. We have already mentioned that the nature of the biomaterial as well as its microstructure and topology are additional critical factors. It should not be forgotten that even in mechanical terms, the microfabrication or biomaterial processing method must be matched to each particular tissue to be engineered. Optimized solutions could be found by combining different RP methods and by following biomimetic design principles through the use of biomaterials, which resemble biological materials as much as possible. This implies the development of hybrid materials and structures with a composite nature and high water content and the integration of two or more RP techniques, for example, with different resolutions and different types of polymers.

4.11   CONCLUSION

An overview of RP methods for biomaterial fabrication has been provided with the aim of illustrating the basic principles behind the scaffold-based tissue engineering. Rather than providing exhaustive technical and comparative details, which are available in several excellent reviews that the interested reader is encouraged to refer to Refs. 2,29,30, we have described aspects which must be taken into consideration when realizing a scaffold such as the resolution time of manufacture ratio, materials employed, and scaffold geometrical design. Furthermore, it is also important for the RP engineer involved in tissue-engineering construct manufacture to be acutely aware of the differences between tissue development and the use of a scaffold to guide cells to appropriate locations on a scaffold. High throughput production of tissue-engineered constructs is still a long way away and not only requires great multidisciplinary effort but also a thorough understanding of the biology, chemistry, and engineering of cells and biomaterials and above all their interaction in complex 3-D environments.

REFERENCES

1. Langer R, Vacanti JP. Tissue engineering. *Science* 260, 920, 1993.
2. Yeong WY, Chua C, Leong KF, Chandrasekaran M. Rapid prototyping in tissue engineering: challenges and potential. *Trends Biotechnol.* 22, 643, 2004.
3. Sachlos E, Reis N, Ainsley C, Derby B, Czernuszka JT. Novel collagen scaffolds with predefined internal morphology made by solid freeform fabrication. *Biomaterials* 24, 1487, 2003.
4. Landers R, Hubner U, Schmelzeisen R, Mulhaupt R. Rapid prototyping of scaffolds derived from thermoreversible hydrogels and tailored for applications in tissue engineering. *Biomaterials* 23, 4437, 2002.
5. Yan Y, Wang X, Pan Y, Liu H, Cheng J, Xiong Z, Lin F, Wu R, Zhang R, Lu Q. Fabrication of viable tissue-engineered constructs with 3D cell-assembly technique. *Biomaterials* 26, 5864, 2005.
6. Tan KH, Chua CK, Leong KF, Cheah CM, Cheang P, Abu Bakar MS, Cha SW. Scaffold development using selective laser sintering of polyetheretherketone–hydroxyapatite biocomposite blends. *Biomaterials* 24, 3115, 2003.
7. Curtis AG, Wilkinson CDW. Reactions of cells to topography. *J. Biomater. Sci. Polymer Edn.* 9, 1313, 1998.
8. Chen CS, Mrksich M, Huang S, Whitesides GM, Ingber DE. Geometric control of cell life and death. *Science* 276, 1425, 1997.
9. Ingber DE. Cellular mechanotransduction: putting all the pieces together again. *FASEB J.* 20, 811, 2006.
10. Francis K, Palssojn BO. Effective inter-cellular communication distances are determined by the relative cytokine secretion and diffusion time constants. *Proc. Natl Acad. Sci.* 94, 12258, 1997.
11. Mattioli-Belmonte M, Vozzi G, Kyriakidou K, Pulieri E, Lucarini G, Vinci B, Pugnaloni A, Biagini G, Ahluwalia A. Rapid-prototyped and salt-leached PLGA scaffolds condition cell morpho-functional behavior. *J. Biomed. Mater. Res. A.* 2007 in press.
12. Vozzi G, Previti A, De Rossi D, Ahluwalia A. Microsyringe based deposition of 2 and 3-D polymer scaffolds with a well defined geometry for application to tissue engineering. *Tissue Eng.* 8, 1089, 2002.
13. Zein I, Hutmacher DW, Tan KC, Teoh SH. Fused deposition modeling of novel scaffold architectures for tissue engineering applications. *Biomaterials* 23, 1169, 2002.
14. Mironov V, Boland T, Trusk T, Forgacs G, Markwald RR. Organ printing: computer-aided jet-based 3D tissue engineering. The layer-by-layer assembly of biological tissues and organs is the future of tissue engineering. *Trends Biotechnol.* 21, 157, 2003.
15. Mikos AG, Sarakinos G, Leite SM, Vacanti JP, Langer R. Laminated three-dimensional biodegradable foams for use in tissue engineering. *Biomaterials* 14, 323, 1993.
16. Giordano RA, Wu BM, Borland SW, Cima LG, Sachs EM, Cima MJ. Mechanical properties of dense polylactic acid structures fabricated by three dimensional printing. *J. Biomater. Sci. Polym. Edn.* 8, 63, 1996.
17. Zeltinger J, Sherwood JK, Graham DA, Mueller R, Griffith LG. Effect of pore size and void fraction on cellular adhesion, proliferation, and matrix deposition. *Tissue Eng.* 7, 557, 2001.
18. Berry E, Brown JM, Connell M, Craven CM, Efford ND, Radjenovic A, Smith MA. Preliminary experience with medical applications of rapid prototyping by selective laser sintering. *Med. Eng. Phys.* 19, 90, 1997.
19. Ciardelli G, Chiono V, Vozzi G, Pracella M, Ahluwalia A, Barbani N, Cristallini C, Giusti P. Blends of poly-(epsilon-caprolactone) and polysaccharides in tissue engineering applications. *Biomacromolecules* 6, 1961, 2005.
20. Dhariwala B, Hunt E, Boland T. Rapid prototyping of tissue-engineering constructs, using photopolymerizable hydrogels and stereolithography. *Tissue Eng.* 10, 1316, 2004.
21. Lee KW, Wang S, Lu L, Jabbari E, Currier BL, Yaszemski MJ. Fabrication and characterization of poly(propylene fumarate) scaffolds with controlled pore structures using 3-dimensional printing and injection molding. *Tissue Eng.* 12, 2801, 2006.
22. Pham QP, Sharma U, Mikos AG. Electrospinning of polymeric nanofibers for tissue engineering applications: a review. *Tissue Eng.* 12, 1197, 2006.
23. Bianchi F, Vassalle C, Simonetti M, Vozzi G, Ahluwalia A, Domenici C. Endothelial cell function on 2D and 3D micro-fabricated polymer scaffolds: applications in cardiovascular tissue engineering. *J. Biomater. Sci. Polym. Edn.* 17(1,2), 37, 2006.

24. Tuzlakoglu K, Bolgen N, Salgado AJ, Gomes ME, Piskin E, Reis RL. Nano- and micro-fiber combined scaffolds: a new architecture for bone tissue engineering. *J. Mater. Sci. Mater. Med.* 16(12), 1099, 2005.
25. Kim TG, Park TG. Biomimicking extracellular matrix: cell adhesive RGD peptide modified electrospun poly(D,L-lactic-*co*-glycolic acid) nanofiber mesh. *Tissue Eng.* 12(2), 221, 2006.
26. Zhang H, Hutmacher DW, Chollet F, Poo AN, Burdet E. Microrobotics and MEMS-based fabrication techniques for scaffold-based tissue engineering. *Macromol. Biosci.* 24, 5(6), 477, 2005.
27. Lysaght MJ, Hazlehurst AL. Tissue engineering: the end of the beginning. *Tissue Eng.* 10, 309, 2004.
28. Hunziker EB. Commentary. *Osteoarthr. Cartilage* 10, 432, 2002.
29. Yang S, Leong K, Zhoahui D, Chua C. The design of scaffolds for use in tissue engineering part II. Rapid prototyping techniques. *Tissue Eng.* 8, 1, 2002.
30. Leong KF, Cheah CM, Chua CK. Solid freeform fabrication of three-dimensional scaffolds for engineering replacement tissues and organs. *Biomaterials* 24, 2363, 2003.

5 Design and Fabrication Principles of Electrospinning of Scaffolds

Dietmar W. Hutmacher and Andrew K. Ekaputra

CONTENTS

5.1 BACKGROUND

Nanotechnology allows for the construction of scaffold and devices that interact at the subcellular level. The application of nanotechnology to biomedical sciences is a rather new and quickly expanding field. The successful use of microscale surface features to study a variety of cellular phenomena has led molecular and cell biologists, in collaboration with material scientists, to engage in the study of how nanoscale cellular extensions (e.g., lammelopodia and filopodia) interact with their environment to effect cell growth, proliferation, and expression. This change in scale (several orders of magnitude lower) is motivated by the various nanoscale structures that comprise the extracellular matrix (ECM). This natural three-dimensional (3-D) topography at the nanoscale causes an increase in the surface area of the ECM of up to three orders of magnitude. This increased area over which cell–surface interactions can take place may give rise to a number of imperative functions in regulating tissue growth. Nanofabricated matrices can play an important role in answering these types of questions through the controlled and reproducible fabrication of substrates that will allow for a systematic study of surface topographies and their effects on a variety of parameters such as cell attachment, migration, and proliferation.

Hence, over the last decade there have been many different techniques employed to create nanoscale topographical features, and several good reviews have also been published. The types of nanotopographical features created on materials can be separated into two main categories: unordered topographies and ordered topographies. Unordered topographies spontaneously occur during processing. Such topographies can be generated using techniques such as polymer demixing, colloidal lithography, electrospinning, and chemical etching. Curtis et al. first performed a comparative study of an ordered topography and an unordered topography. In their experiment, surfaces with various nanoscale ordered patterns were created using electron beam lithography, and surfaces with nanoscale unordered patterns were created using colloidal lithography. Rat fibroblasts showed higher level of adhesion to the surface with an unordered pattern than to both planar surfaces and ordered surfaces. Interestingly, the surfaces with the ordered patterns had even lower levels of adhesion than flat surfaces [1].

Within the biomaterial community there has been a considerable amount of research focused on the design and fabrication of different types of scaffolds for applications in regenerative medicine. Scaffold materials, both natural and synthetic in origin, are being explored with specific tissue engineering applications in mind. An emerging trend in this field is the production and deliberate manipulation of the nanosized features to move toward so-called biomimetic scaffold. Scaffolds that have dimensional similarities to the natural basement membrane can be manufactured by the electrospinning method, and these scaffolds can mimic the fibrous structure of the ECM, thus providing essential cues for cellular organization, survival, and function.

5.1.1 Basic Principles of Scaffold-Based Tissue Engineering

Scaffold-based tissue engineering concepts involve the combination of viable cells, biomolecules, and a structural scaffold combined into a "construct" to promote the repair or regeneration of tissues. The construct is intended to support cell migration, growth, and differentiation, and guide tissue development and organization into a mature and healthy state. The science in this field is still in its infancy and various approaches and strategies are under experimental investigation. It is still not clear what defines ideal scaffold/cell or scaffold/neo-tissue constructs, even for a specific tissue type. The considerations are complex and include architecture, structural mechanics, surface properties, degradation products, and composition of biological components, and the changes of these factors with time *in vitro* or *in vivo* [2].

Scaffolds in tissue-engineered constructs have certain minimum requirements for biochemical as well as chemical and physical properties. Scaffolds must provide sufficient initial mechanical strength and stiffness to substitute for the mechanical function of the diseased or damaged tissue, which it aims at repairing or regenerating. Scaffolds may not necessarily be required to provide complete mechanical equivalence to healthy tissues, but stiffness and strength should be sufficient to at least support and transmit forces to the host tissue site in the context. For example, in skin tissue engineering, the construct should be able to withstand the wound contraction forces. In case of bone engineering, external and internal fixation systems might be applied to give support to the majority load-bearing forces until the bone has matured [3].

After the transplantation, a tissue-engineered construct cell and tissue remodeling are important for achieving stable biomechanical conditions and vascularization at the host site. Hence, the 3-D scaffold/tissue construct should maintain sufficient structural integrity during the *in vitro* or *in vivo* growth and remodeling process. The degree of remodeling depends on the tissue itself (e.g., skin 4–6 weeks, bone 4–6 months), and its host anatomy and physiology. Scaffold architecture has to allow for initial cell attachment and subsequent migration into and through the matrix, mass transfer of nutrients and metabolites, and provision for sufficient space for development and later remodeling of organized tissues. The degradation and resorption kinetics of the scaffold needs to be designed based on the relationships among mechanical properties, molecular weight (M_w/M_n), mass loss, and tissue development.

In addition to these essentials of mechanics and geometry, a suitable construct will possess surface properties, which are optimized for the attachment and migration of cell types of interest (depending on the targeted tissue). The external size and shape of the construct must also be considered, especially if the construct is customized for an individual patient [3]. Furthermore, considerations of scaffold performance based on a holistic tissue engineering strategy and practical considerations of manufacture arise. From a clinical point of view, it must be possible to manufacture scaffolds under Good Manufacturing Practice (GMP) conditions in a reproducible and quality-controlled fashion at an economic cost and speed. To move the current tissue engineering practices to the next frontier, some manufacturing processes will accommodate the incorporation of cells and the growth factors during the scaffold fabrication process.

What follows in this chapter is a description of one of the main fabrication methods that have been used over the last 5 years for creating nanoscale features for scaffolds—electrospinning.

5.2 ELECTROSPINNING

5.2.1 INTRODUCTION

Nanofibrous scaffolds are being exploited in tissue engineering due to their inherently high porosities and surface area-to-volume ratios as well as a wide variety of topographical features to encourage cellular adhesion, migration, and proliferation. Furthermore, the physical properties can be easily altered by altering the fiber size. Thus, there has been an exponential increase in tissue engineering scaffold materials research using the electrospinning technique (Figure 5.1). There are several different methods that have been employed to produce nanofibrous scaffolds for tissue engineering applications. These methods include self-assembly [4] and thermally induced phase separation (TIPS) each with its own benefits and drawbacks in replicating features of the natural ECM. Peptides are used to produce self-assembling scaffolds; however, this method requires highly specific physical and chemical interactions, which can place restrictions on the chemistry and mechanical properties of the scaffold. Phase separation can produce fibers of the same size range as the ECM, and 3-D porous networks can be generated within the scaffold, but it is often difficult to control fiber alignment and diameters. Furthermore a lengthy multistep process encumbers this procedure. Electrospinning provides a convenient approach to fabricate fibers that are within the size range of the ECM. This method allows for the rapid production and manipulation of unique sets of spatial and surface structures on the nano- and microscale and can also be used across a broad range of synthetic and natural polymers and their combinations. These aspects form the focus of this chapter.

5.2.1.1 Electrospinning Principles

Electrospinning, which so far has only been performed with synthetic polymers is now performed using either solutions with synthetic or natural polymers or a polymer melt. Electrospinning commonly results in a nonwoven mat of fibers (Figure 5.2), although other collection techniques are expanding the morphological nature of the scaffolds, particularly in fabricating oriented fibers. Typically, a high (positive or negative) voltage is applied to a polymer solution or melt that is pumped

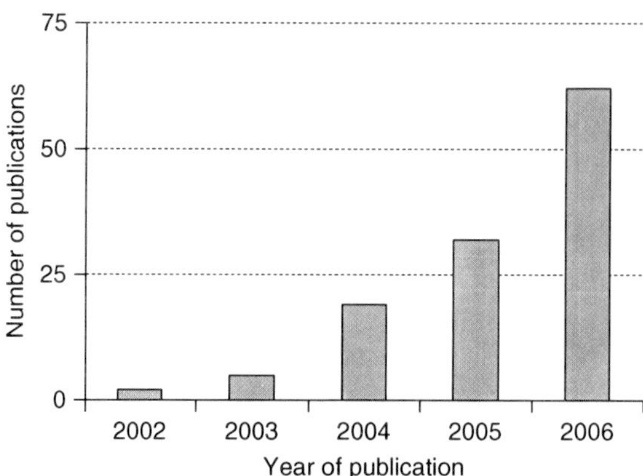

FIGURE 5.1 Number of Pubmed publications over the past 5 years relevant to electrospinning as scaffold fabrication method.

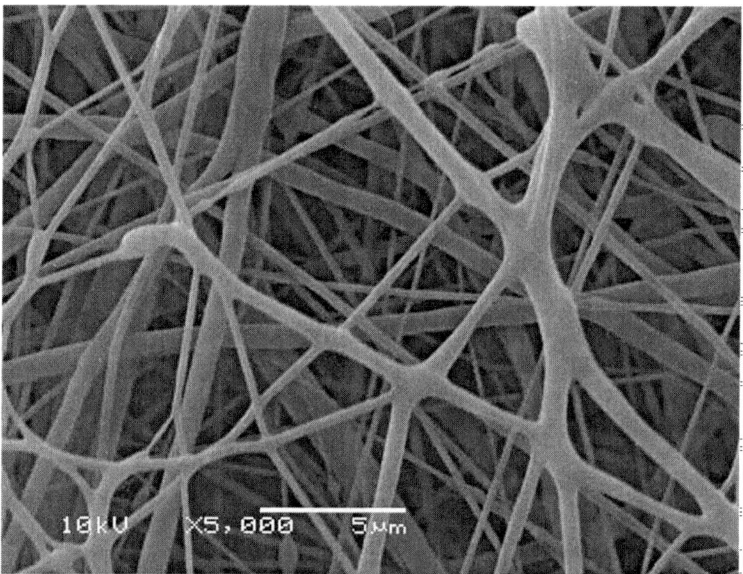

FIGURE 5.2 A typical random mat-like structure of micro- and nanometer-sized polymeric fibers obtained by electrospinning process.

to a spinneret (small orifice, or flat-tipped needle) facing an earthed target, or collector. Upon reaching a critical voltage, the surface tension of the polymer at spinneret tip is counterbalanced by localized charges generated by the electrostatic force, and the droplet elongates and stretches into a (Taylor) cone where a continuous jet is ejected. (*Safety note*: Such high applied voltages need to be safety protected and should only deliver low currents since an exposure to high amperages may result in death.)

A schematic description of the electrospinning process is shown in Figure 5.3. Initially, the polymer jet travels toward the target, but statistical perturbations result in some deviation from the most direct path to the collector. As a charged entity moving across an electric field, a force that is 90°

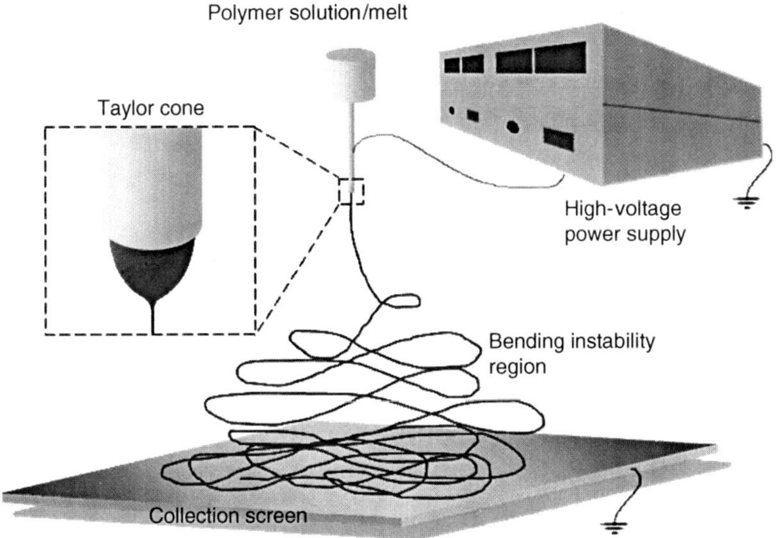

FIGURE 5.3 Schematic drawing of the electrospinning process. As the metal capillary is charged by a high-voltage bias, polymer solution or melt is ejected from the tip forming the Taylor cone. The polymer jet spirals downward while bending and stretching, creating ultrathin fibers. Processing conditions, such as working distance, voltage, and concentration, can be easily adapted to allow for the fabrication of different fiber diameters and orientation. Orientation is changed simply by using different collection devices such as dual rings, rapidly rotating drums, etc.

to the electric field is imparted on the polymer jet, and a spiraling of the jet results. The diameter of the spiral is eventually balanced by the surface tension of the polymer solution or melt; however, the polymer jet undergoes magnitudinal (up to five orders) reduction in diameter as it travels toward the collector. Solvent evaporation or cooling of the polymer prior to landing at the collector results in electrospun fibers with sizes typically between 200 nm and 5 µm, depending on the conditions. The effects of aerodynamics and gravity are small, and electrospinning can be performed with the spinneret(s) and collector(s) in either the vertical or the horizontal axis [5]. Several methods of nanofiber collection systems are shown in Figure 5.4 below.

The path of the polymer jet and the forces involved with it are extremely dynamic and the collection is rapid. It has been determined that the initial polymer jet reaches a speed of 15 m/s before velocimetry data become difficult to interpret due to the bending instabilities. Such high speeds, coupled with long spiraled traveling distances, make accurately controlled deposition of the electrospun fiber technically challenging.

Electrospinning parameters such as applied electric voltage, polymer solution or melt flow rate, needle-to-collector distance, solution concentration, and solvent type affect the resulting fiber morphology and dimensions. Figure 5.5 shows the effect of changes in electric voltage in the resulting dimensions of a poly(caprolactone) (PCL) and collagen (PCL/Col) blend system. It was observed that increasing the voltage from 10 to 20 kV decreased the average diameter of the fibers whereas doubling the flow rate from 0.75 to 1.50 mL/h did not affect the diameter significantly. However, it was reported elsewhere that the relationship might not be linear. Baumgarten revealed that increasing the applied field up to a certain threshold might instead cause incremental increase in the fiber diameter. It was proposed that increasing the electric filed strength causes an increase in volumetric flow rate of the polymer out of the capillary [6].

The effect of polymer concentration in morphology and dimensions of electrospun collagen type I fibers can be observed in Figure 5.6. Bovine collagen was dissolved at varying solution concentration

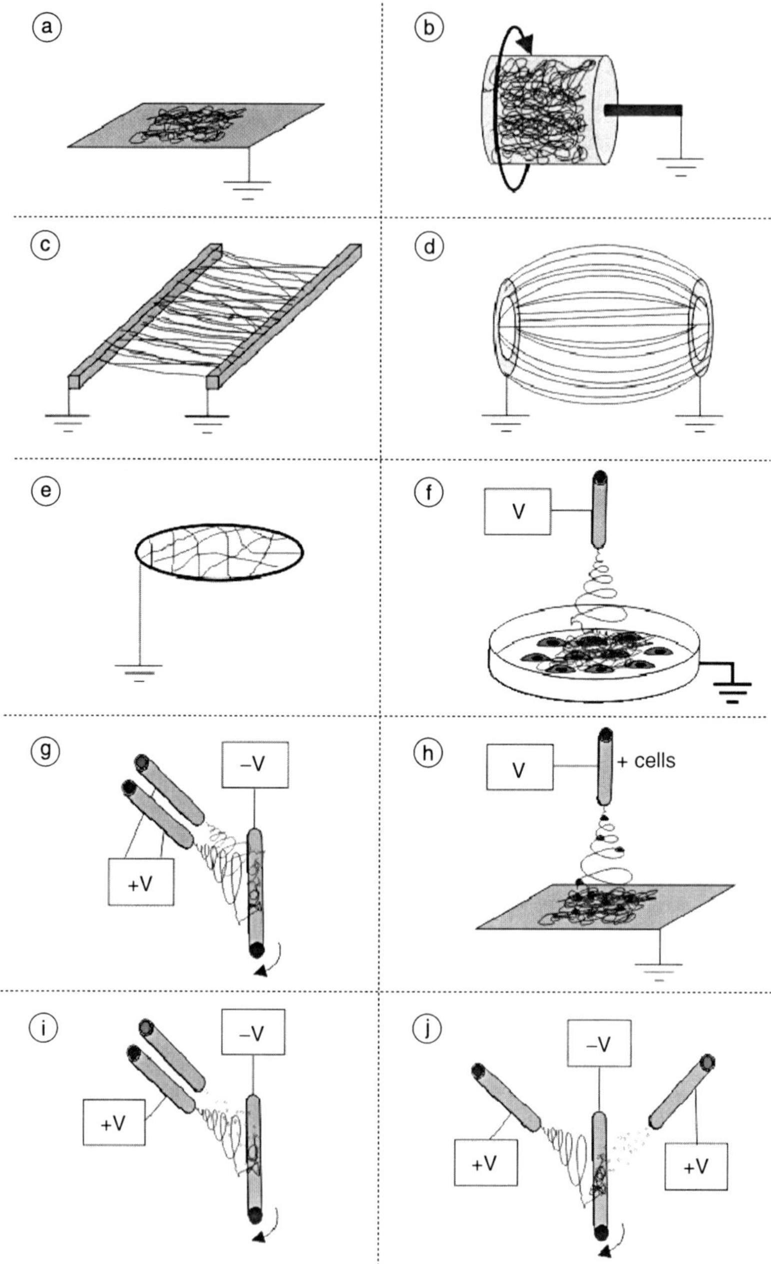

FIGURE 5.4 Selected collection schemes for electrospun fibers (red): (a) single ground, (b) rotating single ground, (c) dual bar, (d) dual ring, (e) single horizontal ring, (f) electrospinning *in vitro* onto cells, (g) dual spinneret electrospinning, (h) electrospinning cells with polymer electrospinning–electrospraying with (i) parallel and (j) perpendicular spinnerets.

from 5% to 15% w/v in 1,1,1,3,3,3-fluoroisopropanol (HFIP) and was electrospun with identical conditions, that is, 10 kV applied voltage, 12 cm tip-to-collector distance, and 0.75 mL/h flow rate. Below 8% solution concentration, the collagen fibers were deposited in wet state. This deposition is due to incomplete evaporation of the solvent during electrospinning and it results in more fusion spots when a fiber comes into contact with another. A concentration of 8–10% produced more uniform and

Electrospinning parameters	Fiber dimension (nm)
10 kV, 0.75 mL/h	513 ± 83
15 kV, 0.75 mL/h	327 ± 60
20 kV, 0.75 mL/h	308 ± 58
10 kV, 1.50 mL/h	466 ± 97
15 kV, 1.50 mL/h	356 ± 63
20 kV, 1.50 mL/h	361 ± 43

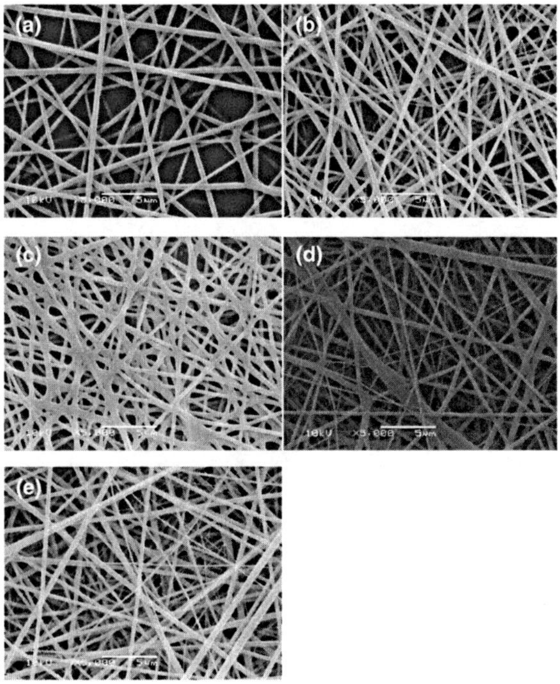

FIGURE 5.5 PCL/Col 20% fibers electrospun with varying voltage and polymer flow rate. Electrospinning distance was kept at 15 cm: (a) 10 kV, 0.75 mL/h, (b) 15 kV, 0.75 mL/h, (c) 20 kV, 0.75 mL/h, (d) 15 kV, 1.5 mL/h, and (e) 20 kV, 1.5 mL/h. Table on the left summarizes the correlation between electrospinning parameters and resulting fiber dimension.

dry fibers with 10% concentration, giving relatively larger diameter fibers and more ribbon formation in the structure. Electrospinning of the collagen became more difficult with concentration above 10% due to viscosity effects. Beading and formation of extremely thick fibers were observed for 15% collagen concentration.

Similar findings were observed with the electrospinning of poly(ethylene oxide) (PEO) as shown in Figure 5.7. The fiber size and morphology of PEO depend on the solution concentrations used for the electrospinning process. At the lower concentration (10%) bead formations were significant although fine fibers were forming as well. Formation of beads is common in polymer solutions with lower concentrations. Viscoelastic forces of polymer jets during the electrospinning process resist fast changes in the fiber shape while surface tension attempts to minimize the surface area. The latter prevails in lower concentration (thus lower viscosity) of polymers while the former is dominant in higher concentration solutions promoting the formation of smooth fibers (Figure 5.7a, 15%, 20%, and 25%). Viscoelastic forces also cause the apparent increase in fiber diameter by resisting the stretching and splaying in the bending instability region.

The morphology of electrospun fibers also depends on the flow rate of polymer to the electrospinning tip. Such effect in the electrospinning of PEO fibers is illustrated in Figure 5.7b. At slower flow rates (0.5 mL/h), polymer mass transfer was not fast enough to maintain a stable jet, which resulted in the formation of beads and broken fibers. Increasing the flow rate improved the stability of the electrospinning jet although beads still formed at 1.0 mL/h and breakages were observed at 1.5 mL/h. At 2.0 mL/h, relatively smooth fibers free of beads and breakages were formed.

Choice of the solvent is one of the critical parameters in electrospinning of polymeric materials. Conductivity, surface tension, dielectric constant, and viscosity are properties of the polymer

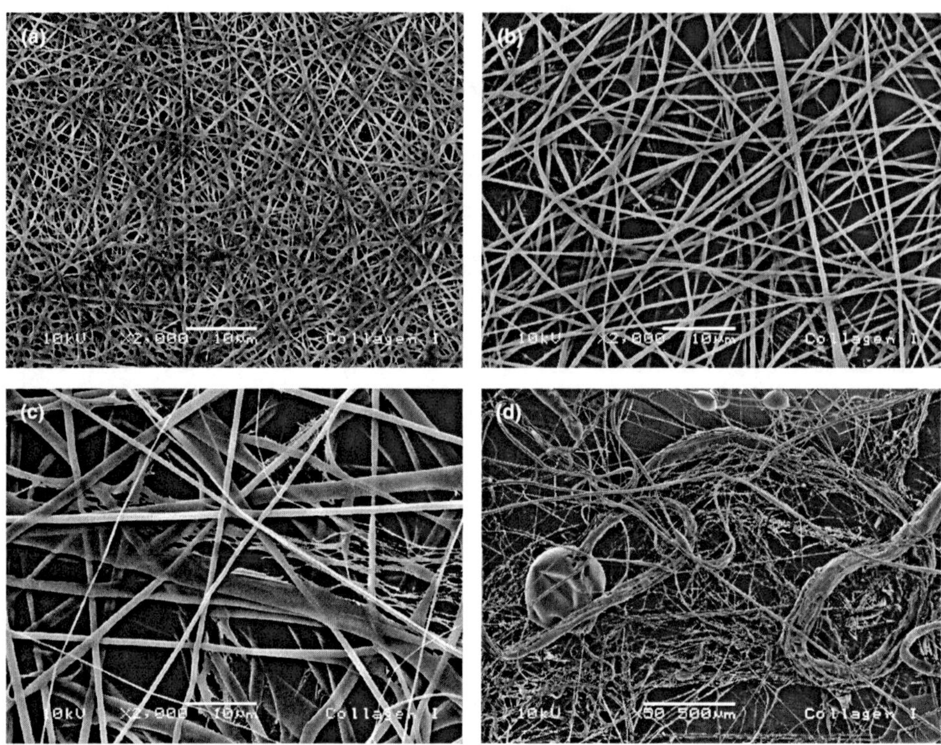

FIGURE 5.6 Electrospun bovine type I collagen with different concentrations: (a) 5% w/v, (b) 8% w/v, (c) 10% w/v, and (d) 15% w/v. Electrospinning voltage, flow rate, and distance were kept at 10 kV, 0.75 mL/h, and 12 cm, respectively. Below 8% concentration, the electrospun fibers were deposited wet while above 10%, formation of submicron-sized fibers was extremely difficult due to high viscosity.

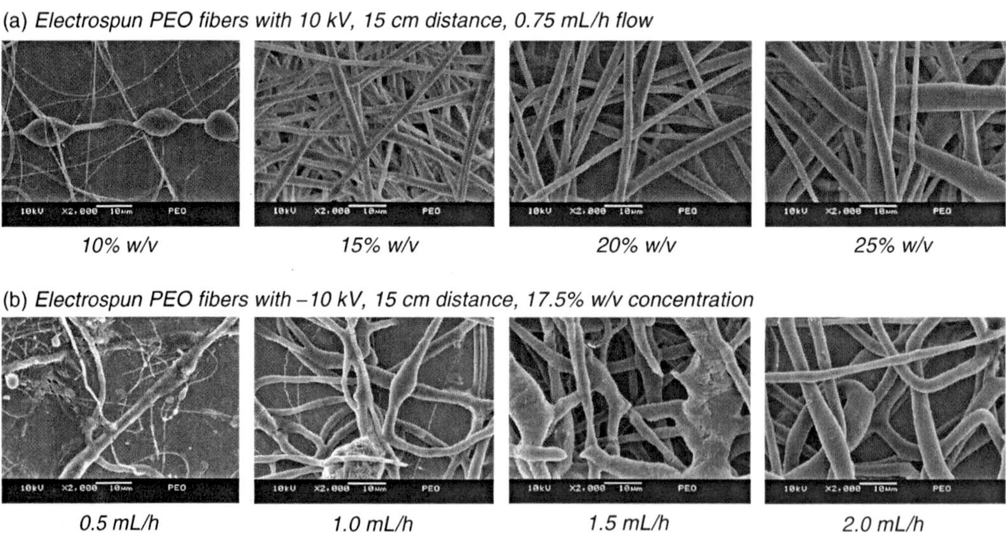

FIGURE 5.7 Electrospun PEO nanofibers obtained with varying parameters. (a) PEO solution concentration affects the final fiber morphology. At lower concentration, beading is more prominent than fibers whereas increasing the concentration results in more uniform and thicker fibers. (b) Variation in morphology due to changes in material flow rate to the capillary. At low material transfer rate, breakages in the fibers occurred while a faster transfer rate allows continuous fiber to be drawn.

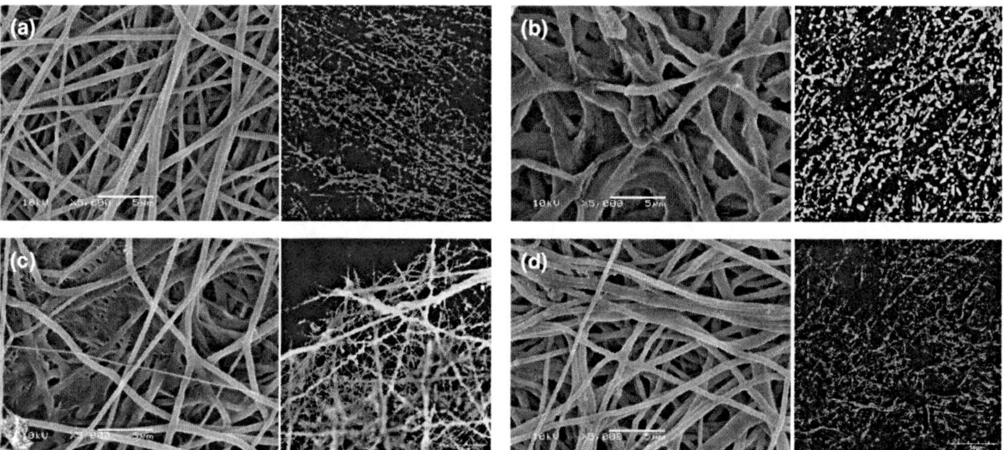

FIGURE 5.8 (a) SEM and fluorescence images of electrospun PCL/Col fibers doped with rhodamine. (b) SEM and fluorescence images of electrospun PEO fibers doped with FITC. (c) Co-electrospinning of PCL/Col and PEO. The two polymers exhibited mixing in the structure with PEO fibers showing more irregular fiber morphology. FITC/rhodamine fluorescence confirmed the mixing of the two fiber species. (d) Leaching of PEO from the structure, leaving only rhodamine-doped PCL/Col.

solution that are directly related to the solvent used. In a study done by Lee et al., morphology of PCL electrospun fibers was highly dependent on the solvent composition. The addition of N,N-dimethylformamide (DMF) into methylene chloride (MC) improved the resulting conductivity of the solution, thus resulting in much finer fibers compared to MC alone [7]. Interaction between the solvent and the polymer chains determines the flexibility of the molecules. Orientation of the polymer molecules and thus stretching of the jet is facilitated during bending instability, resulting in thinner fibers [8].

It is possible to electrospin two or more different species of polymers into a single nanofibrous membrane structure. Figure 5.8 shows co-electrospinning of PCL/Col blend and PEO nanofibers. To visualize the distribution of both fibers, PCL/Col solution was doped with rhodamine dye (Figure 5.8a, red color) and PEO was doped with FITC dye (Figure 5.8b, green color). When they were spun together using a two-syringe electrospinning system and rotating mandrel as a collector, the two fibers were intertwined in the final nanofiber mesh (Figure 5.8c). As PEO is a water-soluble polymer, immersion of the mesh in an aqueous solution resulted in leaching of PEO from the structure leaving only the PCL/Col component (Figure 5.8d).

5.2.1.2 Collection Systems

The collectors may have a range of shapes or configurations. The vast majority of electrospinning systems use a single collection plate to collect the fibers, while grounding a single rotating cylindrical collector can collect fibrous mats, orient the fibers in a thin sheet of fabric, or make a tubular (bilayered) construct. Oriented fibers can also be obtained using dual, grounded collection plates, or rings. In this configuration, the fibers are suspended in a space between the two grounds. Additionally, a ring of wire, when used horizontally as a collector, results in a thin membrane upon which cells can be seeded. Collection systems may also be a hydrogel, water, a confluent layer of cells, or part of a living body.

5.2.1.3 Polymer Solutions

The major parameters controlling the fiber diameter are the concentration of the spinning solution, the electric conductivity of the solution or melt, as well as the feeding rate of the spinning solution. The thickness of the fiber tends to increase with increasing concentration of the solution, and it can be reduced significantly by increasing the electric conductivity, for instance (e.g., by adding salts). Thicker fibers result if the feeding rate, that is, the amount of spinning solution flowing through the die is increased. The magnitude of the applied electric field may also affect the fiber diameter (see Figure 5.5). Fibers with circular cross-section are in most cases formed by electrospinning, yet ribbon-like fibers with a rectangular cross-section have also been manufactured. It is assumed that their formation is the result of a rapid evaporation of the solvent causing skin formation followed by a collapse of the fibers toward a rectangular cross-section. Hollow and porous fibers can also be produced by electrospinning. The electrospinning process itself is characterized by a swift and physically powerful elongational deformation of the spinning jet due to a specific volatility, the so-called whipping instability, which takes place in the course of fiber formation [9].

The whipping mode corresponds to long wavelength oscillations of the centerline of the jet, that is, the jet is subjected to bending modes. The whipping mode tends to dominate for large static charge densities because high charge densities at the surface simultaneously tend to suppress both the decomposition of the jet into individual droplets resulting from the Rayleigh and the axisymmetric modes of instabilities. The corresponding large deformation of the jet gives rise to nanofibers displaying a strong orientation of the chain molecules as well as of the crystals in the fiber, as evident, for instance, from electron diffraction studies [10]. Such orientations cause significant increase in the mechanical stiffness and strength of the fibers. A particular advantage of nanofibers is its high strength due to the low probability of defects on the fiber surface acting as nucleating sites for cracks. A tensile study done on single electrospun PCL fibers revealed that both stress at break and yield stress decreased with increasing fiber diameter whereas strain at break was found to decrease with increasing diameter [11]. To further enhance stiffness and strength, biodegradable polymers are spun to nanofibers displaying liquid crystalline phases. Molecular self-organization effects characterize such phases that are already in the fluid phase, and their signature is the formation of spontaneous orientational orders.

Nanofibers with surface nanopores can also be produced along various routes. Mixed solvents or single solvents causing phase separations into solvent-rich and solvent-poor areas within the jet or ternary solutions containing two different polymers, which phase separate in the fibers, have been used for this purpose. Pore formation can also be induced in highly humid conditions where condensation processes lead to the formation of water islands within the fibers.

Many publications report various polymeric fibers electrospun from solutions, both degradable and nondegradable, and from organic and aqueous solutions. The collected fibers may demonstrate various morphologies, with beads and fused structures, and some with distinct nanotopographies. Nonwoven scaffolds have been fabricated from a large number of polymeric materials, and many different cell types have been deposited onto these with positive results. In addition, some cells seeded on oriented fibrous mats result in oriented cell growth, or demonstrate some guided axonal growth in the case of neurons.

One issue with the use of solvents, which are typically volatile, in electrospinning for TE applications is their toxicity. Electrospun scaffolds from such polymer solutions therefore require solvent removal prior to cell seeding. Electrospun polymeric aqueous solutions necessitate airborne crosslinking prior to collection onto any aqueous-based target to avoid redissolution, with the traveling time between the spinneret and collector being in the order of milliseconds.

5.2.2 Electrospinning of Natural Polymers

5.2.2.1 Collagen/Gelatin

Two methods have been currently adopted for collagen electrospinning. The first method involves the electrospinning of highly concentrated pure collagen dissolved in a highly volatile solvent, commonly utilized 1,1,1,3,3,3-hexafluoro-2-propanol (HFP) and 2,2,2-trifluoroethanol (TFE), and the second involves the electrospinning of a blend of low collagen concentration in acidic solution and a high molecular weight polymer, commonly utilized PEO with M_w of 900 kDa. However, the nanofibrous meshes resulting from these processes are known to dissolve rapidly in water, tissue fluids, or blood and to lack the characteristic D-period of collagen. This property is highly suggestive of denatured collagen or gelatin, a material that is characterized by disrupted fibrillar and triple-helical structure and destroyed peptide chains, without internal structure or configurational order. Furthermore, electrospun collagen scaffolds have been shown to have low cell adhesion levels similar to those of gelatin, possibly attributed to denaturation induced via the electrospinning itself. Shields et al. reported that electrospun collagen type II was able to support attachment and proliferation of chondrocytes, making it a suitable environment for the creation of an articular cartilage repair scaffold [12]. These collagen scaffolds, however, required glutaraldehyde cross-linking prior to *in vitro* cellular assays due to their rapid dissolution in aqueous media.

5.2.2.2 Chitosan

Chitosan is another naturally occurring polymer that has been electrospun into nanofibers. Due to its abundance and relatively good biocompatibility, chitosan has attracted interest in the field of biomedical materials. Ohkawa et al. reported the electrospinning of pure chitosan nanofibers using a variety of solvents and found that trifluoroacetic acid (TFA) and dicholoromethane mixture was a better choice to obtain a homogenous chitosan fibers [13]. In another study using acetic acid as a solvent, Geng et al. found an optimal working acetic acid concentration for the fabrication of uniform, bead-free chitosan fibers [14]. A water-soluble polymer PEO has been reported to be used as a blend with chitosan to improve the size and morphology of the resulting fibers. Bhattarai et al. used a solution comprising of 90/10 chitosan:PEO to fabricate homogenous fibers with diameter of about 40 nm [15].

5.2.2.3 Hyaluronic Acid

Due to its biocompatibility and its abundant presence in the ECM of various tissues such as skin and cartilage, hyaluronic acid (HA) is quickly gaining interest as a scaffolding material in tissue engineering. However, the electrospinning of pure HA has been met with challenges. High viscosity and surface tension of aqueous HA solutions make electrospinning arduous. This issue can be tackled by employing a combination of electrospinning and air blowing technique whereby a flow of hot air is applied to the spinneret assisting the fabrication of nanosized HA fibers with uniform diameters. The hot air flow assists the pulling of fibers from the spinneret, decreases the solution viscosity by elevating the ambient temperature, and increases evaporation rate of the aqueous solvent [16]. A more recent development involves the usage of DMF:water solvent mixture [17] at a volume ratio of 1.5:0.5 DMF to water. This allowed the fabrication of HA and HA/gelatin blend fibers with sizes between 200 and 500 nm without the need for hot air blowing.

An alternative method of the electrospinning of HA fibers is the usage of reactive electrospinning. A low molecular weight derivative of HA, 3,30-dithiobis(propanoic dihydrazide)-modified HA (HA-DTPH), which is thiol-modified, was used in conjunction with a cross-linking agent, poly(ethylene glycol) diacrylate (PEGDA) [18,19]. A dual-syringe mixing technique was used to facilitate the simultaneous cross-linking of the solution and electrospinning, resulting in the deposition of cross-linked HA hydrogel nanofiber system. Utilization of lower molecular weight HA together with PEO as viscosity modifier allowed the fine-tuning of solution properties previously difficult with natural high molecular weight HA. PEO can be subsequently removed from water afterward, and the resulting hydrogel showed good *in vitro* biocompatibility and cellular integration.

5.2.3 ELECTROSPINNING OF SYNTHETIC POLYMERS

Electrospinning has opened new possibilities previously not possible with other methods of synthetic polymer fabrication. Nanofibers of vast number of polymers, for example, poly(lactic acid)

(PLA), poly(ethylene terepthalate) (PET), poly(3-hydroxybutyrate) (P3HB), PCL, etc. have been fabricated using the electrospinning technique and exploited for their potential in tissue engineering. Perhaps the most studied group of polymers is the biodegradable poly(α-hydroxy esters), which are already used in the clinics. Polymers such as PLA or poly(glycolic acid) (PGA) have already found multitude of applications in the biomedical field, which was pioneered by the usage of resorbable sutures. Other polymers such as PCL, poly(anhydrides), poly(orthoesters), and other biodegradable materials have also been electrospun and characterized.

Synthetic materials offer advantages over naturally derived materials since they have less batch-to-batch variations, are more reliable source of raw materials, and can be designed to give a wider range of properties, that is, by fine-tuning the homopolymer and their copolymers. Li et al. studied the mechanical and degradation properties of six groups of electrospun poly(α-hydroxy esters) and their copolymers, that is, PGA, PLGA5050, PLGA8515, PLLA, PDLLA, and PCL. It was revealed that PGA and PLGA polymers were mechanically the stiffest but also more prone to hydrolytic degradation in physiological conditions. PLLA and PCL on the other hand were the more compliant and stable of the group [20]. These groups of electrospun polymers have also often reported to exhibit good capability to support cellular attachment, proliferation, and differentiation. PCL nanofibers show promising potential to be used in cartilage tissue engineering as they were able to sustain the phenotype of chondrocytes and cartilage-like matrix deposition [21]. Furthermore, smooth muscle cells (SMC) and endothelial cells were successfully cultured *in vitro* on PLLA–CL composite electrospun nanofibers indicating potential applications of the polymer in the field of vascular tissue engineering [22].

Badami et al. [23] more specifically investigated the effect of fiber diameter (0.14 and 2.1 μm) of electrospun PLA and poly(ethylene glycol)poly(D,L-lactic acid) (PEG-PLA) block copolymer randomly oriented membranes on the cellular behavior of osteoprogenitor cells (MC3T3-E1). *In vitro* cell studies in the presence of osteogenic factors after 14 days culture showed higher cell densities on larger fibers compared with smaller fibers and the spin-coated controls; however, there was no significant difference in ALP activity. Cell morphology measured by the cell-projected area was not influenced by fiber diameter, but both were significantly smaller than cells cultured on the flat spin–coated controls. However, the aspect ratio of the cells cultured on the 2.1 μm fibers was significantly higher and attributed to increased contact guidance. Focal adhesion contacts occurred predominantly as clusters along the polymer fibers, and the actin stress fibers extended perpendicularly across the polymer fibers and were parallel to each other.

Besides acting as cell delivery agents and tissue scaffolding, electrospun nanofibers have attracted attention as a vehicle of bioactive molecule delivery. Luong-Van et al. incorporated heparin into electrospun PCL nanofiber mats and showed 50% release of the heparin during the first 14 days. The heparin-containing PCL nanofibers exhibited no proinflammatory response, uniform distribution of heparin, and an antiproliferative effect toward SMCs [24]. Another study involved the incorporation of plasmid DNA into electrospun PLGA with PLA–PEG block copolymer. Burst release of DNA after 2 h was observed although release was continued until 20 days of the experiments with up to 80% of the incorporated DNA released. The plasmid DNA was intact as assayed by the expression of the β-Gal gene by MC3T3 cell line [25].

5.2.3.1 Solution Spinning

Electrospinning of synthetic polymers from a solution is the conventional method of obtaining nanofibers. Organic solvents such as chloroform, TFE, DMF, HFIP, and so on are commonly used to dissolve polymers into solutions of known concentrations and viscosity. Dielectric constant, volatility, surface tension, and polymer solubility are aspects of solvents that need to be considered prior to electrospinning. Furthermore, in tissue engineering and biomedical field, toxicity of solvent becomes an increasingly critical issue. Most of the solvents that can be used to dissolve synthetic polymer show some degree of cytotoxicity. Thus it is imperative that solvent must be thoroughly removed from the system prior to any *in vitro* or *in vivo* experimentation. Alternatively, electrospinning of polymers from their molten state can be used to bypass the toxicity issues related to solution spinning.

5.2.3.2 Melt Electrospinning

A very recent aspect of electrospinning is the fabrication of electrospun fibers scaffolds from polymer melts. Melt electrospinning has some technical advantages over polymer solutions for certain tissue engineering applications. It is possible to melt electrospin directly onto cells *in vitro* without issues of solvent toxicity or suitable cross-linking while cell vitality remains unaffected by the process. Figure 5.9a shows the setup of a simple melt electrospinning system and an electron micrograph of a melt-spun PCL-PEG block copolymer. Fibers obtained were slightly larger than solvent electrospinning but uniformity and morphology were comparable. Figure 5.9b shows results of a direct *in vitro* melt electrospinning experiment onto live porcine bone marrow cells previously seeded on a PCL/Col nanofiber mesh. Cells remained viable after 1 week post-spinning. Electron micrograph of the construct revealed that cells adhered to both PCL/Col nanofiber substrate and the melt-spun PCL–PEG polymer. These results indicate nontoxicity and cyto-compatibility of the melt electrospinning process. This is important for fabricating layered tissue–engineering constructs, where cells and electrospun scaffolds are ordered into lamellar structures, and for directly electrospinning onto tissue for *in vivo* applications.

With polymer melts, there is additionally no solvent evaporation at the spinneret compared with the formation of a polymer skin when using volatile solvents. Such defects, which can affect the morphology of the collected electrospun fibers with large-sized structures deposited on top of the smaller fibers, are commonly encountered when electrospinning from polymer solutions is conducted over long time periods. Melt electrospinning has the potential, therefore, to produce more uniform fibers over longer electrospinning times than fibers electrospun from polymer solutions.

5.3 PHYSICAL CHARACTERIZATION OF ELECTROSPUN SCAFFOLDS

The morphology and surface properties of scaffolds strongly influence their interaction with cells. The surface properties of the biomaterials can be categorized into geometric, topographical, and surface chemical properties. Geometric and topographic properties include the roughness of two-dimensional (2-D) polymer surfaces [26–28] as well as the porosity, pore size, and pore size distribution, intrafiber surface roughness and the specific surface area for porous and nonwoven polymer membranes. Surface chemical properties affect the water wettability or hydrophilicity of scaffolds and their energies and can often be manipulated by surface modifications.

5.3.1 Measuring Porosity, Surface Roughness, and Specific Surface Energy of Scaffolds

A traditional method for characterizing the porosity and pore size distribution is mercury porosimetry (Figure 5.10). This method is a liquid intrusion method; it assumes that the pores are cylindrical and pore size is expressed in terms of the diameter of the opening. Pores with diameters smaller than 2 nm, between 2 and 50 nm, and larger than 50 nm are referred to as micropores, mesopores, and macropores, respectively. Mercury has a high surface tension (485.5 dynes/cm at 25°C) and forms large contact angles with most other materials ($\cong 130°$) [29] and does not penetrate pores by capillary action. A positive pressure must be applied to force mercury into the pores. The pore size can be calculated from the pressure applied by the following equation:

$$D = \frac{-4\gamma \cos \theta}{P}$$

where D is the diameter of the pore, γ is the surface tension of mercury, θ is the contact angle between mercury and the solid, and P is the applied pressure. The direct data acquired is the accumulated

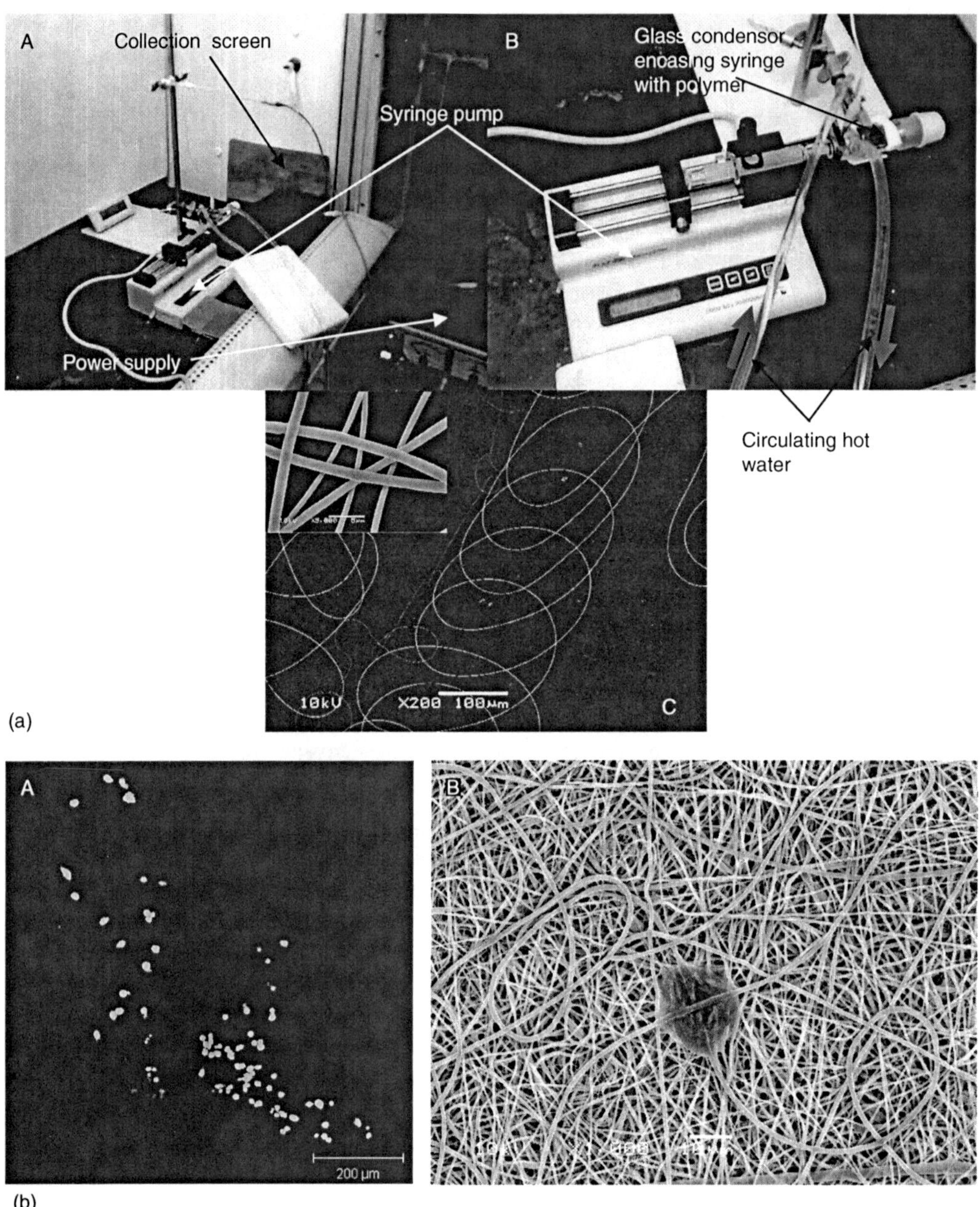

FIGURE 5.9 (a) Setup of electrospinning of polymeric materials from the melt. Basic system consists of a syringe pump, a high-voltage power supply, and a heating circulator to facilitate melting and maintenance of high temperature for the polymer (A and B). The collected melt electrospun fibers are shown in (C). Insert in C shows a higher magnification of the melt-spun fibers. (b) Direct *in vitro* melt electrospinning of PCL-PEG block copolymer onto bone marrow cells pre-seeded on PCL/Col nanofiber mesh. (A) Live-death assay using FDA-PI revealed relatively good viability of the cells after 1 week of culturing post-spinning. (B) Electron micrograph after 1 week culturing post-spinning showing a cell attaching to both PCL/Col nanofiber substrate and melt-spun PCL-PEG.

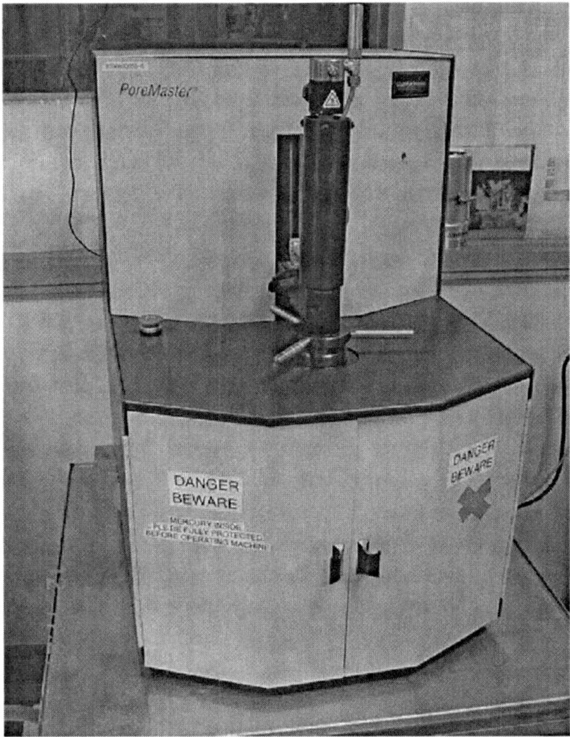

FIGURE 5.10 Mercury porosimeter instrument for the measurement of scaffold porosity.

volume of mercury as it enters the porous system. A pore size distribution curve can then be obtained by relating the accumulated volume to some pore size distribution function. Mercury porosimetry has been used for characterizing the architecture of electrospun nanofiber matrices and to study the effects of processing conditions on the pore size distribution [30–33]. There are, however, some reports suggesting that the pressure applied to polymer samples could cause irreversible structural compression.

Surface roughness is one of the critical surface parameters that not only potentially affects cell response to biomaterials, but also affects the characterization of the material surface. Scanning electron microscopy (SEM) is the most common method employed to qualitatively assess the surface roughness of electrospun scaffolds [27,34]. More quantitative evaluation of surface roughness may be obtained using atomic force microscopy (AFM) (for nanoscale roughness) and a range of contact and noncontact (optical) profilometers (for larger scale roughness).

The contact angle is formed at the junction of three phases (i.e., solid, liquid, and gas) and is linked to the liquid surface tension and the solid surface energy through the Young's equation. The surface energy of a solid is determined by the intermolecular forces, which are of the same origin as those holding atoms and molecules together in the bulk. An isotropic liquid surface provides a special condition for the surface energy to be directly measured. The surface energy of a pure liquid (which has the unit of mJ/m^2, milli-Joules per square meter) is equivalent to surface tension (mN/m, milli-Newtons per meter). For a solid surface, however, there is no established method to directly measure the surface energy. The surface energy of the solid can be estimated by contact angle measurements using liquids with known surface energy.

5.3.1.1 Scanning Electron Microscopy, Atomic Force Microscopy, and Confocal Laser Microscopy

It is important to have a measure of the interfiber distance and fiber diameter of the electrospun scaffolds as these properties influence cell adhesion, migration, differentiation, and proliferation. There are two main methods that are commonly utilized: (1) laser scanning confocal microscopy and (2) SEM. These techniques also have the ability to preserve the structure of any biological material in relation to the fibers.

The characterization of the fibers using laser scanning confocal microscopy requires the usage of some form of fluorescence labeling, for example, doping the polymer solutions with 0.05% w/v of rhodamine or fluorescein. This method may also be employed to characterize colocalization of fibers during multifiber spinning. Furthermore, this technique is particularly useful when immunochemical method is employed to detect specific entities, that is, proteins on the fibers by using dye-labeled antibody. Confocal microscopy can also be used as an *in vitro* tool to assess viability and distribution of cells on the nanofiber membranes. Figure 5.11 shows images of a double-sided seeding of PCL/Col nanofibrous membranes with SMCs. Cells situated on the top and bottom faces of the membrane were stained prior to seeding with cell tracker red and green, respectively. SEM is arguably the simplest method for fiber dimensions analysis. Most SEM systems are equipped with applications that allow point-to-point distance measurements. Immunogold labeling technique can be used in SEM for more specific applications such as detection of a particular matrix protein in the samples.

Jaeger et al. [35] were the first to report that when using AFM to measure the diameters of individual electrospun fibers, values were likely to be overestimated due to the geometry of the AFM tip. Specific surface areas of porous and fibrous polymers can be measured by the BET gas absorption method. The theory behind this method can be found in many classic physical chemistry books [36]. BET gas adsorption has been used to measure specific surface areas of electrospun fibrous membranes [37,38].

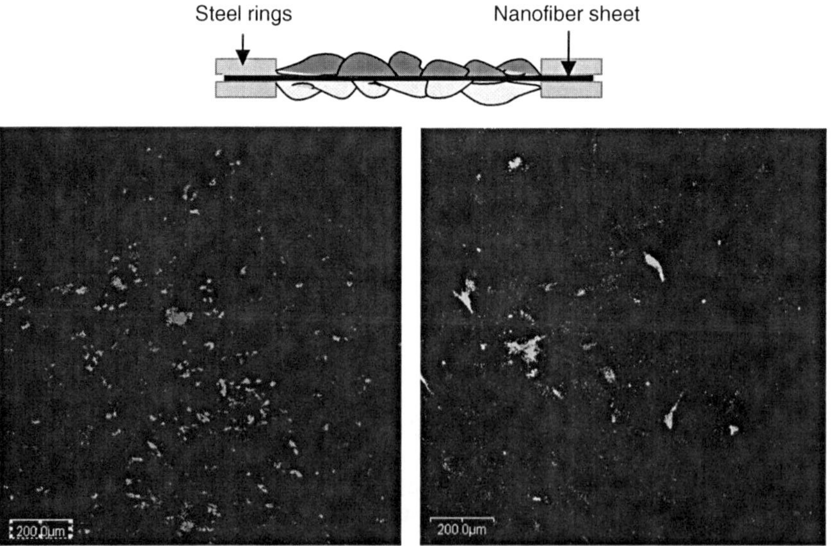

FIGURE 5.11 Schematic drawing showing the double-sided seeding of SMCs on PCL/Col nanofiber sheets using steel rings as an *in vitro* suspension culture method. Viability assays using cell tracker red and green and laser confocal scanning microscopy revealed live cells at the top and bottom surfaces, respectively.

5.3.2 MECHANICAL TESTING

Mechanical behavior is an important parameter in designing and developing new biomaterials. Mechanical and structural integrity of the nanofiber scaffolds are crucial to withstand *in vitro* culture conditions and surgical manipulations. Tensile testing is often used as a method to determine and compare mechanical properties of electrospun nanofiber membranes. As shown in Figure 5.12, composition of the nanofiber mesh is an important parameter in determining its resulting mechanical properties. Collagen incorporation (20% by weight) into the PCL matrix resulted in a mesh with inferior modulus and stress at break although its elongation at break was slightly improved. Physical and chemical interactions between PCL and collagen may have resulted in a weaker composite material with different domains or phases in its structure.

Parameters and conditions at which the mechanical testing was performed may affect the resulting mechanical properties. Temperature and humidity are two factors that might affect a material's behavior under observation. Thus it is imperative to simulate a testing environment, which is relevant to the intended applications of the material. For instance, the tensile tests shown in Figure 5.12 were done at 37°C with PBS immersion. As PCL is a thermoplastic with glass transition temperature of about −60°C and a low melting point of around 60°C, it exists in a rubbery state at ambient temperature. Fluctuation in temperature may affect its mechanical characteristics. Furthermore the intended application of the PCL and PCL/Col nanofiber was for *in vivo* implantation. Hence, 37°C was chosen with complete immersion in saline to better mimic the *in vivo* environment. Room temperature testing may also be carried out in tandem in order to determine and compare ease of handling before the implantation, ease of suturing, etc.

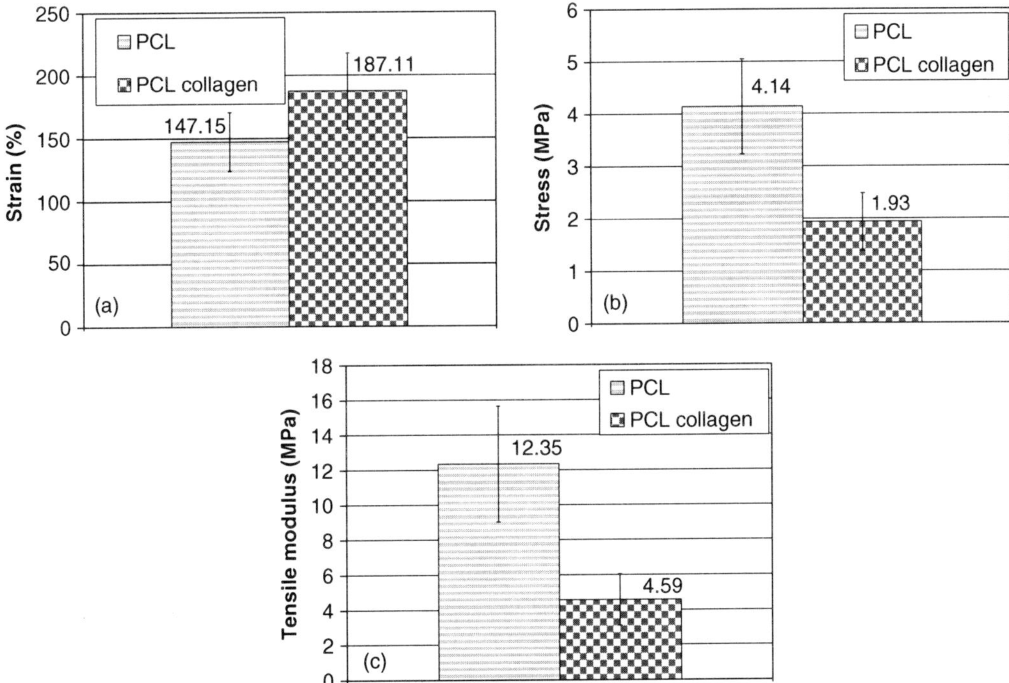

FIGURE 5.12 Mechanical properties comparison of pure PCL and PCL/Col blend electrospun nanofiber membranes. Addition of collagen into the PCL structure resulted in a slight increase in elongation at break (a) and decreases in stress at break and tensile modulus (b and c, respectively). The tensile test was carried out at 37°C in phosphate-buffered saline (PBS) immersion.

5.4 TISSUE ENGINEERING APPLICATIONS BY USING ELECTROSPUN SCAFFOLDS

5.4.1 BONE TISSUE ENGINEERING

Bone is a composite material made from an organic phase of collagen, glycoproteins, and glycosaminoglycans (GAGs) and an inorganic phase primarily consisting of hydroxyapatite (HA) $Ca_{10}(PO_4)_6(OH)_2$ [39]. Bone serves several critical functions including muscular support, production of blood cells and immune cells, and as a mineral reservoir to maintain electrolyte balance in the body. Bone may be lost after trauma, cancer, fractures, periodontitis, osteoporosis, and infectious disease, and presently there are several types and sources used as bone grafts.

Bone is the second most transplanted tissue, second to blood. Current treatment regimes for the reconstruction or enhancement of function of damaged bone rely on autogenous or allogenic tissue grafts. Autogenous bone, by providing an osteoconductive matrix, growth factors, and osteogenic cells (which form the critical elements of bone repair), remains the graft material of choice despite the associated donor site morbidity inflicted on the patient, the potential of infection at the bone harvest site, painful surgical procedure, and the risk of injuring surrounding structures. Surgeons are increasingly facing patient groups, which have limited supply of transplantable autologous bone due to multiple operations, poor bone quality, and patient groups that have limitations for large bone grafts, especially children. The continuing clinical need for improvement of existing treatments for bone disorders ranging from congenital deformity to reconstructive surgery for tumors and trauma repair has resulted in the search for novel approaches to skeletal reconstruction.

Bone tissue engineering aims to heal bone defects with autologous cells and tissues without the donor site morbidity and expense associated with harvesting autogenous bone. One such strategy involves seeding autologous osteogenic cells *in vitro* throughout a biodegradable scaffold to create a scaffold–cell hybrid (TEC). This involves the isolation of a suitable cell population and expansion to a clinically relevant size *ex vivo*, seeding the expanded population onto an appropriate 3-D scaffold, which may be impregnated with appropriate growth factors and other chemical cues to enhance tissue in-growth followed by further culture in a bioreactor and place *in vivo* at the requisite tissue regeneration site. The scaffold is expected to support cell colonization, migration, growth, and differentiation, and to guide the development of the required tissue or to act as a drug delivery device.

Based on this background, approaches are therefore presently being investigated using scaffolds formed by electrospinning. Vacanti's group [40,41] used electrospun PCL membranes (average diameter of 400 ± 200 nm) and investigated their potential for bone tissue engineering. Mesenchymal stem cells (MSCs) were seeded onto the scaffolds and cultured using a combination of static culture and a rotating bioreactor. The MSCs differentiated into osteoblasts and migrated into the scaffold and produced collagen. The scaffold constructs were dimensionally stable and had become noticeably harder after 4 weeks presumably due to mineralization. In a later study, the group cultured MSCs on PCL nanofibrous scaffolds in a rotating bioreactor before implanting them into the omenta of rats. After 4 weeks *in vivo*, the scaffolds maintained their original shape with evidence of mineralization and type I collagen expression within the graft. However, the authors failed to present histological evidence of bone, which is comparable to the natural bone. In addition, no mechanical testing on TEC was performed.

HA–polymer composite scaffolds are increasingly being used for bone tissue engineering in an attempt to create more biomimetic constructs and to improve mechanical properties. Kim et al. investigated HA–gelatin composite nanofibers for bone tissue engineering [42]. Nanocrystals of HA were well distributed throughout the electrospun fibers (average diameter of 200–400 nm) by employing a stepwise process, which involved initial mineralization of HA in the gelatin. Electrospun scaffolds were subsequently cross-linked and up to 40% HA could successfully be incorporated using this technique. Higher amounts of HA resulted in an unstable electrospinning process and bead instead of fiber formation occurred. A preliminary *in vitro* study was performed using MG63 cell line.

HA and bone morphogenetic protein has also been successfully incorporated in electrospun nanofibers of silk fibroin. Li et al. [43] produced aqueous solutions of silk fibroin and electrospun in combination with PEO to increase the viscosity and surface tension thus preventing bead formation. The silk fibroin scaffolds (average fiber diameter of 500–600 nm) allowed attachment of human MSCs and promoted to a certain extent differentiation toward osteogenic lineage. The aqueous electrospinning process allowed the combination of silk fibroin, HAP, and BMP. Hence, this process prevented denaturing of the BMP and it was envisaged that this process could also be used for the delivery of other proteins. Tuzlakoglu et al. [44] investigated electrospun starch–based materials for bone tissue engineering. Nanofibers of starch/PCL blends (30:70), produced by electrospinning, were incorporated between microfibers (produced via a fiber bonding process) of the same material forming "nano-bridges" (average diameter of fibers was 400 nm). The authors state that larger microfibers were incorporated into the structure to increase the pore size and therefore improve cell migration. However, the authors failed to report pore size and size of pore interconnections, which are important parameters. Interestingly, human osteoblast-like osteosarcoma and rat bone marrow stromal cells bridged the microfibers and increased metabolic activity, growth rates, and ALP activity were reported. However, starch is not a biomaterial of first choice and based on its compromised properties, it is least likely to be applied clinically.

Electrospun scaffolds are also currently being investigated for use as membranes to facilitate guided bone regeneration (GBR). GBR membranes prevent epithelial tissue in-growth from the mucosa and ideally should also promote bone growth. However, nondegradable membranes require a second surgical procedure for removal and therefore research has focused on degradable constructs [45].

Fujihara et al. [46] electrospun polycaprolactone/$CaCO_3$ composite nanofibers for GBR. Two compositions of PCL:$CaCO_3$ were produced; 75:25 (900 $\pm$ 450 nm average diameter) and 25:75 (760 $\pm$ 190 nm average diameter). Incorporation of $CaCO_3$ significantly reduced the tensile strength of the membranes, however, this was limited by incorporation of a second electrospun PCL membrane in the construct. The electrospun meshes were surface treated using air plasma to increase the surface hydrophilicity (surface energy not quantified). Human osteoblasts were cultured on the membranes and showed good cell attachment and proliferation and were proportional to the amount of PCL. However, the study had a number of biological limitations and among many other assays, which are needed to prove that the membrane is suitable for GBR, ALP, and osteocalcin expressions were not studied. Electrospun silk fibroin membranes (150–300 nm average fiber diameter) are also currently being investigated for GBR. *In vitro* biocompatibility studies using an osteoprogenitor (MC3T3-E1) showed good cell proliferation with well-defined F-actin stress fibers attached to the nanofibers. Osteocalcin production, which was monitored throughout the 14-day culture, increased, indicating osteoblastic differentiation and calcium phosphate deposition. *In vivo* studies indicated that the membranes induced new bone formation in rabbit calvarial defects.

5.4.2 Cartilage Tissue Engineering

The articular cartilage of joints provides a smooth, near frictionless surface, whilst also mediating load transfer between the joint and the underlying subchondral bone. Cartilage defects typically result from aging, joint injury, and developmental disorder, and can result in pain and immobility. Because it has a very limited capacity to regenerate, there is a requirement to replace or repair the damaged cartilages so as to maintain joint functions. Tissue engineering offers the potential to develop conduits for cell-based replacement and regeneration of articular cartilage. This involves the isolation of articular chondrocytes or MSCs (precursor cells), which are then seeded onto a scaffold before implantation into a damaged joint. The architecture of the scaffold is critical, as it should simulate the ECM of cartilage, thus promoting cellular adhesion, proliferation, differentiation, and migration, whilst also providing resistance to tensile, compressive, and shear stresses.

Numerous materials have been used to electrospin scaffolds for cartilage tissue engineering that include chitosan [47], chitosan/PEO (90/10) [15], PLGA and PLA-PEG [25], PCL [48,49], collagen type II [12], and hyaluronic acid [50].

Sheilds et al. [12] produced cross-linked and uncross-linked electrospun collagen type II scaffolds. The average fiber diameters were 1.46 μm and 496 nm, respectively. Because of the importance of scaffolds withstanding stresses, the average tangent modulus, ultimate tensile strength, and ultimate strain of the uncross-linked samples were measured. Cellular adhesion and proliferation collagen II electrospun scaffolds was evaluated with SEM, showing that chondrocytes infiltrated the interiors of 3-D nanofibrous scaffolds. However, as collagen II scaffolds have limited mechanical properties without severe cross-linking (which decreases cell and tissue compatibility), it is questionable if it offers without reinforcement with a synthetic polymer a foundation for articular cartilage regeneration.

Subramanian et al. [51] generated electrospun chitosan/PEO (90:10) submicron scaffolds that were aligned with slight cross-linking between the parent fibers. The elastic modulus of the electrospun mats was significantly greater than cast films (2.25 MPa compared with 1.19 MPa). These authors assessed the cell compatibility of chitosan/PEO electrospun scaffolds by comparing chondrocyte adhesion, proliferation, and cellular viability with a cast film. After 3 days, the viability of the cells on electrospun mats was 69% to that of the tissue culture plastic (TCP) control, but slightly better than on cast films (63%). Though the chondrocytes grew slowly on the electrospun mats in the first week, the growth rate subsequently increased. By 10 days, the cell number on the electrospun chitosan was almost 82% to that of the TCP, and 56% to that of the cast films.

Li et al. [48] cultured MSCs on randomly orientated PCL electrospun nanofibers ($d = 700$ nm) to examine the capacity for chondrogenesis on these scaffolds. They claim that chondrogenesis was greater when MSCs were seeded onto electrospun scaffolds than for a high-density cell pellet (CP) protocol, suggesting that electrospun scaffolds seeded with MSCs are candidates for cartilage tissue engineering. The significance of this finding was that the CP protocol is currently a system that is widely used to study the chondrogenesis of MSCs, which shows that when the cells are seeded at high density they undergo chondrogenesis, and form tissue that is morphologically and biochemically similar to native cartilage.

5.4.3　Vascular Tissue Engineering

The primary function of the vascular system is to deliver oxygen and nutrients to the tissue and organs, remove CO_2 and other metabolites, and to distribute messenger molecules. Arteriosclerosis results in a thickening of large to medium size arterial walls and is characterized by endothelial dysfunction, inflammation, and eventually calcium and cholesterol plaques. The end result is chronic luminal obstruction leading to a decreased or absent circulation and hence impaired oxygenation of end organs. Coronary artery grafts, using mammary arteries or saphenous veins to bypass these occlusions, is the mainstay of treatments. However, there is frequently a lack of adequate arteries or veins that are suitable for bypass conduits. Furthermore, compliance mismatch between grafts might contribute to myointimal hyperplasia.

Based on the above clinical background, investigations into vascular tissue engineering have been directed at searching for suitable vascular graft substitutes [52]. The challenge is that engineered vascular replacements must withstand pulsation and the high pressure and flow rate of the blood stream. Compliance matching also presents a major challenge and has been addressed by modifying various aspects of graft design such as materials, structure, and fabrication method, without compromising the capacity for cells to form strong attachments and complete monolayer covering of the graft to reduce thrombus. A major reason for grafts failure is the incomplete covering of the graft surface by endothelial cells and the resultant myointimal hyperplasia.

Electrospinning offers the potential of control over composition, mechanical properties and structure of a graft while making it theoretically possible to match the compliance of the synthetic scaffold to the native artery. Therefore it is increasingly used to fabricate vascular grafts and heart tissue constructs [28,53–56].

Topographically aligned submicron fibers have similar circumferential orientations to the cells and fibrils found in the medial layer of the native artery. Because of these similarities between electrospun scaffolds and natural ECM, and because of the large variety of materials that can be used, cell viability is often superior to other scaffold designs.

The choice of material for designing electrospun scaffolds is critical to cell viability, fluid flow, and with respect to pulsations. Boland et al. had electrospun submicron collagen and elastin fibers in an attempt to mimic the native artery [57]. They discounted poly(α-hydroxyl esters) as suitable materials for vascular grafting because it degrades to lactic acid and glycolic acid, the degradation by-products that can cause cell death if their amount becomes too high per volume tissue. Their concern was that a high pH in a local environment would be toxic to the cells and induce an inflammatory response. However, more recently Stitzel et al. discovered that electrospun scaffolds produced with poly(α-hydroxyl esters), in particular PLGA blended with collagen, is biocompatible and without local or systemic toxicity when implanted [53]. Electrospun PLCL can also be designed to pulsate synchronously through changes to the electrospun wall thickness [56]. Thus, because it is "mechano-active" and degradation products seem not to cause any significant cell death and foreign body reaction, materials such as PLCL may actually be a suitable material choice.

There have been many *in vitro* studies to optimize growth, development, and adhesion of cells on electrospun scaffolds produced for vascular grafts. Xu et al. [28] attempted to induce a complete monolayer of SMCs over their electrospun vascular grafts prior to implantation. They cultured human coronary artery SMCs on aligned electrospun PLCL (75:25) nanofibers approximately 500 nm in diameter using polymer films as a control. The SMCs adhered and migrated along the scaffolds in the direction of fiber alignment, and the phenotype was expressed as a "spindle-like contractile." The distribution of the smooth muscle cytoskeleton proteins within the cells was also in the direction of alignment, and the cells adhesion and proliferation was superior on the electrospun scaffold than the films. This study provided promising evidence that a synthetic electrospun matrix on the nanoscale dimensions was capable of mimicking *in vivo* vascular structures making it a suitable vascular graft. The scaffold may have been superior to polymer films because its architecture was similar to the coronary artery, and also because the aligned nanofibers directed proliferation and adhesion via contact guidance.

Similarly Zong et al. found that the engineering of cardiac tissue and function can be manipulated by the chemistry and geometry of the electrospun scaffold [58]. In their experiment, primary cardiomyocytes (CMs) were cultured on electrospun PLLA and PLGA scaffolds of approximately 1 μm in diameter and the cellular attachment, structure, and function were examined. However, they discovered that on porous, nonwoven scaffolds, CMs made use of external cues for isotropic and anisotropic growth. Therefore, it appears that a desirable scaffold for vascular tissue engineering should have aligned fibers to provide contact guidance, but adequate porosity to allow the cells to respond to external cues.

5.4.4 NEURAL TISSUE ENGINEERING

The central nervous system (CNS) is a complex organ with the cells located within a specific region (the nucleus), which are connected to various points of influence via axons. The cell bodies receive axonal inputs via dendrites from multiple regions. A central tenant in neurology is that the CNS does not regenerate new neurons or sprout axons following damage. Consequently injury to the brain or spinal cord by neurodegenerative diseases or trauma is met by limited recovery leading to severe consequences for the patient. The recent recognition that adult neurogenesis does occur, and the potential to exploit fetal and embryonic stem cells in cell-based therapies has offered a more positive outlook. Furthermore, the recognition that adult neurons are prevented from sprouting axons in part by scars and a lack of a relevant cellular matrix has led to the investigation of neural tissue engineering to assist regenerating axons to reconnect the nucleus to points of influence.

There are many different approaches to neural tissue engineering, with most involving attempts at mimicking the natural ECM by fabricating pores, ledges and fibers so as to present the growing axons with appropriate cues and a permissive environment. The tip of the regenerating axon or neurite perceives these cues through a specialized ending known as a growth cone that transduces the cues into intracellular signals for navigation and tip extension. Conventionally, nanostructured scaffolds for neural tissue can be manufacture by a variety of methods. One of the new and most promising techniques involves utilizing electrospinning to fabricate a synthetic EMC from resorbable polymeric fibers.

It may be possible to control neurite outgrowth and cell spreading, adhesion, and proliferation of *in vitro* cultures by manipulating other topographical features of the scaffold [59]. The orientation of electrospun scaffolds can also be easily modified by employing different collection devices. Neurons grown on surfaces with parallel nanoscale ridges form neurites that are aligned with these ridges [60,61]. Similarly, the direction of neuron growth of neural stem cells (NSC) depends on fiber alignment: neurite extension is parallel to the fiber direction when cultured on aligned PLLA nanofibrous scaffolds and is random on nonaligned scaffolds. The rate of differentiation into neurons is also dependent on fiber diameter, with more cells differentiating on aligned nanofibers than on randomly oriented microfibers. The effect of fiber diameter was also shown on scaffolds with minimal fiber alignment. This study supported the idea that nanofibers enhances differentiation of the stem cells and neurite extensions, describing axons of up to 100 μm running parallel to aligned fibers. The authors attributed this encouraging performance to the enhanced contact guidance of neurite extensions with nanofibrous scaffolds, providing a positive guidance cue. However, it also raises many questions. The mechanism that provides directional changes remains unknown and the cells used in the study were not fully phenotyped as a result of which the relative contribution of cell type and structure remains unclear.

5.4.5 ELECTROSPINNING OF CELLS

A major obstacle in creating TEC based on nanofibers is a good integration between the cells and the scaffold. One method of resolving this issue is by electrospinning the cells concurrently with the nanofibers. Stankus et al. [62] coelectrospun SMCs and poly(ester urethane urea) (PEUU) and obtained well-integrated cell–nanofiber constructs. The cells were present across the whole thickness of the constructs and they showed minimal necrosis from the electrospinning process. Townsend-Nicholson and Jayasinghe [63] reported the possibility of electrospinning cells and synthetic polymers using a coaxial spinneret method. A two-chambered capillary was used to electrospin a composite thread comprising of an outer poly(dimethylsiloxane) (PDMS) shell and an inner biosuspension core containing the cells. The cells existed as encapsulated aggregates in the PDMS thread and showed no impairment of viability due to the electrospinning.

5.5 CONCLUSION

Electrospinning is a relatively inexpensive manufacturing technique for submicron and micron diameter fibers from polymer solutions or melts. The process is of interest for scaffold fabrication, as the resulting fibers have similar diameters to that of certain ECM microstructures, particularly the higher ordered collagen microfibrils. The flexibility of the electrospun fibers, due to the very high aspect ratio (length/diameter), is also beneficial as they allow the seeded cells to remodel their surroundings. The size of scale is important in this instance; instead of many cells adhering to one fiber, one cell may adhere to multiple fibers.

It is evident that the response of many cells is significantly different when subjected to nano- and microscale structures and topographies. One line of reasoning for the enhanced response of cells on nanoscale substrates is the dimensional similarities with some of the structural components found in the native ECM and or basement membranes. However, much of the underlying mechanisms for this enhanced response remain unknown and the interactions with nanostructured scaffolds have not yet been fully realized. However there is a clear need for further research on the subject to investigate the effects of nanofiber architecture and interfacial properties on cell behavior, which has just started to be realized.

REFERENCES

1. Curtis, A.S., et al., Substratum nanotopography and the adhesion of biological cells. Are symmetry or regularity of nanotopography important? *Biophysical Chemistry*, 2001, **94**(3): 275–283.
2. Hutmacher, D.W., M. Sittinger, and M.V. Risbud, Scaffold-based tissue engineering: rationale for computer-aided design and solid free-form fabrication systems. *Trends in Biotechnology*, 2004, **22**(7): 354–362.
3. Hutmacher, D.W., Scaffolds in tissue engineering bone and cartilage. *Biomaterials*, 2000, **21**(24): 2529–2543.
4. Silva, G.A., et al., Selective differentiation of neural progenitor cells by high-epitope density nanofibers. *Science*, 2004, **303**(5662): 1352–1355.
5. Reneker, D.H., et al., Bending instability of electrically charged liquid jets of polymer solutions in electrospinning. *Journal of Applied Physics*, 2000, **87**(9): 4531–4547.
6. Baumgarten, P.K., Electrostatic spinning of acrylic microfibers. *Journal of Colloid and Interface Science*, 1971, **36**(1): 71–79.
7. Lee, K.H., et al., Characterization of nano-structured poly(epsilon-caprolactone) nonwoven mats via electrospinning. *Polymer*, 2003, **44**(4): 1287–1294.
8. Lu, C., et al., Computer simulation of electrospinning. Part I. Effect of solvent in electrospinning. *Polymer*, 2006, **47**(3): 915–921.
9. Hohman, M.M., et al., Electrospinning and electrically forced jets. II. Applications. *Physics of Fluids*, 2001, **13**(8): 2221–2236.
10. Dersch, R., et al., Electrospun nanofibers: internal structure and intrinsic orientation. *Journal of Polymer Science Part A—Polymer Chemistry*, 2003, **41**(4): 545–553.
11. Tan, E.P., S.Y. Ng, and C.T. Lim, Tensile testing of a single ultrafine polymeric fiber. *Biomaterials*, 2005, **26**(13): 1453–1456.
12. Shields, K.J., et al., Mechanical properties and cellular proliferation of electrospun collagen type II. *Tissue Engineering*, 2004, **10**(9,10): 1510–1517.
13. Ohkawa, K., et al., Electrospinning of chitosan. Macromolecular rapid communications, 2004, **25**(18): 1600–1605.
14. Geng, X.Y., O.H. Kwon, and J.H. Jang, Electrospinning of chitosan dissolved in concentrated acetic acid solution. *Biomaterials*, 2005, **26**(27): 5427–5432.
15. Bhattarai, N., et al., Electrospun chitosan-based nanofibers and their cellular compatibility. *Biomaterials*, 2005, **26**(31): 6176–6184.
16. Um, I.C., et al., Electro-spinning and electro-blowing of hyaluronic acid. *Biomacromolecules*, 2004, **5**(4): 1428–1436.
17. Li, J.X., et al., Electrospinning of hyaluronic acid (HA) and HA/gelatin blends. Macromolecular rapid communications, 2006, **27**(2): 114–120.
18. Ji, Y., et al., Electrospun three-dimensional hyaluronic acid nanofibrous scaffolds. *Biomaterials*, 2006, **27**(20): 3782–3792.
19. Ji, Y., et al., Dual-syringe reactive electrospinning of cross-linked hyaluronic acid hydrogel nanofibers for tissue engineering applications. *Macromolecular Bioscience*, 2006, **6**(10): 811–817.
20. Li, W.J., et al., Fabrication and characterization of six electrospun poly(alpha-hydroxy ester)-based fibrous scaffolds for tissue engineering applications. *Acta Biomaterialia*, 2006, **2**(4): 377–385.
21. Li, W.J., et al., Biological response of chondrocytes cultured in three-dimensional nanofibrous poly(epsilon-caprolactone) scaffolds. *Journal of Biomedical Materials Research Part A*, 2003, **67A**(4): 1105–1114.
22. Mo, X.M., et al., Electrospun P(LLA-CL) nanofiber: a biomimetic extracellular matrix for smooth muscle cell and endothelial cell proliferation. *Biomaterials*, 2004, **25**(10): 1883–1890.
23. Badami, A.S., et al., Effect of fiber diameter on spreading, proliferation, and differentiation of osteoblastic cells on electrospun poly(lactic acid) substrates. *Biomaterials*, 2006, **27**(4): 596–606.

24. Luong-Van, E., et al., Controlled release of heparin from poly(epsilon-caprolactone) electrospun fibers. *Biomaterials*, 2006, **27**(9): 2042–2050.

25. Luu, Y.K., et al., Development of a nanostructured DNA delivery scaffold via electrospinning of PLGA and PLA-PEG block copolymers. *Journal of Controlled Release*, 2003, **89**(2): 341–353.

26. Huang, Z.M., et al., A review on polymer nanofibers by electrospinning and their applications in nanocomposites. *Composites Science and Technology*, 2003, **63**(15): 2223–2253.

27. Nisbet, D.R., et al., The effect of surface hydrophilicity on the behavior of embryonic cortical neurons. *Journal of Colloid and Interface Science*, 2006, **299**(2): 647–655.

28. Xu, C.Y., et al., Aligned biodegradable nanofibrous structure: a potential scaffold for blood vessel engineering. *Biomaterials*, 2004, **25**(5): 877–886.

29. Webb, P.A. and C. Orr, *Analytical Methods in Fine Particle Technology*. Micromeritics Instrument Corporation, Norcross, GA, 1997.

30. Li, W.J., et al., Electrospun nanofibrous structure: a novel scaffold for tissue engineering. *Journal of Biomedical Materials Research*, 2002, **60**(4): 613–621.

31. Min, B.M., et al., Formation of silk fibroin matrices with different texture and its cellular response to normal human keratinocytes. *International Journal of Biological Macromolecules*, 2004, **34**(5): 281–288.

32. Pham, Q.P., U. Sharma, and A.G. Mikos, Electrospun poly(epsilon-caprolactone) microfiber and multilayer nanofiber/microfiber scaffolds: characterization of scaffolds and measurement of cellular infiltration. *Biomacromolecules*, 2006, **7**(10): 2796–2805.

33. Kwon, I.K., S. Kidoaki, and T. Matsuda, Electrospun nano- to microfiber fabrics made of biodegradable copolyesters: structural characteristics, mechanical properties and cell adhesion potential. *Biomaterials*, 2005, **26**(18): 3929–3939.

34. Xu, C.Y., et al., In vitro study of human vascular endothelial cell function on materials with various surface roughness. *Journal of Biomedical Materials Research Part A*, 2004, **71A**(1): 154–161.

35. Jaeger, R., H. Schonherr, and G.J. Vancso, Chain packing in electro-spun poly(ethylene oxide) visualized by atomic force microscopy. *Macromolecules*, 1996, **29**(23): 7634–7636.

36. Gregg, S.J. and K.S.W. Sing, *Adsorption, Surface Area and Porosity*. 2nd ed., Academic Press, London, 1982, p. 303.

37. Zhang, Y.Z., et al., Fabrication of porous electrospun nanofibers. *Nanotechnology*, 2006, **17**(3): 901–908.

38. Liu, J. and S. Kumar, Microscopic polymer cups by electrospinning. *Polymer*, 2005, **46**(10): 3211–3214.

39. Rhoades, R. and R.G. Pflanzer, *Human Physiology*. 3rd ed., Perennial (HarperCollins), New York, USA, 1996, p. 978.

40. Yoshimoto, H., et al., A biodegradable nanofiber scaffold by electrospinning and its potential for bone tissue engineering. *Biomaterials*, 2003, **24**(12): 2077–2082.

41. Shin, M., H. Yoshimoto, and J.Vacanti, In vivo bone tissue engineering using mesenchymal stem cells on a novel electrospun nanofibrous scaffold. *Tissue Engineering*, 2004, **10**(1,2): 33–41.

42. Kim, H.W., J.H. Song, and H.E. Kim, Nanofiber generation of gelatin-hydroxyapatite biomimetics for guided tissue regeneration. *Advanced Functional Materials*, 2005, **15**(12): 1988–1994.

43. Li, C., et al., Electrospun silk-BMP-2 scaffolds for bone tissue engineering. *Biomaterials*, 2006, **27**(16): 3115–3124.

44. Tuzlakoglu, K., et al., Nano- and micro-fiber combined scaffolds: a new architecture for bone tissue engineering. *Journal of Materials Science-Materials in Medicine*, 2005, **16**(12): 1099–1104.

45. Hutmacher, D., M.B. Hurzeler, and H. Schliephake, A review of material properties of biodegradable and bioresorbable polymers and devices for GTR and GBR applications. *International Journal of Oral and Maxillofacial Implants*, 1996, **11**(5): 667–678.

46. Fujihara, K., M. Kotaki, and S. Ramakrishna, Guided bone regeneration membrane made of polycaprolactone/calcium carbonate composite nano-fibers. *Biomaterials*, 2005, **26**(19): 4139–4147.

47. Subramanian, A. and H.Y. Lin, Crosslinked chitosan: its physical properties and the effects of matrix stiffness on chondrocyte cell morphology and proliferation. *Journal of Biomedical Materials Research Part A*, 2005, **75A**(3): 742–753.

48. Li, W.J., et al., A three-dimensional nanofibrous scaffold for cartilage tissue engineering using human mesenchymal stem cells. *Biomaterials*, 2005, **26**(6): 599–609.

49. Li, D., Y.L. Wang, and Y.N. Xia, Electrospinning of polymeric and ceramic nanofibers as uniaxially aligned arrays. *Nano Letters*, 2003, **3**(8): 1167–1171.

50. Chiu, J.B., et al., Electrospun nanofibrous scaffolds for biomedical applications. *Journal of Biomedical Nanotechnology*, 2005, **1**(2): 115–132.

51. Subramanian, A., et al., Preparation and evaluation of the electrospun chitosan/PEO fibers for potential applications in cartilage tissue engineering. *Journal of Biomaterials Science-Polymer Edition*, 2005, **16**(7): 861–873.

52. Arrigoni, C., D. Camozzi, and A. Remuzzi, Vascular tissue engineering. *Cell Transplantation*, 2006, **15**: S119–S125.

53. Stitzel, J., et al., Controlled fabrication of a biological vascular substitute. *Biomaterials*, 2006, **27**(7): 1088–1094.

54. Williamson, M.R., R. Black, and C. Kielty, PCL-PU composite vascular scaffold production for vascular tissue engineering: attachment, proliferation and bioactivity of human vascular endothelial cells. *Biomaterials*, 2006, **27**(19): 3608–3616.

55. Zong, X., et al., Electrospun fine-textured scaffolds for heart tissue constructs. *Biomaterials*, 2005, **26**(26): 5330–5338.

56. Inoguchi, H., et al., Mechanical responses of a compliant electrospun poly(L-lactide-co-epsilon-caprolactone) small-diameter vascular graft. *Biomaterials*, 2006, **27**(8): 1470–1478.

57. Boland, E.D., et al., Electrospinning collagen and elastin: preliminary vascular tissue engineering. *Frontiers in Bioscience*, 2004, **9**: 1422–1432.

58. Zong, X., et al., Electrospun non-woven membranes as scaffolds for heart tissue constructs. *Polymer Preprints—American Chemical Society*, 2003, **44**(2): 96–97.

59. Khang, G., et al., Interaction of different types of cells on physicochemically treated poly(L-lactide-*co*-glycolide) surfaces. *Journal of Applied Polymer Science*, 2002, **85**(6): 1253–1262.

60. Foley, J.D., et al., Cooperative modulation of neuritogenesis by PC12 cells by topography and nerve growth factor *Biomaterials*, 2005, **26**(17): 3639–3644.

61. Johansson, F., et al., Axonal outgrowth on nano-imprinted patterns. *Biomaterials*, 2006, **27**(8): 1251–1258.

62. Stankus, J.J., et al., Microintegrating smooth muscle cells into a biodegradable, elastomeric fiber matrix. *Biomaterials*, 2006, **27**(5): 735–744.

63. Townsend-Nicholson, A. and S.N. Jayasinghe, Cell electrospinning: a unique biotechnique for encapsulating living organisms for generating active biological microthreads/scaffolds. *Biomacromolecules*, 2006, **7**(12): 3364–3369.

Part II

Drug Delivery Systems

6 Nanoparticles in Cancer Drug Delivery Systems

So Yeon Kim and Young Moo Lee

CONTENTS

6.1 INTRODUCTION

Although the pharmaceutical industry has been successful in discovering many new cytotoxic drugs that are potential candidates for cancer treatment, cancer remains a leading cause of death and is a serious threat to human health. Current anticancer drug therapy results in systemic side effects due to nonspecific uptake by normal, healthy, noncancerous tissues. Many anticancer drugs have marginal selectivity for malignant cells because they target the replicative apparatus in cells with high proliferation rates. Thus, anticancer drugs having the same mechanism of action also have high toxicity against rapidly dividing normal cells [1,2]. Additionally, the side effects associated with chemotherapy limit the dose or cumulative doses that can be administered to patients, which can lead to relapse of the tumor and often to the development of drug resistance [1,2]. Therefore, there have been numerous investigations aimed at developing more efficient systems that improve selective toxicities against cancer cells, that is, therapies that increase efficacy and decrease side effects, resulting in an increase in the therapeutic indices of the anticancer drugs. A successful approach is to use particulate drug carriers to alter the pharmacokinetics and biodistribution of anticancer drugs. Nanoparticle drug carriers can be delivered to specific sites by size-dependent passive targeting or active targeting. Recently, tumor-targeted delivery systems using nanoparticles have become increasingly used in chemotherapeutic engineering of cancer treatments. In the first part of this chapter, we present a short introduction of nanoparticle systems as drug carriers. This review also provides current approaches used in design and optimization of tumor-specific drug delivery systems.

6.2 CHEMOTHERAPY

6.2.1 Tumor Tissues

Current anticancer therapy can only prolong the patient's life but does not cure malignant diseases. Although research efforts to improve anticancer technology have improved patient's survival, cancer remains a leading cause of death. To achieve effective chemotherapy, it is important to recognize the morphological and physiological differences between normal and malignant tissues [1–12]. Cancer is caused by uncontrolled growth and spreading of abnormal cells. Cancerous cells, which can be formed due to external factors (e.g., smoking, chemicals, and infections) or internal factors (e.g., inherited metabolism mutations, hormones, and immune conditions), replicate at a higher rate than other healthy cells, placing strain on nutrient supply and metabolic waste product elimination [2]. Tumor cells will displace healthy cells until the tumor reaches a diffusion-limited maximum size. To grow beyond this size, the tumor must recruit blood vessels to provide the necessary nutrients to fuel continued expansion. Cells at the outer edge of the tumor mass have the best access to nutrients, while cells on the inside that rely on diffusion to deliver nutrients and eliminate waste products die, creating a necrotic core. Thus, tumors exhibit not only densely vascularized regions to acquire adequate supply of nutrients for rapid growth but also necrotic regions or hemorrhages [13].

  Additionally, tumor blood vessels show several abnormalities. Tumors develop a tortuous, chaotic capillary network with a hierarchical branching pattern that is distinguishable from normal vasculature. The capillary vasculature in tumors is often accompanied by occlusions, caused by rapidly proliferating cancer cells. Compression of the vasculature causes hypoxia and eventually necrosis of viable tumor cells. In addition, tumor vasculature exhibits aberrant basement membranes as well as a high proportion of proliferating endothelial cells. Since the fast-growing tumor requires a large amount of oxygen and nutrients, tumor blood vessels show 3–10 times higher permeability [1–5]. The interstitial compartment of a tumor contains a collagen and elastic fiber network, which is immersed in hyaluronate and proteoglycan-containing fluid. The interstitial pressure within the tumor tissue is elevated due to the lack of a lymphatic drainage system. Increased pressure and rapid aberrant cell growth are believed to be responsible for the compression and occlusion of blood and lymphatic vessels in solid tumors and for hindering the extravasations and accumulation of drugs in the tumor tissue [1,2].

6.2.2 Problems of Chemotherapy

Problems of chemotherapy are the high toxicity and lack of tumor specificity of currently used chemotherapeutic drugs. Many anticancer drugs have marginal selectivity for malignant cells because they target the replicative apparatus in cells with high proliferation rates. Thus, anticancer drugs that target the replicating apparatus also have high toxicity against rapidly dividing normal cells, which leads to systemic toxicity causing undesirable severe side effects such as hair loss, and damage to the liver, kidney, and bone marrow. In addition, the dense packing of tumor cells limits the movement of molecules from the vessel into the interstitial compartment [2–5].

The efficacy of anticancer drugs may decrease at times when it is not possible to increase chemotherapeutic dosages or when patients in relapse do not respond to the drug due to an acquired resistance. The lack of tumor response to a drug, drug resistance, can be due to poorly vascularized regions and insufficient accumulation of the drug to a therapeutically effective concentration [10].

While rapid drug internalization by passive diffusion across the plasma membrane produces a sufficient concentration, efflux pumps, which actively pump out a large spectrum of structurally unrelated drugs, counteract the diffusion [5]. Some tumor cells are able to expel intracellular drugs into the external medium, thereby attaining resistance from drug action. This mechanism, called multidrug resistance, is related to the overexpression of transporters from the adenosine triphosphate (ATP)–binding cassette family, including the P-glycoprotein (Pgp) transporter and multidrug resistance protein (MDRP). These transmembrane proteins are capable of pumping out many of the anticancer drugs that diffuse into the plasma membrane [14]. Thus, it is very difficult to achieve and maintain the required effective therapeutic drug concentration in the tumor tissue. Nanoparticles, however, appear to be useful for overcoming certain kinds of drug resistance. Internalized particles bypass the transporter mechanism that recognizes drugs in the plasma membrane, and they are able to release drugs within the cytoplasm or endosomal vesicles, thereby increasing the effectiveness of the drug [14–16]. Several strategies may be employed to achieve drug targeting in tumors, and the method is chosen depending on the tumor type and tissue characteristics, the drug chemical and biological properties, and the rate and time-course of drug application [14–26].

6.3 NANOPARTICLES IN CANCER THERAPY

6.3.1 Particulate Drug Carriers

An approach that overcomes the limitation of chemotherapeutic agents is the targeting of tumors with particulate drug carriers. Particulate drug carriers have become an important area of drug delivery applications due to their ability to deliver a wide range of drugs to varying areas of the body for sustained periods of time [27–40]. Nanoparticles can be defined as colloidal systems with a diameter smaller than 1000 nm. Nanoparticles may or may not be biodegradable and can be defined as solid colloidal particles containing an active substance that are produced by mechanical or chemical means. Nanoparticles are a collective name for nanospheres and nanocapsules. Nanospheres have a matrix-type structure. Drugs may be absorbed at their surface, or entrapped or dissolved within the particle. Nanocapsules are vesicular systems in which the drug is confined to a cavity or inner liquid core surrounded by a membrane. In this case the drugs are usually dissolved in the inner core but may also be adsorbed at their surface [41].

These particles can enter cells, including nuclear compartments, allowing for interaction with DNA and cellular proteins [27]. In addition, nanoparticles can be prepared with different sizes and surface modifications, which will determine their properties in biological systems. Recently, many therapeutic agents including small molecules, proteins, DNAs, and peptides have been combined to form potent and complex agents. Various nanoparticle drug delivery systems, listed in Table 6.1, have been developed using a variety of materials (polymers, liposomes, metals, ceramics, etc.) with unique architectures [27,28,39].

TABLE 6.1
Nanoparticulate Drug Carriers

Nanoparticulate System	Therapeutic Agents	Remarks	Advantages	Limitations
Polymeric nanoparticles	Plasmid DNA, protein, peptides, low-molecular weight compounds	Brain tumor therapy	Sustain localized drug therapeutic agent for weeks	Some polymers exhibit cytotoxicity
Liposomes	Proteins, DNA, anticancer therapeutic agents	Tumor therapy, HIV therapy, vaccine delivery	Effective in reducing system toxicity and can stay longer in targeted tissue	Limited stability
Cationic solid lipid nanoparticles	DNA, proteins, anticancer therapeutic agent	Efficiently bind and transfect plasmid DNA	More stable than liposomes	Limited stability
Metal nanoparticles	Anticancer therapeutic agents, proteins, DNA	Cancer therapy	Extremely small in size with vast surface area to carry large dose	
Polymeric micelles	DNA, anticancer therapeutic agents, proteins	Solid tumor therapy, antifungal treatment	Have hydrophobic core and are suitable carrier for water-insoluble drugs	Limited loading of hydrophilic drugs
Ceramic nanoparticles	Proteins, DNA, anticancer therapeutic agents, high-molecular weight compounds	Photodynamic therapy, liver therapy, diabetes therapy	Ease of preparation Stable in biological environment	Safety of inorganic compounds
Dendrimers	DNA, anticancer therapeutic agents, antibacterial therapeutic agents, antiviral therapeutic agents, high-molecular weight compounds	Tumor therapy, bacterial infection treatment, HIV therapy	Ease of modification at multiple termini	Polymer dependent biocompatibility, biodistribution

Source: Rawat, M., Singh, D., Saraf, S., and Saraf, S., *Biol Pharm Bull* 29, 1790–1798, 2006; Yih, T.C. and Al-Fandi, M., *J. Cell. Biochem.*, 97, 1184–1190, 2006.

One of the major advantages of nanoparticles is their small size, which allows access to capillaries and provides increased resistance to macrophage uptake of the reticuloendothelial system (RES). Another advantage is that therapeutic agents can often be encapsulated, dispersed, or dissolved at a high density within these nanoparticles and engineered to yield different properties and release characteristics for delivery of the required drug concentration [27–32]. When a drug molecule is administered with a carrier, drug clearance decreases (half-life increases), volume of distribution decreases, and the area under the time versus concentration curve increases [27–30].

Due to the versatility of the chemistries and preparations of these systems, nanoparticles can be fabricated to incorporate surface functionalities, which can facilitate attractive properties, such as the attachment of shielding ligands to prolong the circulation of the nanoparticles in the bloodstream or the targeting of ligands for interaction with specific cells or tissues [14].

Nanoparticles have the potential to improve cancer drug delivery, and they provide the following advantages [2,5]: (1) decreased immunogenicity, (2) protection from alteration and inactivation of the active drug, (3) altered biodistribution to reduce systemic toxicity, (4) elimination of multidrug resistance, (5) increased tumor cytotoxicity, (6) passive targeting by enhanced permeability and retention (EPR), and (7) site-specific delivery of drugs by active targeting.

6.3.2 LIPOSOMES

Liposomes, the most intensively investigated family of particulate carriers, are lipid molecules, highly ordered in a lamellar arrangement that encapsulates a fraction of the solvent in which they are suspended [42–47]. Liposomes are considered attractive, harmless drug carriers that can circulate in the bloodstream for an extended time because they are natural materials [11,39]. They may be formulated into small structures to encapsulate hydrophilic drugs in the aqueous interior or hydrophobic drugs within the bilayer [14]. Liposomes can be engineered to yield different properties depending upon the lipid [42–44]. In addition, the liposome surface can be engineered to improve properties. To date, the most noteworthy surface modification is the incorporation of polyethylene glycol (PEG). PEG-modified liposomes show a longer blood circulation period ($T_{1/2} > 48$ h) than that of polymeric micelles ($T_{1/2} < 24$ h). Also, some liposomal formulations, such as Doxil (Alza Co.) and Visudyne (Novartis Co.), have already been approved for clinical use. However, the treatment with Doxil sometimes induces the side effects of the hand–foot syndrome as well as infusion-related reactions. Thus, the patients need to be pretreated with antihistamine or anti-inflammatory agents before the administration of Doxil [27].

PEG can serve as a barrier, preventing interactions with plasma proteins and thus retarding recognition by the RES and enhancing lifetime circulation of the liposome [14]. Liposomes used as particulate drug carriers are homogeneous, unilamellar, and 50–150 nm diameter vesicles [42]. However, there have been major drawbacks to the use of liposomes for targeted drug delivery, most notably due to poor control over drug release from the liposome (i.e., the potential for leakage of the drug into the blood), low encapsulation efficiency and manufacturability at the industrial scale, and poor storage stability [14]. For the liposome to act as a useful drug carrier, it should be able to retain an encapsulated drug for a sufficiently long time after its administration in order to appropriately alter the pharmacokinetics of the drug [48].

TAT or penetratin peptides conjugated to lipid constituents of liposomes have been shown to dramatically improve cellular delivery *in vitro* and to have some potential *in vivo* for gene therapy [3]. Recently, a multicomponent liposomal drug delivery system consisting of doxorubicin and antisense oligonucleotides targeted to MRP1 mRNA and BCL2 mRNA to suppress pump resistance and nonpump resistance, respectively, has been developed. This liposomal system successfully delivered the antisense oligonucleotides and doxorubicin to cell nuclei of multidrug-resistant human lung cancer cells and substantially increased the potential anticancer action of doxorubicin by stimulating the caspase-dependent apoptosis pathway [23,45].

6.3.3 Polymeric Nanoparticles

In the past few decades, there has been intensive research in the development of nanoparticles of biocompatible polymers as an effective drug delivery system for chemotherapy and gene delivery. The drug is either confined to a cavity surrounded by a polymer membrane (nanocapsules) or uniformly dispersed in a matrix (nanospheres) [14,37–39]. Solid, biodegradable nanoparticles have various advantages over liposomes. First, by varying the polymer composition and morphology of the particle, controlled release characteristics can be effectively tuned allowing moderate, constant doses over prolonged periods of time [14].

The early nanoparticles and microparticles were mainly formulated from poly (alkylcyanoacrylate) [36]. Nanoparticles can be prepared by monomer polymerization. Polymeric nanoparticles approximately 200 nm in diameter have been fabricated by mechanically polymerizing dispersed methyl or ethyl cyanoacrylate in an aqueous acidic medium with a surfactant [28].

An increasing requirement for the modulated drug delivery of both conventionally and biotechnology-generated drugs of a high molecular weight and short half-life has received considerable attention in the development of biodegradable polymers and their formulation as a drug delivery system. The use of biodegradable polymers confers the inherent advantage of alleviating the need for surgical removal of the delivery system a later date [49].

Biodegradable polymers used in drug delivery research may be broadly classified as natural or synthetic polymers. The majority of investigations into the use of natural polymers as drug delivery systems has concentrated on the use of proteins (e.g., collagen, gelatin, and albumin) and polysaccharides (e.g., starch, dextran, insulin, cellulose, and hyaluronic acid).

Various synthetic degradable polymers have been investigated for the formulation of controlled drug delivery systems, since they can be synthesized with specific properties to suit particular applications. The most widely investigated biodegradable synthetic polymers are linear aliphatic polyesters based on poly(lactic acid) (PLA), poly(glycolic acid) (PGA), poly(lactic acid-*co*-glycolide) (PLGA), and poly(ε-caprolactone) (PCL). They exhibit important advantages of biocompatibility, predictability of biodegradation kinetics, ease of fabrication, and regulatory approval. Polyanhydride polymers and copolymers have attracted considerable interest for the fabrication of drug delivery system because of their labile anhydride linkages in the polymer structure. In addition, poly(ortho ester)s and polyphosphazenes have received attention for the formulation of nanoparticulate drug delivery system [49,50]. Poly(ortho ester)s have the advantage of undergoing control degradation of some polymeric materials. The degradation of polyphosphazenes and the linkage of reactive drug molecules to the polymer backbone are also controlled by side-group modification [49,50].

The solubility of a hydrophobic drug may be vastly improved by amphiphilic, block copolymer micelles. The micellization of block copolymers in a selective solvent of one of the blocks is a common characteristic of their colloidal properties. When a block copolymer is dissolved in a liquid that is a thermodynamically good solvent for one block and a precipitant for the other, the copolymer chains may reversibly associate to form micellar aggregates with properties resembling those obtained from classical, low molecular weight surfactants. The micelles generally consist of a swollen core of insoluble blocks surrounded by a flexible fringe of soluble blocks. Block copolymeric micelles are typically spherical, nanosized (10–100 nm), supramolecular assemblies of amphiphilic copolymers as shown in Figure 6.1 [40]. The core of these micelles is a loading space that accommodates hydrophobic drugs, and the hydrophilic outer shell facilitates dispersal of micelles in water [26,29,30].

The lower the critical micelle concentration (CMC) value of a given amphiphilic polymer, the more stable the micelles are even at low net concentration of amphiphile in the medium. This is important from the practical point of view, since upon dilution with a large volume of blood, micelles with a high CMC value may dissociate into unimers, and their content may precipitate in the blood [38]. The core compartment of the pharmaceutical polymeric micelle should demonstrate a high loading capacity, a controlled release profile for the incorporated drug, and good compatibility

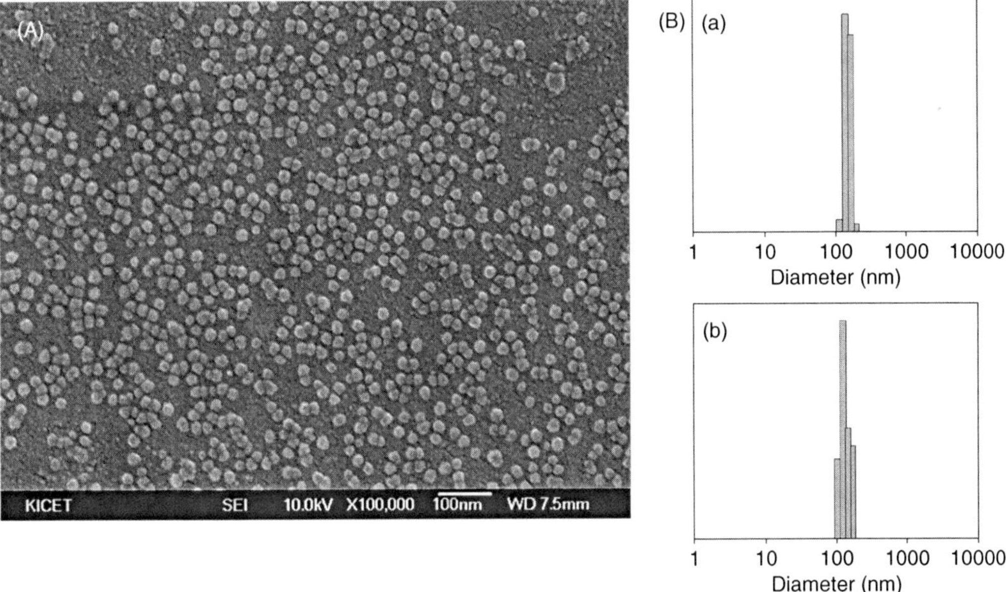

FIGURE 6.1 (A) Biotin-conjugated copolymeric nanoparticles composed of PEG and PCL copolymers observed by field emission scanning electron microscopy. (B) Typical size distribution of biotin-conjugated PEG/PCL block copolymeric nanoparticles determined using a light scattering method after drug loading: (a) biotin-conjugated PEG/PCL nanoparticles, and (b) PEG/PCL nanoparticles without biotin group. (From Kim, S.Y., Cho, S.H., Chu, L.Y., and Lee, Y.M., Macromolecular Research, in press.)

between the core-forming block and the incorporated drug. The micelle corona should provide effective steric protection for the micelle [38]. The molecular weight, polydispersity, charge, and hydrophilic–hydrophobic character of the block polymers influence biodistribution, clearance, biological activity, toxicity, and drug-loading efficiency [5].

Such nanoparticle drug carriers are designed by grafting PEG or polysaccharide chains using the concept of physicochemical steric repulsion to avoid protein adsorption [12]. This approach allows drug carriers to be maintained in the blood circulation for longer periods of time, and the resulting extravasation to the non-RES located cancers may become possible.

PEG-*block*-poly(aspartic acid) (PEG-*b*-P[ASP]) copolymers chemically conjugated with doxorubicin spontaneously form polymeric micelle, which can efficiently entrap free Dox in the inner core, and the optimized formulation called NK911 is now being studied in a phase II clinical trial at the National Cancer Center (NCC) Hospital in Japan [27]. In this formulation, doxorubicin chemically conjugated to the polymer side chain is pharmacologically inactive but contributes to the stable physical entrapment of free doxorubicin into the micellar core through π–π interaction of the anthracycline structure in doxorubicin between the conjugated and unconjugated ones, also allowing its sustained release from the micellar core [27].

The micelles presented by Maysinger et al. likely enter the cell by endocytosis, perhaps after their nonspecific association with the cell surface. The micelle-incorporated small hydrophobic drug can then enter the cytoplasm at a much higher rate by diffusing across the endosomal membrane. In addition, the surfactant nature of the micelle-forming block copolymers may also enhance the permeability of the endosomal membrane or even disrupt it. The detection of micelles in the cytoplasm suggests that the latter mechanism is at least partially responsible [29,51]. Kabanov et al. have demonstrated that Pluronic block copolymers based on PEG-poly(propylene glycol)-PEG can interfere directly with the function of Pgp [29,52].

6.3.4 Other Nanostructures

6.3.4.1 Dendrimers

Dendrimers are highly branched, globular macromolecules with many arms emanating from a central core and are emerging as a new class of polymeric nanosystems with applications in drug delivery. The stepwise synthesis of dendrimers affords molecules with a highly regular branching pattern, a unique molecular weight or low polydispersity index, and a well-defined number of peripheral groups [53–55]. The distinctive star-shaped architecture of dendrimers has contributed to increased interest in their application as drug molecules due to the loading potential in the interior or on the surface [39].

Drug molecules can be associated with dendrimers by physical encapsulation in the void spaces of the interior by incubation, forming a drug network, or prodrugs can be formed from a covalent or noncovalent linkage to the dendrimer surface [23].

Dendrimers are being investigated for drug and gene delivery, as carriers for penicillin, and for use in anticancer therapy. Dendrimers used in drug delivery studies typically incorporate one or more of the following polymers: polyamidoamine (PAMAM), poly(L-glutamic acid) (PG), polyethyleneimine (PEI), poly(propylene imine), and PEG [56].

A comparison of the features of dendrimers with those of linear polymers shows that the dendritic architecture can provide several advantages for drug delivery applications. For example, the controlled multivalency of dendrimers can be used to attach several drug molecules, targeting groups, and solubilizing groups to the periphery of the dendrimers in a well-defined manner. Dendrimer toxicity and immunogenicity should be considered when it is applied for drug delivery. Partial derivatization of the dendrimer surface, such as, a PAMAM dendrimer conjugated with PEG or fatty acids, helps to significantly reduce toxicity and immunogenicity due to a reduction or shielding of the positively charged dendrimer surface [23,57,58]. In addition, the low polydispersity of dendrimers can provide reproducible pharmacokinetics compared with that of some linear polymers, which can have vastly different molecular weights within a given sample [53,54]. Recent progress has been made in the application of biocompatible dendrimers to cancer treatment, including their use as drug delivery systems for anticancer agents such as cisplatin and doxorubicin and as agents for both boron neutron capture therapy and photodynamic therapy (PDT) [53].

PDT is a promising approach for the treatment of malignant tumors and macular degradation. PDT involves the systemic administration of photosensitizers, followed by the local application of a laser with a specific wavelength to the diseased sites. Upon photoirradiation, photosensitizers generate highly reactive singlet oxygen ($^{1}O_2$), thereby inducing light-induced cytotoxicity (photocytotoxicity). In PDT, the development of delivery systems for photosensitizers has recently received much attention to improve the selectivity and effectiveness of PDT as well as prevent the side effects such as skin hypersensitivity [27]. Nishiyama et al. developed an ionic dendritic porphyrin, as potential photosensitizers for PDT, in which the focal core of the porphyrin is surrounded by the third generation of poly(benzyl ether) dendrons with peripheral ionic carboxyl groups. The dendritic framework of the dendritic porphyrins is assumed to sterically prevent the interaction (i.e., self-quenching) of the center porphyrins, ensuring the effective singlet oxygen production from the dendritic porphyrins even at extremely high concentrations [59].

6.3.4.2 Magnetic Nanoparticles

Magnetic nanoparticles can be composed of iron oxide, magnetite, or nickel, cobalt, or neodymium–iron boron oxides. These particles are magnetic or superparamagnetic and range in diameter between 10 and 200 nm. Magnetite (Fe_3O_4) and maghemite (γ-Fe_2O_3) are preferably used since they are biocompatible and nontoxic to humans. Although nickel and cobalt are highly magnetic, they are not suitable for administration to humans due to their toxicity [2,60,61]. Magnetic drug targeting has attracted a great deal of attention. Generally, iron oxide cores are coated with silica, and polymers such as PVA and dextran [60]. Numerous studies are in progress in which tumors are targeted *in vivo* for therapeutic applications such as drug delivery and hyperthermic destruction of tumors. The first clinical magnetic drug trials targeting humans were reported by Lubbe et al. in which a ferrofluid (size about 100 nm) was coated with starch polymers and anionic phosphate groups to load the drug epirubicin. In only approximately 30 min, the ferrofluids were successfully directed to the tumor sites in half of the patients. Similar investigations using liposomes containing magnetic nanoparticles and drugs have also been reported [60]. The efficacy of magnetic therapy is dependent on the applied field strength as well as on the volumetric and magnetic properties of the particles [2].

6.3.4.3 Ceramic Nanoparticles

Inorganic, porous, ceramic nanoparticles have several advantages in cancer therapy. These particles can be easily engineered with the desired size, shape, and porosity, and they are extremely inert. The ceramic materials used are biocompatible and can be easily modified with different functional groups for ligand attachment [62–64]. Thus, growing interest has recently emerged in utilizing ceramic nanoparticles as drug vehicles in cancer therapy, exploring typical biocompatible ceramic nanoparticles, such as silica, alumina, and titania [39].

The luminescent silica nanoparticle has attracted the bioanalysis area recently. Its extensive application is based on the immobilization of various biomolecules such as DNA, antibody, and so forth, onto the surface. Liu et al. introduced amine groups onto the silica nanoparticle surface. Then, mouse monoclonal antihuman CD71 antibody (McAb CD71) and transferrin (Tf) were effectively linked and successfully labeled the receptors in the membrane of fibroblasts [65].

Roy et al. revealed that silica-based nanoparticles doped with photosensitizing drugs can be used for applications in photodynamic therapy. The spherical and highly monodispersed silica-based nanoparticles (size 30 nm) were prepared by controlled hydrolysis of triethoxyvinylsilane in micellar media [62]. Paul et al. developed insulin-loaded porous hydroxyapatite nanoparticles for intestinal delivery. Compared with repeatable injections, the insulin release profile exhibited promising results for orally administered insulin [63]. Recently, silica nanoparticles were used to form ternary complexes with DNA–dendrimer, resulting in a high surface concentration of DNA in the cell culture, and allowing efficient uptake of DNA by an endosomal–lysomal route [64].

6.3.4.4 Metal Nanoparticles

Metal nanoparticles have the ability to carry a relatively high drug dose because they can be fabricated in extremely small sizes (<50 nm) and have a large surface area. Functionalizing the surface of conventional metal nanoparticles such as gold or silver is under investigation for drug delivery molecules [60,66].

Increasing interest in polyelectrolyte multilayer research (PEM) is stimulated by the potential applications of this technology in the area of drug delivery. Microcapsules are fabricated by the layer-by-layer technique through the alternate adsorption of oppositely charged polyelectrolytes on various colloidal templates. Subsequently, the core is dissolved and the remaining shells serve as capsules for materials such as polymers, enzymes, catalysts, and the like. The uniqueness of such microcontainers is that they allow for tailoring the composition of their walls including incorporation of metal nanoparticles. Skirtach et al. proposed a novel method for remote release of encapsulated materials based on real-time monitoring of the capsules under laser light illumination. Laser-mediated remote release of encapsulated fluorescently labeled polymers from nanoengineered polyelectrolyte multilayer capsules containing gold sulfide core/gold shell nanoparticles in their wall is monitored in real time on a single capsule level [67].

Recently, Priyabara et al. demonstrated that gold nanoparticles can be functionalized into a composite system to carry both antiangiogenic and anticancer agents [39,66].

6.3.4.5 Albumin Nanoparticles

Albumin, a major serum protein component, possesses several amino and carboxylic groups, which are available for covalent modification and drug or protein attachment. Albumin nanoparticles can be prepared by a desolvation–crosslinking method, where albumin dissolved in water is desolvated by dropwise addition of ethanol and glutaraldehyde to induce the crosslinking of albumin nanoparticles [23]. Albumin nanoparticles are investigated for DNA delivery because DNA–albumin can avoid opsonization and uptake by the macrophage system encountered by positively charged complexes *in vivo* [68,69]. In January 2005, the FDA approved the use of paclitaxel albumin nanoparticles (~30 nm) (ABI-007 or Abraxane, American Pharmaceutical Partners, Schaumburg, IL) for the clinical treatment of metastatic breast cancer [70]. The overall response rate for Abraxane was 33%, compared with 19% for Taxol [71]. Several methotrexate immunoconjugates and 5-fluoro-2'-deoxyuridine have been prepared with human serum albumin as an intermediate carrier. The conjugates were more cytotoxic *in vitro* (IC_{50} 1.1 ng/mL methotrexate) against osteogenic sarcoma cells than free methotrexate (IC_{50} 2.8 ng/mL) [23].

6.4 *IN VIVO* BIODISTRIBUTION

6.4.1 Biodistribution of Particulate Drug Carriers

The fate of a drug carrier after administration *in vivo* is determined by a combination of several processes: distribution and elimination when given intravenously; absorption, distribution, and elimination when an extravascular route is used. Regardless of the mechanisms involved, each of these processes depends mainly on the physiochemical properties of the drug carrier [49].

Phagocytosis is the defense mechanism of the body that clears invading pathogens, unwanted cells, and small particles. Phagocytic cells primarily consist of circulating polymorphonuclear leukocytes and mononuclear phagocytes. These phagocytes originate from the bone marrow but become fixed in certain tissue sites, primarily the liver, spleen, and bone marrow, to form the mononuclear phagocytic system (MPS) or RES [49]. In the biological environment following intravenous administration, particulate drug carriers will rapidly interact with plasma proteins. The adsorption of these plasma proteins is known as opsonization. Classical examples of opsonic molecules include various subclasses of immunoglobulins, complement proteins like C1q and generated C3 fragments (C3b, iC3b), apolipoproteins, von Willebrand factors, thrombospondins, fibronectins, and mannose-binding proteins [72].

Opsonized particles are recognized by the RES or MPS, which is comprised of macrophages related to liver (Kuffer cells), spleen, lymph nodes (perivascular macrophage), nervous system (microglia), and bones (osteoclasts) [2]. These macrophages internalize the opsonized nanoparticles through phagocytosis and deliver them to the liver, spleen, kidney, lymph nodes, and bone marrow. This clearance can occur within 0.5–5 min, thus removing the active nanoparticles from the circulation and prevent their access to the tumor tissue [2].

Particulate uptake or ingestion proceeds by endocytosis following adhesion to the phagocytes or, alternatively, in the apparent absence of an adhesion step by pinocytosis, whereby small particles are internalized by endocytosis. Once internalized, the endosome or phagosome so formed will fuse with lysosomes, which will expose the carrier to highly active enzyme systems [49]. Such propensity of MPS macrophages for endocytosis or phagocytosis provides an opportunity to efficiently deliver therapeutic agents to these cells using conventional nanoparticles. This biodistribution can be of benefit for the chemotherapeutic treatment of MPS-localized tumors (e.g., hepatocarcinoma or hepatic metastasis arising from digestive tract, gynecological cancers, or bronchopulmonary tumors [primitive tumors or metastasis] including nonsmall cells tumors and small cells tumors, myeloma, and leukemia) [28]. In addition, the modification of surface properties of the nanoparticles and reducing their size to less than 100 nm can mask them so that they are no longer recognized by the MPS and remain in circulation for longer periods of time [2].

6.4.2 PHYSICOCHEMICAL FACTORS INFLUENCING BIODISTRIBUTION OF PARTICULATE DRUG CARRIERS

6.4.2.1 Particle Size

The size of the particulate drug carriers has been proved to be a primary key in determining their biodistribution. Particulate drug carriers with a lower size range are preferable than those in the upper submicron and micron sizes to achieve longer circulation half-lives (reduced MPS uptake) and more efficient celluar uptake (increased internalization) [23]. Generally, particles less than 1 µm generate a phagocytic response. Koval et al. investigated the uptake and transport of IgG-opsonized polystyrene beads of defined size ranging from 0.2 to 3 µm into murine macrophages. They found that phagocytosis uptake was size dependent; more than 30% of 0.2–0.75 µm particles compared with less than 80% of 2–3 µm particles were taken up [73]. Particulate drug carriers should also not exceed 200 nm to prevent substantial entrapment by hepatic and splenic endothelial fenestrations and subsequent clearance [72].

In addition, cellular internalization of drug-loaded particles is likely to play a key role in determining their biological activity. Intracellular uptake of particles can occur by various mechanisms according to the uptake by phagocytic cells, nonphagocytic cells, and drug-resistant cancer cells. The molecular mechanisms mediating the internalization of particles are dependent on the size of the particles. Particles as large as 500 nm can be internalized by nonphagocytic cells through an energy-dependent process, which is inhibited by drugs that affect membrane vesicle formation. Smaller particles with a diameter of less than 200 nm are internalized through clathrin-coated pits, while larger particles are internalized through caveole membrane invaginations [14]. Rejman et al. showed that as particle size increased, internalization was decreased. There was no cellular uptake of particles when they are above 500 nm in size [74]. Tabata and Ikada reported that *in vitro* phagocytosis of polystyrene and polyacolein microspheres by mouse peritoneal macrophages was maximum when the particles were between 1.0 and 2.0 µm in size. When the particle size is reduced below 100 nm, concentration of the carrier can occur in the bone marrow for both radiopharmaceuticals and liposomes [49]. Chemotherapy with small-sized nanoparticles was performed in tumor-bearing animals. Taxol-incorporated polyvinylpyrrolidone nanoparticles with a diameter of 50–60 nm were assayed on a B16F10 murine melanoma transplanted subcutaneously in mice. Mice treated with repeated intravenous injections of taxol-loaded nanoparticles showed a significant tumor regression and higher survival rates than mice treated with free taxol [75].

6.4.2.2 Surface Hydrophobicity

The surface characteristics of particulate drug carriers are also the key for the biological fate of nanoparticles. The importance of surface hydrophobicity in the pathogenicity of bacteria was clearly illustrated by Van Oss and Absolom. If the contact angles (a measure of surface hydrophobicity) were less than those for neutrophils, then phagocytosis was avoided, whereas a more hydrophobic surface led to sequestration. In addition to affecting the extent of ingestion of nonopsonized bacteria, the surface hydrophobicity will also strongly influence the degree of nonspecific IgG adsorption and compartment activation, which promote phagocytic uptake in serum. The adsorption of dysopsonic IgA, however, increased the surface hydrophilicity and hence decreased phagocytosis [49].

Thus, nanoparticles can be coated with biodegradable matrices and become invisible to macrophages. Since the usefulness of conventional nanoparticles is limited by their massive capture by the macrophages of the MPS after intravenous administration, other nanoparticulate devices must be considered to target tumors, which are not localized in the MPS area. Recently, a great deal of work has been devoted to develop so-called Stealth particles, which are invisible to macrophages. These Stealth nanoparticles are characterized by a prolonged half-life in the blood compartment. This property allows them to selectively extravasate in pathological sites like tumors or inflamed regions with leaky vasculature. As a result, such long-circulating nanoparticles are supported to directly target most tumors located outside the MPS region [28].

Tabata and Ikada showed a greater uptake of hydrophobic microspheres compared with hydrophilic microspheres. Extensive investigations have reinforced the apparent link between the *in vitro* surface hydrophobicity and a diminished ability to avoid phagocytic sequestration for a range of surface-modified polystyrene and poly(methylmethacrylate) particles [49]. Hydrophilic coatings are dextran, PEG, polyethylene oxide (PEO), poloxamers and poloxamines, and silicones. PEG coating resulted in enhanced circulation time of the particles and reduced opsonization. Ishiwata et al. showed that PEG coating resulted in suppression of macrophage interaction [2].

Despite these interesting results, the second strategy consisting of the covalent linkage of amphiphilic copolymers is generally preferred for obtaining a protective hydrophilic cloud on nanoparticles, as it avoids the possibility of rapid coating desorption upon dilution or after contact with the blood components. This approach has been employed with amphiphilic copolymers like PLA, PCL, and poly(cyanoacrylate) polymers, which were chemically coupled to PEG [2,28].

6.4.2.3 Surface Charge

The role of surface charge in influencing protein (fibrinogen) adsorption and thus the surface nature of polyamide microcapsules was investigated by Kondo. However, the underlying mechanism was not fully understood, and the evidence for the influence of surface charge on particulate uptake has appeared confusing and often contradictory [49].

Juliano and Stamp [76] reported that the rate of hepatic removal of liposomes was greater when they were negatively charged rather than when they were positively or neutrally charged. However, Park et al. suggested that while some negatively charged liposomes can increase liver and spleen uptake, others could actually avoid uptake leading to prolonged circulation time [49]. Tabata and Ikada showed no differences between negatively and positively charged particles if they had the same absolute value [77]. The same authors also demonstrated that for cellulose microspheres, the extent of phagocytosis increased with increasing negative zeta-potential values [49].

This confusion may reflect the fact that changes in surface charge are also likely to alter other surface properties, such as hydrophobicity, which also influence the opsonization process [49].

6.4.3 Design of Long-Circulating Nanoparticles: PEO-Modified Nanoparticles

There are several reasons why the search for macrophage-evading or long-circulating particles is so extensive [72]. An important reason is to provide a long-circulating drug reservoir from which the drug can be released into the vascular compartment in a continuous and controlled manner. Candidate drugs and therapeutic agents may be those with short elimination half-lives. Therefore, the requirements in terms of drug release from a long-circulating carrier will depend on clearance kinetics of the system as well as a pharmacologically desired free drug profile [72].

During the last 20 years, extensive studies have been carried out on various particulate carriers to serve as long-circulating systems by reducing the uptake by the cells of RES to rapidly remove intravenously applied particulates from the systemic circulation [75].

As mentioned in Section 6.4.2, it has been repeatedly emphasized that the clearance behavior and tissue distribution of intravenously injected particulate drug carriers are greatly influenced by their size and surface characteristics [72]. These physicochemical parameters can control the degree of particle self-association in the blood as well as particle association. The size of particle may change substantially upon introduction into a protein-containing medium (e.g., plasma). Thus, particles and their aggregates should be small enough so that they are not removed from the circulation by simple filtration in the first capillary bed encountered.

The concept of surface modification of particulate carriers to control the opsonization process and the specific interaction of particulate carriers with phagocytic cells as well as the nonspecific interaction with blood components and phagocytic cells raises a question about the optimal surface modification of the particulate carriers [75]. PEO has been the most successful synthetic material used to modify the interactions of solid surfaces with biological media. This fact has been demonstrated for particulate carriers with either grafted PEO or adsorbed amphiphilic PEO-based copolymer, liposomes with incorporated PEO derivatives, and biomedical implants with grafted PEO chains.

It is evident from the results with both nonbiodegradable and biodegradable systems that the surface modification of particulate carriers by the creation of a coating layer composed of PEO chains can result in the avoidance of the physiological processes that would normally occur after parenteral administration of the particles. As injected particles interact with the body components through their surface, the surface properties of the successful model system (e.g., surface chemistry, hydrophilicity, surface charge, coating layer thickness, and arrangements of the PEO chains on the surface) have been extensively studied [75].

The capacity of PEO to repel proteins and not interact with macrophage plasma membrane largely depends on different parameters such as molecular weight, density, and conformation and flexibility of the chains [78]. Illum et al. showed that for the effective stabilization of colloidal drug delivery system, it is essential that the dimensions of the stabilizing polymer chains exceed the range of the van der Waals attraction forces. Many studies showed that the protein adsorption decreased with the increase of molecular weight and an efficient molecular weight in the range of 1500–3500 Da. [79]. A good protection can be obtained after reaching the critical minimum coating layer thickness, which also depends on the size of adsorbed proteins. With this aim, the increase in size of colloidal drug delivery system is generally accompanied by an increase of the molecular weight of the PEO chain. Pavey and Olliff suggested that a more efficient system would be a mixture of PEO lengths because the longer chains would be a mixture of PEG lengths as they would be less inhibited in their movement, and the shorter chains would be interdigitated close to the surface for optimal recovery [80].

Another parameter described as a key factor in the optimization of PEO modification is the density of PEO chains. The higher the density, the faster the proteins are repelled from the polymer structure, the lower the protein adsorption, and the greater the difference of adsorbed protein composition [78]. However, Gref et al. suggested that whatever the thickness or the density of the coating, the qualitative composition of the plasma protein adsorption patterns were very similar, showing that adsorption was mainly governed by interactions with a colloidal drug delivery system. It could be explained that the molecular weight and the density are important criteria that are related to each other and can compensate each other in order to create a sufficient thickness limiting interactions with proteins and macrophages [81].

In addition, the interaction with proteins is influenced by the conformation of the PEO coating. PEO produces a surface that is in a liquid-like state with the polymer chains exhibiting considerable flexibility and mobility. The high mobility of PEO chains has been proposed to repel approaching proteins from the surface because the protein does not have sufficient contact time with the mobile chains to adsorb. Furthermore, the reduced mobility of the PEO chains on a highly crowded surface (produced by grafting of branched PEO derivatives) has been suggested as the reason for higher protein adsorption on this system relative to the surface modified with linear PEO chains [75].

Many studies showed that stealth properties were governed by many interdependent parameters. A parameter can compensate for others and lead to a satisfying system. It could be suggested that in order to have a prolonged time in blood, colloidal drug delivery system must preferentially be small, composed of natural and hydrophilic surface. The coating of hydrophilic polymer chains has to be dense and flexible to reduce all kinds of interactions [78]. But above all, the coating must be organized so as to minimize contact with bare hydrophobic surface of the colloidal drug delivery system, and well-anchored in the colloidal drug delivery system core in order to avoid desorption of chains caused by opsonization [82].

6.5 TARGETED DRUG DELIVERY FOR CHEMOTHERAPY

6.5.1 DRUG TARGETING

Targeted drug delivery by an engineered system is said to be achieved when the time profile of the drug at the target site is optimized, and the burden of drug to other tissues is minimized. This definition assumes that both the activity and toxicity are related to the time profile of the intact drug at the target and toxic sites, respectively. The assessment of targeting can be determined by comparing dose–response curves of the targeted system with the conventional or non-targeted system [48].

Targeted drug delivery has gained recognition in modern therapies, and attempts are being made to explore the potentials of cellular biology–related bioevents in the development of specific, programmed, and target-oriented systems [14–19]. Using nanoparticles to specifically deliver drugs to tumors offers the attractive possibility of avoiding obstacles that occur during conventional, systemic drug administration. Through several targeting strategies, nanoparticles can be selectively accumulated in malignant tissues as opposed to healthy tissues [19–26]. Principal schemes of drug targeting currently being investigated in various experimental and clinical settings include (1) direct application of the drug to the affected sites (organs, tissues); (2) passive accumulation of the drug through leaky vasculature (tumors, infarcts, inflammation); (3) physical targeting of the drug based on abnormal pH and temperature in the target site (tumor, inflammation) and magnetic targeting under the action of an external magnetic field; and (4) use of vector molecules possessing high specific affinity toward the affected site [18].

6.5.2 PASSIVE TARGETING

Functional and morphological differences exist between normal and diseased vasculature, offering therapeutic opportunities and windows for the delivery of therapeutic agents. Rapidly growing cancer cells require quick formation of new blood vessels. The tumor vasculature has many defects, which allows large molecules to easily enter the tumor extravascular space. On the other hand, the lymphatic drainage in cancer cells is undeveloped such that large molecules cannot be released from the tumor [1–5]. Following systemic administration, drugs must be transported through blood vessels across the vascular wall into the surrounding tissues and through the interstitial space. Fluid movement accompanies the extravasation of molecules across leaky vessels by passive diffusion or convection, depending on the hydrostatic and osmotic pressure differences between the blood and interstitial space. As a result of the increased permeability of endothelial barriers in tumor blood vessels and the lack of effective lymphatic drainage from the tumor, passive targeting results in the selective extravasation and accumulation of particulates or other macromolecules in tumor tissues. This phenomenon, termed as the EPR effect, was first described by Maeda et al. in 1986, and it has been confirmed in numerous cases [1–5,14–19].

Passive targeting can result in severalfold increases in drug concentrations within solid tumors relative to concentrations obtained with free drugs. Surface-modified nanoparticles engineered to display an overall positive charge facilitated adhesion to negatively charged arterial walls and have shown about 7–10-fold greater arterial localized drug levels compared with unmodified nanoparticles in different models. Rexin-G, a targeted nanoparticle vector system with a proprietary mutant cell-cycle control gene, has been approved for clinical trials for stage IV metastatic pancreatic cancers [14]. Passive targeting with nanoparticulate drug carriers includes manipulation of the size, hydrophobicity, or other physicochemical properties [15–20].

6.5.3 ACTIVE TARGETING

Active targeting relies on the expression of disease-selective molecular markers, mainly peptide or glycoside receptors and transporters, by either diseased cells or disease-associated cells such as the neoangiogenic endothelium of cancer tissue [14–18]. To achieve active targeting, it is necessary to

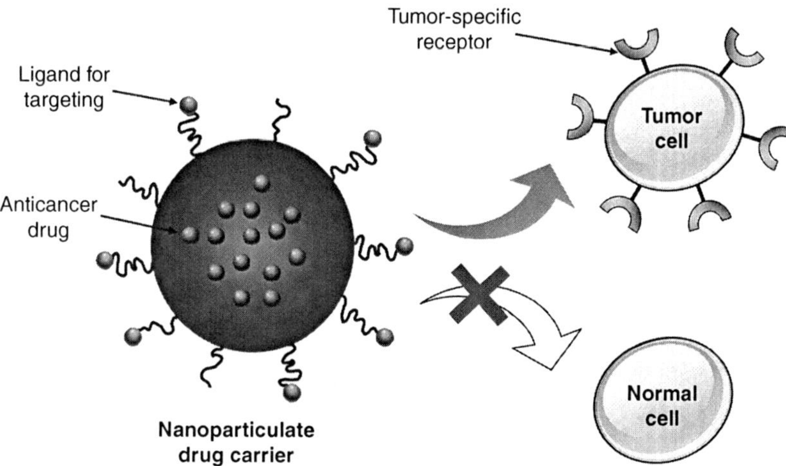

FIGURE 6.2 Schematic representation of ligand-mediated nanoparticulate system for tumor-targeted drug delivery.

(1) define valid targets as markers of disease-associated cells; (2) develop and validate the necessary chemistry to conjugate drugs to cell-selective vectors; (3) release drugs from the vectors at the right place and time; (4) resist hydrostatic, hydrophilic or hydrophobic, and biophysical or biochemical barriers; (5) overcome cellular resistance to treatment; and (6) resist biotransformation, degradation, and clearance mechanisms [14–18,20]. Active targeting is expected to lead to higher intratumoral accumulation and, in the case of targeting with internalizing ligands, to higher intracellular concentrations of the drug (Figure 6.2).

Targets that are employed to achieve tumor-selective localization of particulate drug carriers can be broadly divided into two classes: (1) targets that are overexpressed on tumor cells and (2) targets that are preferentially expressed on endothelial cells of tumor blood vessels [13]. These targets include monoclonal antibody (mAb) immunoconjugates and metabolism-based therapies that seek to exploit increased tumor expression of, for example, proteases, low-density lipoprotein receptors, hormones, and adhesion molecules [14–21]. This review covers the fundamentals of active targeting of particulate drug carriers in tumor therapy, as well as the most recent progress in this field.

6.5.3.1 Tumor-Specific Targeting

Nanoparticle functionalization with targeting agents that bind to tumor cell membrane receptors such as ligands or antibodies facilitate specific and increased uptake into the target cells through receptor-medicated endocytosis, increasing *in vivo* drug specificity [2,14–21] (Figure 6.3). These systems would ideally be dependent on interactions with cells found specifically on the surface of cancerous cells and not on healthy cells.

6.5.3.1.1 Antibodies

A great amount of work has been done with antibodies to target drugs to specific cells, especially for cancer therapy. Theoretically, targeting with antibodies is ideal because antibody–antigen interactions are very specific [48]. There are basically three types of antigens that can be used as targeting moieties for antibodies: organotypic antigens, tumor-associated antigens (TAAs), and tumor-specific antigens. Organotypic antigens would restrict the uptake of the drug–antigen conjugates to one cell type; however, it would not restrict the uptake to the tumor cell. TAAs are present on the surface of embryonic cells and reappear in the course of malignant transformations or exist in small amounts on normal cells and in large amounts on tumor cells [48].

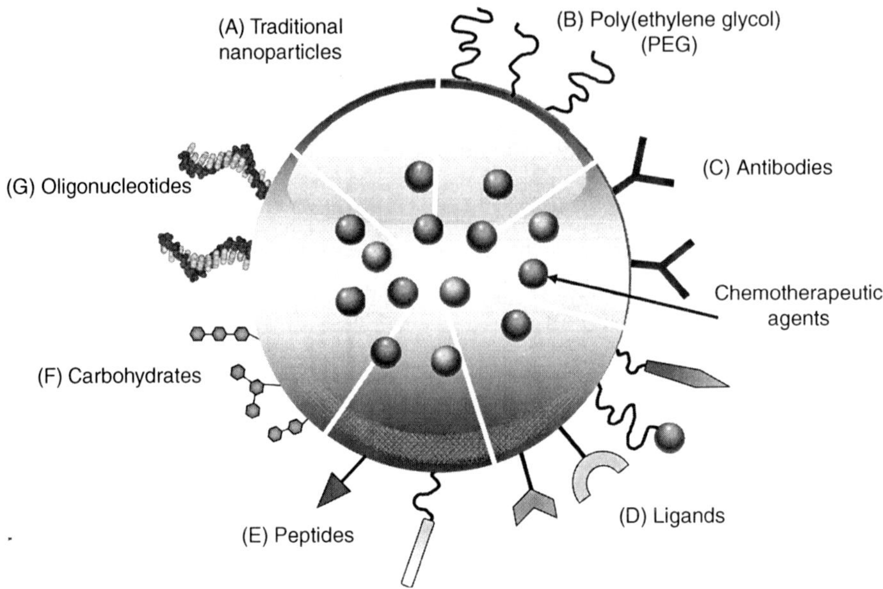

FIGURE 6.3 Schematic representation of nanoparticulate drug carrier structure with site-directing ligands for targeting approaches. Several classes of ligands have been used for targeted chemotherapy: (A) traditional "plain" nanoparticles, (B) long-circulating nanoparticles with surface protecting PEG chain, (C) monoclonal antibody, (D) tumor-specific ligands to cell surface receptor (folate), (E) peptides (RGD, YIGSR, cell membrane-penetrating peptides, etc.), (F) carbohydrates (hyaluronic acid, galactose, etc.), and (G) oligonucleotide aptamers.

Target mAbs were first shown to bind to specific tumor antigens in 1975 [13]. The discovery of antigens that are particularly overexpressed on the cancer cell surface suggests that by using certain antibodies to selectively mark tumor cells, malignant tissues could be distinguished from normal tissues. Monoclonal antibodies that have shown high binding specificity to tumor-specific antigens could fulfill this task. These mAbs could be used as vehicles to selectively deliver cytotoxic drugs to tumor cells. The mAb moiety then binds to the cancer cell antigen, and the conjugate is internalized through receptor-mediated endocytosis followed by the release of the patient drug to restore original activity [19,83–85]. Monoclonal antibodies are being used as imaging vehicles for drug targeting, as drug carriers, and solely as the drug. Early mAb—drug conjugates used mAbs derived from murine hybridomas. Kohler and Milstein described their pioneering work on mAbs by hybridoma technology; however, the therapeutic effects were severely impaired due to the human antimouse antibody (HAMA) response, resulting in the rapid clearance of the immunoconjugates from the bloodstream [86]. Consequently, a recombinant DNA protocol was developed, which produced generations of humanized mAbs generated by grafting the complementary determining region (CDR) from a mouse mAb into a human [19]. In 2000, Mylotarg (gemtuzumab-ozogamicin) was approved by the FDA for the treatment of acute myelogenous leukemia, providing the first in clinic mAb—drug immunoconjugate for the treatment of cancer [19,83–86]. Currently, there are at least nine FDA-approved antibodies for clinical use in cancer, and approximately 20 more are being evaluated in clinical trials (Table 6.2) [6,83–86].

6.5.3.1.2 Transferrin

The Tf family of iron-binding proteins has been the subject of intense investigation since serum transferring was discovered more than 40 years ago. A considerable number of reviews have provided a wide range of functional properties, structures, metal-binding properties, and metal

TABLE 6.2

Therapeutic Antibodies Approved by the FDA for Targeted Cancer Therapy

Generic Name	Trade Name	Type	Molecular Target	Indication	Year of FDA Approval
Monoclonal antibodies					
Rituximab	Rituxan	Chimeric	CD20	Low-grade B-cell non-Hodgkin's lymphoma	1997
Trastuzumab	Herceptin	Humanized	HER2	Metastatic breast cancer	1998
Alemtuzumab	Campath	Humanized	CD52	Chronic lymphocytic leukemia	2001
Bevacizumab	Avastin	Humanized	VEGF	Metastatic colorectal cancer	2004
Cetuximab	Erbitux	Chimeric	EGF receptor	Metastatic colorectal cancer	2004
Immunoconjugates					
Gemtuzumab ozogamicin	Mylotarg	Humanized	CD33	Acute myeloid leukemia	2000
Ibritumomab tiuxetan	Zevalin	Murine	CD20	Relapsed or refractory non-Hodgkin's lymphoma	2002
Tositumomab and ^{131}I tositumomab	Bexxar	Murine	CD20	Non-Hodgkin's lymphoma refractory to Rituximab and relapsed following chemotherapy	2003

Source: Brannon-Peppas, L. and Blanchette, J.O., *Adv. Drug Del. Rev.*, 56, 1649–1659, 2004; Schrama, D., Reisfeld, R.A., and Becker, J.C. *Nat. Rev. Drug Discovery*, 5, 147–159, 2006. Bicknell, R., *Br. J. Cancer*, 92, S2–S5, 2005.

delivery potentials in biomedical processes. The Tfs are typically monomeric glycoproteins with a single polypeptide chain of 670–700 amino acids and a molecular weight of ca. 80 kDa [87].

The transferrin receptor (TfR) assists iron uptake into vertebrate cells through a cycle of endo and exocytosis of Tf. It appears to be expressed in all nucleated cells and has been found in red blood cells, thyroid cells, hepatocytes, intestinal cells, monocytes, brain, the blood–brain barrier, and also in some insects and certain bacteria. Elevated levels of TfR expression in malignant cells is attributed to the requirement of a high iron level for their growth [87,88]. A schematic representation of the endocytosis and recycling cycle for the Tf/TfR complex is given in Figure 6.4. First, Tf binds two Fe^{3+} atoms per molecule. TfR subsequently binds the iron-loaded Tf, and the Tf/TfR complex is internalized through clathrin-coated pits. Tf releases iron in the acidic endosomal environment, and the Tf/TfR is recycled back to the plasma membrane. Then, the iron-free Tf is released from TfR to complete the cycle [88]. Many anticancer agents have been considered for conjugation to Tf by varying methods, including direct chemical linkage, liposomal packaging of toxin, conjugation of DNA–polylysine complexes, and conjugation of liposome–DNA complexes. For example, methotrexate that has been formulated in a liposome complex and conjugated to Tf demonstrated a higher efficiency of cellular uptake and cytotoxicity compared to the control free methotrexate and methotrexate–liposome [46]. Huwyler et al. demonstrated that daunomycin-containing liposomes conjugated to OX26 rat TfR antibody exhibit an increased delivery and uptake in the central nervous system relative to the non-OX26 containing liposomes [47,88].

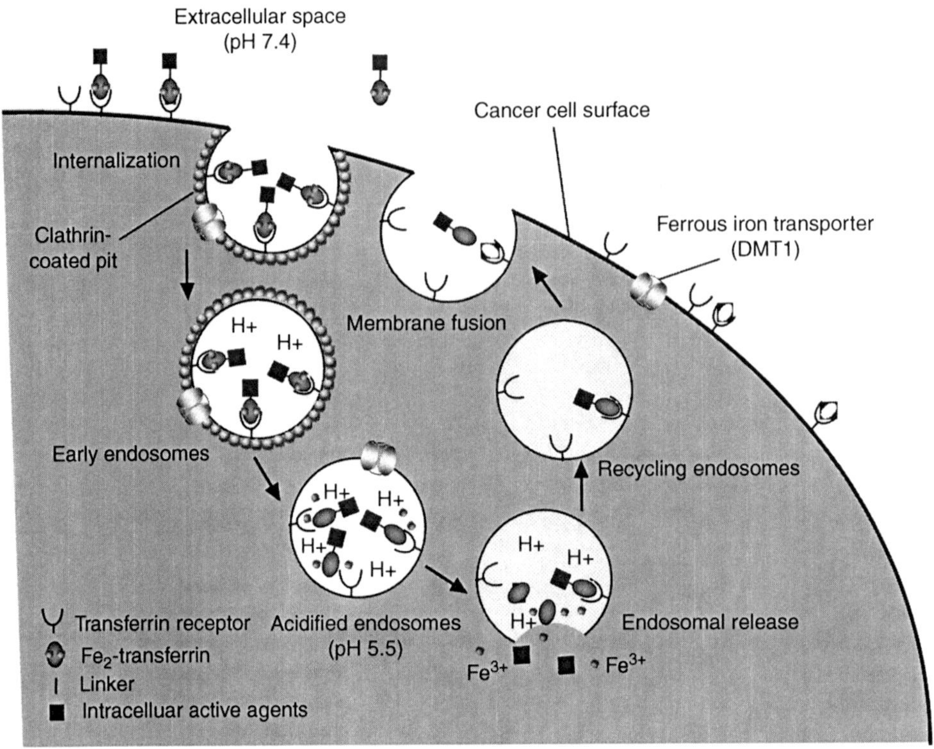

FIGURE 6.4 The cellular uptake pathway of Tf-conjugated nanoparticles through TfR-mediated endocytosis.

6.5.3.1.3 Folate

Folic acid (folate) has become an attractive candidate molecule for targeting cancer cells because it is an essential vitamin for the biosynthesis of nucleotide bases and is consumed in elevated quantities by proliferating cells [89–92]. The folate receptor (FR) is overexpressed in many human cancers, including ovary, brain, kidney, breast, myeloid cells, and lung malignancies. The attractiveness of folate has been further enhanced by the high binding affinity ($K_d \approx 10^{-10}$ M), low immunogenicity, ease of modification, small size ($M_w = 441.4$), storage stability, compatibility with a variety of organic and aqueous solvents, and low cost [19,89–92]. Although the precise mechanism of FR transport into the cells remains unresolved, it is clear that nondestructive folate uptake by mammalian cells occurs via receptor-mediated endocytosis [89].

Lee et al. developed the folate-conjugated, block copolymer nanoparticles composed of PEG and PCL and demonstrated that paclitaxel-loaded, folate-conjugated PEG/PCL nanoparticles exhibited much higher cytotoxicity for cancer cells, such as MCF-7 and HeLa cells, than nanoparticles without the folate group [91,92]. Moreover, Figure 6.5 shows confocal microscopy measurements revealing that as a consequence of FR-mediated endocytosis, folate-conjugated nanoparticles were selectively taken up by MCF-7 cells [92]. FR-mediated uptake of PEG disastearoyl phosphatidylethanolamine (DSPE) liposomes (70–100 nm) loaded with doxorubicin resulted in increased cytosol uptake and release of doxorubicin into the cytoplasm. The drug was released within 2 h *in vivo* in M109-HiFR multidrug-resistant cancer cells. Folate-targeted liposome drug uptake was increased 10-fold compared with free doxorubicin and was more toxic *in vivo* than free doxorubicin [2].

Park et al. investigated that poly(D,L-lactide-*co*-glycolic acid) (PLGA) nanoparticles with anionic surface charge were surface coated with cationic diblock copolymer (poly[L-lysine]-PEG-folate [PLL-PEG-FOL]) conjugate, for enhancing their site-specific intracellular delivery against

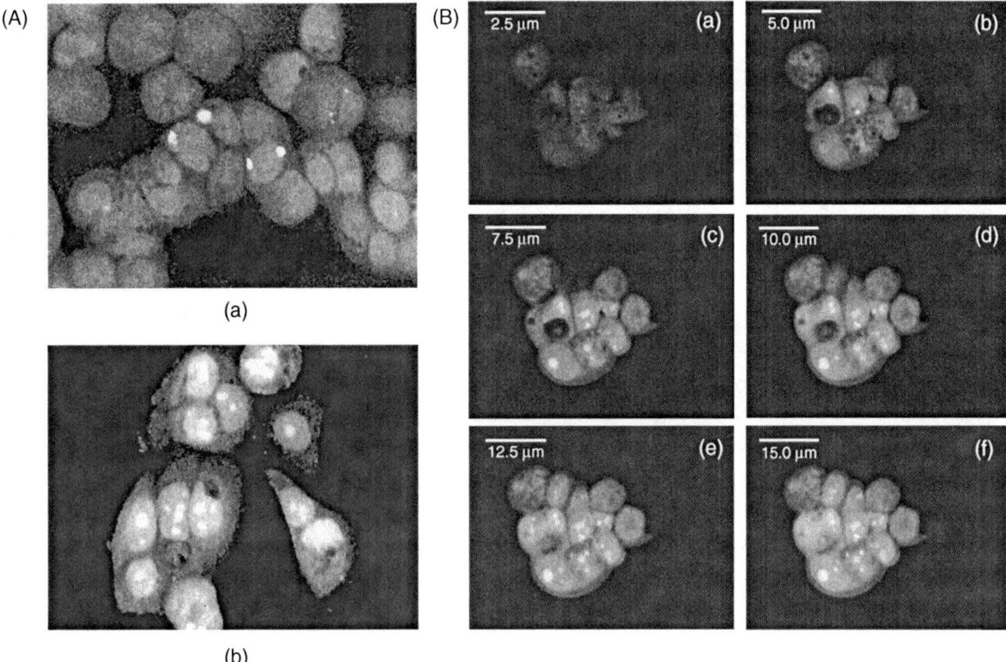

FIGURE 6.5 (A) Confocal fluorescence microscopy images of MCF-7 cells after 15 h *in vitro* exposure to (a) fluorescent paclitaxel-loaded PEG/PCL copolymeric nanoparticles and (b) fluorescent paclitaxel-loaded folate-conjugated PEG/PCL nanoparticles (×1000). (B) A series of representative lateral (*x–y*) confocal fluorescence microscopy images of MCF-7 cells incubated with fluorescent paclitaxel-loaded folate-conjugated PEG/PCL nanoparticles as a function of cell depth. (From Park, E.K., Kim, S.Y., Lee, S.B., and Lee, Y.M. *Journal of Controlled Release* 109, 158–168, 2005.)

FR-overexpressing cancer cells. PLL-PEG-FOL coated PLGA nanoparticles demonstrated far greater extent of cellular uptake to KB cells (A human epidermal carcinoma cell line; folate receptor overexpressing cell line), suggesting that they were mainly taken up by FR-mediated endocytosis. The enhanced cellular uptake was also observed even in the presence of serum proteins, possibly due to the dense-seeded PEG chains [93]. Lee et al. developed folate ligand–coupled DSPE using a PEG linker (folate-PE$_{2000}$-DSPE) to deliver liposome-encapsulated doxorubicin epithelial cancer cells that resulted in a 45-fold increased uptake of encapsulated doxorubicin compared with nontargeted vesicles [42,94,95].

6.5.3.1.4 Hyaluronic Acid

Hyaluronic acid (HA), a negative polysaccharide containing two alternating units of D-glucuronic acid and N-acetyl-D-glucosamine with a molecular weight of 10^5–10^7 Da, is one of the major components of extracellular matrix. HA is responsible for various functions within the extracellular matrix, such as cell growth, differentiation, and migration. Various HA-binding receptors are known, such as cell surface glycoprotein CD44, receptor for HA-mediated motility (RHAMM), HA receptor for endocytosis (HARE), lymphatic vessel endocytic receptor (LYVE-1), and intracellular HA-binding proteins including CDC37, RHAMM/IHABP, P-32, and IHABP4. HA levels are elevated in various cancer cells (epithelial, ovarian, colon, stomach, and acute leukemia), resulting in enhanced binding and internalization of HA [19].

Luo et al. used HA as a tumor-targeting moiety in a drug delivery system with N-(2-hydroxypropyl)methacrylamide (HPMA) polymer. HPMA-HA-doxorubicin bioconjugates with lysosome-degradable peptide linkage showed enhanced internalization and cytotoxicity for the HBL-100 (breast) cell line compared to nontargeting conjugates, while the systemic toxicity of HPMA-HA-doxorubicin bioconjugates in primary murine fibroblasts was very low [96].

Eliaz et al. developed liposomes containing HA and doxoribicin as a tumor targeting drug delivery system. They demonstrated that the binding affinity of liposomes is attributed to the specific CD44–HA interaction, and the degree of HA–liposome uptake by murine melanoma B16F10 tumor cell line was proportional to the loading of HA. The HA–liposomes exhibited almost selective tumor targeting and cytotoxicity [97].

6.5.3.2 Inhibition of Angiogenesis

Angiogenesis, the formation of new capillaries from pre-existing vessels, is essential for tumor progression. Antiangiogenic therapy has proven to be a promising concept by eliminating new tumor vasculature with the destruction of microvasculature. The differentially expressed endothelial cell surface markers in angiogenic tumor vessels should be excellent targets for site-specific therapy [98]. These molecules regulate the proliferative and invasive activity of the endothelial cells that line blood vessels. Some examples of therapeutic strategies include limiting endothelial proliferation and motility, increasing expression of angiogenesis inhibitors, and decreasing the amount of angiogenesis stimulatory factors at the tumor sites. Some of the most prominent angiogenesis stimulatory molecules include vascular endothelial growth factor (VEGF), basic fibroblast growth factor, platelet-derived growth factor, and certain matrix metalloproteinases. Some endogenous angiogenesis inhibitors are the interferon family (α, β, and γ), thrombospondin-1 and -2, certain tissue inhibitors of matrix metalloproteinases, and protein fragments such as angiostatin and endostatin [13,98].

For example, streptavidin-coated fluorescent polystyrene nanoparticles (Fluospheres and Trans-Fluospheres) were used in single color flow cytometry to detect the epidermal growth receptor (EGFR) on A431 human epidermoid carcinoma cells. The results showed that the fluorescent nanoparticles provided a sensitivity 25-fold greater than the conjugate streptavidin–fluorescein [28].

Integrin $\alpha_V\beta_3$ is a molecular target for many solid tumors that is highly expressed in angiogenic endothelial cells. Various $\alpha_V\beta_3$-targeted therapeutic systems have shown remarkable *in vitro* and *in vivo* success [99]. Gao reported the development of multifunctional polymeric micelles with cancer-targeting capability via $\alpha_V\beta_3$ integrins. Doxorubicin and a cluster of superparamagnetic iron oxide (SPIO) nanoparticles were loaded successfully inside the micelle core. The presence of cRGD on the micelle surface resulted in the cancer-targeted delivery to $\alpha_V\beta_3$-expressing tumor cells. *In vitro* MRI and cytotoxicity studies demonstrated the ultrasensitive MRI imaging and $\alpha_V\beta_3$-specific cytotoxicity response of these multifunctional polymeric micelles [34].

6.5.3.3 Vascular Targeting

Unlike the inhibition of angiogenesis, which aims at preventing the growth of new blood vessels, vascular targeting aims at the rapid and selective shutdown and/or damage of the established tumor vasculature, leading to secondary tumor cell death. This strategy shows potential advantages compared with the direct attack of tumor cells [100–102]. It has been known that the endothelium and surrounding stroma in tumors differ from normal tissues. The blood flow through the tumor capillaries is often sluggish due to the disorganized and tortuous tumor vasculature compared with the vasculature in normal organs [103]. The endothelial cell has been shown to respond transcriptionally to all these stimuli, giving rise to the production of new proteins on its surface or surrounding extracellular matrix. Some of these specific markers found either directly on the endothelial cells or secreted into the stroma surrounding the blood vessels could be used as targets for vascular targeting approaches [100].

The first vascular targeting was approved by the FDA in 1999 for the treatment of age-related macular degeneration. In 2003, clinical trials with antiangiogenesis drug Avastin (Genentech) showed prolonged survival of patients with metastatic colorectal cancer. Hood et al. investigated whether gene delivery may also be targeted to neovasculature by coupling lipid-based cationic nanoparticles to integrin $\alpha_V\beta_3$ targeting ligands in tumor-bearing mice. Nontargeted nanoparticles showed limited expression (<0.5 ng/g tissue) in tumor, lung, and heart. For targeted nanoparticles, significant expression was found in the tumor (4 ng/g tissue) and no expression in the lung, liver, or heart [100]. Systemic injection of the cationic nanoparticles coupled with integrin $\alpha_V\beta_3$ targeting ligands resulted in apoptosis of the tumor-associated endothelium, ultimately leading to tumor cell apoptosis and sustained regression of established primary and metastatic tumors [99].

Although the combination of traditional chemotherapy with anti-angiogenesis agents that inhibit blood vessel growth is an emerging model for effective cancer treatments, the implementation of this approach has two major obstacles. First, the long-term shutdown of tumor blood vessels by the antiangiogenesis agent can prevent the tumor from receiving a therapeutic concentration of the chemotherapy agent. Second, inhibiting blood supply drives the intratumoral accumulation of hypoxia-inducible factor-1α (HIF1-α). Overexpression of HIF1-α is correlated with increased tumor invasiveness and resistance to chemotherapy. Recently, Sengupta et al. developed "nanocell," which is composed of nuclear nanoparticles within an extranuclear PEGylated lipid envelope that is preferentially taken up by the tumor [101]. The nanoparticles enable a temporal release of two drugs: the outer envelope first releases an anti-angiogenesis agent, causing a vascular shutdown, and the inner nanoparticles, which are trapped inside the tumor, release a chemotherapy agent. They demonstrated that the focal release within the tumor results in an improved therapeutic index with reduced toxicity [101].

6.5.4 *In Vivo* Studies with Nanoparticulates for Targeted Chemotherapy

Animal tests are critical in determining whether the nanoparticles under a specific design for drug loading could be feasible for clinical administration. Several factors for *in vivo* application that should be considered in the selection of materials and fabrication of nanoparticles are [2,15–18] (1) biocompatibility of particles and coatings, (2) particle size, (3) immunogenicity, (4) surface properties, (5) degradation properties, (6) drug-loading efficiencies, (7) release characteristics, and (8) stability of the drug and fabricated nanoparticles.

The overall therapeutic effects of the system can be determined from plots of the plasma drug concentration versus time. Nanoparticle formulation of the tested drug should be evaluated in comparison with the free drug formulation [3]. Yoo et al. conducted *in vitro* and *in vivo* experiments for controlled release of doxorubicin-loaded PLA nanoparticles. *In vivo* antitumor activity assay showed that a single injection of the nanoparticles had comparable activity with that of free doxorubicin administered by daily injection [104]. Lu et al. investigated the pharmacokinetics of paclitaxel released from long-circulating solid lipid nanoparticles (SLN) in kunming (KM) mice. They found that the nanoparticles exhibited great advantages over the Cremorphor formulation of paclitaxel, with half-lives of 10.06 and 4.88 h, respectively; in comparison, the half-life for the Cremorphor formulation of paclitaxel was 1.36 h [105].

Kim et al. evaluated the *in vivo* distribution of various self-assembled nanoparticles in tumor-bearing mice in order to investigate the mechanisms underlying tumor targeting. Fluorescein isothiocyanate–conjugated glycol chitosan nanoparticles were preferentially localized in perivascular regions, implying extravasation to the tumor through the hyperpermeable tumor vasculature. They showed that the magnitude and pattern of tumoral distribution of self-assembled nanoparticles were influenced by several factors such as *in vivo* colloidal stability, particle size, intracellular uptake of nanoparticles, and tumor angiogenesis [106]. Hashida et al. showed that a sixth generation lysine dendrimer–conjugated PEG exhibited higher retention in blood and lower accumulativeness in organs depending on the rate of polyethlyene glycolation than did intact lysine dendrimer [107].

Yang et al. developed the folate-conjugated block copolymeric nanoparticles containing doxorubicin for targeted delivery [108]. *In vivo* experiments conducted in a 4T1 mouse breast cancer model demonstrated that DOX-loaded micelles had a longer blood circulation time than free DOX

($T_{1/2}$: 140 and 30 min, respectively). In addition, the block copolymeric nanoparticles delivered an increased amount of doxorubicin to the tumor when compared with free DOX [108].

Research performed by Dagor et al. indicated that vasoactive intestinal peptide-targeted liposomes achieve significantly higher intratumoral accumulation than nontargeted counterparts, suggesting that levels of intratumoral accumulation of actively targeted particulates are influenced by the choice of the ligand and by the microenvironment of the individual tumor type. It remains to be established whether noninternalizing ligands will also yield improved therapeutic efficacy compared with passively targeted particulates under conditions of higher intratumoral accumulation [109].

In spite of the limitations in targeting tumor cells in solid tumors, a particulate drug carrier for active targeting has entered clinical trials. MCC465 is a sterically stabilized liposomes containing doxorubicin that selectively targets stomach cancer cells using f(ab')$_2$ human IgG Mab fragment and is currently in Phase I clinical trials [110]. MCC465 demonstrated clinical efficacy and considerably reduced side effects relative to other therapies. Furthermore, an anti-HER2, doxorubicin-incorporating SSL formulation is about to enter clinical development trials [111].

Foarokhzad et al. developed poly(D,L-lactide-*co*-glycolide)-PEG block copolymer nanoparticles conjugated with the A10 RNA aptamer (Apt) that binds to the prostate-specific membrane antigen (PSMA), and they investigated the biodistribution of Apt-conjugated nanoparticle drug carriers in a LNCaP (PSMA+) xenograft mouse model of prostate cancer. The surface functionalization of nanoparticles with the A10 PSMA Apt significantly enhanced delivery of nanoparticles to tumors compared with equivalent nanoparticles lacking the A10 PSMA Apt (a 3.77-fold increase at 24 h) [35].

6.6 CONCLUSIONS

Traditional cancer chemotherapy relies on the premise that rapidly proliferating cancer cells are more likely to be killed by a cytotoxic agent. In reality, however, cytotoxic agents have very little or no specificity, which lead to systemic toxicity, causing severe, undesirable side effects. The current focus in pharmaceuticals is shifting to a "smart drug" paradigm, in which increased efficacy and decreased toxicity are the motivating factors. An attractive strategy to enhance the therapeutic index of drugs is to specifically deliver these agents to the defined target cells, thereby keeping them away from healthy cells, which are sensitive to the toxic effects of the drugs. Many attempts are being made to explore the potential of specific and target-oriented delivery systems. New nanoparticle structures, materials, and new encapsulation methods are continuously being reported. With these dedicated efforts, it seems that the synergistic future of a nanoparticle delivery system holds substantial promise. Engineering the drug loading of nanoparticle drug carriers, controlling the drug release profile, and guiding nanoparticle systems to the desired target are among other challenges that are currently being evaluated. Specifically, ligand receptor–medicated delivery systems have received major attention in the past few years due to the potential of nonimmunogenic, site-specific targeting to ligand-specific sites of the naturally existing ligands and their receptors. There is no doubt that molecularly targeted therapies will revolutionize the treatment of cancer and other diseases. Although major advances have been made in the delivery of cancer chemotherapeutics, much work lies ahead. To accomplish the desired goals of this innovative system, further clinical trials need to be performed as they are the key to the realization and success of the next generation of therapy.

REFERENCES

1. A. El-Aneed, An overview of current delivery systems in cancer gene therapy, *Journal of Controlled Release* 94 (2004) 1–14.
2. C. Leuschner and C. Kumar, Nanoparticles for cancer drug delivery, in *Nanofabrication Towards Biomedical Applications* (Eds.) C. Kumar, J. Hormes, and C. Leuschner, 2005 Wiley-VCH Verlag GmbH & Co., KGaA, Weinheim, Germany, pp. 289–326.

3. S.S. Feng and S. Chien, Chemotherapeutic engineering: Application and further development of chemical engineering principles for chemotherapy of cancer and other diseases, *Chemical Engineering Science* 58 (2003) 4087–4114.
4. G.M. Dubowchik and M.A. Wallker, Receptor-medicated and enzyme-dependent targeting of cytotoxic anticancer drugs, *Pharmacology and Therapeutics* 83 (1999) 67–123.
5. A. Nori and J. Kopecek, Intracellular targeting of polymer-bound drugs for cancer chemotherapy, *Advanced Drug Delivery Reviews* 57 (2005) 609–636.
6. E.S. Kawasaki and A. Player, Nanotechnology, nanomedicine, and the development of new, effective therapies for cancer, *Nanomedicine: Nanotechnology, Biology, and Medicine* 1 (2005) 101–109.
7. R.M. Hughes, Strategies for cancer gene therapy, *Journal of Surgical Oncology* 85 (2004) 28–35.
8. M.J. Vicent and R. Duncan, Polymer conjugates: Nanosized medicines for targeting cancer, *Trends in Biotechnology* 24 (2006) 39–47.
9. M.A. Moses, H. Brem, and R. Langer, Advancing the field of drug delivery: Taking aim at cancer, *Cancer Cell* 4 (2003) 337–341.
10. G. Szakacs, J.K. Paterson, J.A. Ludwing, C. Booth-Genthe, and M.M. Gottesman, Targeting multidrug resistance in cancer, *Nature Reviews Drug Discovery* 5 (2006) 219–234.
11. C.R. Dass and P.F.M. Choong, Carrier-mediated delivery of peptide for cancer therapy, *Peptides* 27 (2006) 3020–3028.
12. P. Couvreur, R. Gref, K. Andrieux, and C. Malvy, Nanotechnologies for drug delivery: Application to cancer and autoimmune diseases, *Progress in Solid State Chemistry* 34 (2006) 231–235.
13. L. Brannon-Peppas and J.O. Blanchette, Nanoparticles and targeted systems for cancer therapy, *Advanced Drug Delivery Reviews* 56 (2004) 1649–1659.
14. T.M. Fahmy, P.M. Fong, A. Goyal, and W.M. Saltzman, Targeted drug delivery, *Nano Today* August (2005) 18–26.
15. V.P. Torchilin, Multifunctional nanocarriers, *Advanced Drug Delivery Reviews* 58 (2006) 1532–1555.
16. A.I. Freeman and E. Mayhew, Targeted drug delivery, *Cancer* 58 (1986) 573–583.
17. K. Petrak, Essential properties of drug-targeting delivery systems, *Drug Discovery Today* 10 (2005) 1667–1673.
18. V.P. Torchilin, Drug targeting, *European Journal of Pharmaceutical Sciences* 11 (2000) S81–S91.
19. S. Jaracz, J. Chen, L.V. Kuznetsova, and I. Ojima, Recent advances in tumor-targeting anticancer drug conjugates, *Bioorganic and Medicinal Chemistry* 13 (2005) 5043–5054.
20. F.J. Toublan, S. Boppart, and K.S. Suslick, Tumor targeting by surface-modified protein microspheres, *Journal of American Chemical Society* 128 (2006) 3472–3473.
21. K.C. Brown, New approaches for cell-specific targeting: Identification of cell-selective peptides from combinatorial libraries, *Current Opinion in Chemical Biology* 4 (2000) 16–21.
22. G. Alvisi, I.K.H. Poon, D.A. Jans, Tumor-specific nuclear targeting: Promises for anti-cancer therapy? *Drug Resistance Updates* 9 (2006) 40–50.
23. O.M. Koo, I. Rubinstein, and H. Onyuksel, Role of nanotechnology in targeted drug delivery and imaging: A concise review, *Nanomedicine: Nanotechnology, Biology, and Medicine* 1 (2005) 193–212.
24. E. Ruoslahti, Drug targeting to specific vascular sites, *Drug Discovery Today* 7 (2002) 1138–1142.
25. E.Y. Zhang, M.A. Phelps, C. Cheng, S. Ekins, and P.W. Swaan, Modeling of active transport systems, *Advanced Drug Delivery Reviews* 54 (2002) 329–354.
26. R.S. Herbst, Role of novel targeted therapies in the clinic, *British Journal of Cancer* 92 (2005) S21–S27.
27. N. Nishiyama and K. Kataoka, Current state, achievements, and future prospects of polymeric micelles as nanocarriers for drug and gene delivery, *Pharmacology and Therapeutics* 112 (2006) 630–648.
28. I. Brigger, C. Dubernet, and P. Couvreur, Nanoparticles in cancer therapy and diagnosis, *Advanced Drug Delivery Reviews* 54 (2002) 631–651.
29. J.A. Hubbell, Enhancing drug function, *Materials Science* 300 (2003) 595–596.
30. A. Rosler, G.W.M. Vandermeulen, and H. Klok, Advanced drug delivery devices via self-assembly of amphiphilic block copolymers, *Advanced Drug Delivery Reviews* 53 (2001) 95–108.
31. G. Riess, Micellization of block copolymers, *Progress in Polymer Science* 28 (2003) 1107–1170.
32. K.K. Jain, Nanoparticles as targeting ligands, *Trends in Biotechnology* 24 (2006) 143–145.
33. J.M. Saul, A.V. Annapragada, and R.V. Bellamkonda, A dual-ligand approach for enhancing targeting selectivity of therapeutic nanocarriers, *Journal of Controlled Release* 114 (2006) 277–287.
34. N. Nasongkla, E. Bey, J. Ren, H. Ai, C. Khemtong, J.S. Guthi, S.F. Chin, A.D. Sherry, D.A. Boothman, and J. Gao, Multifunctional polymeric micelles as cancer-targeted, MRI-ultrasensitive drug delivery systems, *Nano Letters* 6 (2006) 2427–2430.

35. J. Cheng, B.A. Teply, I. Sherifi, J. Sung, G. Luther, F.X. Gu, E. Levy-Nissenbaum, A.F. Radovic-Moreno, R. Langer, and O.C. Farokhzad, Formation of functionalized PLGA-PEG nanoparticles for *in vivo* targeted drug delivery, *Biomaterials* 28 (2007) 869–876.

36. M.L. Hans and A.M. Lowman, Biodegradable nanoparticles for drug delivery and targeting, *Current Opinion in Solid State and Materials Science* 6 (2002) 319–327.

37. M. Rawat, D. Singh, S. Saraf, and S. Saraf, Nanocarriers: Promising vehicles for bioactive drugs, *Biological and Pharmaceutical Bulletin* 29 (2006) 1790–1798.

38. V.P. Torchilin, Targeted polymeric micelles for delivery of poorly soluble drugs, *Cellular and Molecular Life Sciences* 61 (2004) 2549–2559.

39. T.C. Yih and M. Al-Fandi, Engineered nanoparticles as precise drug delivery systems, *Journal of Cellular Biochemistry* 97 (2006) 1184–1190.

40. S.Y. Kim, S.H. Cho, L.Y. Chu, and Y.M. Lee, Biotin-conjugated block copolymeric nanoparticles for tumor-targeted drug delivery systems, Macromolecular Research, in press.

41. C.P. Reis, R.J. Neufeld, A.J. Ribeiro, F. Veiga, Nanoencapsulation II. Biomedical applications and current status of peptide and protein nanoparticulate delivery systems, *Nanomedicine: Nanotechnology, Biology, and Medicine* 2 (2006) 53–65.

42. E. Forssen and M. Willis, Ligand-targeted liposomes, *Advanced Drug Delivery Reviews* 29 (1998) 249–271.

43. B.J. Lestini, S.M. Sagnella, Z. Xu, M.S. Shive, N.J. Richter, J. Jayaseharan, A.J. Case, K. Kottke-Marchant, J.M. Anderson, R.E. Marchant, Surface modification of liposomes for selective cell targeting in cardiovascular drug delivery, *Journal of Controlled Release* 78 (2002) 235–247.

44. T. Terada, M. Iwai, S. Kawakami, F. Yamashita, and M. Hashida, Novel PEG-matrix metallopreoteinase-2 cleavable peptide-lipid containing galactosylated liposomes for hepatocellular carcinoma-selective targeting, *Journal of Controlled Release* 111 (2006) 333–342.

45. R.I. Pakunlu, Y. Wang, W. Tsao, V. Pozharov, T.J. Cook, and T. Minko, Enhancement of the efficacy of chemotherapy for lung cancer by simultaneous suppression of multidrug resistance and antiapoptotic cellular defense: Novel multicomponent delivery system, *Cancer Research* 64 (2004) 6214–6224.

46. M. Singh, Transferrin as a targeting ligand for liposomes and anticancer drugs, *Current Pharmaceutical Design* 5 (1999) 443–451.

47. J. Huwyler, J. Yang, and W.M. Pardridge, Receptors mediated delivery of daunomycin using immunoliposomes: Pharmacokinetics and tissue distribution in the rat, *The Journal of Pharmacology and Experimental Therapeutics* 282 (1997) 1541–1546.

48. R.L. Juliano, *Targeted Drug Delivery*, Springer-Verlag, Berlin Heidelberg, Germany, 1991.

49. P.D. Scholes, A.G.A. Coombes, M.C. Davies, L. Illum, and S.S. Davis, Particle engineering of biodegradable colloids for site-specific drug delivery, in *Controlled Drug Delivery*, K. Park (Ed.), American Chemical Society, Danvers, MA, 1997, pp. 73–106.

50. F. Puisieux, G. Barratt, G. Couarraze, P. Couvreur, J.P. Devissaguet, C. Dubernet, E. Fattal, H. Fessi, C. Vauthier, and S. Benita, Polymeric micro- and nanoparticles as drug carriers, in *Polymeric Biomaterials*, S. Dumitriu (Ed.), Marcel Dekker, Inc., New York, 1994, pp. 749–794.

51. D. Maysinger, O. Berezovska, R. Savic, P.L. Soo, and A. Eisenberg, Block copolymers modify the internalization of micelle-incorporated probes into neutral cells, *Biochimica et Biophysica Acta* 1539 (2001) 205–217.

52. A.V. Kabanov, E.V. Batrakova, and V.Y. Alakhov, Pluronic block copolymers for overcoming drug resistance in cancer, *Advanced Drug Delivery Reviews* 54 (2002) 759–779.

53. E.R. Gillies and J.M.J. Frechet, Dendrimers and dendritic polymers in drug delivery, *Drug Discovery Today* 10 (2005) 35–43.

54. A.K. Patri, J.F. Kukowska-Latallo, and J.R. Barker, Targeted drug delivery with dendrimers: Comparison of the release kinetics of covalently conjugated drug and non-covalent drug inclusion complex, *Advanced Drug Delivery Reviews* 57 (2005) 2203–2214.

55. U. Gupta, H.B. Agashe, A. Asthana, and N.K. Jain, A review of *in vitro–in vivo* investigations on dendrimers: The novel nanoscopic drug carriers, *Nanomedicine: Nanotechnology, Biology, and Medicine* 2 (2006) 66–73.

56. G.A. Hughes, Nanostructure-mediated drug delivery, *Nanomedicine: Nanotechnology, Biology, and Medicine* 1 (2005) 22–30.

57. R. Jevprasesphant, J. Penny, R. Jalal, D. Attwood, N.B. Mckeown, and A. D'Emanuele, The influence of surface modification on the cytotoxicity of PAMAM dendrimers, *International Journal of Pharmaceutics* 252 (2003) 263–266.

58. S.S. Nigavekar, L.Y. Sung, M. Llanes, A. El-Jawahri, T.S. Lawrence, and C.W. Becker, 3H dendrimer nanoparticle organ/tumor distribution, *Pharmaceutical Research* 21 (2004) 476–483.

59. N. Nishiyama, H.R. Stapert, G.D. Zhang, D. Takasu, D.L. Jiang, and T. Nagano, Light-harvesting ionic dendrimer porphyrins as new photosensitizers for photodynamic therapy, *Bioconjugate Chemistry* 14 (2003) 58–66.

60. Y. Gao, Biofunctionalization of magnetic nanoparticles, in *Biofunctionalization of Nanomaterials*, C. Kumar (Ed.), Wiley-VCH Verlag GmbH&Co. KGaA, Weinheim, Germany, 2005.

61. T. Neuberger, B. Schopf, H. Hofmann, M. Hofmann, and B. Rechenberg, Superparamagnetic nanoparticles for biomedical applications: Possibilities and limitations of a new drug delivery system, *Journal of Magnetism and Magnetic Materials* 293 (2005) 483–496.

62. I. Roy, T.Y. Ohulchanskyy, H.E. Pudavar, E.J. Bergey, A.R. Oseroff, and J. Morgan, Ceramic-based nanoparticles entrapping water-insoluble photosensitizing anticancer drugs: A novel drug carrier system for photodynamic therapy, *Journal of American Chemical Society* 125 (2003) 7860–7865.

63. W. Paul and C. Sharma, Porous hydroxyapatite nanoparticles for intestinal delivery, *Trends in Biomaterials and Artificial Organs* 14 (2001) 37–38.

64. R.A. Gemeinhart, D. Luo, and W.M. Saltzman, Cellular fate of a modular DNA delivery system mediated by silica nanoparticles, *Biotechnology Progress* 21 (2005) 532–537.

65. S. Liu, H.L. Zhang, T.C. Liu, B. Liu, Y.C. Cao, Z.L. Huang, Y.D. Zhao, and Q.M. Luo, Optimization of the methods for introduction of amine groups onto the silica nanoparticle surface, *Journal of Biomedical Materials Research* 80A (2006) 752–757.

66. M. Priyabara, B. Resham, and M. Debabrata, Gold nanoparticles bearing functional anti-cancer drug and anti-angiogenic agent: A "2 in 1" system with potential application in therapeutics, *Journal of Biomedical Nanotechnology* 1 (2005) 224–228.

67. A.G. Skirtach, C. Dejugnat, D. Braun, A.S. Susha, A.L. Rogach, W.J. Parak, H. Mohwald, and G.B. Sukhorukov, The role of metal nanoparticles in remote release of encapsulated materials, *Nano Letters* 5 (2005) 1371–1377.

68. S. Rhaese, H. Briesen, H. Rubsamen-Waigmann, J. Kreuter, and K. Langer, Human serum albumin–polyethylenimine nanoparticles for gene delivery, *Journal of Controlled Release* 92 (2003) 199–208.

69. H. Wartlick, B. Spankuch-Schmitt, K. Strebhardt, J. Kreuter, and K. Langer, Tumour cell delivery of antisense oligonucleotides by human serum albumin nanoparticles, *Journal of Controlled Release* 96 (2004) 483–495.

70. M. Ferrari, Cancer nanotechnology: Opportunities and challenges. *Nature Reviews Cancer* 5 (2005) 161–171.

71. K. Garber, Improved paclitaxel formulation hints at new chemotherapy approach, *Journal of the National Cancer Institute* 96 (2004) 90–91.

72. S.M. Moghimi, A.C. Hunter, and J.C. Murray, Long-circulating and target-specific nanoparticles: Theory to practice, *Pharmacological Review* 53 (2001) 283–318.

73. M. Koval, K. Preiter, C. Adles, P.D. Stahl, and T.H. Steinberg, Size of IgG-opsonized particles determines macrophage response during internalization, *Experimental Cell Research* 242 (1998) 265–273.

74. J. Rejman, V. Oberle, I.S. Zuhorn, and D. Hoekstra, Size-dependent internalization of particles via the pathways of clathrin- and caveolae-mediated endocytosis, *Biochemical Journal* 377 (2004) 159–169.

75. S. Stolnik, L. Illum, and S.S. Davis, Long circulating drug carriers, *Advanced Drug Delivery Reviews* 16 (1995) 195–214.

76. R.L. Juliano and D.E. Stamp, The effect of particle size and charge on the clearance rates of liposomes and liposome encapsulated drugs, *Biochemical and Biophysical Research Communications* 63 (1975) 651–658.

77. Y. Tabata and Y. Ikada, Effect of the size and surface charge of polymer microspheres on their phagocytosis by macrophage, *Biomaterials* 9 (1988) 356–362.

78. A. Vonarbourg, C. Passirani, P. Saulnier, and J.P. Benoit, Parameters influencing the stealthiness of colloidal drug delivery systems, *Biomaterials* 27 (2006) 4356–4373.

79. L. Illum, L.O. Jacobsen, R.H. Muller, E. Mak, and S.S. Davis, Surface characteristics and the interaction of colloidal partices with mouse peritoneal macrophages, *Biomaterials* 8 (1987) 113–117.

80. K.D. Pavey and C.J. Olliff, SPR analysis of the total reduction of protein adsorption to surfaces coated with mixtures of long- and short-chain polyethylene oxide block copolymers, *Biomaterials* 20 (1999) 885–890.

81. R. Gref, M. Luck, P. Quellec, M. Marchand, E. Dellacherie, S. Harnisch, T. Blunk, and R.H. Muller, 'Stealth' corona-core nanoparticles surface modified by polyethylene glycol (PEG): Influences of the corona (OEG chain length and surface density) and of the core composition on phagocytic uptake and plasma protein adsorption, *Colloidal and Surfaces B: Biointerfaces* 18 (2000) 301–313.

82. M. Vittaz, D. Bazile, G. Spenlehauer, T. Verrecchia, M. Veillard, F. Puisieux, and D. Labarre, Effect of PEO surface density on long-circulating PLA-PEO nanoparticles which are very low complement activators, *Biomaterials* 17 (1996) 1575–1581.

83. D. Schrama, R.A. Reisfeld, and J.C. Becker, Antibody targeted drugs as cancer therapeutics, *Nature Reviews Drug Discovery* 5 (2006) 147–159.

84. R. Bicknell, The realization of targeted antitumor therapy, *British Journal of Cancer* 92 (2005) S2–S5.

85. Y. Cao and L. Lam, Bispecific antibody conjugates in therapeutics, *Advanced Drug Delivery Reviews* 55 (2003) 171–197.

86. G. Kohler and C. Milstein, Continuous cultures of fused cells secreting antibody of predefined specificity, *Nature* 256 (1975) 495–497.

87. H. Li and Z.M. Qian, Transfferin/transferrin receptor-mediated drug delivery, *Medicinal Research Reviews* 22 (2002) 225–250.

88. A. Widera, F. Norouziyan, and W.C. Shen, Mechanisms of TfR-mediated transcytosis and sorting in epithelial cells and applications toward drug delivery, *Advanced Drug Delivery Reviews* 55 (2003) 1439–1466.

89. Y. Lu and P.S. Low, Folate-mediated delivery of macromolecular anticancer therapeutic agents, *Advanced Drug Delivery Reviews* 54 (2002) 675–693.

90. Y. Lu, E. Sega, C.P. Leamon, and P.S. Low, Folate receptor-targeted immunotherapy of cancer: Mechanism and therapeutic potential, *Advanced Drug Delivery Reviews* 56 (2004) 1161–1176.

91. E.K. Park, S.B. Lee, and Y.M. Lee, Preparation and characterization of methoxy poly(ethylene glycol)/poly(ε-caprolactone) amphiphilic block copolymeric nanospheres for tumor-specific folate-mediated targeting of anticancer drugs, *Biomaterials* 26 (2005) 1053–1061.

92. E.K. Park, S.Y. Kim, S.B. Lee, and Y.M. Lee, Folate-conjugated methoxy poly(ethylene glycol)/poly(ε-caprolactone) amphiphilic block copolymeric micelles for tumor-targeted drug delivery, *Journal of Controlled Release* 109 (2005) 158–168.

93. S.H. Kim, J.H. Jeong, K.W. Chun, and T.G. Park, Target-specific cellular uptake of PLGA nanoparticles coated with poly(L-lysine)-poly(ethylene glycol)-folate conjugate, *Langmuir* 21 (2005) 8852–8857.

94. R.J. Lee and P.S. Low, Delivery of liposomes into cultured KB cells via folate receptor-mediated endocytosis, *The Journal of Biological Chemistry* 269 (1994) 3198–3204.

95. R.J. Lee and P.S. Low, Folate-mediated tumor cell targeting of liposome-entrapped doxorubicin *in vitro*, *Biochimica et Biophysica Acta* 1233 (1995) 134–144.

96. Y. Luo, N.J. Bernshaw, Z.R. Lu, J. Kopecek, and G.D. Prestwich, Targeted delivery of doxorubicin by HPMA copolymer–hyaluronan bioconjugates, *Pharmaceutical Research* 19 (2002) 396–402.

97. R.E. Eliaz and F.C. Szoka, Liposome-encapsulated doxorubicin targeted to CD44: A strategy to kill CD44-overexpressing tumor cells, *Cancer Research* 61 (2001) 2592–2601.

98. M. Shadidi and M. Sioud, Selective targeting of cancer cells using synthetic peptides, *Drug Resistance Updates* 6 (2003) 363–371.

99. J.D. Hood, M. Bednarski, R. Frausto, S. Guccione, R.A. Reisfeld, R. Xiang, and D.A. Cheresh, Tumor regression by targeted gene delivery to the neovasculature, *Science* 296 (2002) 2404–2407.

100. E. Trachsel and D. Neri, Antibodies for angiogenesis inhibition, vascular targeting and endothelial cell transcytosis, *Advanced Drug Delivery* 58 (2006) 735–754.

101. S. Sengupta, D. Eavarone, I. Capila, G. Zhao, N. Watson, and T. Kiziltepe, Temporal targeting of tumor cells and neovasculature with a nanoscale delivery system, *Nature* 436 (2005) 568–572.

102. H. Maeda, J. Fang, T. Inutsuka, and Y. Kitamoto, Vascular permeability enhancement in solid tumor: Various factors, mechanisms involved and its implications, *International Immunopharmacology* 3 (2003) 319–328.

103. G.M. Tozer, S.M. Ameer-Beg, J. Baker, P.R. Barber, S.A. Hill, R.J. Hodgkiss, R. Locke, V.E. Prize, I. Wilson, and B. Vojnovic, Intravital imaging of tumour vascular networks using multi-photon fluorescence microscopy, *Advanced Drug Delivery Review* 57 (2005) 135–152.

104. H.S. Yoo, K.H. Lee, and J.E. Oh, *In vitro* and *in vivo* anti-tumor activities of nanoparticles based on doxorubicin-PLGA conjugates, *Journal of Controlled Release* 68 (2000) 419–431.

105. D.B. Chen, T.Z. Yang, W.L. Lu, and Q. Zhang, *In vitro* and *in vivo* study of two types of long-circulating solid lipid nanoparticles containing paclitaxel, *Chemical and Parmaceutical Bulletin* 49 (2001) 1444–1447.

106. Y.W. Cho, S.A. Park, T.H. Han, D.H. Son, J.S. Park, S.J. Oh, D.H. Moon, K. Cho, C. Ahn, Y. Byun, I. Kim, I.C. Kwon, and S.Y. Kim, *In vivo* tumor targeting and radionuclide imaging with self-assembled nanoparticles: Mechanisms, key factors, and their implications, *Biomaterials* 28 (2007) 1236–1247.

107. T. Okuda, S. Kawakami, N. Akimoto, T. Niidome, F. Yamashita, and M. Hashida, PEGylated lysine dendrimers for tumor-selective targeting after intravenous injection in tumor-bearing mice, *Journal of Controlled Release* 116 (2006) 330–336.

108. S.Q. Liu, N. Wiradharma, S.J. Gao, Y.W. Tong, and Y.Y. Yang, Bio-functional micelles self-assembled form a folate-conjugated block copolymer for targeted intracellular delivery of anticancer drugs, *Biomaterials* 28 (2007) 1423–1433.

109. S. Dagar, A. Krishnadas, I. Rubinstein, M.J. Blend, and H. Onyuksel, VIP grafted sterically stabilized liposomes for targeted imaging of breast cancer: *In vivo* studies, *Journal of Controlled Release* 91 (2003) 123–133.

110. S. Hosokawa, T. Tagawa, H. Niki, Y. Hirakawa, K. Nohga, and K. Nagaike, Efficacy of immunoliposomes on cancer models in a cell-surface-antigen-density-dependent manner, *British Journal of Cancer* 89 (2003) 1545–1551.

111. P. Sapra and T.M. Allen, Ligand-targeted liposomal anticancer drugs, *Progress in Lipid Research* 42 (2003) 439–462.

7 Polymeric Nano/Microparticles for Oral Delivery of Proteins and Peptides

Sajeesh S. and Chandra P. Sharma

CONTENTS

7.1 INTRODUCTION

Recent advancement in the field of pharmaceutical biotechnology and introduction of recombinant DNA technology have led to the production of a number of therapeutic peptides and proteins for the treatment of several life-threatening diseases (Table 7.1). A number of peptide-based therapeutics such as recombinant hormones, cytokines, vaccines, monoclonal antibodies, therapeutic enzymes, and the like have been recently approved for clinical use [1]. However, most of these peptides are administrated by parenteral route. Inherent short half-lives of peptides and chronic therapy requirements in a majority of cases make their repetitive dosing necessary [2]. Frequent injections, oscillating blood drug concentrations, and low patient acceptability make even the simple parenteral administration of these drugs problematic [3,4]. In spite of significant advancement in the field of pharmaceutical research, development of a proper noninvasive delivery system for peptides remains a distant reality. Although there have been reports of successful delivery of various peptide therapeutics across nonoral mucosal routes (such as nasal and buccal), the oral route continues to be the most preferred route for drug administration [5–7]. The oral route, despite enormous barriers that exist in the gastrointestinal tract (GIT), has obvious advantages such as ease of administration, patient compliance, and cost effectiveness [8,9].

TABLE 7.1

Commonly Used Biotech-Derived Pharmaceutical Products

Products	Application
Human insulin	Treatment of diabetes mellitus
Interferon-α	Leukemia, AIDS, and renal cell carcinoma
Interferon-β	AIDS, multiple sclerosis, and cancer
Erythropoietin	Anemia and chronic renal failure
Interleukin-2	Cancer treatment
Streptokinase	Heart attack
Monoclonal antibodies	Cancer treatment and septic shock
Tissue plasminogen activator	Acute myocardial infarction
Human growth hormone	Growth deficiency
Hepatitis B	Hepatitis B vaccine
Calcitonin	Osteoporosis

7.2　BARRIERS TO ORAL DELIVERY OF PROTEINS/PEPTIDES

Peptide-based biotechnology products are subject to the same hostile environment faced by all peptides in the GIT. The major problems associated with oral peptide delivery are the susceptibility to degradation by the hostile gastric environment; metabolism by luminal, brush border, and cytosolic peptidases; and poor permeability across the intestinal epithelium because of size, charge, and hydrophilicity [10,11]. Intestinal epithelium serves as a major barrier for the absorption of orally administered drugs and peptides into the systemic circulation. High-resistance epithelial cell barriers restrict the passage of various hydrophilic compounds from the small intestine into the human body. The high resistance is due to the formation of well-organized tight junctions that connect the cell plasma membranes by a network of apical localized seams. As the name implies, tight junctions exclude the paracellular passage of ions, peptides, and proteins. The paracellular route is the dominant pathway for passive transepithelial solute flow in the small intestine, and its permeability depends on the regulation of intercellular tight junctions. The utility of the paracellular route for oral drug delivery has remained unexplored because of a limited understanding of tight junction physiology and the lack of substances capable of increasing the tight junction permeability without irreversibly compromising intestinal integrity and function. The attempts made so far to find ways to increase paracellular transport by loosening intestinal tight junctions have been hampered by unacceptable side effects induced by the potential absorption enhancers [12]. Physiological considerations, such as gastric transit time, dilution, and interaction with intestinal debris, also influence peptide absorption across the intestinal epithelium. Furthermore, peptides absorbed through the hepatic portal vein have to negotiate with the first-pass metabolism in the liver [9].

The nature of these barriers has now been expanded to include intracellular metabolism by cytochrome P450-3A4 as well as apically polarized efflux mediated by ATP-dependent P-glycoproteins [13]. Although, P-glycoprotein-mediated efflux systems are most commonly observed in tumor cells, they are also present in normal intestinal cells and act to reduce the intracellular accumulation or the transcellular flux of a wide variety of drugs, including peptides. Furthermore, peptides are associated with potential physical and chemical instability, and formulating peptide drugs are much more complex and demanding. Hence formulating a proper delivery system for proteins and peptides with optimal therapeutic effect and shelf life is an elusive goal for pharmaceutical scientists.

7.3 STRATEGY FOR IMPROVED ORAL PROTEIN DELIVERY

Successful oral delivery of protein involves overcoming the barriers of enzymatic degradation, achieving epithelial permeability, and taking steps to conserve bioactivity during formulation processing. The coadministration of enzyme inhibitors and permeation enhancers is an approach used to enhance the bioavailability of oral protein formulations [12,14–16]. Chemical modification of peptides and use of polymeric systems as carriers have also been attempted to overcome the inherent barriers.

Coadministration of protease inhibitors may retard the rate of degradation of peptides [17]. The slow rate of degradation may enhance the amount of peptides available for absorption. Enzyme inhibitors have been associated with systemic intoxication if they are absorbed and may affect the normal digestion of nutritive proteins. Use of absorption enhancers such as fatty acids, surfactants, and bile salts has been proposed to improve drug transport across intestinal epithelium [18–23]. An increase in paracellular transport is mediated by modulating tight junctions of the cells, and an increase in transcellular transport is associated with an increase in the fluidity of the cell membrane. Permeation enhancers that fall into the former category include calcium chelators, and those that fall into the latter category include surfactants and fatty acids. Calcium chelators act by inducing calcium depletion, thereby creating global changes in the cells, including disruption of actin filaments, disruption of adherent junctions, and diminished cell adhesion [18]. Surfactants act by causing exfoliation of the intestinal epithelium, thus compromising its barrier functions [23]. Use of these permeation enhancers has demonstrated that their enhancement is dose- and time-dependent. The utility of this approach for oral drug delivery has remained unexplored because of the limited understanding of tight junction physiology and the lack of substances capable of increasing the tight junction permeability without irreversibly compromising their integrity and function.

Chemical modification using poly(ethylene glycol) (PEG) and fatty acids has been proposed as a promising approach. Site-specific attachment of PEG to proteins such as insulin can significantly enhance the physical and pharmacological properties without negatively affecting its biological potency [24]. Moreover PEGylation may enhance the *in vivo* half-life of proteins, by protecting them from receptor-mediated uptake by the reticuloendothelial system (RES) and preventing recognition and degradation by proteolytic enzymes. However, use of polymer matrixes as carriers of proteins and peptides remains the most promising strategy in oral protein delivery [25]. In this chapter, we discuss the problems and prospects associated with polymeric oral protein-delivery systems.

7.4 POLYMERIC NANO/MICROPARTICLES AS A POSSIBLE ORAL PEPTIDE-DELIVERY SYSTEM

Polymeric drug carriers are particularly useful for formulating new drugs developed using biotechnology, because they can provide protection from degradation in the body and promote their penetration across biological barriers. Numerous attempts were made in the last few decades for formulating a suitable delivery system for peptides and proteins using polymeric carriers [26,27]. Polymeric carriers offer numerous advantages over conventional delivery systems, which include low cost, nonimmunogencity, and versatility. The traditional delivery systems or the so-called first generation polymeric systems are capable of delivering the active ingredient at a specific site in the body. However, application of such systems toward oral peptide delivery has been limited, since the enzymatic and absorption barriers may hinder the uptake of these bioactive agents.

Development of advanced drug-delivery systems, based on polymeric particulate systems, is an emerging area of research. These systems are designed to overcome the enzymatic and absorption barriers in the GIT. Recently much interest has been directed toward the development of small

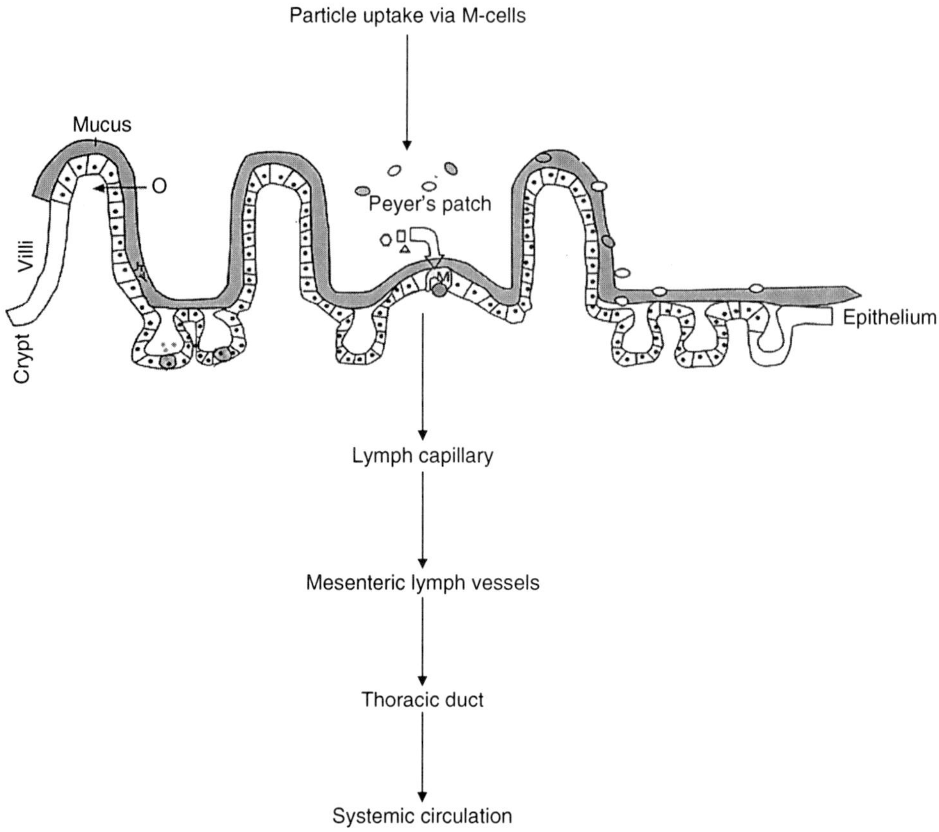

SCHEME 7.1 Particle uptake pathway.

particles (10 µm or less) by oral route [28]. Depending on the nature of the polymer involved, these systems are reported to exhibit interesting properties, which can be exploited for developing oral delivery systems. For instance, polymeric nano/microparticles consisting of hydrophobic biodegradable polymers have been shown to translocate across the intestinal mucosa and hence can facilitate the absorption of peptides and proteins from the gut lumen (Scheme 7.1). M-cells, which are located on the surface of the Peyer's patches, are a possible pathway for transporting the nanoparticles through the epithelium of the gut [29]. On the other hand, particles composed of hydrophilic polymers have restricted movement across the intestinal epithelium under normal circumstances. Some of these materials are effective in enhancing the intestinal permeability and thereby improving the peptide absorption [30]. Net surface charge of the system is also regarded as a factor in deciding the fate of an oral delivery system. Using natural polymers as carriers is another promising prospect in oral peptide delivery. Chitosan, starch, alginate, dextran, and the like, are widely investigated for developing as drug-delivery systems.

Despite of the encouraging potential of polymeric nano/microparticles, formulating a marketable peptide-delivery system still remains a major challenge. In this chapter, we have attempted to review the prospects and problems associated with polymeric nano/microparticles toward oral peptide delivery. Polymers are classified under three different categories: (1) synthetic biodegradable polymers, (2) synthetic nonbiodegradable polymers, and (3) natural- and protein-based polymers (Table 7.2).

TABLE 7.2

Polymers Investigated for Oral Peptide Delivery

Category	Polymers
Synthetic biodegradable polymers	Poly(glycolic acid), poly(lactic acid), and copolymers
	Poly(hydroxy butyrate)
	Poly(anhydrides)
	Poly(cyanoacrylates)
	Poly(ortho esters)
	Poly(phosphazenes)
Nonbiodegradable synthetic polymers	Poly(acrylic acid) and derivatives
	Poly(ethylene glycol)
	Poly(hydroxymethyl methacrylate)
	Poly(vinyl alcohol)/poly(vinyl acetate)
	Poly(vinyl pyrrolidone)
Natural polymers	Chitosan and derivatives
	Alginate
	Cellulose and starch
	Gelatin, casein and collagen
	Pullulan
	Xanthan

7.4.1 SYNTHETIC BIODEGRADABLE POLYMERIC NANO/MICROPARTICLES

A large number of biodegradable polymers have been investigated as carriers in the design of controlled drug-delivery systems. Biodegradable nanoparticles are in much demand nowadays because of their selective uptake by Peyer's patches, which gives them great potential as carriers for oral peptide- or oral vaccine-delivery systems. Biodegradable polymers such as polylactide or glycolide, polyanhydrides, and the like, are capable of moving across intestinal epithelium [31,32]. It was proposed that the use of these nanoparticles would be beneficial for oral delivery because of their control release properties and their ability to protect drugs without exposing them to the gastric and intestinal fluids. However, a major issue with this approach is the insufficient absorption of nanoparticulate drug carriers to achieve an acceptable degree of bioavailability [33].

Drugs administered through the gastrointestinal tract are normally transported into systemic circulation by the portal vein. As a consequence, compounds can sometimes undergo extensive metabolism during the first pass through the liver. First-pass metabolism may result in reduced bioavailability for many drugs compared with the parenteral administration, where drugs are directly released into the systemic circulation. If a drug is absorbed through the lymphatic system rather than by the portal circulation, it will find its way into the blood through the thoracic duct and will, therefore, avoid the first-pass effect [34]. A drug absorbed lymphatically is incorporated into chylomicrons (and other lipoproteins) produced by the fat digestion process. Numerous attempts were made to utilize this route for developing oral peptide-delivery system.

The idea of using biodegradable hydrophobic nanoparticles was proposed as a possible system to deliver proteins through the lymphatic circulation to achieve a higher degree of success. In the 1960s, Volkheimer described intestinal uptake of particulate matter on the absorption of intact starch particles [35]. This description awakened the hopes of achieving peptide and protein delivery using particles as carriers. Thereafter numerous studies were undertaken to establish the phenomenon of particle uptake, and now it is most accepted that the uptake happens mainly through phagocytosis [36]. Further studies carried out using model particles (polystyrene latex, polymethylmethacrylate) in the range of 50 nm to 3 µm revealed that the maximal absorption occurred with particles ranging from 50 to 100 nm in diameter, with particles above 1 µm being trapped in the Peyer's patches. Attempts were further made to study the mechanism responsible for the process and to explore their possible application in drug delivery [37]. It is proposed that M-cells of Peyer's patches are largely responsible for the uptake of these particles [38].

Gut-associated lymphoid tissue (GALT) consists of lymphoid follicles arranged in single or in clusters to form distinct structures called Peyer's patches. The epithelium overlying the follicle is called the follicle-associated epithelium (FAE). This FAE contains specialized antigen sampling cells known as M-cells, which have unique structural features with sparse irregular microvilli on the apical side. In addition, they possess a basolateral cytoplasmic invagination that creates a pocket containing one or more lymphocytes and possibly macrophages. M-cells are thought to sample and transport antigens from the gut lumen to the underlying lymphoid cells and may elicit an immune response. While acting in this immunological surveillance role, it has been suggested that the M-cells absorb particles and consequently may be exploited for the delivery of therapeutic peptides and proteins or vaccines [39–41].

Nanoparticles administered orally are absorbed, not only by way of the membranous epithelial cells (M-cells) of the Peyer's patches, but also by the much more numerous gut enterocytes. The absorption of the Particles is described as crossing either at the level of Peyer's patches or through the enterocyte layer. Usually particles absorbed through the Peyer's patches end up in the lymph and are carried through the mesenteric lymph vessels into the thoracic duct, which are further cleared into the bloodstream. Lymph from the intestinal lymphatic system drains through the thoracic lymph duct into the left internal jugular vein and then to the systemic circulation. Thus, the transport of drug through the intestinal lymphatic system may increase the percentage of drug that can gain access to the systemic circulation [42]. In addition, the process of intestinal lymphatic drug transport often continues over time periods longer than typically observed for drug absorption through the portal vein. Consequently, drug transport through the lymph may be utilized to prolong the time course of drug delivery to the systemic circulation.

The uptake is preceded by the interaction of the particles with the cell surface. Therefore, the nature of the polymer, mainly the hydrophobic or hydrophilic balance and the surface charge, will affect the uptake process to a large extent [28]. Physicochemical properties of particles govern their rate of uptake from the intestinal tract. The two main deciding factors are the size and the nature of the polymer used to make the particles.

Many studies regarding the size effects of nanoparticles absorption by intestinal epithelia have been performed using poly(styrene) standard particle suspensions. Particles with mean diameters of 50 and 100 nm showed a higher uptake in the rat intestine than larger particles [44]. The uptake of the nanoparticles was followed by their appearance in the systemic circulation and distribution to different tissues. After administration of equivalent doses of 33% of the 50 nm and 26% of the 100 nm, nanoparticles were detected in the intestinal mucosa and GALT [45]. In the case of 500 nm nanoparticles, only 10% were localized in intestinal tissues. Nanoparticles with size greater than 1 µm in diameter yielded only little uptake and had exclusive localization in Peyer's patches. Similarly poly(D, L-lactic-co-glycolide) (PLGA) nanoparticles with size 100 nm were uptaken from intestine, and efficiency was higher when compared with larger particles. It was clear from these experiments that the intestinal uptake of particles largely depends on the size [45–47].

Another major factor affecting the particle uptake is the nature of the material used to prepare the particles. Uptake of nanoparticles prepared from hydrophobic polymers seems to be higher than that from particles with more hydrophilic surfaces [32]. Microspheres composed of polystyrene, poly(methylmethacrylate), poly(hydroxybutyrate), poly(D,L-lactide), poly(L-lactide) and poly(D,L-lactide-*co*-glycolide) were absorbed into the Peyer's patches of the small intestine, whereas those composed of ethyl cellulose, cellulose acetate hydrogen phthalate, and cellulose triacetate were not absorbed. Residual poly(vinyl alcohol) in the surface of PLGA nanoparticles significantly reduced the intercellular uptake, in spite of the smaller particle size [48]. Similarly, poloxamer coating of poly(styrene) nanoparticles caused a decrease of gastrointestinal uptake *in vivo*. Moreover, hydrophobic poly(styrene) nanoparticles seem to have a higher affinity for M-cells than for absorptive epithelia [49]. Another factor that influences the particle uptake is the surface charge. Generally, positively charged particles have higher uptake as compared with the negatively or neutrally charged species. Carboxylated poly(styrene) nanoparticles show significantly decreased affinity to intestinal epithelia, especially to M-cells, compared with positively charged and uncharged poly(styrene) nanoparticles [43].

Specific strategies are being proposed to enhance the intestinal uptake of nanoparticles. These strategies include the surface modification of nanoparticles with some targeting ligands such as lectins. Lectins can be defined as proteins of nonimmune origin that bind to carbohydrates specifically and noncovalently. Lectins can increase the adherence of nanoparticles to the intestinal epithelium [50]. After binding to the cells, the lectins undergo cellular uptake and subsequently can also exhibit strong binding to nuclear pore membranes. Polystyrene microparticles coated with tomato lectin were shown to be specifically adhesive to enterocytes [51].

Major questions to be asked here are as follows:

1. Is particle uptake sufficient enough to achieve therapeutic effectiveness?
2. Are biodegradable polymer nanoparticles capable of preserving the delicate structure of sensitive peptide drugs?
3. Are these particle systems safe for long-term therapeutic use?

The first and most important question to be asked here is whether the absorption of drug carriers via normal enterocytes and M-cells is sufficient to allow therapeutic effectiveness. This uptake may be corelated with the low percentage of M-cells present in the gut (0.1% of the epithelial cells), which may be insufficient to get an appreciable amount of bioavailability. Another major issue associated with solid-delivery systems is adsorption of proteins onto these solid-delivery devices [52]. The incorporation of peptides-based pharmaceuticals into solid-delivery matrices exposes them to a high surface to volume environment, creating ample opportunity for adsorption into the delivery devices. Adsorption of proteins may severely limit the amount of free unbound proteins that is available for release. Another major consequence of adsorption may be the surface-induced changes in the three-dimensional (3-D) structure of proteins that could result in loss of biological activity of proteins [53]. This loss of activity may also evoke some immune response in some cases, which in turn can be a major drawback. Several studies have indicated the loss of bioactivity of insulin and salmon calcitonin following the encapsulation onto the biodegradable matrix [52,54].

Another major concern is the *in vivo* fate of these nanoparticles following their uptake by the Peyer's patches. A major aspect is that the exact mechanism of particle uptake is still unclear. A probable mechanism is that the particles absorbed through the Peyer's patches reaches mesenteric duct first and through cystema chyli and thoracic duct reaches bloodstream. A major obstacle is the "RES clearance" of polymeric systems in the body [55]. Particulate carriers in the blood streams may be identified by a group of scavenger cells known as RES, which are located largely in organs such as liver, spleen, lung, and the like. Most colloidal carriers are rapidly removed from the circulation by phagocytic cells in liver and spleen. The recognition of particles by RES is mediated by interactions of blood components with the artificial surface of the carriers (opsonization) leading to activation of the complement system. Moreover, the increase in hydrophobicity or introduction of cationic charges significantly enhances the clearance of these particles from the blood streams [56]. However, these features are some of the prerequisites for the uptake of particles from the GIT. Hence optimization of surface properties or charge without compromising the properties remains a major challenge in this area. A recent area of concern is the long-term effects of these particles on the human body, and more intense investigations are required in this direction.

Linear polyesters of lactides and glycolides, poly(alkyl cyanoacrylates), polyanhydrides, polyphosphazenes are some of the polymers commonly used in the development of polymeric particles.

Polylactic acid (PLA) and PLGA have been used for more than three decades for a variety of medical applications. Extensive research has been devoted to the use of these polymers as carriers for controlled drug delivery of a wide variety of bioactive agents. Mathiowitz and group introduced the concept of bioadhesive oral delivery system based on bioerodible polyanhydrides [57]. Bioerodible materials, which provide a continuously renewable cluster of carboxyl groups, might demonstrate a long duration of bioadhesiveness even though they do not possess flexible polymer chains as found in the case of hydrogels. Poly(fumaric-*co*-sebacic) [P(FA:SA)] was reported as the most bioadhesive polymer system from a series of thermoplastic materials evaluated [58]. Polyanhydride microspheres displayed strong interactions with mucus lining and cellular lining. P(FA:SA) microspheres transverse both mucosal absorptive epithelium and FAE covering the lymphoid tissues of Peyer's patches. This material was proposed as novel oral delivery system for insulin and other peptide drugs. P(FA:SA) microspheres increase the absorption of three model substances of widely varying molecular size: dicumarol, insulin, and plasmid DNA.

Poly(alkyl cyanoacrylate) nanocapsules were successfully used for oral administration of insulin in diabetic rats [59]. Insulin-loaded nanospheres (100 IU/kg of body weight) that were administered perorally in streptozotocin-induced diabetic rats provoked a 50% decrease of fasted-glycemia from the second hour up to 10–13 days. When ^{14}C-labeled nanospheres loaded with ^{125}I insulin were used, it was found that nanospheres increased the uptake of insulin or its metabolites in the GIT, blood, and liver, while the excretion was delayed when compared with ^{125}I insulin nonassociated to nanospheres; in addition, ^{14}C and ^{125}I radioactivities disappeared progressively as a function of time, parallel to the biological effect.

Poly(isobutyl cyanoacrylate) (PIBCA) nanocapsules were dispersed in a biocompatible microemulsion to facilitate the absorption of insulin following intragastric administration to diabetic rats [60]. Insulin-loaded PIBCA nanocapsules were prepared *in situ* in a biocompatible water-in-oil microemulsion by interfacial polymerization. Subcutaneous administration of insulin-loaded nanocapsules to diabetic rats demonstrated that the bioactivity of insulin was retained, and intragastric administration of insulin-loaded nanocapsules resulted in a significantly greater reduction in blood glucose levels of diabetic rats. *In vivo* performance of insulin-loaded PIBCA nanospheres with or without sodium cholate and Pluronic F68 surfactants were studied on alloxan-induced diabetic rats [61]. Administered orally, insulin-loaded (75 IU/kg) nanospheres, in the presence of surfactants, significantly reduced the mean blood glucose level for more than 8 h. These findings suggest the possible application of surfactant-incorporated polymeric nanoparticles for improving gastrointestinal absorption of insulin.

Nanoparticles prepared with a blend of a biodegradable polyester poly(ε-caprolactone) and a polycationic nonbiodegradable acrylic polymer (Eudragit (R) RS) were used for oral administration of insulin [62]. When administered orally by force-feeding to diabetic rats, insulin nanoparticles decreased fasted-glycemia in a dose-dependant manner with a maximal effect observed with 100 IU/kg. These insulin nanoparticles also increased serum insulin levels and improved the glycemic response to an oral glucose challenge for a prolonged period of time. Insulin-loaded poly(lactic-*co*-glycolic acid) nanoparticles were prepared by a double-emulsion solvent evaporation method [63]. After oral administration of 10 IU/kg nanoparticles, the plasma glucose level decreased significantly after 4 h ($p < 0.05$); 10 h later, the glucose level decreased to the lowest (52.4 $\pm$ 10.2%, $p < 0.01$), and the relative pharmacological bioavailability was 10.3 $\pm$ 0.8%. Biodegradable nanoparticles loaded with insulin–phospholipid complex were prepared by a novel reverse micelle-solvent evaporation method in which soybean phosphatidylcholine (SPC) was employed to improve the liposolubility of insulin and biodegradable polymers as carrier materials to control drug release [64]. Intragastric administration of the 20 IU/kg nanoparticles reduced fasting plasma glucose levels to 57.4% within the first 8 h of administration, and this reduction was continued for 12 h. Pharmacokinetic/pharmacodynamics (PK/PD) analysis indicated that 7.7% of oral bioavailability was relative to subcutaneous injection.

7.4.2 NONBIODEGRADABLE SYNTHETIC POLYMERS

Nano/microparticles composed of nonbiodegradable hydrophilic polymers are also of much interest in oral peptide delivery. Polymers such as polyvinyl alcohol (PVA), polyacrylic acid (PAA) and their derivatives, PEG, polyvinyl pyrrolidone (PVP), etc., are widely investigated for drug-delivery applications. Unlike biodegradable particles, these systems have restricted cell permeability under normal circumstances. Most of these systems are designed to release the encapsulated bioactive agent in the favorable regions of the GIT from where they can be absorbed. A very interesting and promising approach in oral peptide delivery is the use of bioadhesive or mucoadhesive polymers. The term bioadhesion refers to the adhesion between two biological materials or between any material and a biological material. Mucoadhesion refers to the interaction of a material with the mucosal surface [65]. It was proposed that if the intestinal transit of a delivery system could be delayed by mucoadhesion, followed by intimate contact at the brush border, might assist the uptake of a peptide or protein even without the intervention of a direct absorption enhancer. The intimate contact between a delivery system and the absorbing cell layer will improve both efficiency and effectiveness of the system. Mucoadhesive nano/microparticles are potential systems for drug-delivery applications, as they offer numerous advantages over conventional delivery systems. They can provide an intimate contact with the mucus layer and thereby enhance bioavailability of the drugs because of a high surface to volume ratio. Mucoadhesive nano/microparticles were proposed as a novel oral delivery system for poorly absorbable drugs such as peptides or proteins [66–68].

GIT is coated with a continuous layer of protective secretions known as mucus. Intestinal mucus layer is composed of water (up to 95% by weight), glycoproteins (0.5–5%), inorganic salts (about 1% by weight), carbohydrates, and lipids. Mucins represent more than 80% of the organic components of mucus, and they are O-linked glycoproteins [69,70]. Mucoadhesive delivery systems can penetrate the mucus layer and bind to the underlying epithelium. Several theories are proposed to explain the process of mucoadhesion; however, the mechanism involved is not fully elucidated yet. There are four main theories that describe the possible mechanisms of mucoadhesion: the electronic, the adsorption, the wetting, and the diffusion theory [71]. The electronic theory assumes that transfer of electrons occurs between the mucus and the mucoadhesive due to the differences in their electronic structures. The electron transfer between the mucus and the mucoadhesive leads to the formation of a double layer of electrical charges at the interface of the mucus and the mucoadhesive. This interaction results in attraction forces inside the double layer. The adsorption theory concerns the attraction between the mucus and the mucoadhesive achieved through molecular bonding caused by secondary forces such as hydrogen and Van der Waals bonds. The resulting attractive forces are considerably larger than the forces described in the electronic theory. The wetting theory correlates the surface tension of the mucus and the mucoadhesive with the ability of the mucoadhesive to swell and spread on the mucus layer and indicates that interfacial energy plays an important role in mucoadhesion. The wetting theory is significant, since the spreading of the mucoadhesive over the mucus is a prerequisite for the validity of all the other theories. The diffusion theory concerns the interpenetration to a sufficient depth and physical entanglement of the protein and polymer chains of the mucus and the mucoadhesive, depending on their molecular weight, degree of cross-linking, chain length, flexibility, and spatial conformation [72–74].

There is no unified theory to explain the process of mucoadhesion. The total phenomenon of mucoadhesion is a combined result of all these theories. First, the polymer gets wet and swells (wetting theory) followed by the noncovalent (physical) bonds created within the mucus–polymer interface (electronic and adsorption theory). Then, the polymer and protein chains interpenetrate (diffusion theory) and entangle together to form further noncovalent (physical) and covalent (chemical) bonds (electronic and adsorption theory). Hydrophilic polymers usually display the property of mucoadhesion because of their large molecular weight and ability to interpenetrate and entangle through mucus gel layer. The presence of hydrophilic functional groups is an important criterion for mucoadhesion. Polymers containing hydrophilic functional groups such as carboxyl, amine, hydroxyl, and sulfate can interact with mucus layer to form noncovalent interactions [75]. Polyanionic polymers such as PAA interacts with mucus by hydrogen and Van der Waals bonds created between the carboxylic groups and the sialic acid residues of mucin glycoproteins [76,77]. On the other hand polycationic polymer such as chitosan exhibits strong mucoadhesive properties due to the formation of hydrogen and ionic bonds between the positively charged amino groups and the negatively charged sialic acid residues of mucin glycoproteins [78]. Polyacrylic acid-based systems (including their commercial forms such as Carbopol, Polycarbophil) are widely used in mucosal drug-delivery applications. Hydrogel microparticles of PAA or polymethacrylic acid (PMAA) prepared by the free radical polymerization of corresponding monomers with bifunctional cross-linking agents, such as ethylene glycol dimethacrylate, or similar bifunctional reagents were investigated for developing mucoadhesive delivery systems [79,80]. It has been proved that use of PEG-based adhesion promoters improves the chain flexibility and mobility of such delivery systems. Peppas and group used the strategy of PEG-grafted PMAA for the development of mucoadhesive drug-delivery systems [81,82].

Recently a novel class of polymers, so-called thiomers, which in fact are capable of forming covalent interactions with mucus layer, was introduced in this area [83]. Thiolated polymers display thiol-bearing side chains and are based on thiol or disulfide exchange reactions, and through a simple oxidation process, disulfide bonds are formed between polymers and cysteine-rich subdomains of mucus glycoproteins. Mucoadhesive polymers such as PAA, alginate, and chitosan were modified with cysteine using water-soluble carbodimide to yield polymer–cysteine conjugate. It is reported that adhesive properties of these polymers were significantly enhanced with the immobilization of thiol groups. Thiolated nano- and microparticles were introduced recently, and these systems seem to be an attractive excipient for oral protein delivery [84,85].

However, a major problem is the absorption of peptides released from the polymer particles. It is reported that some mucoadhesive polymers can enhance the permeability of epithelial tissues by loosening the tight intercellular junctions. Basically there are two types of passive diffusion processes through which a drug can be absorbed from the mucosal site into the bloodstream. The first mechanism is transcellular (intracellular) transport and is used by small molecules. The molecule diffuses from one side of the barrier, through the cell, to the other side. The second mechanism of transport is paracellular transport (intercellular). Paracellular transport is the passage of the molecules through adjacent cells in the layer . This movement is governed by the available space and environment between the cells [78]. Increasing the area available between the cells allows the molecules to move more easily across the layer. Paracellular transport is the primary route used by hydrophilic and charged molecules. The paracellular pathway found along the intestinal wall is an alternative pathway for peptide absorption [86]. This pathway normally does not allow the entry of peptides and nutrients by a specialized regions called "tight junction." In a current model of a tight junction, two major integral membrane proteins are found—occludin and claudin—each with four membrane spanning alpha-helices [87]. The junction depends upon extracellular calcium to maintain integrity. The permeability properties of tight junctions vary considerably in different epithelia, and epithelial cells can transiently alter their tight junctions in order to allow increased flow of solutes and water through breaches in the junction barriers. The tight junctions usually prevent the transport of protein through the paracellular pathway [86].

Among hydrophilic polymers, PAA-based systems turned out to be of particular interest showing the capability of opening epithelial tight junctions, which are mainly responsible for limited paracellular uptake of hydrophilic macromolecules [88,89]. Calcium-binding ability of these polymers seems to be a major reason for such effects. Calcium chelators might disturb cell–cell adhesion by depleting extracellular calcium required for the interaction of components of adherent junctions. Further chelation of calcium may activate intracellular protein kinases, which ultimately can lead to the disruption of junctional integrity. Divalent ion-binding ability of these polymers may also help in reducing the proteolytic degradation of proteins in GIT [90].

Ability of these materials to enhance the intestinal permeability was demonstrated using monolayers of caco-2 cells. Caco-2 cell models are widely used *in vitro* cell culture model for intestinal epithelium. Having originated from human colon adenocarcinoma cells, these cells can differentiate into polarized cells with distinct mucosal (apical) and serosal (basolateral) cell membrane domain. Although they have originated from colon cells, caco-2 cells have many properties of small intestine absorptive cells including microvilli, intercellular junctions, and many of the enzymes nutrient transporters and efflux transporters present in the small intestine. The tightness of the intercellular junctional complex can be characterized by measuring the transepithelial electrical resistance (TER) [91,92].

Numerous investigations using caco-2 cells demonstrated the ability of PAA-based systems to enhance the intestinal permeability. Luessen et al. demonstrated that carbopol and polycarbophil can reduce the TER of caco-2 cells at neutral pH and can improve the transport of hydrophilic markers across the epithelial barrier [89]. Kriwet et al. showed that PAA microparticles could widen the intercellular spaces in the monolayers of the caco-2 cells [93]. Microparticles of poly(methacrylic-*g*-ethylene glycol) hydrogels loaded with insulin and salmon calcitonin demonstrated that the polymer microparticles cause a significant increase in the permeability of these proteins across the cell monolayers [94,95]. This material was also found noncytotoxic and capable of opening the tight junctions in a reversible manner [96].

Another advantage of using PAA-based systems is their pH-dependent release profile because of the protonation or deprotonation of carboxylic acid groups [80]. In acidic media, acid groups remain unionized and remain collapsed, protecting encapsulated drugs from the hostile gastric environment. In the small intestine region, where pH is above the pK_a of PAA, the acid groups get deprotonated and exist in the form of ionized acid groups. Repulsion caused by the adjacent ionized acid group causes the hydrogel network to swell, which in turn leads to the release of the encapsulated material from the system. So protein encapsulated in the particles is protected from the gastric environment and is released in the favorable regions of the intestinal tract [97].

Peppas and his group have made numerous attempts to utilize poly(methacrylic-*g*-ethylene glycol) nano- and microspheres as oral protein-delivery system. Insulin-loaded pH-responsive poly (methacrylic-*g*-ethylene glycol) microspheres were administered orally to both healthy and diabetic Wistar rats. Within 2 h of administration of the insulin-containing polymers, strong dose-dependent hypoglycemic effects were observed in both healthy and diabetic rats up to 8 h [98,99]. Further studies carried out on particles composed of a 1:1 molar ratio of methacrylic acid or ethylene glycol units showed the pronounced hypoglycemic effects following oral administration to healthy rats and achieving a 9.5% pharmacological availability compared with subcutaneous insulin injection [100].

Enteric polymers based on PMAA esters such Eudragit were also studied for developing oral protein-delivery systems. The effectiveness of Eudragit L100 microspheres containing a protease inhibitor was evaluated in normal and diabetic rats [101]. The dosage form based on insulin with protease inhibitor was administered orally with a 20 IU/kg insulin dose by force-feeding. Microspheres without protease inhibitor and with trypsin inhibitor (TI) or chymostatin (CS) produced no marked hypoglycemic response in both groups of rats. A significant continuous hypoglycemic effect was found after oral administration of microspheres containing aprotinin (AP) or Bowman-Birk inhibitor (BBI) in both normal and diabetic rats when compared with controls. The hypoglycemic effect of Eudragit S100 enteric-coated capsules containing sodium salicylate as an absorption promoter was studied in hyperglycemic beagle dogs [102]. This system demonstrated 25–30% reduction in plasma glucose levels and about 12.5% relative to subcutaneous injection of regular soluble insulin.

Eudragit S100 microspheres were prepared using water-in-oil-in-water emulsion solvent-evaporation technique, and their application toward oral insulin delivery was evaluated [103]. Oral administration of PVA-stabilized microspheres in normal albino rabbits (equivalent to 6.6 IU insulin/kg of animal weight) demonstrated a 24% reduction in blood glucose level, with maximum plasma glucose reduction of 76% $\pm$ 3.0% in 2 h, and the effect continued up to 6 h.

7.4.3 Natural and Protein-Based Polymers for Oral Peptide Delivery

Polysaccharides are among the most versatile polymers because of their vast structural diversity and nontoxicity. Among polysaccharides, chitosan, alginate, pectin, hylauronic acid, and dextran have received much attention. Protein-based polymers such as albumin, casein, and gelatin have also been investigated for oral peptide delivery.

Among such materials, chitosan-based systems are of utmost importance. Chitosan ((1-4)-2-amino-2-deoxy-β-D-glucan), which is the deacetylated form of chitin, is of great interest as a functional material of high potential in various fields such as the biomedical field [104,105]. Chitosans have found application as biomaterials in tissue engineering and in controlled drug-release systems for various routes of delivery. Being cationic in nature chitosan possesses mucoadhesive properties. It has unique ability to control the release of active agents, avoids use of organic solvents for the fabrication, and has free amino groups available for cross-linking [106]. Excellent review articles outlining the major findings on the pharmaceutical applications of chitosan-based nano/microparticles have been published in the last few years [107,108]. However, it was Illum who first reported that chitosan can promote the transmucosal absorption of small polar molecules as well as peptide and protein drugs system [109]. Chitosan attracted the attention of pharmaceutical scientists as a mucoadhesive polymer that could be useful for peptide-drug delivery.

When protonated (pH 6.5), chitosan is able to increase the paracellular permeability of peptide drugs across mucosal epithelia. Chitosan in its protonated form is able to interact with the epithelial tight junctions and to provoke their opening allowing for paracellular permeation of hydrophilic macromolecular drugs [110]. Chitosan can bind tightly to the intestinal epithelium, inducing redistribution of F-actin and the tight junction protein ZO-1 [111]. Chitosan nanoparticles were able to demonstrate reduction in TER value in caco-2 experiments [112,113]. However, the major drawback with chitosan is their limited solubility at pH above 6.5. At neutral pH, chitosan exist in nonprotonated form and was found ineffective in improving the permeability of intestinal epithelium [111]. Thanou et al. proposed that the problem of chitosan's ineffectiveness at neutral pH values could be tackled by derivatization at the amine group. Trimethyl chitosan chloride (TMC) was proved to increase substantially the intestinal absorption and bioavailability of peptide drugs. The mechanism by which TMC enhances intestinal permeability is similar to that of protonated chitosan. It reversibly interacts with the components of the tight junctions, leading to the widening of the paracellular routes [114,115].

Chitosan nanocapsules were prepared by the solvent displacement technique using high (450 kDa) and medium (160 kDa) molecular weight chitosan glutamate as well as high-molecular weight chitosan hydrochloride (270 kDa). The nanocapsules were used for the oral delivery of salmon calcitonin [116]. The results of the *in vivo* studies, following oral administration to rats, indicated that chitosan nanocapsules were able to reduce the serum calcium levels significantly and to prolong this reduction for at least 24 h. Bioadhesive polysaccharide chitosan nanoparticles (CS-NP) were prepared by ionotropic gelation of chitosan with tripolyphosphate anions [117]. The ability of CS-NP to enhance intestinal absorption of insulin and increase the relative pharmacological bioavailability of insulin was investigated by monitoring the plasma glucose level of alloxan-induced diabetic rats after oral administration of various doses of insulin-loaded CS-NPs. CS-NP enhanced the intestinal absorption of insulin to a greater extent than the aqueous solution of chitosan *in vivo*. Above all, after administration of 21 IU/kg insulin in the CS-NP, the hypoglycemia was prolonged over 15 h, and the average pharmacological bioavailability relative to subcutaneous (SC) injection of insulin solution was up to 14.9%. Chitosan capsules were also exploited for colon-specific delivery of insulin [118]. Hydroxypropyl methyl cellulose phthalate was used to coat chitosan capsules to achieve colon-specific delivery. Capsules were administrated orally to Wistar rats (20 IU). Hypoglycemic effect started after 6 h and lasted for 24 h. The bioavailability of insulin from the chitosan capsules was 5.3% compared with the intravenous one. Recently application of chitosan-based particles toward developing oral vaccine-delivery systems was demonstrated [119]. *In vivo* uptake of chitosan microparticles prepared by precipitation or coacervation method was studied on murine Peyer's patches using confocal laser scanning microscopy. Microparticles smaller than 10 μm were taken up by Peyer's patches, and chitosan microparticles seem to be the candidate for vaccination systems.

Alginate is another natural polymer of interest in this area [120]. Alginate is a copolymer of D-mannuronic acid and L-guluronic acid, and it can undergo sol–gel transition in the presence of divalent ions such as calcium, zinc, etc. This property has been explored for the fabrication of alginate microparticles. Calcium cross-linked alginate particles can protect peptides from gastric degradation via pH-dependent release mechanism [121]. Alginate-based systems were also found to enhance the paracellular absorption of mannitol across caco-2 cells by about three times [122]. Another important aspect is the formation of polyelectrolyte complex of alginate with polycationic polymers such as chitosan. Hari et al. utilized chitosan–calcium alginate microparticles for oral insulin delivery [123]. Chitosan coating can significantly modulate the release of bioactive agents from the matrix [124].

Alginate microspheres prepared by an emulsion-based process was used for oral insulin delivery. Cyclodextrin-complexed insulin was encapsulated onto these microparticles, and *in vivo* studies were conducted on diabetic albino rats [125]. Radioimmunoassay (RIA) for serum insulin indicated absorption of insulin from the gastrointestinal region following oral administration of insulin formulation. Chitosan-coated alginate nanoparticles containing cyclodextrin–insulin complex demonstrated good glucose-lowering effect in alloxan-induced diabetic rats (unpublished data). Biodegradable microparticles were prepared with alginate by the piezoelectric ejection process, and lectin (wheat germ agglutinin [WGA]) was conjugated to alginate microparticles [126]. The hypoglycemic effects of alginate and WGA-conjugated alginate microparticles were examined after oral administration in streptozotocin-induced diabetic rats. Alginate–WGA microparticles enhance the intestinal absorption of insulin sufficient to drop the glucose level of blood. Ramdas et al. developed an oral formulation for insulin delivery based on liposome encapsulated alginate–chitosan gel capsules. Following oral administration, this formulation delivered insulin in the neutral environment of the intestine, bypassing the acidic media in the stomach, and reduced blood glucose levels in diabetic rats [127].

7.4.3.1 Protein-Based Polymers for Oral Protein Delivery

Some attempts were made to utilize protein-based polymers such as casein, gelatin, and albumin for developing oral delivery systems. However, the major problem associated with these polymers is their degradation caused by the proteolytic enzymes in the GIT. Calcium phosphate–PEG–insulin–casein (CAPIC)-based oral insulin-delivery system was developed by BioSante Pharmaceuticals Inc., and functional activity was tested in a nonobese diabetic (NOD) mice model [128]. Single doses of CAPIC formulation were tested in NOD mice under fasting or fed conditions to evaluate the glycemic activity. Microparticles displayed a prolonged hypoglycemic effect after oral administration to diabetic mice.

7.4.4 Preparation of Nano/Microparticles

With the recent advancement in the pharmaceutical technology, new and innovative techniques are being employed in the fabrication of polymeric nano/microparticles (Table 7.3). A number of review articles and chapters describing various aspects of particle preparation and characterization have been published in the last few decades [129–133]. Hence we are outlining some of the techniques used in the preparation of particles, which are also used for oral peptide delivery. Particles are prepared mainly by two processes. The first process is the *in situ* polymerization of monomer through suitable polymerization process to yield polymeric particulates. The second process is based on the dispersion of well-characterized preformed polymers of synthetic or natural origin using a suitable technique (Scheme 7.2).

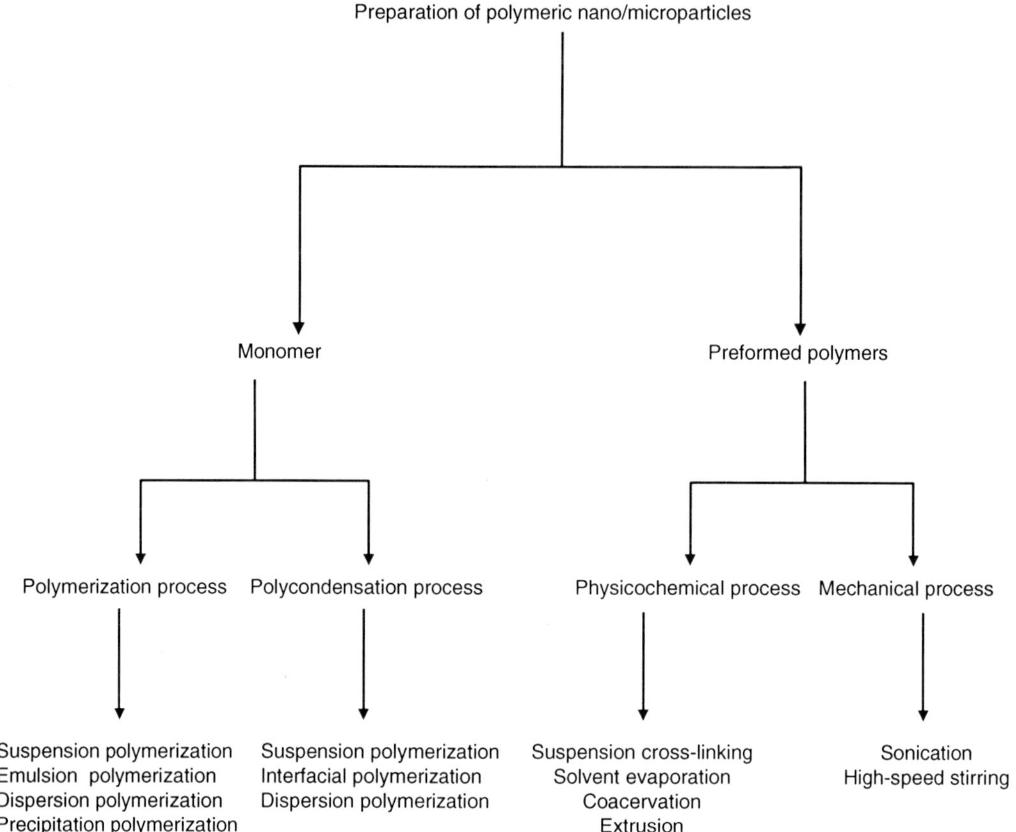

SCHEME 7.2   Commonly employed techniques for the fabrication of polymeric nano/microparticles.

7.4.4.1   Nano/Microparticles Obtained by Polymerization of Monomers

7.4.4.1.1   Emulsion Polymerization

Emulsion polymerization is a widely used method for nanoparticle preparation. This method is classified into two categories based on the nature of the continuous phase in the emulsion. In the first case, the continuous phase is aqueous (o/w emulsion), whereas in the other case continuous phase is organic (w/o emulsion). In either case, the monomer is emulsified in the nonsolvent phase with surfactant molecules. The polymerization takes place in the presence of a chemical or physical initiator. The drug to be encapsulated may be incorporated in the reaction medium during the polymerization or can be subsequently added to the preformed particles. The advantage of this technique is that nanoparticles with smaller size (50–200 nm) can be obtained by this technique. Nanospheres of polymethylmethacrylate, poly(alkyl cyanoacrylate), polyacrylamide, etc., can be prepared by this technique.

7.4.4.1.2   Precipitation and Dispersion Polymerization

In precipitation polymerization technique, the monomer is completely miscible in the polymerization medium, but the medium is a precipitate for the resultant polymer. The polymerization medium will be a homogeneous reaction medium, but the polymerization will lead to the formation of a visible precipitate. Dispersion is similar to the precipitation polymerization, but the addition of one or more stabilizers to the polymerization medium leads to the formation of monodispersed particles.

Donini et al. reported the preparation of poly(methacrylic acid-*g*-polyethylene glycol) nanospheres by solution or precipitation polymerization [134]. The free radical polymerization of

TABLE 7.3

Summary of Particle Manufacturing Techniques and Employed Polymers

Process	Polymers
Emulsion polymerization	Poly(alkyl methacrylate)
	Poly(alkyl cyanoacrylate)
	Poly(styrene)
	Poly(vinyl pyridine)
	Poly(acrolein)
Interfacial polymerization	Poly(alkyl cyanoacrylate)
	Poly(lysine) derivatives
Emulsification evaporation	Poly(lactic acid)
	Poly(lactide-*co*-glycolide)
	Poly(β-hydroxybutyrate)
	Ethyl cellulose
Solvent displacement	Poly(alkyl methacrylate)
	Poly(lactic acid)
	Poly(lactide-*co*-glycolide)
	Poly(1-caprolactone)
Salting out	Cellulose acetate phthalate
	Poly(alkyl methacrylate)
	Ethyl cellulose
	Poly(lactic acid)
	Poly(lactide-*co*-glycolide)
Desolvation and denaturation	Albumin
	Casein
	Gelatin
	Ethyl cellulose
Ionic gelation	Alginate
	Chitosan
	Carboxymethyl cellulose

methacrylic acid with PEG macromer was carried out using a photoinitiator in water. Pluronics-based polymers were used to prevent the aggregation of these nanospheres and to render them redispersion ability.

7.4.4.1.3 Suspension Polymerization

Water-insoluble monomer involves the use of stabilizers and monomer-soluble initiators. This feature leads to the formation of polydisperse monomer droplets in water in the size of about 20–1000 μm followed by polymerization and direct conversion of droplets into corresponding polymer particles of approximately the same size. Skovby et al. described a suspension polymerization technique for the preparation of methacrylic acid using hydroxyapatite and magnesium hydroxide as suspending agents [135,136].

We have recently adopted a novel chitosan-based ionic gelation process for the preparation of PMAA-based microparticles [137–139]. Methacrylic acid was polymerized in the presence of chitosan in aqueous medium, and particles were obtained spontaneously during the polymerization without the addition of any organic solvents and steric stabilizers. PMAA–CS particles displayed good protein encapsulation efficiency and demonstrated pH responsive release behavior at stimulated gastric and intestinal pH. Application of these microparticles toward oral protein delivery was evaluated using insulin and bovine serum albumin (BSA) as model proteins.

7.4.4.2 Particles from Preformed Polymers

7.4.4.2.1 Solvent Evaporation

Solvent evaporation is perhaps the easiest and the most extensively used method of microencapsulation. An organic phase consisting of the polymer solution in solvents such as dichloromethane (or ethyl acetate or chloroform) is mixed with the drug to form the primary water-in-oil emulsion. This emulsion is then added to a large volume of water containing an emulsifier like PVA or PVP to form the multiple emulsions (w/o/w). The so-formed double emulsion is then subjected to stirring until most of the organic solvent evaporates, leaving solid microspheres. The microspheres can then be washed, centrifuged, and lyophilized to obtain the free-flowing and dried microspheres.

There are numerous examples of particles that can be prepared using this technique. PLA and the copolymer of lactic and glycolic acid (PLGA) are the most frequently used particles because of their high biocompatibility. Numerous studies were undertaken to utilize PLGA matrix for oral protein delivery [141].

7.4.4.2.2 Spray Drying

In this process, the drug may be dissolved or dispersed in the polymer solution and spray dried. The quality of spray-dried microspheres can be improved by the addition of plasticizers, for example, citric acid, which promote polymer coalescence on the drug particles and hence promote the formation of spherical and smooth-surfaced microspheres. The size of microspheres can be controlled by the rate of spraying, the feed rate of polymer drug solution, nozzle size, and the drying temperature. This method of microencapsulation is particularly less dependent on the solubility characteristics of the drug and polymer and is simple, reproducible, and easy to scale up.

7.4.4.2.3 Hot Melt Microencapsulation

This method was adopted to prepare polyanhydride copolymer of poly(bis(p-carboxy phenoxy) propane anhydride) with sebacic acid [132]. In this method, the polymer is first melted and then mixed with solid particles of the drug. The mixture is suspended in a nonmiscible solvent (e.g., silicone oil), continuously stirred, and heated to 5°C above the melting point of the polymer. Once the emulsion is stabilized, it is cooled until the polymer particles solidify. The resulting microspheres are washed by decantation with petroleum ether. The primary objective for developing this method is to develop a microencapsulation process suitable for the water-labile polymers, for example, polyanhydrides. Microsphere with diameter of 1–1000 μm can be obtained, and the size distribution can be easily controlled by altering the stirring rate.

7.4.4.2.4 Complex Coacervation

When oppositely charged polyelectrolytes with a relatively low-charge density are mixed at an appropriate temperature and pH concentration, a liquid polyelectrolyte complex called complex coacervate is formed. This technique is widely used in the preparation of polymeric particles.

Sodium alginate is a water-soluble polymer that gels in the presence of multivalent cations such as calcium, zinc, and barium. Alginate particles are usually produced by dropwise extrusion of sodium alginate solution into calcium chloride solution. The preparation of alginate nanoparticles was first achieved in a diluted aqueous sodium alginate solution in which gelation was induced by the addition of a low concentration of calcium. Alginate particles can be prepared by using a modified emulsification or internal gelation. The preparation of alginate nanoparticles by this method does not require specialized equipment and can be performed at an ambient temperature.

Numerous processes are reported for the preparation of chitosan-based particulate system, and excellent review articles have appeared for the same recently. Emulsion cross-linking, coacervation precipitation, spray drying, emulsion droplet coalescence, reverse micellar method, sieving method, ionic gelation process, etc., are widely used in the fabrication of chitosan-based nano- and microparticles. Ionic gelation process has generated much attention since the process involved is simple and mild. Moreover reversible physical cross-linking by ionic interaction between anionic and cationic groups can avoid the use of toxic cross-linkers and organic solvents. Ionotropic gelation method using small molecular weight counterions such as sodium tripolyphosphate and sodium citrate can be employed for the preparation of chitosan particles.

7.4.4.2.5 Thermal Denaturation

A number of water-soluble proteins denature when heated since they are heat-sensitive. The denaturation process causes protein chains to unfold and become chemically cross-linked. This property can be properly modulated to form protein microsphere. BSA microspheres are usually prepared by this technique.

7.5 CONCLUDING REMARKS

Several promising approaches are being developed to improve the efficacy of oral peptide-delivery systems. Polymeric particulate systems undoubtedly have enormous potential toward developing oral drug-delivery systems. Some of these carriers have been shown efficiency in improving the bioavailability of peptides and proteins either by transporting directly through the intestinal epithelium or by enhancing the permeability of the mucosal barriers. In spite of their advantages and shortcomings, polymeric systems continue to be the most promising systems for developing oral formulations for therapeutic peptides. However, most of these studies are still in preclinical phase, and more intense research is required in this direction to make a marketable oral protein formulation.

Another major aspect is that current encapsulation technologies are far from being optimal for a good manufacturing practice (GMP) environment and for making marketable products at industrial scale. Therefore, efforts are currently devoted to developing novel technologies of microencapsulation that can be readily scaled up.

More intense and innovative research is required in the area of polymer drug-delivery systems to render them as a possible solution to the problems associated with protein pharmaceuticals. A better understanding of the mechanisms of action of these novel vehicles will provide a basis for their further optimization, thus opening more exciting opportunities for improving the administration of macromolecules. A positive outcome in this direction will have a direct impact in the society and may help in alleviating human sufferings to a large extent.

REFERENCES

1. Walsh, G. Pharmaceutical biotechnology products approved within the European union. *Eur. J. Pharm. Biopharm.*, 55, 3, 2003.
2. Mcmartin, C. Pharmacokinetics of peptides and proteins: opportunity and challenges. *Adv. Drug Del. Rev.*, 22, 39, 1992.
3. Humphrey, M.J., Ringrose, P.S. Peptides and related drugs: a review of their absorption, metabolism and excretion. *Drug Met. Rev.*, 17, 283, 1986.
4. Meibohm, B. Pharmacokinetics of protein- and nucleotide-based drugs. In *Biomaterials for Delivery and Targeting of Proteins and Nucleic Acid*. Mahato, R.I. (Ed.) CRC Press, USA, 2005, 275.
5. Ingemann, I. et al. Peptide and protein drug delivery systems for non-parenteral routes of administration. In *Pharmaceutical Formulation Development of Peptides and Proteins*. Frokjaer, S. and Hovgaard, L. (Eds.) Taylor & Francis, London, 2000, 189.
6. Edman, P., Bjork, E. Nasal delivery of peptide drugs. *Adv. Drug Del. Rev.*, 8, 165, 1992.
7. Sood, A., Panchagnula, P. Peroral route: an opportunity for protein and peptide drug delivery. *Chem. Rev.*, 101, 3275, 2001.
8. Fix, J.A. Oral controlled release technology for peptides: status and future prospects. *Pharm. Res.*, 13, 1760, 1996.
9. Schen, W.C. Oral peptide and protein delivery: unfulfilled promises? *Drug Dis. Tod.*, 8, 607, 2003.
10. Lee, V.H.L., Yamamoto, Y. Penetration and enzymatic barriers to peptide and protein absorption. *Adv. Drug Del. Rev.*, 4, 171, 1990.
11. Woodley, J.F. Enzymatic barriers for GI peptides and protein delivery. *Cric. Rev. Ther. Drugs*, 11, 61, 1994.

12. Zhou, X.H. Overcoming enzymatic and absorption barriers to non-parentally administrated protein and peptide drugs. *J. Con. Rel.*, 29, 239, 1994.

13. Tandon V.R. P-glycoprotein: pharmacological relevance. *Ind. J. Pharmacol.*, 38, 13, 2006.

14. Fanaso, A. Novel approaches for oral delivery of macromolecules. *J. Pharm. Sci.*, 87, 1351, 1998.

15. Saffran, M. et al. A new approach to the oral administration of insulin and other peptide drugs. *Science*, 233, 1081, 1986.

16. Gomez-Orellana, I. Strategies to improve oral drug bioavailability. *Expert Opin.*, 2, 119, 2005.

17. Bernkop-Schnurch, A. The use of inhibitory agents to overcome the enzymatic barrier to perorally administrated therapeutic peptides and proteins. *J. Con. Rel.*, 52, 1, 1998.

18. Ward, P.D., Tippin, T.K., Thakker, D.R. Enhancing paracellular permeability by modulating epithelial tight junctions. *Pharm. Sci. Tech. Tod.*, 3, 346, 2000.

19. Daugherty, A.L., Mrsny, R.J. Regulation of the intestinal epithelial paracellular barrier. *Pharm. Sci. Tech. Today*, 2, 281, 1999.

20. Aungst, B.J. Intestinal permeation enhancers. *J. Pharm. Sci.*, 89, 429, 2000.

21. Mesiha, M.S., Ponnapula, S., Plakogiannis, F. Oral absorption of insulin encapsulated in artificial chyles of bile salts, palmitic acid and α-tocopherol dispersions. *Int. J. Pharm.*, 249, 1, 2002.

22. Aungst, B.J. et al. Enhancement of the intestinal absorption of peptides and non-peptides. *J. Con. Rel.*, 41, 19, 1996.

23. Anderberg, E.K., Nystrom, C., Artusson, P. Epithelial transport of drugs in cell culture VII: effects of pharmaceutical surfactants excipients and bile acids on transepithelial permeability in monolayers of human intestinal epithelial (caco-2) cells. *J. Pharm. Sci.*, 81, 879, 1992.

24. Katre, N.V. The conjugation of proteins with poly(ethylene glycol) and other polymers altering properties of proteins to enhance their therapeutic potential. *Adv. Drug Del. Rev.*, 10, 91, 1993.

25. Allémann, E., Leroux, J.C., Gurny, R. Polymeric nano- and microparticles for the oral delivery of peptides and peptidomimetics. *Adv. Drug Del. Rev.*, 34, 171, 1998.

26. Couvreur, P., Dubernet, C., Puisieux, F. Controlled drug delivery with nanoparticles: current possibilities and future trends. *Eur. J. Pharm. Biopharm.*, 41, 2, 1995.

27. Soppimath, K.S., Aminabhavi, T.M., Kulkarni, A.R., Rudzinski, W.E. Biodegradable polymeric nanoparticles as drug delivery devices. *J. Con. Rel.*, 70, 1, 2001.

28. Junga, T. et al. Biodegradable nanoparticles for oral delivery of peptides: is there a role for polymers to affect mucosal uptake? *Eur. J. Pharm. Biopharm.*, 50, 147, 2000.

29. Florence, A.T. The oral absorption of micro- and nanoparticulates: neither exceptional nor unusual. *Pharm. Res.*, 14, 259, 1997.

30. Junginger, H.E., Verhoef, J.C. Macromolecules as safe penetration enhancers for hydrophilic drugs—a fiction? *Pharm. Sci. Tech. Tod.*, 1, 370, 1998.

31. Florence, A.T. Nanoparticle uptake by the oral route: fulfilling its potential? *Drug Dis. Tod. Tech.*, 2, 75, 2005.

32. Delie, F., Blanco-Príeto, M.J. Polymeric particulates to improve oral bioavailability of peptide drugs. *Molecules*, 10, 65, 2005.

33. Florence, A.T. Issues in oral nanoparticle drug carrier uptake and targeting. *J. Drug Target*, 12, 65, 2004.

34. Rubas, W., Grass, G.M. Gastrointestinal lymphatic absorption of peptides and proteins. *Adv. Drug Del. Rev.*, 7, 15, 1991.

35. Volkheimer, G., Persorption von mikropartikeln, *Pathologe*, 14, 247, 1993.

36. Shakweh, M. et al. Particle uptake by Peyer's patches; a pathway for drug and vaccine delivery. *Expert Opin. Drug Deliv.*, 1, 141, 2004.

37. Hussain, N. et al. Recent advances in the understanding of uptake of micro particulates across the gastrointestinal lymphatics. *Adv. Drug Deliv. Rev.*, 50, 107, 2001.

38. Clark, M.A., Jepson, M.A., Hirst, B.H. Exploiting M cells for drug and vaccine delivery. *Adv. Drug Del. Rev.*, 50, 81, 2001.

39. Ermak, T.H., Giannasca, P.J. Microparticle targeting to M cells. *Adv. Drug Deliv. Rev.*, 34, 261, 1998.

40. Florence, A.T., Hussain, N. Transcytosis of nanoparticle and dendrimer delivery systems: evolving vistas. *Adv. Drug Deliv. Rev.*, 50, S69, 2001.

41. Brayden, D. Oral vaccination in man using antigens in particles: current status. *Eur. J. Pharm. Sci.*, 14, 183, 2001.

42. Wasan, K.M. The role of lymphatic transport in enhancing oral protein and peptide. *Drug Del. Ind. Pharm.*, 28, 1047, 2002.

43. Jani, P., Halbert, G.W., Langridge, J., Florence, A.T. The uptake and translocation of latex nanospheres and microspheres after oral administer to rats. *J. Pharm. Pharmacol.*, 41, 809, 1989.

44. Jani, P. et al. Nanoparticle uptake by the rat gastro-intestinal mucosa: quantitation and particle size dependency. *J. Pharm. Pharmacol.*, 42, 821, 1990.

45. Desai, M.P., Labhasetwar, V., Amidon, G.L., Levy, R.J. Gastrointestinal uptake of biodegradable microparticles: effect of particle size. *Pharm. Res.*, 13, 1838, 1996.

46. Shakweh, M., Besnard, M., Nicolas, V., Fattal, E. Poly(lactide-*co*-glycolide) particles of different physicochemical properties and their uptake by peyer's patches in mice. *Eur. J. Pharm. Biopharm.*, 61, 1, 2005.

47. Ermak, T.H. et al. Uptake and transport of copolymer biodegradable microspheres by rabbit Peyer's patch M cells. *Cell Tissue Res.*, 279, 2, 1995.

48. Sahoo, S.K., Panyam, J., Prabha, S., Labhasetwar, V. Residual polyvinyl alcohol associated with poly(D,L-lactide-*co*-glycolide) nanoparticles affects their physical properties and cellular uptake. *J. Con. Rel.*, 82, 105, 2002.

49. Jepson, M.A., Simmons, N.L., Hagan, D.T.O., Hirst, B.H. Comparison of poly(DL-lactide-*co*-glycolide) and polystyrene microsphere targeting to intestinal M cells, *J. Drug Targ.*, 1, 245, 1993.

50. Jepson, M.A., Clark, M.A., Hirst, B.H.M. Cell targeting by lectins: a strategy for mucosal vaccination and drug delivery. *Adv. Drug Del. Rev.*, 56, 511, 2004.

51. Hussain, N., Jani, P., Florence, A.T. Enhanced oral uptake of tomato lectin-conjugated nanoparticles in the rat. *Pharm. Res.*, 14, 613, 1997.

52. Sinha, V.R., Tehran, A. Biodegradable microsphere for protein delivery, *J. Con. Rel.*, 90, 261, 2003.

53. Weert, M.V., Hennink, W.E., Jiskoot, W. Protein instability in poly(lactic-*co*-glycolic acid) nanoparticles. *Pharm. Res.*, 17, 1159, 2000.

54. Ibrahim, M.A., Ismail, A., Fetouh, M.I., Gopferich, A. Stability of insulin during the erosion of poly(lactic acid) and poly(lactic-*co*-glycolic acid) microspheres. *J. Con. Rel.*, 106, 241, 2005.

55. Owens, D.E., Peppas, N.A. Opsonization, biodistribution, and pharmacokinetics of polymeric nanoparticles. *Int. J. Pharm.*, 307, 93, 2006.

56. Carstensen, H., Muller, R.H., Muller, B.W. Particle-size, surface hydrophobicity and interaction with serum of parenteral fat emulsions and model-drug carriers as parameters related to RES uptake. *Clin. Nutr.*, 11, 289, 1992.

57. Mathiowitz, E. et al. Biologically erodable microspheres potential oral drug delivery systems, *Nature*, 386, 410, 1997.

58. Chickering, D., Jacob, J., Mathiowitz, E. Poly(fumaric-*co*-sebacic) microspheres as oral drug delivery systems, *Biotechnol. Bioeng.*, 52, 96, 1996.

59. Damge, C., Vranckx, H., Balschmidt, P., Couvreur, P. Poly(alkyl cyanoacrylate) nanospheres for oral administration of insulin. *J. Pharm. Sci.*, 86, 1997, 1403.

60. Watnasirichaikul, S., Rades, T., Tucker, I.G., Davies, N.M. *In-vitro* release and oral bioactivity of insulin in diabetic rats using nanocapsules dispersed in biocompatible microemulsion. *J. Pharm. Pharmacol.*, 54, 473, 2002.

61. Radwan, M.A. Enhancement of absorption of insulin-loaded polyisobutylcyanoacrylate nanospheres by sodium cholate after oral and subcutaneous administration in diabetic rats. *Drug Del. Int. Pharm.*, 9, 981, 2001.

62. Damge C., Maincent P., Ubrich N. Oral delivery of insulin associated to polymeric nanoparticles in diabetic rats. *J. Con. Rel.* 2006 published online Oct 25.

63. Pan, Y. Study on preparation and oral efficacy of insulin-loaded poly(lactic-*co*-glycolic acid) nanoparticles. *Yao Xue Xue Bao.*, 37, 374, 2002.

64. Cui, F. et al. Biodegradable nanoparticles loaded with insulin-phospholipid complex for oral delivery: preparation, *in vitro* characterization and *in vivo* evaluation. *J. Con. Rel.*, 114, 242, 2006.

65. Akiyama, Y., Nagahara, N. Novel formulation approaches to oral mucoadhesive drug delivery systems. In *Bioadhesive Drug Delivery Systems—Fundamentals, Novel Approaches and Development*, Mathiowitz, E., Chickering, D.E., Lehr, C.M. (Eds.) Marcel Dekker, New York, 1998, 477.

66. Vasir, J.K., Tambwekar, K., Garg, S. Bioadhesive microspheres as a controlled drug delivery system. *Int. J. Pharm.*, 255, 13, 2003.

67. Lehr, C.M. Bioadhesion technologies for the delivery of peptide and protein drugs to the gastrointestinal tract. *Cri. Rev. Ther. Drug Carrier Sys.*, 11, 119, 1994.

68. Chowdary, K.P., Rao, Y.S. Mucoadhesive microspheres for controlled drug delivery. *Bio. Pharm. Bull.*, 27, 1717, 2004.

69. Huang, Y., Leobandung, W., Foss, A., Peppas, N.A. Molecular aspects of muco and bioadhesion: tethered structures and site-specific surfaces. *J. Con. Rel.*, 65, 63, 2000.

70. Ahuja, A., Khar, R.K., Ali, J. Mucoadhesive drug delivery systems. *Drug Dev. Ind. Pharm.*, 23, 489, 1997.

71. Dodou, D., Breedveld, P., Wieringa, P.A. Mucoadhesives in the gastrointestinal tract: revisiting the literature for novel applications. *Eur. J. Pharm. Biopharm.*, 60, 1, 2005.

72. Peppas, N.A., Sahlin, J.J. Hydrogels as mucoadhesive and bioadhesive materials: a review. *Biomaterials*, 17, 1553, 1996.

73. Lowman, A.M., Peppas, N.A. Hydrogels. In *Enclyopedia of Controlled Drug Delivery*, Vol. 1, Mathiowitz, E. (Ed.) John Wiley & Sons Inc., New York, 1999, 397.

74. Haas, J., Lehr, C.M. Developments in the area of bioadhesive drug delivery systems. *Expert Opin. Bio. Ther.*, 2, 287, 2002.

75. Leung, S.-H.S., Robinson, J.R. The contribution of anionic polymer structural features to mucoadhesion. *J. Con. Rel.*, 5, 223, 1988.

76. Gu, J.M., Robinson, J.R., Leung, S.H. Binding of acrylic polymers to mucin/epithelial surfaces: structure-property relationships. *Crit. Rev. Ther. Drug Carrier Sys.*, 5, 21, 1988.

77. Park, H., Robinson, J.R. Mechanism of mucoadhesion of PAA hydrogels. *Pharm. Res.*, 4, 457, 1987.

78. Bernkop-Schnurch, A. Chitosan and its derivatives: potential excipients for peroral peptide delivery systems. *Int. J. Pharm.*, 194, 1, 2000.

79. Blanchette, J., Kavimandan, N., Peppas, N.A. Principles of transmucosal delivery of therapeutic agents. *Biomed. Pharmacotherapy*, 58, 142, 2004.

80. Peppas, N.A., Klier, J. Controlled release by using poly(methacrylic acid-g-ethylene glycol) hydrogels. *J. Con. Rel.*, 16, 203, 1991.

81. Ascentiis, A.D., Degrazia, J.L., Bowman, C.N., Colombo, P., Peppas, N.A. Mucoadhesion of P (2-HEMA) is improved when linear PEO chains are added to polymer networks. *J. Con. Rel.*, 33, 197, 1995.

82. Peppas, N.A., Kuys, K.B., Torres-Lugo, M., Lowman, A.M. PEG containing hydrogels in drug delivery. *J. Con. Rel.*, 62, 81, 1999.

83. Leitner, V.M., Walker, G.F., Bernkop-Schnurch A. Thiolated polymers: evidence for the formation of disulphide bonds with mucus glycoproteins. *Eur. J. Pharm. Biopharm.*, 56, 207, 2003.

84. Greindl, M., Bernkop-Schnurch, A. Development of a novel method for the preparation of thiolated polyacrylic acid nanoparticles. *Pharm. Res.*, 23, 2183, 2006.

85. Bernkop-Schnurch, A., Weithaler, A., Albrecht, K., Greimel, A. Thiomers: preparation and *in vitro* evaluation of a mucoadhesive nanoparticulate drug delivery system. *Int. J. Pharm.*, 317, 76, 2006.

86. David, J., Brayden, D.J. O'Mahony, D.J. Novel oral drug delivery gateways for biotechnology products: polypeptides and vaccines. *Pharm. Sci. Tech. Tod.*, 2, 67, 1998.

87. Anderson, J.M., Balda, M.S., Fanning, A.S. The structure and regulation of tight junctions. *Curr. Opin. Cell Bio. Suppl.*, 5, 772, 1993.

88. Borcharel, G. et al. The potential of mucoadhesive polymers in enhancing intestinal peptide drug abs. III: effects of chitosan–glutamate and carbomer on epithelial tight junctions *in vitro. J. Con. Rel.*, 39, 131, 1996.

89. Luessen, H.L. et al. Mucoadhesive polymers in peroral peptide drug delivery. IV polycarbophil and chitosan are potent enhancers of peptide transport across intestinal mucosa *in vitro. J. Con. Rel.*, 45, 15, 1997.

90. Luessen, H.L. et al. Mucoadhesive polymers in peroral peptide drug delivery. II carbomer and poly carbophil are potent inhibitors of intestinal proteolytic enzyme trypsin. *Pharm. Res.*, 12, 129, 1995.

91. Artursson, P., Ungell, A.L., Löfroth, J.E. Selective paracellular permeability in two models of intestinal absorption: cultured monolayers of human intestinal epithelial cells and rat intestinal segments. *Pharm. Res.*, 10, 1123, 1993.

92. Rubas, W. et al. Flux measurements across caco-2 monolayers may predict transport in human large intestinal tissue. *J. Pharm. Sci.*, 85, 165, 1996.

93. Kriwet, B., Kissel, T. Poly(acrylic acid) microparticles widen the intercellular spaces of caco-2 cell monolayers: examination by confocal laser scanning microscopy. *Eur. J. Pharm. Biopharm.*, 42, 233, 1996.

94. Ichikawa, H., Peppas, N.A. Novel complexation hydrogels for oral peptide delivery: *in vitro* evaluation of their cytocompatibility and insulin-transport enhancing effects using caco-2 cell monolayers. *J. Biomed. Mat. Res.*, 67, 609, 2003.

95. Torres-Lugo, M., Garcia, M., Record, R., Peppas, N.A. pH sensitive hydrogels as GI tract absorption enhancers: transport mechanism of salmon calcitonin and other model molecules using caco-2 cell model. *Biotech. Prog.*, 18, 612, 2002.

96. Torres-Lugo, M., García, M., Record, R., Peppas, N.A. Physicochemical behavior and cytotoxic effects of p(methacrylic acid-*g*-ethylene glycol) nanospheres for oral delivery of proteins. *J. Con. Rel.*, 80, 197, 2002.

97. Ranjha, N.M., Doelkar, M. pH sensitive hydrogels for site specific delivery. I. swelling behavior of crosslinked copolymers of acrylic acid and methacrylic acid. *S.T.P Pharm. Sci.*, 9, 335, 1999.

98. Lowman, A.M. et al. Oral delivery of insulin using pH responsive complexation gels. *J. Pharm. Sci.*, 88, 933, 1999.

99. Foss, A.C., Goto, T., Morishita, M., Peppas, N.A. Development of acrylic-based copolymers for oral insulin delivery. *Eur. J. Pharm. Biopharm.*, 57, 163, 2004.

100. Morishita, M. et al. Novel oral insulin delivery systems based on complexation polymer hydrogels: single and multiple administration studies in type 1 and 2 diabetic rats. *J. Con. Rel.*, 110, 587, 2006.

101. Morishita, I. et al. Hypoglycemic effect of novel oral microspheres of insulin with protease inhibitor in normal and diabetic rats. *Int. J. Pharm.*, 78, 9, 1992.

102. Hosny, E.A., Al-Shora, H.I., Elmazar, M.M.A. Oral delivery of insulin from enteric-coated capsules containing sodium salicylate: effect on relative hypoglycemia of diabetic beagle dogs. *Int. J. Pharm.*, 237, 71, 2002.

103. Jain, D., Panda, A.K., Majumdar, D.K. Eudragit S100 entrapped insulin microspheres for oral delivery. *AAPS Pharm. Sci. Tech.*, 6, E100, 2005.

104. Paul, W., Sharma, C.P. Chitosan, a drug carrier for 21st century: a review. *STP Pharm. Sci.*, 10, 5, 2000.

105. Rao, S.B., Sharma, C.P. Use of chitosan as a biomaterial: studies on its safety and haemostatic potential. *J. Biomat. Mat. Res.*, 34, 21, 1997.

106. Berger, J. et al. Structure and interactions in chitosan hydrogels formed by complexation or aggregation for biomedical applications. *Eur. J. Pharm. Biopharm.*, 57, 35, 2004.

107. Kas, H.S. Chitosan: properties, preparations and application to microparticulate systems. *J. Microencap.*, 14, 689, 1997.

108. Agnihotri, S., Mallikarjuna, N.N., Aminabhavi, T.M. Recent advances on chitosan-based micro-and nanoparticles in drug delivery. *J. Con. Del.*, 100, 5, 2004.

109. Illum, L. Chitosan and its use as a pharmaceutical excipient. *Pharm. Res.*, 15, 1326, 1998.

110. Thanou, M., Verhoef, J.C., Junginger, H.E. Chitosan and its derivatives as intestinal absorption enhancers. *Adv. Drug Del. Rev.*, 50, S91, 2001.

111. Schipper, N.G.M. et al. Chitosan as absorption enhancers for poorly absorbable drugs 2: mechanism of absorption enhancement. *Pharm. Res.*, 14, 923, 1997.

112. Artursson, P., Lindmark, T., Davis, S.S., Illum, L. Effect of chitosan on the permeability of monolayer of intestinal epithelial cells (caco-2). *Pharm. Res.*, 11, 1358, 1994.

113. Ma, Z., Lim, L.Y. Uptake of chitosan and associated insulin in caco 2 cell monolayers: a comparison between chitosan molecules and chitosan nanoparticles. *Pharm. Res.*, 20, 1812, 2003.

114. Kotze, A.F. et al. *N*-trimethyl chitosan chloride as a potential absorption enhancer across mucosal surfaces: *in vitro* evaluation in intestinal epithelial cells (caco-2). *Pharm. Res.*, 14, 1197, 1997.

115. Thanou, M. et al. *N*-trimethylated chitosan chloride (TMC) improves the intestinal permeation of the peptide drug buserelin *in vitro* (caco-2 cells) and *in vivo* (rats) *Pharm. Res.*, 17, 27, 2000.

116. Prego, C., Torres, D., Alonso, M.J. Chitosan nanocapsules as carriers for oral peptide delivery: effect of chitosan molecular weight and type of salt on the *in vitro* behavior and *in vivo* effectiveness. *Nanosci. Nanotechnol.*, 6, 2921, 2006.

117. Pan, Y. et al. Bioadhesive polysaccharide in protein delivery system: chitosan nanoparticles improve the intestinal absorption of insulin *in vivo*. *Int. J. Pharm.*, 249, 139, 2002.

118. Tozaki, H. et al. Chitosan capsules for colon drug delivery: improvement of insulin absorption from rat colon, *J. Pharm. Sci.*, 86, 1016, 1997.

119. Lubben, I.M.V. et al. Chitosan microparticles for oral vaccination: preparation characterization and preliminary *in vivo* uptake studies in murine payer's patches. *Biomaterials*, 22, 687, 2001.

120. Tønnesen, H.H., Karlsen, J. Alginate in drug delivery systems. *Drug Dev. Ind. Pharm.*, 28, 621, 2002.

121. Gombotzb, W.R., Wee, S.W. Protein release from alginate matrices. *Adv. Drug Del Rev.*, 31, 267, 1998.

122. Liu, P., Krishnan, T.R. Alginate-pectin-poly-L-lysine particulate as a potential controlled release formulation. *J. Pharm. Pharmcol.*, 51, 141, 1999.

123. Hari, P.R., Chandy, T., Sharma, C.P. Chitosan/calcium alginate beads for oral delivery of insulin. *J. Appl. Pol. Sci.*, 59, 1795, 1996.

124. Dileep, K.J., Roswen M.L., Sharma, C.P. Modulation of insulin from chitosan/alginate microspheres. *Trends Biomat. Art. Organs*, 12, 42, 1998.

125. Jerry, N., Anitha, Y., Sharma, C.P., Sony, P. *In vivo* absorption studies from an oral delivery system. *Drug Del.*, 8, 19, 2001.

126. Kim, B.Y., Jeong, J.H., Park, K., Kim, J.D. Bioadhesive interaction and hypoglycemic effect of insulin-loaded lectin-microparticle conjugates in oral insulin delivery system. *J. Con. Rel.*, 102, 525, 2005.

127. Ramdas, M. et al. Lipoinsulin encapsulated alginate-chitosan capsules: intestinal delivery in diabetic rats. *J. Microencap.*, 17, 405, 2000.

128. Morcol, T. et al. Calcium phosphate-PEG-insulin-casein (CAPIC) particles as oral delivery systems for insulin. *Int. J. Pharm.*, 277, 91, 2004.

129. Arshady, R. Manufacturing methodology of microspheres. In *Microspheres, Microcapusles and Liposomes Vol 1: Preparation and Chemical Applications*, Arshady, R. (Ed.) Citus Book, U.K., 1999, 85.

130. De Jacghere, F., Doelkar, E., Gurny, R. Nanoparticles. In *Encyclopedia of Controlled Drug Delivery Vol II*, Mathowitz, E. (Ed.) John Wiley & Sons Inc. New York, 1999, 641.

131. Barratt, G. et al. Polymeric micro- and nanoparticles as drug carriers. In *Polymeric Biomaterials*, second edition, Dumitriu, S. (Ed.) Marcel Dekker, New York, 2002, 753.

132. Mathiwotiz, E., Kreitz, M.R., Peppas, L.-B. Microencapsulation. In *Encyclopedia of Controlled Drug Delivery Vol II*, Mathowitz, E. (Ed.) John Wiley & Sons Inc. New York, 1999, 493.

133. Allémann, E., Gurny, R., Doelker, E. Drug loaded nanoparticles—preparation methods and drug targeting issues. *Eur. J. Pharm. Biopharm.*, 39, 173, 1993.

134. Donini, C., Robinson, D.N., Colombo, P., Giordano, F., Peppas, N.A. Preparation of poly(methacrylic acid-g-poly(ethylene glycol))nanospheres from methacrylic monomers for pharmaceutical applications. *Int. J. Pharm.*, 245, 83, 2002.

135. Skovby, M.H.B., Kops, J. Preparation by suspension polymerization of porous beads for enzyme immobilization. *J. Appl. Pol. Sci.*, 39, 169, 1990.

136. Keiwet, B., Walker, E., Kissel, T. Synthesis of bioadhesive of poly(acrylic acid) nano and microparticles using an inverse emulsion polymerization method for entrapment of hydrophilic drug candidates. *J. Con. Rel.*, 56, 149, 1998.

137. Sajeesh, S., Sharma, C.P. Cyclodextrin-insulin complex encapsulated polymethacrylic acid based nanoparticles for oral insulin delivery. *Int. J. Pharm.*, 325, 147, 2006.

138. Sajeesh, S., Sharma, C.P. Novel pH responsive polymethacrylic acid-chitosan-polyethylene glycol nanoparticles for oral peptide delivery. *J. Biomed Mat. Res: Appl. Biomat.*, 76B, 298, 2006.

139. Sajeesh, S., Sharma C.P. Novel polyelectrolyte complex microparticles based on polymethacrylic acid-polyethylene glycol for oral peptide delivery. *J. Biomat. Sci.: Polym. Edn.*, 18, 1125, 2007.

140. Sajeesh, S., Sharma, C.P. Interpolymer complex microparticles based on polymethacrylic acid—chitosan for oral insulin delivery. *J. Appl. Pol. Sci.*, 99, 506, 2006.

141. RaviKumar, M.N.V. Nano and microparticles as controlled drug delivery devices. *J. Pharm. Pharmceut. Sci.*, 3, 234, 2000.

8 Nanostructured Porous Biomaterials for Controlled Drug Release Systems

Yang Yang Li, Jifan Li, and Bunichiro Nakajima

CONTENTS

8.1 INTRODUCTION

The advancement in science and technology, especially since 1970, has propelled extensive research in the biomedical field. This research is aimed at discovering effective medicines to prevent disease, promote health, and relieve pain and suffering. After an appropriate drug is identified, determining the method to deliver and release it into the body is as crucial as the therapeutic activity of the drug itself. Controlling the delivery of the drug is a challenging yet essential task in many situations such as the slow release of water-soluble agents, fast release of poor water-soluble agents, localized drug delivery, targeted drug delivery directed at the specific cell tissue or site, coordinated delivery of multiple drugs, and systems based on carriers with a short life time. A drug delivery method that involves a controllable transport path and release rate and is self-regulated and self-reporting is often desirable.[1] This chapter introduces the common biomaterials for controlled drug delivery and then focuses on nanostructured porous materials such as silicon-based photonic and templated materials as examples.

It has been shown that the healing effectiveness of the medicine can often be improved by an optimal drug delivery system. For example, previously, diabetic patients were injected with multiple doses of insulin daily and the effects of this approach were difficult to control. Today, because of the advancement in drug delivery technologies, various formulations are available for insulin treatment. These formulations offer rapid or delayed action over short or long durations, respectively, to meet the needs of different patients to maintain insulin levels within a desired range and to reduce the long-term consequences of diabetes. However, injection remains the main method of delivery, while some alternatives such as the programmable implantable insulin pumps and insulin nasal sprays and mouthwashes are under development to obtain increased patient compliance.[2,3]

Pills, injections, suppositories, patches, topical ointments, and implantable fixtures constitute the common forms of drug administration. Each of these forms of administration imposes its own set of requirements and has its own limits. For example, the oral dosage form is probably the most preferred form but it is not suitable in the case of many drugs (such as proteins and nucleic acids) that degrade or are not absorbed efficiently within the gastrointestinal tract. Drugs that are not deliverable orally are usually administered by intravenous, intramuscular, or subcutaneous injections or implants, depending on the formulations and their applications.

Drug delivery systems must be carefully designed on the basis of the nature of agents and tissue sites to package agents into the systems. The drug delivery systems must be able to a) load the appropriate amount of active agents for optimal availability and therapeutic efficacy, b) avoid any leakage during transport to the target, c) protect the incorporated active agents from degradation before reaching the target, and d) achieve the proper release rate at the target. The release rate of a drug depends on numerous bioenvironmental conditions such as pH, circulation of fluid, viscosity, temperature, ionic strength, adsorption of specific or nonspecific biomolecules, and local redox potential of the surrounding medium. In the case of a self-regulated system, the drug delivery method must integrate the biosensing function with the release system in response to changes in the local bioenvironment. The ideal drug delivery system should also be mechanically strong, simple to administer and remove, and easy to fabricate and sterilize. Finally, the drug delivery system must satisfy long-term toxicological requirements and be comfortable for the patient.

In general, the purpose of controlled drug delivery is to optimize the medicine's effectiveness and eliminate the possibility of underdosing or overdosing. Controlled-delivery systems can help to maintain drug levels within a desired range, reduce the frequency of administrations, and increase patient compliance. In contrast, the potential disadvantages of controlled-delivery systems are toxicity, need for surgery to implant or remove the system, patient discomfort from the delivery device, and higher cost.

Traditional controlled-delivery systems have used a range of polymer materials as key components to achieve both temporal- and distribution-controlled release. Temporal-controlled release is usually achieved by delaying the dissolution of drug molecules, inhibiting the drug outward diffusion, or controlling the flow of drug solutions (Figure 8.1).[4] To achieve distribution control, polymeric drug carriers can simply be applied locally[5] (e.g., a photo-crosslinkable drug-retained wound-healing hydrogel[6]), implanted directly at the site,[7] injected to a localized site and have the polymer form a semisolid drug depot *in situ*[8] (e.g., drug-containing photocrosslinkable hydrogels injected to inhibit subcutaneous tumor growth[9]), or dispensed in the form of either colloidal particles or polymer–drug conjugates, where in either case, the polymer acts solely as a carrier and usually has to adopt the targeting moieties such as immunoglobulins and carbohydrates.[4]

As polymer-based drug carriers are designed, understanding the metabolism of the polymer in the human body is vital in choosing the appropriate carriers for different applications. Nondegradable polymers are acceptable for oral applications in which the polymer passes through the gastrointestinal tract or the delivery systems such as patch or insert that can be removed after drug release. In other applications such as some drug delivery implants,[10] therapeutic aerosols,[3] drug or gene carriers circulating in the blood system,[11] or *in situ* forming drug depot,[8,12] biodegradable polymers are desirable.

Polymers used in drug delivery were originally not intended for biological uses but were borrowed for their suitable properties such as diffusivity, permeability, biocompatibility, solubility, mechanical strength, and environmental sensitivity. For example, polyurethane is used for its elasticity, polysiloxane or silicones for its biocompatibility and insulating ability, and poly(methyl methacrylate) for its physical strength and transparency. Some other nondegradable polymers that are in use or under study for controlled drug delivery include poly(2-hydroxy ethyl methacrylate), poly(*N*-isopropyl acrylamide), poly(*N*-vinyl pyrrolidone), poly(carbophil), poly(vinyl alcohol), poly(ethylene glycol), and poly(acrylic acid). The diffusion, dissolution, permeation, swelling, and stimuli sensitivity characteristics of polymer materials have been used to obtain the constant release of entrapped molecules.[4,13]

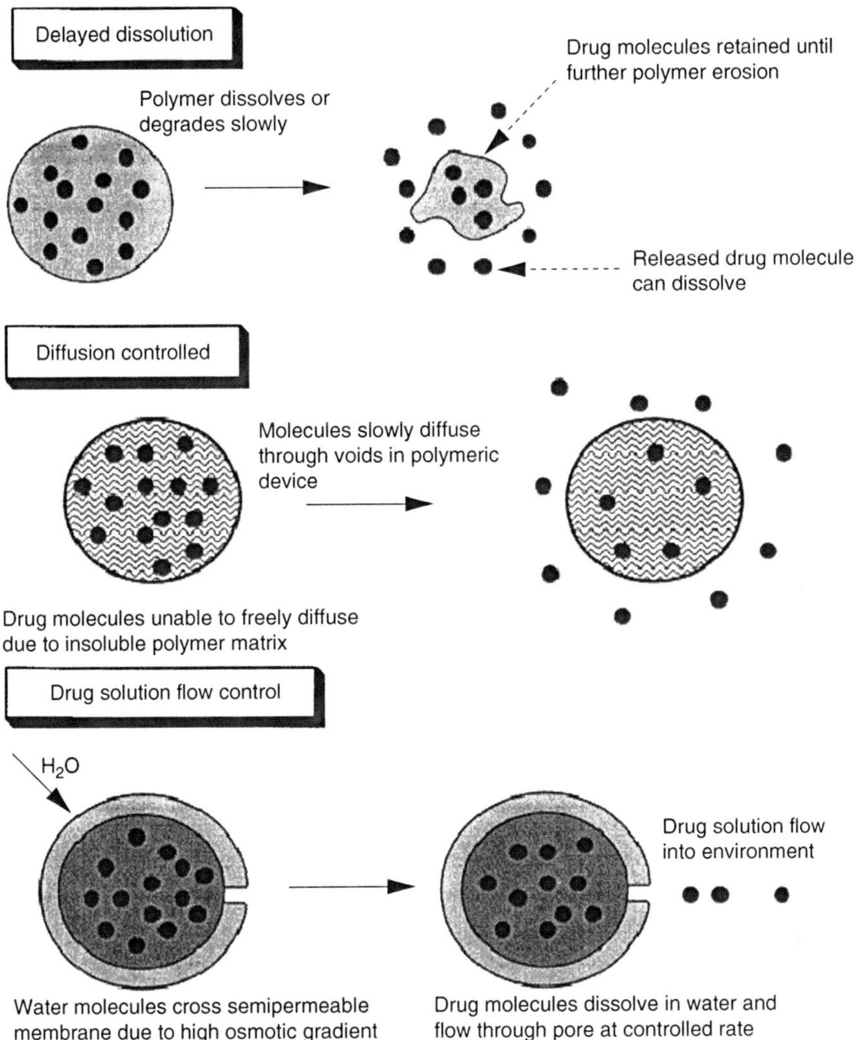

FIGURE 8.1   Examples of mechanisms of temporal-controlled drug release. (Reprinted from Uhrich, K.E. et al., *Chem. Rev.*, 99, 3181, 1999.)

Biodegradable polymers undergo a chemical degradation process in the human body that involves bond cleavage to form smaller molecules. These molecules can then be resorbed or excreted. Natural polymers such as starch, proteins, and chitosan are biodegradable materials with minimum toxicity (this concept of naturally degradable biomaterials was first applied successfully in the biomedical field with catgut sutures).[14] Inspired by these natural materials and realizing their physicochemical limitations, chemists have developed other synthetic biodegradable polymers such as poly(esters), poly(saccharide), poly(amides), poly(anhydride), poly(ortho esters), and poly(saccharide–amide).[4,14] These synthetic biopolymers combine both the biocompatibility and the biodegradability of natural materials and the versatility of synthetic structural design, readily tailorable with mechanical properties to meet specific drug delivery requirements, for instance, the degradation time of synthetic biopolymers can be easily adjusted. Guan and coworkers have demonstrated of a class of hybrid copolymers with good biodegradability and low cytotoxicity. This class of hybrid copolymers was synthesized using natural saccharide and amino acid building blocks, and the potential application of this class in gene-delivery has been demonstrated.[15]

Poly(esters) such as polylactide (PLA) and polyglycolide (PGA) and their copolymers, poly(lactide-*co*-glycolide) (PLGA), are some of the best defined and most extensively employed synthetic biodegradable polymers in clinical applications of controlled drug delivery.[14,16,17] Originally, PLA and PLGA were used as resorbable suture materials (the first patent for the use of PLA as a resorbable suture material was filed in 1967[18]) and, not surprisingly, were later applied in controlled-drug delivery systems. Miscellaneous polyester-based biodegradable delivery systems, for example, injectable drug carriers and implant devices, have been developed.[8,17] Although the primary advantage of biodegradable polymers is that these polymers can be removed from the body through normal metabolic pathways by breaking down into biologically acceptable molecules, biodegradable materials produce degradation by-products and the biodegradable polymers must be tolerated with little or no adverse reaction.

A variety of copolymers consisting of various biodegradable, nonbiodegradable, natural, seminatural, and synthetic components are often designed to fit different drug delivery applications. In an effort to achieve sustained intravesical drug delivery, thermo-sensitive hydrogel formed by poly(ethylene glycol-*b*-[DL-lactic acid-*co* glycolic acid]-*b*-ethylene glycol) (PEG-PLGA-PEG) triblock copolymers has been used for *in situ* gel formation for a depot of hydrophobic and hydrophilic drugs in rats. The triblock copolymer turns from an aqueous solution at room temperature to a viscous gel at body temperature, sustaining the residence time of hydrophobic drugs in rat bladder after its instillation. Nontoxic PEG, glycolic acid, and lactic acid are the products from bioerosion of the triblock copolymer.[19]

8.2 NANOSTRUCTURED POROUS MATERIALS

Nanotechnology is in essence an extension of existing sciences into the nanoscale. Nanotechnology studies phenomena, synthesis, manipulation, and application of materials and devices at the nanoscale by using technology in colloidal science, biology, physics, chemistry, and other scientific fields. Since nanotechnology operates at the same size domain as biology, the tools of nanotechnology are naturally applied to serve the purpose of biomedical development, for example, the effort to design and apply the nanostructured pore-containing biomaterials to offer a degree of control in both the rate and the location of drug delivery.

Although IUPAC defines porous materials into three classes, microporous (<2 nm), mesoporous (2–50 nm), and macroporous (>50 nm),[20] according to their pore sizes, terms such as porous nanomaterials, nanoporous materials, and nanostructured porous materials have been widely used to cover a variety of porous materials studied under nanotechnology. In this chapter, nanostructured pore-containing materials or nanostructured porous materials refer to those materials with pore size ranging from a few nanometers to several microns.

Nanostructured pore-containing materials can be made of various components, including soft materials[21] and inorganic materials. Common soft materials (liposomes, micelles, microemulsions, nanoemulsions, solid lipid nanoparticles, and microgels) used for drug delivery systems are fabricated, polymers,[22] and lipids.[23,24] These nanostructured pore-containing materials can be tailored to provide flexibility in drug loading and release control. By controlling morphological and chemical parameters such as the size and the shape of the material, the number and the volume of the "reservoirs," the wall thickness and the surface chemistry, and the permeability and the resorption rate, we can design more sophisticated systems based on nanostructured pore-containing materials for precise control of drug delivery.

8.2.1 SOFT NANOSTRUCTURED POROUS MATERIALS

Despite the great promise of numerous nanotechnologies, the existing commercial products of nanotechnology have mainly utilized the advantages of nanoparticle additives for applications such as suntan lotion, cosmetics, protective coatings, and stain-resistant textiles. Some other examples of commercial products are nanoclay-reinforced thermoplastics, antistatic and conductive carbon–nanofiber polymer composites, and silver nanoparticle–incorporated antimicrobial resin coatings. Similarly, nanoparticles are the major players among nanomaterials in the biomedical field. In particular, a variety of pore-containing soft colloidal nanoparticles are under extensive study for application in controlled drug delivery, as outlined in Table 8.1.

In general, drug delivery systems using these pore-containing soft nanoparticles have low toxicity. These systems are especially useful in providing efficient protection of labile drugs, improved solubilization for hydrophobic drugs, and encapsulation of water-soluble drugs for increased delivery sufficiency and, often, sustained release. In addition to the adjustable nanostructures for more flexibility in drug loading and release control, the tunable surface chemistry of the nanoparticles enables potential self-regulated drug delivery and site-specific targeting drug delivery. The high ratio of surface area to volume present in these nanoparticles provides further increased sensitivity to surrounding bioenvironmental changes. The small dimensions and the versatile structures of the nanoparticle-based drug carriers facilitate their penetration through tissues and intravenous circulation and open up the possibility of integrating more sophisticated functions. For example, the delivery of haloperidol, a neuroleptic drug, using poly(ethylene oxide) (PEO)-containing block copolymer micelles that are conjugated with cell-specific antibodies shows clearly increased therapeutic effect by selective targeting at brain glial cells.[44] Martin and coworkers demonstrated the precise release of individual drugs and bioactive molecules from the conductive polymer nanotube–deposited microelectrode neural probe at desired points in time by using electrical stimulation of conductive polymer nanotubes (Figures 8.2 and 8.3).[32] The fabrication process involves electrospinning of a drug-incorporated PLA or PLGA biodegardable polymer on the probe tip, followed by electrochemical deposition of a poly(3,4-ethylenedioxythiophene) (PEDOT) conducting polymer coating around the electrospun biodegradable nanofibers. The drug-incorporated fiber templates can be removed or slowly degraded, providing controlled drug delivery. The conducting polymer nanotube-coated microelectrode neural probes were used in the neural prosthetic devices in the nervous systems and showed significantly decreased electrode impedance, which is desirable for obtaining high signal-to-noise ratio because of its well-defined internal and external surface textures providing effective surface area for ionic to electronic charge transfer.[32]

Adding to the tailorable morphology and surface chemistry, polymers with interesting properties provide another dimension of novelty to the nanoporous systems designed for controlled drug delivery. For instance, environment-sensitive hydrogel has been used in a number of smart drug delivery systems; in particular, glucose-sensitive hydrogels that undergo a sol–gel phase transition were used to modulate insulin release. Park and coworkers developed one kind of glucose-sensitive hydrogel by binding glucose to the hydrogel backbone and mixing the glucose-bound hydrogel with concanavalin A (Con A), which is a four-valent lectin that can bind glucose.[45] Insulin was incorporated or trapped in such a composite hydrogel. When the free glucose concentration in the environment is low, the Con A acts as an effective crosslinker and the cross-linking density of the hydrogel is sufficiently high. Thus, the gel pore size is sufficiently low to restrict insulin diffusion. With increased environmental free glucose concentration, there is a competition between the bound glucose and the free glucose for the Con A binding sites, resulting in a less effective cross-linking density of the hydrogel and hence facilitated insulin release. Based on this mechanism, modulated insulin release was achieved using the glucose-sensitive membrane and matrix systems (Figure 8.4).

8.2.2 Inorganic Nanostructured Porous Materials

Rigid inorganic porous nanomaterials are the subject of increasing interest as the potential candidate carriers for controlled drug delivery. In particular, silicon-based porous nanomaterials appear to be promising platforms in this category. As in the case of soft porous nanomaterials, the morphology and the surface chemistry (thanks to the well-studied silicon chemistry) of silicon-based porous

TABLE 8.1

Common Soft Nanomaterials for Drug–Delivery Systems

Material	Properties
Micelles[21] Description: aggregate of surfactant molecules dispersed in a liquid colloid	Easy preparation Good stability Increase the aqueous solubility of hydrophobic drugs Reduce hydrolytic and enzymatic drug degradation Control the drug release rate Permit many administration routes Face risk of disintegration after administration or dilution
Liposomes[25] Size: 25–2500 nm Description: vesicles made from single or multi bilayered phospholipid membranes enclosing an aqueous cavity	Capable of delivery for both water-soluble (e.g., proteins) and oil-soluble drugs by entrapping substances in either the membrane or in the cavity Permit many administration routes Include sufficient PEO derivatives to reduce opsonin adsorption at the surface 17, and, as a result, overcome the following shortcomings with liposome systems: (1) short bloodstream circulation time (2) dose-limiting local toxicity in RES-related tissues, and (3) low bioavailability in tissues other than RES-related ones Biomimetic artificial system (model for cell membranes when made of natural phospholipids) Responsive transitions possible (e.g., temperature-sensitive liposome systems) Complex preparation Suffer from limited physical stability and drug leakage
Solid lipid nanoparticles (SLNs)[24] Size: 50–1000 nm Description: particles made from solid lipids (in contrast to emulsions, where the lipid phase is liquid) with surfactants added as stabilizers	Controlled drug release rate by particle size and composition Excellent tolerability Excellent physical stability Good protection against drug degradation Rare burst release: particularly suitable for cancer therapies to avoid high peak concentrations SLN formulations found to be significantly more efficient than the free drug in solution, suggesting that particle-mediated uptake plays a role Permit many administration routes and are particularly suitable for parenteral drug delivery Insufficient loading capacity Modifications of SLN, the nanostructured lipid carriers (NLC), and the lipid drug conjugate (LDC) nanoparticles, overcome limitations of conventional SLN
Polymer microgels[26,27] Description: polymer gel microparticles and nanoparticles	Swelling–shrinking transitions responding to external stimuli such as pH, temperature, and glucose concentration[28,29] More environment-sensitive for responsive drug release than macroscopic gels High water content, good for sensitive protein drugs

	Permit many administration routes and are particularly suitable for oral and nasal drug delivery Low solubilization capacity for hydrophobic drugs Complex preparation and drug loading
Polymer nanocapsules[30] Size: smaller than 1000 nm Description: single polymeric membrane enclosing an aqueous or oily cavity	Highly responsive Efficient drug protection Controlled release of incorporated drugs Biodegradable Site-specific targeting High water content, good for sensitive protein drugs Suffer from cytotoxicity Low solubilization capacity for hydrophobic drugs Complex preparation and drug loading Difficult large-scale production
Polymer nanofibers and nanotubes[31–35] Description: long polymer fibers with diameters on the micro- or nanoscales	Fiber-based porous scaffold used for tissue engineering and controlled drug release[36] Highly responsive Controlled release of incorporated drugs Biodegradable Site-specific targeting Great design flexibility[37] Compatible with large-scale production
Lipid microtubes[33,38] Size: diameters of a few hundreds of nanometers, wall thicknesses of a few tens of nanometers, lengths of 50 to a few hundred microns Description: planar bilayer sheets rolled up forming microtubes	Low mechanical strength and temperature stability Metallic cladding adds mechanical strength Tube diameter reported tunable with temperature[39] Drug Loaded by absorption and capillary force and released by diffusion Tubule ends able to be covered/uncovered for targeted drug release Self-assemble into a variety of morphologies[40,41] Chemistry and chirality of the lipids controlling the ability to form tubes[42] Limited flexibility with tailoring the microtubes' chemical and physical properties Controlled release of testosterone in living rats[43]
Carbon nanotubes[21]	Potential use for antifungal therapies Loading with both hydrophilic and hydrophobic drugs possible Complex preparation and drug loading Biological response largely unknown Limited administration routes

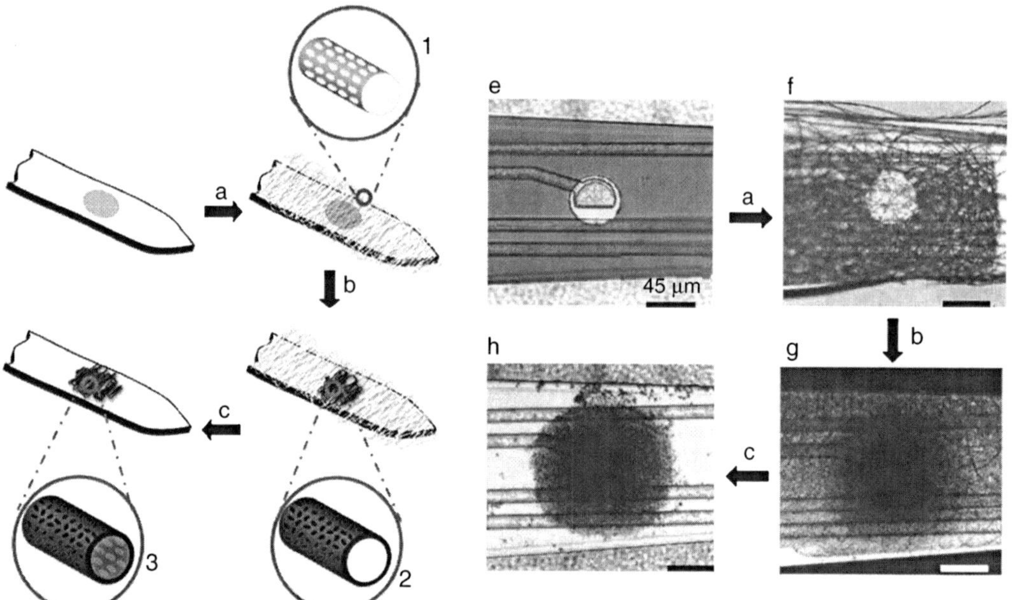

FIGURE 8.2 Schematic diagrams illustrating the fabrication process of surface-modified neural micro-electrodes with nanotubular PEDOT: (a) electrospinning of biodegradable polymer (PLGA) fibers with well-defined surface texture (1) onto the probe tip, (b) electrochemical polymerization of conducting polymers (PEDOT) (2) around the electrospun PLGA fibers, and (c) dissolving the electrospun core PLGA fibers to create nanotubular conducting polymers (3). Optical micrograph of (e) the gold electrode site, (f) the electrode site after electrospinning showing the coverage of the PLGA electrospun nanoscale fibers, (g) the electrode after electrochemical deposition of conducting PEDOT on the gold site and around the electrospun fibers, and (h) the electrode after removal of the core PLGA fiber templates. (Reprinted from Abidian, M.R., Kim, D.H., and Martin, D.C., *Adv. Mater.*, 18, 405, 2006.)

nanomaterials can be tailored toward more sophisticated systems for efficient control of drug delivery. Silicon-based porous nanomaterials include silicon nanowires, porous silica,[46,47] biomimetic siliceous nanocapsules,[48,49] and porous silicon.[50]

8.2.2.1 Mobil Composition of Matter-41 Porous Silica

After the discovery of M41S family at Mobil Corp. in 1992,[51] extensive research interest has been directed at these first synthesized well-ordered mesoporous solids, especially the Mobil Composition of Matter-41 (MCM-41), showing hexagonal arrays of cylindrical mesopores, is prepared by the self-assembly of silica. Surfactant micelles are used as the structuring agent in this process.[52–58] Positively charged surfactants function as templates forming an ordered organic–inorganic composite with the negatively charged silicate species based on the electrostatic interactions. Through calcinations, the surfactant is removed and the porous silicate network is left (Figure 8.5).[59] These materials exhibit well-defined, ordered porosity with a large specific surface area (up to 1000 m^2/g), a large mesoporous volume, and thermal stability. The pore sizes can be controlled during the synthesis and typically range from 15 to 100 Å (Figure 8.6).

In addition to their potential catalytic application, MCM-41 mesoporous materials are used in the drug delivery systems.[60] The silanol-terminated pore walls can be functionalized using convenient chemistry to provide specificity for drug absorption and release schemes.[47,61] Different drug release profiles were obtained depending on the pore size and the interaction between the host matrix and the guest drug molecules. A more complicated gated drug delivery system based on the

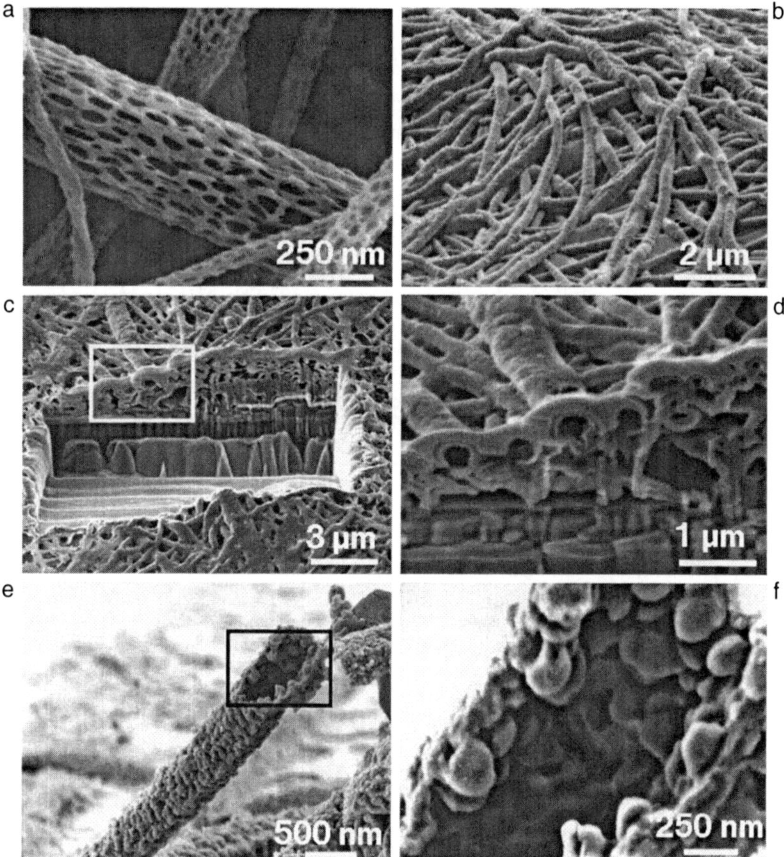

FIGURE 8.3 Scanning electron micrographs of PLGA nanofibers and PEDOT nanotubes. (a) Diameter distribution of the PLGA fibers was in the range 40–500 nm with the majority being between 100 and 200 nm. (b) PEDOT nanotubes on the electrode site of a neural probe tip after removing the PLGA core fibers. (c) A section of (b) cut with a focused-ion-beam showing the silicon substrate layer and PEDOT nanotube coating. (d) Higher magnification image of (c) showing the PEDOT nanotubes crossing each other. (e) A single PEDOT nanotube which was polymerized around a PLGA nanofiber, followed by dissolution of the core PLGA nanofiber. This image shows the external texture at the surface of the nanotube. (f) Higher magnification image of a single PEDOT nanotube demonstrating the textured morphology that has been directly replicated from the external surface of the electrospun PLGA nanofiber templates. The average wall thickness of PEDOT nanotubes varied from 50 to 100 nm, with the nanotube diameters ranging from 100 to 600 nm. (Reprinted from Abidian, M.R., Kim, D.H. and Martin, D.C., *Adv. Mater.*, 18, 405, 2006.)

mesoporous silica MCM-41 was demonstrated by Fujiwara and coworkers.[62,63] Light-sensitive coumarin ligands are attached at the entrance of the pores. These ligands act as gate keepers to control the amount of guest molecules to be released. The gate is shut upon irradiation with light when dimerization of coumarin ligands occurs, and the gate is open upon the removal of the irradiation. In a similar way, Lin and coworkers used CdS[46] or magnetic nanoparticles[64] as the pore caps by attaching them to the entrance of the pores of the mesoporous MCM-41 nanospheres. Controlled reagent release was then triggered by a specific chemical or enzymatic reaction that removed the CdS or magnetic nanoparticle caps (Figures 8.6 and 8.7).[46] Lin's group also developed dendrimer-capped mesoporous silica nanosperes capable of delivery of gene transfection reagents and demonstrated their potential application as a transmembrane carrier for intracellular drug delivery and in imaging (Figure 8.8).[65]

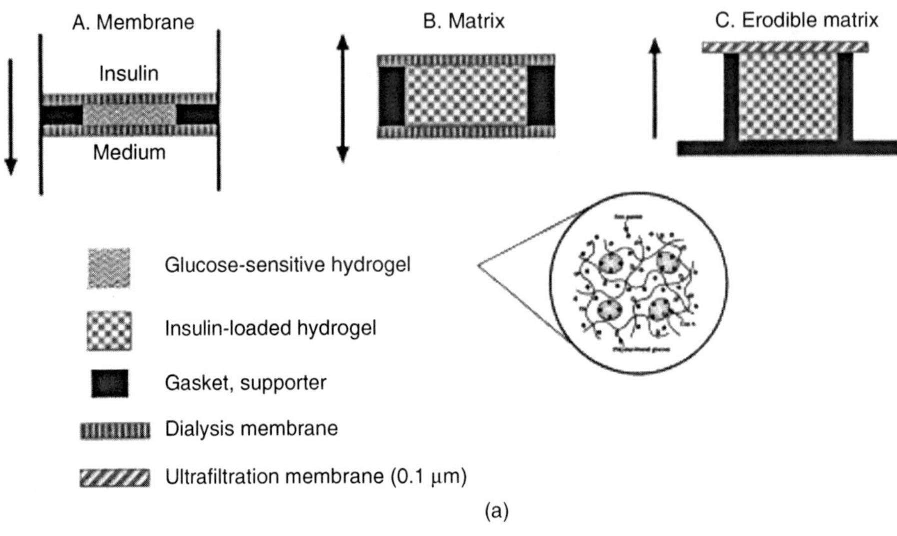

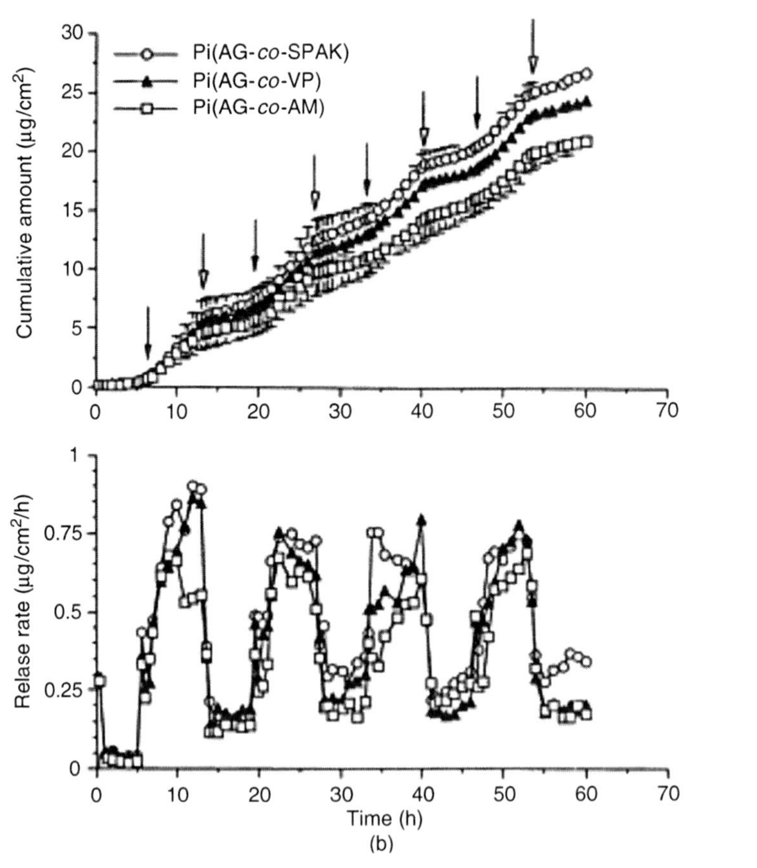

FIGURE 8.4 (a) Schematic representation of modulated insulin–delivery systems using phase-reversible glucose-sensitive hydrogels. Arrows indicate the direction of insulin release from the systems. (b) Cumulative amount of the released insulin and insulin release rate measured as a function of time through glucose-sensitive hydrogel membranes under stepwise changes of the glucose concentration using the glucose-sensitive matrix systems. (Reprinted from Kim, J.J. and Park, K., *J. Contr. Release*, 77, 39, 2001.)

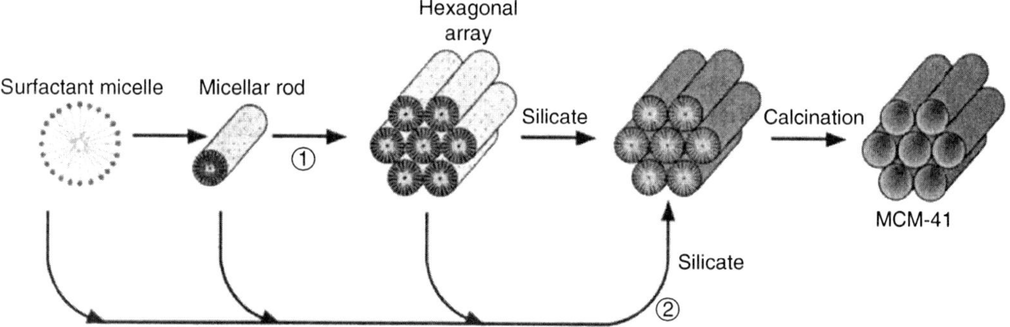

FIGURE 8.5 Two mechanistic liquid-crystal templating pathways for the formation of MCM-41 proposed by Beck et al.: (1) liquid crystal phase initiated and (2) silicate anion initiated. (Reprinted from Beck, J.S. et al., *J. Am. Chem. Soc.*, 114, 10834, 1992.)

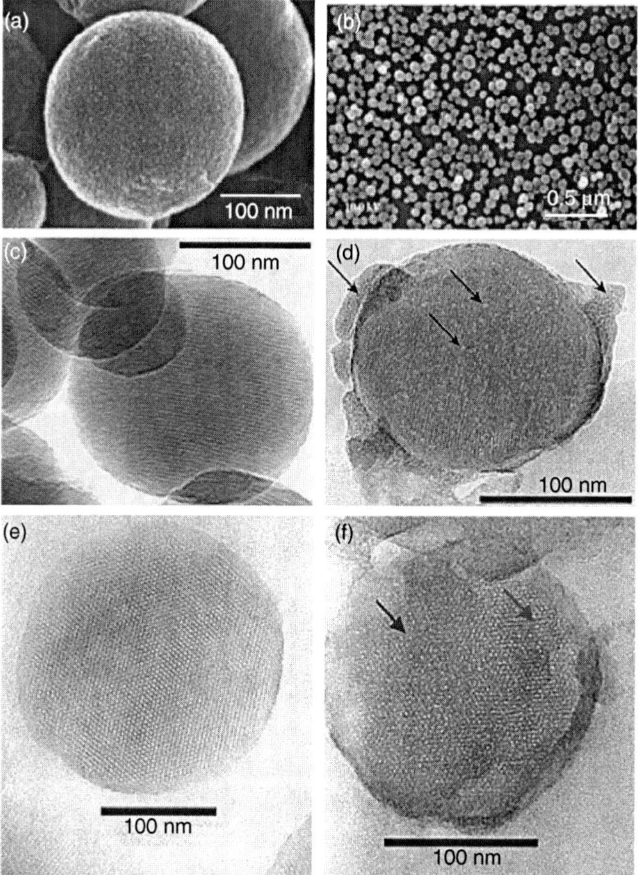

FIGURE 8.6 SEM (a and b) and TEM (300 kV) micrographs of the MCM-41 type mesoporous silica nanospheres (MSNs) with an average particle size of 200 nm (c and e). The N_2 adsorption/desorption isotherms measurement of the material revealed a surface area of 941.0 m^2/g and the average pore diameter of 2.3 nm. The MCM-41 type of mesoporous channel structure of the nanospheres is visualized with the parallel stripes (c) and the hexagonally packed light dots (e) shown in the micrographs. The TEM micrographs (d and f) of the CdS-capped MSNs exhibit aggregations of CdS nanoparticles on the MSN surface, represented by dots in the areas indicated by arrows. The TEM micrographs (d–f) were taken on ultramicrotomed samples with section thickness of 60–80 nm. (Reprinted from Lai, C.Y. et al., *J. Am. Chem. Soc.*, 125, 4451, 2003.)

8.2.2.2 Biomimetic Siliceous Nanocapsules

Biomimetic siliceous nanocapsules are prepared through the hydrolysis and the condensation of a neutral silicon alkoxide precursor by templating surfactants,[66,67] polymers,[68] and phospholipids.[69] A variety of self-assembled organic molecules such as lyotropic lamellar phases and microemulsions[70] can be used as the template. In particular, siliceous liposome nanocapsules or "Liposil" can be synthesized by using liposomes as templates (Figure 8.9).[48,49] Liposil, usually with a diameter of around 100 nm, comprises of a liposome encapsulated in a silica shell, with the silica wall assembled onto the external surface of the liposome. These siliceous liposome nanocapsules exhibit good protection of the drug incorporated, excellent physical stability, which is desirable for long-term storage, and high tolerance to low pH, making them promising drug carriers, especially for oral administration. Slow drug release rate can also be achieved using Liposil.

8.2.2.3 Porous Silicon

Porous silicon, which contains a network of interconnected pores within the crystalline silicon matrix, is usually prepared by anodization of bulk silicon in hydrofluoric acid solution (Figure 8.10). Since the late 1990s, when the pioneering work of Canham and others demonstrated the biocompatibility and the biodegradability of porous Si *in vitro* and *in vivo*,[71–81] porous silicon has been under intensive investigation for biomedical applications, especially as drug carriers. A versatile surface chemistry and an easily adjustable morphology are the other properties of porous silicon that make it suitable for controlled drug delivery. The surface of porous silicon can be conveniently modified with organic or biological molecules, for instance, antibodies.[82] Its pore size can be adjusted, ranging from a few nanometers to a few microns, and its porosity can be easily tuned over 80%, providing a high portion of free volume for drug loading. Swaan and coworkers performed *in vitro* experiments and showed that porous Si particles can be used as efficient delivery vehicles of insulin across intestinal epithelial cells.[83] The drug permeation rate through the membrane was dramatically enhanced when delivered through porous Si particles compared with conventional liquid formulations. Sailor and coworkers demonstrated controlled drug loading and release of a steroid by engineering the surface chemistry and the pore dimensions in porous silicon films.[84] More recently, Vaccari and coworkers investigated the time-dependent drug release of doxorubicin anticancer agent incorporated in the two-layered porous silicon film.[85]

In addition to possessing the adjustable morphological and chemical properties, porous Si is particularly attractive for constructing fluorescent materials[86] and complex optical materials such as Fabry-Pérot films, photonic crystals, dielectric mirrors, and microcavities.[87–98] Both kinds of

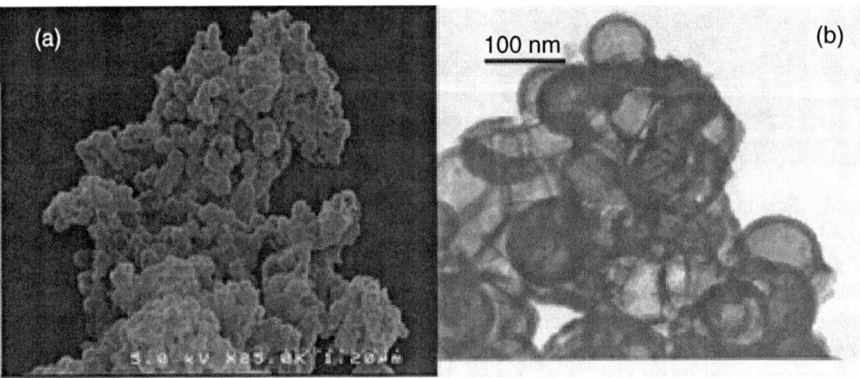

FIGURE 8.9 SEM micrograph (a) and TEM micrograph (b) of aggregated siliceous nanocapsules. (Reprinted from Bégu, S. et al., *Chem. Commun.*, 640, 2003.)

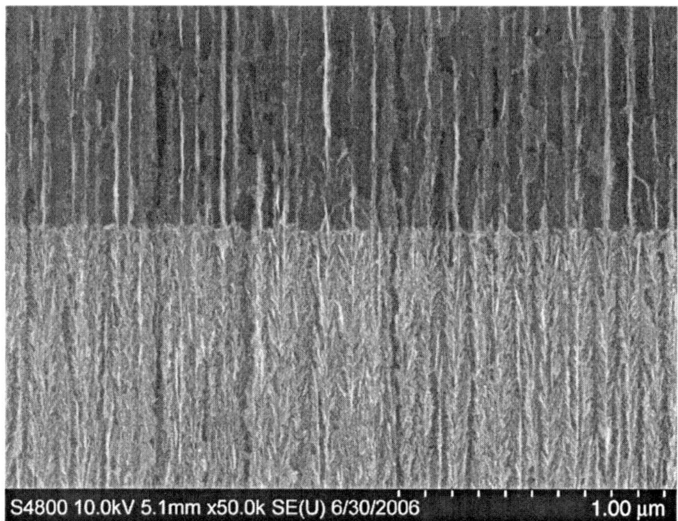

FIGURE 8.10   Cross-sectional SEM micrograph of a double-layered porous silicon film with a large pore layer on top of a small pore layer. The difference of pore size was obtained by simply switching the etching current density during anodization of silicon. Notice the smooth and uniform interface between the two layers. The scale bar is 1 μm.

the porous silicon–based optical materials show excellent sensing properties in responding to the interaction of their porous structures with the guest molecules,[78,99–104] which potentially adds smart functionalities for their biomedical applications. The ease with which porous Si can be integrated into well-established Si microelectronics fabrication techniques should lead to more sophisticated, active medical devices.[81,105,106]

8.2.2.3.1 *Photonic Crystals and Porous Silicon Photonic Crystals*

Photonic crystals are periodic dielectric structures that are ideally infinitely extended with respect to the interacting wavelength.[107] Such structures can diffract light. Photons in photonic crystals behave analogous to electrons in atomic crystals, in the way that forbidden energy gaps form for photons in photonic crystals analogous to electronic band gaps in atomic crystals. Photonic crystals exist in nature and are commonly found in opals abalone shells,[108] beetle shells,[109] butterfly wings,[110] and the King Penguin beak horns.[111] Inorganic photonic crystals are an active area of research for optical switching, optical computing, and other optoelectronic applications,[112] and the capabilities of these materials to act as sensors for chemical or biological compounds have led to a series of developments in the biomedical field. Asher and coworkers demonstrated one of the early applications of the photonic crystals in medicine. By incorporating a photonic crystal into a biocompatible hydrogel matrix, the Asher group demonstrated glucose-sensing contact lenses that change color depending on the concentration of glucose in the user's blood.[113–115]

One-dimensional porous silicon-based photonic crystals are probably the most easily constructed elaborate photonic crystals. These crystals can be conveniently fabricated using a computer-generated periodically varying etching current density.[94,116–118] The resulting structure contains multilayers of alternating indexes of refraction along the direction perpendicular to the surface (z-direction), displaying interesting optical features in its reflectivity spectra corresponding to its energy forbidden gaps for photons. Sensors for proteins, DNA, and small molecules have also been developed based on these and related photonic crystals.[92,102,119,120] Recently, Sailor and coworkers developed a label-free platform based on porous silicon photonic crystals to monitor cellular or enzymatic activities in real-time. This platform can be potentially applied to drug screening and environmental field tests.[121,122]

8.2.2.3.2   *Porous Si Photonic Crystals as Templates for Drug Delivery Materials*

As mentioned earlier in this chapter, MCM-41 and siliceous nanocapsules are constructed by applying templating techniques. The concept of template is in fact applied in many fields of science such as using templates for organic synthesis,[123] preparing porous materials through nanocasting,[124] using silicone stamps as templates for patterning in soft lithography,[125] and using template-imprinted nanostructured surfaces for protein recognition.[126] Templates consisting of microporous membranes,[127,128] zeolites,[57] and crystalline colloidal arrays[129–131] have been used to construct elaborate electronic, mechanical, or optical structures. In particular, the synthesis of materials using microporous membrane templates has emerged as a useful and versatile technique to generate ordered nanostructures.[124] The most commonly used microporous membrane templates are track-etched polymer membranes, porous alumina membranes, and membranes fabricated by lithography and related techniques, although the choice of templating materials is only limited by imagination. Arnold and coworkers demonstrated the synthesis of bifunctional polymer-coated silicon/silica core/shell nanowires from silicon nanowire templates as a way to control the surface properties of nanowires and nanotubes. The surfaces of the nanowires were first modified with polymer initiators, and then methacrylate polymer chains were grown from the surface. After the silicon cores were etched away, the resulting polymer-coated nanotubes with hydrophilic silica cores and hydrophobic polymer shells were obtained.[132]

Recent work has employed other membrane templates such as porous silicon[95,118] to fabricate functional materials. Optical nanostructures consisting of composites of porous Si templates with various polymers have been demonstrated.[118,133,134] Polymers have been placed in a porous Si template by *in situ* polymerization,[134,135] injection molding,[118] or solution casting.[133] The potential of such hybrid materials in sensing and in controlled release drug delivery has been demonstrated.[118] Porous Si is an attractive candidate for use as a template because the porosity and the average pore size can be tuned by adjusting the electrochemical preparation conditions, enabling the construction of photonic crystals, dielectric mirrors, and the more sophisticated optical structures such as microcavities (the first microcavity made entirely out of porous Si was reported in 1995[89]).[90] Elaborate photonic organic and biological polymers have been constructed by using porous silicon photonic crystals as the template.[118] Polymer was infused into the porous silicon template by injection molding[118] or solution casting.[133] Chemical dissolution of the template produces a freestanding porous polymer film.[118] The polymer replicas inherit an inverse of the optical structure of the template. This approach was first demonstrated by using a porous silicon rugate dielectric mirror as the template.[118] A rugate dielectric mirror is a structure that contains a sinusoidal refractive index variation, producing a sharp spectral feature in the optical spectrum. A porous silicon rugate dielectric mirror is prepared by anodic electrochemical etch of a crystalline Si wafer using a pseudo-sinusoidal current–time waveform (Figure 8.11).[87,90–93,116,117] The sharp features in its optical reflectivity spectrum of the porous silicon rugate mirror can be controlled by adjusting the frequency and the amplitude of the sinusoidal current–time waveform.[94]

For many applications, porous Si is limited by its chemical and mechanical stability. The use of porous Si as a template eliminates these issues while providing the means for construction of complex optical structures from flexible materials that are compatible with biological systems or harsh environments.[118] A very promising application of such fabricated materials would be in drug delivery. Such a templating approach enables one to impart the desirable optical features of the porous Si master to a polymer that possesses the required biocompatibility, resorbability, or drug solubility parameters. With the optical features inherited, sensing functionality is enabled for the biopolymer imprints. A self-reporting drug delivery system has been demonstrated using materials fabricated with this templating approach.[118]

A noninvasive, self-reporting drug delivery matrix is desired in many cases. In the case of drug delivery systems implanted in transparent media such as the vitreous body of the eye, if the systems change their spectral properties as they degrade or as they release a loaded drug, the drug delivery status can be monitored using visible light. Similarly, for drug delivery systems implanted in visibly

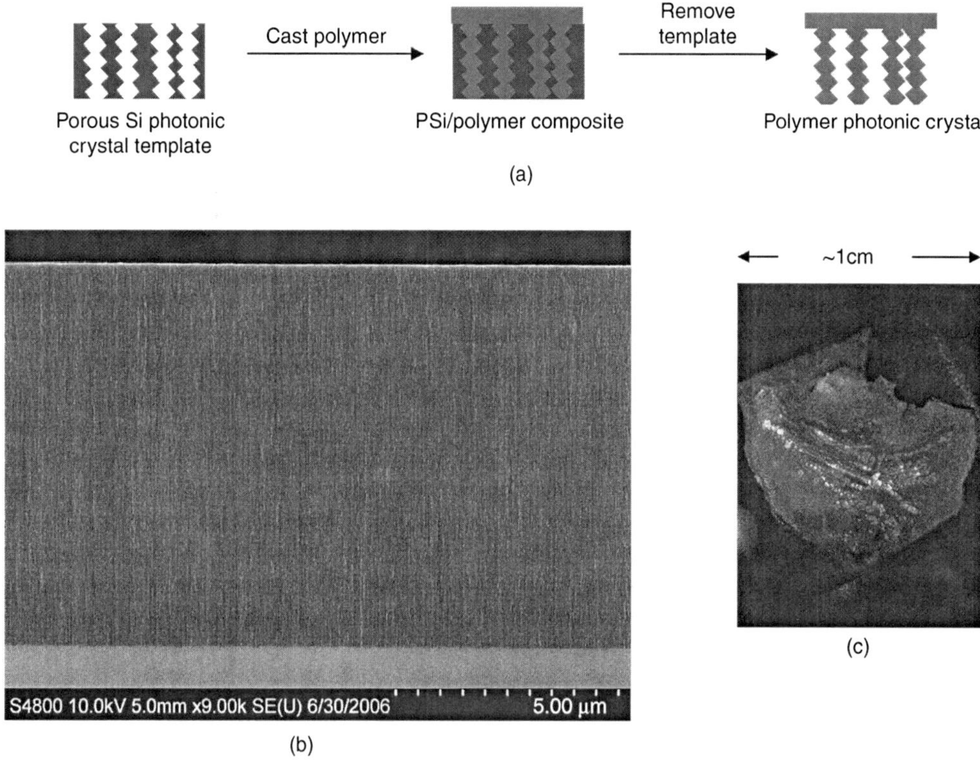

FIGURE 8.11 (a) Schematic illustration of fabrication of polymer photonic materials using porous Si photonic crystal templates. (b) Cross-sectional SEM micrograph of a porous silicon rugate dielectric mirror template showing multi-layers along the z direction, prepared via electrochemical etch of a crystalline Si wafer using a pseudo-sinusoidal current–time waveform. The scale bar is 5 µm. (c) Optical photograph of a polymer photonic crystal fabricated by templating a porous silicon rugate dielectric mirror.

opaque tissue, if the near-infrared, tissue-penetrating spectral features are encoded into the drug delivery material, the fixture conceivably could be probed through the skin or through several millimeters of opaque tissue. This latter concept has been demonstrated with a rugate optical structure made of biodegradable polylactide, impregnated with a test drug.[118] Drug release correlates to the decrease in intensity of the spectral features of the drug loaded rugate structure as expected. By placing the spectral feature of the polylactide imprint within the low-absorbance, near-infrared window of human tissue, a drug delivery matrix that could be read through the skin was demonstrated.[118] With the recently demonstrated encoding ability of porous silicon due to the elaborate optical structure,[94,136] we can design into the material characteristic spectral "bar codes" that enable the fixture to be distinguished from tissue, light scattering centers, or highly colored materials in the body.[117,118]

8.3 SUMMARY AND OUTLOOK

In summary, porous nanostructured systems that can take the form of liposomes, nanospheres, nanocapsules, nanotubes, microspheres, thin films, or other morphologies are intensely studied in laboratories under clinical investigations and some are also commercially available in the market. The preparation of the porous nanostructured systems can be based on diverse methods or mechanisms, following for instance, self-assembly, sol–gel, templating, or soft chemistry routes. Precise control of the nanostructuring and the surface chemistry makes it feasible to achieve functional nanomaterials for optimal performance with desirable optical, magnetic, environment-sensitive, or target-specific properties, leading to controlled delivery patterns such as sustained or environment-responsive release or targeting drug delivery. It should be noted that in addition to those single component porous nanomaterials, composite or hybrid porous nanomaterials are fabricated with multiple components chosen from various soft and inorganic materials,[137,138] which adds more flexibility to the design and engineering of advanced delivery systems. In addition to the controlled drug delivery application, porous nanostructured materials are under extensive investigation for possible use in other biomedical applications such as tissue engineering, imaging, and biosensing. Efforts toward developing multifunctional smart systems suitable for manifold applications are in full swing.[60,96,139–141]

Since 1970, pharmaceutical research has come a long way from drug discovery by empiricism and happenstance to the more sophisticated and rational investigation. Nanotechnology, as a relatively new player in this field, has demonstrated immense potential and brought keen promise for more effective methods of drug and therapy with more sophisticated and smart functionality enabled by engineering at the nanoscale. In addition to the applications discussed above, the possibilities of use of nanomaterials in the pharmaceutical field include superparamagnetic drug-loaded and peptide-coated nanoparticles that not only home into tumors but also amplify their own homing,[139] red blood cell hydrogel mimics with controllable circulating time, near-infrared absorbing metal nanoshells for photothermal cancer therapy and tissue-welding,[142,143] fluorescent quantum dots for diagnostics, and *in vivo* imaging agents during surgery.[144] In all of these systems, the high surface to volume ratio of the nanostructures makes them easily surface modified and thus sensitive for efficient targeting. Advances in nanostructured materials should pave the way for more opportunities in and contributions to diagnostics and therapeutics.

ACKNOWLEDGMENTS

The authors gratefully acknowledge helpful discussions with Prof. Michael J. Sailor of the Department of Chemistry and Biochemistry at the University of California, San Diego.

REFERENCES

1. Wise, D.L. (ed.), *Handbook of Pharmaceutical Controlled Release Technology*, Marcel Dekker Inc., New York, 2000.
2. Saltzman, W.M., *Drug Delivery: Engineering Principles for Drug Therapy*, Oxford University Press, New York, 2001.
3. Edwards, D.A. and Dunbar, C., Bioengineering of therapeutic aerosols, *Annu. Rev. Biomed. Eng.*, **4**, 93, 2002.
4. Uhrich, K.E. et al., Polymeric systems for controlled drug release, *Chem. Rev.*, **99**, 3181, 1999.
5. Ishihara, M. et al., Chitosan hydrogel as a drug delivery carrier to control angiogenesis, *J. Artif. Organs*, **9**, 8, 2006.
6. Obara, K. et al., Acceleration of wound healing in healing-impaired db/db mice with a photocrosslinkable chitosan hydrogel containing fibroblast growth factor-2, *Wound Repair Regen.*, **13**, 390, 2005.
7. Koole, L.H. et al., Sustained local drug delivery from a radiopaque implanted reservoir, *Nat. Biotechnol.*, **16**, 172, 1998.
8. Hatefi, A. and Amsden, B., Biodegradable injectable *in situ* forming drug delivery systems, *J. Contr. Release*, **80**, 9, 2002.
9. Obara, K. et al., Controlled release of paclitaxel from photocrosslinked chitosan hydrogels and its subsequent effect on subcutaneous tumor growth in mice, *J. Contr. Release*, **10**, 79, 2005.
10. St'astny, M. et al., HPMA-hydrogels containing cytostatic drugs. Kinetics of the drug release and *in vivo* efficacy, *J. Contr. Release*, **81**, 101, 2002.
11. Jilek, S., Merkle, H.P. and Walter, E., DNA-loaded biodegradable microparticles as vaccine delivery systems and their interaction with dendritic cells, *Adv. Drug Delivery Rev.*, **57**, 377, 2005.
12. Ishihara, M. et al., Photocrosslinkable chitosan as a dressing for wound occlusion and accelerator in healing process, *Biomaterials*, **23**, 833, 2002.

13. Amass, W., Amass, A. and Tighe, B., A review of biodegradable polymers: Uses, current developments in the synthesis and characterization of biodegradable polyesters, blends of biodegradable polymers and recent advances in biodegradation studies, *Polym. Int.*, **47**, 89, 1998.

14. Gomes, M.E. and Reis, R.L., Biodegradable polymers and composites in biomedical applications: from catgut to tissue engineering, *Intl. Mater. Rev.*, **49**, 261, 2004.

15. Metzke, M. et al., Saccharide-peptide hybrid copolymers as biomaterials, *Angew. Chem. Int. Ed.*, **44**, 6529, 2005.

16. Wang, S.G., Cui, W.J. and Bei, J.Z., Bulk and surface modifications of polylactide, *Anal. Bioanal. Chem.*, **381**, 547, 2005.

17. Jain, R.A., The manufacturing techniques of various drug loaded biodegradable poly(lactide-*co*-glycolide) (PLGA) devices, *Biomaterials*, **21**, 2475, 2000.

18. Schmitt, E.E. and Polistina, R.A., 1967. Surgical sutures. U.S. Patent 3297033, filed Jan. 1967.

19. Giannantoni, A. et al., New frontiers in intravesical therapies and drug delivery, *Eur. Urology*, **50**, 1183, 2006.

20. Sing, K.S.W. et al., Reporting physisorption data for gas/solid systems with special reference to the determination of surface area and porosity, *Pure Appl. Chem.*, **57**, 603, 1985.

21. Malmsten, M., Soft drug delivery systems, *Soft Matter*, **2**, 760, 2006.

22. Soppimath, K.S. et al., Biodegradable polymeric nanoparticles as drug delivery devices, *J. Contr. Release*, **70**, 1, 2001.

23. Heurtault, B. et al., Physico-chemical stability of colloidal lipid particles, *Biomaterials*, **24**, 4283, 2003.

24. Muller, R.H., Radke, M. and Wissing, S.A., Solid lipid nanoparticles (SLN) and nanostructured lipid carriers (NLC) in cosmetics and dermatological preparations, *Adv. Drug Deliv. Rev.*, **54 (Suppl. 1)**, S131, 2002.

25. New, R.R.C. (ed.), *Liposomes a Practical Approach*, Oxford University Press, New York, 1990.

26. Murray, M.J. and Snowden, M.J., The preparation, characterisation and applications of colloidal microgels, *Adv. Colloid Interface Sci.*, **54**, 73, 1995.

27. Lopez, V.C., Hadgraftb, J. and Snowden, M.J., The use of colloidal microgels as a (trans)dermal drug delivery system, *Int. J. Pharm.*, **292**, 137, 2005.

28. Qui, Y. and Park, K., Environment-sensitive hydrogels for drug delivery, *Adv. Drug Delivery Rev.*, **53**, 321, 2001.

29. Kim, J.J. and Park, K., Modulated insulin delivery from glucose-sensitive hydrogel dosage forms, *J. Contr. Release*, **77**, 39, 2001.

30. Brigger, I., Dubernet, C. and Couvreur, P., Nanoparticles in cancer therapy and diagnosis, *Adv. Drug Deliv. Rev.*, **54**, 631, 2002.

31. Burger, C., Hsiao, B.S. and Chu, B., Nanofibrous materials and their applications, *Annu. Rev. Mater. Res.*, **36**, 333, 2006.

32. Abidian, M.R., Kim, D.H. and Martin, D.C., Conducting-polymer nanotubes for controlled drug release, *Adv. Mater.*, **18**, 405, 2006.

33. Martin, C.R. and Kohli, P., The emerging field of nanotube biotechnology, *Nat. Rev. Drug Discovery*, **2**, 29, 2003.

34. Li, D. and Xia, Y., Electrospinning of nanofibers: Reinventing the wheel? *Adv. Mater.*, **16**, 1151, 2004.

35. Chronakis, I.S., Novel nanocomposites and nanoceramics based on polymer nanofibers using electrospinning process—a review, *J. Mater. Process. Technol.*, **167**, 283, 2005.

36. Luu, Y. et al., Development of a nanostructured DNA delivery scaffold via electrospinning of PLGA and PLA-PEG block copolymers, *J. Contr. Release*, **89**, 341, 2003.

37. McCann, J., Marquez, M. and Xia, Y., Highly porous fibers by electrospinning into a cryogenic liquid, *J. Am. Chem. Soc.*, **128**, 1436, 2006.

38. Spector, M.S., Price, R.R. and Schnur, J.M., Chiral lipid tubules, *Adv. Mater.*, **11**, 337, 1999.

39. Douliez, J., Pontoire, B. and Gaillard, C., Lipid tubes with a temperature-tunable diameter, *Chem. Phys. Chem.*, **7**, 2071, 2006.

40. Karlsson, A. et al., Molecular engineering: Networks of nanotubes and containers, *Nature*, **409**, 150, 2001.

41. Lin, Y.C. et al., Manipulating self-assembled phospholipid microtubes next term using microfluidic technology, *Sens. Actuators B*, **117**, 464, 2006.

42. Selinger, J.V. and Schnur, J.M., Theory of chiral lipid tubules, *Phys. Rev. Lett.*, **71**, 4091, 1993.

43. Goldstein, A.S. et al., Testosterone delivery using glutamide-based complex high axial ratio microstructures, *Bioorg. Med. Chem.*, **9**, 2819, 2001.

44. Kabanov, A.V. et al., A new class of drug carriers: Micelles of poly(oxyethylene)-poly(oxypropylene) block copolymers as microcontainers for drug targeting from blood in brain, *J. Contr. Release*, **22**, 141, 1992.

45. Kim, J.J. and Park, K., Modulated insulin delivery from glucosesensitive hydrogel dosage forms, *J. Contr. Release*, **77**, 39, 2001.

46. Lai, C.Y. et al., A mesoporous silica nanosphere-based carrier system with chemically removable CdS nanoparticle caps for stimuli-responsive controlled release of neurotransmitters and drug molecules, *J. Am. Chem. Soc.*, **125**, 4451, 2003.

47. Aiello, R. et al., Mesoporous silicate as matrix for drug delivery systems of non-steroidal antiinflammatory drugs, *Stud. Surf. Sci. Catal.*, **14**, 1165, 2002.

48. Bégu, S. et al., Preparation and characterization of silicious material using liposomes as template, *Chem. Commun.*, 640, 2003.

49. Bégu, S. et al., Characterization of a phospholipid bilayer entrapped into non-porous silica nanospheres, *J. Mater. Chem.*, **14**, 1316, 2004.

50. Canham, L.T. et al., Derivatized porous silicon mirrors: Implantable optical components with slow resorbability, *Phys. Status Solidi A*, **182**, 521, 2000.

51. Kresge, C.T. et al., Ordered mesoporous molecular sieves synthesized by a liquid-crystal template mechanism, *Nat. Biotechnol.*, **359**, 710, 1992.

52. Cieslaa, U. and Schüth, F., Ordered mesoporous materials, *Microporous Mesoporous Mater.*, **27**, 131, 1999.

53. Beck, J.S. and Vartuli, J.C., Recent advances in the synthesis, characterization and applications of mesoporous molecular sieves, *Curr. Opin. Sol. State. Mat. Sci.*, **1**, 76, 1996.

54. Ying, J.Y., Mehnert, C.P. and Wong, M.S., Synthesis and applications of supramolecular-templated mesoporous materials, *Angew. Chem. Int. Ed.*, **38**, 58, 1999.

55. Hüsing, N. and Schubert, U., Aerogels—Airy materials: Chemistry, structure, and properties, *Angew. Chem. Int. Ed.*, **37**, 22, 1998.

56. Sayari, A., Catalysis by crystalline mesoporous molecular sieves, *Chem. Mater.*, **8**, 1840, 1996.

57. Moller, K. and Bein, T., Inclusion chemistry in periodicmesoporous hosts, *Chem. Mater.*, **10**, 2950, 1998.

58. Stein, A., Melde, B.J. and Schroden, R.C., Hybrid inorganic-organic meso-porous silicates-nanoscopic reactors coming of age, *Adv. Mater.*, **12**, 1403, 2000.

59. Beck, J.S. et al., A new family of mesoporous molecular sieves prepared with liquid crystal templates, *J. Am. Chem. Soc.*, **114**, 10834, 1992.

60. Vallet-Regi, M., Ordered mesoporous materials in the context of drug delivery systems and bone tissue engineering, *Chem. Eur. J.*, **12**, 5934, 2006.

61. Tourné-Peteilh, C. et al., The potential of ordered mesoporous for the storage of drugs: the example of a pentapeptide encapsulated in a MSU-Tween 80, *Chem. Phys. Chem.*, **4**, 281, 2003.

62. Mal, N.K., Fujiwara, M. and Tanaka, Y., Photocontrolled reversible release of guest molecules from coumarin-modified mesoporous silica, *Nature*, **421**, 350, 2003.

63. Mal, N.K. et al., Photo-switched storage and release of guest molecules in the pore void of coumarin-modified MCM-41, *Chem. Mater.*, **15**, 3385, 2003.

64. Giri, S. et al., Stimuli-responsive controlled-release delivery system based on mesoporous silica nano-rods capped with magnetic nanoparticles, *Angew. Chem. Int. Ed.*, **44**, 5038, 2005.

65. Radu, D.R. et al., A polyamidoamine dendrimer-capped mesoporous silica nanosphere-based gene transfection reagent, *J. Am. Chem. Soc.*, **126**, 13216, 2004.

66. Zasadzinski, A., Kisak, E. and Evans, C., Complex vesicle-based structures, *Curr. Opin. Colloid Interface Sci.*, **6**, 85, 2001.

67. Kim, S.S., Zhang, W. and Pinnavaia, T.J., Ultrastable mesostructured silica vesicles, *Science*, **282**, 1302, 1998.

68. Coradin, T. et al., Design of silica-coated microcapsules for bioencapsulation, *Chem. Commun.*, **23**, 2496, 2001.

69. Schmidt, H.T. and Ostafin, A.E., Liposome directed growth of calcium phosphate nanoshells, *Adv. Mater.*, **14**, 532, 2002.

70. Hubert, D.H.W. et al., Vesicle-directed growth of silica, *Adv. Mater.*, **12**, 1286, 2000.

71. Anderson, S.H.C. et al., Dissolution of different forms of partially porous silicon wafers under simulated physiological conditions, *Phys. Status Solidi A*, **197**, 331, 2003.

72. Ji, J.M. et al., Use of microcontact printing methods to direct pattern formation of calcified mesoporous silicon, *Adv. Mater.*, **14**, 41, 2002.

73. Jay, T. et al., Autoclaving of porous silicon within a hospital environment: Potential benefits and problems, *Phys. Status Solidi A*, **182**, 555, 2000.
74. Canham, L.T. et al., Derivatized mesoporous silicon with dramatically improved stability in simulated human blood plasma, *Adv. Mater.*, **11**, 1505, 1999.
75. Wainwright, M. et al., Morphological changes (including filamentation) in *Escherichia coli* grown under starvation conditions on silicon wafers and other surfaces, *Lett. Appl. Microbiol.*, **29**, 224, 1999.
76. Canham, L.T. et al., Calcium phosphate nucleation on porous silicon: Factors influencing kinetics in acellular simulated body fluids, *Thin Sol. Films*, **297**, 304, 1997.
77. Bayliss, S.C. et al., Phosphate and cell growth on nanostructured semiconductors, *J. Mat. Sci. Lett.*, **16**, 737, 1997.
78. Bayliss, S.C. et al., The culture of neurons on silicon, *Sens. Actuators A*, **74**, 139, 1999.
79. Bayliss, S.C. et al., The culture of mammalian cells on nanostructured silicon, *Adv. Mater.*, **11**, 318, 1999.
80. Bayliss, S.C. et al., Nature of the silicon-animal cell interface, *J. Porous Mater.*, **7**, 191, 2000.
81. Mayne, A.H. et al., Biologically interfaced porous silicon devices, *Phys. Status Solidi A*, **182**, 505, 2000.
82. Buriak, J.M., Organometallic chemistry on silicon and germanium surfaces, *Chem. Rev.*, **102**, 1272, 2002.
83. Foraker, A.B. et al., Microfabricated porous silicon particles enhance paracellular delivery of insulin across intestinal Caco-2 cell monolayers, *Pharm. Res.*, **20**, 110, 2003.
84. Anglin, E.J. et al., Engineering the chemistry and nanostructure of porous silicon Fabry-Pérot films for loading and release of a steroid, *Langmuir*, **20**, 11264, 2004.
85. Vaccari, L. et al., Porous silicon as drug carrier for controlled delivery of doxorubicin anticancer agent, *Microelectron. Eng.*, **83**, 1598, 2006.
86. Collins, R.T., Fauchet, P.M. and Tischler, M.A., Porous silicon: from luminescence to LEDs, *Phys. Today*, **50**, 24, 1997.
87. Pavesi, L. and Dubos, P., Random porous silicon multilayers: Application to distributed Bragg reflectors and interferential Fabry-Perot filters, *Semicond. Sci. Technol.*, **12**, 570, 1997.
88. Pavesi, L., Panzarini, G. and Andreani, L.C., All-porous silicon-coupled microcavities: Experiment versus theory, *Phys. Rev. B Condens. Matt.*, **58**, 15794, 1998.
89. Mazzoleni, C. and Pavesi, L., Application to optical components of dielectric porous silicon multilayers, *Appl. Phys. Lett.*, **67**, 2983, 1995.
90. Thonissen, M. and Berger, M.G., Multilayer structures of porous silicon, in *Properties of Porous Silicon*, 18th ed, Canham, L. (ed.), Short Run Press Ltd., London, 1997, 30.
91. Lehmann, V. et al., Optical shortpass filters based on macroporous silicon, *Appl. Phys. Lett.*, **78**, 589, 2001.
92. Snow, P.A. et al., Vapor sensing using the optical properties of porous silicon Bragg mirrors, *J. Appl. Phys.*, **86**, 1781, 1999.
93. Vincent, G., Optical properties of porous silicon super lattices, *Appl. Phys. Lett.*, **64**, 2367, 1994.
94. Berger, M.G. et al., Dielectric filters made of porous silicon: Advanced performance by oxidation and new layer structures, *Thin Sol. Films*, **297**, 237, 1997.
95. Matthias, S. et al., Monodisperse diameter-modulated gold microwires, *Adv. Mater.*, **14**, 1618, 2002.
96. Sailor, M.J. and Link, J.R., Smart dust: Nanostructured devices in a grain of sand, *Chem. Commun.*, 1375, 2005.
97. Weiss, S.M. et al., Electrical and thermal modulation of silicon photonic bandgap microcavities containing liquid crystals, *Optic Express*, **13**, 1090, 2005.
98. DeLouise, L.A. et al., Hydrogel-supported optical-microcavity sensors, *Adv. Mater.*, **17**, 2199, 2005.
99. Lin, V.S.Y. et al., A porous silicon-based optical interferometric biosensor, *Science*, **278**, 840, 1997.
100. Sailor, M.J., Sensor applications of porous silicon, in *Properties of Porous Silicon*, 18th ed, Canham, L. (ed.), Short Run Press Ltd., London, 1997, 364.
101. Dancil, K.P.S., Greiner, D.P. and Sailor, M.J., A porous silicon optical biosensor: Detection of reversible binding of IgG to a protein A-modified surface, *J. Am. Chem. Soc.*, **121**, 7925, 1999.
102. Chan, S. et al., Porous silicon microcavities for biosensing applications, *Phys. Status Solidi A*, **182**, 541, 2000.
103. Zangooie, S., Jansson, R. and Arwin, H., Ellipsometric characterization of anisotropic porous silicon Fabry-Perot filters and investigation of temperature effects on capillary condensation efficiency, *J. Appl. Phys.*, **86**, 850, 1999.

104. Tinsley-Bown, A.M. et al., Tuning the pore size and surface chemistry of porous silicon for immunoassays., *Phys. Status Solidi A*, **182**, 547, 2000.
105. Nassiopoulos, A.G. et al., Sub-micrometre luminescent porous silicon structures using lithographically patterned substrates., *Thin Sol. Films*, **255**, 329, 1995.
106. Stewart, M.P. and Buriak, J.M., Photopatterned hydrosilylation on porous silicon, *Angew. Chem. Int. Ed. Engl.*, **37**, 3257, 1998.
107. Krauss, T.F. and De La Rue, R.M., Photonic crystals in the optical regime—Past, present and future, *Prog. Quantum Electron.*, **23**, 51, 1999.
108. Mayer, G. and Sarikaya, M., Rigid biological composite materials: Structural examples for biomimetic design, *Exp. Mech.*, **42**, 395, 2002.
109. Parker, A.R., Mckenzie, D.R. and Large, M.C.J., Multilayer reflectors in animals using green and gold beetles as contrasting examples, *J. Exp. Biol.*, **201**, 1307, 1998.
110. Biró, L.P., et al., Role of photonic-crystal-type structures in the thermal regulation of a Lycaenid butterfly sister species pair, *Phys. Rev. E*, **67**, 021907, 2003.
111. Dresp, B. and Langley, K., Fine structural dependence of ultraviolet reflections in the King Penguin beak horn, *Anat. Rec. A Discov. Mol. Cell Evol. Biol.*, **288**, 213, 2006.
112. Chomski, E. and Ozin, G.A., Panoscopic silicon-a material for all length scales, *Adv. Mater.*, **12**, 1071, 2000.
113. Alexeev, V.L. et al., High ionic strength glucose-sensing photonic crystal, *Anal. Chem.*, **75**, 2316, 2003.
114. Asher, S.A. et al., Photonic crystal carbohydrate sensors: Low ionic strength sugar sensing, *J. Am. Chem. Soc.*, **125**, 3322, 2003.
115. Sharma, A.C. et al., A general photonic crystal sensing motif: Creatinine in bodily fluids, *J. Am. Chem. Soc.*, **126**, 2971, 2004.
116. Schmedake, T.A. et al., Standoff detection of chemicals using porous silicon "smart dust" particles, *Adv. Mater.*, **14**, 1270, 2002.
117. Cunin, F. et al., Biomolecular screening with encoded porous silicon photonic crystals, *Nat. Mater.*, **1**, 39, 2002.
118. Li, Y.Y. et al., Polymer replicas of photonic porous silicon for sensing and drug delivery applications, *Science*, **299**, 2045, 2003.
119. Chan, S. et al., Identification of gram negative bacteria using nanoscale silicon microcavities, *J. Am. Chem. Soc.*, **123**, 11797, 2001.
120. Chan, S. et al., Nanoscale microcavities for biomedical sensor applications, *Proc. SPIE*, **3912**, 23, 2000.
121. Orosco, M.M. et al., Protein-coated porous silicon photonic crystals for amplified optical detection of protease activity, *Adv. Mater.*, **18**, 1393, 2006.
122. Schwartz, M.P. et al., The smart petri dish: a nanostructured photonic crystal for real-time monitoring of living cells, *Langmuir*, **22**, 7084, 2006.
123. Diederich, F. and Stang, P.J. (eds.), *Templated Organic Synthesis*, Wiley-VCH, New York, 2000.
124. Polarz, S. and Antonietti, M., Porous materials via nanocasting procedures: Innovative materials and learning about soft-matter organization, *Chem. Commun.*, **22**, 2593, 2002.
125. Xia, Y. and Whitesides, G.M., Soft lithography, *Angew. Chem. Int. Ed.*, **37**, 550 1998.
126. Cheng, L. et al., Treatment of herpes retinitis in an animal model with a sustained delivery antiviral drug, liposomal 1-O-octadecyl-SN-glycerol-3-phosphonoformate, *Retina*, **19**, 325, 1999.
127. Wirtz, M. et al., Template synthesized nanotubes for chemical separations and analysis, *Chem. Eur. J.*, **16**, 3572, 2002.
128. Hulteen, J.C. and Martin, C.R., A general template-based method for the preparation of nanomaterials., *J. Mater. Chem.*, **7**, 1075, 1997.
129. Reese, C.E. et al., Development of an intelligent polymerized crystalline colloidal array colorimetric reagent, *Anal. Chem.*, **73**, 5038, 2001.
130. Xu, X., Majetich, S.A. and Asher, S.A., Mesoscopic monodisperse ferromagnetic colloids enable magnetically controlled photonic crystals, *J. Am. Chem. Soc.*, **124**, 13864, 2002.
131. Haynes, C.L. and Van Duyne, R.P., Nanosphere lithography: a versatile nanofabrication tool for studies of size-dependent nanoparticle optics, *J. Phys. Chem. B*, **105**, 5599, 2001.
132. Mulvihill, M.J. et al., Synthesis of bifunctional polymer nanotubes from silicon nanowire templates via atom transfer radical polymerization *J. Am. Chem. Soc.*, **127**, 16040, 2005.

133. Li, Y.Y., Kollengode, V.S. and Sailor, M.J., Porous silicon/polymer nanocomposite photonic crystals by microdroplet patterning, *Adv. Mater.*, **17**, 1249, 2005.
134. Yoon, M.S. et al., Covalent crosslinking of 1-D photonic crystals of microporous Si by hydrosilylation and ring-opening metathesis polymerization, *Chem. Commun.*, **6**, 680, 2003.
135. Heinrich, J.L., Lee, A. and Sailor, M.J., Porous silicon used as an initiator in polymerization reactions, *Mat. Res. Soc. Symp. Proc.*, **358**, 605, 1995.
136. Meade, S.O. et al., Porous silicon photonic crystals as encoded microcarriers, *Adv. Mater.*, **16**, 1811, 2004.
137. Boissière, M. et al., Turning biopolymer particles into hybrid capsules: the example of silica/alginate nanocomposites, *J. Mater. Chem.*, **16**, 1178, 2006.
138. Li, D. and Xia, Y., Direct fabrication of composite and ceramic hollow nanofibers by electrospinning, *Nano Lett.*, **4**, 933, 2004.
139. Simberg, D. et al., Biomimetic amplification of nanoparticle homing to tumors, *Proc. Natl Acad. Sci.*, **104**, 932, 2007.
140. Kohli, P. and Martin, C.R., Smart nanotubes for biotechnology, *Curr. Pharm. Biotechnol.*, **6**, 35, 2005.
141. Roy, I. and Gupta, M.N., Smart polymeric materials: Emerging biochemical applications, *Chem. Biol.*, **10**, 1161, 2003.
142. O'Neal, D.P. et al., Photothermal tumor ablation in mice using near infrared absorbing nanoshells, *Cancer Lett.*, **209**, 171, 2004.
143. Gobin, A.M. et al., Near infrared laser tissue welding using nanoshells as an exogenous absorber, *Lasers Surg. Med.*, **37**, 123, 2005.
144. Michalet, X. et al., Quantum dots for live cells, *in vivo* imaging, and diagnostics, *Science*, **307**, 538, 2005.

9 Inorganic Nanostructures for Drug Delivery

Ying-Jie Zhu

CONTENTS

9.1 INTRODUCTION

Nanotechnology has had a significant impact on the development of drug delivery systems over the past decade, leading to the emergence of entirely new research fields [1]. For the pharmaceutical industry, novel drug delivery technologies represent a strategic tool for expanding drug markets, evidenced by the fact that sales of products incorporating a drug delivery system account for approximately 13% of the current global pharmaceutical market. The demand for drug delivery systems in the United States alone is expected to grow by nearly 9% annually, to more than US$ 82 billion by 2007. Controlled drug delivery provides the ability to control the release rate of the drug and the delivery of the drug to a specific location in the body (i.e., targeting). Recently, some reviews on drug delivery were published [1–4]; however, these reviews focused primarily on polymeric systems.

Many organic materials such as polymers [5], liposomes, and micelles have been investigated as drug delivery carriers. However, unsolved problems regarding these organic systems continue to exist. These problems include low chemical stability, swelling, susceptibility to microbiological contamination, and inadequate control over the drug release rate. The release properties of many biodegradable polymer-based drug delivery systems are dependent on the hydrolysis-induced erosion of the carrier structure [2,3]. Such systems usually require the use of organic solvents for drug loading, which could sometimes trigger undesirable modifications of the structure or the function or both of the encapsulated molecules.

In contrast, many inorganic materials are nontoxic, biocompatible, hydrophilic, and chemically stable. These materials hold promise for the development of drug delivery systems, especially for controlled drug delivery. It is possible to produce the stable porous structures of inorganic materials, which can often be tailored to control the drug loading and the drug release rate. In addition, there is no swelling or porosity change under different pH values, which is a common problem encountered when using organic materials. Because of the abovementioned reasons, the research on inorganic nanostructures as drug carriers has gained momentum in recent years and is currently a fast growing field. In this chapter, the recent progress in nanostructured inorganic drug carriers and their drug delivery properties will be briefly reviewed. However, all the literature on this subject will not be reviewed; instead, only some related papers will be included in this chapter. This chapter is divided into three sections: (1) nanostructured silica as drug carriers, (2) nanostructured calcium carbonate and calcium phosphates as drug carriers, and (3) magnetic targeting drug delivery systems.

9.2 NANOSTRUCTURED SILICA AS DRUG CARRIERS

Some papers have been published on the drug carriers of SiO_2 nanoparticles. Barbé et al. [6] reported that bioactive molecules could be encapsulated within silica nanoparticles by combining sol–gel polymerization with either spray-drying or emulsion chemistry. Preliminary *in vivo* experiments revealed the enhanced blood stability of the nanoparticles and the sustained release of antitumor agents, indicating good potential for cancer treatment (Figure 9.1).

Maitra et al. [7] prepared and characterized hydrated silica nanoparticles encapsulating high molecular weight compounds such as [125I]tyraminylinulin (mol. wt. 5 kDa), FITC-dextran (mol. wt. 19.6 kDa), and horse radish peroxidase (mol. wt. 40 kDa). The entrapment efficiency was found to be as high as 80%, and the entrapped compounds showed practically zero leachability for more than 45 days. Enzymes entrapped in these nanoparticles demonstrated Michaelis–Menten kinetics. Peroxidase entrapped in silica nanoparticles showed higher stability toward temperature and pH changes compared with free enzyme molecules.

In recent years, there has been an increasing interest in mesoporous silica materials for their application in controlled drug release because of their nontoxicity, adjustable pore diameter, high specific surface area, and abundant Si—OH bonds on the pore surface and intrinsic hydrophilicity and biocompatibility [8–19]. Many research activities have focused on mesoporous silica, both solid spheres and hollow spheres. These systems exhibit sustained drug release behaviors.

The experimental results show that factors such as crystal structure, pore size, porosity, specific surface area, and functionalization of the pore wall influence the controlled delivery of different drugs. Functionalization is an important influencing factor in the drug adsorption and release rate. It is very important to carefully choose the type of functionalization of the pore wall in agreement with the specific drug to be adsorbed and subsequently released [18].

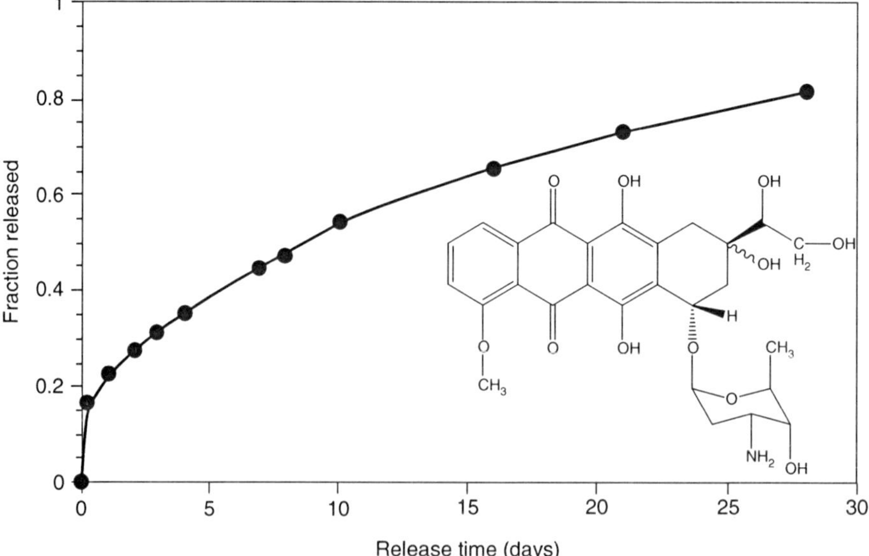

FIGURE 9.1 Release kinetics at pH 6.5–7 for doxorubicin encapsulated in 30 nm SiO_2 nanoparticles. (Reprinted from Barbé, C. et al., *Adv. Mater.*, 16, 1959, 2004.)

A series of micro and mesoporous silica matrices varying in pore size, pore connectivity, and pore geometry were prepared, and their drug loading and release behaviors as carriers were investigated under *in vitro* conditions [19]. Ibuprofen (IBU) was used as a model drug. The loading degree was related to both the surface area and the pore size of the silica matrix. The drug release process could be described as a diffusion-controlled process. The nanostructured silicas that were studied displayed a high degree of drug loading. Depending on the host material, a controlled drug release could be provided for time periods varying from hours to weeks.

Compared with the sustained release system, the stimuli-responsive controlled-release system can achieve a site-selective, controlled release behavior, which can improve the therapeutic efficacy. Till date, only a few reports have been published on stimuli-responsive controlled drug release from mesoporous silica MCM-41 [20,21]. Fujiwara and coworkers realized the photo-controlled reversible release of drug molecules from coumarin-modified MCM-41 [20]. Lin et al. [21] reported the synthesis of a MCM-41 mesoporous silica stimuli-responsive controlled drug release system, which consisted of 2-(propyldisulfanyl) ethylamine functionalized mesoporous silica nanospheres (MSNs) with an average particle size of 200 nm and an average pore diameter of 2.3 nm. The mesopores of the MSNs were used as reservoirs to soak up aqueous solutions of various pharmaceutical drug molecules and neurotransmitters such as vancomycin and adenosine triphosphate (ATP). The openings of the mesopores of the drug/neurotransmitter-loaded MSNs were capped *in situ* by covalently bonding between the pore surface-bound 2-(propyldisulfanyl) ethylamine functional groups and water-soluble mercaptoacetic acid-derivatized cadmium sulfide (CdS) nanocrystals [22] using a reported amidation reaction [23]. The resulting disulfide linkages between the MSNs and the CdS nanoparticles were chemically labile in nature and could be cleaved with various disulfide-reducing agents such as dithiothreitol (DTT) and mercaptoethanol (ME). The release of the CdS nanoparticle caps from the drug/neurotransmitter-loaded MSNs were regulated by introducing various amounts of release triggers. The researchers investigated the stimuli-responsive release profiles, and the delivery efficiency of vancomycin and the ATP encapsulated inside the CdS-capped MSN system. The N_2 adsorption/desorption isotherms revealed a BET isotherm typical of MCM-41 structure (type IV) with a surface area of 941.0 m^2/g and a narrow pore size distribution (average pore diameter of 2.3 nm). In this delivery system, the drug molecules were encapsulated inside the porous framework of the MSN not by adsorption or sol–gel type of entrapment but by capping the openings of the mesoporous channels with size-defined CdS nanoparticles to physically block the drugs/ neurotransmitters of certain sizes from leaching out.

The CdS-capped MSN drug/neurotransmitter delivery system showed less than 1.0% of drug release in 10 mM PBS buffer solutions (pH 7.4) over a period of 12 h (Figure 9.2a), implying a good capping efficiency of the CdS nanoparticles for encapsulation of the vancomycin and ATP molecules [21]. A rapid release of the mesopore-entrapped drug/neurotransmitter was triggered by the addition of disulfide-reducing molecules such as DTT to the aqueous suspension of CdS-capped MSNs. Within 24 h, 85% of the total release was observed. It is very interesting that the release rates of vancomycin and ATP showed similar kinetic profiles, indicating the lack of interaction between these released molecules and the mesoporous silica matrix. However, 53.8% of the encapsulated vancomycin was released after 3 days of the DTT-induced uncapping of the mesopores, while only 28.2% of the entrapped ATP molecules were able to diffuse away. Such a significant difference in the release percentage of vancomycin and ATP implied that ATP molecules were more strongly physisorbed to the organically functionalized mesoporous channels than the vancomycin molecules. Furthermore, in both vancomycin and ATP cases, the amount of drug release after 24 h of the addition of DTT showed similar DTT concentration dependencies (Figure 9.2b), indicating that the release rate was dictated by the rate of removing the CdS caps.

Hollow mesoporous silica spheres are promising candidates as drug carriers. Shi et al. [24] prepared hollow mesoporous silica spheres to enhance the loading capacity for the drugs. These researchers investigated the aspirin storage capacity and release properties of these spheres. The experiments showed that hollow mesoporous silica spheres could store significantly more aspirin

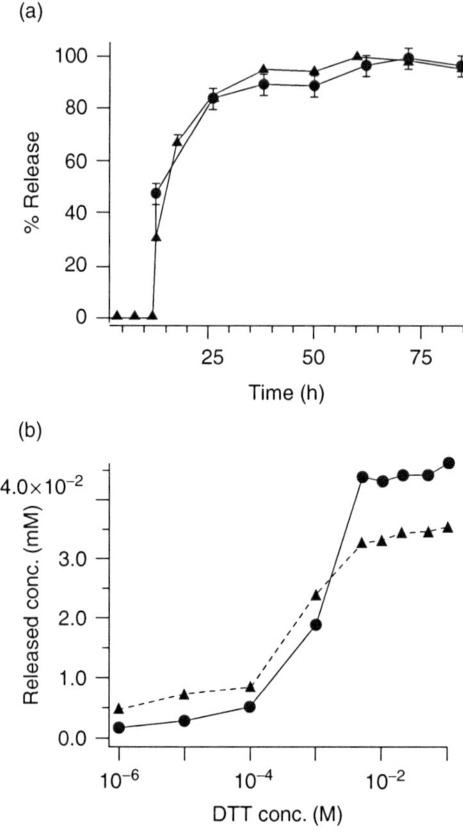

FIGURE 9.2   The DTT-induced release profiles of vancomycin (●) and ATP (▲) from the CdS-capped MSN system: (a) release percentage over time; (b) the DTT concentration-dependent releases. Released analyte concentrations were measured with CdS-MSNs (2.3 mg) in pH 7.4 PBS buffers (0.8 mL) after 24 h of the DTT additions. (Reprinted from Lai, C.Y. et al., *J. Am. Chem. Soc.*, 125, 4451, 2003. © American Chemical Society.)

molecules than the conventional mesoporous MCM-41 and MCM-48 and had sustained drug-release properties. The researchers also prepared hollow mesoporous silica spheres (average diameter of 300–400 nm) with pore channels penetrating from the outside to the inner hollow core (Figures 9.3 and 9.4) [25]. The pH and salt-induced stimuli-responsive function was achieved by polyelectrolyte multilayers (sodium polystyrene sulfonate (PSS) and polycation poly(allylamine hydrochloride) (PAH)) with an average thickness of 14 nm. IBU was used for drug loading and release experiments.

Figures 9.4a and 9.4b show transmission electron microscopy (TEM) micrographs of hollow mesoporous silica spheres with an average diameter of 300–400 nm. The hollow structure can be clearly observed. Figure 9.4c shows a TEM micrograph of a hollow sphere after the adsorption of IBU molecules. No apparent difference can be observed after IBU loading. Figure 9.4d shows a TEM micrograph of an IBU-loaded sphere coated with PAH/PSS multilayers, with a thickness of around 14 nm.

Figure 9.5 shows the cumulative IBU release from the two systems in the release media of pH 1.4 (a simulated gastric fluid) and pH 8.0 (a simulated intestinal fluid). Both systems showed sustained-release properties, and the drug release rates from both the systems were similar in the medium of pH 1.4. The amounts released from the two systems reached about 80% in 48 h. This result implies that the PAH/PSS multilayers had open pathways in the release medium of pH 1.4 and could not cap the openings of the mesoporous channels. When the pH value of the release medium

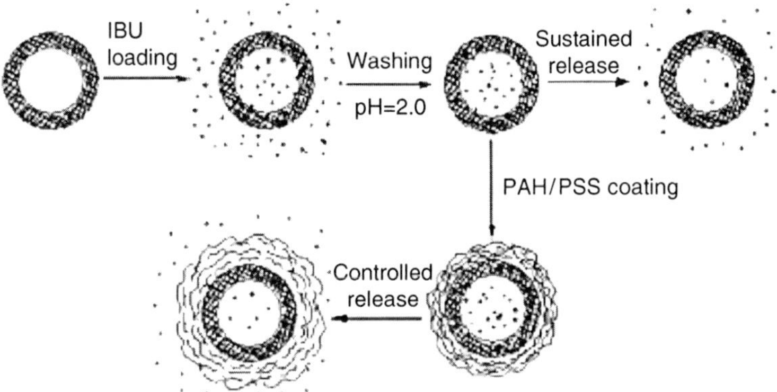

FIGURE 9.3 Schematic illustration of two drug delivery systems that provide different controlled-release patterns. (Reprinted from Zhu, Y.F. et al., *Angew. Chem. Int. Ed.*, 44, 5083, 2005.)

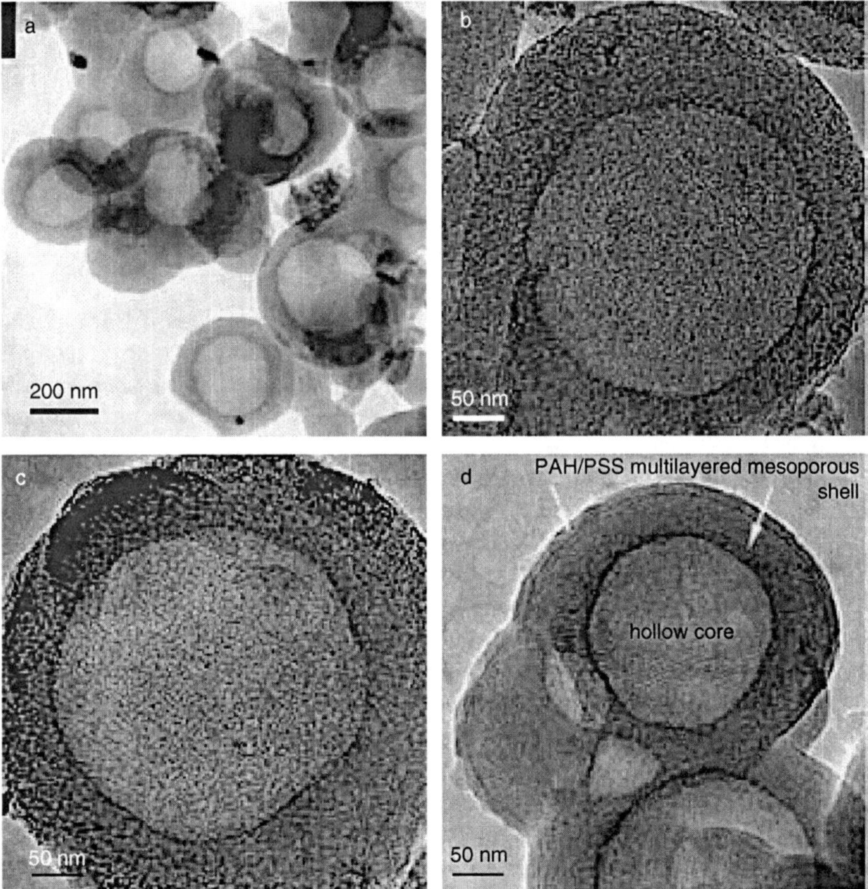

FIGURE 9.4 TEM micrographs: (a and b) hollow mesoporous silica spheres, (c) ibuprofen-hollow mesoporous silica spheres, and (d) ibuprofen-hollow mesoporous silica spheres with polyelectrolyte multilayers. (Reprinted from Zhu, Y.F. et al., *Angew. Chem. Int. Ed.*, 44, 5083, 2005.)

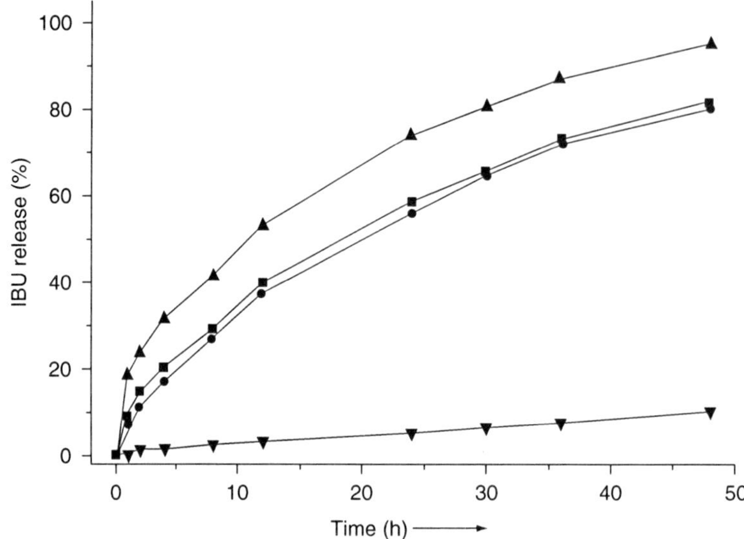

FIGURE 9.5 Cumulative ibuprofen release from the two systems in the release media of different pH values. ■ and ▲: pH 1.4 and 8.0 from hollow mesoporous silica spheres, respectively; ● and ▼: pH 1.4 and 8.0 from PAH/PSS coated hollow mesoporous silica spheres, respectively. (Reprinted from Zhu, Y.F. et al., *Angew. Chem. Int. Ed.*, 44, 5083, 2005.)

increased to 8.0, the drug release rates from both systems were apparently different. The release rate in pH 8.0 release medium was higher than that in the pH 1.4 medium because of the different solubility of IBU in the release media of different pH values. IBU had a lower solubility in low pH (<7) solutions but was readily soluble in high pH (>7) solutions. These results show the good storage and sealing effect of the PAH/PSS multilayer coating on hollow mesoporous spheres in pH 8.0 solution.

Wen and Chen et al. [26] prepared porous hollow silica nanoparticles (PHSNs) with various shell thicknesses in the range of 5–45 nm and a pore diameter of 4–5 nm by a sol–gel route with two different structure-directing templates. The shell thickness was controlled by adjusting the reactant ratio of $Na_2SiO_3 \cdot 9H_2O/CaCO_3$. These researchers investigated the loading and release properties of avermectin in PHSNs and the UV-shielding property. PHSNs carriers had a remarkable loading ability for avermectin (about 60.0% w/w); the amount of loaded avermectin decreased with increasing shell thickness, while the UV-shielding property of PHSNs for avermectin improved as the shell thickness increased. Increasing the shell thickness in the range of 5–45 nm led to a more sustained release by decreasing the release rate of the pesticide from PHSNs, showing that the shell thickness is one of the main controlling factors for the controlled drug release from such systems. Chen et al. [27] prepared PHSNs with a diameter of 60–70 nm and wall thickness of approximately 10 nm by using $CaCO_3$ nanoparticles as the inorganic template. The as-synthesized PHSNs were used as a drug carrier to investigate *in vitro* release behavior of cefradine in simulated body fluid. The experiments showed that cefradine release behavior followed a three-stage pattern and exhibited a delayed release effect.

Prasad et al. [28] reported a novel nanoparticle-based drug carrier for photodynamic therapy, which could provide stable aqueous dispersion of hydrophobic photosensitizers, yet preserve the key step of photogeneration of singlet oxygen, necessary for photodynamic action. Ultrafine organically modified silica-based nanoparticles (diameter of about 30 nm), entrapping water-insoluble photosensitizing anticancer drug 2-devinyl-2-(1-hexyloxyethyl) pyropheophorbide, were synthesized in the nonpolar core of micelles by hydrolysis of triethoxyvinylsilane. The entrapped drug was more fluorescent in aqueous medium than the free drug, permitting the use of fluorescence bioimaging studies. Irradiation of the photosensitizing drug entrapped in nanoparticles with light of suitable wavelength resulted in efficient generation of singlet oxygen. *In vitro* studies showed the active uptake of drug-doped nanoparticles into the cytosol of tumor cells. Significant damage to such impregnated tumor cells was observed upon irradiation with light of wavelength 650 nm.

Lee et al. [29] investigated the controlled release of lidocaine hydrochloride from the doped silica-based xerogels with pore sizes from 0.84 to 1.45 nm and surface area from 95 to 649 m^2/g. In the xerogel preparation, tetraethoxysilane (TEOS), methyltriethoxysilane (MTES), and propyltriethoxysilane (PTES) were used as precursors, and a nonionic surfactant Igepal CO 720 was used as a dopant. The release of lidocaine hydrochloride was controlled by partially substituting TEOS with the organosilanes, and/or by adding the dopant. Adding the organosilane precursors lowered the release of both the drug and the surfactant in the order of TEOS, MTES/ TEOS, and PTES/TEOS xerogels. The release from the PTES/TEOS xerogels was much lower than that from the other xerogels. The release of lidocaine hydrochloride was suppressed by the addition of Igepal CO 720, while the release of Igepal CO 720 was slightly promoted by the addition of the drug. The overall release process was diffusion-controlled.

Drug-loaded silica or titania porous microspheres with complex morphology were prepared by sonication of nanoparticle suspensions confined within aqueous droplets of drug molecules in toluene [30]. The drug molecules were incorporated during the assembly of nanoparticle-containing microspheres. The charge and the amphiphilic nature of the drug molecules had a marked influence on microsphere morphology. As a general rule, when the charge on the drug molecule was the same as that of the inorganic nanoparticles, for example, for negatively silica/IBU or positively charged titania/phenylephrine hydrochloride combinations, the microspheres exhibited smooth outer surfaces perforated with circular apertures that were usually less than a micrometre in diameter. When fractured, these microspheres displayed an elaborate foam-like interior of spherical pores with interconnecting mineralized walls, 50–100 nm in thickness. The strong interactions between the drug molecules and the nanoparticles took place for silica/phenylephrine hydrochloride or titania/ IBU combinations, leading to the inhibition of the formation of the oil-in-water-in-oil micelles. Intact nonperforated microspheres with compact, roughened, and creased surfaces and solid interiors were produced. The release properties of IBU- or phenylephrine-loaded silica microspheres were investigated in simulated body fluid. In both the cases, release of the drugs occurred within 30 min, after which steady-state conditions corresponding to further release of residual drug molecules were observed up to 3 h after immersion.

The nanotubes are highly attractive since it is possible to differentially functionalize the inner and outer surfaces to facilitate drug loading. Lee et al. [31] reported the template synthesis of composite nanotubes containing silica and iron oxide. The inside of nanotubes were differentially functionalized with amino-silane (aminopropyl triethoxysilane, APTS) to generate a polycationic surface for drug loading using ionic interaction between drug molecules and nanotube inner surface. For drug loading, 5-fluorouracil (5-FU), 4-nitrophenol, and IBU were used. The amount of released drug was monitored by measuring changes in absorbance at 264 nm (IBU), 400 nm (4-nitrophenol), and 266 nm (5-FU). Drug release patterns varied with the drugs. For example, 10% of IBU was released in 1 h and 80% was released after 24 h, whereas more than 90% of 5-FU and 4-nitrophenol were released in 1 h. The total release percentage at the same time scale increased in the order of IBU, 4-nitrophenol, and 5-FU.

The recent progress in the design and the development of nanodevices for drug delivery is noteworthy. Sinha et al. [32] developed a high-precision nanoengineered device to yield long-term zero-order release of drugs for therapeutic applications. The device contained nanochannels that were fabricated between two directly bonded silicon wafers and therefore possessed a high mechanical strength. The nanochannels were defined by selectively growing oxide and then etching that oxide (sacrificial oxide), which was grown under dry thermal conditions. It was possible to control the oxide thickness within ±1 nm uniformity; therefore, the nanochannels were fabricated with less than ±1 nm size error. Diffusion through the nanochannels was the rate-limiting step for the release

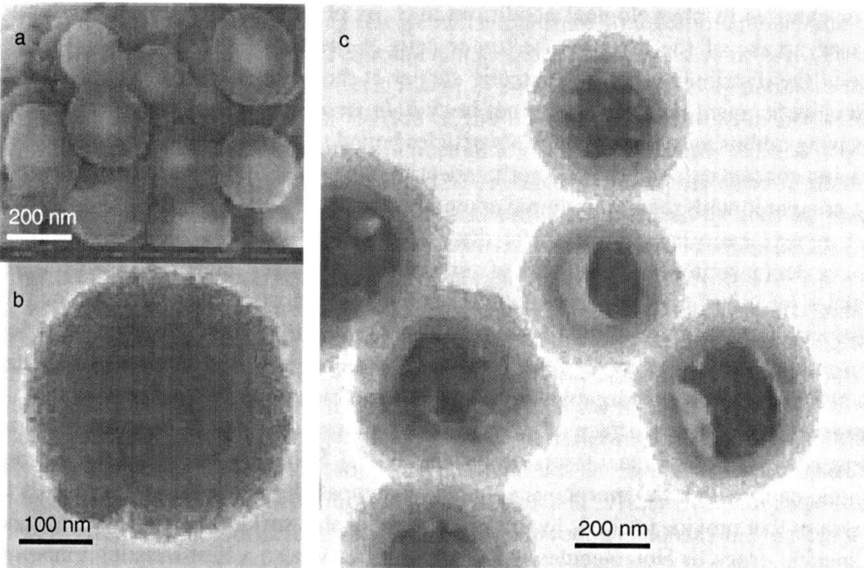

FIGURE 9.8 Backscattered electrons image (a) and TEM micrograph (b) of spheres with a hematite core/ mesoporous silica shell structure, and TEM micrograph (c) of spheres with a Fe_3O_4/Fe core/mesoporous silica shell structure. (Reprinted from Zhao, W.R. et al., *J. Am. Chem. Soc.*, 127, 8916, 2005. © American Chemical Society.)

Fu et al. [53] reported the preparation of microspheres with a core–shell structure. The magnetite nanoparticles were synthesized by a chemical coprecipitation method using ferrous and ferric salts, followed by activation treatment with trisodium citrate. The magnetite nanoparticles were coated by a silica layer, and the magnetic silica nanoparticles (about 30 nm in diameter) were labeled with fluorescein isothiocyanate (FITC). After incorporation of the FITC molecules into the silica layer of the microspheres, another silica layer on these spheres was needed to avoid the aggregation as a result of the introduction of the FITC molecules. Then, the shell of cross-linked poly(*N*-isopropylacrylamide) (PNIPAM) was formed on these spheres (about 200 nm). The experiments indicated that these microspheres exhibited multistimuli-responsive properties, offering promising applications in controlled drug delivery.

Lin et al. [54] reported the synthesis of a controlled-release delivery carrier based on MCM-41-type mesoporous silica nanorods (MSNs) capped with superparamagnetic iron oxide nanoparticles (Figure 9.9). The system consisted of MSNs functionalized with 3-(propyldisulfanyl) propionic acid to provide "linker-MSNs," which had a diameter of 80 nm and length of 200 nm and an average pore diameter of about 3 nm. Fluorescein was used as the guest molecule to be encapsulated inside the linker-MSN. By introducing dry linker-MSNs to an aqueous solution of fluorescein, the mesopores of the MSNs behaved like sponges, soaking up fluorescein molecules. Then, the openings of the mesopores of the fluorescein-loaded linker-MSN were covalently capped *in situ* through amidation of the 3-(propyldisulfanyl)propionic acid functional groups bound at the pore surface with 3-aminopropyltriethoxysilyl-functionalized superparamagnetic iron oxide (APTS-Fe_3O_4) nanoparticles. The disulfide linkages between the MSNs and the Fe_3O_4 nanoparticles were chemically labile and could be cleaved with various cell-produced antioxidants and disulfide reducing agents such as dihydrolipoic acid (DHLA) and dithiothreitol (DTT), respectively.

The experiments showed that less than 1.0% fluorescein in magnet-MSNs were released in the PBS solution (0.1 M, pH 7.4) over a period of 132 h in the absence of trigger molecules, indicating a good efficiency of the Fe_3O_4 nanoparticles to retain fluorescein molecules and prevent undesired

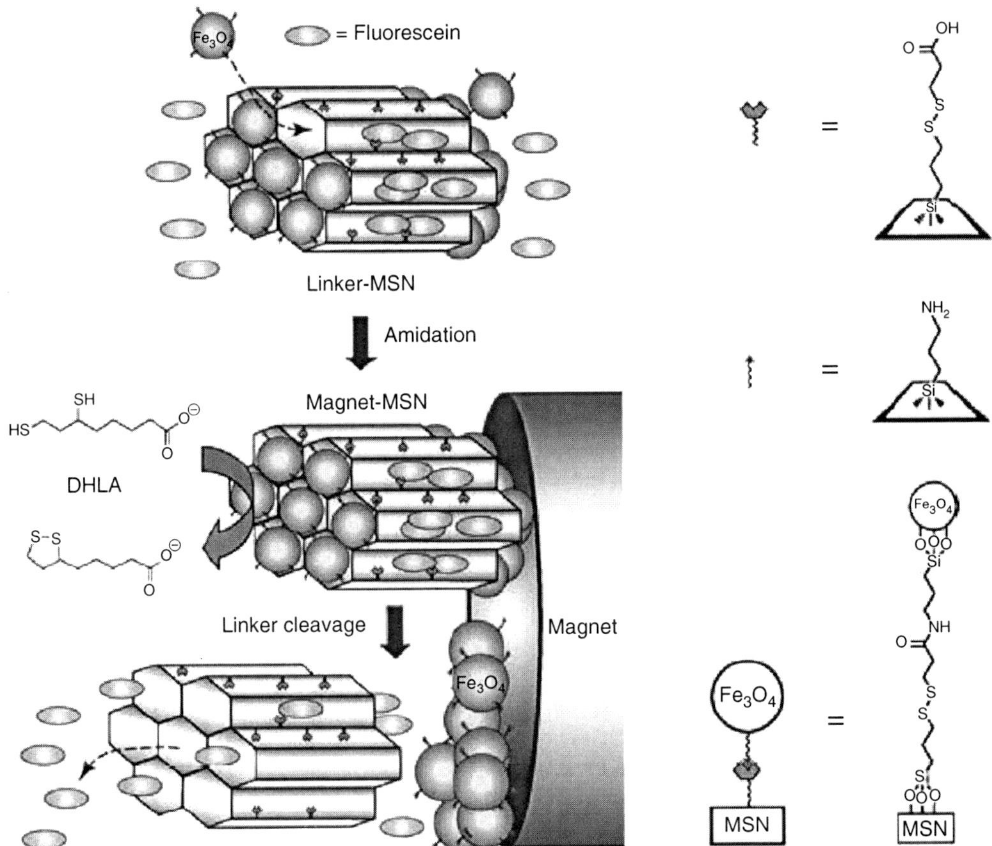

FIGURE 9.9 The schematic of the stimuli-responsive delivery system (magnet-MSN) based on mesoporous silica nanorods capped with Fe_3O_4 nanoparticles. The controlled-release mechanism of the system is based on reduction of the disulfide linkage between the Fe_3O_4 nanoparticle caps and the linker–MSN hosts by reducing agents such as dihydrolipoic acid (DHLA). (Reprinted from Giri, S. et al., *Angew. Chem. Int. Ed.*, 44, 5038, 2005.)

leaching by capping the mesopores [54]. When disulfide reducing agents such as DHLA and DTT were added to a suspension of magnet-MSNs in PBS solution, a rapid release of the mesopore-entrapped fluorescein occurred. Of the total release of fluorescein, 85% (40% of total loading) was attained within 48 h; the maximum extent of release was achieved after 5 days. With DHLA, the maximum percentage of fluorescein released was 31.4% of the total loading. Interestingly, the release rates of fluorescein by the two different triggers showed similar diffusional kinetic profiles, indicating the similar reducing powers of DHLA and DTT. In addition, the magnet-MSNs could be endocytosed by human cervical cancer (HeLa) cells and were biocompatible with HeLa cells *in vitro*, exhibiting promising potential applications in the development of new generations of drug delivery systems.

The hollow tubular structures are very interesting and promising candidates for various applications, including drug delivery [55]. The magnetic tubular structures with drug-friendly interiors and target-specific exteriors are favorable for multifunctional targeted drug delivery. Lee et al. [56] reported the synthesis of magnetic nanotubes and their applications for magnetic field–assisted chemical and biochemical separations, biointeraction, and drug delivery. These researchers synthesized silica nanotubes with a layer of magnetite (Fe_3O_4) nanoparticles on the inner surface of the nanotube using porous alumina film as template (60 and 200 nm pore diameters). Silica nanotubes were prepared in the pores of the template film by the "surface sol–gel" methods [57]. For the differential functionalization of nanotubes, the inner nanotube surface was treated with octadecyltriethoxysilane (C18-silane) while nanotubes were still embedded in the pores of the alumina template. Free-standing magnetic nanotubes were obtained after polishing both sides of the template film mechanically and dissolving the alumina template in NaOH solution. After the template was dissolved completely, magnetic nanotubes were collected by filtration. Both the magnetic nanotubes, with diameters of 60 and 200 nm, respectively, exhibited the superparamagnetic characteristics, and their saturation magnetizations were 2.7 and 2.9 emu/g, respectively. Similar saturation magnetization values were also reported for silica–magnetite nanoparticles [58] and MCM-48–Fe particles [59]. However, this magnitude of saturation magnetization may not be sufficient for the targeting drug delivery, and further work needs to be done to enhance the magnetic property and thus to improve the drug delivery efficiency.

Lee et al. [56] also investigated the drug delivery behavior of magnetic nanotubes. 5-FU, 4-nitrophenol, and IBU were loaded as model drug molecules into the pores of magnetic nanotubes functionalized with amino-silane (aminopropyl triethoxysilane, APTS) to study the effect of the charged hydrogen-bonding interaction between drug and the inner pore surfaces on loading and release. The amine-functionalized magnetic nanotubes were immersed in hexane (IBU) or ethanol (5-FU, 4-nitrophenol) solutions of drugs. The amine functional groups had strong ionic and/or hydrogen-bonding interactions with the acid functional groups of drug molecules. Their experiments showed that $\sim10^7$ IBU molecules per nanotube were loaded, and $\sim10^6$ for 4-nitrophenol and $\sim10^7$ for 5-FU. The value for IBU was about twice the monolayer coverage of the inner surface area of a magnetic nanotube.

Santamaía et al. [60] synthesized nanocomposites consisting of magnetite and FAU zeolite with a high surface area (442.9 m^2/g) by a high-energy milling method. The magnetite nanoparticles had diameters of 20–30 nm and were dispersed within larger zeolite particles (200 nm–1.2 μm long). The resulting magnetic nanoparticles were covered by a thin aluminosilicate coating. The saturation magnetization and coercivity were measured to be 16 emu/g and 94.2 Oe, respectively. The capacity of the magnetite–zeolite composites to adsorb and release a specific drug (doxorubicin) was tested using dispersions of the composites in human plasma. Because the molecular size of doxorubicin used was larger than the mean pore size of the magnetic nanoparticles obtained (0.87 nm), the adsorption occurred on the external surface of the nanocomposites and in the microvoids between the magnetite cores and the zeolite shells. The initial uptake was very fast, with 77% of the initial doxorubicin being adsorbed in 3.1 h. Adsorption of the remaining doxorubicin occurred at a slower rate, and the adsorption process was essentially complete in approximately 25 h, at which time 92% of the initial doxorubicin had been loaded. After removing nonadsorbed doxorubicin by washing, the dried, drug-loaded nanoparticles were redispersed in human plasma. After washing, over 50% of the initial doxorubicin was still adsorbed in the nanoparticles; it was progressively released by desorption and diffusion to the plasma solution, and 77% of the doxorubicin loaded on the nanoparticles was released in 12.6 h.

Wang et al. [61] synthesized tetraheptylammonium-capped nanoparticles of Fe_3O_4, Fe_2O_3, and Ni by the electrochemical deposition method under oxidizing conditions. The synergistic effect of these nanoparticles on the drug accumulation of the anticancer drug daunorubicin in leukemia cells was investigated. The experiments showed that the presence of magnetic nanoparticles could facilitate the drug accumulation of daunorubicin inside leukemia cells and that the enhancement effect of Fe_3O_4 nanoparticles was much stronger than that of the other two magnetic nanoparticles.

Alexiou et al. [62] prepared iron oxide core covered by a layer of starch polymer. The starch layer made the magnetic nanoparticles biocompatible and able to react with various end functional groups for binding other molecules. The drug mitoxantrone was bound to phosphate groups of starch derivatives. A successful application of the magnetic drug targeting was demonstrated by experiments on New Zealand White Rabbits in which VX-2 squamous cell carcinoma was placed at the medial portion of the left hind limb. Typically, 35 days after the treatment, the tumor disappeared completely [47]. No metastases or negative side effects were observed. Both rabbits were treated with mitoxantrone. One rabbit was treated using magnetic drug targeting. Only 20% of the systemic dose was necessary to achieve complete remission of the tumor after 16 days. The second rabbit was treated with conventional local application (femoral artery) of mitoxantrone. To obtain a complete remission of the tumor, 75% of the systemic dose was necessary. However, the side effects of this treatment were atrophy of the left hind limb, alopecia, and ulcerations and weeping inflammation of the skin. The experiments also showed that ferrofluids not only concentrated in the cancer tissue but also penetrated into the tumor cells [62].

Giorgio et al. [63] developed an *in vitro* system to quantify the suitability of superparamagnetic nanoparticles as a site-specific therapeutic vehicle for delivery through fluid- and gel-based systems. The motion of magnetic nanoparticles was induced by an external magnetic field. Magnetic nanoparticles were capped with silica surface coating (135 nm radius) and 300 Da polyethylene glyco (PEG) surface coating (145 and 400 nm radius). PEGylated nanoparticles with a 135 nm radius moved through the extracellular matrix with an average velocity of 1.5 mm/h, suitable for some clinical applications. However, a greater than 1000-fold reduction in magnetic mobility (less than 0.01 mm/h) was observed when the nanoparticle radius was increased to 400 nm while maintaining the same per nanoparticle magnetic susceptibility. The critical influence of nanoparticle size on gel permeation was also observed in silica-coated 135 nm magnetic nanoparticles. Superparamagnetic nanoparticles enabled significant free-solution mobility to specific sites within a cavity and generated sufficient force to penetrate common *in vivo* gels.

9.5 CONCLUDING REMARKS

Inorganic materials are promising for their applications in the development of new controlled drug delivery systems, which constitute a rapidly evolving research field of current interest. As reviewed in this chapter, some interesting work has been done in recent years, and the research activities in this field continue to grow rapidly. In my opinion, one of the main future research directions in this field is the development of multifunctional (controllable drug loading capacity, controllable drug release, targeting ability, biodegradability, etc.) nanostructured inorganic drug carriers with specific structures and morphologies. To prepare such multifunctional nanostructured drug carriers, it is very important to explore new methods that are simple, inexpensive, and environment-friendly. Another important research topic could be exploring new techniques for controllable drug release, which not only control the release rate but more importantly control when and where to release the drug ("start" and "stop" of drug release at the time and the location we want). Biodegradability, which enables the drug-carrier materials to disappear after the drug release is complete, is also an important desirable characteristic for drug carriers. In this case, the influence of the degradation rate on the drug release rate should be investigated, and the degradation rate needs to be considered for the design of the controlled biodegradable drug release systems.

REFERENCES

1. Sahoo, S.K. and Labhasetwar, V., Nanotech approaches to delivery and imaging drug, *Drug Discov. Today*, 8, 1112, 2003.
2. Uhrich, K.E., Cannizzaro, S.M., Langer, R.S., and Shakesheff, K.M., Polymeric systems for controlled drug release, *Chem. Rev.*, 99, 3181, 1999.
3. Langer, R., Polymer-controlled drug-delivery systems, *Accounts Chem. Res.*, 26, 537, 1993.
4. Moghimi, S.M., Hunter, A.C., and Murray, J.C., Long-circulating and target-specific nanoparticles: theory to practice, *Pharmacol. Rev.*, 53, 283, 2001.
5. Li, Y.X. and Kissel, T., Synthesis and properties of biodegradable ABA triblock copolymers consisting of poly(L-lactic acid) or poly(L-lactic-*co*-glycolic acid) A-blocks attached to central poly(oxyethylene) B-blocks, *J. Contr. Release*, 27, 247, 1993.

54. Giri, S., Trewyn, B.G., Stellmaker, M.P., and Lin, V.S.Y., Stimuli-responsive controlled-release delivery system based on mesoporous silica nanorods capped with magnetic nanoparticles, *Angew. Chem. Int. Ed.*, 44, 5038, 2005.

55. Steinle, E.D., Mitchell, D.T., Wirtz, M., Lee, S.B., Young, V.Y., and Martin, C.R., Ion channel mimetic micropore and nanotube membrane sensors, *Anal. Chem.*, 74, 2416, 2002.

56. Son, S.J., Reichel, J., He, B., Schuchman, M., and Lee, S.B., Magnetic nanotubes for magnetic-field-assisted bioseparation, biointeraction, and drug delivery, *J. Am. Chem. Soc.*, 127, 7316, 2005.

57. Kovtyukhova, N.I., Mallouk, T.E., and Mayer, T.S., Templated surface sol–gel synthesis of SiO_2 nanotubes and SiO_2-insulated metal, *Adv. Mater.*, 15, 780, 2003.

58. Yang, H.H., Zhang, S.Q., Chen, X.L., Zhuang, Z.X., Xu, J.G., and Wang, X.R., Magnetite-containing spherical silica nanoparticles for biocatalysis and bioseparations, *Anal. Chem.*, 76, 1316, 2004.

59. Arruebo, M., Galán, M., Navascués, N., Téllez, C., Marquina, C., Ricardo Ibarra, M., and Santamaría, J., Development of magnetic nanostructured silica-based materials as potential vectors for drug-delivery applications, *Chem. Mater.*, 18, 1911, 2006.

60. Arruebo, M., Fernández-Pacheco, R., Irusta, S., Arbiol, J., Ricardo Ibarra, M., and Santamaía, J., Sustained release of doxorubicin from zeolite–magnetite nanocomposites prepared by mechanical activation, *Nanotechnology*, 17, 4057, 2006.

61. Zhang, R.Y., Wang, X.M., Wu, C.H., Song, M., Li, J.Y., Lv, G., Zhou, J., Chen, C., Dai, Y.Y., Gao, F., Fu, D.G., Li, X.M., Guan, Z.Q., and Chen, B.A., Synergistic enhancement effect of magnetic nanoparticles on anticancer drug accumulation in cancer cells, *Nanotechnology*, 17, 3622, 2006.

62. Alexiou, C., Schmid, R.J., Jurgons, R., Kremer, M., Wanner, G., Bergemann, C., Huenges, E., Nawroth, T., Arnold, W., and Parak, F.G., Targeting cancer cells: magnetic nanoparticles as drug carriers, *Eur. Biophys. J.*, 35, 446, 2006.

63. Kuhn, S.J., Hallahan, D.E., and Giorgio, T.D., Characterization of superparamagnetic nanoparticle interactions with extracellular matrix in an *in vitro* system, *Ann. Biomed. Eng.*, 34, 51, 2006.

Part III

Nano Biomaterials and Biosensors

10 Self-Assembly of Nanostructures as Biomaterials

Hua Ai, Yujiang Fan, and Zhongwei Gu

CONTENTS

10.1 INTRODUCTION TO LAYER-BY-LAYER SELF-ASSEMBLY

10.1.1 INTRODUCTION

Nanotechnology has been one of the most important impetuses that accelerated the development of biomaterials, especially third-generation biomaterials, focusing on stimulating specific cellular responses at a molecular level [1]. Layer-by-layer (LbL) self-assembly technique is one of the nanotechnologies that has advanced in the past 10 years. LbL has demonstrated broad applications in electronics, drug delivery, implant coating, and tissue engineering. We cover a few reviews based on LbL self-assembly, including principles [2–4], self-assembled thin films [4–6], and microencapsulation [5,7–9]. The principles of LbL self-assembly will be introduced and applications in biomaterials will be discussed later in this chapter. Generally, to build biomaterials at nanoscale through LbL self-assembly, two methods can be used: assemble ultrathin films in a bottom-up way or encapsulate nanomaterials on micro/nanotemplates. To characterize the assembly process and the self-assembled structures, a few methods such as quartz crystal microbalance technique (QCM), x-ray, and neutron reflectivity measurements can be used.

LbL self-assembly is defined as building multiple layers of charged materials, including particles, polymers, and even small molecules through electrostatic interactions. The concept of the alternate LbL adsorption was first proposed for charged colloidal particles in 1966 by Iler [10]. In 1991, Decher and coworkers developed this concept and later demonstrated various assemblies, mainly using linear polyions, bipolar amphiphiles, or both [2,11–16]. LbL deposition is now recognized as an environmental friendly technology, both in fundamental and applied research [17]. The assembly process is simple and straightforward, with a wide selection of nanoblocks, including natural or synthetic polymers, proteins, lipids, and organic or inorganic nanoparticles. The applications of LbL self-assembly in biomaterials field range from ultrathin coatings in medical implants, tissue engineering, and micropatterning to drug/gene delivery and cell encapsulation.

10.1.2 METHODS FOR LbL SELF-ASSEMBLY

Figure 10.1a depicts a standard LbL self-assembly process on a solid substrate. This principle can also be applied to the encapsulation of micro/nanotemplates (biocolloids) (Figure 10.1b). First, for adsorption of a polyanion layer, a solid support (e.g., slide) with positive surface charge is incubated in a solution containing polyanions for a certain amount of time, usually 30 min. Next, solid supports are rinsed with pure water two or three times to remove excess free polyelectrolyte. Then, the slide is immersed in a solution of cationic polyelectrolytes and a layer is adsorbed. The original surface charge (positive) is restored, and the surface is ready for washing. Generally, the above-mentioned steps are repeated alternately until a film of desired thickness is obtained. One can also assemble biomacromolecules or inorganic nanoparticles onto the precursor film and form a complex structure (Figure 10.1a, last step), for example, polyion/protein multilayer films [18]. More than two components can be used in the assembly with one condition: a proper alternation of positive and negative compounds. The main idea of the method consists of resaturation of polyelectrolyte adsorption, resulting in the alternation of the terminal charge after every subsequent layer deposition. Multilayer films are typically deposited from polyelectrolyte concentrations of several milligrams per milliliter (mg/mL), much higher than the amount that is needed to cover a substrate or a previous layer. Ultrathin ordered films can be designed with "molecular architecture" plans in the range of 5 nm to a few microns, composed of molecular layers even up to a few hundred, with a precision better than 1 nm and a definite knowledge of their molecular composition. In addition, there is no size or shape limitation for substrates that are involved in thin film buildup, and this factor is very important for biocompatible coating because of the wide range of biomedical devices and implants involved. The major driving force for LbL self-assembly is the electrostatic interaction between two adjacent layers, but other interactions such as short-range hydrophobic forces [3], specific interactions between biomolecules [19,20], or hydrogen bonding could also be used [21,22].

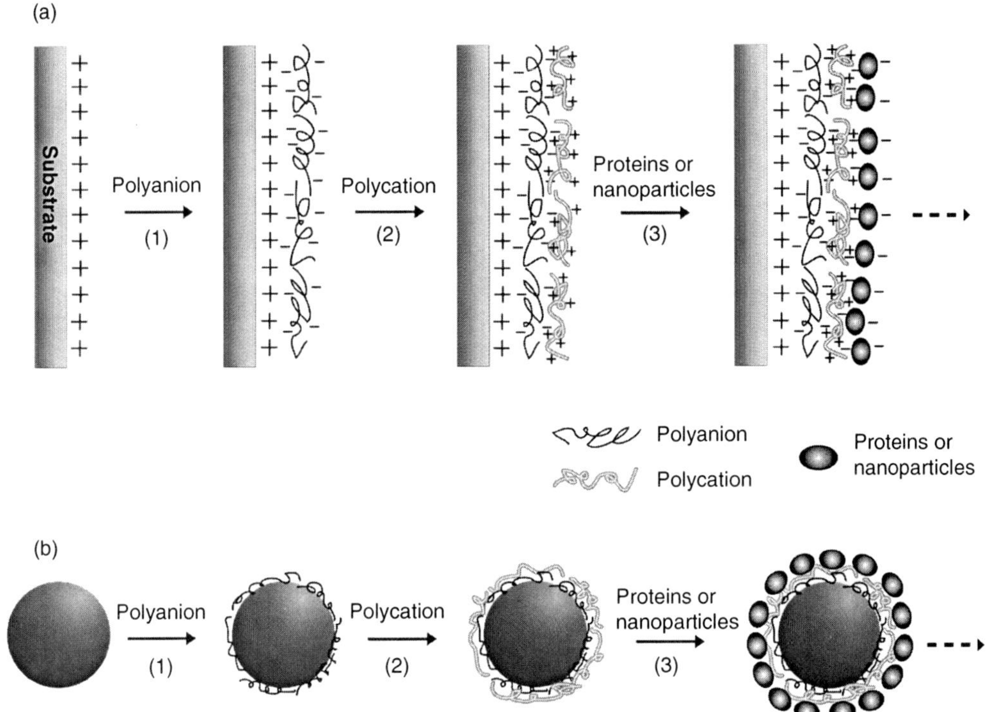

FIGURE 10.1 (a) Schematic illustration of film deposition process through LbL self-assembly on a flat substrate and (b) encapsulation of polyelectrolyte/nanoparticles multilayers on micro/nanotemplates.

To reach a surface charge reversion during linear polyion adsorption one needs a concentration higher than 10^{-5} M [23]. The dependence of polyion layer thickness on concentration is not strong; thus, in the concentration range 0.1–5 mg/mL, polystyrenesulfonate/polyallylamine (PSS/PAH) pair gave a similar bilayer thickness [24]. A large decrease of polyion concentration (using 0.01–0.1 mg/mL) slightly decreases the layer thickness of adsorbed polyion [25,26].

Microencapsulation is the continuation of LbL self-assembly from ultrathin film coating on flat substrates to micro/nano 3-D objects. All kinds of materials, charged or noncharged, including small molecule drug crystals, protein aggregates, inorganic particles, and even biological cells, can be chosen as templates for encapsulation. The coating procedure is simple and straightforward as illustrated in Figure 10.1b. The first step is coincubation of templates with excessive amount of polyelectrolytes, similar to the procedure on 2-D substrates (Step 1, Figure 10.1b). Then, a washing step is required to remove free polymers before coating the second layer. This step can easily be performed through appropriate centrifugation or filtration. By repeating the first two steps, multilayers of polyelectrolytes can be assembled on micro/nanotemplates with precise control of thickness and molecular structures. The modified surface represents new physical and chemical properties, which was designed to fit into different applications.

10.1.3 Materials for LbL Self-Assembly

Among all the charged compounds for LbL self-assembly, polyions are the most important compounds for building biomaterials; especially, while assembling protein and nanoparticle multilayers, an alternation with linear or branched polyion layer is necessary [4]. Flexible polyions can penetrate between protein globules and function as "electrostatic glue," which keeps together neighboring arrays of proteins or nanoparticles. Both synthetic and natural polymers can be chosen for LbL self-assembly. The most commonly used synthetic polymers include polycations such as linear or branched poly(ethyleneimine) (PEI), poly(dimethyldiallyl ammonium) (PDDA), and poly(allylamine) hydrochloride (PAH), and polyanions such as PSS and poly(acrylic acid) (PAA) (Figure 10.2). Most of these polymers are strongly charged and can be used to form LbL films in a wide range of pH environments. These synthetic polymers have been used as substrates for cell adhesion or for building microcapsules for protein encapsulation [27–30]. Incorporation of PEI into LbL self-assembly would be interesting since it has been widely used in gene delivery.

Natural polymers offer great advantages because of their biocompatibility and biodegradability; most of them are water soluble, which are essential for LbL self-assembly. The three major natural polymers are (1) proteins and enzymes (albumin, protamine sulfate, glucose oxidase, etc.); (2) polypeptides (polylysine, poly(α,L-glutamic acid), poly(aspartic acid)); and (3) polysaccharides (hyaluronan (HA), dextran, alginate, heparin, chondroitin, carboxymethyl cellulose, and chitosan [CH]). Modification of natural polymers gives more choices in the self-assembly of biomaterials. For example, HA can be amine-modified to have positive charges [31]. Among all natural polymers, collagen (more than 16 different types) is the most widely available polypeptide, with a unique triple-helical structure, existing in many different tissues. A single molecule of type I collagen has a molecular mass of about 285 kDa, a width of 1.5 nm, and a length of ~300 nm [32]. These molecules can self-assemble into collagen fibrils with diameters ranging from 20 to 200 nm and length of 1–20 μm under various temperatures and assembly time [33]. Collagen-based biomaterials have been widely used in studies on biomaterials and even in clinical applications. Negatively

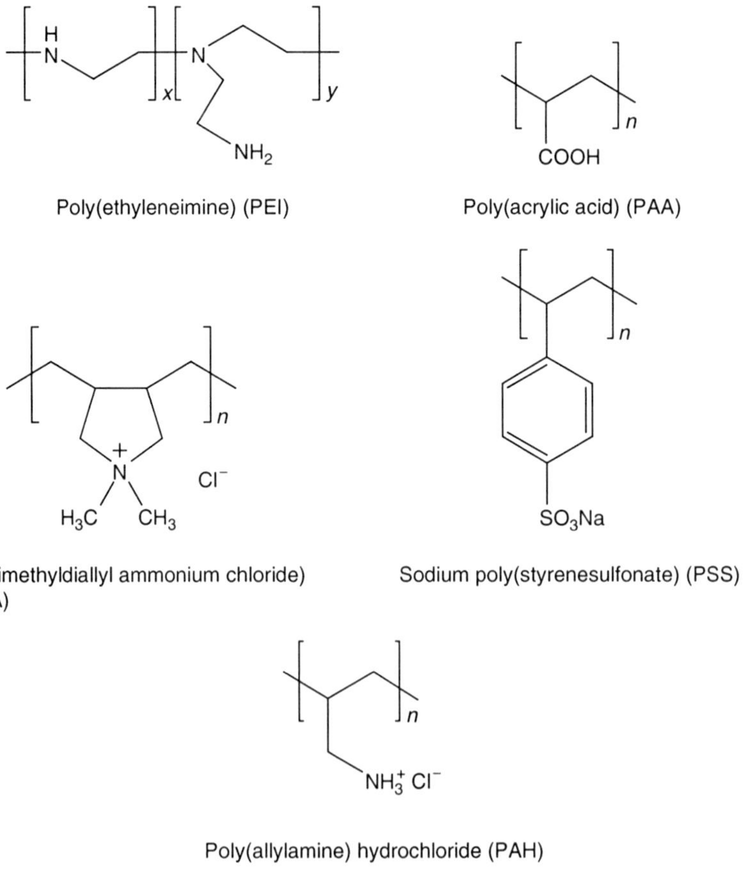

Poly(ethyleneimine) (PEI)

Poly(acrylic acid) (PAA)

Poly(dimethyldiallyl ammonium chloride)
(PDDA)

Sodium poly(styrenesulfonate) (PSS)

Poly(allylamine) hydrochloride (PAH)

FIGURE 10.2	Structural formula of commonly used synthetic polymers.

charged collagen molecules or fibrils can be used to build biocompatible films with polycations through LbL self-assembly [34]. Adjusting assembly pH conditions such as at pH 4, collagen type IV was positively charged and could be alternatively assembled with PAA to form multiple layers for cell attachment [35]. Polysaccharides are abundant in nature and possess excellent biocompatibility and biodegradability. A few commonly used polysaccharides are dextran, CH, alginic acid, hyaluronic acid, and heparin (Figure 10.3). Dextran, a polysaccharide already used as a blood replacement through i.v. injection, has unique properties such as long circulation time due to the least uptake by the reticulo-endothelial system (RES). It may be an appropriate candidate for building LbL self-assembled drug carriers. Also, a wide choice of molecular weight of dextran, from a few thousand to a few million daltons, provides more options for different applications. CH, a positively charged polysaccharide, is widely used for gene delivery and would be useful to build CH/protein or CH/DNA multilayered structures.

Other materials such as lipids and organic and inorganic nanoparticles (magnetite, quantum dot, gold, etc.) can also be incorporated into self-assembled structures. The polyion/nanoparticle hybrid structures are unique and may have physical properties similar to that of natural materials.

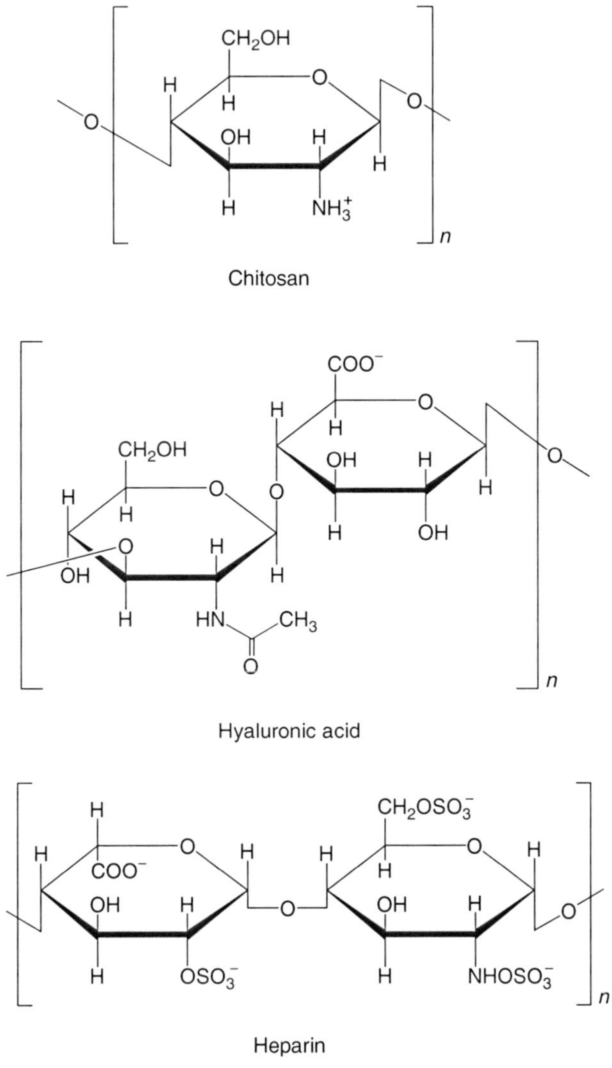

FIGURE 10.3 Structural formula of three polysaccharides: chitosan, hyaluronic acid, and heparin.

For example, alternating PDDA with inorganic montmorillonite clay platelets made it possible to build natural biocomposites such as artificial analogs of nacre [36]. Another type of clay–50 nm diameter halloysite nanotubes—enabled assembly of tubule composites perspective for tissue engineering and as a depot system [37,38].

10.1.4 Characterization of LbL Self-Assembly

To monitor and to study the overall structures in LbL self-assembled biomaterials, the following methods are available: QCM, Fourier transform infrared (FTIR), x-ray and neutron reflectivity, scanning electron microscopy (SEM), transmission electron microscopy (TEM), atomic force microscopy (AFM), confocal laser scanning microscopy (CLSM), contact angle measurement, dynamic light scattering, surface (zeta) potential, ellipsometry, light guiding attenuation, and UV-vis absorbency. Recently, flow cytometry was used to monitor polyelectrolyte multilayer film formation on particles [39].

QCM is a simple, cost-effective, high-resolution mass sensing technique based on the piezoelectric effect [40]. The QCM method is extremely suitable for a time-dependent control of adsorption and monitoring of the assembly *in situ*. The multilayer assemblies can be characterized by the QCM technique in two ways: (1) after drying a sample in nitrogen stream, one can measure the resonance frequency shift and calculate a total amount of adsorbed mass by Sauerbrey equation or (2) by continuously monitoring of resonator frequency during the adsorption process onto one side of the resonator, which is in permanent contact with polyion solutions. For the situation of pure elastic mass added to the surface, the well-known linear Sauerbrey equation (Equation 10.1) was first observed [41] and used to precisely quantify, with ng sensitivity, the quantity of elastic mass added to the surface where Δf is the measured resonant frequency decrease (Hz), f is the intrinsic crystal frequency, Δm is the elastic mass change (g), A is the electrode area, ρ_q is the density of quartz (2.65 g/cm^3), and μ is the shear modulus (2.95 × 10^{11} dyn/cm^2).

$$\Delta f = \frac{-2\Delta m \cdot f^2}{A \cdot \sqrt{\mu \cdot \rho_q}} = -C_f \cdot \Delta m \tag{10.1}$$

$$d(A) \approx -0.16\Delta f \ (\text{Hz}) \tag{10.2}$$

$$d(A) \approx -1.5\Delta f \ (\text{Hz}) \tag{10.3}$$

With the help of dynamic QCM study, it was suggested that polyion adsorption occurs in two stages: quick anchoring to a surface and slow relaxation. The ultrasensitivity of QCM measurement is obvious: for a 9 MHz crystal electrode (USI-System Inc., Japan), 10 Hz frequency change equals 8.7 ng mass adsorption, which for organic films corresponds to ca 0.2 nm [18]. The thin film thickness can be estimated by taking into account the film density (Equation 10.2) [18]. The density was assumed to be 1.2 ± 0.1 g/cm^3 for polyelectrolyte films and 1.2 ± 0.1 g/cm^3 for proteins, while for a 5 MHz quartz crystal electrode (QCM100, Stanford Research System, Inc., Sunnyvale, CA), the relationship between film thickness and frequency shift is given in Equation 10.3 [42].

The internal structure of LbL polyelectrolyte multilayers can be investigated by measuring the x-ray and neutron reflectivity from such a film. X-ray reflectivity measurements of LbL-adsorbed polyelectrolyte films show patterns with profound intensity oscillations (so-called Kiessig fringes, where the steepest gradients in electron density occur, due to interference of x-ray beams reflected from interfaces solid support/film and air/film) [13,43]. From the periodicity of these oscillations, one can calculate the film thickness with the help of Bragg-like equation and taking into account refraction phenomena that are essential at small angles [13,24]. For a poly(vynilsulfate)/poly(allylamine) (PVS/PAH) assembly, x-ray analysis of the film was dried at 20, 26, 32, 39, and 41 cycles of the assembly and showed a linear increase of the film thickness with the number of adsorption cycles [13]. When studying a multilayered PAH/PSS ultrathin film, x-ray reflectivity was sensitive to only the overall structure of the thin polymer film with a large number of Kiessig fringes observed [43]. In contrast to x-rays, neutrons are sensitive to the internal structure of the electrolyte film. For the same film, the neutron reflectivity showed indications of Kiessig fringes and two Bragg reflections. The Bragg reflections resulted from the internal structure of the polymer film, which comprises a superlattice with deuterated PSS as every sixth layer. With the help of x-ray and neutron reflectivity, one could perform systematic investigations to control the microstructure polyelectrolyte films and adjust their structures to certain macroscopic properties. Fourier transform infrared attenuated total internal reflection (FTIR-ATR) technique has been widely used for studying film structural information and the kinetics of film formation [44]. FTIR-ATR has been successfully used in the characterization of LbL self-assembled films. The principle behind FTIR-ATR is using evanescent wave based on total reflection principle. Based on some experimentally collectable data such as the depth of penetration, absorbance, and the effective thickness, the surface adsorption of material of interest can be calculated. For more information on FTIR-ATR, especially application of protein adsorption, please refer to an excellent reference [45]. The growth kinetics of polyelectrolyte multilayers could be followed via this technique [22,46]. Generally, the films were deposited on the surface of an internal reflective element (IRE, such as germanium, ZnSe, Si crystals), and D_2O was used as a solvent to remove the noise of water band. It is preferred that an IRE substrate be constantly thermostated. One application of this technique is to study interactions of polyelectrolytes in assembled films by calculating the adsorbed amount of polymer and the degree of ionization in the film [47]. In addition, the orientation and the conformation of polyions in films can be probed by using polarized light [48]. One can also use this technique to explore the secondary structure information of proteins in multilayers by analyzing the shape and the position of band in Amide I region [49]. FTIR-ATR not only provides quantitative information of surface adsorption on an LbL self-assembled film, but also of interaction between adjacent layers in a film.

To obtain direct visualization of LbL polyelectrolyte film, SEM, TEM, AFM, and CLSM are the four necessary imaging tools. TEM was used to view detailed structures, especially for polyion/nanoparticle assembled films or capsules [36,50]. Similarly, SEM was also a powerful tool to visualize LbL films and shells in the range of tens of nanometers to hundreds of microns, but in a 3-D fashion [18,27,50,51]. AFM has advantages not only in morphology characterization, but also in studying the molecular structure and conformation of polymers. In a tapping mode, AFM is particularly reliable for imaging of flexible long-chain polyelectrolytes without distortion of their native structures [52,53]. In addition, mechanical properties of polyelectrolyte multilayer thin films can be studied. For example, the elasticity of polyelectrolyte multilayer films as a function of polymer charge density during assembly can be successfully probed with force–distance measurements using AFM [54]. CLSM can be used to monitor the buildup process by adding fluorescently labeled polyelectrolytes at different steps of the film construction. Based on this, Picart et al. [55] approved the existence of such a poly-L-lysine diffusion process into the interior of the film. The most important information CLSM can collect is the dynamic behavior of LbL polyion shells in aqueous phase, including shell loading and release of materials [56]. Usually, loading materials (small molecule drug or biomacromolecules) are fluorescently labeled; the processes of encapsulation and release are directly monitored and tuned with different environmental conditions (e.g., pH, ionic strength). It should be noticed that shells smaller than 300 nm may be difficult to study because of the optical limitation.

Other techniques such as contact angle and surface charge measurement are simple and efficient ways of monitoring LbL self-assembly of polyelectrolytes on flat substrates or micro/ nanoparticles. The stepwise switch of hydrophilicity and hydrophobicity of alternate polyelectrolytes can be detected by contact angle measurements through which both surface modification and film growth can be easily monitored [5]. Particle surface zeta-potential measurement is necessary to understand the building of multilayers on micro/nanotemplates, for example, a strongly positively charged PDDA layer has about +40 mV zeta-potential reading, while a polyanion PSS layer is about −37 mV [51].

10.2 MULTILAYERED BIOFILMS THROUGH LbL SELF-ASSEMBLY

10.2.1 INTRODUCTION

As biomaterials, ultrathin films have unique advantages such as precise control over the film's overall "molecular architecture," thickness, surface charge, biocompatibility, and biodegradability. Formulation of appropriate polyion/polyion and polyion/inorganic particles may achieve superior physical and chemical properties that natural materials do not have. The principle of ultrathin films on a flat substrate through LbL self-assembly has been illustrated in Figure 10.1a. A standard approach for film preparation involves the following: (1) taking aqueous solutions of polycation and polyanion at concentration of 0.01 m/L (practically it is 1–3 mg/mL) and adjusting pH in such a way that both polyions are ionized; (2) preparing a substrate of interest carrying a surface charge; (3) carrying out alternate immersion of the substrate in polyion solutions for 30 min with 1 min intermediate water washing. To wash a sample, use a solution of pH that keeps polyions ionized; and (4) drying the sample in a nitrogen stream when it is necessary for ellipsometry, x-ray, UV, QCM, or other analytical methods. It should be mentioned that drying may disturb the assembly process and that it is not necessary for the procedure.

For the applications of LbL self-assembled thin films as biomaterials, we have special interest in their biocompatibility and biodegradability. Understanding these properties would be beneficial to us not only for designing better films for coating medical implants and in tissue engineering, but also useful for constructing polyelectrolyte shells in microencapsulation.

The key to achieve a satisfied biocompatible interface is largely dependent on which material to be used for self-assembly. There are a few natural polymers, including collagen, gelatin, heparin, and CH that are widely used in LbL self-assembly with outstanding biocompatibility [27,34,35,57,58]. The outermost layer largely decides the biocompatibility of a film. For example, in silicone rubber modification, a couple of nonbiocompatible but strongly charged polyelectrolyte layers were first used to form a precursor film, then biocompatible materials such as gelatin or polylysine were further established [27,35,59]. Cell adhesion on those composite nanofilms was successful and no obvious cytotoxicity was observed. Judging the biocompatibility of a multilayered film depends on specific applications, which involve different physiological environments, duration of tissue-material contact, etc. Usually, *in vitro* environment is much simpler and the time frame of application is relatively short. On the contrary, the *in vivo* system is more complicated and may involve systemic immune responses. Some common *in vivo* tests, including hemocompatibility, carcinogenicity, and immune response can be employed to evaluate an LbL composite film. For detailed information on the biocompatibility of biomaterials, please refer to an excellent review by Anderson [60].

10.2.2 MULTILAYERED POLYELECTROLYTE FILMS FOR CELL ADHESION

Cell adhesion, migration, and other behaviors on a biointerface are crucial for both biological studies and biomaterials development. Such a biointerface is usually a thin film deposited on certain substrates. Generally, in LbL assembly of biocompatible coating for cell adhesion, there are two approaches which have to complement one another. In the first method, synthetic polyelectrolytes such as PSS, PAA, and PAH were assembled with such architecture that they gained biocompatible properties [61]. In the second approach, originally biocompatible materials such as polysaccharides, polypeptides, and proteins were used to provide biocompatible patterns and PDDA outermost was used to prevent cell adhesion [27,62]. Table 10.1 summarizes some LbL films that were involved in cell adhesion studies; all the films listed here are well-attached by different cells [27,35,59,63–69]. Self-assembly conditions such as pH value, choice of polyelectrolytes, and crosslinking are important

TABLE 10.1
Summary of Cell Adhesion on Different Polyion Films

Outermost Layer	Alternating Component	Surface Charge at Neutral pH	Cell Types	Reference
PSS	PDDA	Negative	Hepatocyte, fibroblast	65
	PAH	Negative	Smooth muscle cells	67
PAH	PSS	Positive	HUVEC	63
Gelatin	PDL	Negative	Endothelial cells	27
PDL	Fibronectin, laminin	Positive	Neuron	59
	PGA	Positive	HUVEC	63
	Hyaluronic acid	Positive	Fibroblast	64
Collagen	PAA	Negative	Muscle myoblast cells	35
	Hyaluronic acid	Negative	Chondrosarcoma cells	68
Hyaluronic acid	PLL	Negative	Chondrosarcoma cells	66
CH	PSS	Positive	HUVEC	69

factors that control the cell adhesion behavior. Even for the same film, different cells respond differently. For example, from Table 10.1, one can find that hepatocytes, fibroblasts, and smooth muscle cells (SMCs) adhered well on synthetic polyelectrolyte multilayered films with an outermost layer PSS, while HUVEC cells adhered well on a PAH layer. In contrast, poor endothelial cell adhesion was found on a $(PSS/PEI)_8/PSS$ film with the outermost layer PSS [27].

Polydimethylsiloxane (PDMS) (also called silicone rubber) is an interesting substrate for the deposition of LbL thin films and studying cell behavior on such a surface. First, it is used extensively to study cell–substrate interactions because its mechanical properties are easily tuned in physiologically relevant ranges. Second, it can be used to make different medical devices (e.g., intraocular lens, contact lens, catheters, etc.) because of its good biocompatibility and inertness. But the strong hydrophobicity of silicone rubber prevents cell adsorption *in vitro*, and it nonspecifically absorbs proteins *in vivo* with shortened lifetime. How to coat a thin and uniform hydrophilic film on silicone is an important, but not an easy step. Several surface modification methods have already been reported, including chemical immobilization [70], plasma treatment [71,72], and gelatin–glutaraldehyde cross-linking [73]. Plasma treatment could deposit a high-quality thin film, but application was limited to surface areas that can be easily accessed. Tube-shaped vascular grafts are not suitable for plasma deposition. In addition, the adsorption of matrix proteins to silicone rubber substrates through passive adsorption is relatively inefficient [74]. In an earlier attempt, we discovered that polyelectrolyte films can be used to modify silicone rubber surface hydrophobic property and the coating is stable for endothelial cell adhesion and growth [27]. LbL self-assembly of polyelectrolyte was simple and efficient in surface modification of silicone rubber. Without the help of any surface pretreatment, polyelectrolytes can be directly applied onto such a surface through alternate coating of oppositely charged polymers. Usually, highly charged polyelectrolytes PSS and PEI were used as precursor layers in film assembly; polypeptides were further coated to establish biocompatible coatings for cell adhesion. Based on QCM quantification, a PEI/PSS bilayer was about 2–3 nm, and a PDL/gelatin bilayer has a thickness of 5 nm [27]. The thickness of the gelatin/PDL multilayers was linear according to the number of layers. A film composed of $(PEI/PSS)_4/(PDL/gelatin)_{12}$ coated on a QCM electrode was directly observed under SEM without metal coating (Figure 10.4a). The calculated total film thickness was 70 nm, which closely matched with the cross-section thickness of the film in this SEM image. When coating polyelectrolytes on silicone rubber, we found that using PSS as the first layer was more efficient than a PEI layer. The reason is not clear, but we suspect hydrophobic force between silicone rubber and PSS plays a major role here because silicone rubber is not charged.

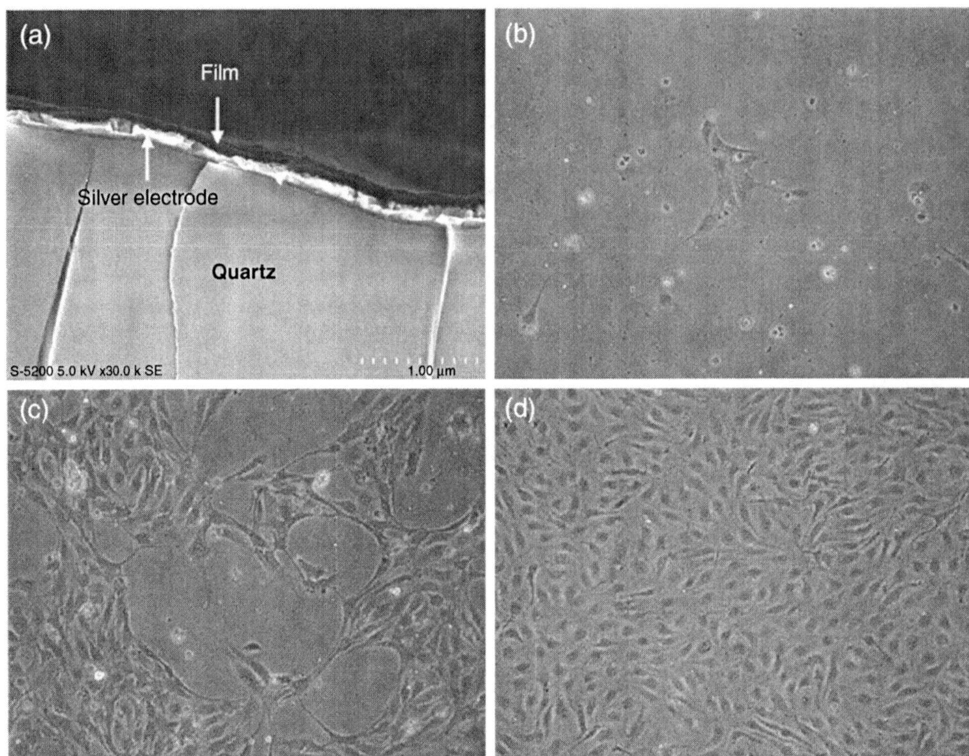

FIGURE 10.4　(a) A SEM photo of [(PEI/PSS)$_4$ + (PDL/gelatin)$_{12}$] film coated on a silver-electrode resonator (cross-section view); (b) endothelial cell adhesion on a (PSS/PEI)$_8$ film at day 3 (100×); (c) endothelial cell adhesion on a [(PSS/PEI)$_8$ + PSS] film at day 3 (100×); and (d) endothelial cell adhesion on a [(PSS/PEI)$_4$ + (gelatin/PDL)$_4$ + gelatin] film at day 3 (100×). (Reproduced from Ai, H., Lvov, Y.M., Mills, D.K., Jennings, M., Alexander, J.S., and Jones, S.A., *Cell Biochem. Biophys.*, 38, 103–114, 2003. With permission.)

This suggestion is consistent with studies of LbL assembly as a method for surface modification of neutral polymer polyethylene terephthalate [75,76].

Few endothelial cells can adhere on silicone rubber substrate. After polyelectrolyte multilayer film deposition, some cells can attach to films with PSS or PEI outermost layers but very few can remain on the surface after 3 days (Figures 10.4b and 10.4c). In comparison, a gelatin outermost layer is friendly for endothelial cell adhesion and growth, and no obvious cytotoxicity was observed (Figure 10.4d). Cell adhesion density on gelatin increased to 11.7 × 10^4 cm^{-2} after 7 days of seeding, which was much higher than PEI (0.4 × 10^4 cm^{-2}) and PSS (2.3 × 10^4 cm^{-2}) outermost layers. In another study, a similar film structure with composition of (PSS/PEI)$_3$/(fibronectin/PDL)$_4$ or (PSS/PEI)$_3$/(laminin/PDL)$_4$ was highly favorable for neuron cell adhesion; both lactate dehydrogenase (LDH) assay and fluorescence cellular metabolism observations demonstrated that the film was biocompatible with those cells [59]. LbL self-assembly and other molecular deposition and lithographic patterning techniques, with nanometer resolution for arranging neuronal-specific molecules, may be useful tools for studying neural cellular communication and signaling [77].

10.2.3　Ultrathin Coatings on Medical Implants

The surface topography and chemistry of a biomaterial are important parameters that influence protein adsorption, cell interaction, and the host response [78]. However, most medical implants lack a reasonable biointerface between the implant and the surrounding tissues. Local nonspecific protein adsorption, inflammation, and infection can interfere with the long-term use of implants. The rationale for surface modification of biomaterials is straightforward: retain the key physical properties while modifying only the outermost surface to influence biointeraction [79]. The ultimate goal of building such an interface is to improve the biocompatibility, reduce tissue–implant reaction, and prolong the lifetime of a device.

As a general rule, nonspecific adsorption of proteins should be minimized and beneficial molecules should become selectively adsorbed onto biomaterials as a result of modifications performed before their implantation [80]. A hydrophilic coating with lubricious property on implants is mostly preferred for prolonging the lifetime of the product. Application of LbL self-assembly to deposit hydrophilic thin films on implants has the following advantages: (1) broad selection of materials; (2) precise control over coating thickness within nanometer range with designed film structure; and (3) no necessity of surface pretreatment in some cases. Ideally, alternation of only the outermost molecular layer (3–10 Å) should be sufficient, but thicker films are required to ensure a full coverage on medical implant [79]. During LbL self-assembly, ordered multilayer films can be built from nanometer to micron range with definite knowledge of their molecular composition. A nonlinear film growth often occurs at the beginning of the alternating assembly process, and the first two to three layers have smaller amounts of adsorbed polyions [24,43]. The film mass of subsequent layers increases linearly with the number of adsorption cycles. The desired film thickness depends on the coating material, implant surface roughness, and biological environment of an implant. Appropriate film thickness is important to provide both biointerface function and maintain the surface morphology and the mechanical property of the implant.

LbL self-assembly has been applied to modify medical devices, and implants include contact lens [81] and vascular stents [57,58]. Here, we are focusing on the thin film coatings on stents. Stent implantation is widely used for the treatment of occlusive blood vessel diseases with the reduction of restenosis. However, stent implantation is also associated with excessive proliferation of vascular SMCs, extracellular matrix synthesis, and chronic inflammatory reaction, which are believed to be initiated by deep vascular injury and further enhanced by the presence of a foreign metallic device [82]. Modified surface should have improved biocompatibility with less thrombogenic and inflammatory reactions. Polysaccharide-based nanocoating of either (PEI/heparin)$_n$ or (CH/HA)$_n$ on endovascular devices was recently developed through LbL self-assembly [57,58]. Both hyaluronic acid (HA) and heparin are glycosaminoglycans. HA is a naturally occurring linear, high-molecular weight anionic polymer ($pK_a = 2.9$) consisting of alternating N-acetyl-β-D-glucosamine and β-D-glucuronic acid residues linked $(1 \rightarrow 3)$ and $(1 \rightarrow 4)$, respectively. Its high-molecular mass and numerous mutually repelling anionic groups make hyaluronate a rigid and highly hydrated molecule, which, in solution, occupies a volume ~1000 times than in its dry state [83]. The inhibitive effects of HA with respect to hyperplasia observed after either systemic or local delivery suggest that the antiproliferative effects of HA may be associated with its antiinflammatory properties [84]. Heparin is a variably sulfated glycosaminoglycan that consists predominantly of alternating $\alpha(1 \rightarrow 4)$-linked residues of D-iduronate-2-sulfate and N-sulfo-D-glucosamine-6-sulfate. It has an average of 2.5 sulfate residues per disaccharide unit, which makes it the most negatively charged polyelectrolyte in mammalian tissues and widely known as an anticoagulant agent [83].

PEI/heparin pairs were used in precursor establishment during LbL self-assembly of polyelectrolytes on stent materials NiTi and 316L stainless steel [57]. It has been found that in PEI/heparin-paired multilayers, the contact angle alternatively shifted from ~59° for a PEI layer to ~25° for a heparin layer. It is a clear indication of film buildup through LbL self-assembly. After immersing the PEI/heparin multilayered film in Tris–HCl buffer (pH 7.35) for 3 weeks, the coating was still stable as verified from electrochemical impedance measurements and contact angle studies. In another study, the contact angle of a HA layer decreased from 40° to 30° when the number of HA layers increased from one to four [58]. Further increase of HA layer numbers did not change the contact angle value. It was suggested that in this case, at least four bilayers were necessary to mask the substrate with respect to the properties of the multilayer–water interface. Linear film growth was observed for both PEI/heparin and CH/hyaluronic acid (CH/HA) multilayer assembly. The in vitro hemocompatibility of CH/HA-coated NiTi surfaces and PEI/heparin-modified 316L stainless steel surfaces were tested through a standard platelet adhesion method [57,58]. Both coatings have shown significant reduction in platelet adhesion compared with unmodified surfaces, indicating better hemocompatibility and a lesser chance of thrombus formation on the implants. Through radiolabeling, quantitative platelet adhesion was measured as $619.7 \pm 258.0 \times 103$ platelets/cm^2 on HA(CH/HA)$_4$-coated metallic versus $1005.9 \pm 97.7 \times 103$ platelets/cm^2 for bare NiTi ($p < 0.05$) [58]. Platelet adhesion is known to be initiated by adsorption of plasma proteins such as fibrinogen. The antifouling properties of HA was believed to be attributable to the hydration layer surrounding HA molecules on the surface [85].

Further application of LbL self-assembly thin film deposition can be extended to tissue repair with advantages including broad selection of materials, precise control over structures at a molecular level, and friendly environment during process. For example, the Tabrizian group recently demonstrated that it was possible to build a nanoscale self-assembled multilayer on damaged arteries through alternating depositions of two polysaccharides, HA and CH [86]. Insulation of the vascular wall by using polyelectrolyte coatings provides a shield against blood components, especially platelets, resulting in a much lower chance of thrombus formation.

10.2.4 Drug Incorporation in Polyelectrolyte Films

Multilayered polyelectrolyte film may provide a passive protection at a certain degree on implant surfaces. Incorporation of active agents in the film with a controlled release fashion will extend the function of biointerface. So far, two approaches have been explored: (1) the multilayer coatings were used as a reservoir for drug storage and delivery [58] and (2) prodrug polyion–drug (HA–paclitaxel) conjugation was assembled into polyelectrolyte films [87].

Sodium nitroprusside (SNP), an anionic nitrous oxide donor used clinically to reduce blood pressure and treat restenosis, has been incorporated into CH/HA polyelectrolyte multilayers following a method used to introduce ionic dyes and proteins within polyelectrolyte multilayers [88]. Briefly, it was doped within the coating during the CH deposition step, as the cationic polysaccharide is able to form a complex with SNP by electrostatic interactions [58]. LbL film growth was not interrupted after introduction of SNP. During *in vitro* hemocompatibility test, incorporation of SNP within the multilayered coating further decreased platelet adhesion by 40% compared with CH/HA-paired multilayers.

The second strategy, "prodrug approach" was used to introduce paclitaxel (PTX) into polyelectrolyte multilayers [87]. Instead of using passive adsorption during LbL self-assembly, the drug PTX was first linked to a HA via a hydrolyzable bond (succinate ester linkage) and later assembled into the film. This methodology has advantages in solubilization of hydrophobic drugs and tunability of the drug pharmacokinetics [89]. A 2′-hemisuccinate derivative of PTX was prepared first, as previously reported [90], activated to the corresponding *N*-hydroxysuccinimide (NHS) ester, and linked to an amine-modified HA. The level of PTX incorporation onto HA was intentionally kept low to preserve the water solubility of the prodrug. Self-assembly of CH and HA-Pac was successful, as higher QCM frequency shifts for CH/HA–Paclitaxel multilayers were noticed than CH/HA coating. It was suggested that the presence of the hydrophobic PTX moieties did not prohibit the construction of multilayers, although the growth mechanism may be affected [87]. The total amount of PTX released was 1.8 µg/cm^2 from HA-Pac(CH/HA-Pac)$_9$ multilayers with 50% and 90% drug release corresponding to 3 and 10 h, respectively. For potential *in vivo* applications, a longer drug release time is preferred (e.g., a few days to a few months).

10.2.5 Micropatterning of Self-Assembled Structures

Micropatterning of biomolecules on a substrate has important applications, including immunoassays, genetic disease screening, chemical and biomedical sensors, drug screening, and tissue engineering. Whitesides et al. were among the first to pattern self-assembled monolayers (SAMs) on gold surfaces [91,92]. In such a process, soft lithography was applied to create patterned surfaces using a combination of SAMs and microcontact printing (μCP). The two key features of soft lithography are the use of elastomeric (i.e., mechanically soft) materials to fabricate the pattern transfer elements by molding and the development of techniques that pattern complex biochemicals [93]. Usually, PDMS was chosen as the stamp material because of its appropriate mechanical properties, transparency, nontoxicity, and hydrophobicity. Efforts were devoted by other groups to increase the accuracy of patterning, easy process, and high resolution in patterns [27,64,94–100]. The patterned materials on a flat substrate usually represent different physical and chemical properties compared with an uncovered space. So far, different materials, including polymers, DNA, nanoparticles, receptors, and extracellular matrix proteins have been patterned.

The combination of SAMs and μCP was able to create patterns consisting of regions that encouraged protein adsorption or cell adhesion, alternated with regions that discouraged such an interaction [92]. However, the process required not only the use of metal coatings, but also alkanethiols or silanes as the ink. In addition, only small areas of micropatterns can be generated through stamping. So, how to create micropatterns on a larger scale is of great interest. Introduction of LbL self-assembly in this field has led to promising progress, especially in the production of large-scale micropatterns on conventional silicon wafers [95,101]. Applying silicon-based lithographical technology has one obvious advantage in that industrial-scale process may be feasible. Three major steps are involved in such a combined process: (1) a photoresist is patterned through a mask by the standard UV-irradiation procedure; (2) the substrate is then entirely covered with polyelectrolyte multilayers and nanoparticles through standard LbL self-assembly process; and (3) micropatterns are created by lifting off polyelectrolyte/nanoparticle film above the photoresist in organic solvent acetone. This method can be compared to the micropatterning of a thiol compound on gold supports and further LbL assembly of multilayers [94]. Both methods gave patterns of approximately the same quality, with clear support surfaces between the pattern features, minimal feature sizes of approximately 1–2 μm, and edge roughness of approx 0.1–0.2 μm. However, the lithographic approach is compatible with existing silicon micromanufacturing technology. For industrial applications, this provides an opportunity to use conventional lithographic technology to produce 4-in. diameter silicon wafers completely covered with LbL self-assembled polyelectrolyte/nanoparticle patterns.

In another attempt, micro/nanostructures were directly patterned on silicone rubber through the μCP method [27]. A PDMS stamp with microchannel structures was first coated with polyelectrolyte/ microparticle multilayers through LbL self-assembly. Pretreatment of PDMS stamp with oxygen plasma or other methods can create a hydrophilic surface for polyelectrolyte layers deposition, but may not be necessary. Next, assembled polyelectrolyte/microparticle multilayers were transferred onto an unmodified silicone rubber surface by contact printing and resulted in well-defined micropatterns. On SEM examination, the resolution, stability, and accuracy of micro/nanosphere patterns correspond to the standard of the μCP technique. Polylysine/gelatin bilayers were further deposited on established micropatterns, and selective adhesion of endothelial cells was observed. The unpatterned area was bare silicone rubber, which had a high-hydrophobicity, representing an unfavorable surface for cell attachment. The mechanism of pattern transfer is not clear, but the most probable explanation is that binding between the hydrophobic surface of silanized glass and proteins is stronger than the adhesion force between the proteins and the silicone rubber surface [102].

In LbL self-assembly-assisted micropatterning for cell adhesion, it is essential to establish a prepattern as the first step. The patterned materials should be hydrophilic and charged for further introduction of biocompatible polyelectrolytes, which are favorable for cell adhesion. The distance between patterned areas can be controlled from tens of micrometers to hundreds of microns depending on a specific application. The unpatterned areas may be modified to seed different cell types, and this was demonstrated in a recent study by the Langer group [64]. In the process, HA patterns were first created on glass substrate with the help of a PDMS mold. Then, addition of fibronectin led to selective deposition on the non-HA areas. Cell type A (fibroblast NIH-3T3) only adhered onto fibronectin-covered area and was rejected by HA-covered patterns. Further coating of positively charged polylysine was adsorbed onto HA patterns, which led to cell type B adhesion onto space not covered by cell type A. Coculture of two different cell lines may provide a novel method for studying cell–cell interactions and tissue engineering.

10.3 POLYELECTROLYTE ENCAPSULATION FOR DRUG/GENE DELIVERY

10.3.1 Introduction

Advanced drug delivery systems are preferred for less administration frequency, fewer side effects, higher drug concentrations at pathological sites, and longer drug bioavailability [103]. A general method to achieve better delivery is through encapsulation of drug inside carriers that are made of biocompatible and biodegradable materials. Polymer microspheres, liposomes, polymer micelles, polymer–drug conjugate, and polymer implants are commonly used drug delivery systems, either under clinical trials or in the market. They have shown promising results in treating cancers and immunological and other diseases that traditional formulations usually fail to match. Still, much improvement is required in drug carrier design and formulation development. A major disadvantage is that chlorinated organic solvents are usually involved in fabrication, and this may lead to organic residues in the system and damage encapsulated materials such as proteins. In addition, incomplete and poorly controlled release is another major limiting factor that affects therapeutic efficacy.

LbL self-assembled polyelectrolyte shells, recognized as one of the nanotechnologies that advanced the field of drug delivery [104], may serve as one of the alternatives to solve the above-mentioned problems. Polyelectrolyte shells present unique advantages such as (1) easy fabrication process; (2) no necessity of chlorinated organic solvent; (3) fine control of permeability through membrane thickness and shell wall pore size. The thickness of the capsule wall can be precisely tuned in the range of a few nanometers by choosing coating materials and number of layers. The pore size on shell wall membrane can be controlled through different polyelectrolyte pairs and assembly conditions; (4) broad selection of shell materials. Not only charged polymers, but also lipids, proteins, and magnetic nanoparticles can be used during shell assembly; (5) shells can be switched between "open" and "closed" states for triggered release. The loading and the release of materials could be controlled by tuning environmental conditions such as pH or magnetic field.

There are two major methods for the encapsulation of therapeutic agents inside polyelectrolyte shells: (1) direct coating of oppositely charged polyelectrolytes onto drug micro/nanoparticles and (2) loading of drug molecules into hollow polyelectrolyte capsules.

Lyophilization is often used to stabilize various pharmaceutical products, including liposomes, virus vaccines, protein, and peptide formulations. Lyophilization of polyelectrolyte-encapsulated drugs are important [105–107]: first, to assure an adequate shelf-life as the majority of physico-chemical reactions, leading to product instability acceleration when stored in aqueous media, and second, to achieve sterility of the dosage form by a suitable terminal sterilization technique (e.g., Gamma radiation). In one recent study, no difference in morphology of polyelectrolyte capsule was observed by SEM examination for the samples resuspended after lyophilization treatment [108]. This satisfies that freeze-dried samples should be restored to their original properties, thus providing opportunities to develop novel pharmaceutical formulations based on LbL self-assembly technique.

10.3.2 Loading Biomacromolecules into Hollow Polyelectrolyte Shells

Currently, there are about 500 biopharmaceuticals that are either approved or in advanced clinical trials [109]. Protein drugs are a major branch and can be divided into monoclonal antibodies, cytokines, hormones, growth factors, and enzymes [110]. More choices are available nowadays than ever because of the fast advance in biotechnology. In comparison, the formulation technology is developing in a relatively slow pace, and the gap between high-therapeutic efficiency demands is getting wider. How to efficiently deliver these protein agents has a direct impact on the potential of protein therapy. Challenges in protein delivery have long been recognized because of the marginal stability of proteins. Unlike low-molecular weight drugs, they possess secondary, tertiary, and, in some cases, quaternary structures with labile bonds and side chains with chemically reactive groups [111]. These structures can be easily modified and even destructed. How to store and deliver these biomacromolecules to target tissues without loss of their functions is a key question that needs to be answered. In addition, we have to consider unfavorable factors existing in conventional administration routes, including subcutaneous, intramuscular, intravenous, inhalation, and oral.

Based on this microencapsulation and further removal of templates (Figure 10.5), a unique micro/nanocarrier system "hollow shells" was first developed in 1998 [50,112,113]. After multilayered polyelectrolytes are adsorbed on templates, the core can be removed mainly by short-time exposure to acids. The capsules are monodisperse in size and the capsule wall serves as a permeable barrier. Ligands, enzymes, and inorganic nanoparticles can be further assembled on shell surface for targeting, bioreaction, and other applications. Polyelectrolyte shells are potential candidates for drug and DNA delivery and may be applied for biosensing when loaded with molecular probes. The interior environment of a polyelectrolyte shell is aqueous, similar to that of liposome and polymer vesicles. Obviously, hydrophilic materials are favorable candidates for loading. In comparison, the hydrophobic core of a polymer micelle is good for encapsulation of hydrophobic drugs or diagnostic agents [114,115]. The advantages of hollow polyelectrolyte shells are as follows: (1) a capsule diameter can be varied from tens of nanometers to tens of microns based on the choice of template; (2) a wide range of sacrificial templates including weakly cross-linked melamine–formaldehyde (MF) particles [50], organic [116] and inorganic crystals [117], metal nanoparticles [17], and biological templates [118] are available; (3) shell materials are not only limited to polymers; other charged materials such as inorganic nanoparticles, lipids, and proteins can also be used; (4) the shell interior environment such as pH value can be adjusted to be different from exterior conditions; (5) the shell wall permeability can be controlled by shell materials and shell thickness; and (6) engineered shells can be responsive to external signals such as low-frequency alternating magnetic field for triggered release of loaded materials [119].

LbL self-assembled hollow polyelectrolyte shells have been studied for encapsulation of different proteins including α-chymotrypsin [120,121], peroxidase [122–124], urease [29], bovine serum albumin (BSA) [125–127], oligonucleotide [128], and insulin [129]. Shells are usually in micron size and subject to "open" and "close" under changes of environmental pH, temperature, solvent, and even magnetic field (Figure 10.5). Basically, shells are switched to "open" in one condition for protein loading and then to "close" for storage. It is important to choose the "close" state similar to the physiological conditions, so proteins will stay inside capsules for long-term storage with minimum initial leakage during administration. Protein release can be triggered passively by pathological conditions or actively by external signals. For example, when capsules are accumulated at tumor site, the low-pH environment [130] would be helpful to passively trigger protein release. We will discuss how to load and release proteins through pH, external magnetic field, and porous particle templates.

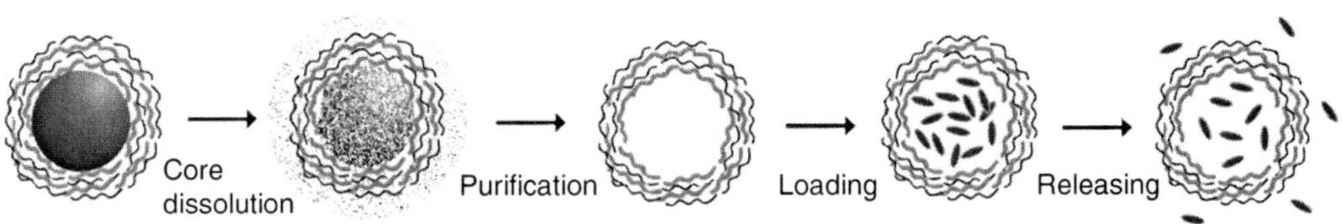

FIGURE 10.5 Scheme of fabrication of functional hollow polyelectrolyte shells and loading of biomacromolecules.

10.3.2.1 pH-Controlled Macromolecule Encapsulation

It has been found that hollow PAH/PSS capsules can open at lower pH values for macromolecule permeation and close at higher pH values for encapsulation [30,120]. The loading process is simple and only requires a few steps of washing. First, proteins and polyelectrolyte capsules are coincubated at a lower pH value at which shells are open for easy penetration of macromolecules. Second, after being mixed for a certain time, the mixture's pH is adjusted to a higher value for closing the capsule. Finally, the capsules are washed a few times, usually through centrifugation at this higher pH environment for removing free proteins.

CLSM is an excellent tool for monitoring capsules "open" and "close" when they are in micron size. Observing the loading procedure of smaller capsules (<200 nm) requires other tools such as AFM or TEM. The opening state of PAH/PSS capsules for a model drug FITC-dextran (MW: 75,000) was observed for pH values up to 6, and most capsules were closed from pH 8 upwards [30]. The surface structure of polyelectrolyte capsules is affected by pH values. Holes up to hundreds of nanometers could be formed in capsule wall when pH was lower than 6.5, which obviously facilitated protein (most in the range of 5–50 nm) penetration into shells [120]. In addition, it was suggested that the opening of the capsule wall presumably occurs as a cooperative process and appears like defect formation [30]. Possibly, changes of the polyelectrolyte charge upon pH variation are able to induce pore formation or loosen the polyelectrolyte network, thus enabling macromolecules to penetrate [30,131]. Further studies are necessary to fully understand the mechanism of pH-induced permeability changes.

In addition to the capsule interior cavity, its membrane also serves as an important reservoir for protein encapsulation. For example, α-chymotrypsin concentration into shells (inside capsule + capsule wall) was in the range of 40–50 mg/mL, which was much higher than the incubation protein concentration of 3.75 mg/mL and even above the solubility limit of α-chymotrypsin (~10 mg/mL) [120]. So the concentration gradient is not the only driving force for protein penetration into shells. After loading, proteins are distributed into two different locations: one is the capsule membrane and the other is inside capsules. The capsule membrane contains 90% loaded proteins because of the high-affinity to proteins and higher capacity and leads to the overall high-protein loading.

A method introduced by Lowry et al. [132] can be used to determine the protein concentration inside shells [120–122,124]. The principle behind the Lowry method of determining protein concentrations lies in the reactivity of the peptide nitrogen[s] with the copper [II] ions under alkaline conditions (pH 10 ~10.5) and the subsequent reduction of the Folin-Ciocalteay phosphomolybdic-phosphotungstic acid to heteropolymolybdenum blue by the copper-catalyzed oxidation of aromatic acids [133]. The Lowry method is sensitive with the protein detection limit as low as 0.005 mg/mL [134]. To avoid any turbidity caused by microcapsules, ultrasonication and purification are necessary before optical measurements.

10.3.2.2 Switch On/Off Capsule Opening through External Magnetic Field

It is of special interest that drug carriers can be triggered to open and release contents upon application of a harmless external magnetic field. This enables one to control a burst release of drugs inside microcapsules at the site of choice when necessary. It has been demonstrated that magnetic nanoparticles and drug can be embedded inside alginate or liposome matrixes, and controlled drug release was achieved when using a low-frequency external magnetic field [135,136]. To apply this methodology to polyelectrolyte capsules, it has to meet two conditions: (1) incorporation of magnetic nanoparticles into the shell wall and (2) movement of magnetic nanoparticles under external magnetic field.

In an earlier attempt, the Lvov group incorporated magnetite nanoparticles into polyelectrolyte shell wall for enhanced bioreaction under external magnetic field [137]. Later, they embedded ferromagnetic cobalt nanoparticles (~3 nm) (Co@Au nanoparticles) into (PSS/PAH)$_n$ polyelectrolyte capsules for capsule wall permeability control and loading of macromolecules [119]. Dextran was used as the model molecule, but the loading procedure can be applied to other macromolecules, including proteins. In that study, shells were built on 5.5 μm diameter $MnCO_3$ particle templates, and the final structure was $(PSS/PAH)_4(PSS/Co@Au)_{1-2}(PSS/PAH)_{2-10}$. To test shell "open" under external magnetic field, $(PSS/PAH)_4(PSS/Co@Au)_1(PSS/PAH)_6$ shells were coincubated with FITC-labeled dextran (MW: 2,000,000, 1 mg/mL) at pH 7.5. Under CLSM observation, the interior of capsules was dark even after 1 h of mixing, indicating little permeability to dextran. In comparison, after applying an alternating electromagnetic field (1200 Oe, 150 Hz) to the capsule/FITC–dextran mixture for 30 min, the capsules became permeable and the fluorescence intensity inside the capsules was similar to bulk solution. It was noticed that the sample temperature increased about 10°C–20°C during the application of an alternating magnetic field. Further thermal tests showed that the temperature's influence on the permeability of capsules was negligible, so it was the external magnetic field contributing to the capsule permeability change.

The influence of frequencies (100–1000 Hz) of electromagnetic fields on the permeability of capsule walls was investigated at a fixed magnetic field of 1200 Oe. For lower frequencies (<300 Hz), there is a tendency for faster diffusion of FITC-dextran. While higher frequencies (>300 Hz) have only negligible effects on the diffusion of FITC-dextran into capsules, even after keeping the mixture for 1 h in the magnetic field. It was possible that the increase of frequency reduced agitation effects of the magnetic field on the Co@Au nanoparticles embedded in the capsule walls and could not influence the permeability of the magnetic capsules. It was suggested that magnetostatic interactions inside the magnetic nanoparticle aggregations would lead to the appearance of a fairly large demagnetizing field [119]. In such a field, they will try to align their easy axis along the direction of the external magnetic field, and this may result in the formation of rather large stresses inside the capsule walls. Such stresses can lead to an increase of pore size in the capsule walls and the release of encapsulated macromolecules. Under a resonant frequency, the stress may be drastically enhanced and even rupture the shell walls.

10.3.2.3 Porous Particles for Protein Encapsulation

Porous polymer microparticles with optimal aerodynamics (lower particle density and larger particle size) were ideal candidates for pulmonary drug delivery [138,139]. In addition, inorganic particles with porous structures provide a unique way of loading and delivering macromolecules. Recently, the Sukhorukov group reported using porous $CaCO_3$ microparticles, with the help of LbL self-assembly, for the encapsulation of biomacromolecules [126,127]. Inorganic porous particles were used as sacrificial templates for protein loading, and there were two general strategies involved. In the first strategy, the $CaCO_3$ microparticle was consecutively coated with oppositely charged polymer layers, resulting in adsorption of the polyelectrolytes not only on the surface of the template but also inside pores. Afterwards, the core material could be dissolved in the presence of 0.1 M EDTA and polyelectrolyte complexes were left inside capsules. Finally, biomacromolecules could be spontaneously loaded into capsules through binding to those polyelectrolyte complexes. In the second strategy, proteins were first entrapped inside porous particles because of the high-surface area (8.8 ± 0.3 m²/g) and reasonably large pore size (20–60 nm). Then, alternate coating of polyelectrolyte was used to form protein–polyelectrolyte complexes before core dissolution. One obvious advantage of using $CaCO_3$ porous particles is that particle dissolution in EDTA, which is relatively friendly to proteins than the acids used in the capsule "open" and "close" process aforementioned.

Upon core dissolution, either gel-like matrix or clusters of polyelectrolyte complex were observed inside shells [126,127]. The shell-loading capacity was impressive; an 11 pg $(PSS/PAH)_3$ shell can encapsulate about 12 pg BSA. For a capsule with 8 bilayers, the weight was 24 pg and the amount of BSA adsorbed was found to be 63% of the total mass. Taking into account that 15 pg of BSA was adsorbed into a microcapsule with an average diameter of 4.5–5.0 μm, the protein concentration per capsule was approximately 250 mg/mL, which is much higher than the protein solubility [127]. It indicates that the adsorbed proteins were formed complex with polyelectrolytes instead of in a free state.

10.3.2.4 Protection of Polyelectrolyte Capsules

10.3.2.4.1 Penetration Barrier

Polyelectrolyte capsules not only serve as carriers for proteins, they also provide protection for the loaded materials. In an enzyme (α-chymotrypsin) encapsulation experiment, Tiourina et al. [120] discovered that only 40% enzymatic activity was lost after coincubation with its inhibitor basic pancreatic trypsin inhibitor (BPTI) (30 min, [BPTI]/[enzyme] = 2). The native protein was completely inhibited after 5 min incubation with even a smaller [BPTI]/[enzyme] ratio = 1. Proteins that bind to wall materials may have better thermal and pH stability than free ones. For example, the glucose oxidase/PEI multilayer was active up to 60°C compared with the 50°C glucose oxidase activity limit in solution [140]. Silica multilayer shell was also used as protection against ultraviolet radiation [141].

10.3.2.4.2 Active Catalytic Defense

Polyelectrolyte capsules are highly permeable to small molecules in aqueous solution. This may present a chance for oxidation of loaded proteins with the existence of radicals in solution. Incorporation of enzymes such as catalase into a LbL film can protect underneath protein/polyelectrolyte multilayers [142]. A similar system was established to explore how to preserve encapsulated proteins from oxidation [125]. In this study, the goal was to preserve albumin inside PAH/PSS shells from oxidation caused by H_2O_2. Three types of modified polyelectrolyte capsules were tested, including (PAH/PSS)$_4$–PAH microcapsules, (PAH/PSS)$_4$–PAH capsules surface engineered with magnetite nanoparticles, and (PAH/PSS)$_4$–PAH microcapsules covered with enzyme catalase. Magnetite nanoparticles or catalase on shell surface served as a catalyst layer for H_2O_2 decomposition to H_2O and less active O_2. For (PAH/PSS)$_4$–PAH microcapsules, shell materials (PAH, PSS) were oxidized and thus led to the loss of shell integrity, resulting in the destruction of the polyelectrolyte shell wall structures. In comparison, modification of the polyelectrolyte shell with catalase led to much less damage to shell wall and encapsulated proteins. This shielding catalyzes H_2O_2 decomposition to O_2, results in a drastic increase of the antioxidant properties of the shell, and decreases the number of carbonyl groups in encapsulated BSA after H_2O_2 treatment. The most effective protection is the magnetite nanoparticle layer. The catalase-modified polyelectrolyte capsules are 1.5 times less effective compared with Fe_3O_4-modified ones, possibly due to partial deactivation of enzymes after adsorption on PAH. The stability and the integrity of the capsule shell are better preserved, benefiting from addition of the active outer layer.

10.3.3 MICROENCAPSULATION FOR GENE DELIVERY

Principally, the aim of gene delivery is the same as protein delivery: protect the loaded materials during delivery and release them at the target locations. Viral and nonviral (polymer-based) gene delivery have achieved exciting success in recent years. However, a lack of high-enough efficiency of encapsulation and needs to engineer the structure and properties of protective shell on nanometer scale provide an avenue for further efforts in this direction. Polyelectrolyte shells are potential candidates for solving the above problems.

The Lvov group was the first to introduce DNA into LbL self-assembled polyelectrolyte capsules [143]. The loading process is different from those discussed previously. Biocompatible polyelectrolytes chondroitin sulfate (PG)/poly(L-arginine) (PA) capsules of 4 μm diameter were developed for encapsulation of DNA molecules. First, highly polymerized DNA molecules were deposited by controlled precipitation of DNA/sperimidine (Sp) complex onto a surface of template microparticles. Then, biocompatible coatings of (PA/PG)$_4$/PA were further assembled as a protection shell with thickness of 40 nm through QCM measurements. Next, $MnCO_3$ template particles were dissolved in de-aerated 0.01 M HCl and washed for purification. Finally, these capsules were treated with

0.1 M HCl for 10 min, which led to the decomposition of DNA/Sp complex formed in aqueous solution at neutral pH [144]. As a result, low-molecular weight sperimidine was released and further removed from the capsule interior. DNA may be released through high-salt solutions since DNA/Sp pairs fall apart in such an environment due to high-ionic strength [144]. The estimated average concentration of DNA encapsulated via DNA/Sp complex is 0.4 mg/mL. Shells were examined under CLSM before and after dissolution of the inner DNA/Sp complex (Figure 10.6). Figure 10.6a illustrates a typical fluorescence image of (DNA/Sp)PA/PG capsules immediately after dissolution of template, and the fluorescence signal is caused by presence of Rhodamine-labeled DNA in the capsule wall. In comparison, the capsule filled with freely floating DNA molecules had fluorescence signal from the whole capsule volume with even distribution (Figure 10.6b). The circular dichroism (CD) spectrum also demonstrated successful loading of active DNA inside capsules. The CD spectrum of a double-stranded DNA has a strong signal in the 230–350 nm range [145]. After decomposition of the DNA/Sp complex, the CD spectrum of DNA captured inside PA/PG microcapsules reveals minor changes (~90% of the helicity preserved) compared with initial DNA. Shchukin et al. suggested that sperimidine and polyarginine partially compensate in capsule volume and reduce the negative effect of low-pH, forming pH gradient across the capsule shell.

10.3.4 Direct Coating on Protein Aggregates

Protein crystal formulation is preferred in pharmaceutical industry for its advantages in handling, stability, bioavailability, and controlled release [146]. Furthermore, protein crystals have shown

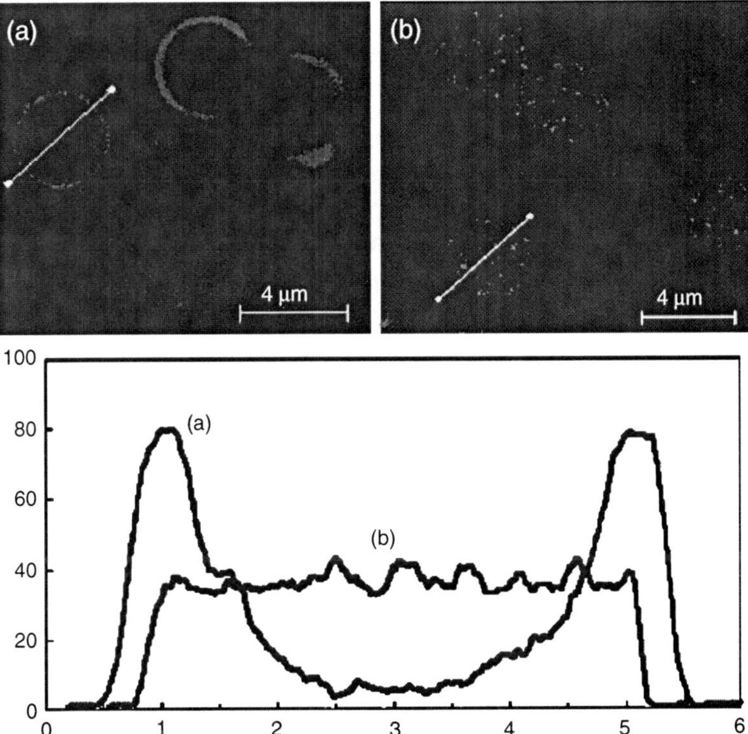

FIGURE 10.6 Fluorescence confocal microscopy images of the DNA-containing capsules composed of four PA/PG bilayers just after decomposition of template core (a) and after dissolution of the inner DNA/Sp complex (b). Areas under the curves are similar. The inset demonstrates the fluorescence profile for both cases. (Reproduced from Shchukin, D.G., Patel, A.A., Sukhorukov, G.B., and Lvov, Y., *J. Am. Chem. Soc.*, 126, 3374–3375, 2004. With permission.)

greater protection against proteolytic enzymes compared with their amorphous counterparts. The most common and easy form of protein crystals are naked crystals, which have shown controlled release and desirable pharmaceutical properties such as good resuspendability. The major barrier for using naked crystals is the limited release profile, usually within a day [147]. Encapsulation of these crystals in biocompatible and biodegradable polymer systems may not only extend the release to a much longer time, but also increase the protein stability to a higher degree. Unfortunately, the manufacturing methods used for encapsulating protein in polymeric systems often adversely affect protein stability because of exposure to organic solvent, hydrophobic surfaces, and vigorous agitation [148].

Direct LbL self-assembly of polyelectrolytes onto protein crystals serves as a simple and easy method for encapsulation. Similar to encapsulation of small-molecule drug crystals, this self-assembly process has advantages including no exposure to organic solvent, less agitation, wide selection of coating materials, precise release rate control, and high-loading density. It has been found that either electrostatic or hydrophobic interactions can facilitate the first layer growth on protein crystals [149]. Further layers can be assembled following standard LbL self-assembly coating process on colloidal particles. Interestingly, the efficiency of protein (α-chymotrypsin) encapsulation (the ratio of loaded protein amount over the protein content in solution before the coating process) was reduced with more layers of coating. The estimated efficiency was 73%, 50%, 40%, and 33% for 3-, 5-, 7-, and 11-layer PSS/PAH-paired microcapsules (with PSS as the first layer), respectively. It was suggested that partial protein aggregates dissolution and loss of microcapsules during washing steps may be the major reasons [149]. The encapsulation also provides a good protection of loaded materials. For example, small molecule enzyme inhibitor phenylmethane sulfonyl fluoride (MW: 174) can penetrate into the $(PAH/PSS)_n$ shells and reduce the enzymatic activity by about 69%, while high-molecular weight inhibitor BPTI (MW: 6500) can only suppress 13% activity [149].

10.3.5 Encapsulation of Small-Molecule Drug Micro/Nanoparticles

It is well-recognized that poor aqueous solubility is the major obstacle in small-molecule drug discovery and development. Many drug candidates cannot be further developed mainly because of the very low water solubility [150]. Even some drugs in clinical use are barely soluble in water. The most direct method to increase the solubility is through salt generation but this can not be applied to nonionizable compounds. Instead, preparing drug crystals in nano or microsizes provides a promising future for delivery of poorly soluble drugs. There are various methodologies including milling, emulsification solvent evaporation, pH-controlled precipitation, and supercritical fluid-processing for generating drug nanoparticle formulations [151,152]. Next, to prevent drug micro/nanocrystal agglomeration or aggregation when dispersed in water, stabilizers are used to promote particle size reduction process and generate physically stable formulations [151]. But excess amount of stabilizer can induce Ostwald ripening. How to stabilize drug crystals in a simple and an efficient way is of great interest. Direct LbL self-assembly of polyelectrolyte on drug crystals may serve as an alternative with two functions: (1) stabilize drug crystal dispersion in aqueous environment and (2) control drug release rate.

Some preliminary work has demonstrated the feasibility of direct self-assembly of polyelectrolyte layer on drug microcrystals and controlled of release [108,153–155]. A few conditions must be satisfied before elaboration of coating: (1) a favorable pH environment for stabilizing drug crystals and maintaining polyelectrolytes charged. For example, ibuprofen is 16 times less soluble in pH 5 than pH 7.4 [156]. In this case, we would prefer to use pH 5 to stabilize drug crystals as this gives a much better loading efficiency. Appropriate pairs of polyelectrolytes should be chosen so that at such a pH both polycation and polyanion be well charged and (2) enabling surface charge of drug crystals at that pH value. Some drugs are weakly charged in aqueous environment, but others are neutral without charges. To impart charge on particle surface, ionic surfactants, phospholipids, or

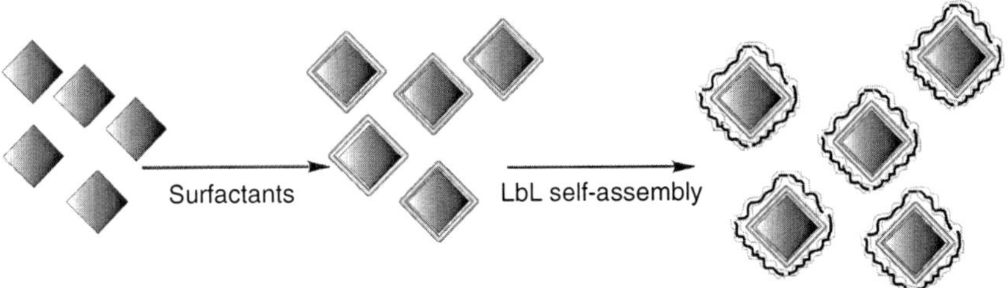

FIGURE 10.7 Scheme of direct coating of polyelectrolytes onto small molecule drug crystals. Surfactants could be used to impart charges onto noncharged drug crystals and followed by LbL self-assembly of polyelectrolytes.

charged amphipathic polymers could be used first (Figure 10.7). It has been demonstrated that a model drug pyrene crystals exposed to didodecyldimethylammonium bromide (positively charged) showed a zeta-potential of +50 mV, while sodium dodecyl sulfate (negatively charged) dispersed another model drug fluorescein diacetate crystal exhibited a value of −50 mV [157]. Once charged, polyanions and polycations can be further applied for shell encapsulation (Figure 10.7).

The next important step is to choose appropriate polymers for LbL self-assembly. Natural polymers are preferable because of their excellent biocompatibility and biodegradability. Commonly used hydrophilic materials in pharmaceutical applications include polysaccharides (e.g., CH), polypeptides (e.g., poly[aspartic acid]), and proteins (e.g., gelatin). Besides, synthetic biocompatible and biodegradable polymers are also good candidates. For example, poly(α-[4-aminobutyl]-L-glycolic acid) (PAGA), a novel poly-L-lysine analog, containing both a degradable ester linkage and a positively charged backbone, provides good biocompatibility and degradability for gene and interleukin delivery [158,159]. Poly(β-amino ester), a cationic and degradable polymer, when built with heparin multilayers, showed tunable drug release upon hydrolytic degradation of the polymers [160].

The drug release rate can be directly controlled by varying the number of layers of coating [153,154,161,162]. In a model drug study experiment, fluorescein dye microcrystals were used as templates, and multilayers of PSS and PAH were self-assembled on particle surface [116]. For 8 to 18 layers, the permeability value decreased from 7×10^{-9} to 2×10^{-9} m/s. The permeability can be converted into a diffusion coefficient (D) by means of multiplying the permeability with the shell wall thickness. Assuming 3 nm for each individual polyelectrolyte layer, the calculated diffusion coefficients ranged from 1.7×10^{-16} to 1×10^{-16} m²/s. The Mohwald group has discovered that there is a limitation when increasing film thickness to reduce the shell permeability, that is, permeability can no longer be changed after a certain number of layers have been assembled [162]. For example, after 16 bilayers of PAH/PSS assembly on ibuprofen drug crystals were achieved, further shell thickness increase did not reduce shell permeability. This phenomenon can be explained by film homogenization after coating certain number of layers [162]. Basically, pores or defects may exist in the films at the beginning of LbL self-assembly because of incomplete coverage by polyelectrolytes. It can be expected that the permeation through these pores or defects will give rise to the permeability of the films. With the number of coating layers increased, the pores or defects could be reduced or completely closed. As a result, the film permeability decreases and eventually reaches a constant value when the films are structurally homogeneous.

Another parameter to control shell permeability is choosing different materials for shell assembly. On encapsulation with 15 bilayers of polysaccharides, CH and dextran sulfate, the half-release time of ibuprofen ($t_{1/2}$) was about twice as bare drug microcrystals at pH 7.4 [154]. Only five bilayers of PAH/PSS coating prolonged the half-release time about 6 times longer than bare microcrystals [162]. Using gelatin led to even much slower drug release; it has been demonstrated that at pH 7.4, six bilayers of gelatin and PSS prolonged half drug release time about 300 times compared with uncoated furosemide microcrystals [153]. Similarly, slower drug release from gelatin-containing capsules was observed compared with dextran/CH-paired polyelectrolytes [108]. Gelatin is a weakly charged polyelectrolyte with low-charge density. This may result in formation of a loopy conformation at coating conditions and lead to adsorption of several monomolecular protein layers [153]. The suggestion was verified during QCM study of gelatin/PSS assembly, because the averaged frequency shift was 483 Hz for each gelatin layer, which corresponds to a thickness of 8 nm. Obviously, a single gelatin layer is much thinner than this.

Most polyelectrolyte shells are composed of one weak base and one strong acid (e.g., PAH/PSS, CH/dextran sulfate). It should be observed that permeability of shells built on these paired polyelectrolytes would not change much upon pH variations. For example, PAH/PSS multilayers have slightly higher (1.5 times) permeability at pH 1.4 than that at pH 7.4 [154]. The possible reason is that the charge of weak base PAH is relatively stable at different pH values, and interactions with PSS are not significantly affected. Similarly, CH/dextran sulfate is weak base–strong acid combination and obvious pH effects were not observed. When strong acid was replaced by weak acids such as carboxymethyl cellulose sodium salt or alginate, similar release profiles were noticed at pH 7.4. This indicates that the strength of the ionic groups on the polymer chains may not significantly influence the permeability of the polysaccharide multilayers [154]. The pH stability of above formulations may be advantageous in oral administration because of insensitivity to GI tract's pH variation.

10.3.6　Carrier Surface Functionalization

10.3.6.1　PEGylation of Polyelectrolyte Shells

Poly(ethylene glycol) (PEG), a noncharged hydrophilic polymer, is well-accepted in pharmaceutical industry for drug formulation. When incorporated onto liposomes, it has shown the effects to prolong blood circulation time and improve drug pharmacokinetics [163]. Polyelectrolyte shells represent certain charges on their surfaces that may not be ideal for intravenous injection because of hemocompatibility concerns and sequestration by the mononuclear phagocytic system (MPS) in liver and spleen. PEGylation on shell surface provides a reasonable solution. It has been demonstrated that PEG can be linked to polycation PAH outermost layer as a last step during drug crystal coating process [155]. This modification was accomplished by the covalent attachment of mPEG–SPA to a PAH layer of the encapsulated drug particles via the reaction between the hydroxysuccinimidyl (NHS) moiety of mPEG–SPA with an amine on PAH. The requirement for this reaction to take place is keeping the pH of the buffered solution between 8.2 and 8.5. At this basic pH, the protonated amine of the PAH layer becomes deprotonated and PEG can be covalently attached to this secondary amine. Consequently, incorporation of PEG to the nanoshell of the encapsulated drug particle created neutralization in charge of the nanoparticle. Successful PEG conjugation was verified as the particle surface zeta-potential dropped from positive 25 mV to near zero. XPS study further demonstrated the conjugation of PEG to PAH as apparent increase in C—(O,N) (286.34 eV) peak area and decrease in C=O, C—F (287.64 eV) peak area compared with PAH-coated drug crystals.

In a study of cell interactions with LbL capsules, PEGylation reduced nonspecific protein adsorption onto polyelectrolyte capsule surface [51]. PEI–PEG copolymers with PEI/PEG graft ratios (1, 5, and 10) were synthesized and used as the outermost layers for shell assembly. Compared with PEI outermost layer covered capsules, all PEI–PEG covered ones had much less changes in surface zeta-potential after serum contact. It indicated that the shielding property of PEG could effectively deter protein adsorption [164].

10.3.6.2　Active Targeting of Capsules

Effective delivery of therapeutic agents to the diseased site requires that the carriers have targeting moieties, which recognize highly expressed antigens or receptors on cell surface. One strategy to achieve cancer-targeted drug delivery is the utilization of unique molecular markers overexpressed at the cancerous tissues. Antibodies and specific ligands are good candidates for such a purpose.

Recently, two studies have demonstrated that either monoclonal antibody or peptide ligand can be deposited onto polyelectrolyte capsule surface with successful *in vitro* targeting. Suslick group chose a small tripeptide turn sequence arginine-glycine-aspartic (RGD) as the targeting ligand, which recognizes highly expressed $\alpha V\beta 3$ receptors on tumor endothelial cells [165]. Different peptides with an RGD motif embedded at the ends or in the middle of a highly positively charged, polylysine sequence were synthesized: at the amino terminus, RGDKKKKKK; in the middle, KKKKRGDKKK; and at the carboxy terminus, KKKKKKKRGD. An additional decapeptide polylysine K10 was prepared as a control. The positively charged lysine residues electrostatically secure the RGD motif to the surface of the microspheres. Human colon tumor cells (HT29), over expressing of integrins, were used to test the efficacy of the RGD-modified microspheres in tumor targeting. The fluorescence microscopy revealed that binding of RGD-modified microspheres is increased relative to the unmodified ones, especially the RGDKKKKKK peptides exhibit the best binding to the tumor cells, with the KKKKRGDKKK peptide binding the least. In the other study led by the Caruso group, humanized A33 monoclonal antibody (HuA33 mAb), labeled on LbL shells, were tested to recognize A33 antigen-expressing LIM1215 colorectal cancer cells *in vitro* [166]. Both flow cytometry and fluorescence microscopy studies showed increased cell binding of shells tagging with HuA33 mAb. To determine the effectiveness of polyelectrolyte capsules as novel colloidal delivery systems, *in vivo* targeting experiment is necessary.

10.4 POLYMERIC MICELLES FOR DRUG AND GENE DELIVERY

10.4.1 INTRODUCTION

In recent years, nano-sized particles have been receiving much attention in the field of drug delivery systems because of their special drug-loading abilities and their unique distribution characteristics in the body. Polymeric micelles, formed by the self-assembly of either amphiphilic or oppositely charged copolymers in aqueous solution, are one of the most studied nanocarriers for both drug and gene delivery applications. These micelles have characteristic core–shell architecture and, generally, narrow size distribution. In the micelles, hydrophobic or oppositely charged segments aggregate because of either the hydrophobic interaction or the electrostatic interaction to form an inner core, while the shell of the micelles is formed by a hydrophilic segments that are covalently connected with the core segments. Hydrophobic drugs or ionic compounds are loaded through hydrophobic interaction or electrostatic interaction into the core of the micelles, which are surrounded by the hydrophilic corona that barrier the contact of the drug with the surrounding environments. The distribution of the drug-loaded micelles in the body are thus mainly determined by the size of the micelles and also the surface properties of the micelles shell, but less influenced by the nature of the loaded drug.

The use of nano-sized polymeric micelles as drug carriers has many advantages. These particles are ultrafine sized; thus, they can penetrate the capillary and move to desired place inside the body. They are of high-loading capacity, and, particularly, they are powerful vehicles that provide a particular mechanism to disperse water-insoluble drugs into aqueous media.

10.4.2 AMPHIPHILIC BLOCK COPOLYMER MICELLES: PEO-PPO-PEO BLOCK COPOLYMER (PLURONIC)

Among the polymeric micelles, those composed of the amphiphilic block copolymers are well-studied nanoparticles that showed high potential in drug delivery. The increasing interest in amphiphilic block copolymer in the biomedical field arises mainly because of their ability to form micelles with core–shell architecture. The amphiphilic block copolymers are generally defined as macromolecules with linear arrangements of two or more different blocks of hydrophilic and lipophilic segments. The self-assembly of these amphiphilic block copolymer to form the core in aqueous solution is based on the hydrophobic interaction between the lipophilic polymer segments. The hydrophobic core is sterically stabilized by a hydrophilic palisades formed from the hydrophilic segments of the block copolymer. The palisades are dense enough to avoid the core from contacting with the aqueous environment. Thus, the amphiphilic block copolymer micelles are capable of encapsulating hydrophobic molecules in the core through nonpolar or hydrophobic interaction between the lipophilic polymer segments and the hydrophobic drugs. This can increase the concentration and the stability of hydrophobic drugs in the aqueous environments. The potential of using amphiphilic block copolymers as colloidal vectors provides the possibility of delivery of many newly developed highly efficacious therapeutic compounds that are water-insoluble.

Beyond increasing the solubility of water-insoluble drugs, the amphiphilic block copolymer micelles also act like other kinds of nanodrug carriers, elongating the blood cycling time of drugs and targeting the payload drug to specific tissue or organism through ether passive or active pathways. In this section, typical amphiphilic block copolymer PEO-PPO-PEO block copolymer (Pluronic) micelles are discussed, including their composition, structure, preparation, and biomedical applications as drug carriers.

Pluronics are ABA type tri-block copolymers of polyethylene oxide (PEO) and polypropylene oxide (PPO) with the PPO segments at the center and PEO segments at both ends of the polymeric chain. The commercial available Pluronics are generally synthesized from the anionic polymerization ring-opening polymerization of ethylene oxide initiated from the hydroxyl groups at both ends of PPO chain. Therefore, Pluronics always have controlled molecular architecture and narrow molecular weight distribution.

Pluronics have been investigated as vectors for drug and gene delivery *in vitro* and *in vivo* and were demonstrated to have high efficiency for both the drug and gene transfer *in vivo* [167–170]. The incorporation of drugs into Pluronic micelles results in increased solubility and stability of drugs. In addition, the enhanced swallow of the Pluronic micelles by the cell has been well–known [169,171]. Consequently, the micelles are used for delivery of bioactive low-molecular weight compounds in the body.

Pluronic was used for delivery of ATP into cells. In an intact Jurkat cells culture system, no participation of the exogenous γ-32P ATP in phosphorylation of intracellular proteins could be observed, because the negatively charged ATP could not penetrate cell plasma membrane. Whereas considerable increase of protein phosphorylation was obtained by adding of γ-32P ATP solubilized in positively charged Pluronic micelles to cells (the positively charged micelles were obtained by adding of dodecylamine). The Pluronic micelles showed good biocompatibility, not influencing the viability of cells and permeabilize cell plasma membrane under the experimental condition [172].

To target the micelles into the cell, cell targeting ligands can be conjugated with the Pluronic molecule. The conjugates are incorporated into the micelle by preparing the micelles from the mixture of Pluronics and the conjugates. The incorporation of ligands capable of receptor-mediated endocytosis can result in enhancement of the efficiency of cell loading of the micelles. Using this concept, the micelles of pluronic P85 incorporated with *Staphylococcus aureus* enterotoxin B (SEB) ligands were used as microcontainers for *in vitro* delivery of the fluorescent dye into Jurkat and MDCK cells. Enhanced fluorescence radiation was observed compared with the non-SEB micelles. At 4°C, under the condition in which endocytosis is abolished, there is no enhancement of fluorescence, indicating that the increase of fluorescence is attributed to the enhanced swallow of the SEB-incorporated micelles [173].

Pluronic block copolymer micelles are also useful in the delivery of anticancer agents, e.g., doxorubicin (DOX), PTX, and platinum compound, into tumor cells [171,174–176]. In the presence of Pluronic micelles, the obviously increased uptake of these drugs by tumor cells were observed, apparently due to the effect of the polymeric micelles on cell membrane permeability. One example of the drug/Pluronic formulation employed PTX as the cytotoxic agent. The spherical PTX-loaded micelles with a mean size of approximately 25 nm and narrow size distribution showed two- to threefold higher cytotoxicity than that of free PTX. In addition, increased uptake of the PTX-loaded micelles in the plasma, ovary and uterus, lung, and kidney were observed, whereas the uptake in the liver and brain decreased. These results indicate the high promise that Pluronic micelles can effectively solubilize PTX, prolong blood circulation time, and modify the distribution of PTX [175]. The broad specificity for other drugs of block copolymer micelles might be a valuable property for developing new drug delivery systems to increase drug accumulation in cancer organs by encapsulating the drug in micelles to prevent unwanted interactions with healthy cells.

Recently, the enhanced uptake of anticancer drugs into the tumor cell induced by ultrasound was reported [177,178]. Pruitt and coworkers reported a stable Pluronic micelles by core-cross-linking. The micelles were able to sequester the DOX and protect cells from the drug at low concentrations for approximately 12 h. Application of low-frequency ultrasound resulted in a synergistic killing effect with DOX and low concentrations of stabilized Pluronic due to release of DOX and permeabilization of the cell membrane [179]. One animal experiment that applied the drug-encapsulated Pluronic micelles in ovarian cancer-bearing mice indicated that ultrasonic irradiation locally to the tumor significantly enhanced accumulation of Pluronic micelles in the tumor cells. The degree of targeting was enhanced by a local tumor sonication [180].

This enhancement is considered to possibly have two independent mechanisms that work in concert. The first one is related to the acoustically triggered drug release from micelles that results in higher concentration of the free drug in the incubation medium. The second mechanism is based on the perturbation of cell membranes that results in the increased uptake of the micellar-encapsulated drug. Under the radiation of ultrasound, the micellar-encapsulated drug tends to release from the micelle due to micelle perturbation; meanwhile, the ultrasound induces a series of cellular changes that enhance the accessibility of various cellular structures to drug, making it easier for the drugs to achieve intracellular distribution. An important advantage offered by ultrasound is that the same degree of the intracellular drug uptake may be achieved at a substantially lower drug concentration in the incubation medium [181,182].

During the treatment of tumor with antitumor agents, the human multidrug transporter MDR1 P-glycoprotein and the multidrug resistance proteins MRP1 and MRP2 transport a range of cytotoxic drugs, thus often resulting in multidrug resistance in tumor cells [183]. Incorporating Pluronic block copolymer in the cancer therapy, the micelles can sensitize multidrug-resistant (MDR) cancer cells, increasing the cytotoxic activity of antitumor agents. This effect is attributed to the inhibition of the most clinically relevant P-glycoprotein through the combined ATP depletion and inhibition of P-glycoprotein ATPase activity [184]. DOX is often observed to induce the MDR of tumor organs. In the study employing DOX/Pluronic formulation, the treatment of the cells with DOX/Pluronic formulation significantly enhanced the proapoptotic activity of the drug and prevented the activation of the antiapoptotic cellular defense, thus inducing apoptosis in the resistant cancer cells more efficiently than free Dox [185]. The high-frequency ultrasound showed positive effects on DOX uptake by MDR cells from DOX/Pluronic micelles. It was observed that even a short exposure to high-frequency ultrasound significantly enhanced the intracellular DOX uptake [186].

Pluronic triblock copolymers were used to enhance the cytotoxicity of carboplatin, a metallic anticancer agent, to rat tumor cell. Compared with control groups receiving carboplatin alone, the great enhancement of carboplatin cell cytotoxicity with induced Pluronic were observed. The experimental data demonstrate that Pluronic P85 is a optimal agent for increased cytotoxicity of carboplatin in the DHB/K12/TRb rat colorectal carcinoma cell line. This study implies that the Pluronic may act as a potential drug delivery scheme for carboplatin in cancer therapy [176].

10.4.3 Amphiphilic Block Copolymers Based on Aliphatic Polyesters

Aliphatic polyesters are biodegradable hydrophobic polymers. PEO-polyester block copolymers are thus composed of hydrophilic PEO segment and hydrophobic polyester segment. The PEO-polyester amphiphilic block copolymers are generally prepared by polymerization of cyclic lactones or lactide initiated from the end hydroxyl group of PEO. They self-assemble into micelles in aqueous solution. The formation of micelle inner core is due to the hydrophobic interaction of the biodegradable polyester chains. Hydrophobic drugs are physically entrapped in the hydrophobic core through nonpolar interaction, stabilized by the highly hydrophilic and low-toxic PEO palisade. The micelles collapse after the degradable core-segment, and the left PEO segment finally permeated through kidney and was eliminated from the body. Therefore, the PEO segments employed in PEO-polyester micelles are generally low-molecular weight products with M_n less than 10,000. The typical polyester segment composed of poly (ε-caprolactone) (PCL) and poly (D,L-lactide) (PDLLA).

The micelles composed of PEO-polyester block copolymers were found to be internalized into cells within a short culture period (several hours). The internalization process was found to be time-, temperature-, pH-, and energy-dependent, fulfilling the basic criteria for endocytotic uptake. In addition, there are other results that provide the evidence to support the endocytosis of the micelles by cells. Thus, nowadays, it is widely ratified that the mode of cellular internalization of PEO–polyester micelles is endocytotic [187–189].

Hydrophobic anticancer drugs and other compounds are encapsulated into the PEO–polyester micelles for delivery into the tumor cells and organs [190]. The copolymer derived from PDLLA of M_w 1866 and PEG of M_w 3300–4000 can obtained through the drug-loading micelles with the maximum drug-loading ability if 12 mg/g. The drug release from these micelles was reported as mainly "degradation controlled" [191]. A PCL-PEO copolymer micelle was reported to be capable of encapsulating DOX in the hydrophobic cores in aqueous solutions. The micelle diameter is adjustable, increasing with the increase of PCL block length in the copolymer composition. Compared with free DOX, the DOX-loaded micelles can provide hemolysis in the blood. Different from free DOX, these DOX-loaded micelles accumulate mostly in cytoplasm instead of cell nuclei [192]. Amphiphilic diblock copolymers based on methoxy PEG (MPEG) and poly(δ-valerolactone) (PVL) (MPEG-PVL) that can load PTX was reported. At a certain composition, micelles of 31 nm in diameter with a narrow size distribution can be formed, which improve the apparent aqueous solubility of PTX by more than 9000-fold, and show excellent biological activity in human MCF-7 breast and A2780 ovarian cancer cells [193].

In addition to PEG, other hydrophilic polymers are used as shell component of polymeric micelles. Polymeric micelles based on amphiphilic block copolymers of poly(2-ethyl-2-oxazoline) (PEtOz) and PCL were reported as a nanocarrier for the delivery of PTX using dialysis method. Their loading content was in the range of 0.5–7.6 wt.%, varying mainly with the block composition of block copolymers. The hydrodynamic diameters of PTX-loaded micelles were in the range 18.3–23.4 nm with narrow size distribution. PTX-entrapped polymeric micelles exhibited comparable activity to that observed with Cremophore EL-based PTX formulations in inhibiting the growth of KB cells [194].

The stability of the drug-loaded micelles is modified by crosslinking of either the core-segment or the shell segment. Double bonds were introduced into the PCL blocks, and cross-linkable PEG-PCL di- and triblock copolymers were synthesized. The nanoscale micelles containing hydrophobic PTX in their hydrophobic cores were cross-linked by radical polymerization to enhance their thermodynamic stability. It was reported that the PTX loading did not obviously affect the micelle size or size distribution, and the drug-loading efficiency of micelles was enhanced significantly upon micelle core-cross-linking. The cross-linked micelles exhibited a significantly enhanced thermodynamic stability against dilution with aqueous solvents [195]. Xu et al. reported a new type of highly stable core-surface-cross-linked polymer micelles made from amphiphilic brush copolymers with PCL cores and PEG or poly[2-(N,N-dimethylamino)ethyl methacrylate] (PDMA) shell. An anticancer agent, cisplatin, could be loaded in the micelle with high-loading efficiency (approximately 90%). This drug-loading micelle could be easily taken up by SKOV-3 ovarian cancer cells. It was found that cisplatin encapsulated in the micelle had much enhanced cytotoxicity to the cancer cells compared with free cisplatin. It seems that the positive charges on the micelle surface promoted the cellular internalization of the nanoparticles, resulting in higher cytotoxicity of cisplatin [196].

The modification of the micelles surface with biofunctional ligands or antibodies is considered as an effective approach that strengthens the targeting of the micelles into the tumor site and penetrates the membrane of cancer cells. Nasongkla et al. developed a RGD-functionalized DOX-loading PEG-PCL micelle. They at first prepared a micelle of PEG–PCL-containing PTX. At the surface of the micelle, reactive maleimide groups were connected to the PEG molecule chain end. Then, the cell-recognized peptide RGD was encapsulated on the surface. The dynamic diameter of the micelles increased from 20.9 nm for the RGD-free micelle to 24.4 nm for the RGD-conjugated micelles. The internalization of the RGD-functionalized micelles was found to be greatly enhanced. The cell uptake of the RGD-functionalized micelle increased 30-fold compared with the RGD-free micelle [197].

It is known that folate receptor overexpressed in some tumor cell membranes. Thus, folate-conjugated micelles were expected to have specific interaction with the tumor cell. Park et al. reported that amphiphilic block copolymers composed of MPEG and PCL with the folic acid conjugated at the surface to produce a folate-receptor-targeted drug carrier for tumor-specific drug delivery. PTX was encapsulated into the micelle in the size range of about 50–130 nm. PTX-loaded folate-conjugated MPEG/PCL micelles exhibited much higher cytotoxicity for cancer cells than micelles without the folate group. The folate-functionalized PTX-loaded micelles were receptor-mediated endocytosed into cancer cells through the interaction with overexpressed folate receptors on the surface of the cancer cells [198].

Amphiphilic block copolymers based on amorphous polyesters are also be used for the delivery of other drugs and bioactive molecules. An injectable formulation of rapamycin was prepared using amphiphilic block copolymer micelles of PEO-PCL with less than 100 nm in diameter and contained rapamycin at 7% to 10% weight (>1 mg/mL) [199]. PEG-PCL was also investigated as a drug delivery vehicle for dihydrotestosterone (DHT). The micelles were found to have a high-loading capacity for DHT, and the release profile of the drug from the micelle solution was found to be a slow steady release, which continued over a 1-month period. The biological activity of the micelle-incorporated DHT was found to be fully retained [200]. PEG-PCL micelles with encapsulated fenofibrate were prepared for the purpose of control release. The size of the fenofibrate-loaded PEG-PCL micelles is less than 50 nm, and can encapsulate up to more than 90% of the initial loading level of fenofibrate at a polymer concentration of 1.0 mg/ml [201]. Indomethacin-loaded polymeric nanospheres with an average diameter in the range of less than 200 nm were prepared from amphiphilic PEG-PGA diblock copolymers with different molar compositions. Indomethacin continuously released from the nanospheres without any burst effect. Compared with unloaded free drug, these PEG-PG copolymer nanospheres could remarkably reduce cell damage [202].

A highly stable polymer micelles, core-surface-cross-linked nanoparticles (SCNPs) made from amphiphilic poly(ε-caprolactone)-b-PEG brush copolymers, were reported to be able to carry cisplatin, an anticancer drug with low solubility in water. Cisplatin was loaded in the SCNPs with high-loading efficiency (approximately 90%). *In vitro* experiments gave out the result that SCNPs containing cisplatin could be easily taken up by ovarian cancer cells. Much enhanced cytotoxicity of the cisplatin encapsulated in the SCNPs, compared with free cisplatin, was observed for the cancer cells. A surface positive charged SCNPs, derived from PCL and (PDMA), was found to have higher uptake in tumor cells, probably due to the surface positive charge that promoted the cellular internalization of the nanoparticles, thus resulting in higher cytotoxicity of cisplatin [196].

10.4.4 BLOCK COPOLYMERS BASED ON POLY L-AMINO ACID (PLAA)

Micelles self-assembled from block copolymers of poly(L-amino acid) (PLAA) and water-soluble polymer blocks have some unique advantages and are used for drug delivery for specific purposes such as prolonging circulation time, introducing targeting moieties, and modifying the drug-release profile [167,203]. As water-soluble blocks, the most widely investigated and used ones are PEO and PEG, the commonly used nonionic water-soluble polymers. The property of the hydrophobic segment of PLAA varies from the amino acid that composed the polymer backbone. The multiform nature of the core-forming PLAA blocks provides a feasible approach to optimize the properties of the PLAA micelles for encapsulation of various kinds of drugs, peptides, proteins, and genes in the micelles core for delivery proposes. Because of the existence of reactable functional groups on the side chain of the amino acids, the PLAA copolymers not only form micelles that encapsule hydrophobic drugs through the physical hydrophobic interaction, but also form block copolymer–drug conjugates that aggregate in aqueous phase to form micelles. These micelles are functionally similar to the biological carriers, namely lipoproteins and viruses. The amino acids originate naturally from living creatures, thus making the micelles based on PLLA core advantageous for safety, stability, and easy to scale-up.

Block copolymers of PEG and poly(beta-benzyl-L-aspartate) were synthesized (PEG–PBLA) by Kataoka and coworkers. Anticancer agent DOX was physically encapsulated into the core of the micelles with a substantial drug-loading level (15–20 w/w%). The size of these DOX-loaded micelles ranged about 50–70 nm, with narrow size distribution. The DOX was considered to possibly interact with the benzyl residues of PBLA blocks through π–π resonance, to facilitate the stability of the micelles and the release behaviors. At the beginning of the DOX release, an initial boost was observed. This was followed by a slow and long-lasting release of DOX. The encapsulation of DOX into the PEG–PBLA micelle carrier greatly elongated the DOX blood circulation period because of the reduced reticuloendothelial system uptake of the micelles through a steric stabilization mechanism. Compared with free DOX, the micelle drug delivery system showed a considerably higher *in vivo* antitumor activity in the animal experiment using mouse as the model animal [204,205].

Platinum compounds are potent anticancer agents that are clinically employed in cancer chemotherapeutics. However, the poor water solubility of these compounds limits their application. Some efforts have been made to improve the solubility by encapsulating these compounds in polymeric micelles [176,196]. Because of the various types of PLAA, the various side chains of the polymer can be obtained by using different amino acids as the starting material. Some PLLA with carboxylic side groups were found to form complex with platinum compounds that were stable enough to aggregate as the core of micelles. Thus, block copolymers of these PLLA with PEG or other hydrophilic polymer block form the micelles with platinum compounds that act as drug delivery system.

Cabral et al. reported a block copolymer of PEG–poly(glutamic acid) [PEG–P(Glu)]. A platinum compound, dichloro(1,2-diaminocyclohexane)platinum(II) (DACHPt), was mixed with the copolymer in distilled water to prepare the metal–complex micelles through polymer–metal complex formation. As a result, the micelles sized approximately 40 nm with narrow distribution were obtained. The initial size of the micelles remained unchanged even after 240 h, suggesting that the micelles were very stable. DACHPt-loaded micelles showed a sustained release rate of platinum after an induction period of 12 h. They exhibited considerable *in vitro* cytotoxicity against murine colon adenocarcinoma 26 (C-26) cells. The cytotoxicity increased with exposure time as a result of the release of platinum complexes from the micelle. *In vivo* biodistribution assay performed on tumor-bearing mice demonstrated that the micelle had prolonged blood circulation due to its high-stability and high-tumor accumulation for a prolonged time [206].

Copolymers of poly(aspartic acid) and PEG were also used to prepare metal–complex micelles with platinum compounds to achieve the delivery of the metal anticancer agent to the tumor cell. The pharmacological activity and the pharmacokinetics of a clinical anticancer agent, cisplatin (CDDP)-loaded polymeric micelles were examined by Nishiyama et al. using PEG–poly(aspartic acid) block copolymer as the carrier. *In vivo* investigation in Lewis lung carcinoma-bearing mice revealed that compared with the free CDDP, the micelles exhibited 5.2- and 4.6-fold higher concentration of Pt in the plasma and tumor, respectively, suggesting prolonged circulation of Pt and specific accumulation in the tumor. The micelles did not increase the plasma BUN at the concentration that free CDDP induced a remarkable increase. Thus, CDDP-loaded micelles are considered to restrain nephrotoxicity, the dose-limiting factor of CDDP, while exhibiting tumor-specific accumulation [207].

DNAs are negatively surface charged and are difficult to be delivered into cells because of the cell surface charge counteraction. Polycations can form ion complexes with DNA, preventing the degradation of *in vivo* enzymes and providing the facility for penetrating the cell membrane by changing the surface charge of the complex [208]. Thus, polycations, such as polyethylene imine (PEI), are usually employed as nonvirus vectors for *in vivo* gene delivery [209,210]. Poly(L-amino acid) with positive charge at the side chain, poly(L-lysine) (PLL), is also a commonly adopted gene carrier in gene therapy. The positive charge of PLL makes it possible to form an ion complex with the negatively charged DNA, thus preventing the gene from being degraded by the enzymes *in vivo* [211].

Block copolymer consisting of PLL and PEG forms polyion complex micelles with DNA, resulting in nano-sized core-shell particles with PEG hydrophilic outer shells. As the same concept described above, the PEG outer shells can keep the particles stable in blood circulation, preventing the uptake of micelles from the RES *in vivo*. This kind of formulation is possibly a potential nonvirus gene delivery vector [212]. Thus, the polyion complex micelles of DNA and block copolymer of PLL and PEG having self-assembling core-shell structures were prepared. These micelles were spherical nano-particles with small absolute values of zeta-potential. The micelles with shorter PLL lengths showed lower stability in the blood stream. After intravenous injection of the micelles having the charge ratios of 1:4, supercoiled DNA was observed for 30 min and open circular or linear DNA was seen for 3 h. The micelles were found to be efficiently transfect into HepG2 cells. This gene delivery system is considered to be intrinsically efficient.

The polyion complex micelles derived from different polycations and PEG were further modified by attaching so-called signal molecules at the surface to improve the active targeting behaviors. Proteins [209], lactose [213], and galactose [214] are employed as the targeting molecules. The PEGs here not only act as the hydrophilic layer to stabilize the micelles, but also act as a spacer for the targeting molecules that need to move freely to attach the receptor site of the tumor cell surface.

10.4.5 "Smart" Micelles for Drug Delivery Application

The so-called "smart" micelles mean those that respond to the environmental changes or to the adscititious physical or physiological processes to regulate the behavior of the micelles themselves and the release behaviors of the drugs from the micelles. The affected part of the body generally suffers some kinds of physiological changes such as higher temperature, lower pH value, and specific type of proteins compared with the normal tissues. Making use of this unconventionality, scientists designed and developed special drug delivery systems to control the drug release processes that specifically respond to certain kinds of diseases. On the other hand, adscititious processes can also be applied to certain affected sites of the body to enhance the accumulation of drug-loaded carriers and accelerate the release of the drugs from the carriers, thus to tone up the curative effect. Here, some examples of the "smart" micelle drug delivery systems are introduced.

In a polymeric micelle drug delivery design, DOX was chemically conjugated to the terminal end of a di-block copolymer of PLLA and PEG via two acid-cleavable linkages. DOX was connected to the terminal group of PLLA block in the block copolymer through a hydrazone bond and a *cis*-acotinyl bond. Micelles were prepared by self-assembly of the DOX-conjugated PLLA-PEG block copolymers in aqueous solution. The size of the micelle was about 89.1 nm. The critical micelle concentration (CMC) was about 1.3 mg/ml. In an acidic condition, which is typical in the endosomes after the micelle uptake by the tumor cell endocytosis process, the conjugated DOX in the hydrazone linkage was readily cleaved, releasing the intact drug from the micelles. This micelle drug delivery system was more potent in cell cytotoxicity than free DOX [215].

Another intracellular pH-sensitive polymeric micelle drug carrier that controls the systemic, local, and subcellular distributions of pharmacologically active drugs was reported by Bae et al. [216]. The micelle carriers composed of the block copolymers of PEG and poly(aspartic acid). The anticancer drug, adriamycin, was conjugated to the side carboxylic acid groups of poly(aspartic acid) block through acid-sensitive hydrazone linkers. Under physiological conditions (pH 7.4), the hydrophobic interaction of DOX induces the poly(aspartic acid) block aggregates to form a core-structure and the PEG segments the shell structure. The micelles can stably preserve drugs in this formation. When the micelles uptake was through endocytosis of the cell, the drugs were released by sensing the intracellular pH decrease in endosomes (pH 5–6). The experimental data clearly showed that this system has intracellular pH-triggered drug release capability, can be enrolled into tumor cells, and effectively fordo tumor cells with extremely low side effects.

pH-sensitive polymeric mixed micelles were prepared by mixing poly(L-histidine) (polyHis)-PEG block copolymer and PLLA-PEG block copolymers. The micelles showed accelerated DOX release as the pH decreased. The blending of PLLA-PEG block copolymer with polyHis-PEG block copolymer shifted the triggering pH of the DOX to a lower value. Depending on the amount of PLLA-PEG, the triggering pH for adriamycin release from the mixed micelles was destabilized range of 7.2–6.6. The micelles were further conjugated with folic acid, resulting more effective tumor cell killing due to folate receptor–mediated tumor uptake. The polyHis can promote effective cytosolic ADR delivery into cell plasma by virtue of fusogenic activity [217].

Many other pH-sensitive micelles were designed from dendritic polymers [218], block copolymer of PEG and polyacrylates [219], and block copolymers of PEG and hydrophobic poly ethers [220], and other kinds of block copolymers have been reported. These systems aimed at forming stable micelles in aqueous solution at physiological neutral pH but to disintegrate to release the loaded drugs at mildly acidic pH following the break of pH-sensitive bonds that conjugate the drugs with the carriers. In general, these formulations showed exciting results in the *in vitro* evaluation using tumor cells or cell lines [204,221,222]. Some of these systems showed improved release control over *in vivo* examinations using animal model bearing tumor tissue. Their promise as a new generation of advanced drug delivery carriers has attracted the interest of scientists and researchers working on drug delivery systems and in pharmaceutical science, polymeric science, and other related research fields.

Temperature-sensitive micelles are another extensively investigated series of "smart" micelle carriers. Poly(*N*-isopropylacrylamide) (PNIPAAm) showed thermally sensitive phase transfer from hydrophobic to hydrophilic with the increase of temperature. Copolymer of PNIPAAm and other blocks can be synthesized through RAFT, ATRP, and other kinds of living radical copolymerization. One concept of the thermo-sensitive micelles utilizes the phase transfer of PNIPAAm. PNIPAAm acts as hydrophilic blocks at lower temperature. As the temperature rises, the PNIPAAm is transferred into hydrophobic and the micelles shrink to release the drugs. The infected sites or tumor tissues generally have some thermo phenomena and higher temperature than normal tissues; when the temperature-sensitive micelles are transferred into these positions, the drugs are accelerated to release, while the release might be rather lower in the normal tissue and blood circulation where the temperature is at the normal physiological level.

Liu et al. reported thermally sensitive block copolymers of PNIPAAm-c-PDMAAm and PLGA with different compositions and lengths of PLGA block. DOX was loaded into the copolymer micelles by a membrane dialysis method for targeted anticancer drug delivery. The micelles are spherical and have clear core-shell structure with size below 200 nm. The lower critical solution temperature (LCST) of the micelles observed from the various polymers is around 39°C in phophate-buffered solution (PBS). The DOX-loaded micelles are stable in PBS containing serum at 37°C. When temperature rises to 39.5°C, the micelles disappear, triggering the release of DOX. At 37°C, the micelles penetrate the cell membrane by endocytosis and accumulate mostly in cytoplasm. At a temperature above the LCST, more DOX molecules release from the micelles and enter the nuclei compared with the temperature below the LCST, thus showing greater cytotoxicity at a temperature above the LCST [223].

Chung et al. prepared DOX-loaded micelles from block copolymers of PNIPAAm and poly(butylmethacrylate) (PBMA). The micelle inner core is formed by self-aggregates of PBMA blocks with loaded drug (DOX), and the outer shell is formed from PIPAAm chains. The thermal-sensitive PNIPAAm outer shell plays a stabilizing role at physiological temperature and initiates micellar thermo-response at higher temperature. This system is expected to be able to achieve a combination of spatial specificity in a passive manner with a stimuli-responsive targeting mechanism. After optimizing the conditions of synthesis and micelle formation fabrication, the outer shell hydrophilicity can be suddenly switched to hydrophobic at a specific site by local temperature increase beyond the LCST (32.5°C). The DOX-loaded micelles showed a dramatic thermo-responsive on/off switching behavior for both drug release and *in vitro* cytotoxicity [224].

10.5   ENCAPSULATION OF BIOLOGICAL CELLS

Microencapsulation of cells has applications in cell transplantation [225], cell-based drug delivery [226], gene delivery [227], and culture in bioreactors [228]. Before encapsulation of the cells, the idea was tested by microencapsulation of cell lysates in aqueous environment through semiper-meable nylon microcapsules [229]. Later, living cells and tissues were successfully encapsulated in biocompatible capsules (e.g., alginate/polylysine), and they were still able to grow and flourish [230]. The commonly used techniques for cell encapsulation include ionic gelation, interfacial phase inversion, *in situ* polymerization, and complex coacervation [231]. Obviously, microcapsules need to be biocompatible and semipermeable, and permeability should be controlled during fabrica-tion for different applications. It has been found that multilayered microcapsules can give a better environment for cell functions than a single layer encapsulation [225,232].

LbL self-assembly offers a simple and easy method in producing multilayered shells for encap-sulation of biological cells and even viruses. Advantages of this technique include capsule perme-ability control, a broad choice of biopolymers, and precise control shell structures at a molecular level. We have demonstrated that polyelectrolytes, nanoparticles, and antibodies can be assembled on biological cells, for example, bovine platelets [233]. In that study, bovine platelets were coated with 78 nm silica nanoparticles, 45 nm fluorescent nanospheres, or bovine immunoglobulin G (IgG) through LbL assembly by alternate adsorption with oppositely charged linear polyions. It is known that platelets are covered with different glycoproteins, most of which are negatively charged at physiological pH environment [234]. Sequential deposition on platelet surfaces of cationic PDDA and anionic PSS was followed by adsorption of nanoparticles or immunoglobulin. A platelet coated with a shell of [PDDA/PSS/PDDA + (silica/PDDD)$_2$] was viewed under a transmission electron microscope (Figure 10.8). Clearly, the platelet was fully covered with 78 nm silica nanoparti-cles. Successful labeling of bovine IgG on platelets through LbL self-assembly was verified with antibovine IgG-FITC labeling.

For immune protection of artificial tissue, LbL microencapsulation of pancreatic islet was tested to avoid life-long immune suppression [235]. Krol et al. demonstrated that different polyca-tions (PAH or PDDA) could be alternatively attached on human pancreatic islets with PSS. All synthetic polyelectrolyte solutions were prepared with a concentration of 2 mg/mL by solving it in RPMI 1640 medium 1 day in advance. During encapsulation process, the islet pellets were collected by low-speed centrifugation and the medium was exchanged with polyelectrolyte solution. Release of insulin and immune assay were used to characterize the function of the islets after encapsulation as well as the permeability of the capsule, and the protection capability of the capsule was proved. Thus, LbL self-assembly technique may provide an effective alternative for artificial tissue nano-encapsulation with immune protection.

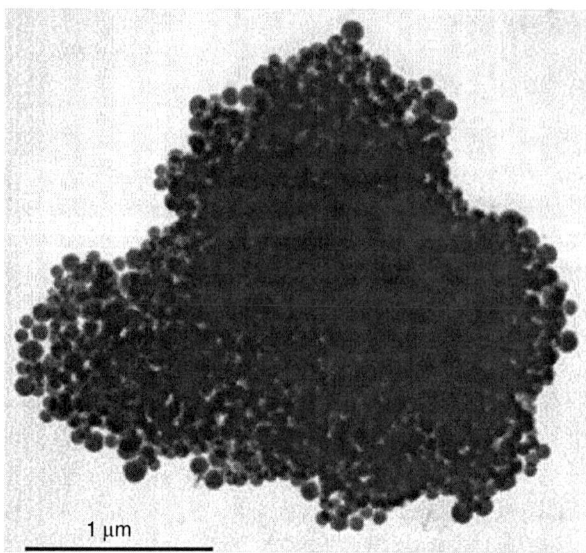

FIGURE 10.8   TEM image of a bovine platelet covered with PDDA/PSS/PDDA + (silica/PDDD)$_2$ indicating the platelet surface is totally covered with 78 nm silica. (From Ai, H., Fang, M., Jones, S.A., and Lvov, Y., *Biomacromolecules*, 3, 560–564, 2002. With permission.)

10.6   CONCLUSIONS

1. LbL self-assembly is a simple and reliable method for nanocoating of any surfaces with organized multilayers of known architectures with precisely located layers of polymers, proteins, nanoparticles, and DNA. A film thickness may be from five to hundreds of nanometers, and they may be deposited on surfaces of any shape and area. Such coating may modify the surface of a support, for example, to vary its wettability from super-hydrophobic to super-hydrophilic. Specific features to provide biocompatibility and promotion or prevent cell growth can be developed. This approach is prospective for coating of nonhomogenous biological surfaces, including blood vessels and bones, as well as for biocompatible coating of medical implants.

2. An application of LbL self-assembly to micro- and nano-cores allowed encapsulation of tiny cores such as drug microparticles, biological cells, and viruses. Therefore, such coating enables the controlled release of materials from microcores (drug) and the changing of their surface properties, providing enhanced colloidal stability and protection of the interior against microbial attacks, proteolytic agents, and oxidation.

3. An LbL assembly of shells on microcores that are later dissolved (weakly cross-linked cores or inorganic cores such as $MnCO_3$) enabled production of empty microshells with semipermeable walls of 20–100 nm thickness and diameter from 50 to 5000 nm. This micro- or nanocapsules may be loaded with proteins or DNA for targeted and controlled delivery. Besides, polymeric replicas of biological cells and viruses may be produced.

4. Architectural micro- and nanoshell sensors based on smart location design of fluorescent indicators (usually in the core) and enzymatic detection layers (usually in the outer shell) enabled production of simple biocolloids capable for semiquantitative detection of glucose, lactose, urea, and other materials, which are specific substrates for the corresponding biocatalytical reactions.

5. Polymeric micelle drug delivery carriers provide possible therapies for many diseases that are difficult to treat. The carrier materials used for preparing micelles include not only amphiphilic block copolymers, but synthetic and natural materials such as polysaccharides and proteins. New concepts and functions are under investigation to make micelle carriers more intelligent and effective. Besides traditional cytotoxic agents, micelles are used to incorporate genes, photodynamic agents, antibodies, peptides, and proteins.

ACKNOWLEDGMENTS

H. Ai acknowledges support from a Chinese National 973 Project (No. 2005CB623903) and CNSF funding (30570514 & 50603015).

REFERENCES

1. L. L. Hench and J. M. Polak, *Science* **295**, 1014 (2002).
2. G. Decher, *Science* **277**, 1232 (1997).
3. N. A. Kotov, *NanoStruct. Mater.* **12**, 789 (1999).
4. Y. Lvov, in *Protein Architecture: Interfacing Molecular Assemblies and Immobilization Biotechnology* Y. Lvov, H. Mohwald, Eds., Marcel Dekker, New York, 2000, pp. 125–168.
5. H. Ai, S. A. Jones and Y. M. Lvov, *Cell. Biochem. Biophys.* **39**, 23 (2003).
6. T. Salditt and U. S. Schubert, *J. Biotechnol.* **90**, 55 (2002).
7. D. G. Shchukin, G. B. Sukhorukov and H. Mohwald, Angew. *Chem. Int. Ed. Engl.* **42**, 4472 (2003).
8. G. Ibarz, L. Dahne, E. Donath and H. Mohwald, *Adv. Mater.* **13**, 1324 (2001).
9. C. S. Peyratout and L. Dahne, *Angew. Chem. Int. Ed. Engl.* **43**, 3762 (2004).
10. R. K. Iler, *J. Colloid Interf. Sci.* **21**, 569–594 (1966).
11. G. Decher and J.D. Hong, Ber. Bunsenges. *Phys. Chem.* **95**, 1430 (1991).
12. G. Decher, Y. Lvov and J. Schmitt, *Thin Solid Films* **244**, 772 (1994).
13. Y. Lvov, G. Decher and H. Mohwald, *Langmuir* **9**, 481 (1993).
14. Y. Lvov, G. Decher and G. B. Sukhorukov, *Macromolecules* **26**, 5396 (1993).
15. Y. Lvov, H. Haas, G. Decher, H. Mohwald and A. Kalachev, *J. Phys. Chem.* **97**, 12835 (1993).
16. Y. Lvov, H. Haas, G. Decher, H. Mohwald, A. Michailov, B. Mtchedlishvily, E. Morgunova and B. Vainshtain, *Langmuir* **10**, 4232 (1994).
17. G. Schneider and G. Decher, *Nano Lett.* **4**, 1833 (2004).
18. Y. Lvov, K. Ariga and T. Kunitake, *J. Am. Chem. Soc.* **117**, 6117 (1995).
19. G. Decher, B. Lehr, K. Lowack, Y. Lvov and J. Schmitt, *Biosens. Bioelectron.* **9**, 677 (1994).
20. M. Sano, Y. Lvov and T. Kunitake, *Annu. Rev. Mater. Sci.* **26**, 153 (1996).
21. W. B. Stockton and M. F. Rubner, *Macromolecules* **30**, 2717 (1997).
22. S. A. Sukhishvili, *Macromolecules* **35**, 301 (2002).
23. P. Berndt, K. Kurihara and T. Kunitake, *Langmuir* **8**, 2486 (1992).
24. Y. Lvov and G. Decher, *Crystallogr. Rep.* **39**, 628 (1994).
25. J. H. Cheung, A. F. Fou and M. F. Rubner, *Thin Solid Films* **244**, 985 (1994).
26. M. Ferreira and M. F. Rubner, *Macromolecules* **28**, 7107 (1995).
27. H. Ai, Y. M. Lvov, D. K. Mills, M. Jennings, J. S. Alexander and S. A. Jones, *Cell Biochem. Biophys.* **38**, 103 (2003).
28. C. Boura, S. Muller, D. Vautier, D. Dumas, P. Schaaf, J. C. Voegel, J. F. Stoltz and P. Menu, *Biomaterials* **26**, 4568 (2005).
29. Y. Lvov, A. Antipov, A. Mamedov, H. Mohwald and G. B. Sukhorukov, *Nano Lett.* **1**, 125 (2001).
30. G. B. Sukhorukov, A. Antipov, A. Voigt, E. Donath and H. Mohwald, *Macromol. Rapid Commun.* **22**, 44 (2001).
31. A. Schneider, C. Picart, B. Senger, P. Schaaf, J. C. Voegel and B. Frisch, *Langmuir* **23**, 2655 (2007).
32. M. E. Nimni and R. D. Harkness, in *Collagen Vol. I Biochemistry* M. E. Nimni, Ed. (CRC Press, Boca Raton, FL, 1988), vol. I, pp. 1–79.
33. K. E. Kadler, D. F. Holmes, J. A. Trotter and J. A. Chapman, *J. Biochem.* **316 (Pt 1)**, 1 (1996).
34. G. Grant, D. S. Koktysh, B. Yun, R. L. Matts and N. A. Kotov, *Biomed. Microdev.* **3**, 301 (2001).

35. V. A. Sinani, D. S. Koktysh, B. Yun, R. L. Matts, T. C. Pappas, M. Motamedi, S. N. Thomas and N. A. Kotov, *Nano Lett.* **3**, 1177 (2003).
36. Z. Tang, N. A. Kotov, S. Magonov and B. Ozturk, *Nat. Mater.* **2**, 413 (2003).
37. D. Kommireddy, Y. Lvov and D. K. Mills, *J. Biomed. Nanotech.* **3**, 286 (2005).
38. Y. Lvov, R. Price, B. Gaber and I. Ichinose, *Colloids Surf.* A **198**, 375 (2002).
39. A. P. Johnston, A. N. Zelikin, L. Lee and F. Caruso, *Anal. Chem.* **78**, 5913 (2006).
40. K. A. Marx, *Biomacromolecules* **4**, 1099 (2003).
41. G. Z. Sauerbrey, *Z. Phys.* **155**, 206 (1959).
42. P. Rajagopalan, C. J. Shen, F. Berthiaume, A. W. Tilles, M. Toner and M. L. Yarmush, *Tissue Eng.* **12**, 1553 (2006).
43. J. Schmitt, T. Grünewald, K. Kjaer, P. Pershan, G. Decher and M. Lösche, *Macromolecules* **26**, 7058 (1993).
44. P. A. Suci, J. D. Vrany and M. W. Mittelman, *Biomaterials* **19**, 327 (1998).
45. K. K. Chittur, *Biomaterials* **19**, 357 (1998).
46. A. F. Xie and S. Granick, *Macromolecules* **35**, 1805 (2002).
47. E. Kharlampieva and S. A. Sukhishvili, *Macromolecules* **36**, 9950 (2003).
48. M. Muller, B. Kessler and K. Lunkwitz, *J. Phys. Chem.* B **107**, 8189 (2003).
49. M. Debreczeny, V. Ball, F. Boulmedais, B. Szalontai, J. Voegel and P. Schaaf, *J. Phys. Chem.* B **107**, 12734 (2003).
50. E. Donath, G. B. Sukhorukov, F. Caruso, S. A. Davis and H. Mohwald, *Angew. Chem. Int. Ed. Engl.* **37**, 2201 (1998).
51. H. Ai, J. J. Pink, X. Shuai, D. A. Boothman and J. Gao, *J. Biomed. Mater. Res.* **73A**, 303 (2005).
52. M. Schneider, M. Zhu, G. Papastavrou, S. Akari and H. Mohwald, *Langmuir* **18**, 602 (2002).
53. M. Zhu, S. Akari and H. Mohwald, *Nano Lett.* **1**, 569 (2001).
54. O. Mermut, J. Lefebvre, D. G. Gray and C. J. Barrett, *Macromolecules* **36**, 8819 (2003).
55. C. Picart, J. Mutterer, L. Richert, Y. Luo, G. D. Prestwich, P. Schaaf, J. C. Voegel and P. Lavalle, *Proc. Natl Acad. Sci. U.S.* A **99**, 12531 (2002).
56. G. Ibarz, L. Dahne, E. Donath and H. Mohwald, *Chem. Mater.* **14**, 4059 (2002).
57. Q. Tan, J. Ji, M. A. Barbosa, C. Fonseca and J. Shen, *Biomaterials* **24**, 4699 (2003).
58. B. Thierry, F. M. Winnik, Y. Merhi, J. Silver and M. Tabrizian, *Biomacromolecules* **4**, 1564 (2003).
59. H. Ai, H. Meng, I. Ichinose, S. A. Jones, D. K. Mills, Y. M. Lvov and X. Qiao, *J. Neurosci. Methods* **128**, 1 (2003).
60. J. Anderson, *Annu. Rev. Mater. Res.* **31**, 81 (2001).
61. M. C. Berg, S. Y. Yang, P. T. Hammond and M. F. Rubner, *Langmuir* **20**, 1362 (2004).
62. J. S. Mohammed, M. A. DeCoster and M. J. McShane, *Biomacromolecules* **5**, 1745 (2004).
63. C. Boura, P. Menu, E. Payan, C. Picart, J. C. Voegel, S. Muller and J. F. Stoltz, *Biomaterials* **24**, 3521 (2003).
64. A. Khademhosseini, K. Y. Suh, J. M. Yang, G. Eng, J. Yeh, S. Levenberg and R. Langer, *Biomaterials* **25**, 3583 (2004).
65. S. Kidambi, I. Lee and C. Chan, *J. Am. Chem. Soc.* **126**, 16286 (2004).
66. L. Richert, F. Boulmedais, P. Lavalle, J. Mutterer, E. Ferreux, G. Decher, P. Schaaf, J. C. Voegel and C. Picart, *Biomacromolecules* **5**, 284 (2004).
67. D. S. Salloum, S. G. Olenych, T. C. S. Keller and J. B. Schlenoff, *Biomacromolecules* **6**, 161 (2005).
68. J. Zhang, B. Senger, D. Vautier, C. Picart, P. Schaaf, J. C. Voegel and P. Lavalle, *Biomaterials* **26**, 3353 (2005).
69. Y. Zhu, C. Gao, T. He, X. Liu and J. Shen, *Biomacromolecules* **4**, 446 (2003).
70. T. Okada and Y. Ikada, *J. Biomater. Sci. Polym. Ed.* **7**, 171 (1995).
71. G. H. Hsiue, S. D. Lee, C. C. Wang and P. C. Chang, *J. Biomater. Sci. Polym. Ed.* **5**, 205 (1993).
72. S. D. Lee, G. H. Hsiue, C. Y. Kao and P. C. Chang, *Biomaterials* **17**, 587 (1996).
73. H. Ai, D. K. Mills, A. S. Jonathan and S. A. Jones, *In Vitro Cell Dev. Biol. Anim.* **38**, 487 (2002).
74. J. J. Cunningham, J. Nikolovski, J. J. Linderman and D. J. Mooney, *Biotechniques* **32**, 876 (2002).
75. W. Chen and T. J. McCarthy, *Macromolecules* **30**, 78 (1997).
76. J. Levasalmi and T. J. McCarthy, *Macromolecules* **30**, 1752–1757 (1997).
77. G. A. Silva, *Nat. Rev. Neurosci.* **7**, 65 (2006).
78. B. D. Ratner and S. J. Bryant, *Annu. Rev. Biomed. Eng.* **6**, 41 (2004).
79. B. D. Ratner, *Biosens. Bioelectron.* **10**, 797 (1995).
80. B. D. Ratner, *J. Biomed. Mater. Res.* **27**, 837 (1993).

81. Y. Qiu, L. C. Winterton, J. M. Lally and Y. Matsuzawa, U. S. P. Office, Ed. (Novartis AG, U.S.A., 2005), vol. 6, 896, 926.
82. M. N. Babapulle and M. J. Eisenberg, *Circulation* **106**, 2734 (2002).
83. D. Voet and J. G. Voet, *Biochemistry*, John Wiley & Sons, Inc., New York, 2nd Edition, 1995, pp. 264–265.
84. B. Heublein, E. G. Evagorou, R. Rohde, S. Ohse, R. R. Meliss, S. Barlach and A. Haverich, *Int. J. Artif. Organs* **25**, 1166 (2002).
85. M. Morra, *J. Biomater. Sci. Polym. Ed.* **11**, 547 (2000).
86. B. Thierry, F. M. Winnik, Y. Merhi and M. Tabrizian, *J. Am. Chem. Soc.* **125**, 7494 (2003).
87. B. Thierry, P. Kujawa, C. Tkaczyk, F. M. Winnik, L. Bilodeau and M. Tabrizian, *J. Am. Chem. Soc.* **127**, 1626 (2005).
88. K. Ariga, M. Onda, Y. Lvov and T. Kunitake, *Chem. Lett.* **26**, 25 (1997).
89. R. Duncan, *Nat. Rev. Drug Discov.* **2**, 347 (2003).
90. K. C. Nicolaou, C. Riemer, M. A. Kerr, D. Rideout and W. Wrasidlo, *Nature* **364**, 464 (1993).
91. H. A. Biebuyck and G. M. Whitesides, *Langmuir* **10**, 2790 (1994).
92. R. Singhvi, A. Kumar, G. P. Lopez, G. N. Stephanopoulos, D. I. Wang, G. M. Whitesides and D. E. Ingber, *Science* **264**, 696 (1994).
93. G. M. Whitesides, E. Ostuni, S. Takayama, X. Jiang and D. E. Ingber, *Annu. Rev. Biomed. Eng.* **3**, 335 (2001).
94. K. Chen, X. Jiang, L. Kimerling and P. T. Hammond, *Langmuir* **16**, 7825 (2000).
95. F. Hua, T. Cui and Y. Lvov, *Langmuir* **18**, 6712 (2002).
96. S. Liu, R. Maoz, G. Schmid and J. Sagiv, *Nano Lett.* **2**, 1055 (2002).
97. B. Michel, A. Bernard, A. Bietsch, E. Delamarche, M. Geissler, D. Juncker, H. Kind, J. P. Renault, R. Rothuizen, H. Schmid, P. Schmidt-winkel, R. Stutz and H. Wolf, *IBM J. Res. Dev.* **45,** 697 (2001).
98. V. Santhanam and R. P. Andres, *Nano Lett.* **4**, 41 (2004).
99. M. H. V. Werts, M. Lambert, J.P. Bourgoin and M. Brust, *Nano Lett.* **2**, 43 (2002).
100. S. Y. Yang and M. F. Rubner, *J. Am. Chem. Soc.* **124**, 2100 (2002).
101. F.Hua, J. Shi, Y. Lvov and T. Cui, *Nano Lett.* **2**, 1219 (2002).
102. H. D. Inerowicz, S. Howell, F. E. Regnier and R. Reifenberger, *Langmuir* **18**, 5263 (2002).
103. R. Langer, *Nature* **392**, 5 (1998).
104. D. A. LaVan, D. M. Lynn and R. Langer, *Nat. Rev. Drug Discov.* **1**, 77 (2002).
105. A. M. Klibanov and J. A. Schefiliti, *Biotechnol. Lett.* **26**, 1103 (2004).
106. S. C. Tsinontides, P. Rajniak, D. Pham, W. A. Hunke, J. Placek and S. D. Reynolds, *Int. J. Pharm.* **280**, 1 (2004).
107. W. Wang, *Int. J. Pharm.* **203**, 1 (2000).
108. D. B. Shenoy and G. B. Sukhorukov, *Eur. J. Pharm. Biopharm.* **58**, 521 (2004).
109. G. Walsh, *Nat. Biotechnol.* **21**, 865 (2003).
110. J. L. Cleland, A. Daugherty and R. Mrsny, *Curr. Opin. Biotechnol.* **12**, 212 (2001).
111. T. Arakawa, S. J. Prestrelski, W. C. Kenney and J. F. Carpenter, *Adv. Drug. Deliv. Rev.* **46**, 307 (2001).
112. F. Caruso, R. A. Caruso and H. Mohwald, *Science* **282**, 1111 (1998).
113. G. Sukhorukov, in *Dendrimers, Assemblies, Nanocomposites* R. Arshady, A. Guyot, Eds., Citus Books, London, 2002, vol. 5, pp. 111–147.
114. K. Kataoka, A. Harada and Y. Nagasaki, *Adv. Drug Deliv. Rev.* **47**, 113 (2001).
115. V. P. Torchilin, *Adv. Drug Deliv. Rev.* **54**, 235 (2002).
116. A. Antipov, G. B. Sukhorukov, E. Donath and H. Mohwald, *J. Phys. Chem. B* **105**, 2281 (2001).
117. A. I. Petrov, A. V. Gavryushkin and G. B. Sukhorukov, *J. Phys. Chem. B* **107**, 868 (2003).
118. E. Donath, S. Moya, B. Neu, G. B. Sukhorukov, R. Georgieva, A. Voigt, H. B. Pumler, H. Kiesewetter and H. Mohwald, *Chem. Eur. J.* **8**, 5481 (2002).
119. Z. Lu, M. D. Prouty, Z. Guo, V. O. Golub, C. S. S. R. Kumar and Y. M. Lvov, *Langmuir* **21**, 2042 (2005).
120. O. P. Tiourina, A. Antipov, G. B. Sukhorukov, N. I. Larionova, Y. Lvov and H. Mohwald, *Macromol. Biosci.* **1**, 209 (2001).
121. O. P. Tiourina and G. Sukhorukov, *Int. J. Pharm.* **242**, 155 (2002).
122. N. G. Balabushevich, O. P. Tiourina, D. V. Volodkin, N. I. Larionova and G. B. Sukhorukov, *Biomacromolecules* **4**, 1191 (2003).
123. C. Gao, X. Liu, J. Shen and H. Mohwald, *Chem. Commun.* **17**, 1928 (2002).
124. H. Zhu and M. J. McShane, *Langmuir* **21**, 424 (2005).
125. D. G. Shchukin, T. Shutava, E. Shchukina, G. B. Sukhorukov and Y. Lvov, *Chem. Mater.* **16**, 3446 (2004).

126. D. V. Volodkin, N. I. Larionova and G. B. Sukhorukov, *Biomacromolecules* **5**, 1962 (2004).
127. D. V. Volodkin, A. I. Petrov, M. Prevot and G. B. Sukhorukov, *Langmuir* **20**, 3398 (2004).
128. A. N. Zelikin, Q. Li and F. Caruso, *Angew. Chem. Int. Ed. Engl.* **45**, 7743 (2006).
129. S. Ye, C. Wang, X. Liu, Z. Tong, B. Ren and F. Zeng, *J. Control. Release* **112**, 79 (2006).
130. I. F. Tannock and D. Rotin, *Cancer Res.* **49**, 4373 (1989).
131. J. D. Mendelsohn, C. J. Barret, V. V. Chan, A. J. Pal, A. M. Mayes and M. F. Rubner, *Langmuir* **16**, 5017 (2000).
132. O. H. Lowry, N. J. Rosebrough, A. L. Farr and R. J. Randall, *J. Biol. Chem.* **193**, 265 (1951).
133. M. J. Dunn, in *Protein Purification Methods*, E. L. V. Harris, S. Angal, Eds., IRL Press, Oxford, 1992.
134. N. C. Price, *Proteins Labfax*, Academic Press, Oxford, 1996, pp. 27–30.
135. M. Babincova, P. Cicmanec, V. Altanerova, C. Altaner and P. Babinec, *Bioelectrochemistry* **55**, 17 (2002).
136. J. Kost, J. Wolfrum and R. Langer, *J. Biomed. Mater. Res.* **21**, 1367 (1987).
137. M. Fang, P. S. Grant, M. J. McShane, G. B. Sukhorukov, V. O. Golub and Y. M. Lvov, *Langmuir* **18**, 6338 (2002).
138. D. A. Edwards, A. Ben-Jebria and R. Langer, *J. Appl. Physiol.* **85**, 379 (1998).
139. D. A. Edwards, J. Hanes, G. Caponetti, J. Hrkach, A. Ben-Jebria, M. L. Eskew, J. Mintzes, D. Deaver, N. Lotan and R. Langer, *Science* **276**, 1868 (1997).
140. M. Onda, K. Ariga and T. Kunitake, *J. Biosci. Bioeng.* **87**, 69 (1999).
141. J. Yuan, S. Zhou, B. You and L. Wu, *Chem. Mater.* **17**, 3587 (2005).
142. T. G. Shutava, D. S. Kommireddy and Y. M. Lvov, *J. Am. Chem. Soc.* **128**, 9926 (2006).
143. D. G. Shchukin, A. A. Patel, G. B. Sukhorukov and Y. Lvov, *J. Am. Chem. Soc.* **126**, 3374 (2004).
144. C. Schuler and F. Caruso, *Biomacromolecules* **2**, 921 (2001).
145. D. M. Gray, R. L. Ratliff and M. R. Vaughan, *Methods Enzymol.* **211**, 389 (1992).
146. A. Jen and H. P. Merkle, *Pharm. Res.* **18**, 1483 (2001).
147. S. K. Basu, C. P. Govardhan, C. W. Jung and A. L. Margolin, *Expert Opin. Biol. Ther.* **4**, 301 (2004).
148. A. L. Daugherty and R. J. Mrsny, *Expert Opin. Biol. Ther.* **3**, 1071 (2003).
149. N. G. Balabushevitch, G. B. Sukhorukov, N. A. Moroz, D. V. Volodkin, N. I. Larionova, E. Donath and H. Mohwald, *Biotechnol. Bioeng.* **76**, 207 (2001).
150. C. Lipinski, *Am. Pharm. Rev.* **5**, 82 (2002).
151. E. Merisko-Liversidge, G. G. Liversidge and E. R. Cooper, *Eur. J. Pharm. Sci.* **18**, 113 (2003).
152. B. E. Rabinow, *Nat. Rev. Drug Discov.* **3**, 785 (2004).
153. H. Ai, S. A. Jones, M. M. de Villiers and Y. M. Lvov, *J. Control. Release* **86**, 59 (2003).
154. X. Qiu, S. Leporatti, E. Donath and H. Mohwald, *Langmuir* **17**, 5375 (2001).
155. A. S. Zahr, M. M. de Villiers and M. V. Pishko, *Langmuir* **21**, 403 (2005).
156. A. Avdeef, C. M. Berger and C. Brownell, *Pharm. Res.* **17**, 85 (2000).
157. F. Caruso, W. Yang, D. Trau and R. Renneberg, *Langmuir* **16**, 8932 (2000).
158. Y. B. Lim, S. O. Han, H. U. Kong, Y. Lee, J. S. Park, B. Jeong and S. W. Kim, *Pharm. Res.* **17**, 811 (2000).
159. A. Maheshwari, R. I. Mahato, J. McGregor, S. Han, W. E. Samlowski, J. S. Park and S. W. Kim, *Mol. Ther.* **2**, 121 (2000).
160. K. C. Wood, J. Q. Boedicker, D. M. Lynn and P. T. Hammond, *Langmuir* **21**, 1603 (2005).
161. Z. An, G. Lu, H. Mohwald and J. Li, *Chemistry* **10**, 5848 (2004).
162. X. Qiu, E. Donath and H. Mohwald, *Macromol. Mater. Eng.* **286**, 591 (2001).
163. M. C. Woodle, *Adv. Drug Deliv. Rev.* **32**, 139 (1998).
164. K. L. Prime and G. M. Whitesides, *Science* **252**, 1164 (1591).
165. F. J. Toublan, S. Boppart and K. S. Suslick, *J. Am. Chem. Soc.* **128**, 3472 (2006).
166. C. Cortez, E. Tomaskovic-Crook, A. Johnston, B. Radt, S. Cody, A. Scott, E. Nice, J. Heath and F. Caruso, *Adv. Mater.* **18**, 1998 (2006).
167. M. L. Adams, A. Lavasanifar and G. S. Kwon, *J. Pharm. Sci.* **92**, 1343 (2003).
168. C. F. van Nostrum, *Adv. Drug Deliv. Rev.* **56**, 9 (2004).
169. A. V. Kabanov and V. Y. Alakhov, *Crit. Rev. Ther. Drug Carrier Syst.* **19**, 1 (2002).
170. A. V. Kabanov, E. V. Batrakova and V. Y. Alakhov, *J. Control. Release* **82**, 189 (2002).
171. E. V. Batrakova, S. Li, D. W. Miller and A. V. Kabanov, *Pharm. Res.* **16**, 1366 (1999).
172. V. I. Slepnev, L. E. Kuznetsova, A. N. Gubin, E. V. Batrakova, V. Alakhov and A. V. Kabanov, *Biochem. Int.* **26**, 587 (1992).
173. A. V. Kabanov, V. I. Slepnev, L. E. Kuznetsova, E. V. Batrakova, V. Alakhov, N. S. Melik-Nubarov, P. G. Sveshnikov and V. A. Kabanov, *Biochem. Int.* **26**, 1035 (1992).

174. N. Y. Rapoport, J. N. Herron, W. G. Pitt and L. Pitina, *J. Control. Release* **58**, 153 (1999).
175. L. M. Han, J. Guo, L. J. Zhang, Q. S. Wang and X. L. Fang, *Acta Pharmacol. Sin.* **27**, 747 (2006).
176. A. A. Exner, T. M. Krupka, K. Scherrer and J. M. Teets, *J. Control. Release* **106**, 188 (2005).
177. G. A. Husseini, D. A. Christensen, N. Y. Rapoport and W. G. Pitt, *J. Control. Release* **83**, 303 (2002).
178. Y. C. Chen, H. D. Liang, Q. P. Zhang, M. J. Blomley and Q. L. Lu, *Ultrasound Med. Biol.* **32**, 131 (2006).
179. J. D. Pruitt and W. G. Pitt, *Drug Deliv.* **9**, 253 (2002).
180. Z. Gao, H. D. Fain and N. Rapoport, *Mol. Pharm.* **1**, 317 (2004).
181. A. Marin, M. Muniruzzaman and N. Rapoport, *J. Control. Release* **75**, 69 (2001).
182. A. Marin, M. Muniruzzaman and N. Rapoport, *J. Control. Release* **71**, 239 (2001).
183. R. Evers, M. Kool, A. J. Smith, L. van Deemter, M. de Haas and P. Borst, *Br. J. Cancer* **83**, 366 (2000).
184. D. W. Miller, E. V. Batrakova and A. V. Kabanov, *Pharm. Res.* **16**, 396 (1999).
185. T. Minko, E. V. Batrakova, S. Li, Y. Li, R. I. Pakunlu, V. Y. Alakhov and A. V. Kabanov, *J. Control. Release* **105**, 269 (2005).
186. A. Marin, H. Sun, G. A. Husseini, W. G. Pitt, D. A. Christensen and N. Y. Rapoport, *J. Control. Release* **84**, 39 (2002).
187. C. Allen, Y. Yu, A. Eisenberg and D. Maysinger, *Biochim. Biophys. Acta* **1421**, 32 (1999).
188. L. Luo, J. Tam, D. Maysinger and A. Eisenberg, *Bioconjug. Chem.* **13**, 1259 (2002).
189. A. Mahmud and A. Lavasanifar, *Colloids Surf. B. Biointerfaces* **45**, 82 (2005).
190. R. T. Liggins and H. M. Burt, *Adv. Drug. Deliv. Rev.* **54**, 191 (2002).
191. E. Piskin, X. Kaitian, E. B. Denkbas and Z. Kucukyavuz, *J. Biomater. Sci. Polym. Ed.* **7**, 359 (1995).
192. X. Shuai, H. Ai, N. Nasongkla, S. Kim and J. Gao, *J. Control. Release* **98**, 415 (2004).
193. H. Lee, F. Zeng, M. Dunne and C. Allen, *Biomacromolecules* **6**, 3119 (2005).
194. S. C. Lee, C. Kim, I. C. Kwon, H. Chung and S. Y. Jeong, *J. Control. Release* **89**, 437 (2003).
195. X. Shuai, T. Merdan, A. K. Schaper, F. Xi and T. Kissel, *Bioconjug. Chem.* **15**, 441 (2004).
196. P. Xu, E. A. Van Kirk, S. Li, W. J. Murdoch, J. Ren, M. D. Hussain, M. Radosz and Y. Shen, *Colloids Surf. B. Biointerfaces* **48**, 50 (2006).
197. N. Nasongkla, X. Shuai, H. Ai, B. D. Weinberg, J. Pink, D. A. Boothman and J. Gao, *Angew. Chem. Int. Ed. Engl.* **43**, 6323 (2004).
198. E. K. Park, S. Y. Kim, S. B. Lee and Y. M. Lee, *J. Control. Release* **109**, 158 (2005).
199. M. L. Forrest, C. Y. Won, A. W. Malick and G. S. Kwon, *J. Control. Release* **110**, 370 (2006).
200. C. Allen, J. Han, Y. Yu, D. Maysinger and A. Eisenberg, *J. Control. Release* **63**, 275 (2000).
201. K. K. Jette, D. Law, E. A. Schmitt and G. S. Kwon, *Pharm. Res.* **21**, 1184 (2004).
202. S. Y. Kim, I. G. Shin and Y. M. Lee, *Biomaterials* **20**, 1033 (1999).
203. A. Lavasanifar, J. Samuel and G. S. Kwon, *Adv. Drug Deliv. Rev.* **54**, 169 (2002).
204. K. Kataoka, T. Matsumoto, M. Yokoyama, T. Okano, Y. Sakurai, S. Fukushima, K. Okamoto and G. S. Kwon, *J. Control. Release* **64**, 143 (2000).
205. K. Kataoka, A. Harada and Y. Nagasaki, *Adv. Drug Deliv. Rev.* **47**, 113 (2001).
206. H. Cabral, N. Nishiyama, S. Okazaki, H. Koyama and K. Kataoka, *J Control Release* **101**, 223 (2005).
207. N. Nishiyama, Y. Kato, Y. Sugiyama and K. Kataoka, *Pharm. Res.* **18**, 1035 (2001).
208. D. Putnam, *Nat. Mater.* **5**, 439 (2006).
209. S. Vinogradov, E. Batrakova, S. Li and A. Kabanov, *Bioconjug. Chem.* **10**, 851 (1999).
210. H. Y. Tian, C. Deng, H. Lin, J. Sun, M. Deng, X. Chen and X. Jing, *Biomaterials* **26**, 4209 (2005).
211. J. H. Jeong and T. G. Park, *J. Control. Release* **82**, 159 (2002).
212. M. Harada-Shiba, K. Yamauchi, A. Harada, I. Takamisawa, K. Shimokado and K. Kataoka, *Gene Ther.* **9**, 407 (2002).
213. D. Wakebayashi, N. Nishiyama, Y. Yamasaki, K. Itaka, N. Kanayama, A. Harada, Y. Nagasaki and K. Kataoka, *J. Control. Release* **95**, 653 (2004).
214. B. Frisch, M. Carriere, C. Largeau, F. Mathey, C. Masson, F. Schuber, D. Scherman and V. Escriou, *Bioconjug. Chem.* **15**, 754 (2004).
215. H. S. Yoo, E. A. Lee and T. G. Park, *J. Control. Release* **82**, 17 (2002).
216. Y. Bae, N. Nishiyama, S. Fukushima, H. Koyama, M. Yasuhiro and K. Kataoka, *Bioconjug. Chem.* **16**, 122 (2005).
217. E. S. Lee, K. Na and Y. H. Bae, *J. Control. Release* **91**, 103 (2003).
218. E. R. Gillies, T. B. Jonsson and J. M. Frechet, *J. Am. Chem. Soc.* **126**, 11936 (2004).
219. V. P. Sant, D. Smith and J. C. Leroux, *J. Control. Release* **97**, 301 (2004).
220. M. Hruby, C. Konak and K. Ulbrich, *J. Control. Release* **103**, 137 (2005).

221. E. R. Gillies and J. M. Frechet, *Chem. Commun. (Camb).* 1640 (2003).
222. M. C. Jones, M. Ranger and J. C. Leroux, *Bioconjug. Chem.* **14**, 774 (2003).
223. S. Q. Liu, Y. W. Tong and Y. Y. Yang, *Biomaterials* **26**, 5064 (2005).
224. J. E. Chung, M. Yokoyama, M. Yamato, T. Aoyagi, Y. Sakurai and T. Okano, *J. Control. Release* **62**, 115 (1999).
225. S. Schneider, P. J. Feilen, V. Slotty, D. Kampfner, S. Preuss, S. Berger, J. Beyer and R. Pommersheim, *Biomaterials* **22**, 1961 (2001).
226. J. J. Vallbacka, J. N. Nobrega and M. V. Sefton, *J. Control. Release* **72**, 93 (2001).
227. I. T. Tai and A. M. Sun, *FASEB J.* **7**, 1061 (1993).
228. A. Bader, E. Knop, K. Boker, N. Fruhauf, W. Schuttler, K. Oldhafer, R. Burkhard, R. Pichlmayr and K. F. Sewing, *Artif. Organs* **19**, 368 (1995).
229. T. Chang, *Science* **146**, 524 (1964).
230. F. Lim and R. D. Moss, *J. Pharm. Sci.* **70**, 351 (1981).
231. H. Uludag, P. De Vos and P. A. Tresco, *Adv. Drug Deliv. Rev.* **42**, 29 (2000).
232. S. M. Chia, A. C. Wan, C. H. Quek, H. Q. Mao, X. Xu, L. Shen, M. L. Ng, K. W. Leong and H. Yu, *Biomaterials* **23**, 849 (2002).
233. H. Ai, M. Fang, S. A. Jones and Y. M. Lvov, *Biomacromolecules* **3**, 560 (2002).
234. J. L. McGregor, K. J. Clemetson, E. James, E. F. Luscher and M. Dechavannne, *Biochim. Biophys. Acta* **599**, 473 (1980).
235. S. Krol, S. delGuerra, M. Grupillo, A. Diaspro, A. Gliozzi and P. Marchetti, *Nano Lett.* **6**, 1933 (2006).

11 Electrohydrodynamic Processing of Micro- and Nanometer Biological Materials

Yiquan Wu and Robert Lewis Clark

CONTENTS

11.1 INTRODUCTION

Electrohydrodynamic processing, in which a solution with a controlled flow rate is pumped into a nozzle to initiate aerosol jets under an electric field, is a novel and cost-effective technique capable of producing particles in a range of micrometer to nanometer scales by altering the processing parameters. Instead of using the inertial forces, a uniform electrohydrodynamic force is used to break up the liquids into fine jets when the charge density on the droplet surface exceeds a critical value known as the Rayleigh limit [1–4]. This process has recently attracted the attention of many researchers, because this technique has been used to prepare both micro- and nanometer architectures with application to patterned materials, bioactive films and coatings, drug-delivery carriers, and particles with controllable structures [5–10].

In a typical electrohydrodynamic process, a liquid precursor is fed through a nozzle and a droplet forms at the nozzle. When a strong electric field is applied over this droplet, a charge is induced on the surface of the droplet. Influenced by the electrostatic field, the droplet at the tip of the nozzle forms a conical-shaped jet. When the electrostatic field is sufficiently strong, the charges on the droplet surface will overcome the surface tension and break up into many charged jets having a controllable size within a narrow distribution [11,12]. This kind of electrohydrodynamic process is called electrospraying.

The atomization modes of electrohydrodynamic processing can be divided into two groups [13]. The first group includes modes in which only fragments of liquid are ejected from the nozzle. This group comprises the dripping mode, microdripping mode, spindle mode, multispindle mode, and ramified-meniscus mode. The second group includes modes in which the liquid ejects from the nozzle in the form of a long continuous jet, which disintegrates into droplets only at some distance from the tip of the nozzle. This group contains cone-jet mode, oscillating-jet mode, procession mode, multijet mode, and ramified-jet mode. The modes of spraying are classified and characterized in terms of the jet and droplet formations. These atomization modes are complicated functions of the applied voltage, the flow rate of the liquid, the nozzle diameter, and the physical properties of the precursors. As the applied field strength increases, the atomization modes can be transformed through a cone jet from a dripping mode to a multijet mode. The single cone-jet mode is the preferred spraying mode because it can offer a uniform, stable, and continuous spraying pattern with a controllable jet size. An outstanding feature of electrospraying is its ability to generate monodispersed droplets, the size of which may vary from hundreds of micrometers to tens of nanometers through optimizing the processing parameters.

11.2 ELECTROSPRAYING

11.2.1 Definition

Electrospraying is a process of generating very fine aerosol droplets through electrostatic charging instead of mechanical forcing. During electrospraying, a liquid solution is pushed through a small capillary or needle that is connected to the positive electrode of a power supply. The power supply electrically charges the liquid to a high voltage and aggregates more and more charge on the droplets. When this charge reaches a critical point, the droplets cannot hold any more electrical charge and therefore become unstable. Eventually, the charged droplets are emitted out of the tip of the capillary or needle and, due to the repelling nature of the charge, form a flume of fine aerosol droplets. These fine droplets are less than 1 µm in diameter and are attracted to an oppositely charged component. When the charged liquid droplets are attracted to the oppositely charged electrode, they shrink rapidly as the solvent evaporates. Therefore, the charge density on the droplet increases to a critical value at which the droplets break up into the tiny aerosol droplets because of the repulsive Coulombic forces. This process can be repeated in the same way until the charge density on the tiny droplets is no longer strong enough to break up the droplets. Figure 11.1 demonstrates the basic principle of electrospraying.

Electrospraying in cone-jet mode is a process in which an electric stress resulting from the surface charges on the liquid droplet transforms the droplet into a conical shape. This transformation occurs when a liquid solution is pumped through a needle at an appropriate flow rate [14]. The liquid droplets form a conical shape because a cylindrical shape can hold more charges than a sphere.

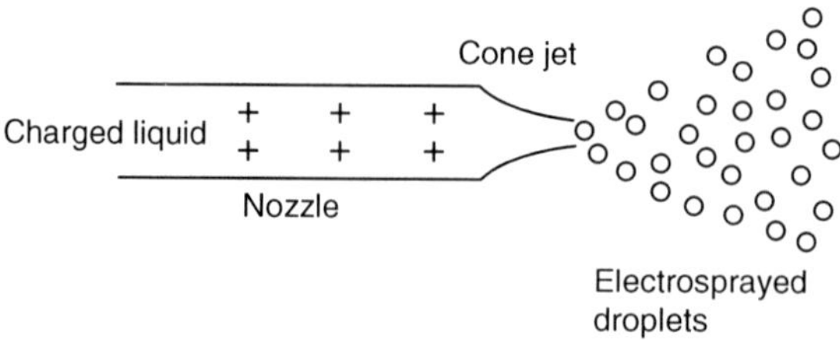

FIGURE 11.1 An illustration of the basic principle of electrospraying.

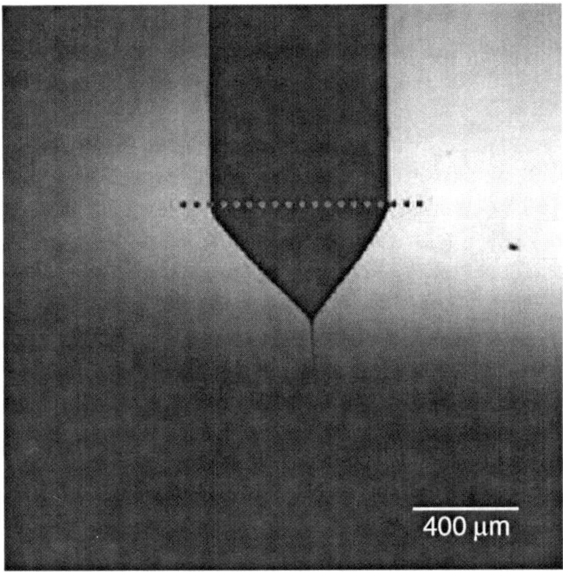

FIGURE 11.2   A photograph of the cone-jet electrospraying pattern. (Reprinted from Samarasinghe, S.R. et al., *Gold Bull.*, 39, 48, 2006. © World Gold Council. With permission.)

Therefore, the applied voltage accelerates the surface charge toward the cone apex so that a jet with a high charge density will be formed at the cone apex. Figure 11.2 shows a diagram of a cone-jet electrospraying pattern. The liquid at the conical tip is emitted into a fine jet, which then becomes unstable and breaks up into a mist of fine aerosol droplets. The aerosol droplets repel each other vigorously, as they are highly charged with the same electrical charge. Consequently, the droplets break into a number of primary and secondary droplets. Electrospraying is a technique used to atomize a liquid solution into charged fine droplets, which allows the generation of aerosol droplets with a controllable droplet size in a narrow size distribution [15].

11.2.2   Background

Rayleigh derived the phenomenon and theory of atomization of liquids into small charged droplets by an electrostatic field a hundred years ago [16]. He found that a charged droplet is unstable and causes the Coulomb fission of the liquid droplet into smaller droplets when the electrohydrodynamic forces caused from the electrostatic charges overcome the balance of the surface tension forces. There is a maximum limit of surface charge density, termed the Rayleigh limit. The relationship between the maximum charge, Q_R, on a droplet and the size of a droplet, d, can be described as follows [17]:

$$Q_R = 8\ \pi(\varepsilon_0 \sigma d^3)^{1/2} \tag{11.1}$$

where ε_0 is the dielectric constant of the liquid and σ is the surface tension of the liquid.

Zeleny was the first researcher to study the electrospraying phenomenon systematically using a capillary-plate experimental configuration in 1917 [18]. He experimented with different electrospraying modes, including the dripping mode, cone-jet mode, and multijet mode with ethanol and glycerin. He was also the first person to take photographic images of electrospraying and provide the first solid scientific description of the process. However, Zeleny did not establish the general rules for boundary values of the processing parameters, such as electrical conductivity, surface tension, and viscosity of electrosprayed solution, as these parameters affect the electrospraying process interactively. He found that it was difficult to establish a cone-jet electrospraying pattern using undistilled water as the electrosprayed precursor but was successful with alcohol, lubricating oil, and distilled water. This is attributed to the low electrical conductivity of alcohol and distilled water.

In between Zeleny's pioneering studies on electrospraying early last century and the research work carried out in 1952 by Vonnegut and Neubauer, who reported the generation of monodispersed aerosol droplets produced by electrospraying, very little knowledge was developed in the field of electrospraying [19]. In 1964, Taylor gave the first explanation and theoretical description of the conical shape of the droplet at the capillary exit by investigating the hydrostatic balance between electrical and surface tension forces [20]. The cone jet is also referred to as a Taylor cone in honor of his contribution to the understanding of electrospraying. In 1982, Joffre et al. developed a mathematical model for calculating the conical shape of a stable droplet at the tip of a capillary under electrospraying, which demonstrated consistency between the experimental data and the modeled results [21]. The equations are based on the balance of the inner pressure of the droplet and the electrical potential distribution between the capillary and a counter-electrode plate. Since then, there have been a number of experiments on the stability limits of the cone-jet mode and on the influences of the liquid properties and the processing parameters. Experiments have also covered the electrostatic conditions of current and the droplet size emitted from an electrified conical point [22–24]. In 1979, Mutoh et al. estimated the upper conductivity limit for a cone jet to be 10^{-5} S/m [25]. Smith, however, investigated the stability of the cone shape based on the onset potential, capillary radius, and liquid conductivity and viscosity and established the upper conductivity limit of a cone jet at 10^{-1} S/m [26]. In 1999, Hartman et al. developed a model to calculate the shape of a cone jet [27]. This model is also capable of calculating surface charge density and the values of the electric field both inside and outside the cone jet.

The electric current of the electrospraying system can be calculated from the developed model. In particular, Tang et al. experimentally defined the stability of the cone jet in the voltage–liquid flow rate $(V - Q)$ plane in 1994 [28]. For a given liquid, the voltage and the liquid flow rate are the two primary independent variables. In 1994, Fernandez et al. studied the electric current and the cone-jet droplet size based on the liquid properties, the flow rate of the solution, the electric potentials, and the configuration of the system [29]. They established the following equation to describe the relationship coupling the electric current I of the electrospraying with the flow rate of solution Q and the physical properties of the solution:

$$I = f(\varepsilon)(\gamma Q K/\varepsilon)^{1/2} \tag{11.2}$$

where K is the electrical conductivity of the solution, ε the relative permittivity of the solution, γ the surface tension of the solution, and the function $f(\varepsilon)$ is experimentally determined.

In 1997, Gañán et al. carried out an experimental measurement of the current and the size of the primary droplets by electrospraying a variety of liquids with different electrical conductivities, surface tension, permittivities, densities, and viscosities [30]. They derived scaling laws for the spray currents as well as the charges and sizes of the droplets based on a theoretical model of charge transport. Their results show that the current and size of the droplets generated through electrospraying solutions with higher viscosity and conductivity exhibit different behavior from those liquids with lower viscosity and conductivity. These experimental results fit theoretical predictions very well. The separation between both behaviors is governed by the dimensionless parameters determined by the liquid viscosity, conductivity, and surface tension of the solution:

$$D = \left[\frac{\gamma^3 \varepsilon_0^2}{\mu K^2 Q}\right]^{1/3} \tag{11.3}$$

where γ is the liquid surface tension, ε_0 the permittivity of the vacuum, μ the liquid viscosity, K the liquid electrical conductivity, and Q the liquid flow rate. Gañán found a square root dependence of

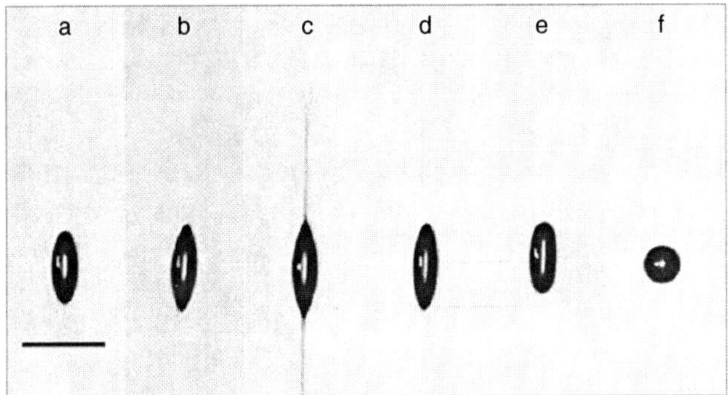

FIGURE 11.3   The disintegration process of levitated microdroplets. Scale bar—100 µm. (Reprinted from Duft, D. et al., *Nature*, 421, 128, 2003. © Nature Publishing Group. With permission.)

the current from the flow rate of the solution $(I \sim Q^{1/2})$ when $D < 1$ (high conductivity and viscosity liquids) and a fourth root dependence of the current from the flow rate $(I \sim Q^{1/4})$ when $D > 1$ (low conductivity and viscosity).

The multijet electrospraying mode has been observed by Shtern et al., Jaworek et al., and others [31–35]. Only Jaworek et al. developed a stability map in the voltage–flow rate $(V - Q)$ plane. Such tremendous research studies have attracted the attention of many researchers who are interested in the principles and potential application of electrospraying. In 1994, Cloupeau et al. described and explained the different electrospraying patterns in terms of the electric potentials, the physical properties and the flow rate of the liquid, and the setup geometry of the system [36]. When the physical properties of the solution and the parameters of the process are proper, a conical meniscus is formed at the exit of the capillary to produce fine aerosol jets. In 2003, Duft et al. visualized the Rayleigh droplet breakup using a high-speed camera [37]. Figure 11.3 shows high-speed imaging of the disintegration of a levitated droplet charged to the Rayleigh limit. The results revealed that an ethylene glycol droplet with an initial radius of 58 µm was captured using the camera, and the droplet became unstable and emitted fine jets when it reached the size of 24 µm because of evaporation. The liquid jets disintegrated into small droplets as the evaporation continued, and the inherent instabilities of the jets ultimately led to its breakup into fine droplets.

11.2.3   Mechanisms and Modes of Electrospraying

It has been mentioned that electrospraying makes use of uniform electrohydrodynamic force rather than inertial force to break liquid up into aerosols of fine droplets. When a high voltage is applied over the droplet, the electric field will induce free charge on the surface of the liquid droplets. The free charge can be transported through two ways into the droplet [27,38]: either through conduction due to the electric fields or through charge convection. This free charge consists of ions that are accelerated toward the cone apex by the electric field because of a tangential electric stress on the free ions in the liquid. Therefore, the electric stress occurs on the surface of the droplets and produces a downward longitudinal force, transforming the shape of the droplet into a conical one. This in turn results in a high charge density at the cone apex of the liquid jet. In a certain range of applied voltage and flow rate—when the radial force exceeds the shear force—the liquid jet will break into highly charged droplets with a narrow size distribution in a steady and special regime.

Theoretically, if a large potential is gradually applied to a capillary in an electrospraying process, the dripping rate of the drops increases and the size of the liquid drops decreases. The jet is formed by the stripping of the drop surface rather than by the pulling of the liquid from the bulk of the drop, or the detachment of small droplets from the liquid apex [39]. At a certain potential and flow rate, the droplets at the tip of the capillary can form different atomization modes, depending in part on the

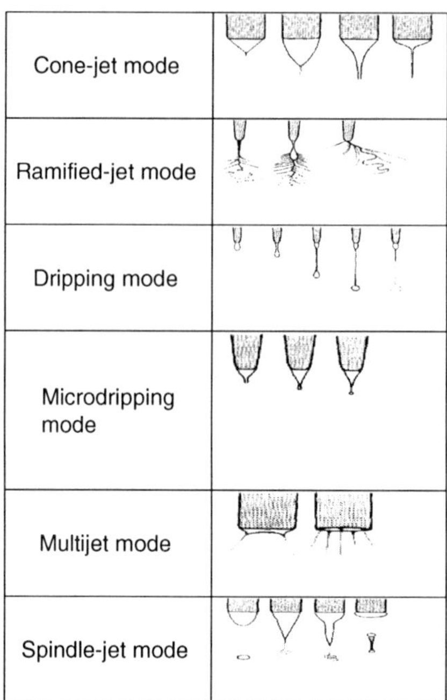

FIGURE 11.4   Electrospraying patterns for different modes. (Reprinted from Cloupeau, M. and Prunetfoch, B., *J. Electrostat.*, 25, 165, 1990. © Elsevier Science. With permission.)

properties of the solution, such as viscosity, concentration, electrical conductivity, electrical permittivity, and surface tension. These atomization modes include microdripping, spindle, cone-jet and multijet, dripping, and ramified-jet modes, which are determined by the physical properties of the suspension, the strength of the electric field, and the flow rate of the liquid. Figure 11.4 shows different modes of the electrospraying pattern. In the cone-jet mode, a jet forms at the tip of the capillary and later propagates into spraying. The droplet size distribution produced in the cone-jet mode depends on the diameter and the breakup of the jet. The applications of charged droplets with cone-jet spraying pattern can be established to control the droplet size and particle transport by using a designed and controlled external electric field. For every solution with different physical properties, there is a minimum flow rate at which the jet breaks up because of the axisymmetric instabilities [40].

When the flow rate is below a certain minimum value, a stable cone-jet mode cannot be formed. However, at higher flow rates, the current through the cone-jet liquid will increase, resulting in an increased surface charge on the jet. Moreover, the jet breakup will also be influenced by lateral or azimuthal instabilities of the jet above a certain surface charge. When the influence of these instabilities increases, the size distribution of the electrosprayed droplets becomes wide. Electrospraying in a cone-jet mode can essentially be described in three different processes [27]. The first process is the acceleration of the liquid in the cone jet, which is a result of the balance of liquid pressure, liquid surface tension, gravity, electric stresses in the liquid surface, the liquid inertia, and the liquid viscosity. Figure 11.5 shows the various forces in electrospraying for a cone-jet mode. The second process is the breakup of the jet into droplets. The third process is the development of the electrospray after the droplet formation in the cone-jet mode.

11.2.4   PROCESSING PARAMETERS

In terms of the application of electrospraying, a main objective of the research is to obtain the scaling laws for the electrosprayed droplet charge and size as functions of the processing parameters, which can guide the electrospraying process and the transformation of solutions into electrosprayed

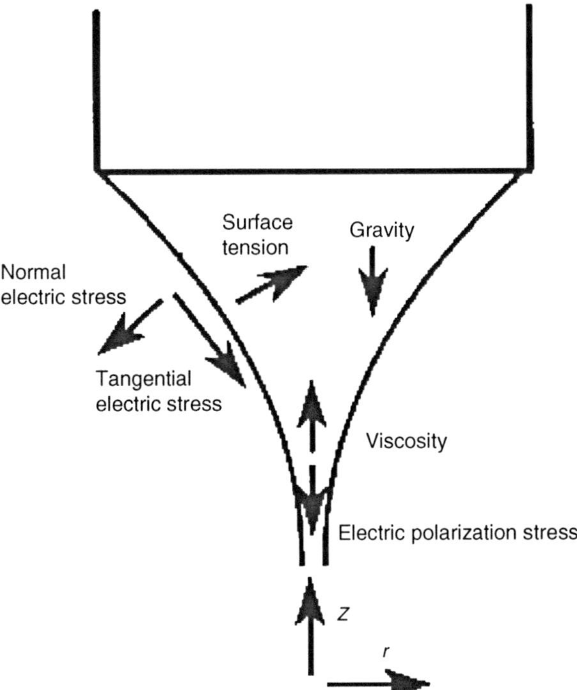

FIGURE 11.5 An illustration of the forces occurring during electrospraying in a cone-jet mode. (Reprinted from Hartman, R.P.A. et al., *J. Aerosol Sci.*, 30, 823, 1999. © Elsevier Science. With permission.)

particles. The main parameters include solution viscosity, electrical conductivity, surface tension, dielectric constant, applied electric potential, flow rate, and solution concentration. If conductivity and viscosity of the solution are high enough, the axial momentum is very efficiently transmitted across the jet section through a viscous diffusion. The axial velocity profile of the liquid becomes almost flat so that the surface stress acts upon the entire cross-section as a volumetric force [27,29]. If the conductivity and viscosity of the solution are low, the liquid mass needs a long axial length to be accelerated so that the tangential stress acts on the liquid through a surface boundary layer along most of the length of the jet.

The following equations were originally proposed to estimate the droplet diameter and the current emitted through the liquid cone. These equations are called the scaling laws for electrospraying in a cone-jet mode and are only valid for liquid with a flat radial profile of the axial liquid velocity in the jet [29]:

$$d_\mathrm{d} = b_1(\varepsilon_r)\left(\frac{Q\,\varepsilon_0\,\varepsilon_r}{K}\right)^{1}_{3} + C_1 \quad I = b_2(\varepsilon_r)\left(\frac{\gamma Q K}{\varepsilon_t}\right)^{1/2} + C_2 \tag{11.4}$$

where d_d is the droplet diameter, Q the liquid flow rate, K the electrical conductivity, γ the surface tension, ε_r the relative permittivity of the liquid, ε_0 the permittivity of a vacuum, I the current, b_1 and b_2 the functions of the liquid permittivity, and C_1 and C_2 are the constants.

However, a revised scaling law of current and droplet size has been proposed by giving new relations for b_1 and b_2 and introducing constants C_1 and C_2. These equations are shown as follows [23]:

$$d_\mathrm{d} = 3.78 \cdot \pi^{-2/3} \cdot 0.6 \cdot Q^{1/2}\left(\frac{\rho \varepsilon_0}{\gamma K}\right)^{1/6} \tag{11.5}$$

$$I = 4.25\left[\frac{(QK\gamma)}{\ln\left((Q/Q_0)^{1/2}\right)}\right]^{1/2} \tag{11.6}$$

where Q is the liquid flow rate, K the electrical conductivity, γ the surface tension, ε_0 the permittivity of a vacuum, ρ the density of the solution, and Q_0 is the characteristic flow rate and is equal to $\rho K/\varepsilon_0 \gamma$.

It is observed that the droplet size is dependent on the liquid flow rate and the liquid properties such as electrical conductivity, surface tension, and density. The experimental results have revealed that when the electrical conductivity of the liquid is too low, such as in the range of 10^{-8} to 10^{-10} S/m, the liquid cannot be electrosprayed in a cone-jet mode because of an insufficient current of the droplets [41]. However, if the electrical conductivity is too high, an unstable mode of electrospraying in a polydispersity will occur. A solution with a high surface tension is difficult to electrospray in a cone-jet mode, and this high electrical potential is needed to overcome the surface tension to break up the droplets. On the other hand, when the flow rate of the solution is too low, a stable cone-jet mode cannot be formed because of the insufficient current. However, when the flow rate is too high and more liquid leaves the capillary, the charges and current needed to form a stable cone-jet spraying mode become insufficient. The relationship between the current and the droplet size can be found from Equation 11.7 and is only valid for liquid with a low viscosity and electrical conductivity, which suggests that the droplet size will decrease as the flow rate of the solution increases [2,27]:

$$d = c\left(\frac{\rho\varepsilon_0 Q^4}{I^2}\right)^{1/6} \tag{11.7}$$

where d is the droplet size, c a constant, ρ the density of the liquid, Q the flow rate of the liquid, ε_0 the permittivity of vacuum, and I is the current of the droplets and a function of the flow rate, surface tension, and electrical conductivity of the liquid.

Gañán-Calvo et al. proposed universal scaling laws of the electrospraying current as well as the charge and size of the droplets in a cone-jet mode from a theoretical model of the charge transport and through experimentation [30]. The two scaling laws are applicable to different solutions—those with relatively high viscosity and electrical conductivity and those with low viscosity and electrical conductivity. This variation will depend on the dimensionless parameter, which governs the liquid acceleration process and ultimately the electrospraying current and droplet size. The dimensionless parameter is defined as follows [30]:

$$\delta\mu \cdot \delta^{1/3} = \left[\frac{\gamma^3 \varepsilon_0^2}{\mu^3 K^2 Q}\right]^{1/3} \tag{11.8}$$

where Q is the flow rate of liquid, ε_0 the permittivity of vacuum, K the electrical conductivity, γ the surface tension, and μ the viscosity of the solution.

If $\delta\mu \cdot \delta^{1/3} \leq 1$, the current I and size of the droplet d in a cone-jet electrospraying mode are as follows:

$$I/I_0 = 6.2[Q/(\beta - 1)^{1/2} \cdot Q]^{1/2} \tag{11.9}$$

$$d/(\beta - 1)^{1/3} d_0 = 1.6[Q/(\beta - 1)^{1/2} Q_0]^{1/3} - 1.0 \tag{11.10}$$

If $\delta\mu \cdot \delta^{1/3} \geq 1$, the current I and size of the droplet d in a cone-jet electrospraying mode are as follows:

$$I/I_0 = 11.0[Q/Q_0]^{1/4} - 5.0 \tag{11.11}$$

$$d/d_0 = 1.2[Q/Q_0]^{1/2} - 0.3 \tag{11.12}$$

where $I_0 = (\varepsilon_0 \gamma^2/\rho)^{1/2}$, $Q_0 = \varepsilon_0 \gamma/(\rho K)$, and $d_0 = [\gamma\varepsilon_0^2/(\rho K^2)]^{1/3}$.

$$= \frac{4k^2 r_{\text{jet}}^2}{(8 + k^2 r_{\text{jet}}^2)} \left[1 - k^2 r_{\text{jet}}^2 - 2R_{\text{Es}} \left\{ 1 + kr_{\text{jet}} \left(\lim_{m \to n} \frac{I'_m(kr_{\text{jet}}) - I'_{-m}(kr_{\text{jet}})}{I_m(kr_{\text{jet}}) - I_{-m}(kr_{\text{jet}})} \right) \right\} \right] \tag{11.28}$$

$$\omega' = \frac{\omega r_{\text{jet}}^{1.5} \rho^{0.5}}{\gamma^{0.5}}; \quad \text{Oh} = \frac{\mu}{(\gamma \rho d_{\text{jet}})^{1/2}}; \quad k' = kr_{\text{jet}}; \quad R_{\text{Es}} = \frac{\sigma^2 r_{\text{jet}}}{2\gamma \varepsilon_0} \tag{11.29}$$

where μ is the absolute liquid viscosity, ρ the liquid density, and I_m is a Bessel function.

The Oh is a ratio of loss of energy resulting from viscosity over the potential energy of the jet because of surface tension, k' the ratio of the jet radius over the wavelength times 2π, and R_{Es} is the ratio of the electric stress over the surface tension stress. The normalized growth rate ω' can be calculated as a function of the dimensionless numbers of Equation 11.29 by using Equation 11.28.

11.2.6 BASIC ELECTROSPRAYING SYSTEM

In a typical instrumental setup, the electrospraying is generated by pumping liquid into a conductive capillary at a high potential relative to a grounded surface. When the liquid emerges from the capillary, the droplet is distorted by a strong electrical field and forms a conical spraying mode commonly known as a Taylor cone. Figure 11.8 shows basically the experimental setup, which is composed of a capillary, a high-voltage power supply, a syringe pump, and a collector. The solution is forced from a syringe reservoir by a syringe pump through a plastic tube attached to the capillary, which can be designed to have different outer and inner diameters. The flow rate of the solution can be controlled through a programmable syringe pump. The capillary is maintained at a high potential by connecting it to a high-voltage power supply. The strength of the electric field and its patterns can be generated and controlled using a programmable high-voltage power supply. A collector, held a specified distance from the capillary, is either grounded or negatively charged. In some cases, to obtain the spraying patterns and the dynamic behaviors of electrosprayed droplets under an applied electric field, the electrospraying process can be monitored through a controlling system, which consists of a high-speed charge-coupled device (CCD) camera with a magnifying lens, a synchronized strobe lamp, and an integrated frame-grabber or image-processor.

11.2.7 CHARACTERISTICS OF ELECTROSPRAYING

Experiments have demonstrated electrospraying to be capable of generating micro- or nanometer droplets. These highly charged droplets result in self-repelled particles without coalescence. By selecting the proper processing parameters, the electrosprayed droplets can be produced in a narrow size distribution. It is conceptually easy to control the size of electrosprayed particles from nanometer to micrometer by varying the flow rate of the solution, the applied voltage, the spraying

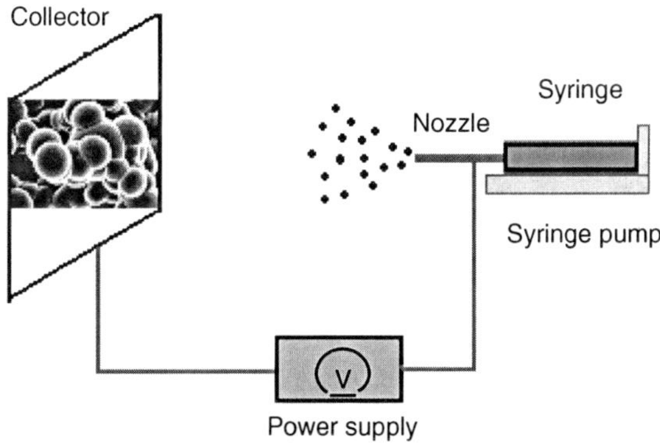

FIGURE 11.8 A basic electrospraying setup.

distance, and the physical properties of the solution. The unique characteristics of electrospraying for atomizing a liquid offer several advantages over other techniques. These characteristics include [3,45–47] (1) the relatively easy instrumental setup; (2) ability to perform in an open atmosphere without the need of a sophisticated chamber; (3) the generation of controllable particle sizes in a narrow distribution; (4) high production efficiency due to the direct ejection of charged particles onto the collector under an electric field; and (5) well-dispersed particles due to the self-repellence resulting from the electric charges on the particles.

11.2.8 Fabrication of Biological Materials

11.2.8.1 Drug Delivery Carriers

Significant effort has recently been devoted to the development of novel technologies for preparing drug delivery carriers by either localized or targeted delivery in a cost-effective, versatile way. These technologies offer suitable means for delivering small molecular weight drugs as well as macromolecules such as proteins, peptides, or genes [48–50]. Traditional drug-delivery carriers are not the most efficient formulations for a given product and novel delivery carriers are required to optimize efficiency and minimize side effects of the delivered agents to the tissues [51]. Biodegradable micro- and nanoparticles have attracted significant attention as carriers for delivering low–molecular mass drugs and macromolecule proteins. These particles in a micrometer or nanometer size range can be prepared by using solvent-evaporation emulsion and spray-drying methods [52,53]. The methods using ultrasound and air pressure can result in the agglomeration of the biodegradable polymer particle, making it difficult to control bead size and uniformity. Electrospraying has been considered as a promising technique for preparing drug-delivery carriers. It is a simple and cost-effective method for preparing polymer particles with controllable microstructures in a desired particle size. The biodegradable particles prepared using electrospraying have a fairly narrow size distribution and are well-dispersed because of the electrical repellence. Compared with conventional methods for preparing drug-delivery carriers, electrospraying is capable of preparing micro- and nanoparticulate drug-delivery systems such as microsphere and microcapsules in which the biological agents are encapsulated into biodegradable polymer particles.

11.2.8.1.1 Drug Delivery

Drug delivery remains an important challenge in medicine and various fabrication techniques have been used to develop novel processing to generate size-controllable and well-dispersed delivery carriers with high encapsulation efficiency in the last decade. The micro- and nanometer deliveries through novel technologies for small molecules, proteins, and DNA, among other things, have advanced the development of new and efficient therapeutic treatment.

Ding et al. prepared poly(ε-caprolactone) (PCL) particles encapsulated with the anticancer drug Taxol using the electrospraying technique [7]. PCL has been used as the polymer matrix of controlled drug-release devices because of its biodegradable, biocompatible, and highly crystalline properties. The solution was prepared by dissolving PCL in dichloromethane solvent. The mixed precursor containing PCL solution and Taxol was injected into a chamber through a spraying nozzle using a syringe pump at a constant flow rate. A schematic diagram of the setup is shown in Figure 11.9. High voltages were applied to the spray nozzle (V_n) and the copper ring (V_r) around the nozzle to generate a high electric field to electrospray the precursor for generating fine droplets. The function of the grounded corona needle was to supply the ions to discharge the droplets or particles. The electrosprayed droplets were transported to the collection filter by a cross flow of nitrogen. PCL particles prepared using electrospraying have a smooth surface and uniform morphology with a uniform size distribution, as shown in Figures 11.10a and 11.10b. Particles collected from the side wall of the chamber, grounded needle, or spraying nozzle usually have a similar morphology and microstructure as those collected from the filter, as shown in Figures 11.10e and 11.10f. The morphology of particles became comparatively smoother with an increase in concentration of the

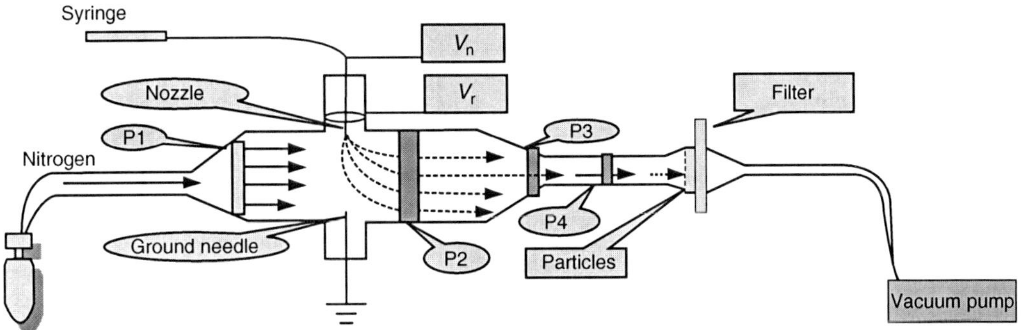

FIGURE 11.9 Schematic diagram of electrospraying apparatus. (Reprinted from Ding, L., Lee, T., and Wang, C.H., *J. Contr. Release*, 102, 395, 2005. © Elsevier Science. With permission.)

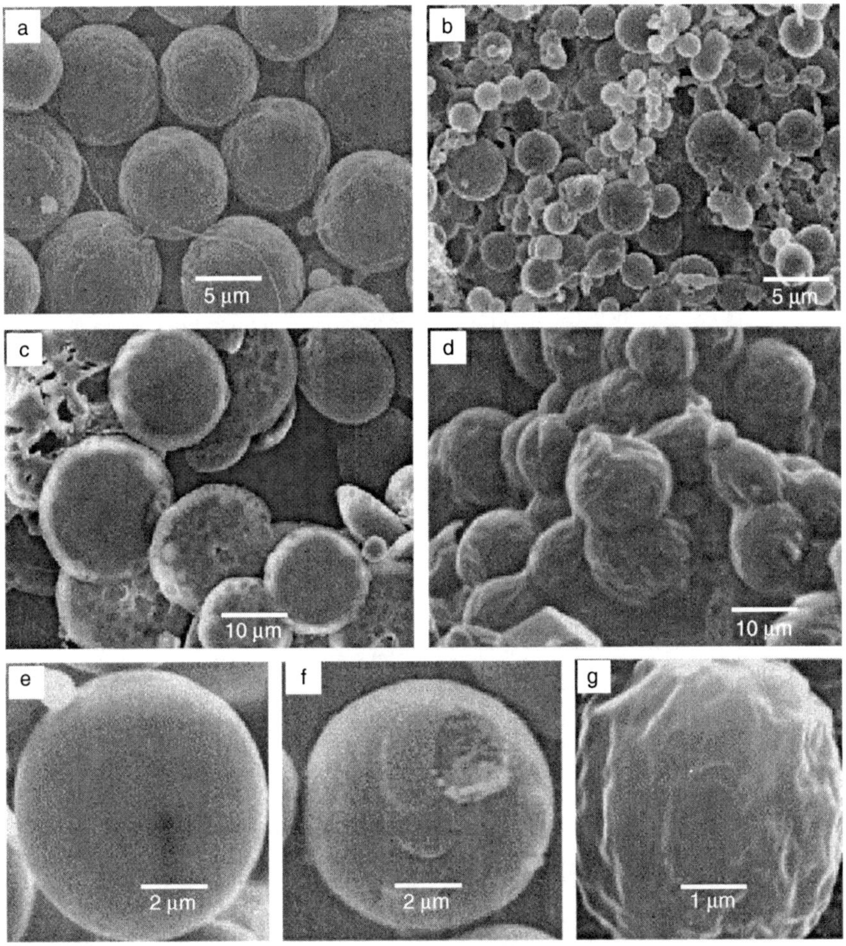

FIGURE 11.10 SEM images of PCL particles: (a) particles collected from filter, (b) particles prepared using spray-drying, (c) particles collected from side wall, (d) particles after 45 days *in vitro* release, (e) morphology of particles collected from filter, (f) morphology of particles collected from side wall, and (g) same as (f) except PCL/DCM concentration is 3% g/mL. The drug loading for all samples were 1%. PCL/DCM concentration is 7.5% g/mL. (Reprinted from Ding, L., Lee, T., and Wang, C.H., *J. Contr. Release,* 102, 395, 2005. © Elsevier Science. With permission.)

polymer solution, as shown in Figures 11.10e through 11.10g. PCL particles collected from the areas close to the spraying zone sometimes stuck to each other. Figure 11.10c shows the ultrasonic treatment of these particles. The scanning electron microscopy (SEM) image revealed that the particles were shaped as thick disks with visible pores and that the diameters of such thick disks were larger than those of the microspheres collected from other locations.

The release profile revealed that the drug released within 45 days amounted to less than 40% of the total drugs encapsulated in the particles for all samples. It was attributed to the semicrystalline structure of PCL and the hydrophobic characteristics of Taxol. From SEM image in Figure 11.10d, it can be seen that the outer shell of the PCL particle has no sign of significant erosion after a 45-day release. This feature may be attributed to the highly crystalline structure of PCL, which resulted in the slow degradation of polymer. Cell uptake features of electrosprayed PCL particles were investigated to determine how the particles could be localized within the tumor cell and how well the anticancer drug Taxol could be absorbed and affected the viability of the tumor cell. The results showed the uptake efficiencies of the three samples to be around 60% after a 2 h experiment. This result demonstrates that particles generated using the electrospraying technique can have an efficient uptake. By modifying the processing parameter and collection method, the yields of the drug encapsulation can reach about 80%, demonstrating a practical technique for fabricating fine drug carrier particles.

Xu and Hanna prepared bovine serum albumin (BSA)–loaded poly(lactide) acid (PLA) particles using the electrospraying technique [54]. PLA has been used as a biomaterial because of its biodegradability and biocompatibility as well as because of its approved regulatory status. The PLA solution was prepared by dissolving 300 mg of PLA in 10 mL of 1,2-dichloroethane (DCE) and stirring for 8 h at room temperature. Specified amounts of BSA previously dissolved in distilled water were mixed with PLA solutions and emulsified by a sonication for 10 min. A schematic illustration of the electrospraying setup is shown in Figure 11.11. A positive electrode from a high-voltage power supply was connected to the needle, and a negative electrode was placed in the collection solution 10 cm away from the needle. The precursor was electrosprayed at an applied voltage of 12.5 kV and at a flow rate of 1.0 mL/h to a receiving beaker containing distilled water (the collection solution). The PLA particles were separated from the collecting solution by filtering and drying at room temperature. The size of the PLA particles ranged from 0.84 ± 0.18 to 3.95 ± 0.51 μm, and increased

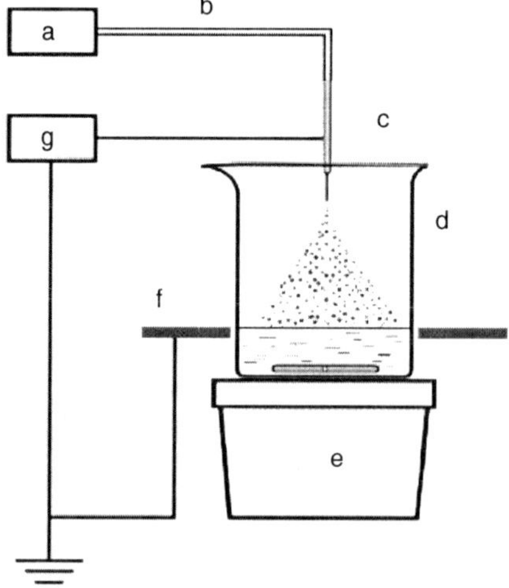

FIGURE 11.11   A schematic diagram of the electrospraying setup (a) pump, (b) feeding line, (c) needle, (d) collecting solution, (e) magnetic stirrer, (f) copper collector ring, and (g) high-voltage power supply. (Reprinted from Xu, Y.X. and Hanna, M.A., *Int. J. Pharm.*, 320, 30, 2006. © Elsevier Science. With permission.)

with the increase in the organic phase ratio. The size of the particles did, however, first decrease and then increase as the BSA/PLA weight ratio decreased from 1:2 to 1:6. The spherical shape of the particles was lost with a decreasing organic phase ratio and BSA amount. The particle yield was in the range of 64.3–80.1%, and the BSA loading capacities were in the range of 74.2–91.4%. The BSA encapsulation efficiency that ranged between 22.9 and 80.6%, increased with an increasing organic/aqueous phase ratio and decreased with an increasing BSA/PLA ratio. In the last stage, high BSA/PLA ratio significantly increased the BSA release rate, but a high organic/aqueous phase ratio decreased the BSA release rate. The results showed that the physicochemical properties of electrosprayed BSA-loaded PLA particles were affected by the organic/aqueous phase volume ratio and the BSA/PLA weight ratio as well as the physical properties of emulsions.

Xie et al. applied the electrospraying technique to produce biodegradable polymeric micro- and nanoparticles for pharmaceutical productions [42]. The solutions were prepared by dissolving poly-lactic-*co*-glycolic acid (PLGA) polymer in acetonitrile (2–16%, w/v) with and without certain amounts of paclitaxel (0–10%, w/w), surfactants Pluronic F127 (0–16%, w/w), and didodecyldimethylammonium bromide (0–2 mM). Three different experimental setups designed to study the effects of particle formation are shown in Figure 11.12. In the configurations, setup (a) did not use a ring electrode under the nozzle, and setup (b) did not use a glass chamber, but setup (c) was designed with a glass chamber to control the solvent evaporation rate and to improve the collection rate of the particles through a pneumatic conveying method. High voltages in the ranges of 5–10 kV and 0–10 kV were applied to the nozzle and the ring, respectively. By varying the processing parameters, PLGA particles with a controllable morphology and size can be achieved through this technique. PLGA particles with an approximate size of 250 nm can be produced by adding organic salts to increase the solution conductivity for electrospraying at a relatively high flow rate. The ability to control the size of encapsulated drug particles provides a means to control the drug release properties. SEM images in Figure 11.13 show the effects of polymer concentration on the particle morphology and size. The size of the PLGA particles prepared by electrospraying decreased with a reduction in the flow rate of the solution. The flow rates from 0.15 mL/h onward would form a stable cone-jet spraying mode and produce particles with an approximate size of 900 nm in diameter. Organic salt would increase the conductivity of the solution. With 1% salt concentration in the solution, PLGA particles with an approximate size of 300 nm were produced to have relatively good morphology at a flow rate of 0.2 mL/h. Higher flow rates could still produce PLGA particles in a nanometer scale when a higher organic salt concentration was used to increase the conductivity. Surfactant concentration had marginal effects on the size of particles and then was added in small amounts to form nonagglomerated particles. The solution concentration did not affect the particle size dramatically, except where the concentration was higher than 10%. Higher solution concentrations also gave better surface morphology.

Ijsebaert et al. used electrospraying technique also to prepare pharmaceutical particles for inhalation purposes [55]. Methylparahydroxybenzoate (MPHB) was used as a model drug in the initial experiments and beclomethasone dipropionate (BDP) was used as a drug for inhalation purpose. The solution was prepared by dissolving MPHB and BDP in the ethanol solvent. Table 11.1 shows the influence of the liquid flow and drug concentration on the particle size and width of the distribution for the MPHB solution. The results showed that the size of the particles increased with an increasing flow rate, and at the equal flow rates the particle size increased when the concentration was increased from 0.5% to 3%. At a flow rate of 1.0 mL/h and a concentration of 0.5%, the electrosprayed MPHB particles had an average size of 1.58 µm with a geometric standard deviation (GSD) of 1.18. However, at a flow rate of 3.0 mL/h and a concentration of 3%, the average particle size was 4.55 µm with a GSD of 1.29. The experiments showed that BDP resulted in similar particle sizes to MPHB, and the mass of BDP was in the range of 1.42–6 µg/L air. The experiment demonstrated that the electrospraying technique is a promising method to deliver antiasthma drugs to patients. The key advantages of electrospraying a drug solution for the purpose of inhalation are the ease of aerosol production and the narrow particle size distribution.

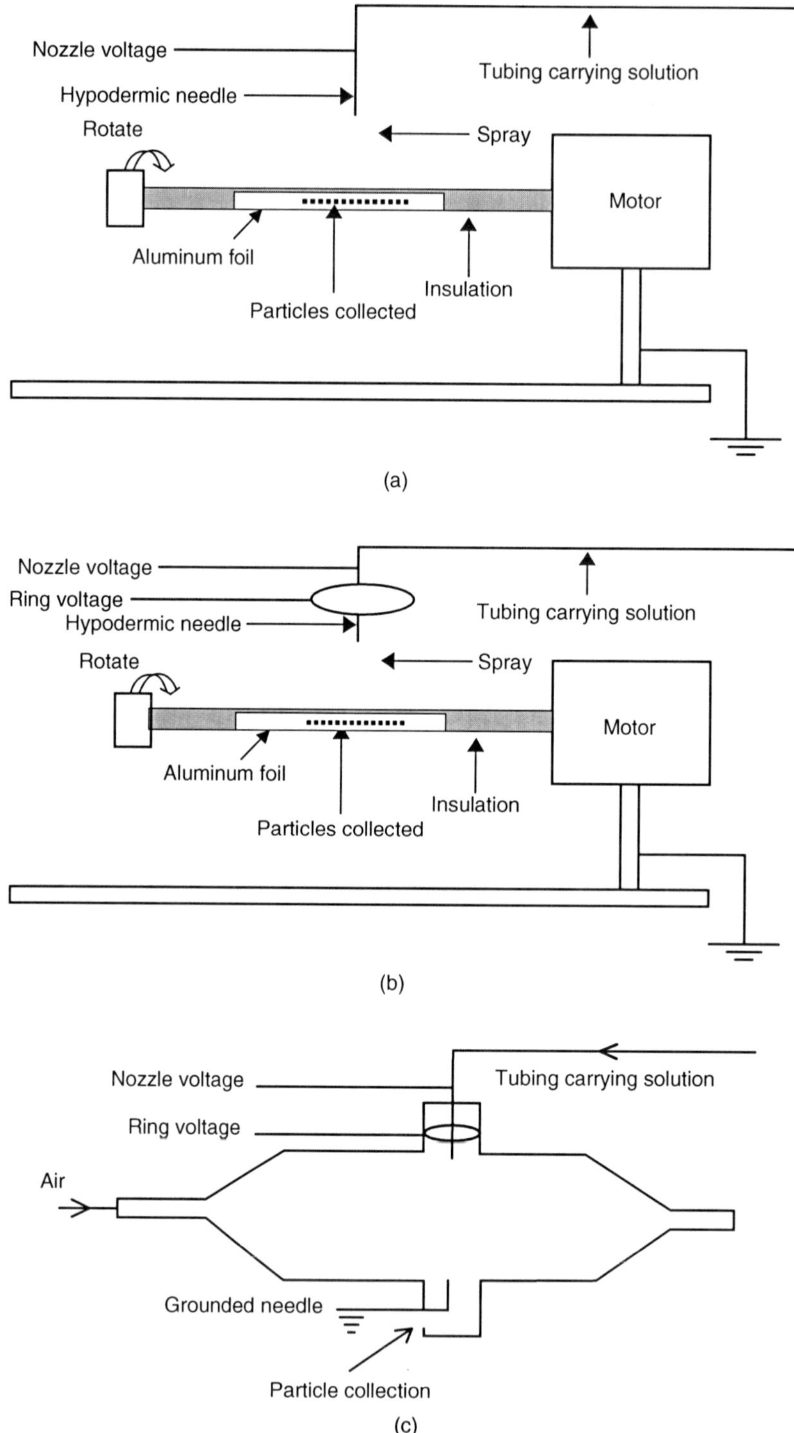

FIGURE 11.12 Diagrams of difficult setups for particle preparation. (Reprinted from Xie, J.W. et al., *J. Colloid Interface Sci.*, 302, 103, 2006. © Elsevier Science. With permission.)

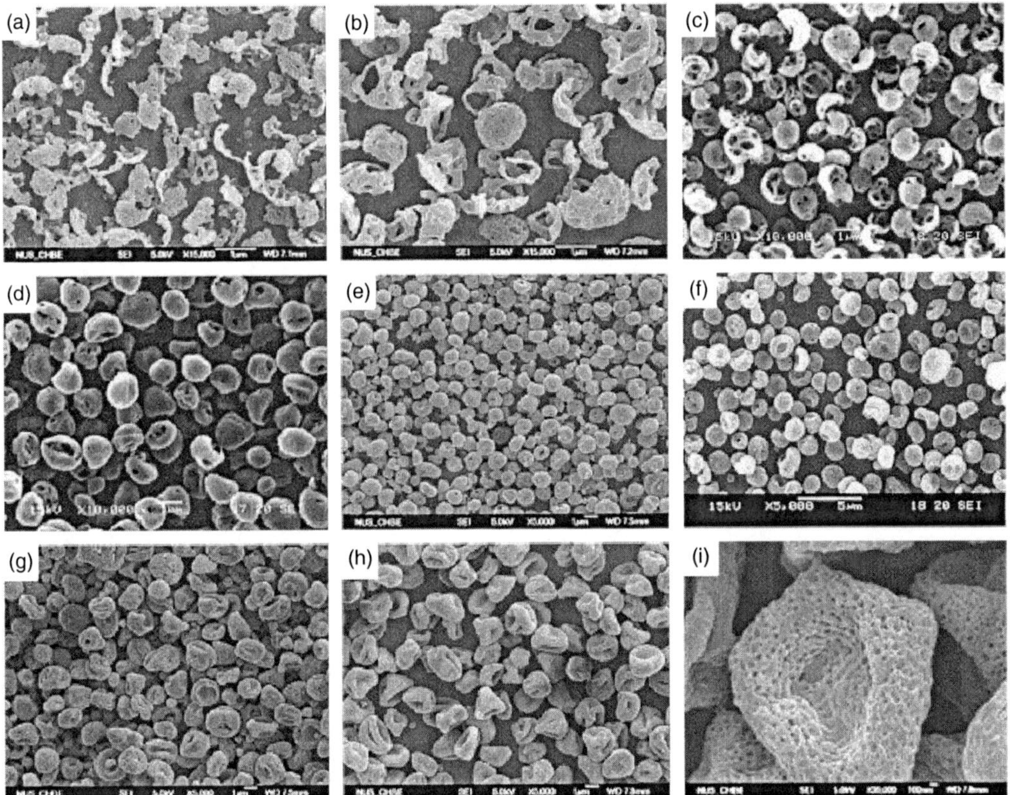

FIGURE 11.13   The effect of concentration on the particle morphology with setup b is as follows: (a) 1%, (b) 2%, (c) 4%, (d) 6%, (e) 8%, (f) 10%, (g) 12%, (h) 14%, and (i) high magnification of (h) (acetonitrile, paclitaxel = 5%, flow rate = 0.25 mL/h, V_n = 10 kV and V_r = 7.5 kV). (Reprinted from Xie, J.W. et al., *J. Colloid Interface Sci.*, 302, 103, 2006. © Elsevier Science. With permission.)

TABLE 11.1

Influence of the Liquid Flow Rate and Drug Concentration on Particle Size

MPHB Concentration in Ethanol (%)	Flow Rate					
	1 mL/h		2 mL/h		3 mL/h	
	MMAD (µm)	GSD	MMAD (µm)	GSD	MMAD (µm)	GSD
0.5	1.58 ± 0.05	1.18 ± 0.03	2.07 ± 0.07	1.17 ± 0.02	2.51 ± 0.07	1.23 ± 0.03
2.0	2.22 ± 0.02	1.18 ± 0.03	3.04 ± 0.03	1.22 ± 0.03	3.43 ± 0.17	1.28 ± 0.01
3.0	2.69 ± 0.05	1.37 ± 0.02	3.98 ± 0.05	1.37 ± 0.02	4.55 ± 0.05	1.29 ± 0.05

Values are means ± SD of 10 consecutive measurements at 1 min intervals. Each measurement shows a mass median aerodynamic diameter (MMAD) and GSD, and they were considered as independent aerosol parameters. The mean with its SD was calculated for both parameters.

Reyderman et al. generated excipient-free microspheres of cholesterol using electrospraying with a melting precursor under atmospheric pressure and controlled temperature [56]. Cholesterol was chosen as the model compound to study the behavior of melts during the electrospraying. Moreover, the chemical structure of cholesterol is analogous to diverse steroids, suggesting that the melt-electrospraying can be used to prepare water-insoluble steroid microspheres for a sustained

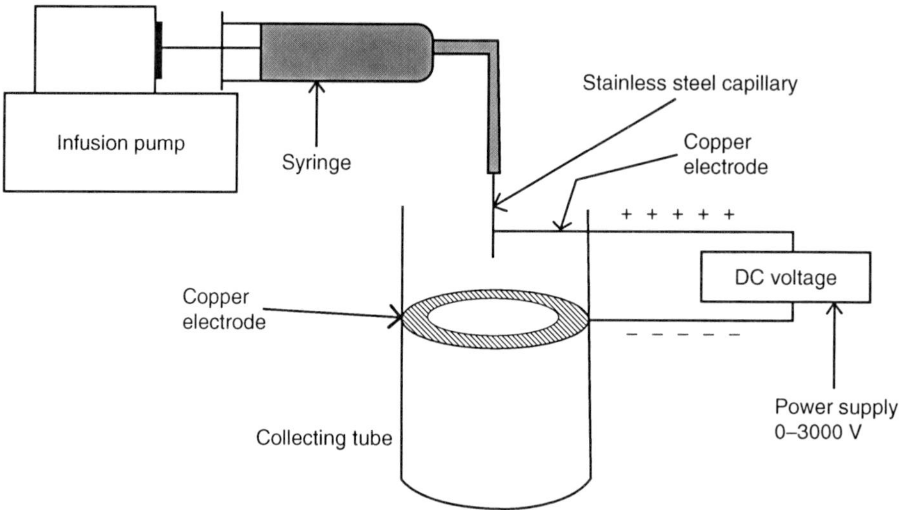

FIGURE 11.14 A schematic representation of electrospraying equipment. (Reprinted from Reyderman, L. and Stavchansky, S., *Int. J. Pharm.*, 124, 75, 1995. © Elsevier Science. With permission.)

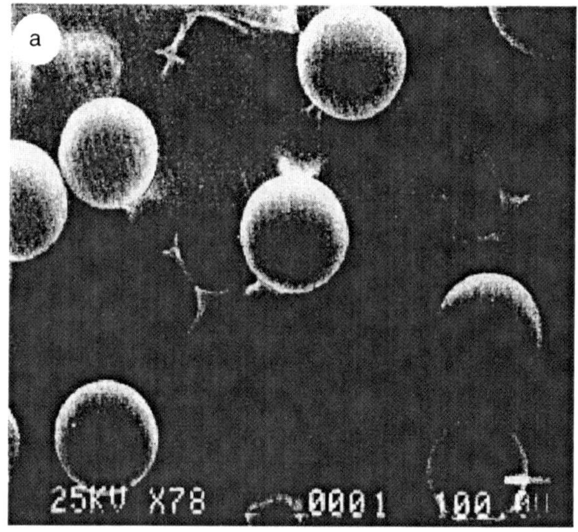

FIGURE 11.15 SEM of cholesterol microspheres prepared using electrospraying. (Reprinted from Reyderman, L. and Stavchansky, S., *Int. J. Pharm.*, 124, 75, 1995. © Elsevier Science. With permission.)

release formulation upon intramuscular or intradermal administration. A schematic diagram of the apparatus used in the work is shown in Figure 11.14. The apparatus consisted of an infusion pump, a glass syringe, a stainless steel capillary, and a power supply. The electrodes were positioned 0.2 cm apart, one of them being at the tip of the capillary. A heating mantle controlled by a thermostat was positioned around the syringe extending down to the capillary and upper electrode to maintain cholesterol in the molten state and to provide uniform flow for electrospraying cholesterol in a molten state. SEM image revealed that the cholesterol microspheres prepared using a 3 kV voltage source had a mixture of spherical particles of 150–250 µm, as shown in Figure 11.15. The experiments demonstrated that electrospraying has another potential use in spraying a melt for producing microspheres in a uniform size. However, considerations need to be placed on the thermal stability of drugs and the polymorphic changes taking place during the electrospraying of melts, as well as the moisture entrapment during the solidification process.

11.2.8.1.2 Targeted Drug Delivery

Targeted drug delivery directs a therapeutic agent in a site-specific manner, which embodies the delivery of the therapeutic agent to a specific organ or location in the body [57–59]. The targeted drug delivery utilizes a specific carrier–site interaction to seek its cellular target. The micro- and nanometer delivery particles prepared using electrospraying can be allowed to pass through small intercellular openings to target the tissues or organs easily. Furthermore, the antibodies can be coupled onto the electrosprayed particles to achieve more efficient targeting. The recent development of nanotechnology has resulted in a variety of new processes to prepare targeted drug delivery, focusing on formulating therapeutic agents in biocompatible nanocomposites, which in general can be applied to provide targeted delivery of drugs, proteins, peptides, and genes in a specific tissue or in organs. Electrospraying can be considered as a promising technique to prepare targeted delivery carriers due to the controllable size and efficient encapsulation of biomedical agents.

Polymer-based particles with two distinct phases were recently prepared by electrospraying two polymer solutions by Roh et al. [60]. The individual phase was independently loaded with biomolecules or selectively modified with model ligands. During the processing experiment, a laminar flow of two distinct polymer solutions was pumped at suitable flow rates through a modified nozzle with side-by-side geometry, as shown in Figure 11.16a. A micrograph of the outlet region of the nozzle is shown in Figure 11.16b, revealing the biphasic character of the jetting liquid. Each jetting solution was prepared by dissolving the components in distilled water. In this experiment, dilute aqueous solutions of polyethylene oxide (PEO) and polyacrylic acid (PAA) were prepared with added dye or molecules in a certain concentration to reveal the biphasic structure. The transmission electron microscopy (TEM) images showed that most of the PEO-based particles had diameters between 100 and 400 nm, and the PAA-based particle had an average diameter of 170 nm. Particles made of PEO were spindle-like and had a relatively narrow size distribution, whereas PAA particles had almost perfect spherical morphology and were discontinuous.

Electrospraying was also applied to prepare particles with surface-selective chemical modification. These particles will be developed to targeted delivery carriers. Figure 11.17a shows single-phasic nanocolloids prepared by electrospraying solutions composed of PEO and amino-dextran. The free amine groups of the particles were subsequently modified with 4,4-difluoro-5,7-dimethyl-4-bora-3a,4a-diaza-s-indacene-3-propionic acid, succinimidyl ester (BODIPY) ligands. After chemical modification, the amino-modified nanocolloids showed homogenously distributed green

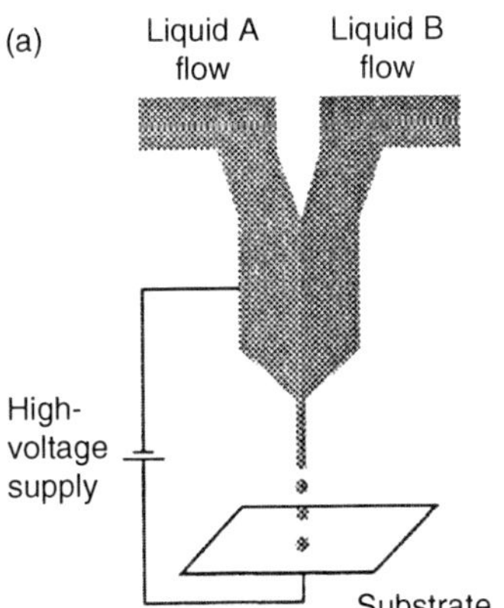

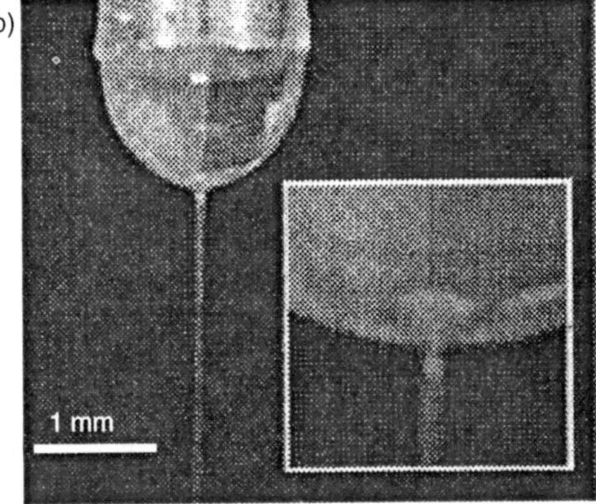

FIGURE 11.16 Biphasic electrified jetting using side-by-side dual capillaries. (Reprinted from Roh, K.H., Martin, D.C., and Lahann, J., *Nat. Mater.*, 4, 759, 2005. © Nature Publishing Group. With permission.)

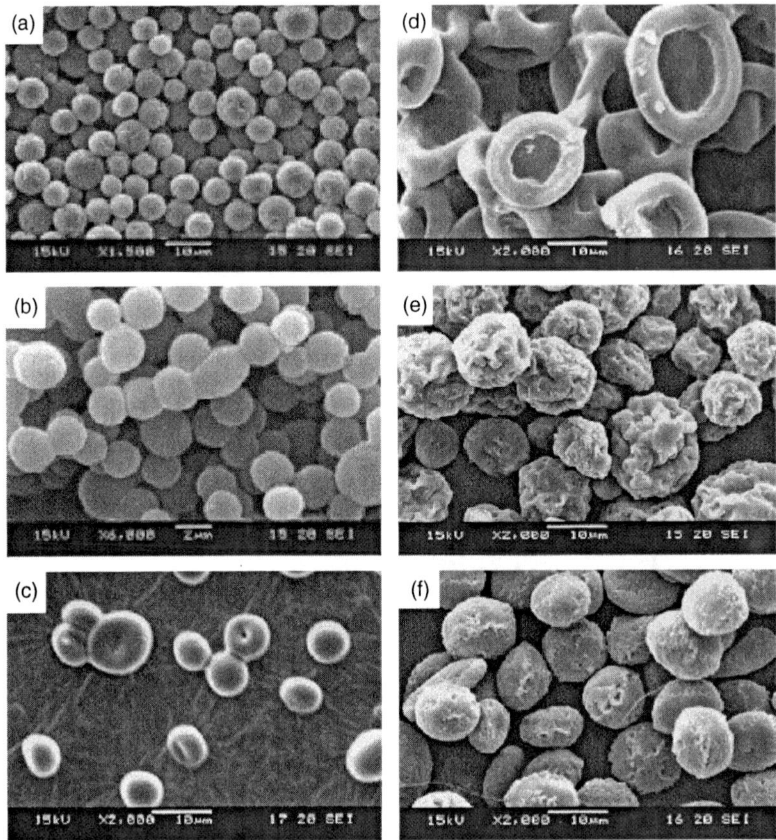

FIGURE 11.19 SEM images of particles fabricated with different organic solvents and different polymers: (a) DCM, (b) acetonitrile, (c) THF, (d) EVAC, (e) PLGA, and (f) PDLA. (Polymer, PCL; airflow rate, 20 L/min; concentration, 3%; flow rate, 3 mL/h; needle size, 0.34 mm; voltages of nozzle and ring, 8.8 and 7.1 kV). (Reprinted from Xie, J.W., Marijnissen, J.C.M., and Wang, C.H., *Biomaterials*, 27, 3321, 2006. © Elsevier Science. With permission.)

Bioceramic coatings or films, regarded as the attractive substitute materials in the orthopedic fields, have been deposited onto the metal shaft of hip implant and dental screws to promote cellular ingrowth and also to reduce the mechanical mismatch between the devices and new tissues. The bioactive surface coatings or films can help integrate the implants into the body. Some biopolymeric films or coatings have been deposited on the electrode surface of biosensors to enhance biocompatibility. For example, a protein of the extracellular matrix, collagen, has been successfully deposited to the metallic biomaterial surface to enhance the bioactivity and biocompatibility [66,67]. Native biomaterials such as starch, protein, and other biomolecules have also been prepared as film and coating materials in the fields of genomic, proteomic, and clinical analyses, as well as in various food and pharmaceutical applications.

11.2.8.2.1 Bioceramic Materials

Electrostatic spray deposition, a coating technique developed from electrospraying, was used by Leeuwenburgh et al. [68] to deposit calcium phosphate (CaP) coatings with a variety of chemical properties. In the biomedical fields, bioceramic coatings are frequently deposited onto the surface of metallic dental or orthopedic implants to improve the biological performance. The CaP bioceramics are considered as a suitable class of biomaterials for use as a surface coating on titanium metals because of its similarity to the inorganic component of bone and teeth. It can form bonds between the implant materials and surrounding osseous tissue, resulting in a strong interface between the implant surface and bone [69]. Currently, plasma spraying is often used to coat titanium implants with synthetic CaP films and coatings. However, the CaP phases like carbonate apatite, which resembles the composition and crystallinity of bone minerals, is difficult to be deposited because of the extremely high processing temperatures [9,70]. Electrospraying has already been developed as a novel coating technique to overcome the above-mentioned drawback. The experimental results showed that the chemical properties of CaP coatings prepared using electrospraying technique were strongly dependent on the chemical and physical properties of the precursor solution. Various crystal phases and phase mixtures were formed, such as carbonate apatite, β-TCP, Mg-substituted whitlockite, monetite, β/γ-pyrophosphate, and calcite, by varying the relative Ca/P solution ratio, absolute precursor concentration, acidity of the precursor solution, and the type of Ca precursor salt. The results showed that carbonate played an essential role in the chemical mechanism for the formation of CaP coatings. Depending on the processing parameters of electrospraying, there were three reactions for carbonate anions: (1) reaction with acidic phosphate groups, (2) incorporation into apatitic CaP phases, and (3) reaction with excessive Ca^{2+} cations in case of phosphate-deficient precursor solutions.

Leeuwenburgh et al. also investigated the fabrication of CaP coatings with defined chemical properties through electrospraying [71]. The relationships between various processing parameters and the chemical properties of CaP coatings were studied to prepare the CaP coatings with tailored chemical characteristics. The experimental results showed that the chemical properties of the CaP coatings could be determined by the physical and chemical properties of solutions, as well as the apparatus-related factors. Figure 11.20 shows a schematic diagram of the setup. Ca and P precursors were prepared by dissolving $Ca(NO_3)_2 \cdot 4H_2O$ or $CaCl_2 \cdot 2H_2O$ and H_3PO_4 in butyl carbitol ($C_8H_{18}O_3$) or ethanol. A two-component nozzle with separate inlets for Ca and P precursor solutions was used as a standard nozzle to avoid premature precipitation of precursors prior to the spraying generation. By varying the processing parameters, the chemical properties of CaP coatings can be tailored to have defined crystal phases ranging from the carbonate-free phases to carbonate-containing phases. The experiment demonstrated that electrospraying was an appropriate technique to prepare coatings with a large variety of chemical properties, which is especially suitable to the research focused

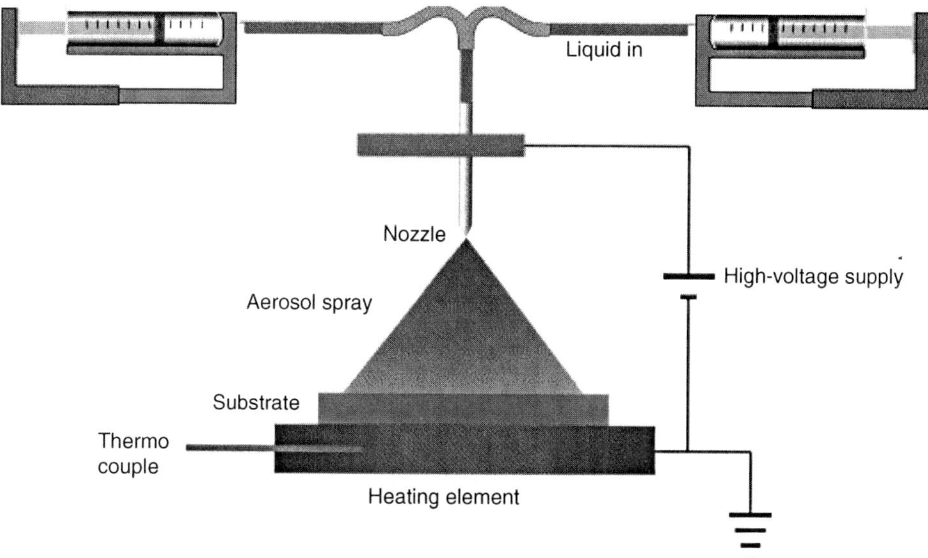

FIGURE 11.20 A diagram of the setup of the electrospraying for two solutions. (Reprinted from Leeuwenburgh, S.C.G. et al., *J. Eur. Ceram. Soc.*, 26, 487, 2006. © Elsevier Science. With permission.)

on the fundamental relationships between the characteristics of CaP coating and the biological performance.

The dissolution and precipitation behaviors of porous CaP coatings prepared using electrospraying technique were investigated *in vitro* by soaking the coatings in simulated body fluid for 2, 4, 8, and 12 weeks, and also *in vivo* after subcutaneous implantation of CaP-coated implants in the back of goats for identical time periods [72]. The CaP coatings had a unique microstructure characterized by a three-dimensional (3-D) and interconnected pore-network with variable pore size, which offered the advantage of creating an implant surface with a controllable surface area. Figure 11.21 shows SEM image of porous CaP coatings prepared using electrospraying deposition. The experimental results showed that *in vitro* all apatitic coatings induced the formation of homogeneous and adherent CaP precipitation layers, and *in vivo* no adverse tissue reactions (toxic effects or inflammatory cells) were observed. A dense and fibrous tissue capsule surrounded all coatings after implantation. The biological characterization demonstrated that electrospraying was a versatile technique for manufacturing bioceramic coatings with a wide variety of controlled surface properties in terms of the chemical properties and the morphology of coatings.

Kim et al. prepared hydroxyapatite bioactive films by using the sol–gel-assisted electrospraying technique with calcium nitrate and phosphoric acid as the starting materials [73]. Hydroxyapatite, the CaP-based bioceramics, has been applied in medicine and dentistry for the last 20 years (such as in bioceramic coatings for orthopedic and dental implants, alveolar ridge augmentation, maxillofacial surgery, and scaffolds for bone growth). In this work, the sol–gel process was combined with electrospraying to obtain hydroxyapatite films with the stoichiometry and precise control of the film composition because the sol–gel process has been proved to be a promising method for preparing films on a variety of substrates because of its precise control of chemical composition. $Ca(NO_3)_2 \cdot 2H_2O$ and H_3PO_4 were used as reactants for the preparation of hydroxyapatite films. The sol was diluted with methanol to adjust the concentration and the viscosity for depositing hydroxyapatite films using electrospraying technique. The SEM image of hydroxyapatite film prepared by sol–gel-assisted electrospraying is shown in Figure 11.22. The amorphous as-deposited films prepared at 80°C can be transformed to the hydroxyapatite films at 500°C heat treatment. The microstructure of the hydroxyapatite films showed a crack-free and dense structure, while the surface of the films deposited at lower or higher temperature than the boiling point of methanol exhibited cracks and agglomeration. The experimental results showed that the temperature, similar to the boiling point of solvent, was an ideal depositing temperature for preparing smooth and dense hydroxyapatite films using electrospraying.

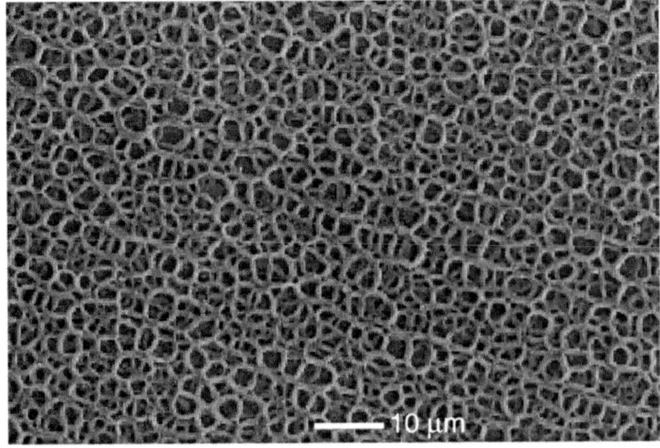

FIGURE 11.21 SEM of CaP coating deposited by electrospraying technique. (Reprinted from Leeuwenburgh, S.C.G. et al., *J. Eur. Ceram. Soc.*, 26, 487, 2006. © Elsevier Science. With permission.)

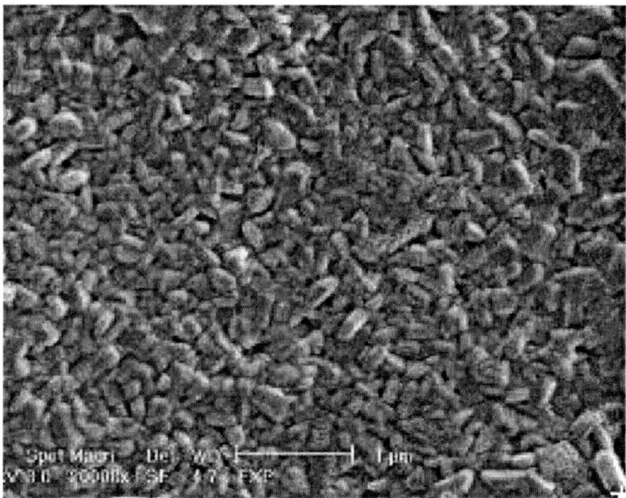

FIGURE 11.22 SEM of hydroxyapatite (HAP) films deposited using electrospraying at 80°C. (Reprinted from Kim, B.H., 33, 119, 2007. © Elsevier Science. With permission.)

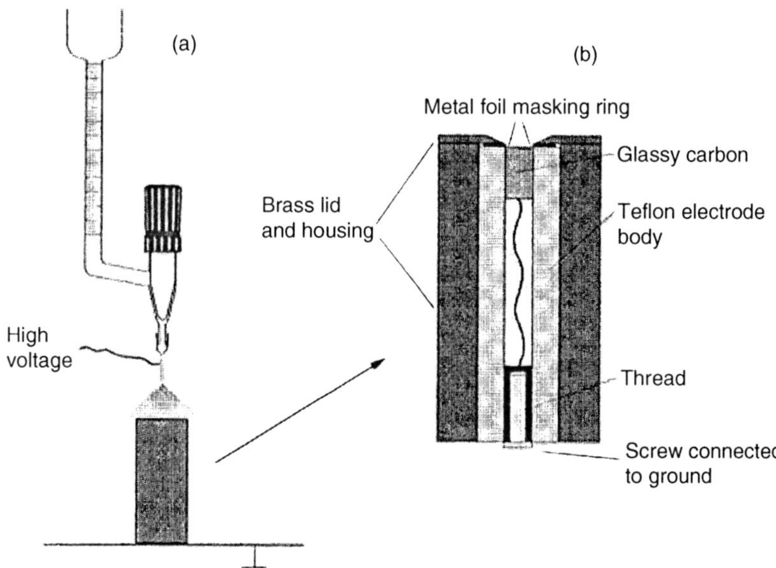

FIGURE 11.23 A schematic diagram of electrospraying coating setup (a) and cross-section of electrode (b). (Reprinted from Hoyer, B. et al., *Anal. Chem.*, 68, 3840, 1996. © American Chemical Society. With permission.)

11.2.8.2.2 Biopolymer Materials

Hoyer et al. deposited biological cellulose acetate (CA) membranes on carbon electrodes using electrospraying [74]. The spraying solution consisted of 20 g of acetone, 0.250 mL of pore-former solution, and 0.05 g of CA. The purpose of the CA membrane prepared by electrospraying was to prevent fouling of the electrode surface by discriminating against macromolecular species, which often cause severe absorption interferences when complex samples are analyzed by electrochemical methods. The schematic diagram of an electrospraying apparatus for preparing CA coating is shown in Figure 11.23. The precursor was fed to the needle from a grounded glass capillary with a screw-type Teflon stopcock whose tip was conical-shaped to allow easy pressure mounting of standard injection needles. Before electrospraying, the carbon electrode was inserted into a cylindrical brass housing shown in Figure 11.23b. The results have shown that electrospraying can produce CA membranes with a high quality and uniform thickness, which is important for a biological membrane.

Morota et al. generated nanostructured PEO films using electrospraying from an aqueous solution [75]. The films fabricated through electrospraying can find wide application in the fields of biosensors, microfluidic devices, antifouling, and biocompatible layers for medical devices. In this study, the influences of the applied voltage and the solution properties (viscosity, surface tension, conductivity, and molecular weight) on the microstructure of the PEO films were thoroughly investigated. It was the first comprehensive study on the control of nanostructured PEO polymer thin films prepared using electrospraying. By varying the applied voltage and the solution properties, the microstructure of PEO films is changed from nanospherical to nanofibrous. The study results demonstrated several conclusions: (1) a higher applied voltage tended to produce fibrous microstructures; (2) a higher polymer concentration tended to produce fibrous microstructures; (3) a higher electrical conductivity tended to produce fibrous microstructures; (4) a higher molecular weight tended to produce a fibrous structure, which suggested that the configuration of the polymer chains and their entanglement in solution contributed to the formation of the fibrous structure. The SEM images of the electrosprayed PEO films with various molecular weights are shown in Figure 11.24. These experimental results can provide systematic information for the preparation of nanostructured PEO-based thin films using electrospraying.

Berkland et al. developed a modified electrospraying technique, named flow-limited field-injection electrostatic spraying (FFESS) to prepare poly(D,L-lactide-*co*-glycolide) (PLG) films with various controllable micro- and nanostructures [76]. The technique provided enhanced control of surface microstructure of the PLG films by injecting charge into the PLG solution using a nanosharpened tungsten electrode. A schematic diagram of a comparison between conventional electrospraying (CES) and FFESS is shown in Figure 11.25. The advantage is field-ionization of the polymer solution through charge injection so that an insulating solution can still be electrosprayed in a stable and uniform jet-spraying mode through emission from a smooth glass nozzle. By varying the flow rate, the solution concentration, the applied voltage, and the electrospraying distance, a wide variety of structures—from smooth films to uniform nanoparticles—were produced using FFESS. The surface structure discretely changed from smooth to increasingly porous to distinct particles is shown in Figure 11.26. The ability to produce biodegradable PLG polymer

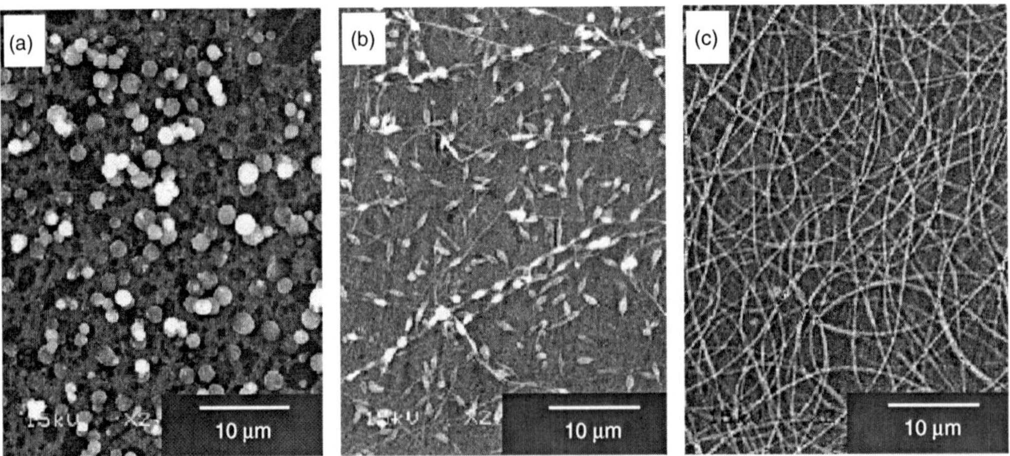

FIGURE 11.24 SEM images of electrospraying PEO films from polymer with different molecular weights are as follows: (a) 20,000, (b) 500,000, and (c) 4,000,000. (Reprinted from Morota, K. et al., *J. Colloid Interface Sci.*, 279, 484, 2004. © Elsevier Science. With permission.)

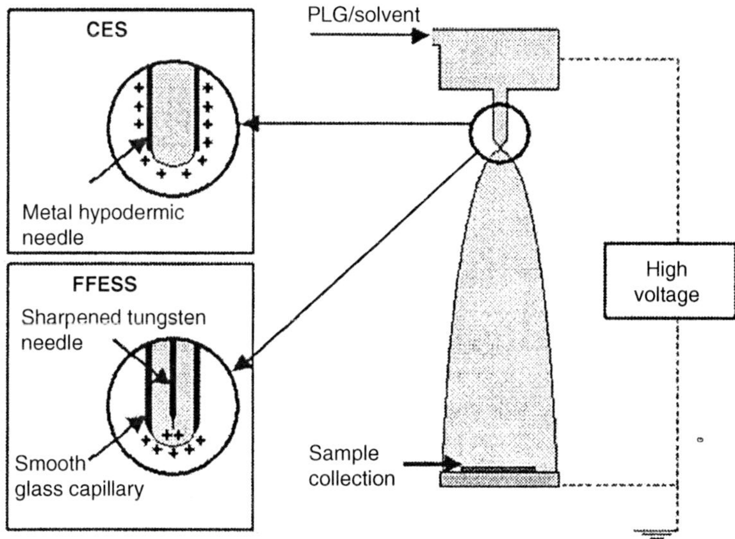

FIGURE 11.25 Schematic diagrams of FFESS and CES. (Reprinted from Berkland, C., Pack, D.W., and Kim, K., *Biomaterials*, 25, 5649, 2004. © Elsevier Science. With permission.)

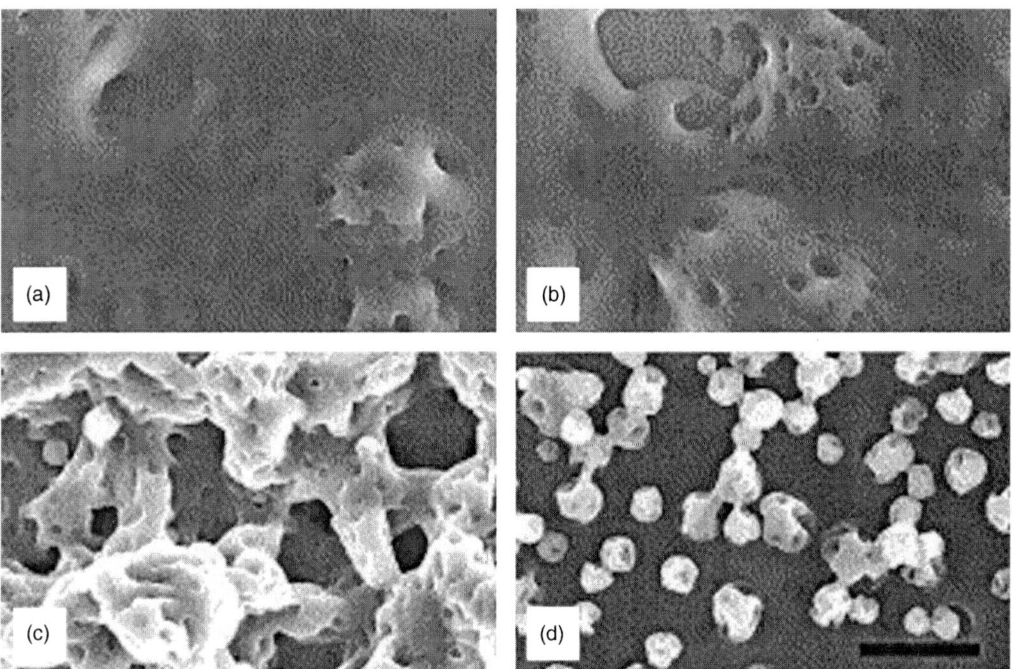

FIGURE 11.26 SEM images of films prepared using different voltages are as follows: (a) 4 kV, (b) 5 kV, (c) 6 kV, and (d) 9 kV. Scale bar—5 µm. (Reprinted from Berkland, C., Pack, D.W., and Kim, K., *Biomaterials*, 25, 5649, 2004. © Elsevier Science. With permission.)

with definable micro- and nanostructures provides an opportunity to develop enhanced biological and medical devices, which may lead to enhanced performance of devices such as vascular grafts, tissue scaffolds, and templates for guided tissue regeneration. There are two differences between the CES and the FFESS processes. Firstly, the FFESS relied on a charge-injection electrode to charge the solution surface and resulted in reproducible charging and stable axisymmetric electrospraying. Secondly, at high voltages the charge injection was dominated by field injection because of the sharp electrode, and thus generated finer particles and fibers.

11.2.8.2.3 Native Biomaterials

The manufacturing of protein and other biomolecule biomaterial films onto an electrode surface is a necessary step in the fabrication of enzyme electrodes and other types of biosensors for biomedical application. Morozov and Morozova were the first to prepare functionally active protein films using electrospraying [77]. A schematic diagram of the setup for depositing protein is shown in Figure 11.27. They used a solution prepared by dissolving a commercial dry powder of alkaline phosphates in water. In the experiment, three different designs of the capillaries for electrospraying were studied. The first design, as shown in Figure 11.27a, was a glass capillary coated with a silver layer on the external surface of a glass capillary. A conductive wire that is in contact with the coated capillary was connected with a high-voltage power supply. In the second design, as shown in Figure 11.27b, the metal electrode was not exposed to a gas phase in order to reduce the risk of corona discharge at high voltage, which was a glass capillary with an inner electrode. In the third version of the capillary design, as shown in Figure 11.27c, a liquid bridge between the electrode and the solution was introduced to avoid any contact of the metal electrode with the protein solution. The external surface of the stainless steel tube was used as an electrode exposed to the interior of the large external glass capillary, whereas the internal thin plastic capillary was used to supply protein solution. The setup for depositing protein materials is shown in Figure 11.28. The experimental results showed that the functional activity of alkaline phosphates could completely survive the electrospraying process. Electrospraying neither destroyed the compact native structure of alkaline phosphates protein molecules nor irreversibly inactivated them. It is definitely a feasible technique to fabricate biologically specific film materials for biosensors, libraries, and diagnostic assays.

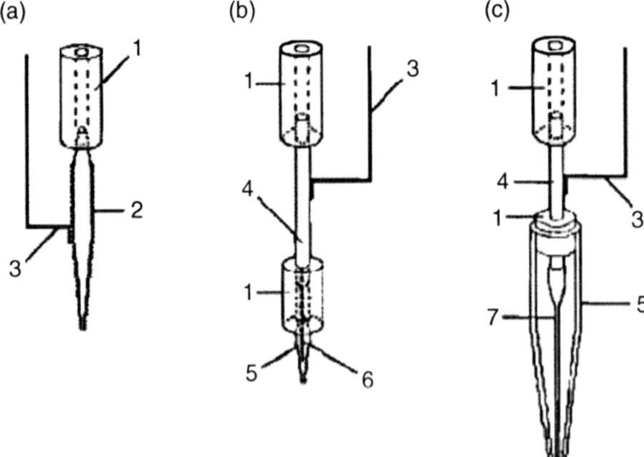

FIGURE 11.27 Types of capillaries used for electrospraying: (a) capillary with external electrode, (b) capillary with internal electrode, and (c) capillary with a liquid bridge. (1) Plastic tubing, (2) glass capillary coated with the silver layer, (3) contact wire, (4) stainless steel tube, (5) glass capillary, (6) internal tungsten or stainless steel electrode, and (7) plastic capillary. (Reprinted from Morozov, V.N. and Morozova, T.Y., *Anal. Chem.*, 71, 1415, 1999. © American Chemical Society. With permission.)

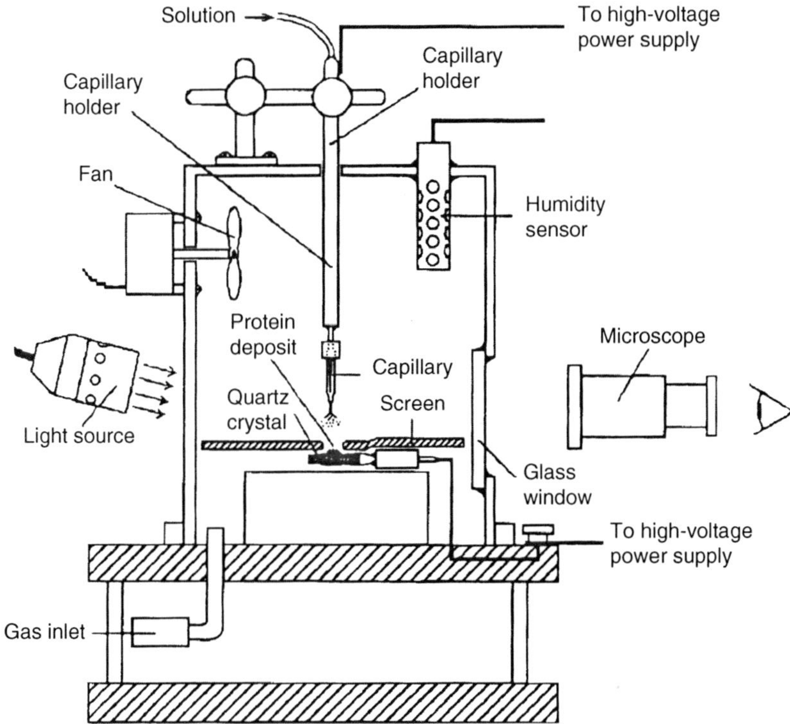

FIGURE 11.28 A schematic diagram of the setup to deposit protein by electrospraying. (Reprinted from Morozov, V.N. and Morozova, T.Y., *Anal. Chem.*, 71, 1415, 1999. © American Chemical Society. With permission.)

Uematsu et al. prepared α-lactalbumin (α-LA) protein films from aqueous solutions of α-LA at different concentrations using electrospraying [78]. α-LA is present in mammalian milk and functions as a specific modifier of the enzyme galactosyltransferase. The schematic diagram of the setup is shown in Figure 11.29. The biological activities of the cross-linked α-LA protein films prepared by electrospraying were tested by the mechanochemical method. Figure 11.30 shows the microstructures of the α-LA films prepared through electrospraying with different initial concentrations. The response to Ca^{2+} ion demonstrated that the biological activity of the films was preserved. The postdeposition cross-linking enabled the fabrication of freestanding α-LA protein films that were insoluble in water, which could open a new direction in the application of protein-based biomaterials. The results of the experiment demonstrated that the electrospraying technique is potentially useful for the fabrication of porous and dense protein thin films with biological activities.

Lee et al. [79] successfully electrosprayed transparent iron-free cytochrome *c* (Cyt *c*) protein film in which the heme was covalently linked with apo-protein matrix. The photochemically active Cyt *c* protein film can be cross-linked covalently through the proto-porphyrin IX and iron-free Cyt *c*. The electrospraying instrument is schematically illustrated in Figure 11.31. A glass capillary with internal platinum electrode of 50 μm in diameter was used as a nozzle for electrospraying. To control the humidity and the environment air, the instrument was installed in a chamber. Iron-free Cyt *c* desalted with PD-10 column to reduce their electrical conductivity was electrosprayed on an ITO-glass substrate and then cross-linked with the vapor of 70% glutaraldehyde aqueous solution. The prepared protein films still preserved the functional properties of the molecules from damage upon electrospraying and found higher thermal stability of the burned holes of the proto-porphyrin IX (PPIX) in

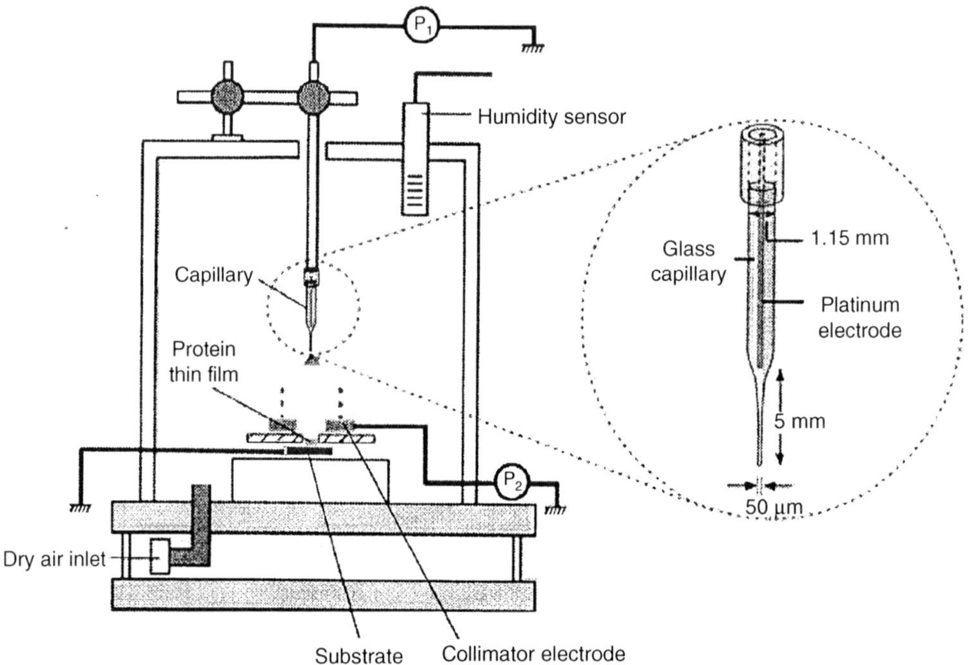

FIGURE 11.29 A schematic diagram of the electrospraying device. (Reprinted from Uematsu, I. et al., *J. Colloid Interface Sci.*, 269, 336, 2004. © Elsevier Science. With permission.)

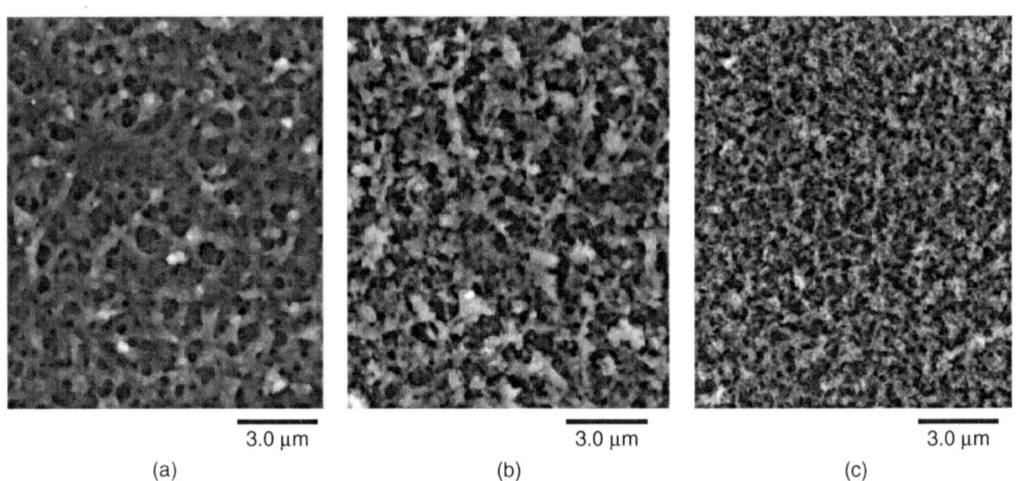

FIGURE 11.30 Surface SEM images of electrospray-deposited protein thin film using different concentrations: (a) 0.5 mg/mL, (b) 1.25 mg/mL, and (c) 2.5 mg/mL. (Reprinted from Uematsu, I. et al., *J. Colloid Interface Sci.*, 269, 336, 2004. © Elsevier Science. With permission.)

Cyt *c* than in the synthetic polymer. Electrospraying can be successfully applied in the manufacture of bioactive films or coatings in various fields, including molecular memory devices as frequency-domain optical memory for molecular computing and the electrodes in biodevices.

Research has also demonstrated the significant impact of the topography of 3-D implants, such as the pore size, porosity, and roughness on the cell interactions, and the biocompatibility with the tissues. To facilitate the implant integration with the tissue, 3-D porous microstructured biopolymer

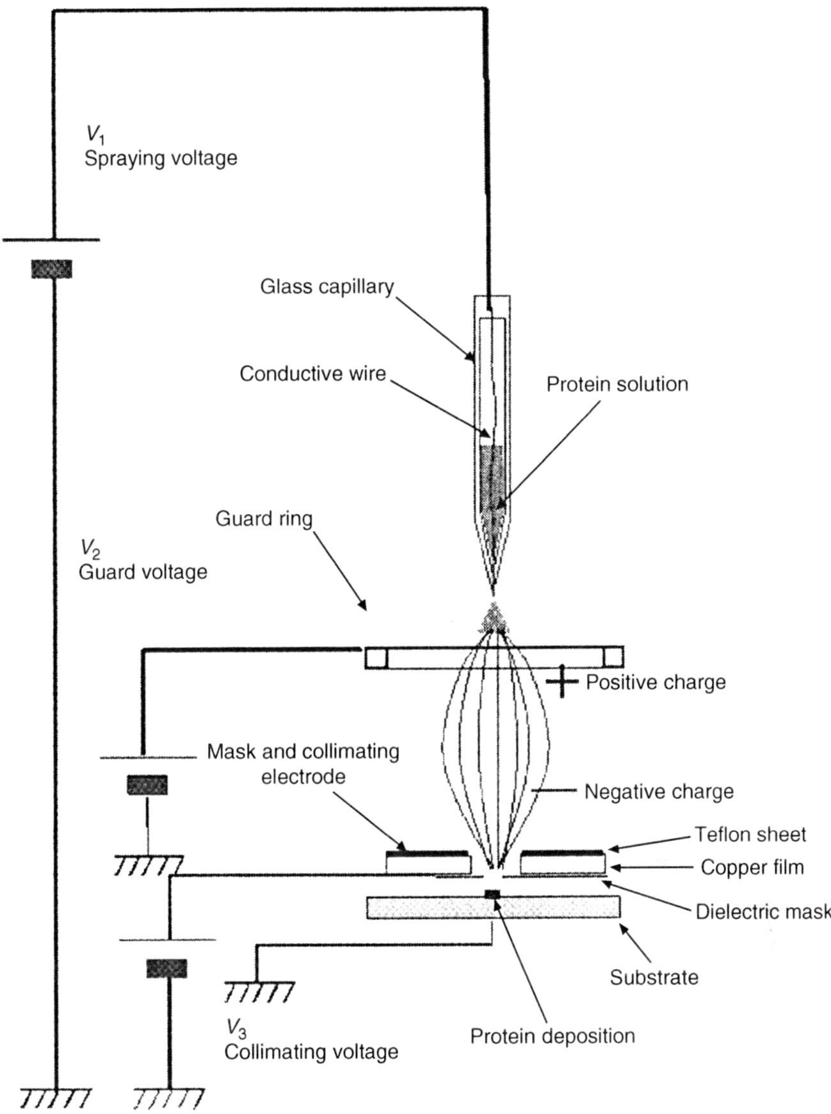

FIGURE 11.31 A schematic diagram of the electrospraying setup for fabricating protein films. (Reprinted from Lee, B. et al., *Biomaterials*, 24, 2045, 2003. © Elsevier Science. With permission.)

films or coatings are deposited on the surface of implants. For example, genetically engineered protein coatings were intended to improve the performance of implantable neural prosthetic devices. Buchko et al. [80] prepared native biopolymer coatings on the silicon substrate using electrospraying in terms of the processing parameters and the microstructure of coatings. The solution was prepared by dissolving the protein silk-like polymer with fibronectin functionality (SLPF) in formic acid. In the study, the protein coatings deposited on the silicon substrate with varied topography were used as models for providing a means for the quantitative exploration of the topography effects on the performance of the neural prosthetic devices and biocompatibility. The SLPF coatings were made from biosynthesized polypeptides designed to contain the structural stability of natural silk and the biofunctional properties of proteins native to the body. The image of porous SLPF film is shown in Figure 11.32.

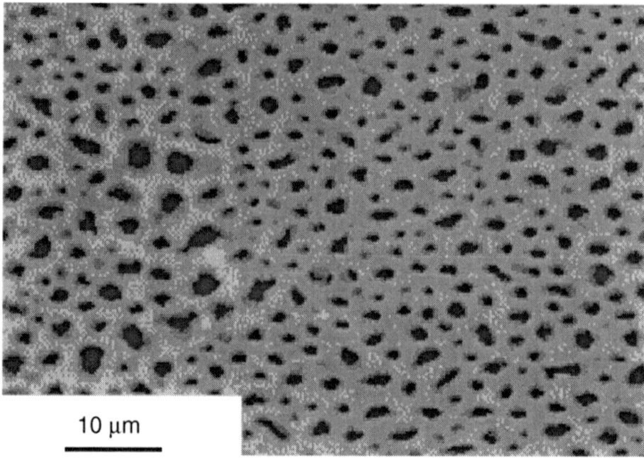

FIGURE 11.32   An image of protein-thin films prepared using electrospraying. (Reprinted from Buchko, C.J., Kozloff, K.M., and Martin, D.C., *Biomaterials*, 22, 1289, 2001. © Elsevier Science. With permission.)

11.2.8.3   Patterned Nanostructure Biomaterials

11.2.8.3.1   Controllable Deposition of Biomaterials

The ability to deposit biological materials in a controllable fashion with a resolution ranging from micrometers to nanometers is becoming increasingly important in the biomedical and engineering fields. This is because there is an increasing need for miniaturized biodevices to reduce the amount of biomaterials needed and to decrease the analysis time. For example, patterned biomaterials and other biomolecules generated using controllable deposition techniques can be widely applied in proteomics, drug discovery, and tissue engineering [81–83]. Electrospraying has been developed as a technique to deposit biomaterials on substrates in a controllable way, allowing the deposition of various biomaterials dissolved in a solution.

Blake et al. [84] and Ouyang et al. [85] applied electrospraying technique to ionize and then deposited proteins selected individually by mass/charge ration (m/z) at different positions in a controllable way. This technique was designed to be a possible method for the separation of biological materials from mixtures and controllable deposition in the array format for increased throughput of biomedical analysis in the proteomics and biotechnology fields. Figure 11.33 shows a schematic diagram of the setup, which consisted of an electrospraying ionization source and vacuum interface, ion optics, a mass analyzer, associated electronics, as well as a surface positioning system. The whole system was housed in a single vacuum chamber. This technique exhibited good spatial resolution in the deposition of biological materials through a computer-controlled XYZ platform, because the electrosprayed ion-beam spots can be controlled to achieve micrometer dimensions. In the experiment, a mixture of four proteins—Cyt c, lysozyme, insulin, and apomyoglobin was separated and deposited on a substrate using electrospraying ionization technique. The results showed that the deposition efficiency of native proteins did not depend on the selected charge state of the proteins. Other examples that have an ability to prepare arrays of different biomaterials from a mixture of proteins are illustrated in Figure 11.34. The analysis of the results for individual array spots demonstrated the success of the controlled deposition of biological materials using electrospraying and mass-selective techniques from the mixture components, and none of the individual spectra of the array spot contained more than one protein.

Welle et al. developed a process, which combined electrospraying technique and electric-force directing deposition, to deposit biological materials onto a desired area on a substrate [86]. The process applied the electrospraying technique to atomize the biological materials from a liquid into a gas phase, and employed the global and localized electric fields to direct and deposit the electrosprayed biomaterials onto the desired locations on a substrate. Figure 11.35 shows an illustration of the deposition system, which included an electrospraying ionization module and an electric field–assisted

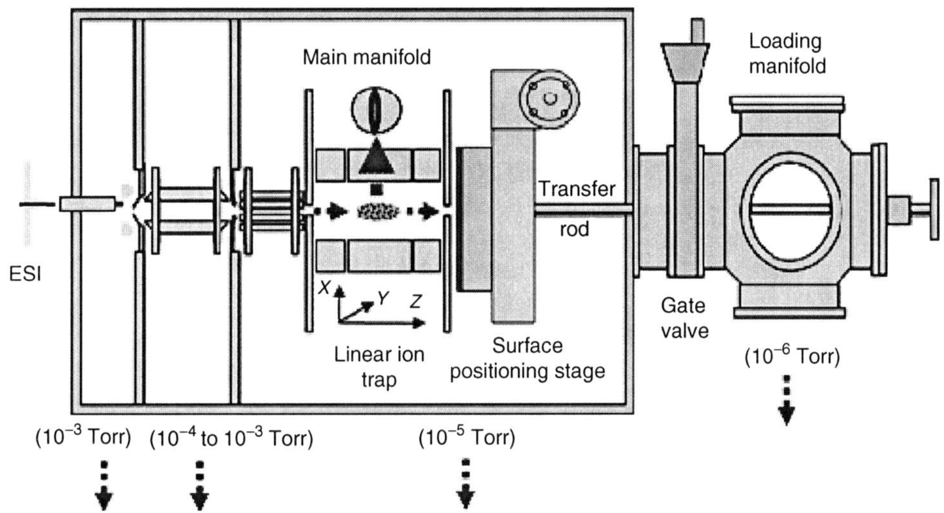

FIGURE 11.33 A schematic of soft-landing instrument including electrospraying setup. (Reprinted from Blake, T.A. et al., *Anal. Chem.*, 76, 6293, 2004. © American Chemical Society. With permission.)

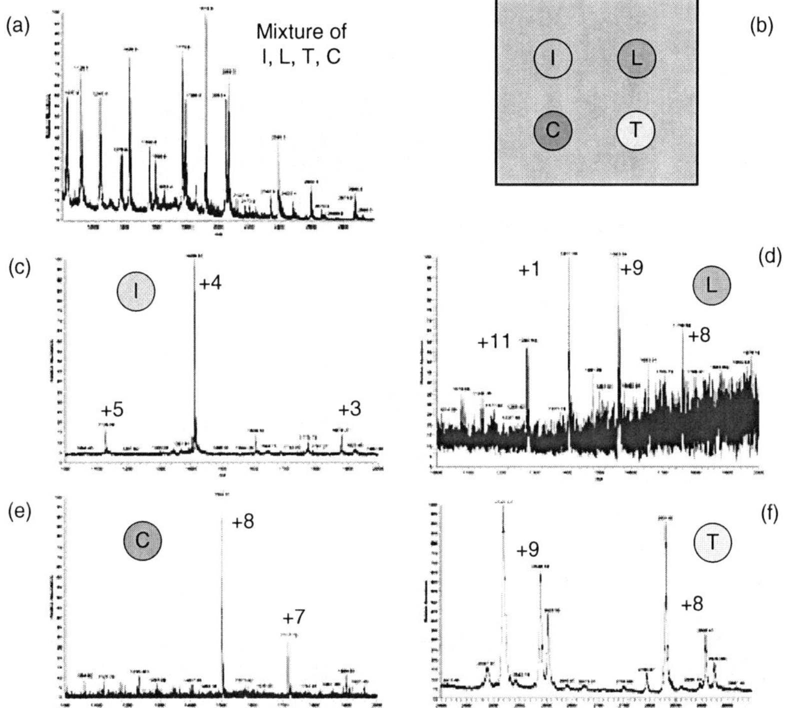

FIGURE 11.34 An array of different spots prepared using electrosprayed ion soft landing from a protein mixture: (a) spectrum of the four proteins insulin (I), lysozyme (L), trypsin (T), and cytochrome *c* (C); (b) deposition of protein array; (c)–(f) spectrum of individual protein spot. (Reprinted from Blake, T.A. et al., *Anal. Chem.*, 76, 6293, 2004. © American Chemical Society. With permission.)

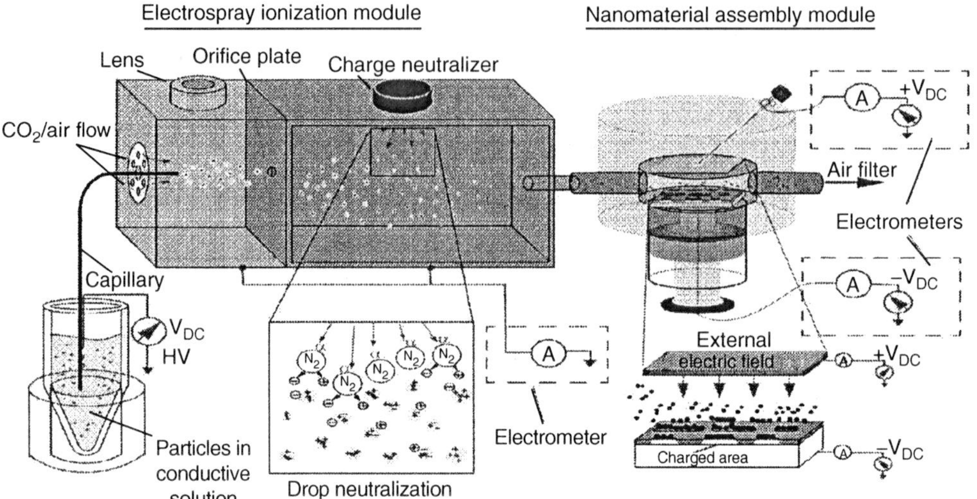

FIGURE 11.35 A schematic diagram of electrospraying technique for controllable deposition. (Reprinted from Welle, A.M. and Jacobs, H.O., *Appl. Phys. Lett.*, 87, 263119, 2005. © American Institute of Physics. With permission.)

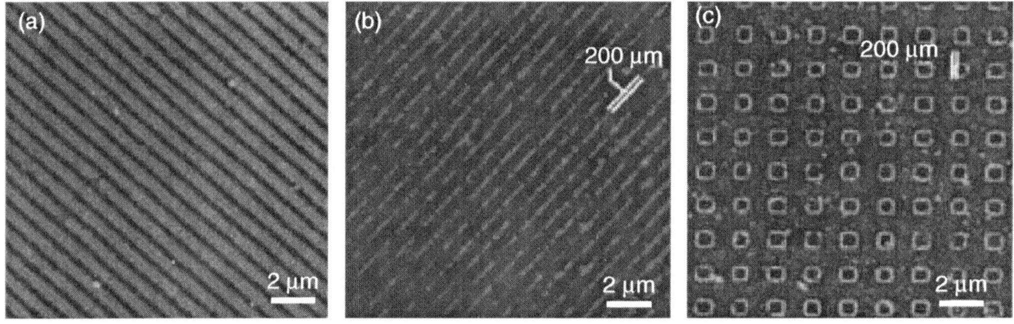

FIGURE 11.36 Fluorescent microscope images of printed proteins are as follows: (a) albumin FITC bovine, (b) avidin sulforhodamine, and (c) albumin FITC bovine. (Reprinted from Welle, A.M. and Jacobs, H.O., *Appl. Phys. Lett.*, 87, 263119, 2005. © American Institute of Physics. With permission.)

assembly module. The electrospraying system, which consisted of a high-voltage source, a pressure regulator and chamber, a capillary, and a neutralization chamber, can provide a greater control to monitor the electrospraying currents. An electrometer was used to monitor the electrospraying current, which varied depending on the flow rate, the solution properties, and the electrospraying voltage. The highly charged primary droplets entered a neutralization chamber and formed aerosol, which was introduced to an assembly module through an opening. An electric field was applied to bring charged biological materials into close proximity of the charged patterned substrate to attract the oppositely charged biomaterials in an assembled way. Figure 11.36 shows fluorescent micrographs taken from different types of proteins deposited on substrates using electrospraying. All images show patterned microstructures generated through a controlled deposition. Figure 11.36a shows albumin fluorescein isothiocyanate (FITC) bovine deposited onto negatively charged lines. The albumin FITC bovine was electrosprayed in a positive ion mode to generate positively charged protein aerosol, and then a positive potential was applied to the top electrode in the assembly module while the substrate was kept at ground to direct the positively charged proteins to the substrate surface in a controllable way. Figure 11.36b shows positively charged avidin assembled onto negatively charged lines using the same technique. Figure 11.36c shows albumin FITC bovine that was assembled onto negatively charged squares.

11.2.8.3.2 Biochip Manufacturing

Techniques for manufacturing biological materials in microarrays have attracted great interest, as microarrays are indispensable for genetics, medical diagnostics, and pharmaceutical analyses to enable the parallel tests of many compounds [87–90]. Therefore, there is a demand for the biochip manufacturing technologies with which a variety of proteins in infinitesimal amounts can be prepared in small spots to enhance the screening throughput without losing their biological activity. Electrospraying has been developed as a method to prepare biochips of biological materials to meet the requirements. It is a method of generating very fine droplets from a solution by means of electrostatic charging and is an effective technique for immobilizing biological materials with a very small amount of samples. During the electrospraying process, the dehydration process for biological materials is extremely quick, and thus the activity loss of bioactive materials is low. Moreover, the electrospraying can allow a spontaneous deposition of many identical arrays with a remarkable spatial resolution.

Morozov and Morozova applied electrospraying technique as a method for mass fabrication of mono- and multicomponent microarrays of biological and biologically active substances on certain areas of a substrate [91]. Microarrays of protein and DNA can be deposited simultaneously through an array of holes in a dielectric mask covering a slightly conductive substrate. Multicomponent microarrays can be manufactured by shifting the mask with respect to the substrate and then depositing a new substance on a desired area. A schematic illustration is shown in Figures 11.37a and 11.37b. The basic setup included a glass capillary connected to a power supply, a dielectric mask with an array of holes, a ground electrode, a conducting substrate, and a chamber. The microarrays on a biochip can be produced by attracting electrosprayed substances onto the specified substrate areas under the control of a local electrostatic field. One way to form such a field was to cover a conducting substrate with a dielectric mask containing an array of holes, as shown in Figure 11.37a. Another way was to locally increase conductivity of a photoconductive substrate by illuminating it through an appropriate photomask to attract charged substances onto the illuminated areas, as illustrated in Figure 11.37b.

Proteins (bovine intestinal AP, horseradish peroxidase, HHb, HSA, BSA, OA, the IgG fraction of a goat anti-HSA antiserum and mouse monoclonal antibiotin AP conjugate) were deposited from water solutions with concentrations of 0.1–1.0 mg/mL. The processing parameters for depositing the proteins were as follows: a voltage of 3.0–4.0 kV, a current of 5–50 nA, a humidity of 30–70%, and a flow rate of 0.1–0.2 µL/min. The precursor solutions were dialyzed for 12–24 h before electrospraying in order to reduce their electrical conductivity. The results demonstrated that dots in a micrometer range were fabricated using this electrospraying technique. Importantly, the proteins and DNA biochip retained their ability to specifically bind antibodies and match DNA probes, which enabled the fabrication of matrices in dot immunobinding (DIB) and in DNA hybridization assays. The results also provided additional evidence for the preservation of functional properties of the electrosprayed biological molecules, such as antigenic and enzyme catalytic properties of proteins and the hybridization ability of DNA molecules. By using the electrospraying technique, enzymes can be deposited on the surface of redox or pH electrodes to design multicomponent enzyme biosensors. Different antibodies or DNA molecules can also be deposited onto an array of quartz resonators used in a plasmon resonance detector.

Lee et al. used electrospraying to prepare protein microarrays for immunoassay [92]. In the work, an antibody-based protein microarray for high-throughput immunoassay was fabricated by an electrospraying method using a quartz mask with holes. The protein was deposited under the control of a local electrostatic field, which was formed by masking a conducting substrate using a dielectric mask with holes. Therefore, the electrosprayed protein was attracted and deposited onto specified substrate areas through the holes in the mask. An anti-immunoglobulin (IgG) antibody solution was electrosprayed onto a glass substrate using parameters of 3.0–4.0 kV and humidity 20–30%. After the

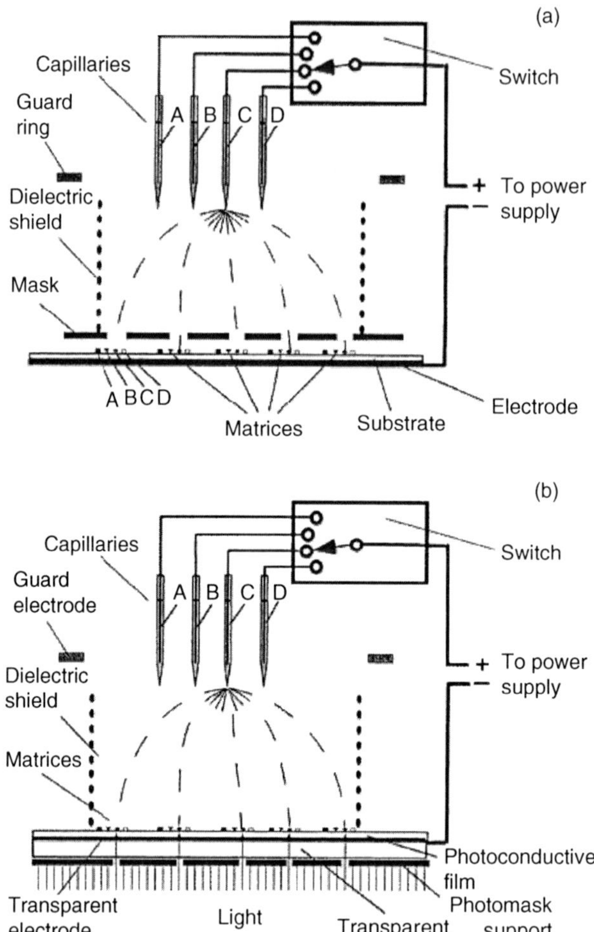

FIGURE 11.37 A schematic diagram of fabrication of biochip using electrospraying. (Reprinted from Morozov, V.N. and Morozova, T.Y., *Anal. Chem.*, 71, 3110, 1999. © American Chemical Society. With permission.)

electrospraying, the deposited anti-IgG antibody arrays were blocked with 2% skimmed milk in phosphate buffer solution (PBS) for 2 h at room temperature, then the plates were incubated with appropriate quantities of horseradish peroxidase (HRP) or FITC-conjugated IgG antigens (100 ng/mL) for 1 h at 37°C. The excess antigens were washed away with PBS/0.1% Tween 20 and PBS solution. Finally, a protein multimicroarray with several kinds of IgG antibodies was manufactured. Figure 11.38 shows the electrospraying-deposited spots of anti-mouse IgG. The multimicroarray biochips fabricated using electrospraying technique showed neither nonspecific absorption nor nonspecific binding. These electrosprayed protein spots were still biologically active, which was advantageous to the reproducible quantification of antigens. The experiment demonstrated that this technique is applicable in protein array biochip manufacturing, allowing the spontaneous deposition of many identical arrays.

Moerman et al. applied a miniaturized electrospraying technique to produce microarrays of reproducible micrometer-sized biomaterial spots [93]. In the process, the charged jet from the capillary tip broke into a spray of charged droplets and deposited in the form of uniform spots at 220–400 μm on a substrate. The study demonstrated that electrospraying in a stable cone-jet mode at <400 μm spraying distance was a powerful technique to produce spots in a micrometer-sized range. After a spot was prepared, the distance between the capillary tip and the substrate was increased

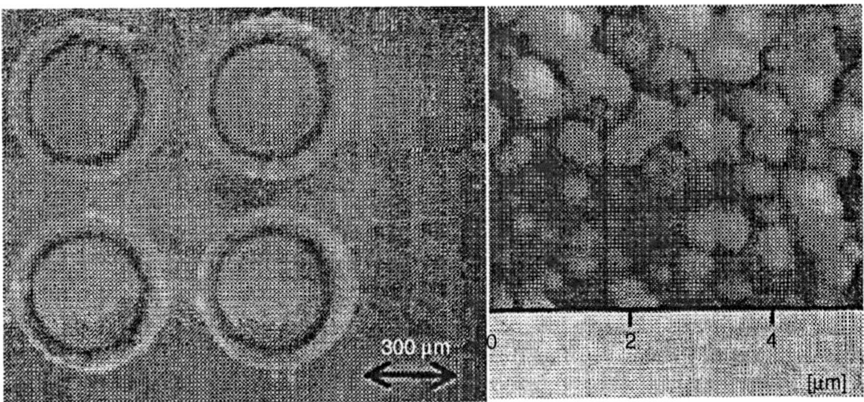

FIGURE 11.38   SEM images of electrosprayed protein spots. (From Lee, B. et al., *J. Chem. Eng. Jpn*, 36, 1370, 2003. © Society of Chemical Engineers, Japan. With permission.)

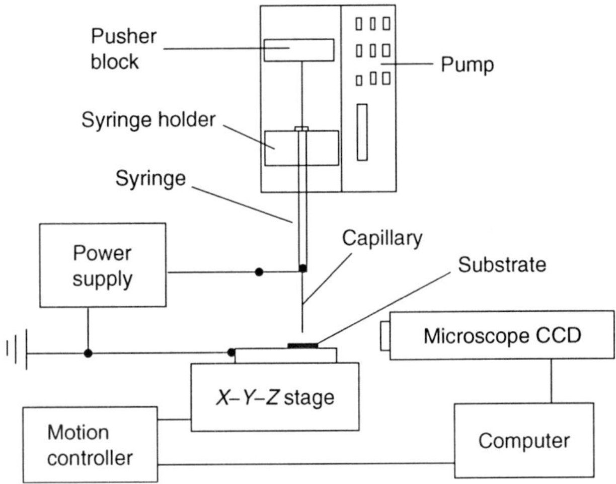

FIGURE 11.39   A schematic diagram of electrospraying for producing microarrays. (Reprinted from Moerman, R. et al., *Anal. Chem.*, 73, 2183, 2001. © American Chemical Society. With permission.)

more than 400 µm, which stopped the spraying instantaneously. Then, a rapid shift of the substrate sideways and a decrease of the electrospraying distance were performed to resume the electrospraying again, because of the increased electric field strength, which resulted in the deposition of a second spot. A microarray biochip can be manufactured by repeating the process automatically. A schematic diagram of the setup is shown in Figure 11.39. The syringe displaced liquid through the connected stainless steel capillary, which was connected to a power supply. The aluminum substrate fixed on a grounded metal holder was accurately positioned and moved relative to the capillary using an X–Y–Z table. Solutions containing biological materials were electrosprayed in the form of spots by repeatedly moving the substrate 100 µm downward (spraying stops), 400 µm sideways (to the next target area in <150 ms), and 100 µm upward (spraying), as shown in Figure 11.40. The applied voltage and the flow rate were kept constant during the electrospraying of array spots. The spot diameter was mainly determined as a function of the flow rate, liquid properties, applied voltage, spraying distance, and deposition time.

Figure 11.41 shows the microarrays of uniform spots that were prepared by electrospraying a liquid solution consisting of 20 U/mL of lactate dehydrogenase (LDH), 0.5 wt.% of trehalose,

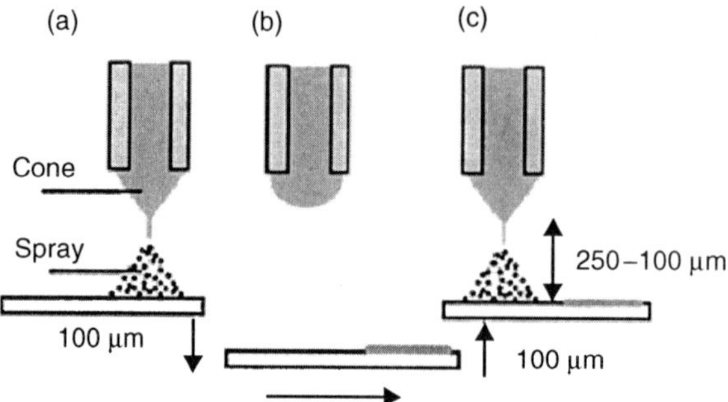

FIGURE 11.40   Schematic diagram of the cone-jet electrospraying mode (a), electrospraying stops due to an increase of the distance between the tip and substrate (b), and electrospraying resumes (c). (Reprinted from Moerman, R. et al., *Anal. Chem.*, 73, 2183, 2001. © American Chemical Society. With permission.)

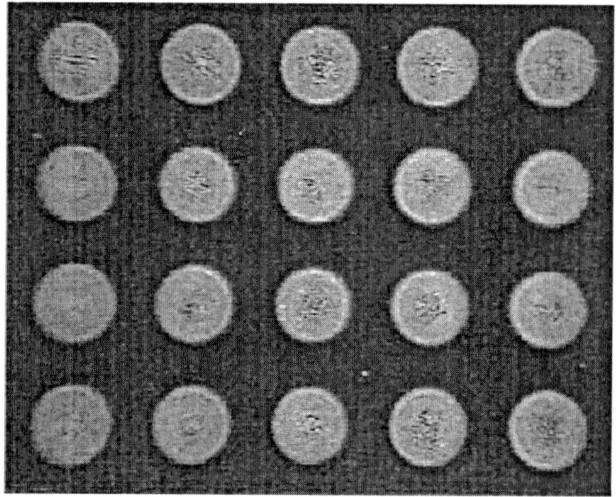

FIGURE 11.41   Images of protein spots manufactured by miniaturized electrospraying. Spot diameter—260 µm. (Reprinted from Moerman, R. et al., *Anal. Chem.*, 73, 2183, 2001. © American Chemical Society. With permission.)

0.5 wt.% of Brij 35, and 0.05 M triethanolamine (TEA). A spraying time of 1 s and a spraying voltage of 1.3 kV were used. The effects of electrospraying on the activities of the relatively labile enzymes LDH, glucose-6-phosphate dehydrogenase (G6P-DH), and pyruvate kinase (PK) were analyzed in a quantitative manner. The experiment revealed that electrospraying of LDH, G6P-DH, and PK on a liquid layer resulted in a complete preservation of their activities. Particularly, when multiple analytes need to be studied simultaneously and quantitatively, a biochip device is needed to allow for parallel dispensing of small liquid volumes accurately without cross-contamination. A miniaturized electrospraying in the cone-jet mode was proved to be a powerful and promising technique for manufacturing biochip microarrays of active enzyme spots. The biological activities can be completely preserved after electrospraying at the moderate processing parameters with an appropriate solution.

11.2.8.4   Encapsulated Electrospraying of Biomaterials

Encapsulation technology for preparing microbeads and microcapsules has been used in many fields [94–98]. For example, microparticles encapsulated with cells were applied for cell transplantation therapy in medicine for the treatment of several diseases and for protecting cells from shear damage. Electrospraying technique has recently been investigated as a method for preparing encapsulated particles and beads in a controllable size. The encapsulated substances can be imbedded into the microparticles by mixing the living cells or biological materials with the precursor or by reacting to the electrosprayed droplets with a collecting solution to form microbeads.

11.2.8.4.1 Biomolecule-Encapsulated Biomaterials

Amsden et al. has studied electrospraying for generating polymeric microbeads loaded with solid protein particles [99]. This method involved electrospraying a suspension of protein particles within a polymer solution under an electric field. The electric force effectively atomized the droplet off the end of the needle and generated a series of smaller droplets. The electrosprayed droplets formed microbeads by reacting with a collecting solution. In the work, a solution of BSA particles suspended in a mixture of ethylene vinyl acetate (EVA) and dichloromethane was used for electrospraying. Figure 11.42 shows the experimental setup for the microbead production. The mixed solution was poured into a stirring sealed flask. The agitated protein and dissolved EVA suspension was forced through a needle by air pressure, which was regulated to ensure that the flow rate of the suspension was kept at 0.5 mL/min. A positive electrode was connected to the needle while a ground was applied to the collecting solution, which was 4 cm below the needle. The collecting solution consisted of methanol cooled to $-75°C$ using a dry ice/methanol bath contained in a Dewar flask so that the EVA promptly gelled and then slowly precipitated upon entering the solution. The electrosprayed EVA/protein microbeads were kept in the cold methanol for 5 min and then transferred along with the methanol into a glass dish, which was stored in a $-20°C$ environment for 2 days. After that, the microbeads were placed in a vacuum at room temperature for 1 day to remove the solvent completely. The experimental results illustrated that the microbead size and size distribution were controlled primarily by the strength of the electric field, the gauge of the needle, and the EVA concentration. Figure 11.43 shows a diagram of the electrosprayed bead diameter distributions using a 15% w/v EVA concentration and an applied voltage of 4.0 kV. The smaller microbeads can be formed by using a higher electric field and a smaller internal diameter needle. Protein was effectively incorporated into the microbeads, which was demonstrated by its release from the microbeads into a saline solution. The critical volumetric loading for the microbeads was dependent on the size

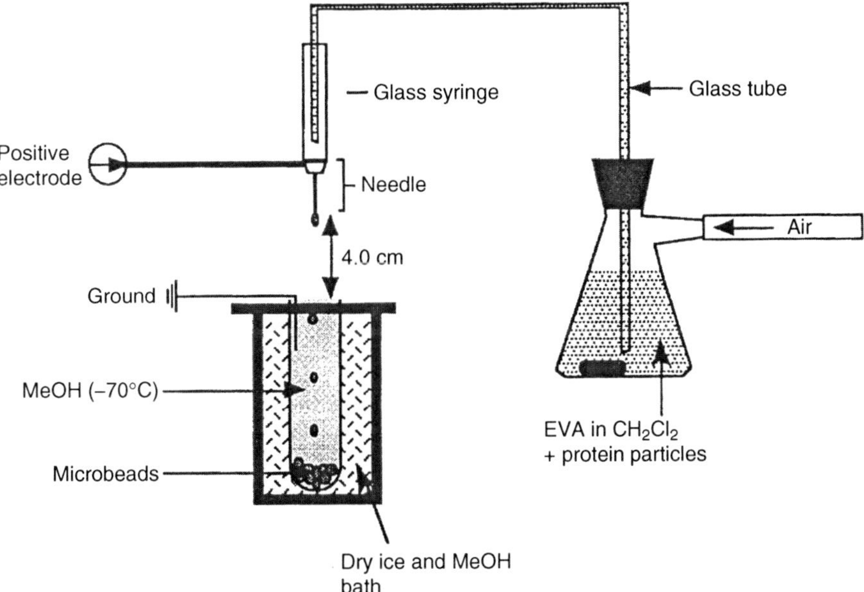

FIGURE 11.42 A schematic diagram of microbead production electrospraying apparatus. (Reprinted from Amsden, B.G. and Goosen, M.F.A., *J. Contr. Release*, 43, 183, 1997. © Elsevier Science. With permission.)

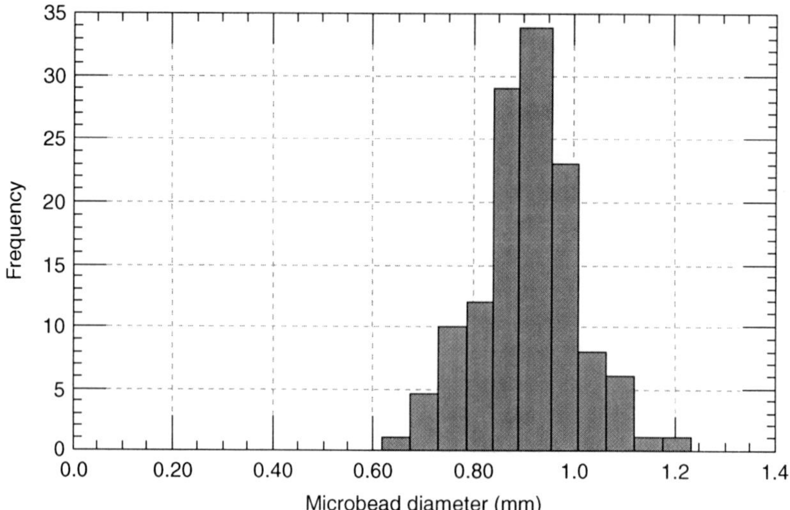

FIGURE 11.43 Electrosprayed bead diameter distributions at a 15% w/v EVA concentration and 4.0 kV applied voltage. (Reprinted from Amsden, B.G. and Goosen, M.F.A., *J. Contr. Release*, 43, 183, 1997. © Elsevier Science. With permission.)

of the incorporated particle and was approximately 0.40 and 0.45 for the encapsulated protein with an average size of 92 and 26 μm, respectively. The experiments demonstrated that electrospraying is capable of producing protein-loaded hydrophobic polymeric microbeads from a suspension of protein particles in a polymer–organic solvent solution at varying protein volumetric loadings.

Watanabe et al. prepared immobilized enzyme–gel particles with high catalytic effectiveness using an electrospraying atomization technique [100]. In the work, an aqueous sodium-alginate solution containing enzymes was electrosprayed into a $CaCl_2$ solution to prepare gel beads. Sodium alginate, calcium chloride, sucrose, and invertase were used as an immobilizing matrix, a gelling agent, a substrate of enzyme reaction, and an immobilized enzyme, respectively. Figure 11.44 shows the experimental apparatus for electrospraying atomization. A sodium-alginate solution with a concentration of 10–30 g/L containing 1.0 g/L enzyme was flown out from a nozzle electrode. The high DC voltages in a range of 0–5 kV were applied between the nozzle and the grounded electrodes. The electrosprayed droplets of the precursor were ejected into $CaCl_2$ aqueous solution with a concentration of 5–20 g/L. After the gelation in $CaCl_2$ solution, particles immobilizing the enzyme were incubated at 277 K for 24 h to stabilize the gel matrices. The particles were then filtered using a sheet of nitrocellulose membrane with an average pore size of 1.0 μm. The optimum immobilization conditions were (1) an applied voltage of 5.0 kV, (2) a sodium-alginate solution concentration of 30 g/L, and (3) a flow rate of 1.33×10^{-2} mL/min. The relationship between the Ca-alginate bead diameter and the applied voltage is shown in Figure 11.45. It can be seen that the decrease in the diameter was not so sensitive to the applied voltages exceeding V_c. The results also showed that the diameter of microbeads was directly proportional to the power of the volumetric flow rate. The experiments demonstrated that Ca-alginate beads were prepared with a minimum diameter of 100 μm, which was one order smaller than that attained by the conventional dropping methods. In terms of the efficiency based on the encapsulated enzyme, the immobilized enzyme particles had higher effectiveness factors than those prepared by the conventional methods. Electrospraying technique has been proved to be useful for enhancing the performance of immobilized enzyme particles by producing particles with a smaller diameter.

Xu et al. used electrospraying to encapsulate BSA protein with PLA [101]. Principally, an electrosprayed PLA droplet was generated by applying an electric field to a nozzle from which the PLA/BSA solution was pumped. The solutions were prepared by dissolving PLA in 10 mL of

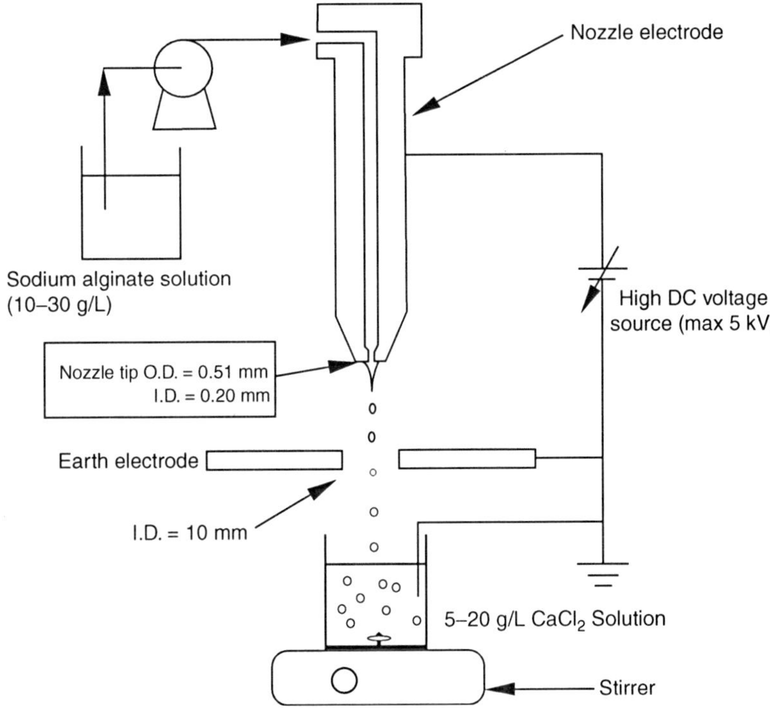

FIGURE 11.44 A schematic diagram of experimental apparatus for electrospraying. (Reprinted from Watanabe, H., Matsuyama, T., and Yamamoto, H., *Biochem. Eng. J.*, 8, 171, 2001. © Elsevier Science. With permission.)

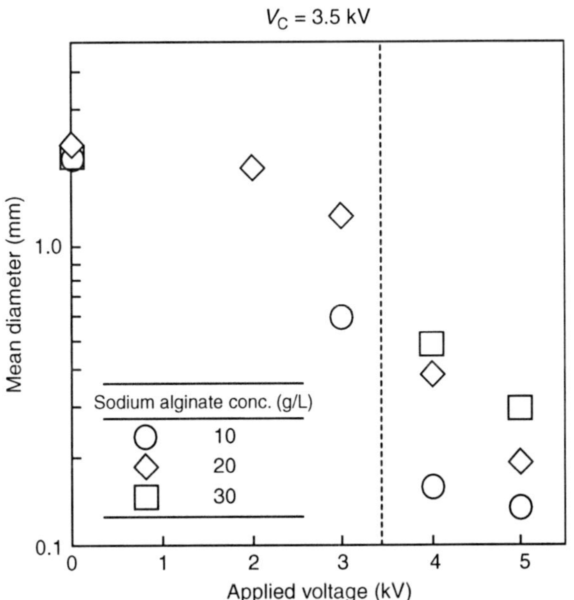

FIGURE 11.45 Dependency of diameter of Ca-alginate beads on applied voltage. (Reprinted from Watanabe, H., Matsuyama, T., and Yamamoto, H., *Biochem. Eng. J.*, 8, 171, 2001. © Elsevier Science. With permission.)

different solvents or solvent mixtures and stirred for 8 h at room temperature. Specific amounts of BSA, previously dissolved in 0.5 mL of distilled water, were mixed with the PLA solutions and emulsified by sonication for 10 min. The emulsion was drawn into a syringe with an 18-gauge metal needle, which was applied at a voltage in a range of 0–30 kV. Different solvents had different effects on the morphology of particles when the voltage and flow rate were fixed at 12.5 kV and 1.0 mL/h, respectively. The experimental results showed that BSA-loaded PLA particles prepared with dichloromethane solvent were spherical with smooth surfaces and had an average diameter of 4.68 ± 1.35 μm. The BSA-loaded particles using 1,2-DCE solvent were also spherical with smooth surfaces and had an average diameter of 4.77 ± 1.97 μm. The average diameter of the electrosprayed particles using 1,2-DCE/acetone solvents was 1.64 ± 0.51 μm, significantly smaller than that using 1,2-DCE. However, the PLA particles were no longer spherical. The results revealed that the spherical particles cannot be achieved from a concentration of 1% PLA, but spherical particles were formed from 2% emulsion. Fully spherical particles were produced at a concentration of 3% emulsion. Further increasing the concentration to 4% resulted in the formation of a mixture of beads and fibers. The experiment also showed that the average diameter of the particles decreased as the applied voltage was increased from 10 to 15 kV, but increased as the flow rate was increased from 0.5 to 3 mL/h.

11.2.8.4.2 Cell-Encapsulated Biomaterials

Electrospraying technique was employed by Zhou et al. to achieve a scalable encapsulation of hepatocytes in the microcapsules formed by complex coacervation between the cationic methylated collagen and the anionic terpolymer of hydroxylethyl methacrylate, methyl methacrylate, and methylacrylic acid (HEMA–MMA–MAA) [102]. Figure 11.46 shows a schematic illustration of the setup for hepatocyte microencapsulation. The system consisted of a syringe pump equipped with a syringe, a rotator, and a high-voltage power supply. For generating encapsulated microbeads, a cell–collagen suspension was electrosprayed into a terpolymer solution (5% w/v) through a syringe fixed on the rotator. This rotator was used to prevent the hepatocyte sedimentation in the collagen solution. It consisted of a shaft with a bearing and an impulse-generator motor, which moved clockwise and counterclockwise repeatedly. The cell–collagen suspension was electrosprayed into tiny droplets using the processing parameters: a high voltage of 5–15 kV between the nozzle and grounded collecting plate and a spraying distance of 3.7 cm between the tip of the nozzle and the collection plate. The microcapsules were exchanged in PBS solution by sedimentation for cell culture and the subsequent characterizations. The encapsulated particles prepared using electrospraying had a diameter in the range of 200–800 μm with a narrow size distribution (standard deviation of 5–28%). The experimental results proved that the microcapsule sizes were dependent on several

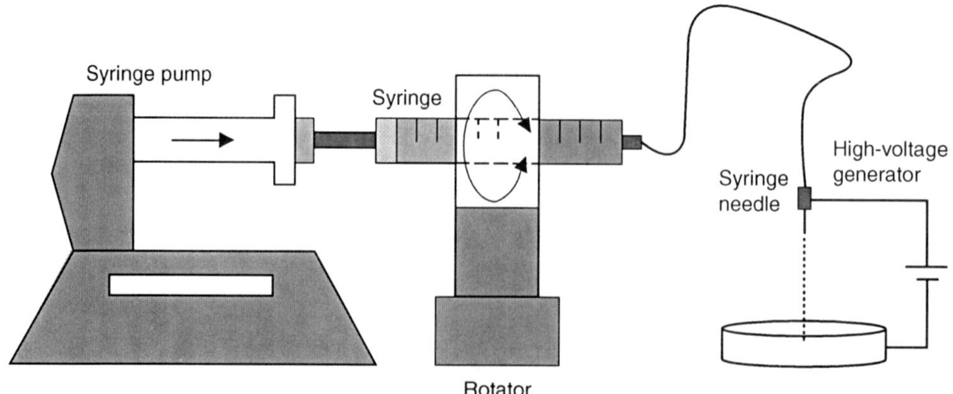

FIGURE 11.46 A schematic diagram of electrospraying for microencapsulation. (Reprinted from Zhou, Y. et al., *J. Biotechnol.*, 117, 99, 2005. © Elsevier Science. With permission.)

important parameters, including the diameter of the nozzle, the flow rate, and the applied voltage. The parameters also influenced the hepatocyte viability and functions. By using appropriate parameters, large quantities of microcapsules can be produced with a practical encapsulation rate of up to 55 mL/h providing good support for hepatocyte viability and functions and maintaining cell viability (>87%) and mechanical stability. The microcapsules formed by this method exhibited good physical properties and hepatocyte biofunctions, which can meet the requirements in bioartificial, liver-assisted device applications. A multiple electrospraying system can be developed for mass production of microencapsulated hepatocytes or other sensitive cells for various cell-based therapeutic applications. This system could represent a practical and scalable method of production for the encapsulation of cell-containing microcapsules.

Al-Hajry et al. used electrospraying to encapsulate callus cells in alginate microparticles [103]. The encapsulation and growth of callus tissue in alginate particles prepared by electrospraying was investigated, as was the mechanism of alginate-encapsulated droplet formation. The encapsulation generation system, as shown in Figure 11.47, consisted of a syringe, a syringe pump, a needle, a high-voltage power supply, and a collecting solution. The positive electrode wire was connected to the needle, and the ground wire was attached to the $CaCl_2$ dehydrate collecting solution. When the alginate solution was pumped through the needle by the syringe pump, the droplets were electrosprayed by the action of electric forces. In some experiments, the needle was removed and the positive electrode wire was inserted directly into the alginate solution. The sodium alginate solutions were prepared first by placing 300 mL of distilled water in a beaker in a boiling water bath, and then alginate powder (3–18 g) was added to this beaker and stirred until the powder got dissolved. After that, the alginate solution was placed in a sealed bottle and stored at 4°C. In the cell immobilization studies, the alginate solutions were autoclaved at 120°C and 15 psi for 20 min before use. For encapsulating the callus cells, the dissociated callus cells of 200 mg were added to a 5 mL of sodium alginate solution with different concentrations of 2%, 4%, and 6% so that the cell loading was approximately 20% (volume of cells/volume of alginate solution). The suspension was electrosprayed into the collecting solution to form encapsulated particles using the processing parameters: an applied voltage of 5.0–10.0 kV, a spraying distance of 6–10 cm, and a flow rate of 36 mL/h. The experiment revealed that callus cells were successfully immobilized by using electrospraying, and the average size of alginate microbeads was as small as 500 ± 50 μm in diameter. The callus cells encapsulated in 2% sodium alginate and cultured on agar gel still retained viability over a 2-month culture period. The encapsulation cell microbeads aided in the germination and growth of callus tissue by enhancing higher cell densities and protecting cells from shear damage in culture media.

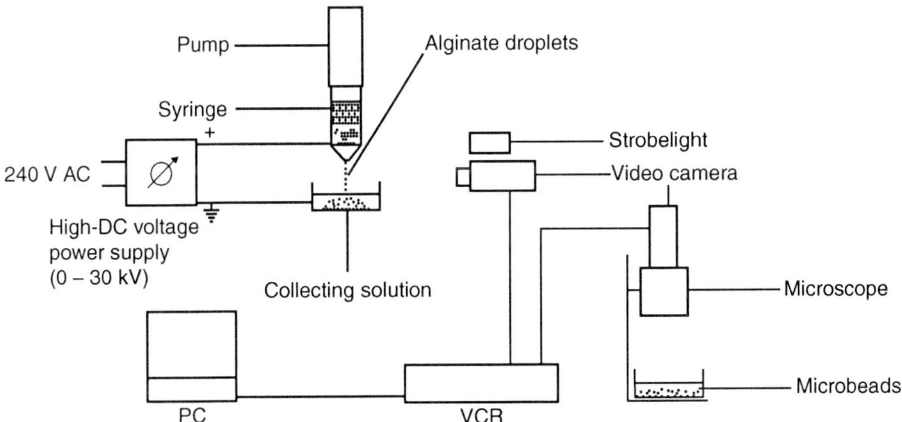

FIGURE 11.47 An electrospraying droplet generator and a video image analysis system. (Reprinted from Al-Hajry, H.A. et al., *Biotechnol. Progr.*, 15, 768, 1999. © American Chemical Society. With permission.)

Orive et al. employed electrospraying to prepare alginate–agarose microcapsules encapsulated with an antivascular endothelium (VE)–cadherin antibody secreting 1B5 hybridoma cells for the inhibition of angiogenesis [104]. Tumor growth and lethality are dependent on angiogenesis, and VE-cadherin is a key factor in the last step of angiogenesis. Therefore, there is much interest in using antiangiogenesis agents to inhibit tumor expansion. By using the electrospraying technique, hybridoma cells can be encapsulated into biocompatible and semipermeable microparticles as a living drug-delivery system that permits the exit of anti-VE-cadherin monoclonal antibodies but not the entry of cellular immune mediators. In the process, the 1B5 hybridoma cells were suspended with 1.68% alginate–agarose (1:1) solutions (5×10^6 cells/mL). The cell–gel suspension was pumped through a needle from a peristaltic pump and was electrosprayed into 55 mM anhydrous calcium chloride–collecting solution as a gelling agent (pH 7.4) at a flow rate of 2.1 mL/h. The collecting solution containing the microbeads was maintained in an ice bath for 20 min to provoke thermal gelation of the agarose. The microcapsules-encapsulated 1B5 hybridoma cells were suspended in 0.05% poly-L-lysine (PLL) solution for 3 min and then were coated again with another layer of 0.1% alginate for 3 min. Finally, the cell-encapsulated microcapsules were washed twice using saline and transferred to a complete RPMI-1640 medium under normal culture conditions. Figures 11.48a through 11.48d show the optical microscopic images of microcapsules encapsulated with 1B5 hybridoma cells on various days of postencapsulation (day 1, 9, 12, and 19). The results showed that the microcapsules were spherical with an intact and defined membrane made of PLL and alginate. The 1B5 hybridoma cells grew gradually within the microcapsules and formed small aggregates, but some beads presented large aggregates because of a high cell density. The 1B5 hybridoma cells secreted anti-VE-cadherin antibodies during 9 days of culture, reaching a cumulative concentration of 1.7 µg/mL. The results revealed that the antibody concentration inhibited microtubule formation (reached 87%) in the *in vitro* angiogenesis Matrigel assay and the antiangiogenic effects depended

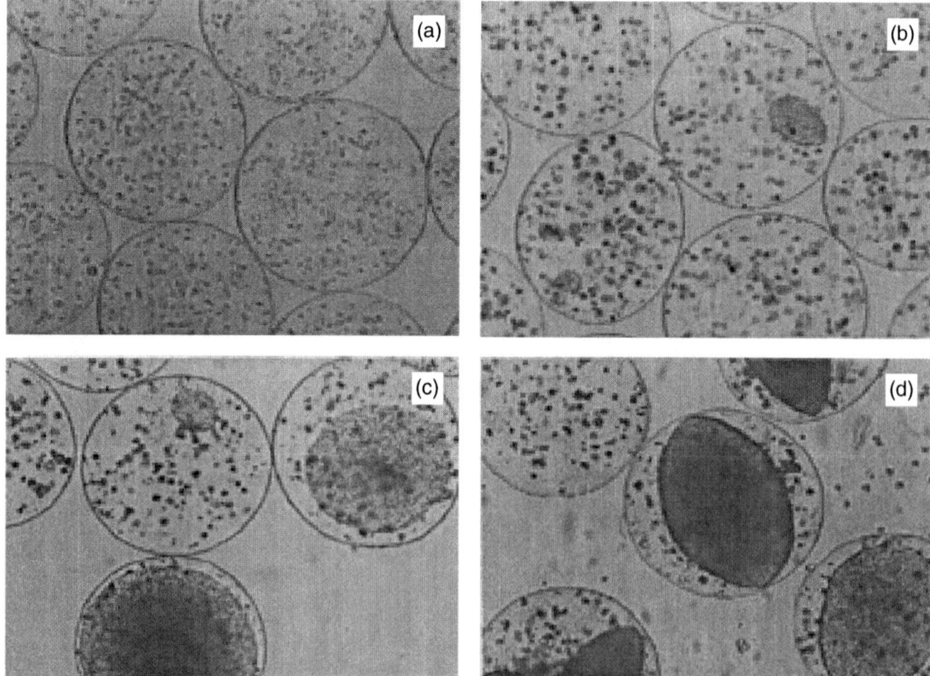

FIGURE 11.48 Images of growth profile of 1B5 hybridoma cells encapsulated in alginate–agarose microcapsules on various days (a) day 1, (b) day 9, (c) day 12, and (d) day 19. Average diameter of beads—618 ± 17 µm. (Reprinted from Orive, G. et al., *Biotechnol. Bioeng.*, 76, 285, 2001. © John Wiley & Sons Inc. With permission.)

on the antibody concentration. These findings could open a new alternative for the prevention of angiogenesis, demonstrating the feasibility of using microencapsulated cells as a control drug-delivery system through an electrohydrodynamic processing technique.

11.2.8.5 Aerosolization of Biomaterials

Electrospraying has recently been explored for aerosolizing biorelated materials. The technique is applied as a processing route for atomizing biological substances on a micrometer to nanometer size. For example, the aerosol drug delivery offers a route for inhaling biomedicines as a therapeutic treatment for diseases [105–107]. Moreover electrohydrodynamic process is a soft way to aerosolize cell suspension to generate and deposit fine droplets containing living cells.

11.2.8.5.1 DNA and Protein Biomolecule

Pareta et al. employed electrospraying to aerosolize BSA protein [108]. The solution for electrospraying was prepared by dissolving BSA in a mixture of 10 vol.% ethanol in deionized water with a concentration of 5, 20, and 50 mg/mL. The solutions were filtered using a CA membrane to get rid of any undissolved BSA. The apparatus used for aerosolizing BSA protein consisted of a syringe, a syringe pump, a stainless steel nozzle, and a power supply. The spraying distance between the nozzle and the ground electrode was 10 mm. A high-speed camera was used to observe the jet modes and capture the spraying images. Two BSA solutions were electrosprayed at a voltage of 6.5 kV and a flow rate of 8×10^{-11} m³/s for a concentration of 5 mg/mL, and a voltage of 6.5 kV and a flow rate of 4×10^{-11} m³/s for 20 mg/mL. The electrosprayed droplets of the BSA were collected just below the ring ground electrode on a carbon-coated aluminum stub for a characterization by SEM. The SEM image in Figure 11.49 shows that the size of the electrosprayed BSA relics were in the range of 10–20 μm, and the aggregated relics contained clusters of small protein. The size of the small BSA protein was a few micrometers. The experimental results revealed that a stable cone-jet electrospraying mode for aerosolizing BSA protein could be achieved at the processing parameters: electrospraying voltage <6.5 kV and flow rate $<2 \times 10^{-10}$ m³/s for a concentration of 5 mg/mL. The study demonstrated that electrospraying is a viable method for aerosolizing and encapsulating proteins in biomedicines.

Davies et al. applied electrospraying technique to aerosolize plasmid DNA [109]. It was the first experiment to investigate the feasibility of electrospraying for the aerosol delivery of naked DNA *in vivo*, because the naked plasmid DNA (pDNA), a potential gene transfer agent for lung gene therapies, cannot be aerosolized without a degradation using the conventional nebulization devices. Unlike the conventional nebulizers that continually recycle aerosol, the electrosprayed pDNA was

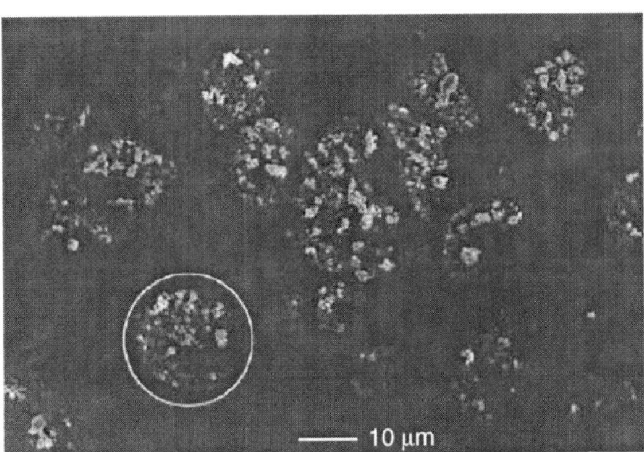

FIGURE 11.49 SEM image of BSA particles aerosolized by electrospraying. (Reprinted from Pareta, R. et al., *J. Mater. Sci. Mater. Med.*, 16, 919, 2005. © Springer Science and Business Media. With permission.)

generated by passing the sprayed biomaterials through the electrohydrodynamic atomization instrument, and the pDNA was exposed to shear damage only once. Therefore, electrospraying is a more appropriate technique for the aerosolization of delicate macromolecules such as a naked DNA. A schematic diagram of the setup for aerosolizing pDNA is shown in Figure 11.50. Electrosprayed pDNA was generated using a 3 mm cylinder of stainless steel with a central bore of 1 mm and a polyacetyl cap with a 500 μm spraying aperture. The application of −5 kV to the nozzle using a high-voltage power supply generated cone-jet spraying. The solution consisting of 80% ethanol, 20% water, 1 mM ethanoic acid, and pDNA was pumped to the nozzle at different liquid flow rates using a syringe pump. The aerosolized pDNA was collected by bubbling the aerosol through a Dreschel bottle containing 30 mL of chloroform. The plasmid DNA was separated by centrifugation of the chloroform and extraction of the aqueous supernatant.

A formulation of 80% ethanol and 20% water was chosen for stable electrospraying in the work because the aqueous pDNA solution was difficult to be aerosolized in a stable mode due to high surface tension and the relatively high conductivity of pDNA formulated. The stability of electrospraying can be increased by the addition of 1 mM ethanoic acid. A stable electrosprayed aerosol containing up to 1 mg/mL of pDNA was generated by using this formulation. Figure 11.51a shows the size of the electrosprayed droplets generated using various concentrations of plasmid pCIKLux. The electrosprayed aerosols containing 1 mg/mL pDNA were stable at flow rates up to 1.4 μL/s. Figure 11.51b shows that at a flow rate of 0.4 μL/s, the pDNA aerosol had a volume median diameter (VMD) of 3.45 μm, and a GSD of 0.61. Over 95% of droplets had a smaller diameter than 5 μm. The experiment revealed that very little degradation of the aerosolized pDNA was observed when compared with nonaerosolized pDNA. Aerosolization studies *in vivo* showed detectable levels of pDNA deposition and measurable luciferase reporter gene expression in the lungs of exposed mice. This study demonstrates that the respirable aerosols of naked pDNA can be generated without plasmid degradation through electrospraying technique, which has been proved to be an appropriate technique for the aerosolization of delicate gene transfer agents.

Gomez et al. produced insulin protein nanoparticles through aerosolizing a solution by electrospraying [110]. The technique was sufficiently good enough to provide no fragmentation of the macromolecules and was gentle enough to aerosolize insulin protein. The investigation demonstrated the feasibility of producing monodispersed and biologically active insulin particles using electrospraying. Figure 11.52 is a schematic illustration of the apparatus, which consisted of a gravity-controlled feed-line to adjust the flow rates, a disposable syringe, a needle with a tapered end, and high-voltage power supply. The needle was perpendicularly positioned to the ground electrode and was kept approximately 3 cm apart from the collecting electrode. A voltage of 5 kV was applied between the two electrodes to establish a necessary electric field to form a stable conical spraying.

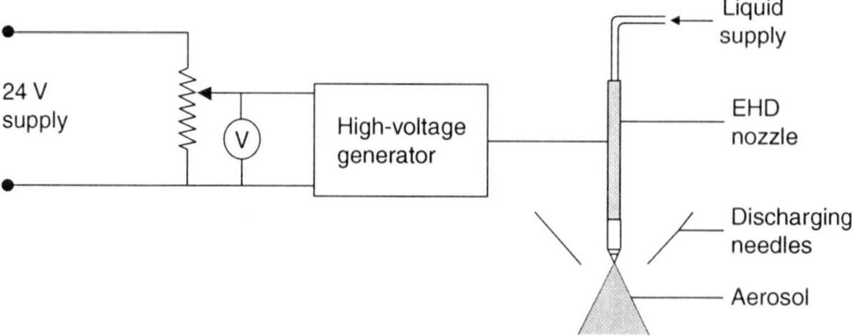

FIGURE 11.50   A schematic diagram of electrospraying apparatus for aerosolization of DNA. (Reprinted from Davies, L.A. et al., *Pharmaceut. Res.*, 22, 1294, 2005. © Springer Science and Business Media. With permission.)

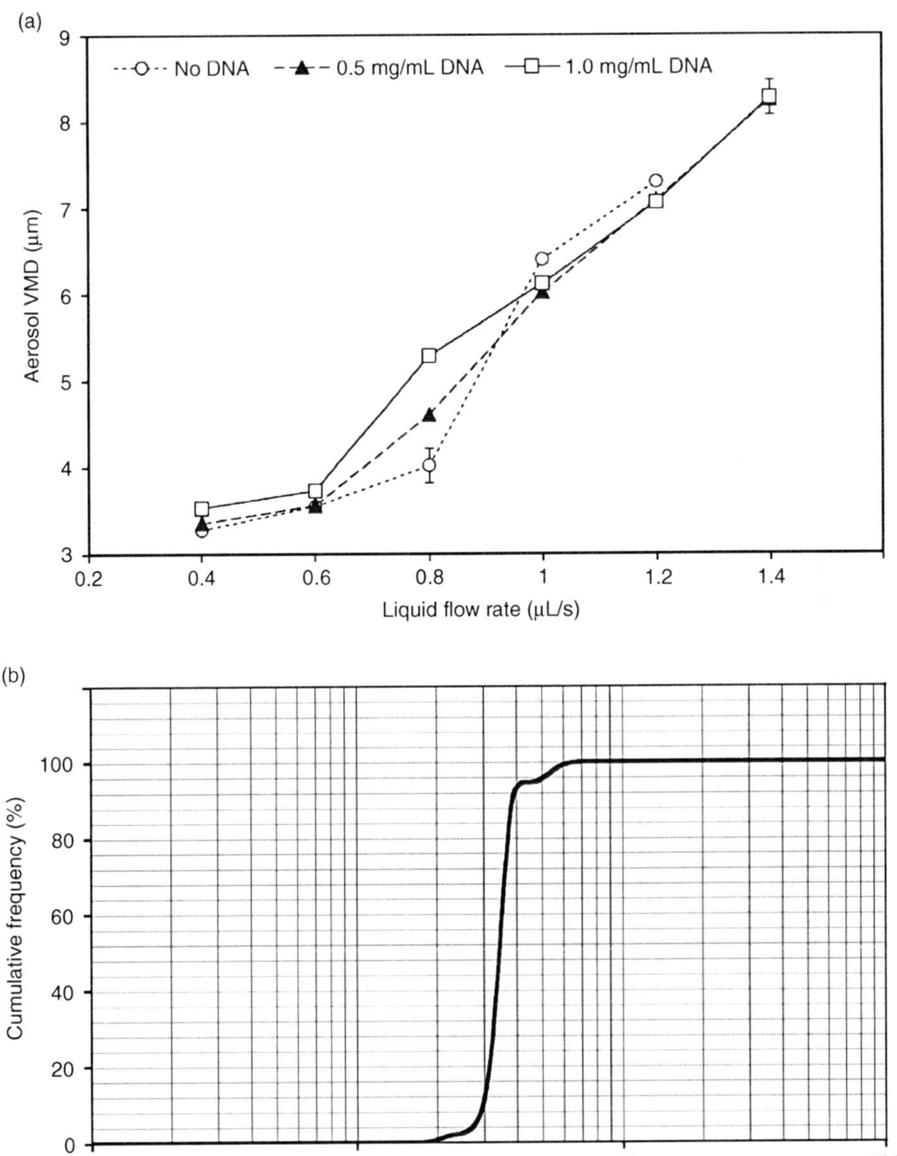

FIGURE 11.51   Electrosprayed aerosol properties are as follows: (a) aerosol size with liquid delivery rate and (b) production of monodispersed DNA aerosols. (Reprinted from Davies, L.A. et al., *Pharmaceut. Res.*, 22, 1294, 2005. © Springer Science and Business Media. With permission.)

Solution was sonicated for 3 min to remove any bubbles that might cause spray instabilities before being transferred into the reservoir syringe.

The results showed that the highest flow rate at which a stable electrospraying was sustained was 0.38 µL/min, which corresponded to a production rate of about 0.23 mg/h. At a flow rate of 2.2 µL/min, it was still possible to stabilize the conical meniscus but was difficult to achieve monodispersed spraying mode. The higher feed rates resulted in unstable behavior of the conical meniscus. Figure 11.53 shows SEM images of particles produced using a flow rate of 0.17 mL/min. The microstructure revealed that the electrosprayed protein particles were typically shaped as doughnuts, and some

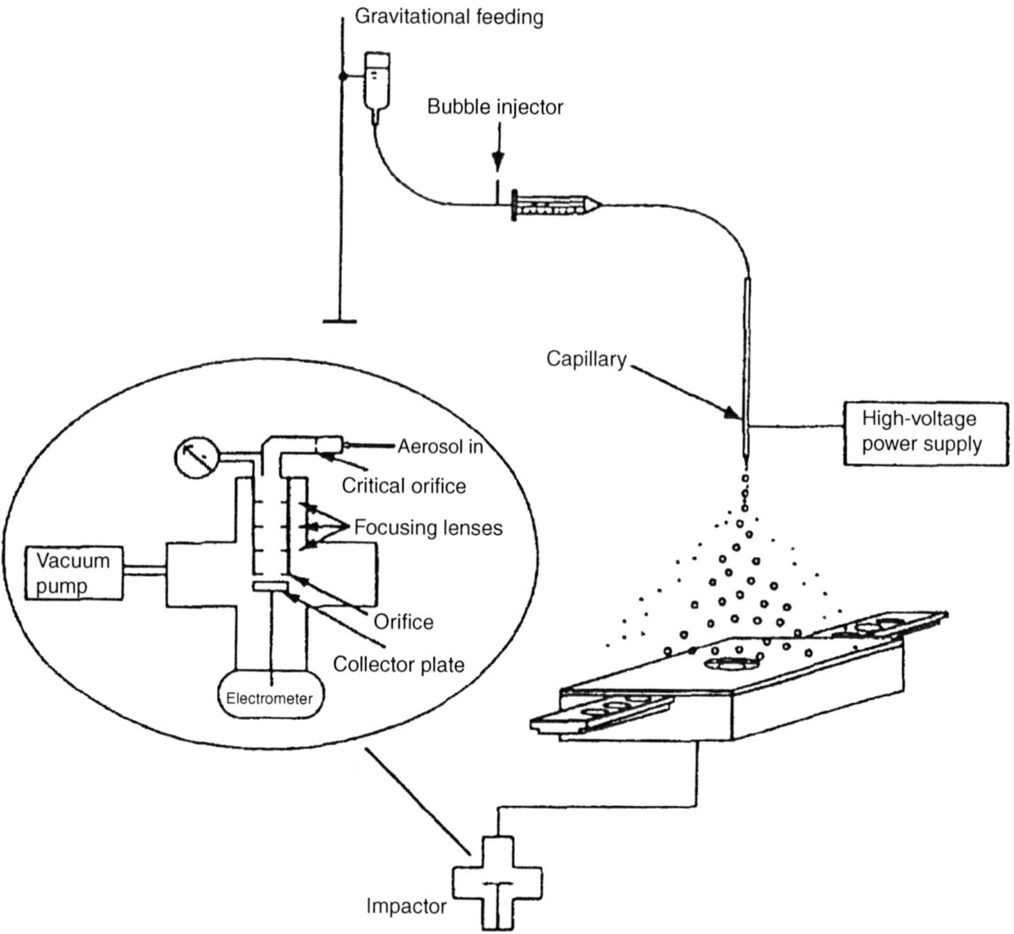

FIGURE 11.52   A schematic diagram of electrospraying for aerosolizing protein. (Reprinted from Gomez, A. et al., *J. Aerosol Sci.*, 29, 561, 1998. © Elsevier Science. With permission.)

of them exhibited horseshoe morphology. The microstructure analysis yielded an average particle size of 98 nm with a SD of 19 nm. The analysis of a similar microstructure obtained at a flow rate of 0.38 μL/min yielded an average diameter of 117 nm with a SD of 27 nm. The stability and the spraying mode in terms of the electrosprayed droplet size and monodispersity were primarily determined by the electrical conductivity and the concentration of the solution. The biological activity of the electrosprayed insulin particles was confirmed by comparing the binding properties on insulin receptors with a control sample. The experiment demonstrated that the electrospraying technique was sufficiently "gentle" so as not to hinder the insulin biological activity during the aerosolization process. Although the maximum production rate for monodispersed insulin nanoparticles prepared using electrospraying is low, the overall production can be increased by multiplexing the nozzles. Meanwhile, the production rate can also be increased by using a higher flow rate, which would result in larger particle sizes.

11.2.8.5.2   Living Cells and Drugs

Jayasinghe et al. applied the electrospraying technique to aerosolize the living Jurkat cell suspension for the first time [111]. In the investigation, electrospraying was used to aerosolize and deposit living cells onto the surface, and the results demonstrated that the living cells were viable and continued to

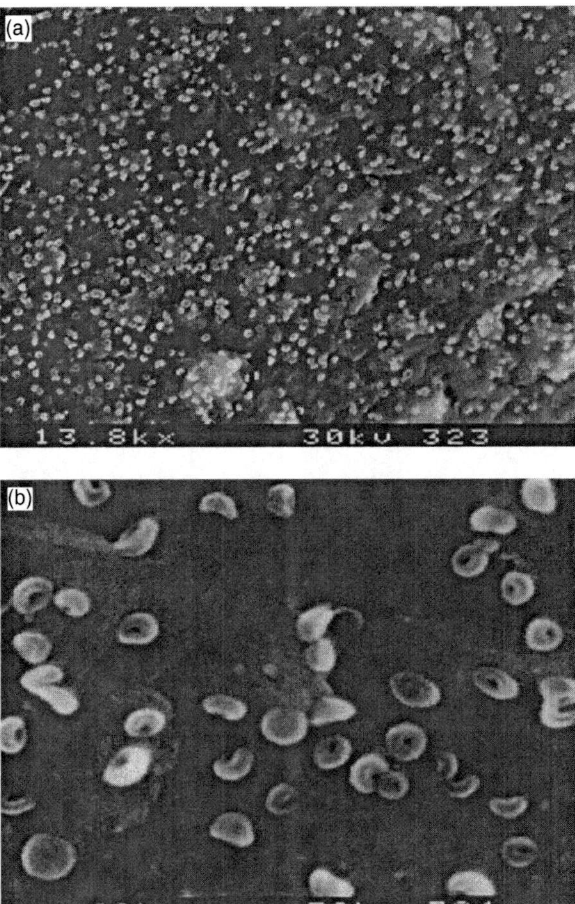

FIGURE 11.53 SEM images of insulin particles aerosolized by electrospraying. Average particle diameter—98 ± 19 nm. (Reprinted from Gomez, A. et al., *J. Aerosol Sci.*, 29, 561, 1998. © Elsevier Science. With permission.)

divide normally after electrospraying. No adverse effects on living cells have been observed when they were processed with this technique. Jurkat cells were grown for 48 h in RPMI 1640 growth medium with 10% fetal calf serum in an incubator at 37°C and 4% CO_2. Cell viability was assessed by staining with Trypan blue, and viable cells were counted by using a bright-field hemocytometer with a phase microscope. A cell suspension in 2–5 mL containing 1–2 × 10^6 cells/mL was used for each electrospraying experiment. In the process, Jurkat cell suspension was syringed through a needle, which initiated the aerosolization of the suspension. The flow rate and the applied voltage were varied over a rather large parametric range to establish a stable spraying mode, but electrospraying of the Jurkat cell suspension occurred in an unstable mode, resulting in a polydispersed distribution of droplets. This feature was attributed to the high electrical conductivity and the high surface tension of the solution. Figure 11.54 shows the unstable spraying mode. In the investigation, electrospraying of Jurkat cell suspension was carried out at an applied voltage of 8.5 kV and a flow rate of 10^{-8} m^3/s. Figure 11.55 shows the observed results of the electrosprayed cells. The living cells were observed by optical microscopy for about 2 h after the electrospraying. No signs of cellular damage were seen as the result of this processing route. Cells changed their morphology over time (cells X and Y), and in some cases the cells underwent cytokinesis (cell Q) as shown in Figures 11.55b through 11.55f. This experiment has elucidated the ability to successfully

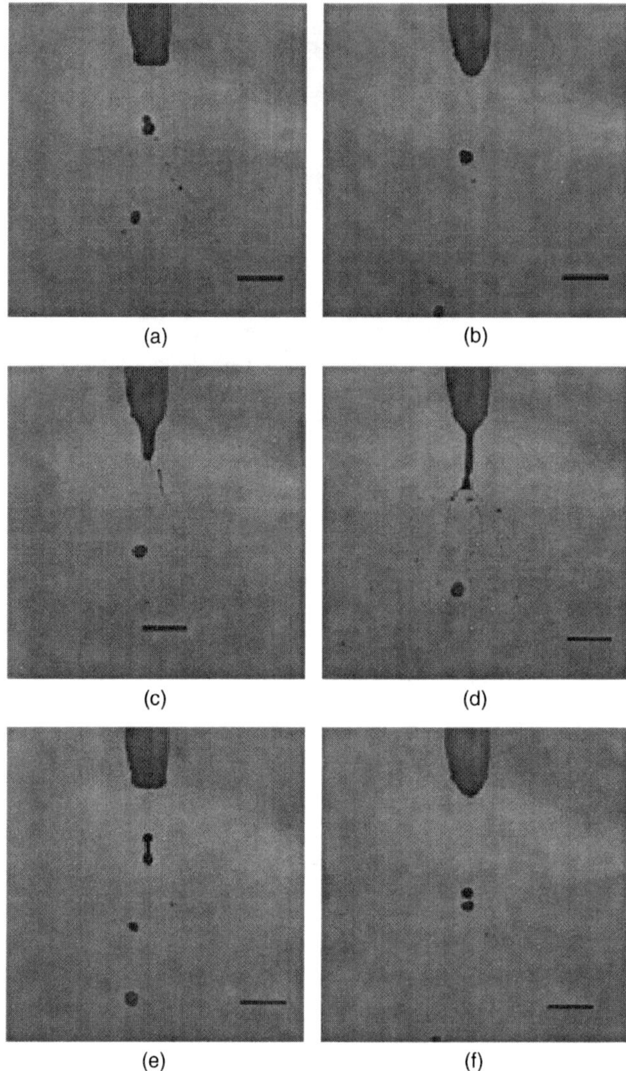

(a)   (b)

(c)   (d)

(e)   (f)

FIGURE 11.54 Images of electrospraying patterns for Jurkat cell suspension. (Reprinted from Jayasinghe, S.N., Qureshi, A.N., and Eagles, P.A.M., *Small*, 2, 216, 2006. © John Wiley & Sons Inc. With permission.)

aerosolize living cells using electrospraying without harming cell integrity. This demonstrates that the technique is a novel method for atomizing living cells. The potential of the preliminary findings has wide implications for the aerosolization and deposition of a range of living cellular materials.

Li et al. investigated the capability of electrospraying for aerosolizing drug particles [112]. Aspirin is one of the most popular drugs in the world and has been selected as a model compound in the study because of its functions in the relief of headaches, muscle, and joint aches. A cone-jet spraying mode was used to generate monodispersed distribution of droplet relics, leading to the formation of particulate aspirin crystals in this study. A stable cone-jet mode of aerosolization was determined by the surface tension, the density, the electrical conductivity, the viscosity, and the relative permittivity of the solution. The solutions were prepared by dissolving the aspirin powder into an ethanol solvent with a continuous stirring at 37°C. The concentration of aspirin powder completely soluble in ethanol was found to be 200 g/L. The equipment used for aerosolizing the aspirin

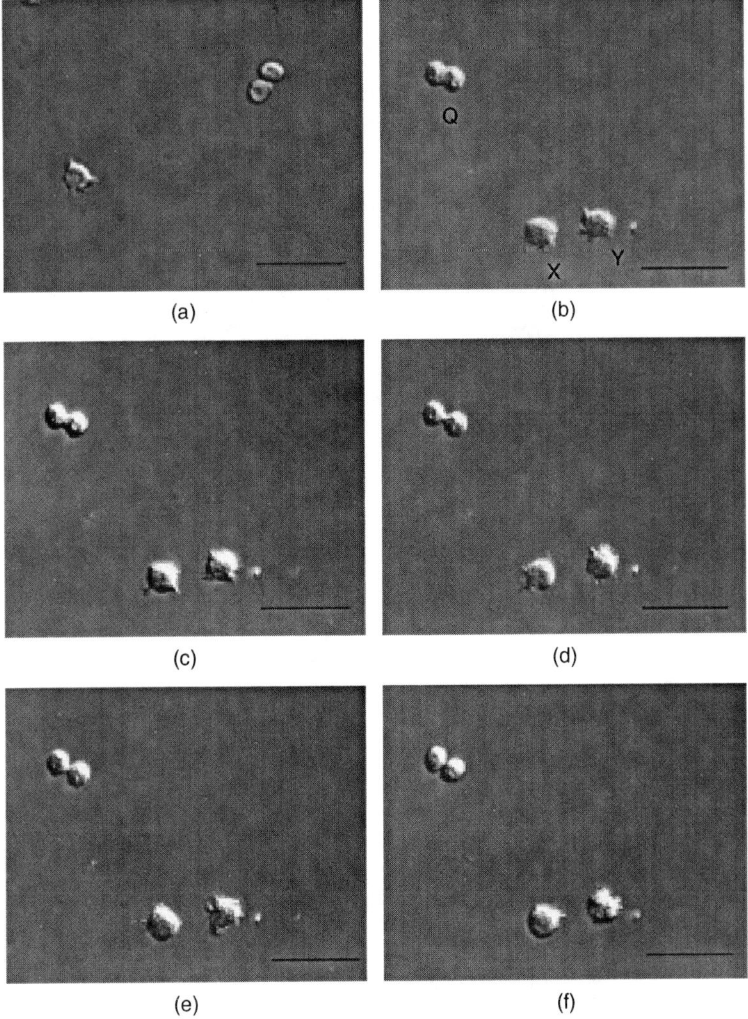

FIGURE 11.55 Morphologies of optical micrographs of electrosprayed Jurkat cells. Scale bar—20 μm. (Reprinted from Jayasinghe, S.N., Qureshi, A.N., and Eagles, P.A.M., *Small*, 2, 216, 2006. © John Wiley & Sons Inc. With permission.)

particles basically consisted of a stainless steel needle connected to a high-voltage power supply and a ring ground electrode. The needle was connected to a programmable syringe pump to allow the flow rate to be varied between 10^{-6} and 10^{-17} m³/s. The spraying distance between the needle and the ring was kept at ~11 mm. In this work, an aspirin solution was aerosolized to generate droplets at a flow rate of 10^{-10} m³/s under an electric filed of 0.36 kV/mm. The flow rate was minimized to obtain the finest droplets. However, if the flow rate is too low, a stable cone-jet electrospraying cannot be formed. A stable cone-jet mode can be achieved in the range of 3.5–4.2 kV, as shown in Figure 11.56. A saturated solution of aspirin in ethanol was capable of forming aspirin droplets in the size range of 0.3–20 μm from a needle with an orifice of ~200 μm. The droplets viewed immediately after deposition were remarkably uniform in size, and the electrosprayed particulate crystals were in the size range of 5–10 μm. The morphology of the crystals was considerably more regular when compared with those formed without using an electrospraying technique. Figure 11.57 shows the aspirin crystals generated using electrospraying. The experiment demonstrated that the electrospraying could aerosolize drugs to release an effective inhalation stream of fine drug droplets.

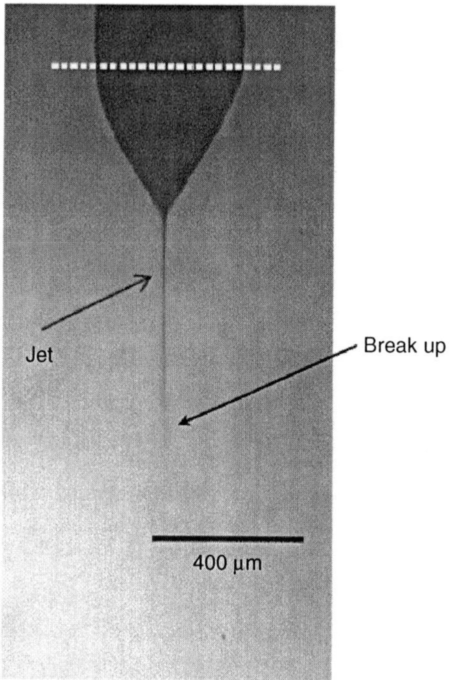

FIGURE 11.56 An image of stable cone-jet electrospraying for aerosolizing aspirin solution. (Reprinted from Li, S.W., Jayasinghe, S.N., and Edirisinghe, M.J., *Chem. Eng. Sci.*, 61, 3091, 2006. © Elsevier Science. With permission.)

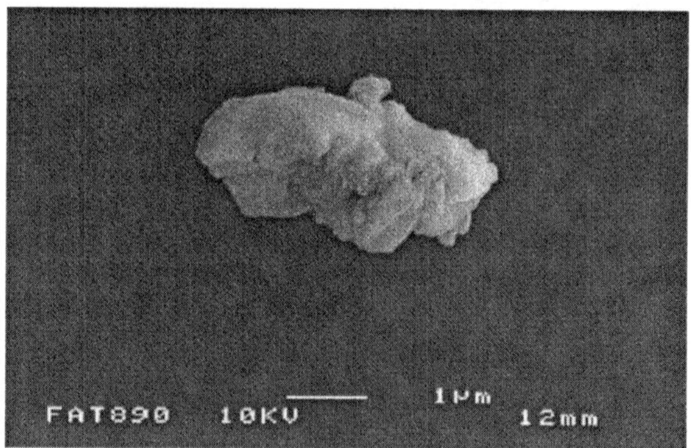

FIGURE 11.57 SEM image of aspirin relics aerosolized using electrospraying. (Reprinted from Li, S.W., Jayasinghe, S.N., and Edirisinghe, M.J., *Chem. Eng. Sci.*, 61, 3091, 2006. © Elsevier Science. With permission.)

Eagles et al. employed electrospraying also to aerosolize the mouse neuronal cells [113]. The research explored the feasibility of atomizing the neuronal cell suspension into fine droplets, because the patterns of these cells would enable studies on neuronal networking, interactions, and biochemical communications to be initiated. The Cath.a-differentiated (CAD) cell was chosen as a model biomaterial, because it can differentiate and behave like a primary neuron when it is deprived of serum. CAD cells were grown for 96 h in 100 mL of Dulbecco's modified Eagle's medium (DMEM) /Ham's F-12 growth medium with 10% (v/v) fetal-calf serum in an incubator at 37°C and 4% (v/v) CO_2. The cell viability was assessed by staining cells with Trypan Blue. They

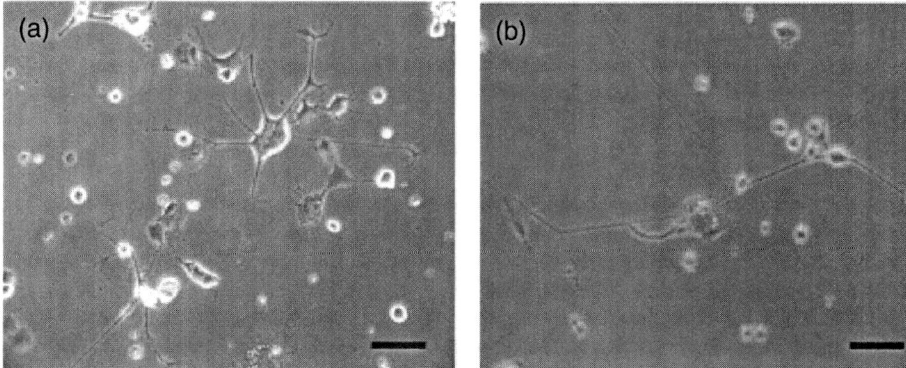

FIGURE 11.58 Optical micrographs taken 1 month after the cells were jetted (a) control CAD cells and (b) CAD cells that were jetted at 7 kV. Scale bar—100 µm. (Reprinted from Eagles, P.A.M., Qureshi, A.N., and Jayasinghe, S.N., *Biochem. J.*, 394, 375, 2006. © Elsevier Science. With permission.)

were then counted using a haemocytometer under a phase-contrast microscope. A 2–5 mL portion of cell suspension containing $(1-2) \times 10^6$ cells/mL was used for electrospraying. The CAD cell suspension was electrosprayed at an electric field strength of 0.47–0.67 kV/mm. The results showed that CAD cells can be aerosolized and still remain viable at applied voltages in a range of 7–10 kV. The cells appeared normal and continued to divide at rates similar to those shown by control samples. When placed in a serum-free medium, the cells can undergo differentiation for at least 1 month. Figure 11.58a illustrates the control CAD cells and Figure 11.58b shows the electrosprayed CAD cells at 7 kV after 1-month incubation, demonstrating that the electrosprayed cell retained the ability after electrospraying. The results showed that at the applied voltages of 7 and 10 kV, the average diameter of the spots ranged from approximately 300–1000 µm. There were a greater proportion of droplets with either no cells or small numbers of cells at an applied voltage of 7 kV. It is concluded from the research that the electrospraying technique could be used to aerosolize and deposit neuronal cells in droplets with a controllable resolution. The investigation opens up the possibility of using a novel approach to deposit small numbers of living nerve cells in the fabrication of biological tissues as well as in the production of biochips and biosensors for a range of bioengineering applications.

11.3   SUMMARY

This chapter has reviewed the electrohydrodynamic process as an efficient and versatile technique to prepare biomaterials in terms of their principles, processing parameters, and biomedical applications, with the emphasis on the influences of processing parameters on the microstructures of the final products. The biological particles, coatings, and microarrays in micrometer and nanometer scales were successfully produced using electrohydrodynamic processing—electrospraying. The biological materials prepared through electrospraying with the easy processability can establish a useful starting point for utilizing these biomaterials in the drug delivery, biointerface, and biochip applications, which would have a significant impact on the production of micro- or nanostructured biomaterials for biomedical applications. These preliminary research results have demonstrated the capability and merits of electrohydrodynamic processing for manufacturing materials applied in the biomedical fields with designed microstructure. However, in order to advance the applications of electrospraying as an innovative technique to prepare biomaterials, the researches will require more collaborative interdisciplinary from the different areas, such as material scientists, biological scientists, and engineers.

REFERENCES

1. Lefebvre, A., *Atomization and Sprays*, Taylor & Francis Inc., Hemisphere Publishing, New York, 1989.
2. Hartman, R.P.A. et al., Jet break-up in electrohydrodynamic atomization in the cone-jet mode, *Journal of Aerosol Science*, 31, 65, 2000.
3. Grace, J.M. and Marijnissen, J.C.M., A review of liquid atomization by electrical means, *Journal of Aerosol Science*, 25, 1005, 1994.
4. Borra, J.P. et al., A new production process of powders with defined properties by electrohydrodynamic atomization of liquids and post-production electrical mixing, *Journal of Electrostatics*, 633, 40, 1997.
5. Lee, J.G. et al., Electrohydrodynamic (EHD) dispensing of nanoliter DNA droplets for microarrays, *Biosensors and Bioelectronics*, 21, 2240, 2006.
6. Chen, D.R. and Pui, D.Y.H., Electrospraying of conducting liquids for monodisperse aerosol generation in the 4 nm to 1.8μm diameter range, *Journal of Aerosol Science*, 27, 646, 1996.
7. Ding, L., Lee, T., and Wang, C.H., Fabrication of monodispersed taxol-loaded particles using electrohydrodynamic atomization, *Journal of Controlled Release*, 102, 395, 2005.
8. Samarasinghe, S.R. et al., Printing gold nanoparticles with an electrohydrodynamic direct-write device, *Gold Bulletin*, 39, 48, 2006.
9. Leeuwenburgh, S. et al., Electrostatic spray deposition (ESD) of calcium phosphate coatings, *Journal of Biomedical Materials Research A*, 66A, 330, 2003.
10. Siebers, M.C. et al., Electrostatic spray deposition (ESD) of calcium phosphate coatings, an *in vitro* study with osteoblast-like cells, *Biomaterials*, 25, 2019, 2004.
11. Ku, B.K. and Kim, S.S., Electrohydrodynamic spraying characteristics of glycerol solutions in vacuum, *Journal of Electrostatics*, 57, 109, 2003.
12. Borra, J.P., Ehouarn, P., and Boulaud, D., Electrohydrodynamic atomisation of water stabilised by glow discharge—operating range and droplet properties, *Journal of Aerosol Science*, 35, 1313, 2004.
13. Cloupeau, M. and Prunetfoch, B., Electrostatic spraying of liquids-main functioning modes, *Journal of Electrostatics*, 25, 165, 1990.
14. Gañan-Calvo, A.M. and Barrero, A., A global model for the electrospraying of liquids in steady cone-jet mode, *Journal of Aerosol Science*, 27, S179, 1996.
15. Barrero, A. and Gañan-Calvo, A.M., Taylor cone electrohydrodynamics: the minimum and maximum flow rates in electrospraying, *Journal of Aerosol Science*, 30, 973, 1999.
16. Rayleigh, L., On the instability of jets, *Proceedings of the London Mathematical Society*, 11, 4, 1878.
17. Rayleigh, L., On the conditions of instability of electrified drops, *Proceedings of the Royal Society*, 29, 71, 1879.
18. Zeleny, J., Instability of electrified liquid surface, *Physical Review*, 10, 1, 1917.
19. Vonnegut, B. and Neubauer, R.L., Production of monodisperse liquid particles by electrical atomization, *Journal of Colloid Science*, 7, 616, 1952.
20. Taylor, G.I., Disintegration of water drops in an electric field, *Proceedings of the Royal Society of London Series A Mathematical and Physical Sciences*, 280, 383, 1964.
21. Joffer, G. et al., Deformation of liquid menisci under the action of an electric-field, *Journal of electrostatics*, 13, 151, 1982.
22. Noymer, P.D. and Garel, M., Stability and atomization characteristics of electrohydrodynamic jets in the cone-jet and multi-jet modes, *Journal of Aerosol Science*, 31, 1165, 2000.
23. Gañan-Calvo, A.M., Cone-jet analytical extension of Taylor's electrostatic solution and the asymptotic universal scaling laws in electrospraying, *Physical Review Letters*, 79, 217, 1997.
24. Gañan-Calvo, A.M., The size and charge of droplets in the electrospraying of polar liquids in cone-jet mode and the minimum droplet size, *Journal of Aerosol Science*, 25, 309, 1994.
25. Mutoh, M., Kaied, A.S., and Kamimura, K., Convergence and disintegration of liquid jets induced by an electrostatic-field, *Journal of Applied Physics*, 50, 3174, 1979.
26. Smith, D.P.H., The electrohydrodynamic atomization of liquids, *IEEE Transactions on industry applications*, 22, 527, 1986.
27. Hartman, R.P.A. et al., Electrohydrodynamic atomization in the cone-jet mode physical modeling of the liquid cone and jet, *Journal of Aerosol Science*, 30, 823, 1999.
28. Tang, K. and Gomez, A., On the structure of an electrostatic spray of monodisperse droplets, *Physics of Fluids*, 6, 2317, 1994.
29. Delamora, J.F. and Loscertales, I.G., The current emitted by highly conducting Taylor cones, *Journal of Fluid Mechanics*, 260, 155, 1994.

30. Gañan-Calvo, A.M., Dávila, J., and Barrero, A., Current and droplet size in the electrospraying of liquids: scaling laws, *Journal of Aerosol Science*, 28, 249, 1997.

31. Shtern, V. and Barrero, A., Striking features of fluid-flows in Taylor cones related to electrospray, *Journal of Aerosol Science*, 25, 1049, 1994.

32. Jaworek, A. and Krupa, A., Forms of the multijet mode of electrohydrodynamic spraying, *Journal of Aerosol Science*, 27, 979, 1996.

33. Yoon, S.S. et al., Modeling multi-jet mode electrostatic atomization using boundary element methods, *Journal of Electrostatics*, 50, 91, 2001.

34. Duby, M.H. et al., Stabilization of monodisperse electrosprays in the multi—jet mode via electric field enhancement, *Journal of Aerosol Science*, 37, 306, 2006.

35. Wilhelm, O. and Madler, L., Cone-jet and multijet electrospray: transport and evaporation, *Atomization and Sprays*, 16, 83, 2006.

36. Cloupeau, M. and Prunetfoch, B., Electrohydrodynamic spraying functioning modes-A critical review, *Journal of Aerosol Science*, 25, 1021, 1994.

37. Duft, D. et al., Coulomb fission—Rayleigh jets from levitated microdroplets, *Nature*, 421,128, 2003.

38. Bailey, A.G., *Electrostatic Spraying of Liquid*, John Wiley & Sons, New York, 1988.

39. Hayati, I., Bailey, A.I., and Tadros, T.F., Mechanism of stable jet formation in electrohydrodynamic atomization, *Nature*, 319, 41, 1986.

40. Hartman, R.P.A., The evolution of electrohydrodynamic sprays produced in the cone-jet mode, a physical model, *Journal of Electrostatics*, 47, 143, 1999.

41. Kelly, A.J., Charge injection electrostatic atomization modeling, *Aerosol Science and Technology*, 12, 526, 1990.

42. Xie, J.W. et al., Electrohydrodynamic atomization for biodegradable polymeric particle production, *Journal of Colloid and Interface Science*, 302, 103, 2006.

43. Hartman, R.P.A., Marijnissen, J.C.M., and Scarlett, B., Electrohydrodynamic atomization in the cone-jet mode: a physical model of the liquid cone and jet, *Journal of Aerosol Science*, 28, S527, 1997.

44. Melcher, J.R., *Field-Coupled Surface Waves,* MIT Press, Cambridge, MA. 1962.

45. Rosenbaum, S. and Clasen, R., Electrospraying of glasses—preparation of glass coatings on glass, *Journal of Aerosol Science*, 30, 975, 1999.

46. Chen, C.H. et al., Electrostatic sol-spray deposition of nanostructured ceramic thin films, *Journal of Aerosol Science*, 30, 959, 1999.

47. Jaworek, A. et al., Spectroscopic studies of electric discharges in electrospraying, *Journal of Electrostatics*, 63, 635, 2005.

48. Moinard-Checot, D. et al., Nanoparticles for drug delivery: review of the formulation and process difficulties illustrated by the emulsion-diffusion process, *Journal of Nanoscience and Nanotechnology*, 6, 2664, 2006.

49. Sinha, R. et al., Nanotechnology in cancer therapeutics: bioconjugated nanoparticles for drug delivery, *Molecular cancer Therapeutics*, 5, 1909, 2006.

50. De Gaetano, F. et al., Sol-gel processing of drug delivery materials and release kinetics, *Journal of Materials Science-Materials in Medicine*, 16, 261, 2005.

51. Langer, R., Drug delivery and targeting, *Nature*, 392, 5, 1998.

52. Soppimath, K.S. et al., Biodegradable polymeric nanoparticles as drug delivery devices, *Journal of Controlled Release*, 70, 1, 2001.

53. Re, M.I., Formulating drug delivery systems by spray drying, *Drying Technology*, 24, 433, 2006.

54. Xu, Y.X. and Hanna, M.A., Electrospray encapsulation of water-soluble protein with polylactide—Effects of formulations on morphology, encapsulation efficiency and release profile of particles, *International Journal of Pharmaceutics*, 320, 30, 2006.

55. Ijsebaert, J.C. et al., Electrohydrodynamic atomization of drug solutions for inhalation purposes, *Journal of Applied Physiology*, 91, 2735, 2001.

56. Reyderman, L. and Stavchansky, S., Electrostatic spraying and its use in drug delivery-cholesterol microspheres, *International Journal of Pharmaceutics*, 124, 75, 1995.

57. Poste, G. and Kirsh, R., Site-specific targeted drug delivery in cancer-therapy, *Biotechnology*, 1, 869, 1983.

58. Lu, Z.R. et al., Design of novel bioconjugates for targeted drug delivery, *Journal of Controlled Release*, 78, 165, 2002.

59. Barbe, C. et al., Silica particles: a novel drug-delivery system, *Advanced Materials*, 16, 1959, 2004.

60. Roh, K.H., Martin, D.C., and Lahann, J., Biphasic Janus particles with nanoscale anisotropy, *Nature Materials*, 4, 759, 2005.
61. Xie, J.W., Marijnissen, J.C.M., and Wang, C.H., Microparticles developed by electrohydrodynamic atomization for the local delivery of anticancer drug to treat C6 glioma *in vitro, Biomaterials*, 27, 3321, 2006.
62. Leeuwenburgh, S.C.G. et al., Influence of deposition parameters on morphological properties of biomedical calcium phosphate coatings prepared using electrostatic spray deposition, *Thin Solid Films*, 472, 105, 2005.
63. Leeuwenburgh, S.C.G. et al., Morphology of calcium phosphate coatings for biomedical applications deposited using electrostatic spray deposition (ESD), *Thin Film Solid*, 503, 69, 2006.
64. Yu, Y. et al., Highly porous spongelike ceramic films with bimodal pore structure prepared by electrostatic spray deposition technique, *Aerosol Science and Technology*, 39, 276, 2005.
65. Chen, C.H. et al., Morphology control of thin $LiCoO_2$ films fabricated using the electrostatic spray deposition (ESD) technique, *Journal of Materials Chemistry*, 6, 765, 1996.
66. Rammelt, S. et al., Coating of titanium implants with collagen, RGD peptide and chondroitin sulfate, *Biomaterials*, 27, 5561, 2006.
67. Brodie, J.C. et al., Osteoblast interactions with calcium phosphate ceramics modified by coating with type I collagen, *Journal of Biomedical Materials Research A*, 73A, 409, 2005.
68. Leeuwenburgh, S.C.G. et al., Influence of precursor solution parameters on chemical properties of calcium phosphate coatings prepared using electrostatic spray deposition (ESD), *Biomaterials*, 25, 641, 2004.
69. LeGeros, R.Z., Biodegradation and bioresorption of calcium phosphate ceramics, *Clinic Materials*, 14, 65, 1993.
70. Layrolle, P., De Groot, K., and Van Blitterswijk, C.A., Biomimetic hydroxyapatite coating on Ti6Al4V induced by pre-calcification, *Bioceramics*, 11, 465, 1998.
71. Leeuwenburgh, S.C.G. et al., Deposition of calcium phosphate coatings with defined chemical properties using the electrostatic spray deposition technique, *Journal of the European Ceramic Society*, 26, 487, 2006.
72. Leeuwenburgh, S.C.G. et al., *In vitro* and *in vivo* reactivity of porous, electrosprayed calcium phosphate coatings, *Biomaterials*, 27, 3368, 2006.
73. Kim, B.H., Hydroxyapatite layers prepared by sol–gel assisted electrostatic spray deposition, *Ceramics International*, 33, 119, 2007.
74. Hoyer, B. et al., Electrostatic spraying: a novel technique for preparation of polymer coatings on electrodes, *Analytical Chemistry*, 68, 3840, 1996.
75. Morota, K. et al., Poly(ethylene oxide) thin films produced by electrospray deposition: morphology control and additive effects of alcohols on nanostructure, *Journal of Colloid and Interface Science*, 279, 484, 2004.
76. Berkland, C., Pack, D.W., and Kim, K., Controlling surface nano-structure using flow-limited field-injection electrostatic spraying (FFESS) of poly(D,L-lactide-*co*-glycolide), *Biomaterials*, 25, 5649, 2004.
77. Morozov, V.N. and Morozova, T.Y., Electrospray deposition as a method to fabricate functionally active protein films, *Analytical Chemistry*, 71, 1415, 1999.
78. Uematsu, I. et al., Surface morphology and biological activity of protein thin films produced by electrospray deposition, *Journal of Colloid and Interface Science*, 269, 336, 2004.
79. Lee, B. et al., Fabrication of a protein film by electrospray deposition method and investigation of photochemical properties by persistent spectral hole burning, *Biomaterials*, 24, 2045, 2003.
80. Buchko, C.J., Kozloff, K.M., and Martin, D.C., Surface characterization of porous, biocompatible protein polymer thin films, *Biomaterials*, 22, 1289, 2001.
81. Matsuzawa, M., Krauthamer, V., and Potember, R.S., Directional guidance of neurite outgrowth using substrates patterned with biomaterials, *Biosystems*, 35, 199, 1995.
82. Biebricher, A. et al., Controlled three-dimensional immobilization of biomolecules on chemically patterned surfaces, *Journal of Biotechnology*, 112, 97, 2004.
83. Gates, B.D. et al., New approaches to nanofabrication: molding, printing, and other techniques, *Chemical Reviews*, 105, 1171, 2005.
84. Blake, T.A. et al., Preparative linear ion trap mass spectrometer for separation and collection of purified proteins and peptides in arrays using ion soft landing, *Analytical Chemistry*, 76, 6293, 2004.
85. Ouyang, Z. et al., Preparing protein microarrays by soft-landing of mass-selected ions, *Science*, 301, 1351, 2003.

86. Welle, A.M. and Jacobs, H.O., Printing of organic and inorganic nanomaterials using electrospray ionization and Coulomb-force-directed assembly, *Applied Physics Letters*, 87, 263119, 2005.
87. Petrik, J., Diagnostic applications of microarrays, *Transfusion Medicine*, 16, 233, 2006.
88. Templin, M.F. et al., Protein microarrays: promising tools for proteomic research, *Proteomics*, 3, 2155, 2003.
89. Kallioniemi, O.P., Biochip technologies in cancer research, *Annals of Medicine*, 33, 142, 2001.
90. Jain, K.K., Applications of biochips: from diagnostics to personalized medicine, *Current Opinion in Drug Discovery and Development*, 7, 285, 2004.
91. Morozov, V.N. and Morozova, T.Y., Electrospray deposition as a method for mass fabrication of mono- and multicomponent microarrays of biological and biologically active substances, *Analytical Chemistry*, 71, 3110, 1999.
92. Lee, B. et al., Fabrication of protein microarrays for immunoassay using the electrostatic spray deposition (ESD) method, *Journal of Chemical Engineering of Japan*, 36, 1370, 2003.
93. Moerman, R. et al., Miniaturized electrospraying as a technique for the production of microarrays of reproducible micrometer-sized protein spots, *Analytical Chemistry*, 73, 2183, 2001.
94. Khani, Z. et al., Alginate/carbon composite beads for laccase and glucose oxidase encapsulation: application in biofuel cell technology, *Biotechnology Letters*, 28, 1779, 2006.
95. Desai, T.A., Microfabrication technology for pancreatic cell encapsulation, *Expert Opinion on Biological Therapy*, 2, 633, 2002.
96. Visted, T., Bjerkvig, R., and Enger, P.O., Cell encapsulation technology as a therapeutic strategy for CNS malignancies, *Neuro-Oncology*, 3, 201, 2001.
97. Uludag, H., De Vos, P., and Tresco, P.A., Technology of mammalian cell encapsulation, *Advanced Drug Delivery Reviews*, 42, 29, 2000.
98. Colton, C.K., Engineering challenges in cell-encapsulation technology, *Trends in Biotechnology*, 14, 158, 1996.
99. Amsden, B.G. and Goosen, M.F.A., An examination of factors affecting the size, distribution and release characteristics of polymer microbeads made using electrostatics, *Journal of Controlled Release*, 43, 183, 1997.
100. Watanabe, H., Matsuyama, T., and Yamamoto, H., Preparation of immobilized enzyme gel particles using an electrostatic atomization technique, *Biochemical Engineering Journal*, 8, 171, 2001.
101. Xu, Y.X., Skotak, M., and Hanna, M., Electrospray encapsulation of water-soluble protein with polylactide. I. Effects of formulations and process on morphology and particle size, *Journal of Microencapsulation*, 23, 69, 2006.
102. Zhou, Y. et al., Scalable encapsulation of hepatocytes by electrostatic spraying, *Journal of Biotechnology*, 117, 99, 2005.
103. Al-Hajry, H.A. et al., Electrostatic encapsulation and growth of plant cell cultures in alginate, *Biotechnology Progress*, 15, 768, 1999.
104. Orive, G. et al., Microencapsulation of an anti-VE-cadherin antibody secreting 1B5 hybridoma cells, *Biotechnology and Bioengineering*, 76, 285, 2001.
105. Terzano, C. and Allegra, L., Importance of drug delivery system in steroid aerosol therapy via nebulizer, *Pulmonary Pharmacology and Therapeutics*, 15, 449, 2002.
106. Sweeney, L.G. et al., Spray-freeze-dried liposomal ciprofloxacin powder for inhaled aerosol drug delivery, *International Journal of Pharmaceutics*, 305, 180, 2005.
107. Corcoran, T.E. and Gamard, S., Development of aerosol drug delivery with helium oxygen gas mixtures, *Journal of Aerosol Medicine-Deposition Clearance and Effects in the Lung*, 17, 299, 2004.
108. Pareta, R. et al., Electrohydrodynamic atomization of protein (bovine serum albumin), *Journal of Materials Science—Materials in Medicine*, 16, 919, 2005.
109. Davies, L.A. et al., Electrohydrodynamic comminution: a novel technique for the aerosolisation of plasmid DNA, *Pharmaceutical Research*, 22, 1294, 2005.
110. Gomez, A. et al., Production of protein nanoparticles by electrospray drying, *Journal of Aerosol Science*, 29, 561, 1998.
111. Jayasinghe, S.N., Qureshi, A.N., and Eagles, P.A.M., Electrohydrodynamic jet processing: an advanced electric-field-driven jetting phenomenon for processing living cells, *Small*, 2, 216, 2006.
112. Li, S.W., Jayasinghe, S.N., and Edirisinghe, M.J., Aspirin particle formation by electric-field-assisted release of droplets, *Chemical Engineering Science*, 61, 3091, 2006.
113. Eagles, P.A.M., Qureshi, A.N., and Jayasinghe, S.N., Electrohydrodynamic jetting of mouse neuronal cells, *Biochemical Journal*, 394, 375, 2006.

12 Fabrication and Function of Biohybrid Nanomaterials Prepared via Supramolecular Approaches

Katsuhiko Ariga

CONTENTS

12.1   INTRODUCTION

Various functional devices have been developed on the basis of recent rapid progress in nanotechnology, which is a methodology to provide nanostructures for fabrication of fine devices such as mechanical machines and information converters, with nanometer-scale structural precision. Miniaturization of electronic and photonic devices has had an enormous impact on technology and fueled many important research efforts in the field of materials science. Successful advances in silicon nanotechnology, such as very large scale integrated circuitry (VLSI) and ultra large scale integrated circuitry (ULSI), are results of the downscaling of metal oxide semiconductor (MOS) transistors. Our daily life is actually supported by a variety of nanodevices whose functions depend upon such highly integrated electronic circuits.

However, in some aspects, current artificial technologies are quite inferior to those seen in naturally occurring systems. For example, a dog can smell and a bat can hear more sensitively than most artificial sensors. Information conversions of brain and nerve systems are much more sophisticated than that of modern computers. We must learn much from biological systems. Biomimetic approaches in supramolecular chemistry are indispensable for the future direction of our technology. Hybridizing functional biomaterials with artificial nanostructures, which has developed in the recent decades, is one of the wisest strategies to utilize natural functions that have been developed for billions of years (Figure 12.1).

Immobilization of fragile biomaterials into rigid nanostructures can be a highly useful methodology for the stable entrapment of biofunctions, leading to practical usage of biomaterials under severe conditions. For example, proteins immobilized in mechanically strong nanostructures often exhibit enhanced stability. The advantage of hybridization of biomaterials with nanostructures is not limited to such technological aspects. Biomolecules entrapped in nanostructures would experience

"

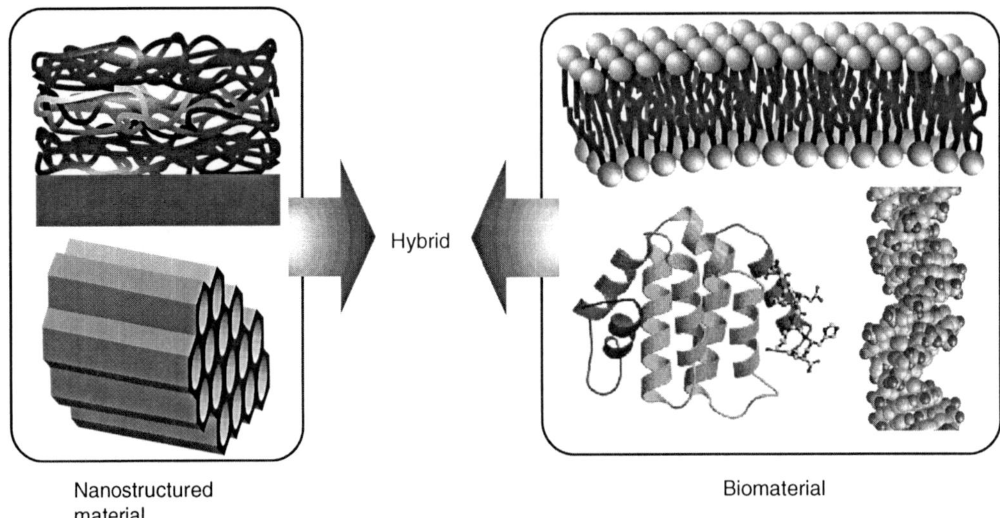

FIGURE 12.1 Hybridization between nanostructured materials and biomaterials.

restricted freedom in their motions, conformational changes, and selected access to external signals, including chemical and physical stimuli. The latter scientific aspects would be much more worthy of research, because many sciences still remain unexplored for biomolecules in nanostructured media.

Since nanofabrication methods based on top–down approaches such as photolithography are expected to encounter fabrication size limitations in the near future, bottom–up approaches based on supramolecular assemblies are now receiving much attention as novel techniques to obtain precisely structured materials [1–4]. In contrast to the processes in silicon-based nanofabrication, these approaches are suitable for hybridization of biomaterials with simple procedures under rather mild conditions. In this background, several examples of biohybrid nanomaterials prepared by supramolecular approaches are introduced in this chapter. This chapter describes fabrication strategies and outstanding functions of three kinds of biohybrid nanomaterials, lipid-based hybrid nanomaterials, hybrid nanomaterials with other small bioactive molecules, and hybrid nanomaterials with proteins.

12.2 LIPID-BASED HYBRID NANOMATERIALS

The simplest but most important biocomponents can be lipids and their families, which are the major components of cell membranes. A cell membrane is mainly formed through the spontaneous assembly of lipids, proteins, oligosaccharides, and others. The basic structure of the cell membrane is the lipid-bilayer membrane and it is mimicked often by supramolecular chemistry, as seen in liposome and vesicle structures [5–7]. In these structures, the lipid bilayer structure extends two-dimensionally and forms the "skin" of a closed sphere that has a water pool inside. The lipid-bilayer structures are known to behave as a thermotropic liquid crystal. At low temperature, the lipid bilayer is in a gel (or crystalline) state with motional freezing of the alkyl chains. As the temperature rises, the alkyl chains melt and attain a flexible motional state, though the bilayer structure is maintained. Since permeability of the small molecules through the lipid-bilayer membranes depends much on the states of the lipid bilayer, permeation control upon the gel (or crystalline)–liquid crystalline phase transition of the lipid bilayer membrane are extensively researched, which is sometimes aimed at development of drug delivery systems (DDS) [8,9]. However, the lipid-bilayer membranes themselves are mechanically weak supermolecules, which characteristic is not always advantageous in practical usage. In order to overcome such a weak feature of the lipid bilayer membranes, hybridization of the lipid bilayer membranes with mechanically stable supporting materials have been widely investigated. One of the examples is

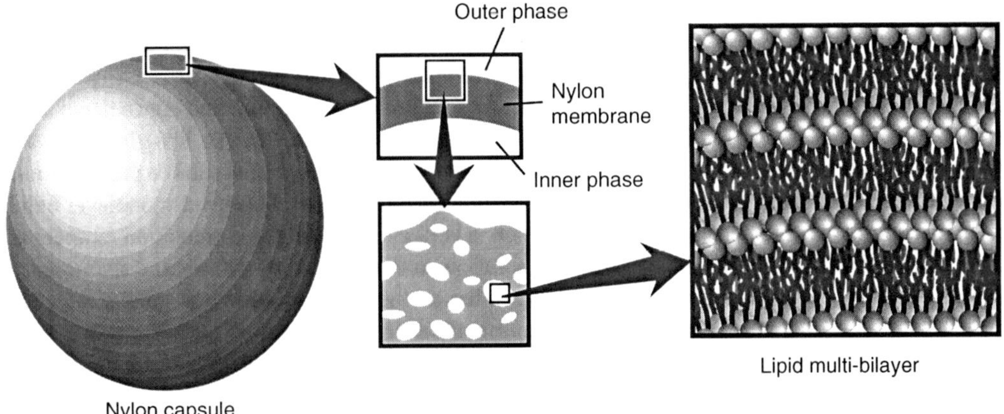

FIGURE 12.2 Lipid-bilayer-corked capsule.

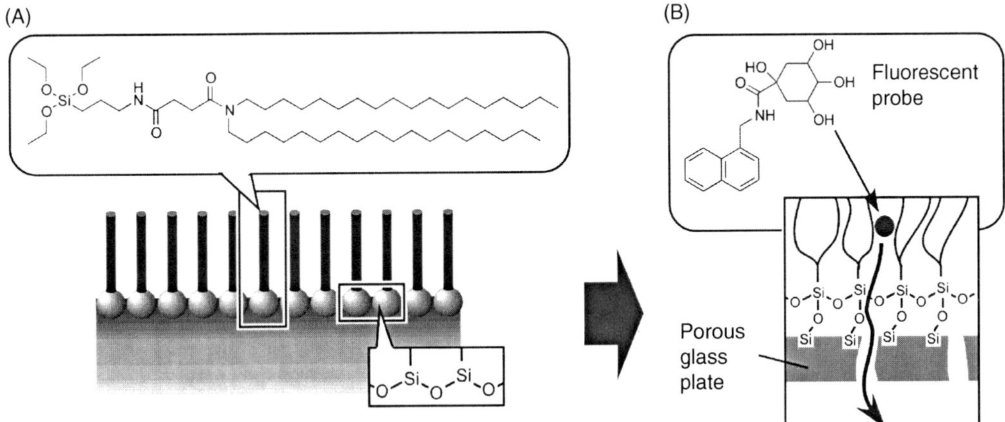

FIGURE 12.3 (A) A Langmuir monolayer of dialkylorganosilane. (B) Permeation control of fluorescence molecular probe through the monolayer-immobilized porous glass plate.

shown in Figure 12.2, in which a lipid-bilayer-corked capsule is illustrated [10]. As reported by Okahata and coworkers, nylon capsules with diameter of 2 mm and membrane thickness of 1 μm were prepared by interfacial polycondensation using ethylenediamine and 1,10-*bis*(chlorocarbonyl)decane. Surface membranes of the capsules have porous structures and are capable of stable accommodation of multibilayer structures of lipids, as illustrated in Figure 12.2. Target drug molecules were dissolved in inner water pool, from where permeation of the entrapped drugs was monitored. Systematic measurement by changing ambient temperatures revealed that the permeation coefficient of the drug through the multibilayer membranes could be discontinuously altered around phase transition temperature of the lipid membrane. Such controls of drug release can be successfully driven by the other stimuli such as application of external electric fields [11].

The same research group also demonstrated permeation control through a much thinner supramolecular film, that is, they realized permeation control through a single monolayer of amphiphile (Figure 12.3) [12,13]. A monolayer of dialkylorganosilane was prepared at the air–water interface and transferred onto a porous glass plate through Langmuir–Blodgett (LB) technique. By using this hybrid nanostructure, material permeation through the monolayer on glass was successfully regulated. The dialkylorganosilane compounds were polymerized through the formation of Si–O–Si linkages on the acidic aqueous surface, and covalently immobilized on glass surface by reaction

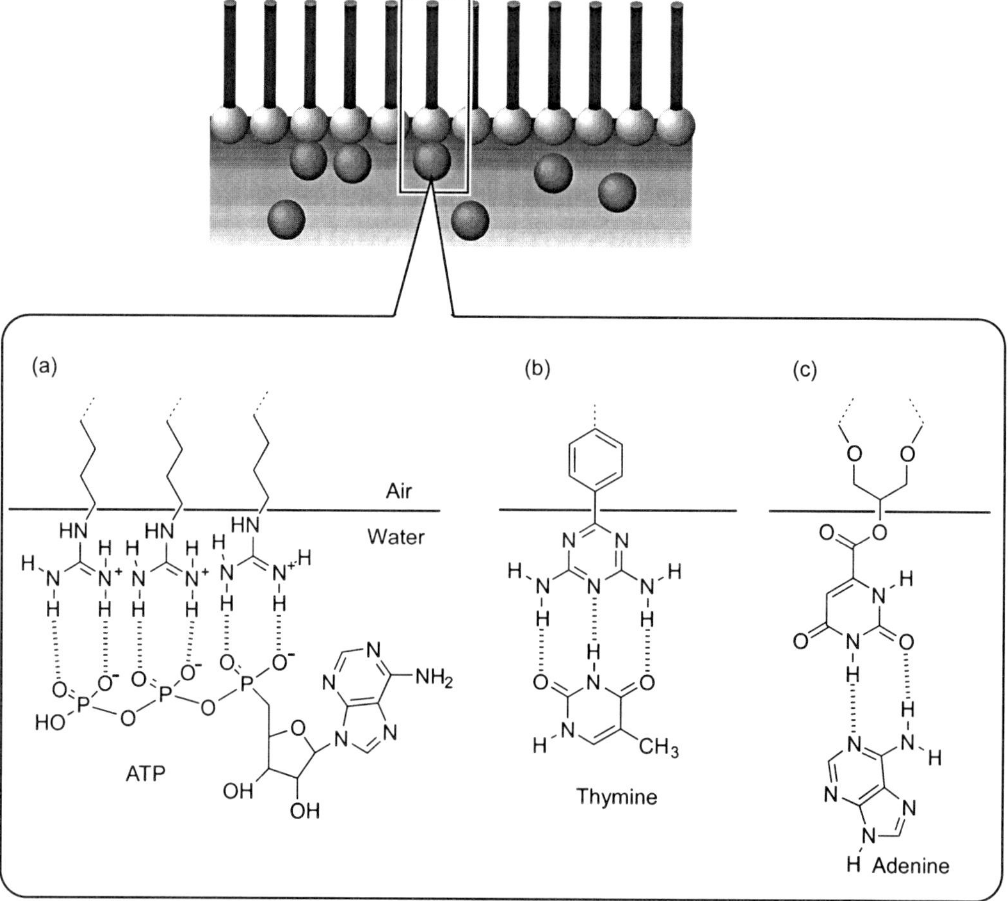

FIGURE 12.7   Molecular recognition at the air–water interface: (a) ATP recognition, (b) thymine recognition, and (c) adenine recognition.

FAD molecule binds two guanidinium molecules at phosphate groups, one orotate molecule at adenine sites, and diaminotriazine at isoalloxiazine ring [51]. Such multipoint binding of aqueous biomolecule to Langmuir monolayer leads to a novel strategy for molecular pattern formation in a two-dimensional 2-D plane, as illustrated in Figure 12.8 [52–54], where two kinds of amphiphiles, guanidinium-amphiphile and orotate-amphiphile, were used for pattern formation (Figure 12.8A). The monolayer transferred on a mica surface was observed by AFM. Repeated height differences in the angstrom range were observed for the orotate or guanidinium-mixed monolayer transferred from aqueous FAD solution as a resulting molecular pattern (Figure 12.8B). As illustrated in a molecular model in Figure 12.8A, the binding of FAD with the orotate or guanidinium-mixed monolayer would dispose two functional units at the same level, resulting in a height difference between the two terminal methyl groups. The methodology to prepare artificial patterns in 2-D planes has not been well developed so far, especially in molecular size, and the approach demonstrated above would lead to develop novel fabrication in 2-D molecular patterning.

The formation of complicated recognition sites upon self-assemblies of several components is a useful strategy for biomolecular hybridization. Similar concepts have been already accomplished by biological polymers such as enzymes and antibodies. For example, the immune system can treat numerous antigens by genetically tuning the recognition sites in antibodies. A variation of the amino acid sequence in several small hypervariable regions provides diversity in antigen-binding sites.

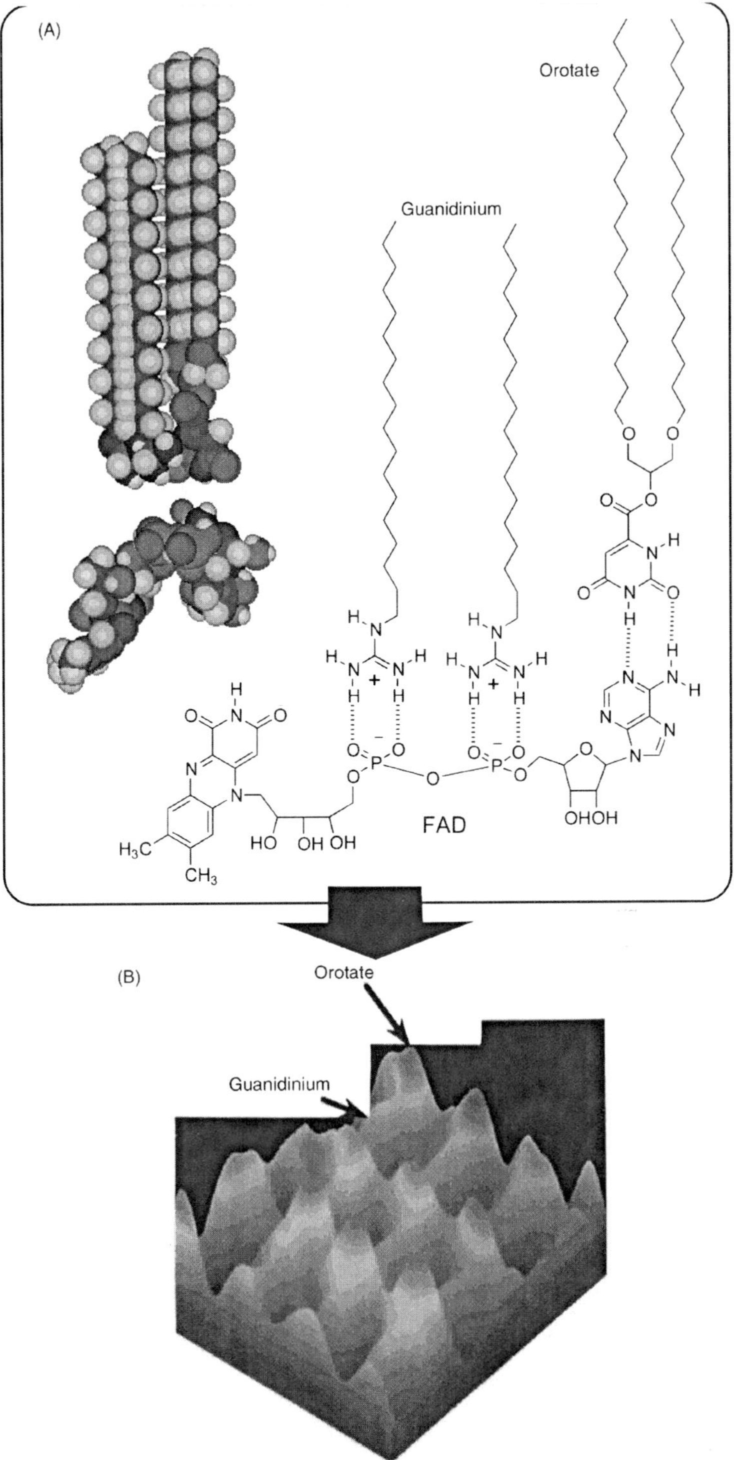

FIGURE 12.8 Two-dimensional molecular patterning through molecular recognition at the air–water interface: (A) recognition pair of guanidinium-amphiphile and orotate-amphiphile with FAD and a model of formed complex and (B) an AFM image of the formed pattern. (Reprinted from Oishi, Y., et al., *Langmuir*, 13, 519, 1997. © American Chemical Society. With permission.)

A similar situation can be recreated by an appropriate design of monolayer of amphiphilic peptides. Exposing an array of peptide segments or amino acid residues creates a protein-like surface that becomes recognition-systems adaptable for various kinds of aqueous guests. As illustrated in Figure 12.9, effective peptide binding, together with guest selection, was observed in monolayers of dialkyl peptide amphiphiles, where the dialkylamine moiety was connected with the glycylglycinamide head group via the terephthaloyl unit [55]. Binding efficiencies of various dipeptides were compared at a given guest concentration, resulting in an apparent difference in binding efficiency between GlyLeu and LeuGly. Favorable interaction between the benzene planes of the host-amphiphile and hydrophobic side chain induced C-terminal insertion with antiparallel β-sheet-type hydrogen bonding for GlyLeu (Figure 12.9A), and N-terminal insertion with parallel β-sheet-type hydrogen bonding for LeuGly (Figure 12.9B). The parallel interpeptide hydrogen bonding is not as stable as its antiparallel cousin, because hydrogen bonding between the parallel peptide chains cannot be linearly extended.

This approach can be extended to the formation of more elaborate structures of recognition sites through introduction of additional host functional groups. The latter functional group can interact with guest C-terminal or N-terminal of guest peptides, which would enhance the binding efficiency. As shown in Figure 12.10, mixed monolayer of glycylglycinamide-amphiphile and benzoic acid-amphiphile can bind GlyLeu guest efficiently [56,57]. This mixed monolayer has a binding constant of 475 M^{-1} to GlyLeu guest, while the binding constant of a single component monolayer to the same guest remains only 35 M^{-1}. Because the benzoic-acid moiety can interact with both C-terminal and N-terminal of the guest peptides, efficient binding to the mixed monolayer was observed for both GlyLeu and LeuGly. The introduction of a guanidinium-amphiphile as a second amphiphile selectively results in the C-terminal insertion of the aqueous dipeptides due to strong interaction between guanidinium and carboxylate [58].

As described in the former section (12.2), hybridization of biomolecules to rigid inorganic supports is undoubtedly an important approach for practical application. The strategy used for immobilization of the lipid monolayer to a porous glass plate was applied to fabricate a novel type of vitamin-functionalized electrode (Figure 12.11) [59]. The vitamin B_{12} mimics having a core that

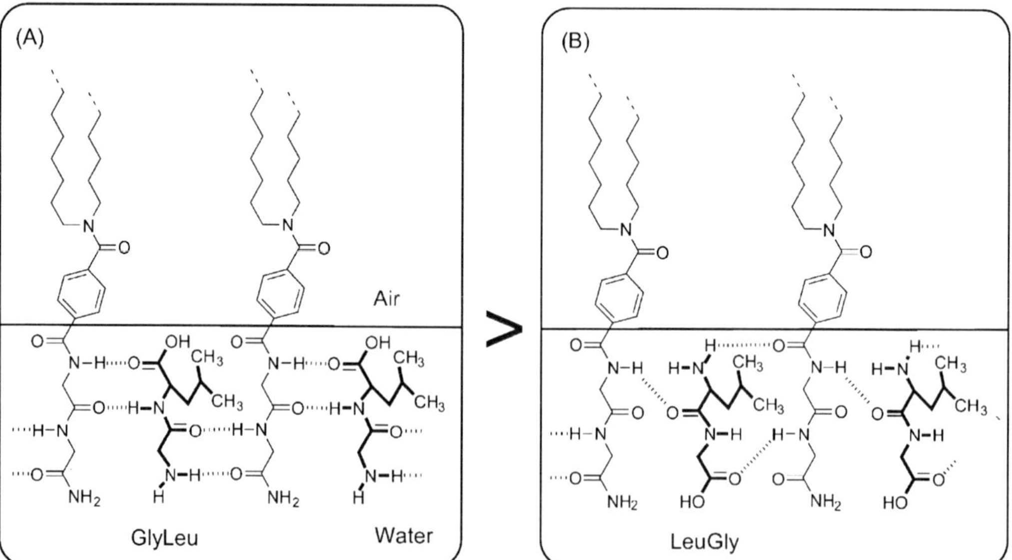

FIGURE 12.9 Recognition of aqueous dipeptides ((A) GlyLeu and (B) LeuGly) by the monolayer of glycylglycinamide-amphiphile. Binding of GlyLeu with antiparallel β-sheet-type hydrogen bonding is more effective than binding of LeuGly with parallel β-sheet-type hydrogen bonding.

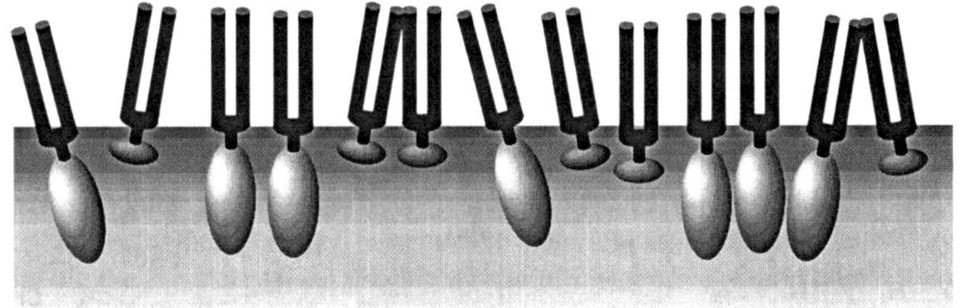

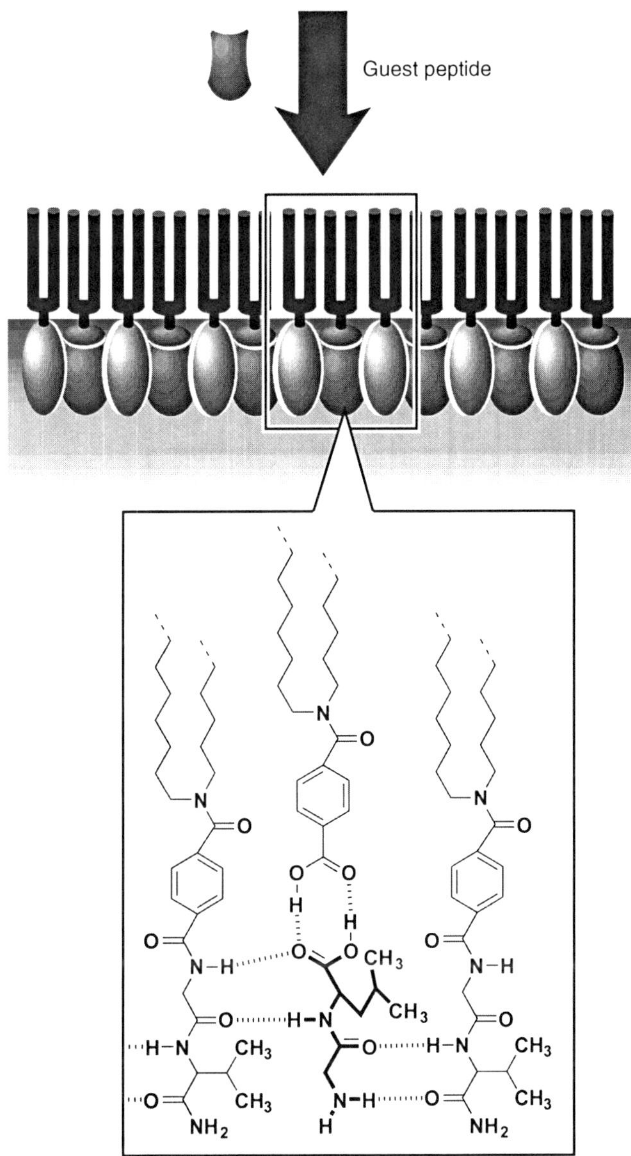

FIGURE 12.10 Binding of GlyLeu by the mixed monolayer of glycylglycinamide-amphiphile and benzoic acid-amphiphile.

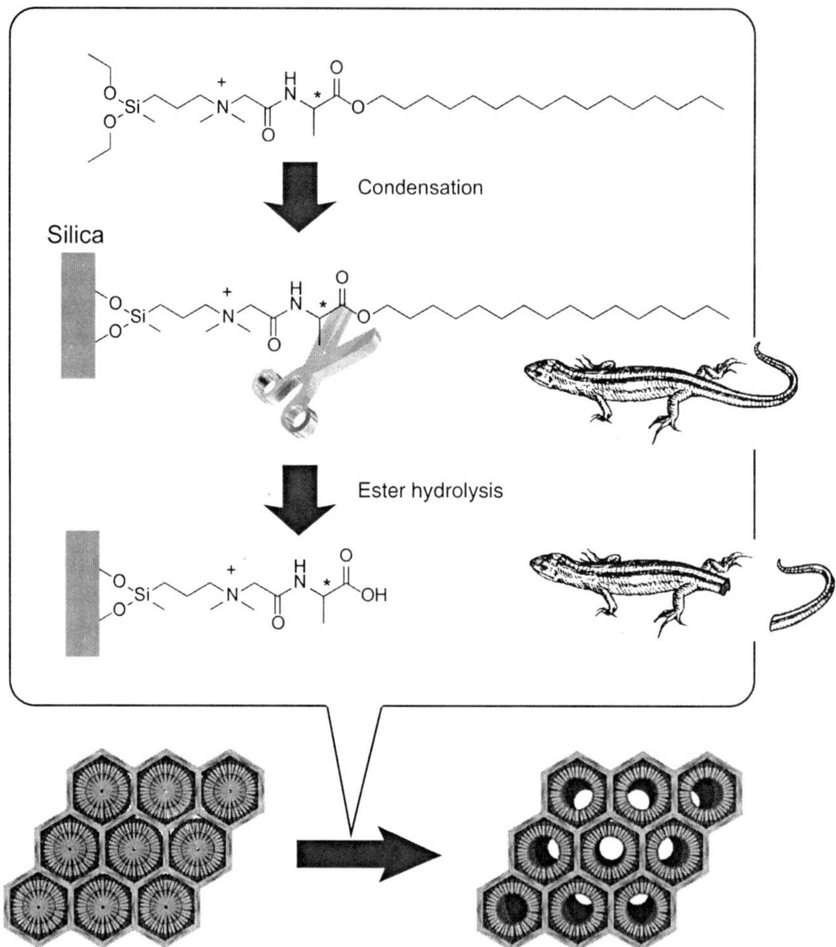

FIGURE 12.14 Conceptual illustration of lizard templating method dense hybridization of alanine residues in mesopore inside wall. (Reprinted from Zhang, Q., et al., *J. Am. Chem. Soc.*, 126, 988, 2004. © American Chemical Society. With permission.)

on protein adsorption onto mesoporous materials [101–106]. Figure 12.15A displays adsorption isotherm of lysozyme onto three mesoporous silica materials (C_{12}-MCM-41, C_{16}-MCM-41, and SBA-15) at pH 10.5 [107]. All the isotherms obeyed Langmuir-type behavior with adsorption capacity of 13.4, 28.1, and 35.3 μmol g^{-1} for C_{12}-MCM-41, C_{16}-MCM-41, and SBA-15, respectively. These values depend significantly on structural parameters of pores: pore volume (C_{12}-MCM-41, 0.70 cm^3 g^{-1}; C_{16}-MCM-41, 0.86 cm^3 g^{-1}; SBA-15, 1.25 cm^3 g^{-1}) and pore diameter (C_{12}-MCM-41, 3.54 nm; C_{16}-MCM-41, 4.10 nm; SBA-15, 10.98 nm). The obtained results strikingly demonstrate the importance of pore structures on the protein adsorption capability. Protein adsorption behaviors can also be regulated by selection of ambient conditions. Especially, the effect of pH on the protein adsorption is a subject worthy of detailed investigation, because charged states of both the proteins and silicate depend significantly on surrounding pH. Figure 12.15B shows adsorption isotherms of lysozyme onto SBA-15 at various pH conditions [107]. The maximum adsorption capability of lysozyme to SBA-15 was obtained at pH 10.5, which is very close to the isoelectric point of lysozyme. Electric repulsion among the protein molecules near the isoelectric point of the protein is significantly suppressed, which may allow the proteins to pack densely in confined spaces. Protein

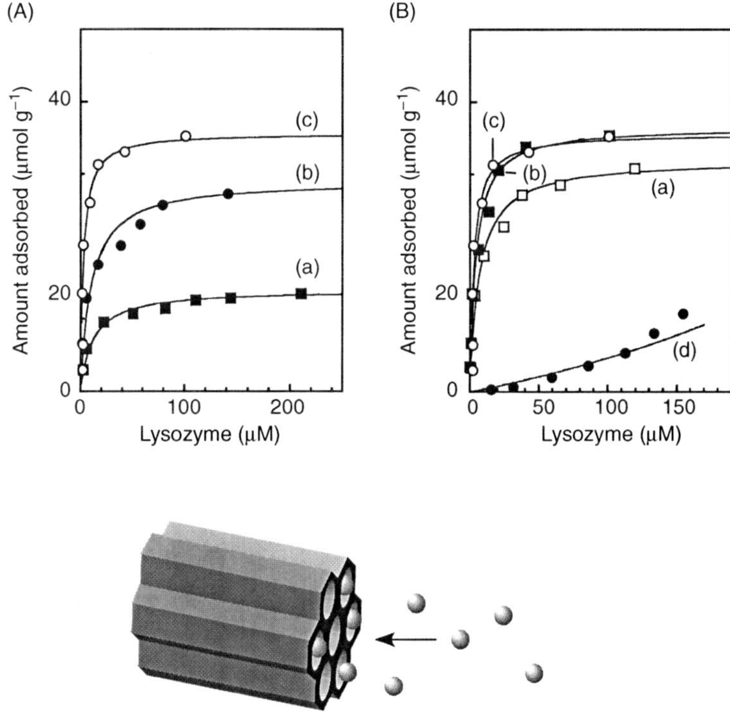

FIGURE 12.15 (A) Adsorption isotherms of lysozyme onto mesoporous silica materials at pH 10.5: (a) C_{12}-MCM-41, (b) C_{16}-MCM-41, and (c) SBA-15. (B) Adsorption isotherms of lysozyme onto SBA-15 at various pH conditions: (a) pH 6.5, (b) pH 9.6, (c) pH 10.5, and (d) pH 12.0. (Reprinted from Vinu, A., et al., *J. Phys. Chem. B*, 108, 7323, © American Chemical Society. With permission.)

molecules tend to be compacted at zero net charge. The area per molecule of lysozyme in solution having a pH near the isoelectric point was reported to be similar to that in its crystallized state (13.5 nm^2), whereas it is 26.6 nm^2 at a solution pH of 4 [108]. Smaller occupied area in the former case may result in larger monolayer adsorption capacity.

The structural stability of the mesoporous silica adsorbent under aqueous condition is relatively poor because of the hydrolysis of their siloxane bridges. Therefore, mesoporous materials, which are much stabler than mesoporous silica, have to be applied for the immobilization of biomaterials in application requiring usage under rather harsh conditions. The mesoporous carbon CMK-3 families prepared through carbonization of carbon source using mesoporous silica as removable SBA-15 replicas (see Figure 12.16A), would be powerful candidates as adsorbents for protein immobilization, because mesoporous carbon has perfect stability against hydrolytic aqueous conditions. Adsorption of lysozyme onto various mesoporous carbon materials was investigated by Vinu and coworkers, in which four kinds of pore-engineered CMK materials, CMK-3-150, CMK-3-130, CMK-3, and CMK-1, were used as adsorbents [109]. The obtained adsorption capacities are plotted as functions of three kinds of pore structural parameters, specific surface area (graph (a) in Figure 12.16B), specific pore volume (graph (b) in Figure 12.16B), and pore diameter (graph (c) in Figure 12.16B). The adsorption capacity did not show clear relevance with the specific surface area. In contrast, positive correlation was obviously observed between the adsorption capacity and the pore volume. This relation sounds reasonable from the viewpoint of pore filling by the lysozyme molecules. Unavoidable negative deviation from the expected line can be detected for the adsorption capacity to the mesoporous carbon with the smallest pore diameter (CMK-1). This result would be explained by the size exclusion effect at mesoporous

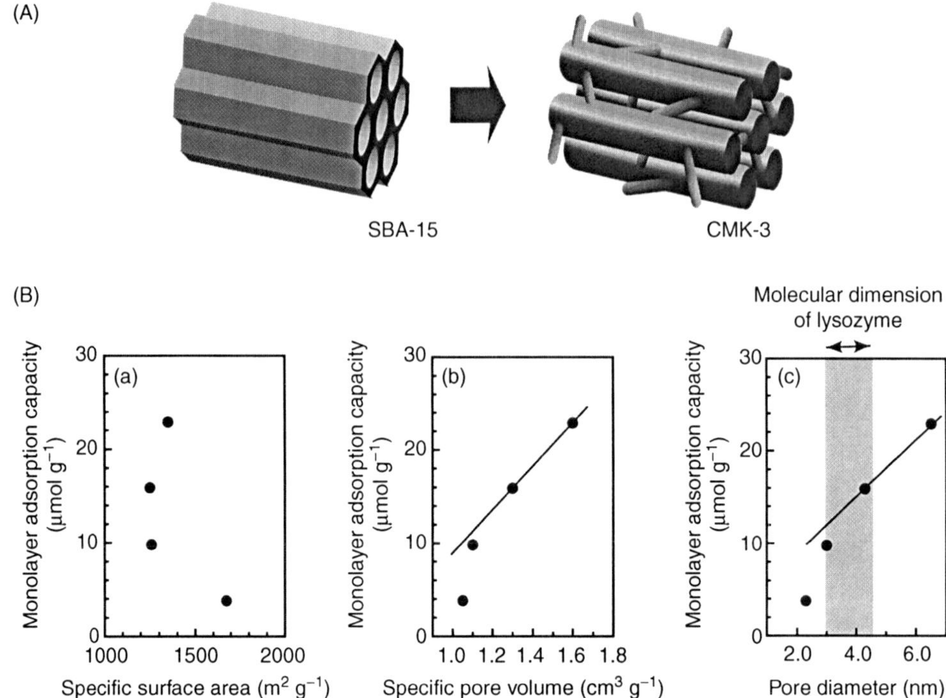

FIGURE 12.16 (A) Conceptual illustration of synthesis of CMK-3 from SBA-15. (B) Effect of structural parameters on monolayer adsorption capacities of lysozyme onto mesoporous carbon materials: (a) specific surface area, (b) specific pore volume, and (c) pore diameter.

media. In order to confirm the structural stability of lysozyme after adsorption on the mesoporous carbon, FT-IR spectra were recorded for the lysozyme molecules loaded mesoporous adsorbents CMK-3 in comparison to unloaded lysozyme. The intensity ratio between amide I and amide II bands did not virtually alter upon adsorption of lysozyme onto the mesoporous carbon, indicating the absence of serious denaturation accompanying changes in secondary structures through the adsorption process. The adsorbent was also characterized by nitrogen adsorption–desorption isotherms after the lysozyme adsorption. This investigation was to ascertain whether the lysozyme molecule enters the mesopore of CMK-3. The amount of nitrogen adsorbed was decreased by increasing the amount of the lysozyme adsorption. The reduction in the specific mesopore volume after the lysozyme adsorption clearly indicates that the lysozyme molecules are adsorbed inside the mesopores of CMK-3 adsorbent.

Vinu and coworkers have recently synthesized more advanced materials like novel nanocarbon, "carbon nanocage" [110–112], through replica synthesis using 3-D large cage-type face-centered cubic mesoporous silica materials (KIT-5) [113], as inorganic templates. The image of the synthesis of carbon nanocage is illustrated in Figure 12.17. It should be however noted that these illustrations show just a rough idea of the obtained materials. The textural characteristics of the carbon nanocage materials determined by nitrogen adsorption–desorption measurement apparently exceed those of the conventional mesoporous carbon CMK-3. The specific surface area of 1600 m² g⁻¹ and specific pore volume of 2.1 cm³ g⁻¹ were obtained for carbon nanocage synthesized under optimized conditions. These values are apparently larger than those reported for conventional mesoporous carbon and CMK-3 (surface area, 1260 m² g⁻¹; pore volume, 1.1 cm³ g⁻¹). A further analysis with the method proposed by Ravikovitch et al. [114] provided the cage diameter of 15 nm for the corresponding carbon nanocage, which has pore diameter of 5.2 nm. Integrated

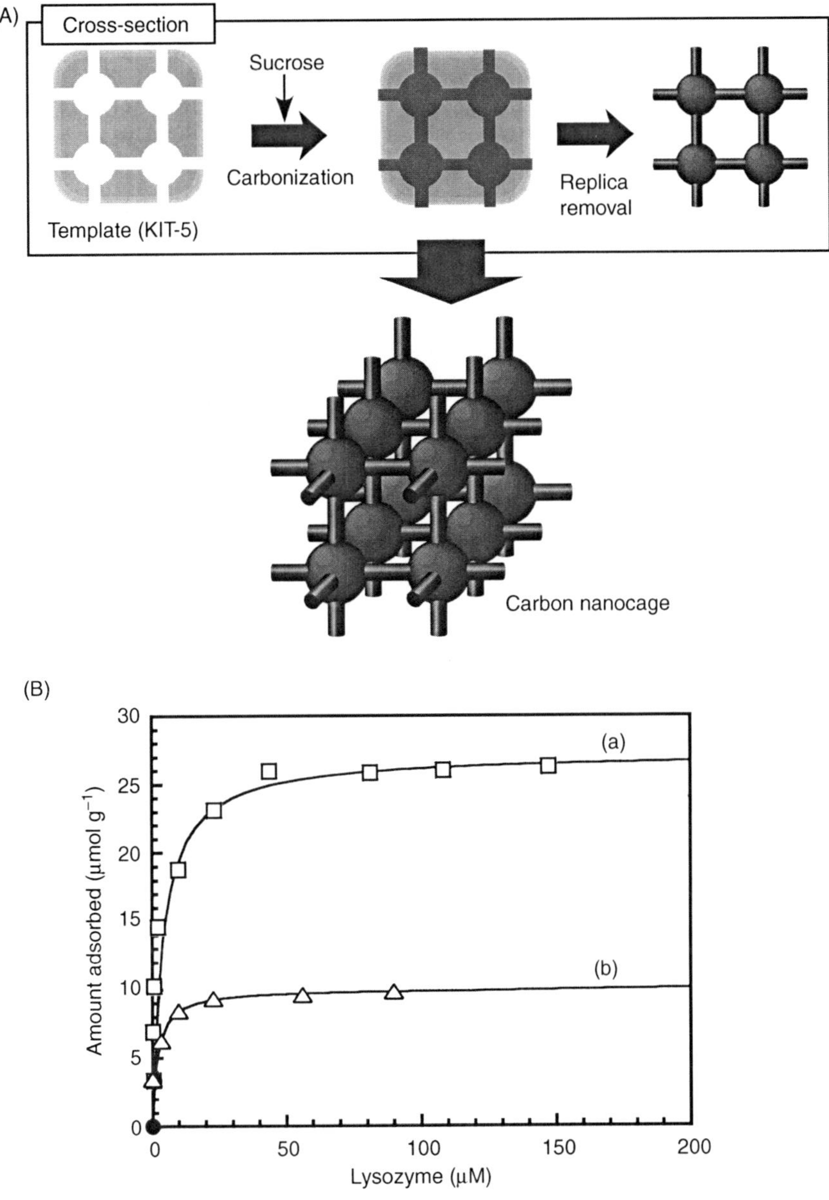

FIGURE 12.17   (A) Conceptual illustration of synthesis of carbon nanocage from KIT-5. (B) Binding isotherms of lysozyme to mesoporous materials: (a) carbon nanocage and (b) mesoporous carbon CMK-3. (Reprinted from Vinu, A. et al., *J. Mater. Chem.*, 15, 5122, 2005. © Royal Society of Chemistry. With permission.)

structures with large differences between pore size and cage size would result in huge values of the surface area and pore volume. Because of the large pore volume of the carbon nanocage, it would show superior capability in the biomaterials adsorption. As a simple demonstration, adsorption behaviors of lysozyme to the carbon nanocage materials were compared with those of conventional mesoporous carbon (Figure 12.17B). The maximal monolayer adsorption capacity of carbon nanocage was 26.5 µmol g^{-1}, while that of CMK-3 is assigned to only 9.8 µmol g^{-1}. Not limited to protein adsorption, carbon nanocage would have superior capability in molecular adsorption, extraction, and removal, which are currently being investigated in our research group.

Another productive approach is the hybridization of proteins onto organic thin films. For example, immobilization of proteins as molecular thin films using LB technique is attractive, but proteins sometimes suffer denaturation by high surface tension on the water surface. In order to overcome this disadvantage, Okahata and coworkers prepared LB films of lipid-coated enzyme (Figure 12.18A) that could be obtained as a precipitate by mixing aqueous solutions of the enzyme (glucose oxidase [GOD] in this case) [115]. Covering GOD with lipids successfully prevented the denaturation of the proteins, even at the air–water interface. The lipid-coated enzymes were obtained as precipitates by mixing aqueous solutions of the enzyme and the lipid, and the resulting lipid-coated enzymes are soluble only in organic solvent. Therefore, the monolayer of the lipid-coated enzymes can be prepared by spreading organic solution of the complex. The formed monolayer can be transferred onto a solid support by the conventional LB technique. Glucose sensing by a Pt electrode modified by the LB films of lipid-coated GOD was demonstrated (Figure 12.18B) [116,117]. This method has an advantage in economizing on the amount of protein. However, the disadvantage of the LB film can

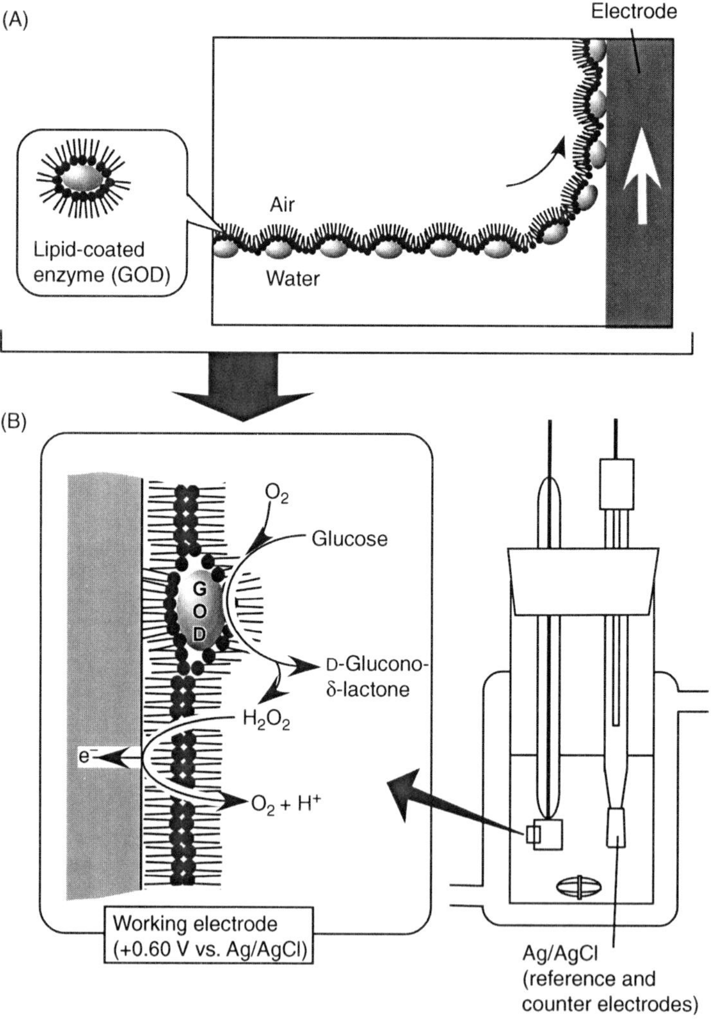

FIGURE 12.18 (A) Transfer of monolayer of lipid-coated glucose oxidase (GOD) onto an electrode by Langmuir–Blodgett (LB) technique. (B) Glucose sensor using the electrode modified with lipid-coated GOD films.

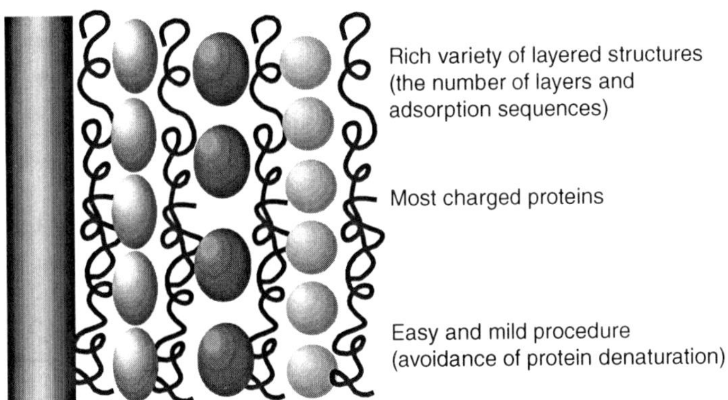

FIGURE 12.19   Advantageous features of protein immobilization by LbL technique.

be seen in the slow diffusion of substrates through the film when rather thick films were used. This disadvantage may originate from dense packing of the lipid molecules in LB films.

Unlike LB films, LbL films are less dense component molecules [118]. Most proteins, especially water-soluble proteins, have charged sites on their surface, and thus the electrostatic LbL adsorption is quite useful for the construction of various protein organizations. It was actually demonstrated that a large number of water-soluble proteins were assembled in combination with oppositely charged polyelectrolytes. As summarized in Figure 12.19, several advantages exist in the LbL assembly of proteins and a wide variety of layered structures can be prepared. For example, the number of layers and the layering sequence are easily modified. Most charged proteins are applicable in this assembling technique. Protein denaturation would be minimized because the adsorption process is conducted under mild conditions.

In order to demonstrate the advantage of the LbL method concerning wide freedom in structural designs, a multienzyme reactor was prepared (see Figure 12.20) [119]. The adsorption behaviors of the two kinds of enzyme, GOD and glucoamylase (GA), were quantitatively evaluated using a QCM technique, because the resonant frequency of the QCM sensitively changes due to the mass adsorption on its electrodes. Systematic QCM analyses revealed that adsorption of both the proteins can be done with appropriately selected counterionized polyelectrolytes, and that layered sequences can be freely modified between these enzymes without causing any interference in the amount of adsorption. Multienzyme films with GOD and GA were prepared on porous filter paper that was immobilized at the bottom of solution container [119]. Substrate (starch) solution was added on the multienzyme film and the solution containing the products was collected as filtrate. The reaction scheme of the multienzyme reactor is shown in Figure 12.20B. Hydrolysis of the glycoside bond in starch by GA produces glucose. Glucose is converted to gluconolactone by GOD, with H_2O_2 as a coproduct. An aqueous solution of water-soluble starch in 0.1 M PIPES buffer (pH 7.0) was placed on the enzyme-immobilized ultrafilters in the upper cup. Filtration was started by applying pressure to the upper cups with a syringe. The filtrate was added to a mixed solution of peroxidase (POD) and indicator dye DA67, and the concentration of the resulting H_2O_2 was evaluated from the change in absorbance at 665 nm. The concentration of unreacted starch was assayed by the iodostarch reaction. However, unreacted starch was not detected in the filtrate at all. Starch cannot pass through the filter, thus it allows separation of substrate and products without additional procedures. Systematic research on reactor performance using LbL films in various layer designs was carried out, revealing the importance of layered order of the two enzymes and appropriate separation of the enzyme layers for efficient material conversion. The advantages of the multienzyme reactor preparation by the LbL technique can be described as follows. The most pronounced advantage is freedom in film construction, and various film structures are easily obtainable by quite simple procedures, that is, a change in the dipping sequences provides films with desirable layering structures. The simplicity of the

13. Ariga, K. and Okahata, Y., Polymerized monolayers of single-chain, double-chain, and triple-chain silane amphiphiles and permeation control through the monolayer-immobilized porous glass plate in aqueous solution, *J. Am. Chem. Soc.*, 11, 5618, 1989.

14. Katagiri, K., Ariga, K., and Kikuchi, J., Preparation of organic-inorganic hybrid vesicle "cerasome" derived from artificial lipid with alkoxysilyl head, *Chem. Lett.*, 661, 1999.

15. Katagiri, K., Hamasaki, R., Ariga, K., and Kikuchi, J., Preparation and surface modification of novel vesicular nano-particle "Cerasome" with liposomal bilayer and silicate surface, *J. Sol-Gel Sci. Techn.*, 26, 393, 2003.

16. Decher, G., Hong, J.D., and Schmitt, J., Build-up of ultrathin multilayer films by a self-assembly process 3. Consecutively alternating adsorption of anionic and cationic polyelectrolytes on charged surfaces, *Thin Solid Films*, 210, 831, 1992.

17. Lvov, Y., Ariga, K., and Kunitake, T., Layer-by-layer assembly of alternate protein polyion ultrathin films, *Chem. Lett.*, 2323, 1994.

18. Lvov, Y., Ariga, K., Ichinose, I., and Kunitake, T., Assembly of multicomponent protein films by means of electrostatic layer-by-layer adsorption, *J. Am. Chem. Soc.*, 117, 6117, 1995.

19. Lvov, Y., Ariga, K., Ichinose, I., and Kunitake, T., Layer-by-layer architectures of concanavalin A by means of electrostatic and biospecific interactions, *J. Chem. Soc. Chem. Comm.*, 2313, 1995.

20. Lvov, Y., Ariga, K., Ichinose, I., and Kunitake, T., Formation of ultrathin multilayer and hydrated gel from montmorillonite and linear polycations, *Langmuir*, 12, 3038, 1996.

21. Onda, M., Lvov, Y., Ariga, K., and Kunitake, T., Sequential actions of glucose oxidase and peroxidase in molecular films assembled by layer-by-layer alternate adsorption, *Biotechnol. Bioeng.*, 51, 163, 1996.

22. Lvov, Y., Ariga, K., Ichinose, I., and Kunitake, T., Molecular film assembly via layer-by-layer adsorption of oppositely charged macromolecules (linear polymer, protein and clay) and concanavalin A and glycogen, *Thin Solid Films*, 285, 797, 1996.

23. Lvov, Y., Ariga, K., Onda, M., Ichinose, I., and Kunitake, T., Alternate assembly of ordered multilayers of SiO_2 and other nanoparticles and polyions, *Langmuir*, 13, 6195, 1997.

24. Ariga, K., Lvov, Y., and Kunitake, T., Assembling alternate dye-polyion molecular films by electrostatic layer-by-layer adsorption, *J. Am. Chem. Soc.*, 119, 2224, 1997.

25. Ariga, K., Lvov, Y., Onda, M., Ichinose, I., and Kunitake, T., Alternately assembled ultrathin film of silica nanoparticles and linear polycations, *Chem. Lett.*, 125, 1997.

26. Ariga, K., Onda, M., Lvov, Y., and Kunitake, T., Alternate layer-by-layer assembly of organic dyes and proteins is facilitated by pre-mixing with linear polyions, *Chem. Lett.*, 25, 1997.

27. Onda, M., Lvov, Y., Ariga, K., and Kunitake, T., Molecularly flat films of linear polyions and proteins obtained by the alternate adsorption method, *Jpn. J. Appl. Phys.*, 36, L1608, 1997.

28. Decher, G., Fuzzy nanoassemblies: toward layered polymeric multicomposites, *Science*, 277, 1232, 1997.

29. Lvov, Y., Onda, M., Ariga, K., and Kunitake, T., Ultrathin films of charged polysaccharides assembled alternately with linear polyions, *J. Biomater. Sci. Polymer. Ed.*, 9, 345, 1998.

30. Caruso, F., Furlong, D.N., Ariga, K., Ichinose, I., and Kunitake, T., Characterization of polyelectrolyte-protein multilayer films by atomic force microscopy, scanning electron microscopy, and fourier transform infrared reflection-absorption spectroscopy, *Langmuir*, 14, 4559, 1998.

31. Ariga, K., Lvov, Y., Ichinose, I., and Kunitake, T., Ultrathin films of inorganic materials (SiO_2 nanoparticle, montmorillonite microplate, and molybdenum oxide) prepared by alternate layer-by-layer assembly with organic polyions, *Appl. Clay Sci.*, 15, 137, 1999.

32. Lvov, Y., Ariga, K., Onda, M., Ichinose, I., and Kunitake, T., A careful examination of the adsorption step in the alternate layer-by-layer assembly of linear polyanion and polycation, *Colloid. Surface. Physicochem. Eng. Aspect.*, 146, 337, 1999.

33. Caruso, F., Nanoengineering of particle surfaces, *Adv. Mater.*, 13, 11, 2001.

34. Hammond, P.T., Form and function in multilayer assembly: new applications at the nanoscale, *Adv. Mater.*, 16, 1271, 2004.

35. Katagiri, K., Hamasaki, R., Ariga, K., and Kikuchi, J., Layer-by-layer self-assembling of liposomal nanohybrid "cerasome" on substrates, *Langmuir*, 18, 6709, 2002.

36. Katagiri, K., Hamasaki, R., Ariga, K., and Kikuchi, J., Layered paving of vesicular nanoparticles formed with cerasome as a bioinspired organic-inorganic hybrid, *J. Am. Chem. Soc.*, 124, 7892, 2002.

37. Kitano, H. and Ringsdorf, H., Surface behaviors of nucleic -acid base-containing lipids in monolayer and bilayer systems, *Bull. Chem. Soc. Jpn.*, 58, 2826, 1985.

38. Kurihara, K., Ohto, K., Tanaka, Y., Aoyama, Y., and Kunitake, T., Molecular recognition of sugars by monolayers of resorcinol cyclotetramer, *J. Am. Chem. Soc.*, 113, 444, 1991.

39. Kurihara, K., Ohto, K., Honda, Y., and Kunitake, T., Efficient, complementary binding of nucleic acid bases to diaminotriazine-functionalized monolayers on water, *J. Am. Chem. Soc.*, 113, 5077, 1991.

40. Ikeura, Y., Kurihara, K., and Kunitake, T., Molecular recognition at the air-water interface: specific binding of nitrogen aromatics and amino acid by monolayers of long-chain kemp acid, *J. Am. Chem. Soc.*, 113, 7342, 1991.

41. Sasaki, D.Y., Kurihara, K., and Kunitake, T., Self-assembled multifunctional receptors for nucleotide at the air-water interface, *J. Am. Chem. Soc.*, 114, 10994, 1992.

42. Ariga, K., Kamino, A., Koyano, H., and Kunitake, T., Recognition of aqueous flavin mononucleotide on the surface of binary monolayers of guanidinium and melamine amphiphiles, *J. Mater. Chem.*, 7, 1155, 1997.

43. Ariga, K. and Kunitake, T., Molecular recognition at air-water and related interfaces: complementary hydrogen bonding and multisite interaction, *Accounts Chem. Res.*, 31, 371, 1998.

44. Ariga, K., Nakanishi, T., and Hill, J.P., A paradigm shift in the field of molecular recognition at the air-water interface: from static to dynamic, *Soft Matter*, 2, 465, 2006.

45. Onda, M., Yoshihara, K., Koyano, H., Ariga, K., and Kunitake, T., Molecular recognition of nucleotides by the guanidinium unit at the surface of aqueous micelles and bilayers. A comparison of microscopic and macroscopic interfaces, *J. Am. Chem. Soc.*, 118, 8524, 1996.

46. Springs, B. and Haake, P., Equilibrium constants for association of guanidinium and ammonium ions with oxyanions: effect of charging basicity of oxyanion, *Bioorg. Chem.*, 6, 181, 1977.

47. Sasaki, Y., Kurihara, K., and Kunitake, T., Specific, multi-point binding od ATP and AMP to a guanidinium-functionalized monolayer, *J. Am. Chem. Soc.*, 113, 9685, 1991.

48. Sakurai, M., Tamagawa, H., Furuki, T., Inoue, Y., Ariga, K., and Kunitake, T., Theoretical interpretation of remarkable enhancement of intermolecular binding at the lipid-water interface, *Chem. Lett.*, 1001, 1995.

49. Sakurai, M., Tamagawa, H., Inoue, Y., Ariga, K., and Kunitake, T., Theoretical study of intermolecular interaction at the lipid-water interface 1. Quantum chemical analysis using a reaction field theory, *J. Phys. Chem. B*, 101, 4810, 1997.

50. Tamagawa, H., Sakurai, M., Inoue, Y., Ariga, K., and Kunitake, T., Theoretical study of intermolecular interaction at the lipid-water interface 2. Analysis based on the Poisson-Boltzmann equation, *J. Phys. Chem. B*, 101, 4817, 1997.

51. Taguchi, K., Ariga, K., and Kunitake, T., Multisite recognition of flavin adenine dinucleotide by mixed monolayers on water, *Chem. Lett.*, 701, 1995.

52. Tamagawa, H., Sakurai, M., Inoue, Y., Ariga, K., and Kunitake, T., Two-dimensional molecular patterning through molecular recognition, *Chem. Lett.*, 411, 1996.

53. Oishi, Y., Torii, Y., Kato, T., Kuramori, M., Suehiro, K., Ariga, K., Taguchi, K., Kamino, A., Koyano, H., and Kunitake, T., Molecular patterning of a guanidinium/orotate mixed monolayer through molecular recognition with flavin adenine dinucleotide, *Langmuir*, 13, 519, 1997.

54. Ariga, K., Template-assisted nano-patterning: from the submicron scale to the submolecular level, *J. Nanosci. Nanotechno.*, 4, 23, 2004.

55. Cha, X., Ariga, K., Onda, M., and Kunitake, T., Molecular recognition of aqueous dipeptides by noncovalently aligned oligoglycine units at the air-water interface, *J. Am. Chem. Soc.*, 117, 11833, 1995.

56. Cha, X., Ariga, K., and Kunitake, T., Multi-site binding of aqueous dipeptides by mixed monolayers at the air-water interface, *Chem. Lett.*, 73, 1996.

57. Cha, X., Ariga, K., and Kunitake, T., Molecular recognition of aqueous dipeptides at multiple hydrogen-bonding sites of mixed peptide monolayers, *J. Am. Chem. Soc.*, 118, 9545, 1996.

58. Ariga, K., Kamino, A., Cha, X., and Kunitake, T., Multisite recognition of aqueous dipeptides by oligoglycine arrays mixed with guanidinium and other receptor units at the air-water interface, *Langmuir*, 15, 3875, 1999.

59. Ariga, K., Tanaka, K., Katagiri, K., Kikuchi, J., Shimakoshi, H., Ohshima, E., and Hisaeda, Y., Langmuir monolayer of organoalkoxysilane for vitamin B_{12}-modified electrode, *Phys. Chem. Chem. Phys.*, 3, 3442, 2001.

60. Yanagisawa, T., Shimizu, T., Kuroda, K., and Kato, C., The preparation of alkylammonium kanemite complex and their conversion to microporous materials, *Bull. Chem. Soc. Jpn.*, 63, 988, 1990.

61. Inagaki, S., Fukushima, Y., and Kuroda, K., Synthesis of highly ordered mesoporous materials from layered polysilicate, *J. Chem. Soc. Chem. Comm.*, 680, 1993.

62. Kresge, C.T., Leonowicz, M.E., Roth, W.J., Vartuli, J.C., and Becj, J.S., Ordered mesoporous molecular sieves synthesized by a liquid-crystal template mechanism, *Nature*, 359, 710, 1992.
63. Beck, J.S., Vartuli, J.C., Roth, W.J., Leonowicz, M.E., Kresge, C.T., Schnitt, K.D., Chu, C.T.W., Olson, D.H., Shepard, E.W., McCullen, S.B., Higgins, J.B., and Schlenker, J.L., A new family of mesoporous molecular shieves prepared with liquid-crystal templates, *J. Am. Chem. Soc.*, 114, 10834, 1992.
64. Vartuli, J.C., Schmitt, K.D., Kresge, C.T., Roth, W.J., Leonowicz, M.E., McCullen, S.B., Beck, J.S., Schlenker, J.L., Olson, D.H., and Sheppard, E.W., Effect of surfactant silica molar ratios on the formation of mesoporous molecular sieves: inorganic mimicry of surfactant liquid-crystal phase and mechanistic implications, *Chem. Mater.*, 6, 2317, 1994.
65. Dubos, M., Gulik-Krzywicki, T., and Cabane, B., Groeth of silica polymers in a lamellar mesophase, *Langmuir*, 9, 673, 1993.
66. Tanev, P.T. and Pinnavaia, T.J., Neutral templating route to mesoporous molecular sieves, *Science*, 267, 865, 1995.
67. Bagshaw, S.A., Prouzet, E., and Pinnavaia, T.J., Templating of mesoporous molecular sieves by nonionic polyethylene oxide surfactant, *Science*, 269, 1242, 1995.
68. Corma, A., From microporous to mesoporous molecular sieve materials and their use in catalysis, *Chem. Rev.*, 97, 2373, 1997.
69. Zhao, D., Feng, J., Huo, Q., Melosh, N., Fredrickson, G.H., Chmelka, B.F., and Stucky, G.D., Triblock copolymer syntheses of mesoporous silica with periodic 50 to 300 angstrom pores, *Science*, 279, 548, 1998.
70. Zhao, D., Huo, Q., Feng, J., Chmelka, B.F., and Stucky, G.D., Nonionic triblock and star diblock copolymer and oligomeric surfactant syntheses of highly ordered, hydrothermally stable, mesoporous silica structures, *J. Am. Chem. Soc.*, 120, 6024, 1998.
71. Davis, M.E., Ordered porous materials for emerging applications, *Nature*, 417, 813, 2002.
72. Schmidt-Winkel, P., Lukens, Jr., W.W., Zhao, D., Yang, P., Chmelka, B.F., and Stucky, G.D., Mesocellular siliceous foams with uniformly sized cells and windows, *J. Am. Chem. Soc.*, 121, 254, 1999.
73. Okabe, A., Fukushima, T., Ariga, K., and Aida, T., Color-tunable transparent mesoporous silica films: immobilization of one-dimensional columnar charge-transfer assemblies in aligned silicate nanochannels, *Angew. Chem. Int. Ed.*, 41, 3414, 2002.
74. Okabe, A., Fukushima, T., Ariga, K., Niki, M., and Aida, T., Tetrafluoroborate salts as site-selective promoters for sol-gel synthesis of mesoporous silica, *J. Am. Chem. Soc.*, 126, 9013, 2004.
75. Vinu, A., Hossain, K.Z., and Ariga, K., Recent advances in functionalization of mesoporous silica, *J. Nanosci. Nanotechno.*, 5, 347, 2005.
76. Jin, H., Liu, Z., Ohsuna, T., Terasaki, O., Inoue, Y., Sakamoto, K., Nakanishi, T., Ariga, K., and Che, S., Control of morphology and helicity of chiral mesoporous silica, *Adv. Mater.*, 18, 593, 2006.
77. Lee, J., Yoon, S., Oh, S.M., Shin, C.H., and Hyeon, T., Development of a new mesoporous carbon using an HMS aluminosilicate template, *Adv. Mater.*, 12, 359, 2000.
78. Ryoo, R., Joo, S.H., Kruk, M., and Jaroniec, M., Ordered mesoporous carbons, *Adv. Mater.*, 13, 677, 2001.
79. Vinu, A. and Ariga, K., Preparation of novel mesoporous carbon materials with tunable pore diameters using directly synthesized AISBA-15 materials, *Chem. Lett.*, 34, 674, 2005.
80. Ryoo, R., Joo, S.H., and Jun, S., Synthesis of highly ordered carbon molecular sieves via template-mediated structural transformation, *J. Phys. Chem. B,* 103, 7743, 1999.
81. Jun, S., Joo, S.H., Ryoo, R., Kruk, M., Jaroniec, M., Liu, Z., Tetsu Ohsuna T., and Terasaki, O., Synthesis of new, nanoporous carbon with hexagonally ordered mesostructure, *J. Am. Chem. Soc.*, 122, 10712, 2000.
82. Vinu, A., Ariga, K., Mori, T., Nakanishi, T., Hishita, S., Golberg, D., and Bando, Y., Preparation and characterization of well-ordered hexagonal mesoporous carbon nitride, *Adv. Mater.*, 17, 1648, 2005.
83. Vinu, A., Terrones, M., Golberg, D., Hishita, S., Ariga, K., and Mori, T., Synthesis of mesoporous BN and BCN exhibiting large surface areas via templating methods, *Chem. Mater.*, 17, 5887, 2005.
84. Vinu, A., Hossain, K.Z., Satish Kumar, G., Sivamurugan, V., and Ariga, K., Adsorption of amino acid on mesoporous molecular sieves, *Stud. Surf. Sci. Catal.*, 156, 631, 2005.
85. Vinu, V., Hossain, K.Z., Satish Kumar, G., and Ariga, K., Adsorption of L-histidine over mesoporous carbon molecular sieves, *Carbon*, 44, 530, 2006.
86. Hartmann, M., Vinu, A., and Chandrasekar, G., Adsorption of vitamin E on mesoporous carbon molecular sieves, *Chem. Mater.*, 17, 829, 2005.

87. Chandrasekar, G., Vinu, A., Murugesan, V., and Hartmann, M., Adsorption of vitamin E on mesoporous silica molecular sieves, *Std. Surf. Sci. Catal.*, 158, 1169, 2005.

88. Zhao, J., Gao, F., Fu, Y., Jin, W., Yang, P., and Zhao, D., Biomolecule separation using large pore mesoporous SBA-15 as a substrate in high performance liquid chromatography, *Chem. Comm.*, 752, 2002.

89. Vallet-Regi, M., Rámila, A., del Real, R.P., and Pérez-Pariente, J., A new property of MCM-41: drug delivery system, *Chem. Mater.*, 13, 308, 2001.

90. Mal, M.K., Fujiwara, M., and Tanaka, Y., Photocontrolled reversible release of guest molecules from coumarin-modified mesoporous silica, *Nature*, 421, 350, 2003.

91. Mal, N.K., Fujiwara, M., Tanaka, Y., Taguchi, T., and Matsukata, M., Photo-switched storage and release of guest molecules in the pore void of coumarin-modified MCM-41, *Chem. Mater.*, 15, 3385, 2003.

92. Ariga, K., Zhang, Q., Niki, M., Okabe, A., and Aida, T., Proteosilica: mesoporous silicates densely filling amino acid and peptide assemblies in their nanoscale pores, *Stud. Surf. Sci. Catal.*, 146, 427, 2003.

93. Ariga, K., Silica-supported biomimetic membranes, *Chem. Rec.*, 3, 297, 2004.

94. Ariga, K., Aimiya, T., Zhang, Q., Okabe, A., Niki, M., and Aida, T., "Proteosilica" a novel nanocomposite with peptide assemblies in silica nanospace: photoisomerization of spiropyran doped in chiral environment, *Int. J. Nanosci.*, 1, 521, 2002.

95. Zhang, Q., Ariga, K., Okabe, A., and Aida, T., High-density modification of mesoporous silica inner walls with amino acid function by residue transfer from template, *Stud. Surf. Sci. Catal.*, 146, 465, 2003.

96. Zhang, Q., Ariga, K., Okabe, A., and Aida, T., A condensable amphiphile with a cleavable tail as a "lizard" template for the sol-gel synthesis of functionalized mesoporous silica, *J. Am. Chem. Soc.*, 126, 988, 2004.

97. Diaz, J.F. and Balkus, K.J., Enzyme immobilization in MCM-41 molecular sieve, *J. Mol. Catal. B-Enzym.*, 2, 115, 1996.

98. Takahashi, H., Li, B., Sasaki, T., Miyazaki, C., Kajino, T., and Inagaki, S., Catalytic activity in organic solvents and stability of immobilized enzymes depend on the pore size and surface characteristics of mesoporous silica, *Chem. Mater.*, 12, 3301, 2000.

99. Yiu, H.H.P., Wright, P.A., and Botting, N.P., Enzyme immobilisation using SBA-15 mesoporous molecular sieves with functionalised surfaces, *J. Mol. Catal. B-Enzym.*, 15, 81, 2001.

100. Lai, C.-Y., Trewyn, B.G., Jeftinija, D.M., Jeftinija, K., Xu, S., Jeftinija, S., and Lin, V.S.Y., A mesoporous silica nanosphere-based carrier system with chemically removable CdS nanoparticle caps for stimuli-responsive controlled release of neurotransmitters and drug molecules, *J. Am. Chem. Soc.*, 125, 4451, 2003.

101. Vinu, A., Streb, C., Murugesan, V., and Hartmann, M., Adsorption of cytochrome c on new mesoporous carbon molecular sieves, *J. Phys. Chem. B*, 107, 8297, 2003.

102. Vinu, A., Murugesan, V., Tangermann, O., and Hartmann, M., Adsorption of cytochrome c on mesoporous molecular sieves: influence of pH, pore diameter, and aluminum incorporation, *Chem. Mater.*, 16, 3056, 2004.

103. Vinu, A., Miyahara, M., Hossain, K.Z., Nakanishi, T., and Ariga, K., Adsorption of lysozyme over mesoporous carbons with various pore diameters, *Stud. Surf. Sci. Catal.*, 156, 637, 2005.

104. Miyahara, M., Vinu, A., Hossain, K.Z., Nakanishi, T., and Ariga, K., Adsorption study of heme proteins on SBA-15 mesoporous silica with pore-filling models, *Thin Solid Films*, 499, 13, 2006.

105. Vinu, A., Miyahara, M., and Ariga, K., Assemblies of biomaterials in mesoporous media, *J. Nanosci. Nanotechno.*, 6, 1510, 2006.

106. Miyahara, M., Vinu, A., and Ariga, K., Immobilization of lysozyme onto pore-engineered mesoporous AISBA-15, *J. Nanosci. Nanotechno.*, 6, 1765, 2006.

107. Vinu, A., Murugesan, V., and Hartmann, M., Adsorption of lysozyme over mesoporous molecular sieves MCM-41 and SBA-15: influence of pH and aluminum incorporation, *J. Phys. Chem. B*, 108, 7323, 2004.

108. Su, T.J., Lu, J.R., Thomas, R.K., Cui, Z.F., and Penfold, J., The effect of solution pH on the structure of lysozyme layers adsorbed at the silica-water interface studied by neutron reflection, *Langmuir*, 14, 438, 1998.

109. Vinu, A., Miyahara, M., and Ariga, K., Biomaterial immobilization in nanoporous carbon molecular sieves: influence of solution pH, pore volume, and pore diameter, *J. Phys. Chem. B*, 109, 6436, 2005.

110. Vinu, A., Miyahara, M., Sivamurugan, V., Mori, T., and Ariga, K., Large pore cage type mesoporous carbon, carbon nanocage: a superior adsorbent for biomaterials, *J. Mater. Chem.*, 15, 5122, 2005.

111. Vinu, A., Miyahara, M., and Ariga, K., Preparation and pore size control of cage type mesoporous carbon materials and their application in protein adsorption, *Stud. Surf. Sci. Catal.*, 158, 971, 2005.

112. Vinu, A., Miyahara, M., Mori, T., and Ariga, K., Carbon nanocage: a large pore cage-type mesoporous carbon material as an adsorbent for biomolecules, *J. Porous Mater.*, 13, 379, 2006.

113. Kleitz, F., Liu, D., Anilkumar, G.M., Park, I.-S., Solovyov, L.A., Shmakov, A.N., and Ryoo, R., Large cage face-centered-cubic Fm3m mesoporous silica: synthesis and structure, *J. Phys. Chem. B*, 107, 14296, 2003.

114. Ravikovitch, P.I. and Neimark, A.V., Density functional theory of adsorption in spherical cavities and pore size characterization of templated nanoporous silicas with cubic and three-dimensional hexagonal structures, *Langmuir*, 18, 1550, 2002.

115. Okahata, Y. and Ijiro, K., A lipid-coated lipase as a new catalyst for triglyceride synthesis in organic solvents, *J. Chem. Soc. Chem. Comm.*, 1392, 1988.

116. Okahaya, Y., Tsuruta, T., Ijiro, K., and Ariga, K., Langmuir-Blodgett films of an enzyme-lipid complex for sensor membranes, *Langmuir*, 4, 1373, 1988.

117. Okahaya, Y., Tsuruta, T., Ijiro, K., and Ariga, K., Preparation of Langmuir-Blodgett films of enzyme lipid complexes: a glucose sensor membrane, *Thin Solid Films*, 180, 65, 1989.

118. Onda, M., Ariga, K., and Kunitake, T., Activity and stability of glucose oxidase in molecular films assembled alternately with polyions, *J. Biosci. Bioeng.*, 87, 69, 1999.

119. Onda, M., Lvov, Y., Ariga, K., and Kunitake, T., Sequential reaction and product separation on molecular films of glucoamylase and glucose oxidase assembled on an ultrafilter. *J. Ferment. Bioeng.*, 82, 502, 1996.

120. Kikuchi, J., Ariga, K., and Ikeda, K., Signal transduction mediated by artificial cell-surface receptors: activation of lactate dehydrogenase triggered by molecular recognition and phase reorganization of bile acid derivatives embedded in a synthetic bilayer membrane, *Chem. Comm.*, 547, 1999.

121. Kikuchi, J., Ariga, K., Miyazaki, T., and Ikeda, K., An artificial signal transduction system. Control of lactate dehydrogenase activity performed by an artificial cell-surface receptor, *Chem. Lett.*, 253, 1999.

122. Fukuda, K., Sasaki, Y., Ariga, K., and Kikuchi, J., Dynamic behavior of a transmembrane molecular switch as an artificial cell-surface receptor, *J. Mol. Catal. B-Enzym.*, 11, 971, 2001.

123. Kikuchi, J., Ariga, K., Sasaki, Y., and Ikeda, K., Control of enzymic activity by artificial cell-surface receptors, *J. Mol. Catal. B-Enzym.*, 11, 977, 2001.

124. Shimizu, T., Kogiso, M., and Masuda, M., Vesicle assembly in microtubes, *Nature*, 383, 487, 1996.

125. Ariga, K., Yamada, N., Naito, M., Koyama, E., and Okahata, Y., AFM observation of a supramolecular rod-like structure of bilayer membrane formed from tripeptide-containing amphiphiles, *Chem. Lett.*, 493, 1998.

126. Yamada, N., Ariga, K., Naito, M., Matsubara, K., and Koyama, E., Regulation of β-sheet structures within amyloid-like beta-sheet assemblage from tripeptide derivatives, *J. Am. Chem. Soc.*, 120, 12192, 1998.

127. Ariga, K., Kikuchi, J., Narumi, K., Koyama, E., and Yamada, N., Formation of mesoscopic patterns with molecular-level flatness by simple casting of chloroform solutions of tripeptide-containing amphiphiles, *Chem. Lett.*, 787, 1999.

128. Yamada, N. and Ariga. K., Formation of beta-sheet assemblage with a view to developing an amyloid model, *Synlett*, 575, 2000.

129. Ariga, K., Kikuchi, J., Naito, M., Koyama, E., and Yamada, N., Modulated supramolecular assemblies composed of tripeptide derivatives: formation of micrometer-scale rods, nanometer-size needles, and regular patterns with molecular-level flatness from the same compound, *Langmuir*, 16, 4929, 2000.

130. Yamada, N., Matsubara, K., Narumi, K., Sato, Y., Koyama, E., and Ariga, K., Lyotropic aggregate of tripeptide derivatives within organic solvents: study on dynamic property of molecular assembling, *Colloid Surf. A-Physicochem. Eng. Asp.*, 169, 271, 2000.

131. Ariga, K., Kikuchi, J., Naito, M., and Yamada, N., FT-IR, TEM, and AFM studies of supramolecular architecture formed by tripeptide-containing monoalkyl amphiphiles, *Polym. Advan. Technol.*, 11, 856, 2000.

132. Shimizu, T., Masuda, M., and Minamikawa, H., Supramolecular nanotube architectures based on amphiphilic molecules, *Chem. Rev.*, 105, 1401, 2005.

13 Polypyrrole Nano- and Microsensors and Actuators for Biomedical Applications

Yevgeny Berdichevsky and Yu-Hwa Lo

CONTENTS

13.1 INTRODUCTION

The conducting polymer polypyrrole (PPy) possesses many interesting properties that make it an attractive material for a variety of applications. In particular, this polymer undergoes reversible redox reactions in electrolyte with applied voltage that allow control over many material properties such as conductivity, ion exchange, hydrophobicity, and even the material dimensions. The control of ion exchange properties of the polymer is important in the design of selective sensors, while voltage control over material geometry makes PPy a particularly suitable material for the design of actuators. Furthermore, the controllable ion exchange and volume change are material properties of PPy and can be utilized at any dimension ranging from macroscale, or devices with the size of several centimeters, to nanoscale, or devices with the size of several tens of nanometers. This flexibility allows the design of a great variety of PPy devices, including "artificial muscles" intended for medical prosthetics, microactuators for lab-on-a-chip integrated systems and microrobotics, and electrochemical sensors for various biological molecules.

In this chapter, the focus is on the devices fabricated from PPy doped with dodecylbenzenesulfonate (DBS), which are capable of operating in aqueous environments ranging from sea water to blood plasma. DBS-doped PPy has long-term stability in water solutions and operates by uptake or expulsion of small positive ions during voltage-controlled reduction or oxidation, respectively, from or to the surrounding electrolyte. This property makes the PPy(DBS) devices particularly suitable for biomedical applications in which the environment consists of an electrically conducting aqueous solution containing a number of small positive ions such as Na^+, K^+, and Ca^{2+}. Therefore, a PPy actuator device that operates on the principle of volume change due to the movement of sodium ions can use the biological solution such as extracellular fluid or blood plasma as a supporting electrolyte without the need for device encapsulation.

Several micro- and nanosized devices based on the properties of PPy have been developed by a number of laboratories for biomedical applications. Devices described in this chapter include microvalve designs based on a PPy volume change for use in microfluidics and drug delivery, a microrobotic device that uses PPy–gold bilayers as actuators, PPy nanowires capable of reversible length change with the applied voltage, PPy-coated nanosensor for detection of catecholamine neurotransmitters, which displays nanomolar sensitivity and improved time response, and PPy coatings for cell growth substrates and microelectrodes used in neuroscience.

Section 13.2 begins with a description of PPy electrochemistry and principles of PPy synthesis and reversible volume change that occurs during electrochemical cycling of the polymer. Section 13.3 describes how this volume change has been harnessed by several laboratories to design and fabricate microdevices for biological applications. In Section 13.4, the steps toward the fabrication and characterization of PPy nanoactuators are reported, and Section 13.5 reviews PPy microscale biosensors and the use of PPy in tissue and cell cultures.

13.2 POLYPYRROLE ACTUATORS—SYNTHESIS AND PRINCIPLES OF OPERATION

13.2.1 INTRODUCTION

Conducting polymer actuators are well suited for applications in both biological and medical microsystems.[1] These actuators can change their volume due to an electrochemically induced redox reaction, with attendant movement of ion and solvent in and out of the polymer matrix. The resulting volume change can be as large as 30% with only a few volts of applied voltage.[2] Low-voltage requirement, large relative displacement, and ability to operate in aqueous environments make conducting polymer actuators promising candidates for microfluidics,[3] micromachined biological sensors, and lab-on-chip devices for manipulation of cells and organelles. Of further interest is their ability to microfabricate conducting polymer structures on semiconductor substrates, leading to intriguing possibilities of integrating actuator functionality with optical modulation or optical power transfer. Furthermore, conducting polymer nanostructures can also be fabricated with suggested applications in areas such as biosensors, bioencapsulation, and drug delivery.[4]

13.2.2 POLYPYRROLE ELECTROCHEMISTRY

PPy is one of the conducting polymers that have been used as actuators or "artificial muscles." PPy can be fabricated by electrochemical synthesis on a conducting substrate.[5] Various dopants can be used to endow the material with customized properties, but the focus here is on PPy doped with DBS^- anions. When voltage is applied to this polymer in an aqueous solution containing a small positive ion, such as Na^+, the PPy undergoes a redox reaction:

$$PPy^+(DBS^-) + e^- + Na^+(aq) \leftrightarrow PPy^0(DBS^-Na^+) \tag{13.1}$$

Insertion of Na^+ and its hydration shell causes swelling of polymer matrix, while expulsion of Na^+ ions results in contraction of the polymer. Reliance on a ubiquitous small positive ion such as Na^+ allows PPy to function in a variety of aqueous environments such as blood, urine, cell culture media, and even seawater.

13.2.2.1 Electropolymerization of Polypyrrole

PPy can be polymerized by either purely chemical or electrochemical means by oxidizing the monomer pyrrole. Electrochemical polymerization is achieved by applying a voltage (or current) between the working electrode (WE) and the counter electrode (CE) (a reference electrode [REF] can be in a three-electrode electrochemical cell configuration to ensure the correct voltage drop at the WE). This voltage is anodic enough to oxidize pyrrole monomers in contact with the WE by removing electrons from the pyrrole molecules, which then dimerize, trimerize, and eventually polymerize into PPy chains. These chains then precipitate out of the solution onto the WE surface. The thickness of the deposited PPy is controlled by the time of the deposition; for large area WE (>1 cm^2), the deposition rate is approximately 1 μm/h. Films with thickness of 40 μm can be deposited with this method. The color of the deposited films changes depending on the thickness for films thinner than 1 μm, for thicker films the color is black. Smooth glossy films with thickness up to 10 μm can be produced; however, the roughness of the film surface tends to increase with increased thickness.

13.2.2.2 Polypyrrole Conductivity

PPy is considered as a conducting polymer due to its conjugated backbone (Figure 13.1). The electrons shown schematically as double bonds in the chemical structure of PPy are mobile and can

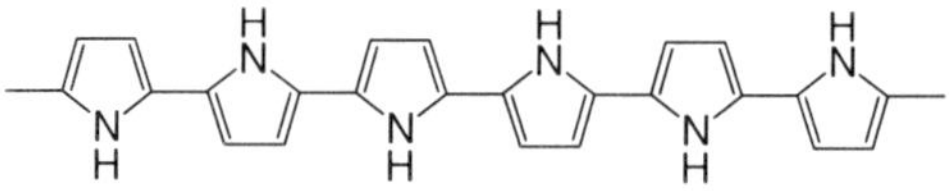

FIGURE 13.1 Polypyrrole chemical structure.

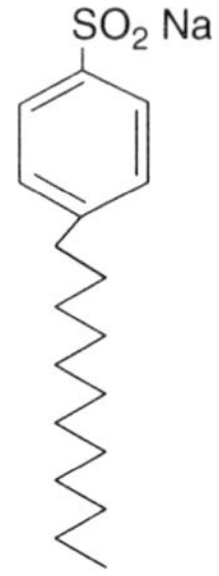

FIGURE 13.2 Chemical structure of sodium dodecylbenzenesulfonate (NaDBS).

move from one pyrrole unit to the other on the chain. If there are defects in the synthesized PPy, or if there are intentionally introduced dopant ions, such as the DBS$^-$ ion in this work, the double bonds can become ionized (electrons removed or added) to form structures known as solitons, polarons, and bipolarons. In PPy, the conduction mechanism is "bipolaron hopping" along the polymer chain. In a heavily doped polymer, the presence of many bipolarons generates bipolaron conduction bands in the material band-gap, and the polymer becomes conductive. In the case of PPy doped with DBS, the conductivity is on the order of 10 Ω/cm, depending on the oxidation state and temperature.[6]

13.2.2.3 Doping of Polypyrrole with DBS Ions

The presence of sodium dodecylbenzenesulfonate (NaDBS) in the synthesis solution serves several functions: first, NaDBS functions as a conducting electrolyte to allow oxidation of pyrrole monomers; second, NaDBS is an amphiphilic surfactant that allows a high concentration of hydrophobic pyrrole monomer to be dissolved in an aqueous solution; and third and most important, the DBS$^-$ ion becomes incorporated into the polymer matrix during synthesis and serves as a dopant ion. DBS is a large molecule with a long hydrophobic tail (Figure 13.2).

Due to its size and the favorable hydrophobic–hydrophobic interactions with the PPy, DBS ion becomes permanently embedded in the polymer matrix, acting as a permanent dopant and also altering the polymer nanostructure, as discussed in Section 13.4. The degree of the doping is far higher in PPy than the typical doping in inorganic semiconductors; in PPy, there is roughly one DBS ion per four pyrrole units.

13.2.2.4 Electrochemical Cycling of PPy(DBS)

For electrochemical testing of PPy doped with DBS ions, the experimental setup shown in Figure 13.3 can be used with an NaDBS aqueous electrolyte.

The voltage range versus the Ag/AgCl reference is 0 to -1 V, corresponding to approximately 0 to -2.5 V measured between WE and CE. This range ensures complete oxidation (at 0 V versus Ag/AgCl) and reduction (at -1 V versus Ag/AgCl) of the PPy without undesirable effects such as irreversible overoxidation or electrolysis that begin to occur at more positive or negative voltages. The reversible reaction is described in Equation 13.1, where the left side, PPy$^+$(DBS$^-$) represents the polymer in its oxidized state, while the right side, PPy^0(DBS$^-$Na$^+$) represents the reduced polymer. As the application of negative voltage adds electrons to the polymer backbone (reduction), charge

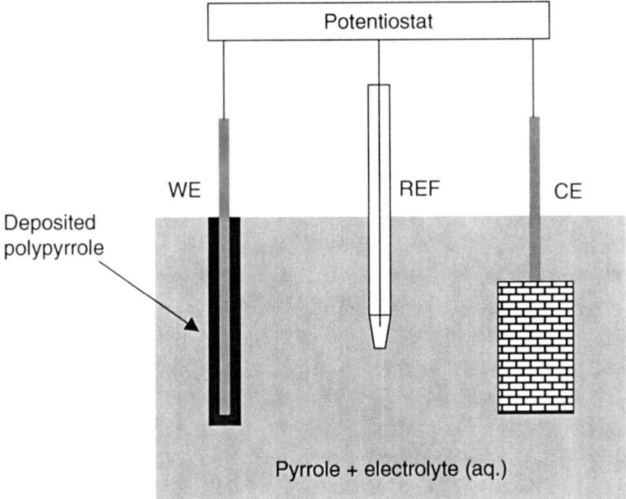

FIGURE 13.3 Experimental setup: WE, working electrode; REF, reference electrode; CE, counter electrode; deposited polypyrrole is shown in black covering the working electrode.

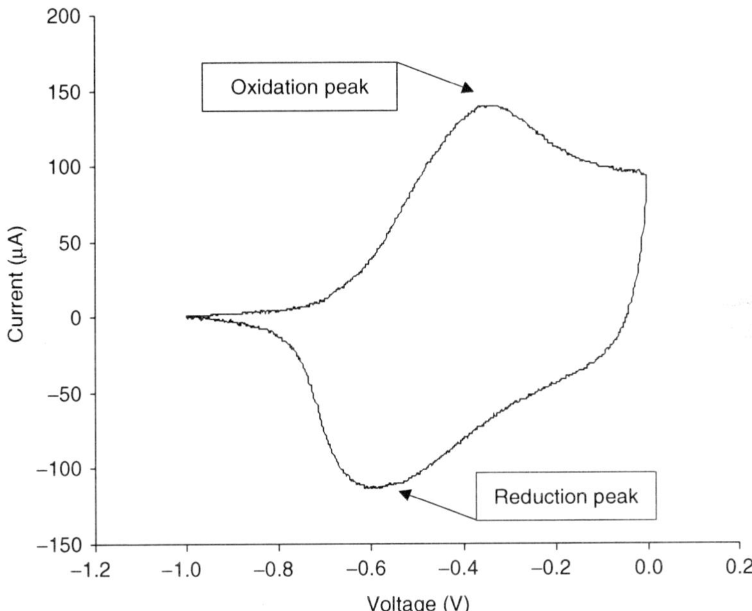

FIGURE 13.4 Cyclic voltammogram of PPy(DBS) in 0.1 M NaDBS electrolyte at 50 mV/s voltage scan.

neutrality is preserved by the movement of sodium ions from the surrounding electrolyte into the polymer matrix to compensate for the negative charge of the immobile DBS^- dopant ions. When oxidizing voltage is applied to the polymer (0 V versus Ag/AgCl), electrons are removed from PPy, resulting in a positively charged polymer matrix that pushes mobile sodium ions out to the surrounding solution to preserve charge neutrality. This reaction is reversible and can be carried out by applying a voltage ramp to the polymer while measuring the oxidizing/reducing currents, as shown in Figure 13.4.

This electrochemical method is known as cyclic voltammetry. It allows determination of the voltages at which oxidation and reduction reactions take place. Tracing the voltammogram from 0 V through the reduction peak to −1 V and back through oxidation peak to 0 V, the following events take place: the polymer starts out in the oxidized state, and as the voltage is lowered, the potential barrier for adding electrons onto the polymer backbone is overcome, and the current due to polymer reduction begins to flow. The reduction current reaches its peak at -0.6 V and begins to taper off as the polymer matrix becomes fully reduced. This reduction is accompanied by simultaneous movement of Na^+ ions from the electrolyte into the polymer to compensate the negative charge on DBS^- dopant ions. At -1 V, the current has reached its minimum, signifying that the reduction of the polymer is complete. If the voltage is lowered further, the current would begin to increase again due to water electrolysis, which would damage the polymer. Therefore, the applied voltage is limited to -1 V, as this voltage is low enough to reduce the polymer without negative effects of electrolysis. As the voltage is then increased on the return scan, oxidation current can be observed due to the electrons being removed from the polymer and the corresponding movement of Na^+ ions out of the PPy matrix. The peak occurs at -0.35 V, and the current reaches a minimum at 0 V, corresponding to a complete oxidation of the PPy. At higher voltages, an irreversible oxidation of the polymer occurs, accompanied by chemical changes to the PPy structure. If allowed, this higher voltage would render PPy unusable; therefore, the applied oxidation voltage is limited to 0 V.

13.2.2.5 Volume Change Due to Reversible Electrochemical Redox Reaction of PPy(DBS)

As the polymer is electrochemically cycled between 0 and -1 V, movement of Na^+ in and out of the PPy matrix occurs as described in Section 13.2.2.4. Each Na^+ ion is accompanied by a solvation shell of several water molecules, and, in addition, osmotic pressure causes more water molecules to enter the polymer alongside the sodium ions.[7] The additional volume of Na^+ ions and water that have entered the PPy film causes conformational changes of the PPy molecules and in the overall dimensions of the deposited PPy (Figure 13.5).

As seen in the figure, the applied voltage and the entering sodium ions and water molecules cause a conformational change of the PPy chains (dotted lines), with the resulting volume change of the film. If the film has length L and thickness H, the expansion of the film under reducing voltage can be as high as $\Delta L/L = 2-3\%$ and $\Delta H/H = 30\%$. The increase in length is used in so-called bilayer actuators in which a PPy film is laminated to a thin film of another material that does not undergo volume changes with applied voltage; this modification allows the magnification of the relatively small changes in the length of PPy film and results in large-scale movement. The reversible increase in thickness, on the other hand, is relatively large compared with the size of the synthesized film and can be used directly in micro- and nanoactuators discussed in Sections 13.3 and 13.4. The strong anisotropy of the volume change in PPy(DBS) films is likely due to the layered orientation of the polymer chains and the dopant anions. It heavily depends on the synthesis conditions, with implications for the fabrication of micro- and nanostructures. The evidence for the layered structure of

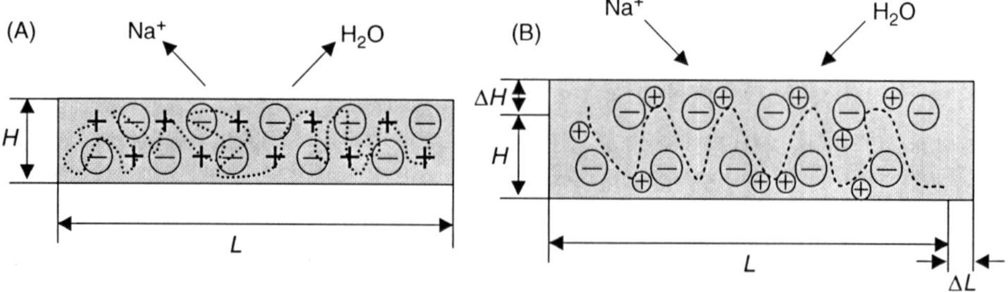

FIGURE 13.5 Schematic cross-section of a polypyrrole film. (A) Oxidized film (V versus Ag/AgCl $= 0$ V) with sodium ions and water expelled from the polymer matrix, polymer backbone charged positive (+ signs), compensating the charge on immobile DBS^- ions (encircled ($-$) signs). (B) Reduced film with the neutral polymer backbone and Na^+ ions entering the film (encircled (+) signs) to compensate the charge on DBS^- ions.

PPy films doped with large alkyl sulfonates is presented in Section 13.4 in which the implications of the synthesis parameters of PPy nanowires on polymer morphology are examined with x-ray diffraction.

13.2.2.6 Time Response of the Polypyrrole Films

A PPy-film chronoamperogram, or current response to applied voltage steps plotted versus time, is shown in Figure 13.6.

The experimental setup used to perform chronoamperometry is the same as the one described above for cyclic voltammetry. A defined voltage is applied between the WE and the REF while current is measured between the WE and the CE. WE is kept at 0 V prior to the start of the experiment, reducing voltage of -1 V versus Ag/AgCl is applied at $t = 0$ s, and an oxidizing voltage of 0 V versus Ag/AgCl is applied at $t = 60$ s. In Figure 13.6, the current response to the voltage steps can be observed: first, there is a large current spike that corresponds to charging of the double-layer capacitance, and then the current begins to decay as the polymer becomes reduced or oxidized, and ions diffuse in and out of the polymer matrix, respectively. However, the time response of the current is not purely due to ion diffusion. An inflection point can be seen clearly in the reducing current, and the oxidizing current is not a simple exponential decay that could be expected as the remaining ions leave the polymer by diffusion. The change in conformation of PPy chains, which occurs during both reduction and oxidation, introduces further time delay into the course of the current response.[8] In the oxidized PPy, polymer chains are in a "compacted" conformation, packed close together as there is neither water nor sodium ions in the polymer matrix. When a reducing voltage is applied, the chains take some time to rearrange their conformation state, which is likely to be driven by electrostatic repulsion of the dopant DBS^- ions whose negative charge is no longer being compensated by the positive charge on the polymer. As the PPy chains move further apart, the structure of the film becomes less dense, allowing ion and water diffusion into the polymer. The current–time response is, therefore, a summation of two processes—the conformational changes of the PPy chains in response to applied voltage and the diffusion of sodium ions and water molecules to maintain charge neutrality. These two processes combine to produce the inflection in the measured current at the point where the film structure becomes fully open and ion diffusion takes over as the current-limiting factor.

A more quantitative analysis of the PPy electrochemical time response is impeded and complicated by the presence of other processes that take place during the reversible redox reaction: changes in conductivity of the PPy film as it passes from an oxidized to a reduced state, current due

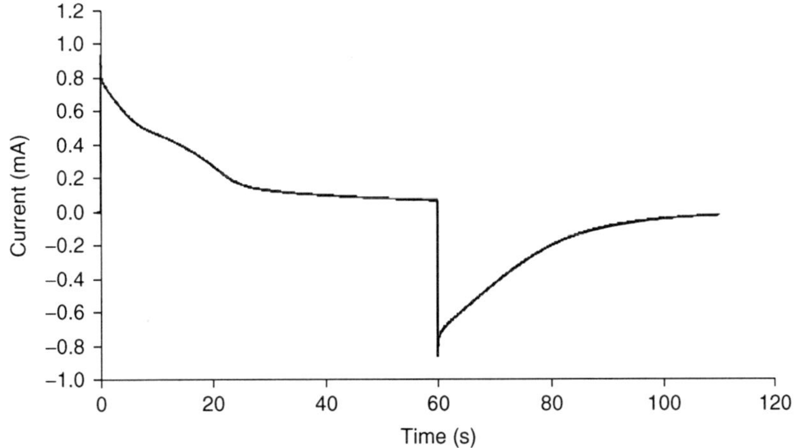

FIGURE 13.6   Chronoamperogram of a large area (>1 cm^2) 30 μm thick polypyrrole film.

to the capacitive charging of the double layer throughout the polymer (which can be viewed as a conductive porous electrode), the contribution of electric field–driven ion migration[9] to the apparent diffusion constants of Na^+ ions and their water solvation shells, and the uncompensated solution resistance between the electrodes in the electrochemical cell, which can introduce a significant voltage drop and effectively lower the applied voltage at the film–solution interface. A theoretical analysis of the diffusion contribution to the time course of PPy doping/undoping is discussed in Section 13.4 in which the role of PPy device geometry (shape and size) in the electrochemical time response is examined.

13.2.3 · Actuation of Polypyrrole Microstructures

13.2.3.1 Microfabrication of the Polypyrrole Test Lines

To evaluate the ability of PPy microstructures to function as actuators due to electrochemically induced changes in thickness, PPy micro-test lines of varying width were fabricated using photolithographic techniques and tested in solution using a profilometer and an optical microscope. The fabrication sequence is shown schematically in Figure 13.7.

Voltage of 0.55 V versus Ag/AgCl was applied to all Au/Ti lines simultaneously for 7 h to produce a film of 6.5–7 μm thickness coating the metal (Figure 13.8). Since PPy growth occurs isotropically, a widening of the Au/Ti patterns occurred. The thickness was uniform over the metal except the edges, where the PPy coating was thicker by approximately 1 μm than in the middle of the metal strip line. This edge thickness is caused by nonuniformity in the electric field and the improved pyrrole monomer diffusion at the edges of the metal lines, which act as WEs.

13.2.3.2 Measurement of Electrochemically Controlled Thickness Change of Polypyrrole Test Lines

Experimental setup for the evaluation of electrochemically induced thickness changes in the PPy test lines is shown schematically in Figure 13.9.

Two methods were used to evaluate the thickness changes of the PPy test lines induced by applied voltage: a mechanical profilometer measurement and optical imaging. The profilometer has the advantage of higher sensitivity and precision, but due to the physical constraints of the equipment used, a very shallow electrolyte bath was used. A gold CE had to be fabricated on the same substrate as WE, while REF was excluded. Therefore, the voltage was applied between

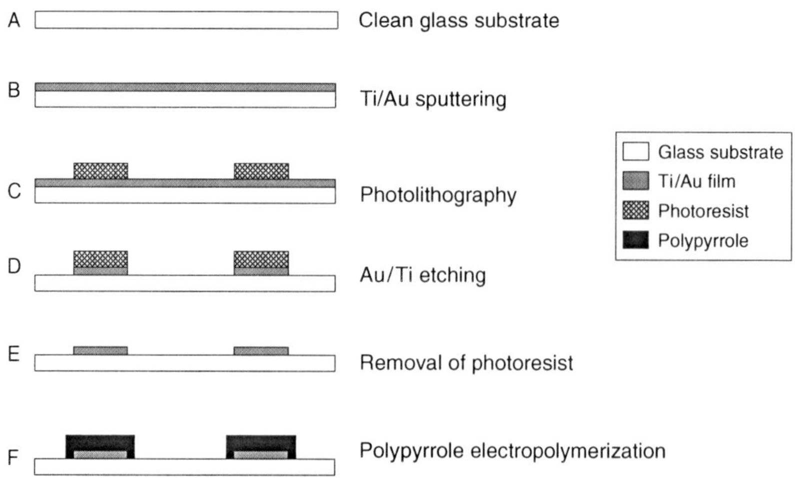

FIGURE 13.7   Steps for the microfabrication of polypyrrole test lines.

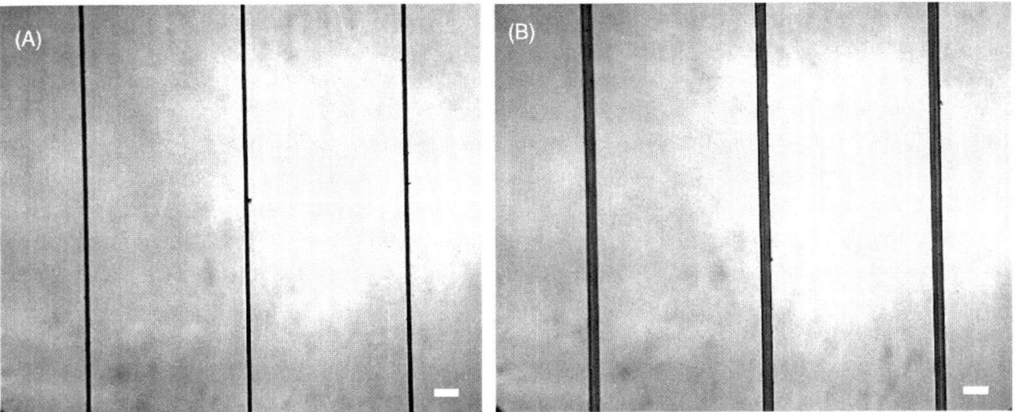

FIGURE 13.8 Optical micrographs of polypyrrole test lines: (A) 5 μm wide PPy lines and (B) 25 μm wide PPy lines. The scale bars in both images represent a distance of 50 μm.

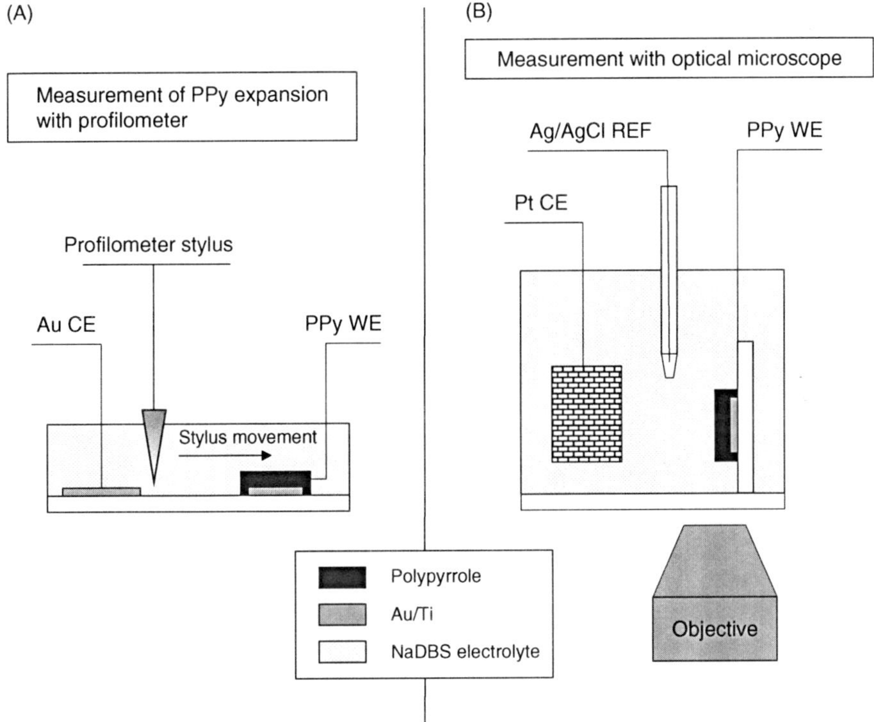

FIGURE 13.9 Experimental setup for the measurement of electrochemically controlled volume change of polypyrrole test structures. (A) A profilometer is used to measure the change in thickness of polypyrrole electropolymerized on an Au/Ti line. (B) An inverted optical microscope is used to observe the profile of a polypyrrole test line, allowing measurement of the thickness change. WE, working electrode; CE, counter electrode; REF, reference electrode.

WE and CE, with the same values as measured between WE and CE in the three-electrode setup (0 V for oxidizing voltage, −2.5 V for reducing voltage). The inverted optical microscope allowed the use of a larger volume electrolyte bath with three electrodes; however, the resolution of this imaging was lower than that of the profilometer. This low resolution was due to the relatively long distance between the objective and the measured PPy line, limiting the imaging to lower power or long-working distance objectives. Nevertheless, optical imaging has the added advantage of allowing video microscopy with easy visualization of the time course of PPy thickness change.

The change of PPy line thickness with voltage applied between PPy WE and gold CE, measured with profilometry and confirmed with optical microscopy, is shown in Figure 13.10.

The measurement shown in Figure 13.10 is taken after the PPy has been electrochemically cycled at least three times. This procedure is used because the first expansion of a PPy is generally much larger than that on later cycles. The original thickness of the PPy film in Figure 13.10 was 6.5 μm just after synthesis, and as seen in the figure, the thickness of the film does not return to this value once it has been subjected to a redox cycle.

An important issue that becomes apparent after PPy test lines have been reduced and oxidized a few times involves adhesion failure between PPy and gold seed layer. There is no covalent attachment between the gold film and the electropolymerized PPy, and the polymer tends to detach from gold after a few redox cycles due to its linear expansion of a few percent, which is relative to the supporting electrode. This is the same problem that also plagues the designers of bilayer actuators, and several solutions involving increased roughness of the gold (through varying parameters of gold electrochemical deposition) or other electrode materials have been proposed in the literature.[10,11] We have used a novel electrode geometry that was used to prevent adhesion failure between PPy and gold in the microvalve design (Section 13.3).

13.2.4 INTEGRATION OF POLYPYRROLE MICROSTRUCTURES WITH SILICON DEVICES

PPy test lines described in Section 13.2.3.2 have been fabricated using photolithography on a planar substrate. This fabrication methodology is fully compatible with semiconductor microfabrication with the implication that PPy microstructures can be potentially integrated on the same substrate with such semiconductor devices, transistors, and optical diodes. Such integration opens up a realm of interesting possibilities of using PPy actuators as mechanically active elements integrated on a single chip with electronic control circuitry and optical remote communications and power delivery with potential applications in microrobotics. A proof-of-concept integration of PPy test lines with electrochemically controlled thickness and a silicon pn junction that can function as a photodiode is described in Sections 13.2.4.1 and 13.2.4.2. Connection to the pn junction allowed optical control of actuation, potentially enabling microfluidic and lab-on-chip devices, which could be remotely controlled by a laser or a photodiode across a layer of biological fluid.

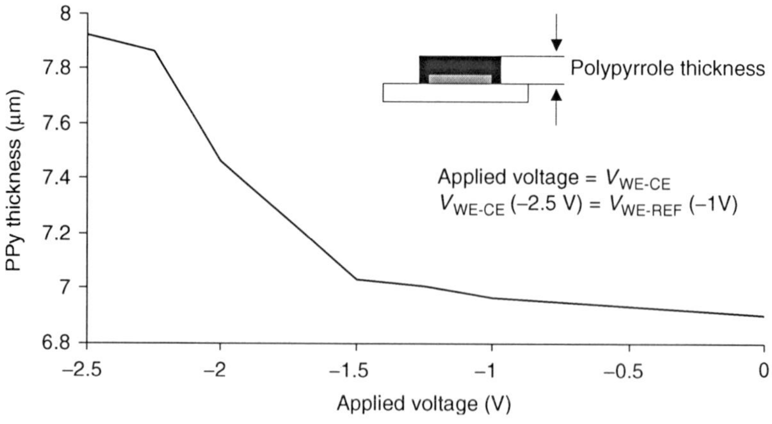

FIGURE 13.10   Change in thickness of polypyrrole with applied voltage measured by profilometry.

### 13.2.4.1	Fabrication of an Optically Controlled Polypyrrole Microstructure

An n-type Si wafer with an implanted p-type top layer was used as a substrate. A thin metal film was deposited and patterned on the back and front sides of the substrate. A thin layer of SiO_2 was then sputtered and patterned on the front side of the wafer to protect exposed Si surface from contact with the electrolyte solution (Figure 13.11). A second layer of metal was deposited and patterned into 50 μm wide strips on top of the oxide layer to provide a seed layer for PPy deposition. The two metal layers and oxide layer were patterned such that both metal films were electrically connected, thus providing PPy with an electrical contact to the p-doped side of the photodiode. PPy was electrochemically deposited on the seed layer from an aqueous solution of pyrrole monomer to a thickness of 4 μm.

### 13.2.4.2	Operation of the Device

The finished device was placed in an aqueous solution of NaDBS and biased at $V_{bias} = 2.25$ V. The displacement of the PPy in the direction normal to substrate surface was then measured by a profilometer as incident light was first switched on and then switched off (Figure 13.12).

The maximum contraction or expansion of the actuator due to light modulation (T_{max}) was measured to be ~90 nm, which is ~2% of the PPy thickness as deposited. As seen from

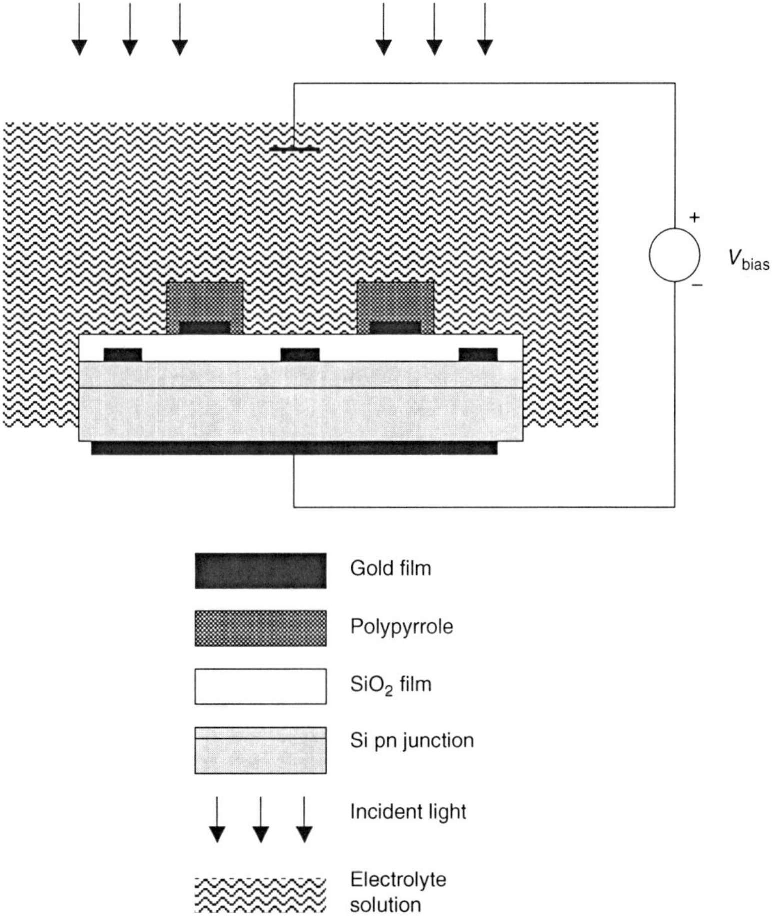

FIGURE 13.11	Operation of PPy microactuator integrated with Si photodiode.

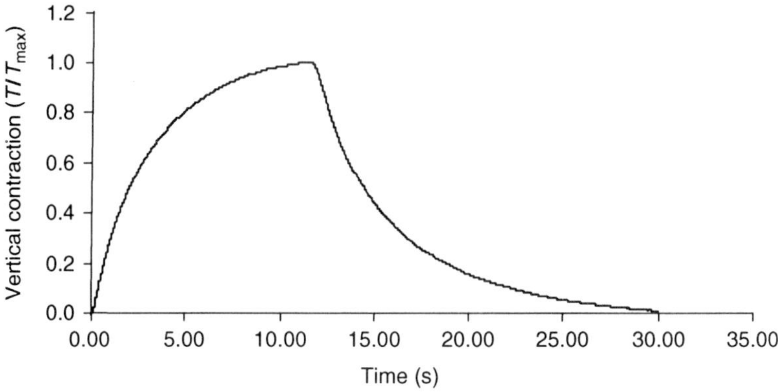

FIGURE 13.12 Modulation of PPy expansion or contraction with incident light.

Figure 13.12, the time response of the microactuator (τ) is approximately 10 s. The time response of the electrochemically actuated PPy depends primarily on mass transport through the polymer matrix, in this case diffusion of Na^+ ions. It follows that if the actuator is scaled down, the diffusion time should decrease as well. In Section 13.4, a method to fabricate PPy rods with a diameter of 200 nm is described. These structures have a time constant (for complete electrochemical oxidation or reduction) at least two orders of magnitude smaller than the microactuator, bringing it closer to the time response of biological muscle (10–100 ms).

13.3 POLYPYRROLE MICROACTUATORS

13.3.1 BILAYER ACTUATORS

A significant amount of progress has been made in the design of devices utilizing micromuscles of a bilayer PPy(DBS) and gold for operation in aqueous electrolytes.[1,12] These devices are based on the application of planar photolithographic microtechnology to fabricate microstructures similar to the process outlined in Section 13.2. Thin films of PPy are electropolymerized on patterned gold films, which either have a weak adhesion to the substrate or are detached from the substrate by dissolution of a sacrificial thin film underlying the gold.[5] Bilayer films fabricated in this manner can remain attached to the substrate at one end, while the other end can carry a useful load such as a silicon or a polymer rigid plate. They have been utilized in devices ranging from microvalves to microrobots. An interesting application of this technology is the design of "cell clinic," which is a micromachined well that can be opened and closed with a microlid mounted on a PPy/Au microactuator. The authors expect to use this device for confinement and the study of individual cells, including electrical impedance measurements and optical observation of cellular response to mechanical stress. Microbilayer technology was also used to make more complex robotic device such as the microarm capable of gripping and moving small objects in an electrolyte.[12] Several individually controlled microactuators were used to control the movement of the robotic "hand" to pick up and move small objects such as glass microbeads.

The ability to fabricate and control many microactuators simultaneously is an important feature that makes PPy micromuscles suitable as active components of microfluidic systems. A typical microfluidic system for such applications as a lab-on-a-chip or remote sensing will utilize relatively long microchannels with width and depth of only a few tens of micrometers or less. Typical fabrication materials include glass, quartz, silicon, as well as polymer materials such as polycarbonate and polymethylmethacrylate (PMMA).[13] Also, a high number of microfluidic devices are fabricated using polydimethylsiloxane (PDMS), which is a transparent elastomer.[14] This material has many attractive optical and mechanical properties and can be easily molded and bonded at temperatures less than 100°C.

A valve utilizing a surface micromachined PPy bilayer actuator[15] has been reported, where PPy–Au hinge moved a rigid plate of benzocyclobutene (BCB) polymer to open or block a microfluidic channel fabricated with SU-8 photosensitive epoxy and PDMS. However, there are a few problems associated with the bilayer mode of actuation. The mechanical force that can be applied by the tip of the bilayer, which is the point that undergoes the most physical displacement, is very small—some orders of magnitude smaller than the pressure generated in the PPy film. Also, delamination of the polymer from the substrate is very common, since the bonding between the polymer film and the electrode is mostly due to noncovalent interactions.[10] As discussed in Section 13.2, PPy electropolymerized in the presence of NaDBS can undergo reversible volume change of 30% or more in the direction normal to the substrate.[16] This volume change, if realized in a thick micropatterned PPy film, can be directly applied in a variety of micromechanical systems. Fabrication and operation of a microvalve utilizing anisotropic volume change of PPy(DBS) and PDMS microfluidics is described in Section 13.3.2.

13.3.2 DIRECT-MODE POLYPYRROLE–PDMS MICROVALVE

A property of PDMS that is particularly useful in the design of a microvalve is that it is possible to fabricate thin PDMS membranes by spin-coating technique. These membranes are very flexible and form a nonpermanent watertight seal when pressed against another smooth surface. A valve design[3] implemented with a PDMS microfluidic system consists of two chambers: working channel for biological or chemical analyte separated by a thin PDMS membrane from the electrolyte bath containing the PPy microactuator and a gold CE (see Figure 13.13). This valve operates as follows: an application of voltage between WE, consisting of PPy(DBS) deposited on a gold conductor, and CE, which is a patterned gold film, produces a redox reaction involving Na^+ ions in the electrolyte. As ions move into the polymer, it swells and pushes the membrane separating two chambers into the working channel. This action seals the working channel completely and results in a closed state for the valve. Under application of reverse voltage, polymer shrinks, allowing the PDMS to come back into original position, thus opening the working channel.

As mentioned above, polymerizing PPy(DBS) on a flat gold electrode results in a very significant problem. After two or three cycles, the polymer completely delaminates from the electrode due to swelling parallel to the substrate, which happens simultaneously with volume change that is normal to the substrate. As discussed earlier, this lateral volume change is far smaller than the one in the vertical direction, but it is enough to detach the polymer from the substrate. For this reason, PPy was deposited on electroplated gold posts of 8–9 μm height (see Figure 13.14). These posts were electroplated through photoresist wells, resulting in a T-shaped cross-section.

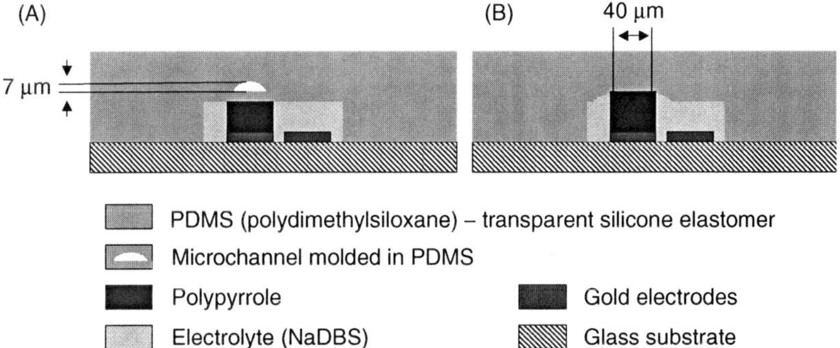

FIGURE 13.13 Microvalve design. Working channel is open (A) and is closed by the expanding polypyrrole (B).

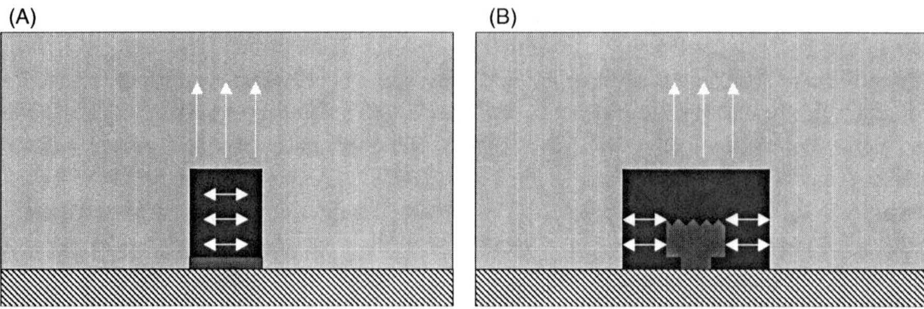

FIGURE 13.14 Forces exerted by expanding polypyrrole are represented as arrows. (A) The lateral forces are not countered and will result in delamination after few cycles. (B) The lateral forces are countered by Au post.

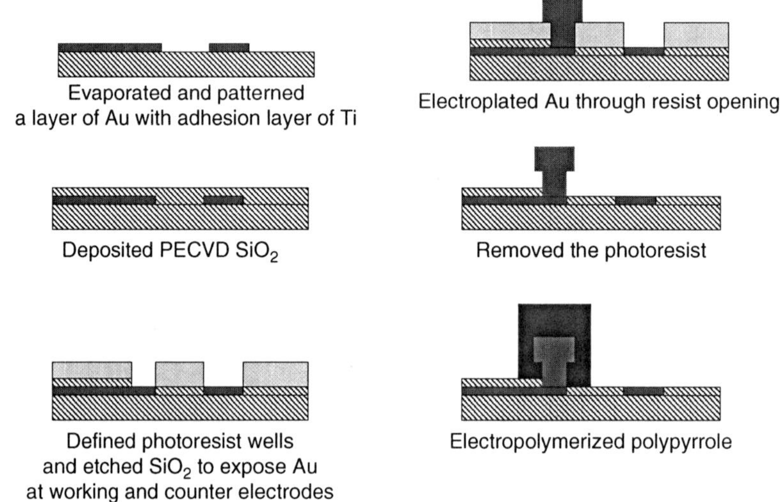

FIGURE 13.15 Microfabrication process for polypyrrole actuator—the active component in a microfluidic valve.

PPy was then electropolymerized on these posts, completely surrounding them, which reduced the possibility of delamination during operation. In addition, the gold posts were left with a rough top surface, which further improved adhesion between gold and PPy.

13.3.2.1 Microfabrication of the Active Part of the Microvalve

The active component in this microvalve is the PPy microactuator. The microfabrication process sequence on a glass substrate is as follows (see Figure 13.15).

First, an adhesion layer of Ti (10 nm) is thermally evaporated onto a glass substrate. Then, a conducting film of gold of 400 nm thickness is thermally evaporated on top of Ti, and both metals are photolithographically patterned to form WE and CE as well as metal traces to contact pads. An insulating silicon dioxide film of 500 nm thickness is deposited via plasma enhanced chemical vapor deposition (PECVD). SU-8(5) photoresist is then spin-coated onto the oxide to a thickness of 2 μm, exposed and developed to open up resist wells over the electrodes. The exposed area of the WE is a 40 μm square while the exposed area of the CE is a 40 μm wide semicircular strip surrounding the WE. Oxide in these wells is etched away, and more gold is electroplated in the

WE well to produce the round T-shape with rough surface discussed above. It was experimentally determined that electroplated Au posts need to be at least 8–9 μm high to provide good mechanical support for the PPy. The photoresist is then stripped away using oxygen plasma etching, and the chip is ready for electropolymerization of PPy. An aqueous solution of 0.04 M pyrrole and 0.04 M NaDBS is prepared, and the PPy is deposited onto the WE at 0.62 V (versus Ag/AgCl CE) using a potentiostat. Polymerization time is 4.3 h, resulting in a PPy(DBS) thickness of 34 μm on top of the gold post. PPy grows laterally as well, at roughly the same rate, producing a pattern width of around 110 μm (gold post width is 40 μm and has ~35 μm of PPy surrounding it). This growth is not uniform, and the resulting pattern is not symmetrical. Rather, it appears that PPy growth follows slight imperfections in the substrate surface.

13.3.2.2 Microfabrication of the Passive Microfluidic Component

A technique known as soft lithography was utilized in the fabrication of PDMS microchannels. Briefly, the working channel was made by photolithographically defining a positive photoresist of 6.2 μm thickness into 50 μm wide and 20 mm long strips making a Y-shape on silicon substrate. The photoresist was then reflowed at 150°C for 20 min, producing a spherical cross-section (the resist cross-section was originally rectangular, see Figure 13.16D). A prepolymer of PDMS was then mixed with a cross-linking agent, degassed in vacuum, and poured onto the silicon wafer with photoresist pattern. After a curing step, the fully cross-linked PDMS was peeled off the silicon mold master by hand, and cut into chip-sized pieces.

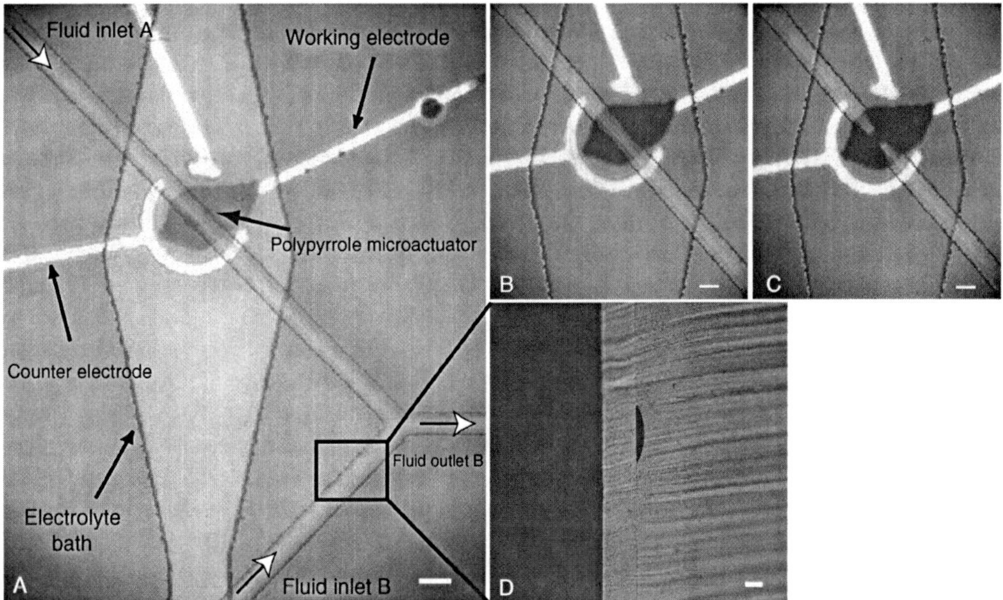

FIGURE 13.16 Micrograph of the top view of the fully assembled microvalve including the active component with electrodes and metal traces (bright lines), rhombus-shaped electrolyte bath, and Y-shaped working channel (A). The valve is placed under one of the arms of the Y, preventing or allowing the analytes flowing in that channel from merging with contents of the other arm. (B) Valve is open. (C) Valve is closed. Expanding polypyrrole (dark material between Au traces) can be seen to pinch off the working channel in (C). The bar represents a distance of 50 μm. (D) The cross-section of the working microfluidic channel molded against reflowed photoresist and sealed with PDMS membrane. Bar represents a distance of 50 μm in (A)–(C) and a distance of 15 μm in (D).

An analogous method was used to make the microchannel that would act as an electrolyte bath. SU-8(50) photoresist was spin-coated onto a silicon wafer with 41 μm thickness. The photoresist was then patterned according to the parameters that the manufacturer supplied, making 100 μm wide and 20 mm long strips with a wider area (0.5 mm at the widest point) in the middle to accommodate the actuator with CE and electrolyte bath. PDMS was then mixed as described above, spin-coated onto this mold master at 1000 rpm, and then heat-cured as above. This treatment produces a PDMS membrane about 85 μm thick in the resistance-free areas and 44 μm thick on top of the SU-8(50) pattern.

The PDMS chip containing the Y-shaped working channel was then bonded to the PDMS membrane still on the silicon wafer by both exposing to oxygen plasma and pressing them together after visual alignment on a mechanical stage. The PDMS assembly was then demolded from the second silicon master.

The final step of the process was to drill fluid access openings into the PDMS assembly and align it with the active PPy actuator on the glass substrate (see Figure 13.16).

Plasma bonding was not used in this step, since pressing PDMS against a glass surface produces a reversible watertight seal and enables reuse of either passive or active part of the device. The electrolyte channel was then filled up with 0.1 M aqueous solution of NaDBS, and voltage was applied between WE and CE to produce a change in volume of the PPy(DBS) actuator.

13.3.2.3 Microvalve Operation

Actuation was carried out between $V_{WE}-V_{CE} = -2.6$ V and $V_{WE}-V_{CE} = 0.0$ V, which roughly correspond to -1 and 0 V versus an Ag/AgCl reference. Voltage was limited to these values because hydrogen bubbles start to form below -2.6 V, and it is possible to permanently damage the polymer above 0 V. It became apparent that it would be highly desirable to have a REF-integrated on-chip next to the microactuator to enable application of accurate voltages, as the voltage between WE and CE drifted occasionally. Nevertheless, despite the lack of integrated REF, it was possible to close and open the working channel (see Figures 13.16B and 13.16C). As seen from the micrographs, the hemispherical cross-section of the channel enabled a complete seal at the maximum volume increase in the PPy(DBS) actuator. The operation was then quantitatively verified under a profilometer using an open PDMS electrolyte bath with no microchannel, allowing access for the profiling stylus. The actuation proceeded as follows: first, the polymer expanded to the thickness of 45 μm from the original thickness of 34 μm with 32% vertical volume change, after application of $V_{WE-CE} = -2.6$ V. Under subsequent application of $V_{WE-CE} = 0.0$ V, the PPy returned to the thickness of 41 μm. It was then possible to reversibly alternate the height of the microactuator between 41 and 45 μm by alternating the voltage between -2.6 and 0 V (although not always returning to the same height due to voltage drifts in the absence of REF). Thus, the reversible volume change in direction normal to the substrate is 12% of the original volume. This volume change took 10–15 s. This volume change was significantly lower than that reported for a continuous thick PPy film or a micropatterned thinner film (1–1.5 μm)—80% nonreversible original volume change and 30% subsequent reversible volume change. The difference in measured volume change is likely due to the fabrication method used—instead of polymerizing the PPy on a flat substrate, PPy was deposited onto a protruding gold post to prevent delamination. It is possible to hypothesize that anisotropic morphology of PPy is oriented normal to the substrate and is thus actually oriented parallel to the wafer surface in PPy surrounding the post while oriented normal to the wafer surface in PPy on top of the post. The large volume change then occurs not only in the normal direction but also in the lateral direction in the Au post design. This characteristic was confirmed by video microscopy, which showed reversible lateral volume expansion increasing the diameter of PPy actuator by 4 μm, or about 6% half of the volume expansion in the normal direction but still much larger than the lateral expansion in PPy films that was grown conventionally on a flat substrate.

13.4　POLYPYRROLE NANODEVICES

13.4.1　INTRODUCTION

In recent years, intensified effort was launched to create nanosized devices capable of carrying out mechanical work. The work reported in the literature has ranged from top-down fabrication of nanoelectromechanical actuators with ultraviolet or electron-beam lithography and scanning-probe microscopy manipulation to bottom-up chemical synthesis of molecular machines and DNA motors and harvesting natural biomotors.[17–19] Applications of successful nanomachines are potentially numerous and far-reaching, including advances in computation and communications through the use of rapidly switching nanoactuators coupled to mirrors or magnetic storage elements. Nanorobotic devices capable of operating in a fluid environment could be used in biomedical sciences and in health care, allowing small-scale manipulation of flows and particles. Some of the problems encountered in fabrication and operation of nanomechanical devices include potential for mass production, ease of control, and restrictions on operating environment. For example, the use of electron-beam lithography is suitable for fabricating components one at a time, in a serial fashion, and hence creating large numbers of nanoactuators with this method could be prohibitively expensive. On the other hand, chemical synthesis or utilization of naturally occurring nanomotors could allow simultaneous fabrication of large numbers of these devices; however, these motors can be difficult to control and require very restricted operating environments.

In this section, a different approach to nanowire fabrication is described. Template synthesis in nanoporous membranes can be used to create PPy nanowires[20] that can be operated as electrically controlled nanoactuators in an aqueous fluid environment. A template synthesis method has been used to shrink the dimensions of a conducting polymer (PPy) actuator to nanoscale to simultaneously synthesize $>10^8$ (pore density of an anodized alumina template can range from 10^8 to $10^{12}/cm^2$) artificial muscle nanowires capable of electrically controlled reversible expansion and contraction. The fabrication methodology, performance evaluation, and characterization of PPy nanoactuators are described in this section (13.4) in detail.

13.4.2　POLYPYRROLE NANOWIRE ELECTROPOLYMERIZATION AND EVALUATION OF THE ELECTROCHEMICALLY CONTROLLED VOLUME CHANGE

13.4.2.1　Removal of Hollow Region of Synthesized Polypyrrole Nanowires by Mechanical Lapping

PPy films can be synthesized on a conducting surface by electropolymerization, and various dopant ions can be incorporated into the polymer altering many of its properties. In template synthesis of PPy(DBS) nanowires, one side of a nanoporous membrane is coated with conducting material, and then the PPy is electropolymerized through the pores. We used a 60 µm thick alumina membrane with 200 nm diameter pores, resulting in nanowires of the same diameter with a length controlled by polymerization time.[21] As seen in Figure 13.17A, the top portion of the nanofibers is hollow with very thin sidewalls (<20 nm) and probably unsuitable for mechanical actuation. To remove the hollow tube portion of the nanofiber, the following procedure was used: PPy nanofibers of 40 µm length were electropolymerized in the alumina template as above, but before the alumina was dissolved, an extra step was added to the fabrication sequence. The alumina membrane with PPy nanofibers was subjected to mechanical lapping to remove the top 10–15 µm of the nanofibers (Figure 13.18, sample 1). The alumina was then dissolved in 0.2 M NaOH (aq.) solution, and the nanofibers were imaged with a scanning electron microscope (SEM). In Figure 13.17B, it can be seen that the remaining lower portions of the nanofibers are solid and more suitable for actuation, and only the top few micrometers of the PPy(DBS) nanofibers were hollow.

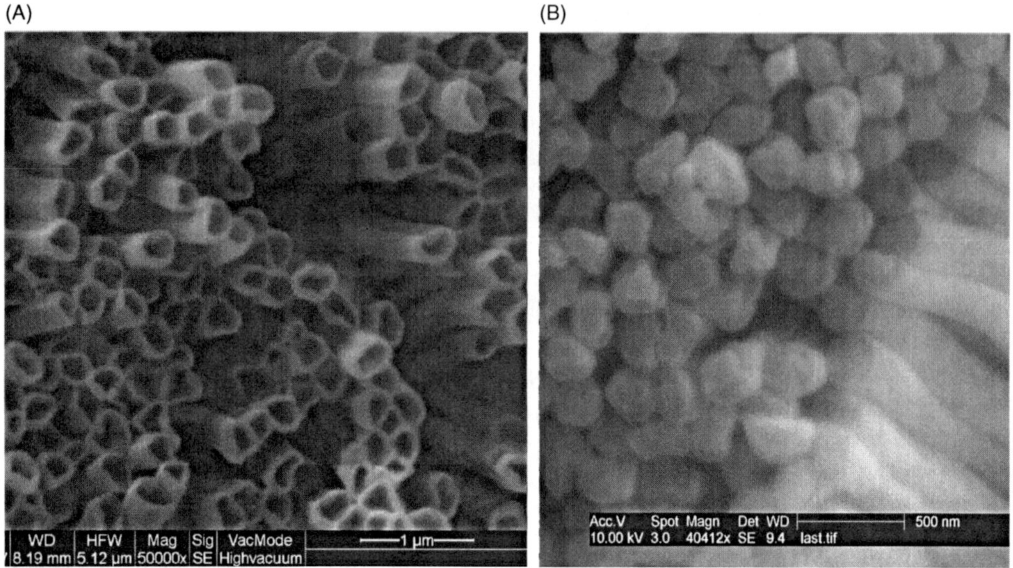

FIGURE 13.17 SEM top view of the PPy(DBS) nanowires: (A) the hollow top portion of the nanowires can be clearly seen and (B) the nanowires have been mechanically lapped.

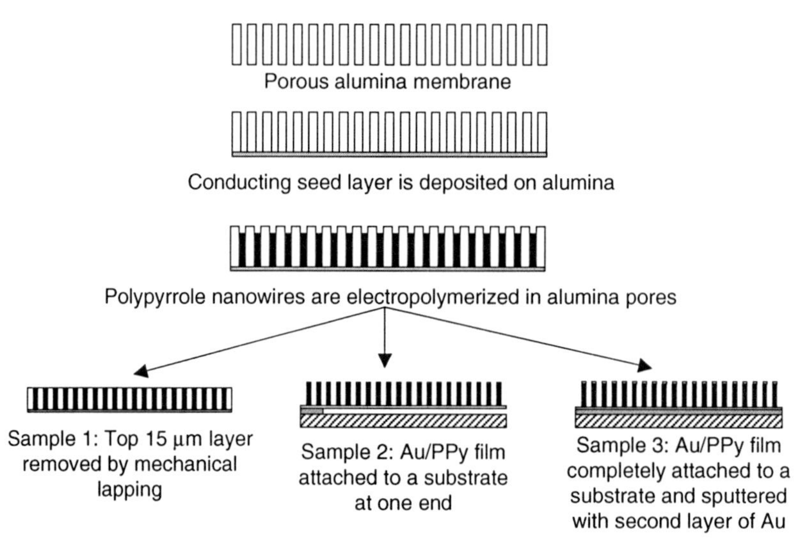

FIGURE 13.18 Schematic representation of the process flow seen in cross-section.

13.4.2.2 SEM Evidence of Electrochemically Induced Volume Change in Polypyrrole Nanowires

The ability of the PPy nanowires to act as actuators was initially examined by SEM imaging. The nanowires were left embedded in the alumina membrane and then subjected to mechanical lapping to remove the top 10–15 µm (Figure 13.18, sample 1). The top surface was imaged with a SEM (Figure 13.19A). As seen from the figure, the surface is smooth since the upper surfaces of the nanowires are even with the top surface of the alumina membrane. This assembly (lapped alumina membrane with embedded PPy nanowires) was placed in the NaDBS electrolyte with a platinum

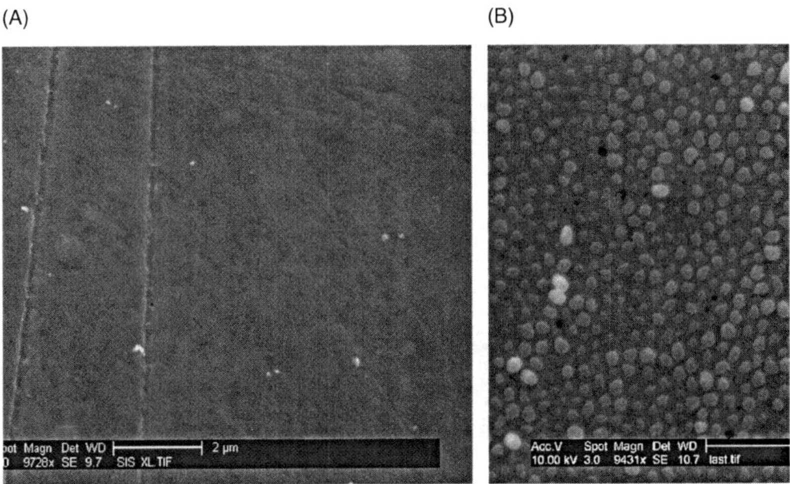

FIGURE 13.19   SEM image (A) shows the lapped and polished surface of alumina with top ends of PPy nanowires even with the surface; image (B) shows a similar sample after electrochemical reduction cycle in NaDBS electrolyte, with nanowires visibly expanding with the influx of sodium ions. Scale bars represent a distance of 2 μm.

CE and an Ag/AgCl REF to complete the three-electrode electrochemical cell. A voltage of −1 V versus the REF was then applied between WE and CE to induce reduction of PPy accompanied by the movement of sodium ions, which in turn resulted in the expansion of nanowires. The membrane was then taken out of solution, dried, and imaged with SEM (Figure 13.19B). The PPy nanowires were clearly protruding from alumina surface as the result of ion influx and polymer swelling. Unfortunately, it was very hard to quantitatively evaluate the actuation with this method, since the sample had to be taken out of the electrochemical cell and dried to image the surface. However, it provided clear qualitative evidence of nanowire actuation.[22]

13.4.2.3   Real-Time Optical Microscopy of Nanowire Actuation

Two real-time experiments were carried out using an optical microscope to detect reversible actuation of nanowires in both lateral and normal directions relative to electrode surface.[23] First, we dissolved the alumina membrane, leaving a 5 mm × 5 mm gold film covered with PPy nanowires. The film was attached at one end to a substrate and mounted so that the cross-section could be observed with an inverted optical microscope (Figure 13.18, sample 2). The assembly was then immersed in electrolyte solution, and the electrodes were connected as before. Upon cycling the WE voltage between 0 and −1 V relative to the REF, the composite film bent away and toward the substrate, respectively (Figure 13.20). Since PPy(DBS) contracts when oxidized (0 V) and expands when reduced (−1 V), the film's behavior is consistent with a bimorph interaction between PPy nanowires and gold. This effect is somewhat surprising since nanowires are discrete; however, it seems that there is enough interaction between individual nanowires to behave similar to homogeneous PPy films.

To detect whether the nanowires could also expand or contract in the direction normal to the gold film (along the nanowire length), the gold/PPy nanowire film was completely attached to the substrate (Figure 13.18, sample 3). A thin layer of gold was then sputtered on top of the PPy nanowires to make optical measurement more precise. The substrate was subsequently sectioned and mounted in such a manner that the cross-section was visible in the objective of the microscope. The ends of the nanowires were clearly marked by the original gold seed layer on one side and the sputtered thin gold layer on the other side (Figure 13.21 inset).

(A)   (B)

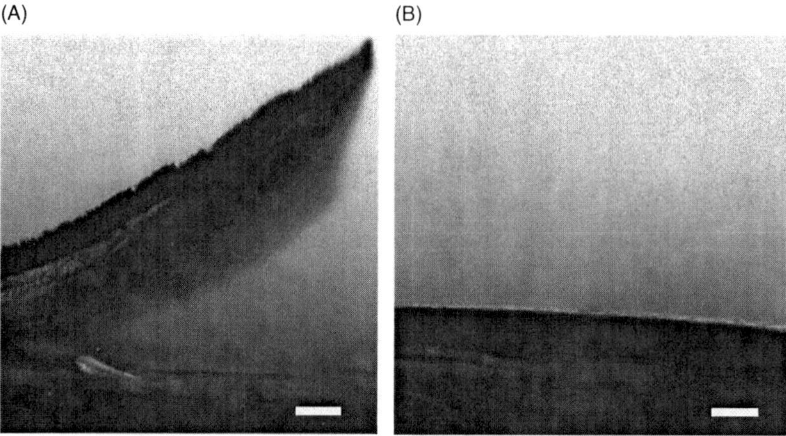

FIGURE 13.20   Micrograph (A) shows curving bimorph of polypyrrole nanowires (on top) and Au film (on the bottom). The bimorph was attached on the left to a substrate, and polypyrrole was oxidized (V versus Ag/AgCl = 0 V) in NaDBS electrolyte, contracting the nanowires and curving the bimorph upward. Image (B) shows the same bimorph with swelled polypyrrole nanowires in an electrochemically reduced state (V versus Ag/AgCl = −1 V). The scale bars represent 50 µm.

(A)   (B)

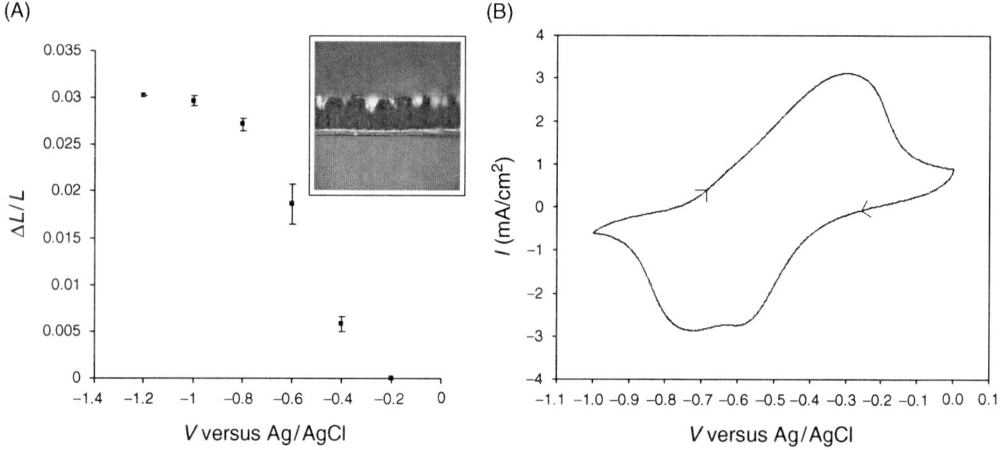

FIGURE 13.21   (A) Expansion of polypyrrole nanowires is shown as a function of voltage, starting with polypyrrole in an oxidized state and applying a voltage from −0.2 to −1.2 V versus the reference electrode. Original length of the nanowires L = 43 µm. The inset is an optical micrograph of the cross-section of the sample. The scale bar represents 50 µm. (B) A cyclic voltammetry of the same sample is shown, where an oxidation peak at −0.3 V and split reduction peaks at −0.61 and −0.73 V can be seen.

The actuation was carried out as above, and the opposing gold films were seen to move apart by ~1.3 µm when the nanowires (43 µm long originally) were reduced at −1 V and then move back to the original position upon oxidation at 0 V. The setup was put through more than 20 cycles, and the magnitude of expansion or contraction remained the same. Cyclic voltammetry curve for the sample used in this experiment is shown in Figure 13.21B with prominent oxidation and reduction peaks.

13.4.2.4   Discussion of Optical Microscopy and Cyclic Voltammetry Data

There is a strong correlation between the electrochemical behavior of the PPy nanowires and the observed lengthwise expansion. When a negative reducing voltage is applied to an oxidized PPy, positive ions move into the polymer matrix from the surrounding electrolyte to maintain charge neutrality, causing the polymer to swell. However, the geometrical changes are not linear with voltage and can be explained by the cyclic voltammetry data. The reduction peaks occur after the voltage reaches -0.6 V with the attendant increase in expansion at the same voltage. After -0.8 V, the expansion reaches its near maximum value, corresponding to a drop in current in the cyclic voltammetry curve as reduction of the nanowires is nearly complete.

It was observed that the time response of the nanoactuators depended on their position in the sample. The nanowires at the edge tended to respond much faster than those in the middle of the sample, with response times (oxidation to reduction and back to oxidized state) ranging from 2 s for the edge to more than 40 s for the middle of the sample (determined from measurements of current versus time). Since the response time is diffusion limited and defined by the position of a nanowire on the sample, we can conclude that the mass transport of sodium ions from the solution to the nanowires (as opposed to diffusion of ions inside the PPy) and the current density achieved at an individual nanowire are the limiting factors in our experiments. The switching speed of an isolated nanowire with no close neighbors is much faster than 2 s as the concentration of ions and the current density are maximized, which is examined further in this section.

The PPy(DBS) nanowires retain actuation behavior of films prepared from the same material; however, some important changes can be seen. The vertical expansion (normal to electrode surface) of the films can be as high as 30% of the thickness of the film, but the same mode of expansion in nanowires produces displacements of only ~3% of nanowire length. It is not likely that this change is due to the damage the nanowires sustained during dissolution of alumina, since the nanowires display very good electrochemical redox behavior. A more likely reason for this difference is that the PPy(DBS) nanowires do not retain the same internal morphology as the PPy(DBS) films. As reported in the literature, PPy films synthesized with surfactant dopants such as DBS$^-$ display a columnar structure oriented perpendicular to the conducting seed substrate where the nucleation and subsequent growth of the polymer film starts.[24] In this case, a template of nanosized pores causes the polymerization process to occur in a somewhat different manner. It has been mentioned earlier that the polymer nanowires appear as nanotubes when viewed from above with a SEM. Then the top portion of these 40 µm long nanowires is removed by mechanical lapping to investigate whether the hollow center region extends to the conducting seed layer. It was found that only the top 1–2 µm portion is, in fact, a nanotube while the remaining length is a solid nanowire. This result suggests that the polymer growth starts both on the metal seed layer and on the pore walls, which is quite different from the case of the film, which grows in only one direction. The difference in polymerization conditions induced by these very different geometries is likely the reason behind the different actuation performance of PPy(DBS) films and nanowires. This conclusion is further supported by the difference in redox-induced geometric changes of PPy(DBS) microactuators when compared with films of similar thickness as described in Section 13.3. Together, the evidence from fabrication of micro- and nano-PPy structures led to undertake a closer examination of the morphological changes accompanying different synthesis conditions of PPy(DBS) devices.

13.4.3 Polypyrrole Nanowire Morphology

PPy films doped with DBS undergo anisotropic volume change when undergoing electrochemical redox reactions. The anisotropy is significant: PPy(DBS) films undergo lateral length change (along the plane of the film) of 2–3%, while the thickness change (normal to the plane of the film) can be as high as 30%.[2,16] The authors hypothesized that the large relative difference in expansion modes can be attributed to an anisotropic morphology of the PPy(DBS) films. X-ray diffraction (XRD) data in the literature supports this hypothesis: PPy films doped with n-alkyl sulfonate ions have a strong scattering peak at low-diffraction angles ($2° < 2\theta < 5°$) in addition to the broader diffraction peak at larger angles ($15° < 2\theta < 25°$) that is characteristic of the distance between pyrrole units in the polymer chains. The low-angle peak is attributed to the presence of parallel planes that are normal to z-direction, or in-plane of the polymer film, and cause a Bragg reflection at an angle that is related to the spacing between the planes. It was found that the "lattice spacings" d are related to the size of the dopant ions according to the linear relationship:

$$d(n) = (0.19n + 1.2) \text{ nm}$$

where n is the number of carbon atoms in the hydrophobic tail of the n-alkyl sulfonate dopant. This feature led authors to the conclusion that the morphology of the PPy doped with large amphiphilic ions such as n-alkyl sulfonates is that of alternating planes of polymer chains and dopant ions stacked tail to tail, and the interplane distance is related to the size of the dopant ion.[25] XRD results for chemically synthesized PPy doped with dodecylbenzenesulfonic acid included a sharp peak at $2\theta = 3.34°$, corresponding to d-spacing of 26.4 Å,[26] while XRD data for electropolymerized PPy doped with different isomers of DBS were as follows: $d = 39.2, 31.7, 24.2$ Å for PPy-(1D)BS, PPy-(2D)BS, and PPy-(6D)BS, respectively.[27]

The XRD data from the literature give weight to the hypothesis that PPy(DBS) film morphology is strongly anisotropic, made up of alternating planes of polymer chains, and dopant ions that lie in the plane of the film. The XRD reflection data from large area thick PPy(DBS) films on Au/Ti conducting seed layer electropolymerized in our laboratory are shown in Figure 13.22. A peak at $2\theta = 3.7°$ is clearly visible and corresponds to $d = 23.9$ Å ($\lambda = 2d \sin \theta$, $\lambda = 1.54$ Å). This peak is somewhat broad, most likely due to the presence of different isomers in the DBS that is available commercially and is in agreement with the published data. It is likely that the anisotropy in the volume change of PPy film undergoing electrochemical redox is related to the morphological

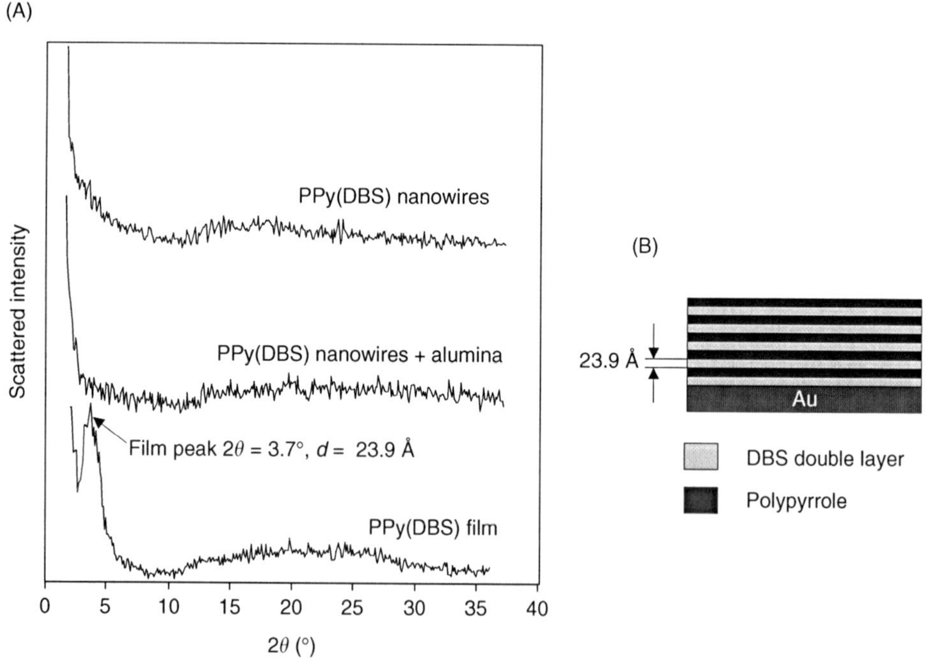

FIGURE 13.22 (A) XRD data for large area PPy(DBS) film (50 μm thick, bottom spectrum), PPy(DBS) nanowires (50 μm long) embedded in alumina (middle) and with alumina removed (top). (B) Schematic representation graphically shows the layered structure of PPy(DBS) films, corresponding to the bottom XRD spectrum on the left.

anisotropy, as the sodium ions and water molecules that enter the polymer matrix will tend to follow the layered structure of the film.

From the data shown in Figure 13.22 for PPy(DBS) nanowires, it can be readily seen that the small angle peak is absent while the broad diffraction due to pyrrole–pyrrole spacing is still present. Therefore, it must be concluded that the nanowires do not possess the layered plane structure in the z-direction (along the nanowire axis, or growth direction) that the PPy(DBS) films possess. The reason for this conclusion was not readily apparent, since the electropolymerization conditions were identical for both the films and the nanowires but must be related to the nanoscale geometry. A possible cause involves surface interactions during polymerization between the precipitating PPy chains and the walls of the alumina pore, which disrupt the formation of the layered plane structure. Some evidence for this mechanism can be gathered from Figure 13.17B, where the mechanical lapping of the top portion of the nanowires gives some idea of the nanowire cross-section. It can be seen that the cross-section is not homogeneous but consists of two phases—the circumference and the center regions of the nanowire, supporting the assumption that the surface interactions with the alumina pore walls affect nanowire morphology.

The internal morphology of the PPy(DBS) material has a strong effect on the anisotropy of the volume change and therefore on the magnitude of the volume change in a given direction. The reversible expansion of the PPy films in lateral direction, where there is no alternating plane structure, is approximately 3% of the original size. This expansion is closely mirrored by 3% reversible length change of PPy(DBS) nanowires, which similarly lack layered plane structure in this direction as evidenced by x-ray diffraction experiments. It can be inferred from this data that the smaller, than expected, actuation magnitude of PPy nanowires is due to the morphology change of PPy when synthesized in nanowire geometry.

13.4.4 TIME RESPONSE OF ISOLATED NANOWIRES

13.4.4.1 Actuation Speed in High-Density Nanowires

The speed of nanowire actuation, as observed with optical microscopy, varied depending on the position of the nanowires in the sample. Specifically, the nanowires at the edges of the sample responded significantly faster (2 s) than those closer to the middle of the sample (30–40 s). The likely reason for the slower actuation is the impeded ion diffusion in the nanowires with close neighbors. As seen in the SEM images, the number of nanowires per unit area or nanowire density is quite high, and for the nanowire in the middle of the sample, the ion diffusion proceeds from top to bottom rather than from the nanowire wall to the center. Thus, the characteristic diffusion length is not 100 nm radius of the nanowire, but rather 43 μm length of the nanowire. The significantly longer ion diffusion slows down the actuation speed (and current response) of the nanowires and makes the determination of true time constant of single nanowire difficult.

13.4.4.2 Fabrication of Isolated (Low-Density) Nanowires

To measure the time response of the nanowires unimpeded by negative effects of high density, a novel fabrication method was employed to increase the space between the nanowires. An alumina membrane with 20 nm pore size was used as a template for Au electrode electroplating (Figure 13.23).

As the first step in the fabrication of electrodes, a suspension of 0.5 μm polystyrene beads in water was deposited onto the alumina membrane. The membrane was then air-dried, and a 50 nm film of SiO_2 was sputtered onto the side of the membrane with the microbeads. The beads were then removed by ultrasonication followed by sputter deposition of 10 nm Ti and 200 nm Au films to form a conductive seed layer for electroplating. The SiO_2 layer completely covered the 20 nm pores, preventing access of the electroplating solution to the seed layer below. On the other hand, the removal

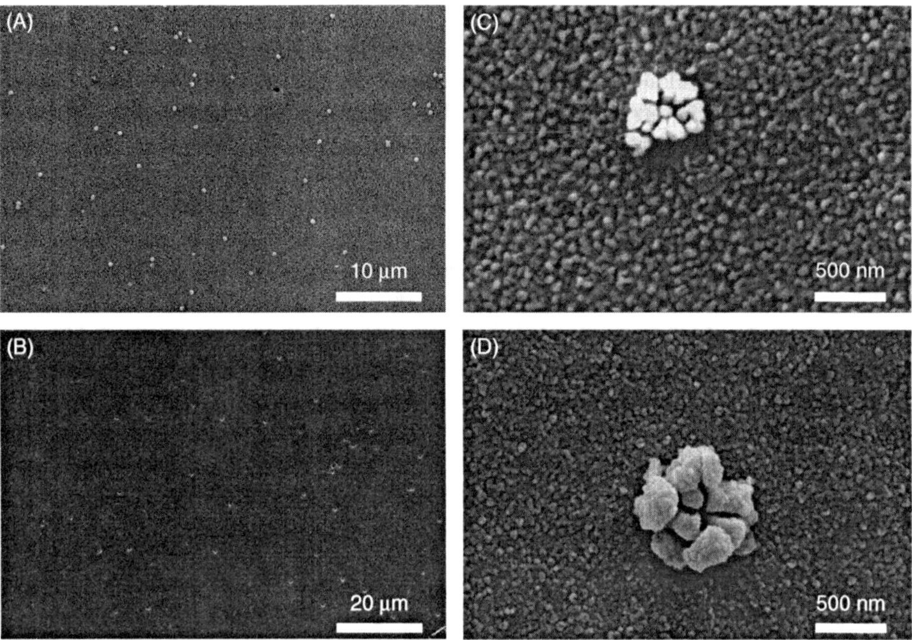

FIGURE 13.29 Scanning electron microscope (SEM) images at different stages of the fabrication: (A) polystyrene microbeads dispersed on the alumina membrane; (B) openings in the oxide film after the beads have been removed; (C) single electrode composed of a group of electroplated Au nanoposts; and (D) the electrode with the deposited *o*-PPy coating.

the configuration of the electrodes can be controlled in terms of both overall diameter and density of electrodes on the substrate. In this work, the nanostructured electrodes are connected with each other, allowing the recording of a single signal from a large area. However, in applications requiring parallel recording from small areas of a brain slice, the Ti/Au seed layer can be micropatterned to allow multiple electrical connections.

To provide selectivity in detection, particularly when a large concentration of other oxidizable molecules such as AA is present in the solution, as in the case with the extracellular fluid found in mammalian brain, the electrodes are coated with a thin film of *o*-PPy. Overoxidized PPy is a positively charged polymer that rejects ascorbate anions at physiological pH[52] while allowing dopamine molecules to reach the underlying conducting electrode surface.

The electrodes were tested in a phosphate-buffered solution (PBS) (pH 7.4) with a 100 μM AA background to simulate physiological conditions. Electrodes were kept at a constant anodic potential (0.5 V), and the change in current was monitored while small concentrations of dopamine were sequentially added to the solution. The arrows in Figure 13.30 correspond to an addition of a defined concentration of dopamine to the solution (25, 50, 100 nM increase in concentration of dopamine in the sample solution) and cause a corresponding step in the current. The size of the current step is plotted against the increase in concentration in the inset in Figure 13.30. There is a linear relationship between changes in concentration and current, demonstrating the suitability of nanoelectrodes for quantitative measurements of changing the dopamine levels against an AA background of more than a thousand times higher concentration than that of dopamine.

In addition to current measurements at a constant potential, a variety of other voltammetric techniques can be used for the detection of electrochemically oxidizable species of interest. One such technique is DPV, where the applied potential consists of a voltage ramp with superimposed

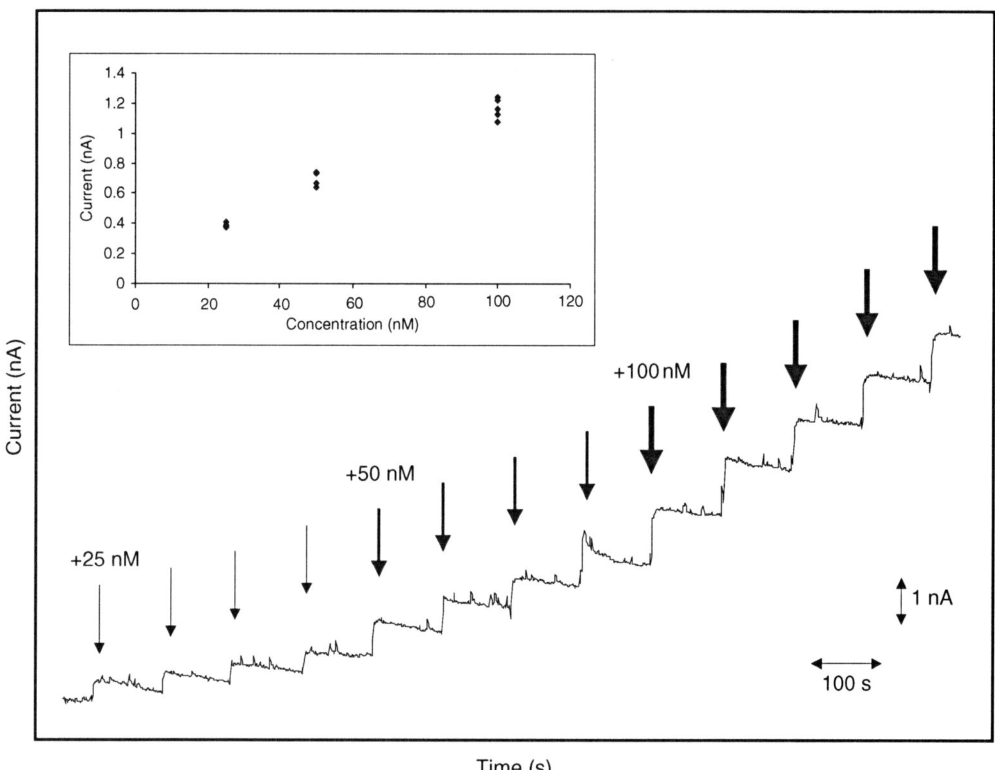

FIGURE 13.30 Current response due to the addition of small concentrations of dopamine. Thin arrows represent additions of 25 nM of dopamine to solution, medium arrows 50 nM additions, and thick arrows 100 nM additions of dopamine. The inset shows the change in current when a defined concentration of dopamine is added.

small amplitude potential pulses. The current is measured before each pulse and is subtracted from the current value at the end of the pulse. The recorded current is, therefore, in differential form, which is plotted against a voltage range. Different chemical species oxidize at slightly different voltages, resulting in current peaks centered at a characteristic voltage value for each molecule and providing more specific detection than amperometry. Furthermore, DPV keeps the residual current (due to the charging of double-layer capacitance) low, increasing the sensitivity. An accumulation step can be used with DPV, preconcentrating the analyte at the electrode surface prior to applying oxidizing potential, which also results in an improvement in sensitivity. Unfortunately, the increased sensitivity is accomplished at the expense of time resolution, as the voltage scan requires about 80 s,[45] while the preconcentration step takes another 100 s[47] to achieve the sensitivity required for measuring dopamine levels as low as 5 nM. This constraint makes real-time experiments measuring dopamine release due to external stimulation very difficult. Therefore, electrodes with a faster time response (due to decreased size as discussed above) can be particularly suitable for scanning voltammetric techniques such as DPV or differential pulse stripping voltammetry (DPSV, or DPV with the added accumulation step). In Figure 13.31, the nanoelectrode DPSV scan of 2.5 nM dopamine in PBS solution is shown with the background current digitally subtracted. The accumulation time was reduced to only 5 s, but the dopamine peak is still clearly visible. This shows that nanoelectrodes with improved time response can have an important role to play in speeding up the voltage scan times that are used with the high-sensitivity voltammetric techniques.

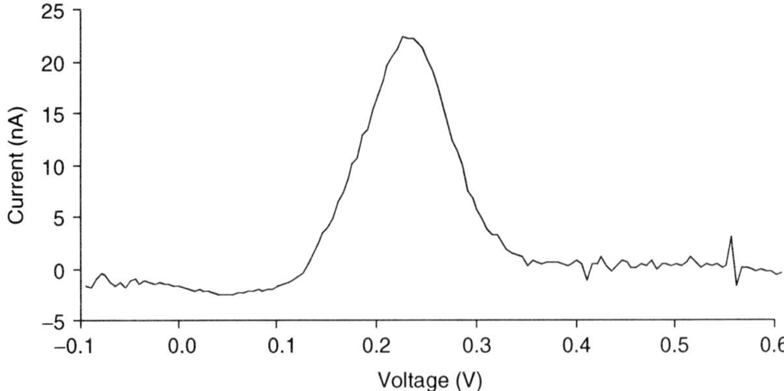

FIGURE 13.31 Differential pulse stripping voltammetry of 2.5 nM dopamine in PBS solution. The current is shown with the background digitally subtracted, and the dopamine peak is clearly visible.

REFERENCES

1. Immerstrand, C. et al., Conjugated-polymer micro- and milliactuators for biological applications, *MRS Bull.*, 27(6), 461, 2002.
2. Smela, E. and Gadegaard, N., Volume change in polypyrrole studied by atomic force microscopy, *J. Phys. Chem. B*, 105(39), 9395, 2001.
3. Berdichevsky, Y. and Lo, Y.H., Polymer microvalve based on anisotropic expansion of polypyrrole, *Mat. Res. Soc. Symp. Proc.*, 782, A4.4.1, 2004.
4. Martin, C.R., Template synthesis of electronically conductive polymer nanostructures, *Acc. Chem. Res.*, 28, 61, 1995.
5. Smela, E., Microfabrication of PPy microactuators and other conjugated polymer devices, *J. Micromech. Microeng.*, 9, 1, 1999.
6. West, K. et al., Electronic conductivity of polypyrrole-dodecyl benzene sulfonate complexes, *J. Phys. Chem. B*, 108, 15001, 2004.
7. Bay, L. et al., Mechanism of actuation in conducing polymers: osmotic expansion, *J. Phys. Chem. B*, 105, 8492, 2001.
8. Otero, T.F., Grande, H.J., and Rodriguez, J., Reinterpretation of polypyrrole electrochemistry after consideration of conformational relaxation processes, *J. Phys. Chem. B*, 101, 3688, 1997.
9. Ren, X. and Pickup, P.G., Ion transport in polypyrrole and a polypyrrole/polyanion composite, *J. Phys. Chem.*, 97, 5356, 1993.
10. Cui, X. and Martin, D.C., Fuzzy gold electrodes for lowering impedance and improving adhesion with electrodeposited conducting polymer films, *Sensor Actuat. A*, 103, 384, 2003.
11. Pyo, M. et al., Direct strain measurement of polypyrrole actuators controlled by the polymer/gold interface, *Chem. Mater.*, 15, 916, 2003.
12. Jager, E.W.H., Smela, E., and Inganas, O., Microfabricating conjugated polymer actuators, *Science*, 290, 1540, 2000; Jager, E.W.H., Inganas, O., and Lundstrom, I., Microrobots for micrometer-size objects in aqueous media: potential tools for single-cell manipulation, *Science*, 288, 2335, 2000.
13. Madou, M.J., *Fundamentals in Microfabrication*, CRC Press, Boca Raton, FL, 1997.
14. Duffy, D. et al., Rapid prototyping of microfluidic systems in poly(dimethylsiloxane), *Anal. Chem.*, 70, 4974, 1998.
15. Pettersson, P.F., Jager, E.W.H., and Inganas, O., Surface micromachined polymer actuators as valves in PDMS microfluidic system, in 1st IEEE-EMBS Special Topic Conference on Microtechnologies in Medicine and Biology, 2000.
16. Smela, E. and Gadegaard, N., Surprising volume change in PPy(DBS): an atomic force microscopy study, *Adv. Mater.*, 11(11), 953, 1999.
17. Fennimore, A.M. et al., Rotational actuators based on carbon nanotubes, *Nature*, 424, 408, 2003.
18. Craighead, H.G., Nanoelectromechanical systems, *Science*, 290, 1532, 2000.

19. Requicha, A., Nanorobots, NEMS, and nanoassembly, *Proc. IEEE*, 91, 1922, 2003.
20. Martin, C.R., Template synthesis of electronically conductive polymer nanostructures, *Acc. Chem. Res.*, 28, 61, 1995.
21. Berdichevsky, Y. and Lo, Y.H., Fabrication of polypyrrole nanowires, *Proc. SPIE*, 5759, 268, 2005.
22. Berdichevsky, Y. and Lo, Y.H., Fabrication and evaluation of conducting polymer nanowire heterostructures, *Mat. Res. Soc. Symp. Proc.*, 872, J13.4.1, 2005.
23. Berdichevsky, Y. and Lo, Y.H., Polypyrrole nanowire actuators, *Adv. Mater.*, 18, 122–125, 2006.
24. Naoi, K. et al., Electrochemistry of surfactant-doped polypyrrole film(I)—formation of columnar structure by electropolymerization, *J. Electrochem. Soc.*, 142, 417, 1995.
25. Wernet, W., Monkenbusch, M., and Wegner, G., A new series of conducting polymers with layered structure: polypyrrole n-alkylsulfates and n-alkylsulfonates, *Makromol. Chem. Rapid Commun.*, 5, 157–164, 1984.
26. Song, M.K. et al., Synthesis and characterization of soluble polypyrrole doped with alkylbenzenesulfonic acids, *Synthetic Met.*, 141, 315, 2004.
27. West, K. et al., Electronic conductivity of polypyrrole-dodecyl benzene sulfonate complexes, *J. Phys. Chem. B*, 108, 15001, 2004.
28. Daum, P. et al., Diffusional charge transport through ultrathin films of radiofrequency plasma polymerized vinylferrocene at low temperature, *J. Am. Chem. Soc.*, 102, 4649, 1980.
29. Crank, J., *The Mathematics of Diffusion*, Clarendon Press, Oxford, UK, 1975.
30. Oglesby, D.M., Omang, S.H., and Reilley, C.N., Thin layer electrochemical studies using controlled potential or controlled current, *Anal. Chem.*, 37, 1312, 1965.
31. Ariza, M.J. and Otero, T.F., Ionic diffusion across oxidized polypyrrole membranes and during oxidation of the free-standing film, *Colloid. Surface. A*, 270–271, 226–231, 2005.
32. Gerard, M., Chaubey, A., and Malhotra, B.D., Application of conducting polymers to biosensors, *Biosens. Bioelectron.*, 17, 345, 2002.
33. Santhanam, K.S.V., Conducting polymers for biosensors: rationale based on models, *Pure Appl. Chem.*, 70, 1259, 1998.
34. Bartlett, P.N. and Birkin, P.R., The application of conducting polymers in biosensors, *Synthetic Met.*, 61, 15, 1993.
35. Genies, E.M. and Marchesiello, M., Conducting polymers for biosensors, application to new glucose sensors, *Synthetic Met.*, 55–57, 3677, 1993.
36. Koopal, C.G.J., Eusma, B., and Nolte, R.J.M., Chronoamperometric detection of glucose by a third generation biosensor constructed from conducting microtubules of polypyrrole, *Synthetic Met.*, 55–57, 3689, 1993.
37. Kros, A., Nolte, R.J.M., and Sommerdijk, N.A.J.M., Conducting polymers with confined dimensions: track-etch membranes for amperometric biosensor applications, *Adv. Mater.*, 14, 1779, 2002.
38. Bidan, G. et al., Conducting polymers as a link between biomolecules and microelectronics, *Synthetic Met.*, 102, 1363, 1999.
39. Wong, J.Y., Langer, R., and Ingber, D.E., Electrically conducting polymers can noninvasively control the shape and growth of mammalian cells, *Proc. Natl Acad. Sci. USA*, 91, 3201, 1994.
40. Williams, R.L. and Doherty, P.J., A preliminary assessment of poly(pyrrole) in nerve guide studies, *J. Mater. Sci. Mater. Med.*, 5, 429, 1994.
41. Schmidt, C.E. et al., Stimulation of neurite outgrowth using an electrically conducting polymer, *Proc. Natl Acad. Sci. USA*, 94, 8948, 1997.
42. George, P.M. et al., Fabrication and biocompatibility of polypyrrole implants suitable for neural prosthetics, *Biomaterials*, 26, 3511, 2005.
43. Cui, X. et al., Electrochemical deposition and characterization of conducting polymer polypyrrole/PSS on multichannel neural probes, *Sensor Actuat. A*, 93, 8, 2001.
44. Kawagoe, K.T., Zimmerman, J.B., and Wightman, R.M., Principles of voltammetry and microelectrode surface states, *J. Neurosci. Meth.*, 48, 225, 1993.
45. Stamford, J.A. and Justice, J.B, Probing brain chemistry, *Anal. Chem.*, 68, A359, 1996.
46. Zhang, X. et al., Over-oxidized polypyrrole-modified carbon fibre ultramicroelectrode with an integrated silver/silver chloride reference electrode for the selective voltammetric measurement of dopamine in extremely small sample volumes, *Analyst*, 121, 1817, 1996.
47. Robinson, D.L. et al., Detecting subsecond dopamine release with fast-scan cyclic voltammetry *in vivo*, *Clin. Chem.*, 49(10), 1763, 2003.
48. Fleischmann, M. et al., Eds., *Ultramicroelectrodes*, Datatech Systems, Morgantown, NC, 1987.

49. Tanaka, K. and Kashiwagi, N., *In vivo* voltammetry with and ultramicroelectrode, *J. Electroanal. Chem.*, 275, 95, 1989.
50. Kasai, N. et al., Real-time multisite observation of glutamate release in rat hippocampal slices, *Neurosci. Lett.*, 304, 112, 2001.
51. Zhu, G. et al., Dysfunction of M-channel enhances propagation of neuronal excitability in rat hippocampus monitored by multielectrode dish and microdialysis systems, *Neurosci. Lett.*, 294, 53, 2000.
52. Olivia, H. et al., Selective amperometric detection of dopamine using OPPy-modified diamond microsensor system, *Analyst*, 127, 1572, 2002.

14 Processing of Biosensing Materials and Biosensors

Yingchun Zhu, Yu Yang, and Yanyan Liu

CONTENTS

Biosensors play an important role in clinical detection, environment monitoring, food analysis, and also in some other fields. The advancement of biomaterials has profound direct impacts on the development of biosensors. On one hand, the application of biorecognition materials determines the function and use of biosensors based on their biological nature. On the other hand, the introduction of intermedia biomaterials impacts on properties and efficiencies of biosensors because of their effects on biorecognition material immobilization and signal transferring. In this chapter, we have summarized most of the biorecognition materials such as enzymes, microbes, DNA, and antigens–antibodies that have been used in biosensors, and some special biomaterials mentioned as intermedia materials in biosensors have been listed. We described processing techniques to prepare biorecognition materials and intermedia materials and assemble them as functional biosensors.

14.1 BIORECOGNITION MATERIALS

14.1.1 ENZYMES

Enzymes have been used as analytical reagents for selective detection of special materials since 1940s because of their special catalysis to substrates and selective recognition of coenzymes and inhibitors correspondingly. Enzymes are the preferred sensitive materials for the preparation of biosensors. Clark [1] first put forward the principle of the measurement of substrates of enzymes by combining the specificity of enzymes with electrodes.

Enzyme biosensors use enzymes as molecular recognition elements immobilized on signal transducers such as electrochemical electrode, optical fiber, and field-effect transistor (FET) facility. Being reagentless, speedy, precise, and even inexpensive, enzyme biosensors are now widely used in the fields of clinical detection, environment monitoring, process controlling, and also in pharmaceutical biochemical research [2].

Most of the enzymes belong to the family of proteins, so they possess some basic properties of proteins such as low active temperature, narrow effective pH range, denaturation or devitalization in strong acids, alkalies, and heavy metallic salts (physicochemical properties of some enzymes are listed in Table 14.1). These properties severely limit the application of enzymes in biosensors. It is one of the most important tasks to overcome these restrictions in the development of enzyme biosensors.

Up to now, many enzymes such as glucose oxidase (GOD), cholesterol oxidase (COD), acetylcholinesterase (AChE), horseradish peroxidase (HRP) that have been used in relatively mild condition in the area of biosensors are described in the following sections.

14.1.1.1 Glucose Oxidase

GOD (β-D-glucose: oxygen 1-oxidoreductase, E.C. 1.1.3.4) is the first enzyme used by Updike and Hicks in 1967 to prepare biosensors [3]. Due to the broad pH range, high catalytic activity, and relatively wide action temperature, GOD is the most widely used enzyme in biosensor construction.

TABLE 14.1

Physicochemical Properties of Some Enzymes

Enzymes	Molecular Weight (kDa)	Isoelectric Point (IEP) (pI)	Stable pH Range	Optimal pH	Optimal Temperature (°C)
Glucose oxidase (GOD) (*Aspergillus niger*)	150–186	~4.9	3.5–6.5	5.6	30–50
Cholesterol oxidase (COD) (*Pseudomonas*)	60	5.1–5.4	4.0–11.0	7.0	4–60
Acetylcholinesterase (AChE)	260	—	7.5–8.5	8.0	~30
Horseradish peroxidase (HRP)	~42	7.2	4–10	6.5	~40
Lactate dehydrogenase (LDH) (heart muscle)	135	4.5–4.8	—	8.75–9.0	~32
Pyruvate oxidase (PyOD) (*Lactobacillus plantarum*)	260	—	—	5.7	30

TABLE 14.2

Special Catalytic Property of GOD to the Oxidation of β-D-Glucose

Substrates	Relative to Glucose[a] (%)
β-D-Glucose	100
2-Deoxy-D-glucose	25–30
4-*O*-methyl-D-glucose	15
6-Deoxy-D-glucose	10
4-Deoxy-D-glucose	2
2-Deoxy-6-fluoro-D-glucose	1.85
3,6-Methyl-D-glucose	1.85
4,6-Dimethyl-D-glucose	1.22
3-Deoxy-D-glucose	1
6-*O*-methyl-D-glucose	1
α-D-Glucose	0.64
Mannose	0.2, 1
Altrose	0.16
Galactose	0.08
Xylose	0.03
Idose	0.02

[a] Activity relative to β-D-glucose in percentage.

Source: Leskovac, V., Trivić, S., Wohlfahrt, G., Kandrač, J., and Peričin, D., *Int. J. Biochem. Cell. B.*, 37, 731, 2005. With permission.

GOD is a flavin-containing glycoprotein. The fungal enzyme is a homodimer made up of two identical subunits of molecular weight (kDa) approximately 80,000 Da each [4]. Dissociation of subunits is possible only under denaturing conditions accompanied by the loss of the coenzyme flavin adenine dinucleotide (FAD) [5].

GOD has a special property to catalyze the oxidation of β-D-glucose [6] (detailed in Table 14.2). This oxidation is a representative two-step process of enzyme reaction [7] including oxidation of

TABLE 14.3

Examples of All Kinds of Glucose Biosensors

	Signal Transducers	Immobilization Method of GOD	Ref.
Amperometric glucose biosensor	Pt electrode	GOD was entrapped into the polypyrrole (PPy) film during an electrochemical polymerization process	11
	Screen-printed Ag–carbon strip two-electrode	GOD was covalently immobilized in the membranes prepared by condensation of both β-cyclodextrin polymer (β-CDP) and carboxymethylated β-cyclodextrin polymer (β-CDPA)	12
	Pt electrode	GOD was dropped onto the Pt/(CHIT/PAA)$_n$ layer, and then chitosan solution was placed on the surface; after being dried at room temperature, glutaraldehyde (GA) slowly spread over the chitosan film	13
	Glassy carbon electrode (GCE)	GOD was immobilized on the negatively charged surface of carbon nanotubes (CNTs) by alternatively assembling a cationic polydiallyldimethylammonium chloride (PDDA) layer and a GOD layer	14
	Ni electrode	GOD was immobilized by a glutaraldehyde (GA)/bovine serum albumin (BSA) cross-linking procedure on the surface of an alkali nickel hexacyanoferrate thin film	15
	Cu-dispersed ceramic–graphite biocomposite electrode	GOD was immobilized into a copper-dispersed sol–gel-derived ceramic–graphite composite	16
	Pt electrode	GOD was entrapped in a polyacrylamide microgel	17
	Screen-printed electrode	GOD was genetically modified by adding a polylysine chain at the C-terminal with a peptide linker inserted between the enzyme and the polylysine chain	18
	Indium–tin oxide (ITO)-coated glass electrode	GOD was immobilized in layer-by-layer (LbL) films, adsorbed alternately with poly(allylamine) hydrochloride (PAH) layers	19
	Nanoelectrode array (NEA) Pt electrode	GOD was immobilized on the NEA electrode by a physical adsorption	20
	Pt electrode	GOD was immobilized into a poly(o-phenylenediamine) (POPD) film by simple one-step electropolymerization procedure	21
	Ink-printed gold film electrode	GOD was modified with ferrocene derivatives as the electron transfer mediator	22
	Pt electrode	GOD was immobilized in a PPy layer on the electrode	23
	GCEs modified by processible polyaniline (PANI)	GOD was suspended by 0.25–0.3% neutralized Nafion, and the complex was syringed onto the surface of the electrode	24
Optical glucose biosensor	Oxygen-sensitive optode membrane	GOD was covalently immobilized on an eggshell membrane	25
	Oxygen transducer of [Ru(dpp)$_3$][(4-Clph)$_4$B]$_2$	GOD was immobilized on a bamboo inner shell membrane with GA as a cross-linker	26
	Spectrophotometer	GOD was linked onto Prussian blue (PB) film chemically	27
	Optical oxygen transducer	GOD was entrapped within the xerogel that was derived from tetraethylorthosilicate and hybridized with hydroxyethyl carboxymethyl cellulose polymer	28

The total reaction can be expressed as follows:

$$\text{Cholesterol} + O_2 \xrightarrow{\text{COD}} \text{cholest-4-en-3-one} + H_2O_2 \tag{14.12}$$

Based on Reaction 14.12, COD can also be used to prepare amperometric biosensor, potentiometric biosensor, and optical biosensor for cholesterol detection. Furthermore, biosensors constructed with the combination of COD and CEH can be used for the detection of cholesteryl ester. Examples of biosensors prepared by COD or by the combination of CEH and COD are listed in Table 14.4.

Biosensors composed of COD or CEH/COD can be used to detect the contents of cholesterol in serum and sterol medicines. In addition, they are involved in the tracking measurement of Zn^{2+} and other heavy metal ions in water with high facility and efficiency [44].

14.1.1.3 Acetylcholinesterase (AChE)/Choline Oxidase

AChE (E.C. 3.1.1.7) is an important component of cholinergic synapses in the peripheral and central nervous systems, which are partly responsible for terminating the actions of the neurotransmitter acetylcholine in all the vertebrates and invertebrates [45].

AChE splits into four subunits in the presence of guanidine and mercaptoethanol, and each subunit has one-fourth of the molecular weight of the original enzyme. Examination of the C-terminal residues by two independent methods, namely hydrazinolysis and enzymatic hydrolysis by carboxypeptidase A, revealed that there were two types of polypeptide chains in AChE. This examination suggests that AChE has a dimeric hybrid structure, with two α and two β chains [46].

AChE can catalyze the hydrolysis of acetylcholine to produce choline and acetic acid specifically as in Reaction 14.13:

$$\text{Acetylcholine} + H_2O \xrightarrow{\text{AChE}} \text{choline} + CH_3COOH \tag{14.13}$$

Choline oxidase (ChOD, E.C. 1.1.3.17) can be extracted from *Cylindrocarpon didymium* M-1 [47], *Alcaligenes* sp. [48], and *Arthrobacter globiformis* [49]. Based on amino acid sequence comparisons, the enzyme ChOD can be grouped in the glucose-methanol-choline (GMC) oxidoreductase enzyme superfamily [50], which utilizes FAD as cofactor for catalysis and uses nonactivated primary alcohols as substrate.

ChOD catalyzes the four-electron oxidation of choline to glycine betaine (*N,N,N*-trimethylglycine, betaine), while molecular oxygen acts as the primary electron acceptor in Reaction 14.14 [49].

$$\text{Choline} + 2O_2 + H_2O \xrightarrow{\text{ChOD}} \text{glycine betaine} + H_2O_2 \tag{14.14}$$

ChOD is an important enzyme in Reaction 14.15 because glycine betaine is one of the limited compatible solutes that accumulate to high levels in the cytoplasm of cells to prevent dehydration and plasmolysis in adverse hyperosmotic environments [51].

Especially, organophosphorus (OP) pesticide is similar to acetylcholine in molecular morphology, which can combine the active ester locus of AChE and then restrain the activity of the enzyme. There is a fine linear relationship between the concentration of OP pesticide and the inhibition degree of AChE, while the activity of AChE decides the outcome of choline and acetic acid. Based on this character, potentiometric and optical biosensors can be prepared for the detection of OP pesticide by measuring the decrease of H^+ concentration. When ChOD is coworked with AChE, the Reaction 14.14 will be weakened by OP pesticide, so amperometric biosensor for OP pesticide detection can also be constructed on the basis of monitoring the decrease of hydrogen peroxide. Biosensors composed of AChE or AChE/ChOD for OP pesticide detection are listed in Table 14.5.

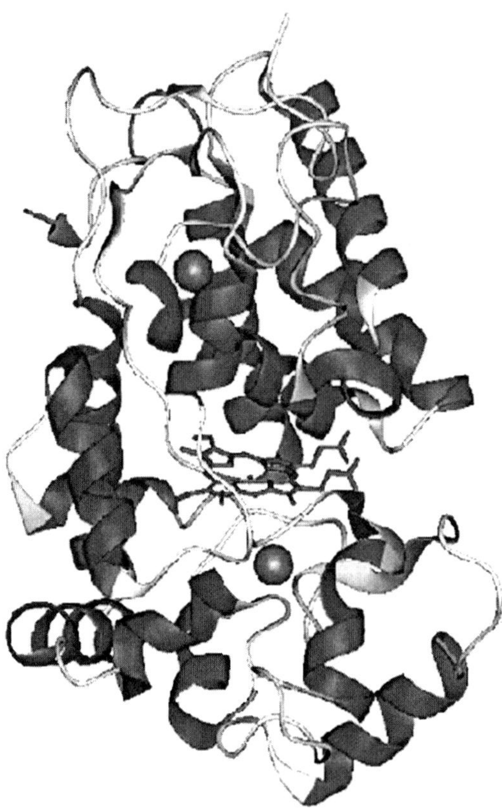

FIGURE 14.1 Three-dimensional representation of the x-ray crystal structure of HRP isoenzyme C. The heme group is located between the distal and proximal domains, each of which contains a calcium atom. (From Veitch, N.C., *Phytochem.*, 65, 249, 2004. With permission.)

Moreover, HRP usually works together with oxidases to construct biosensors, since it can catalyze the redox reaction of H_2O_2 generated by oxidases at a relatively low potential. For example, HRP is coimmobilized with GOD for glucose detection [72], with COD for cholesterol detection [73], and with L-glutamate oxidase (GLOD) for the detection of L-glutamate and alanine aminotransferase in blood [74].

14.1.1.5 Lactate Dehydrogenase

Lactate dehydrogenase (LDH, E.C. 1.1.1.27) is a kind of dehydrogenase that widely exists in the tissues of animals and cells of all kinds of microorganisms. LDH is a large sulfhydryl oligomeric enzyme consisting of four subunits [75]. These subunits can be classified into two types, that is, M type and H type. These two types can be assembled into five tetramers of H4, H3M, H2M2, HM3, and M4. Therefore, there are five isoenzymes of LDH, expressed as LDH1, LDH2, LDH3, LDH4, and LDH5, respectively. Though the molecular structures and physicochemical properties of such five enzymes are different from each other, they catalyze the same reversible conversion between lactate and pyruvate, with concomitant redox between the cofactor NAD^+ and nicotinamide adenine dinucleotide (NADH) (14.16).

$$\text{Lactate} + NAD^+ \xrightarrow{\text{LDH}} \text{pyruvate} + NADH \qquad (14.16)$$

Both sides of this reversible reaction can induce the electron transfer in the presence of some mediators (Med). For example, when lactate is oxidized by NAD^+ with the catalysis of LDH, the

TABLE 14.6
Examples of Biosensors Prepared by HRP

Substrates	Signal Transducers	Immobilization Method of Enzyme	Type	Ref.
Phenolic compounds: Phenol Hydroquinone o-Aminophenol o-Chlorophenol Resorcinol o-Cresol	Au electrode	HRP was immobilized on the precursor film of poly(allylamine hydrochloride) (PAH)/Poly(sodium-p-styrene-sulfonate) (PSS)/PAH with PAH based on a layer-by-layer method	Amperometric	63

(Continued)

TABLE 14.6 (Continued)
Examples of Biosensors Prepared by HRP

p-Nitrophenol	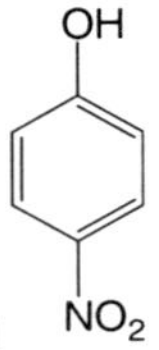
o-Nitrophenol	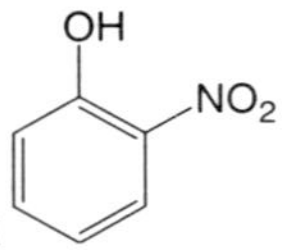
Phytomelin	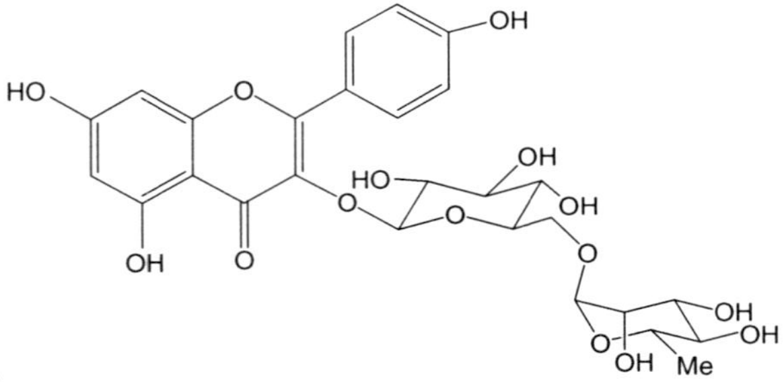
Quercitrin	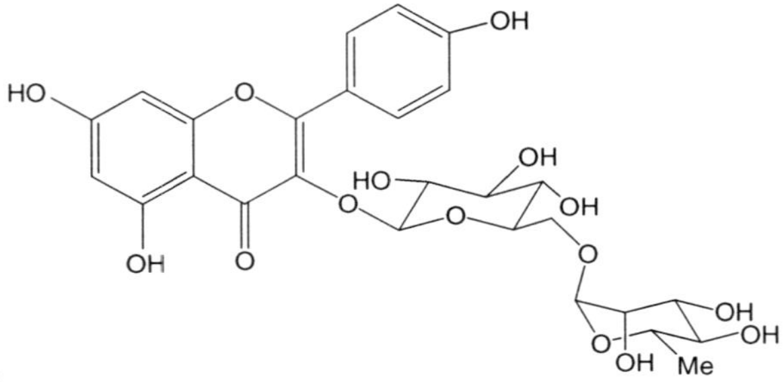

Clozapine (a dibenzoxazepine drug)	Solid carbon-paste electrode	HRP was immobilized on the magnetized silica-based microparticles (MMPs) with high-density nanopores	Amperometric	64
Human serum chorionic gonadotropin (HCG)	GCE	HRP was immobilized with the labeled HCG antibody on a HCG/TiO$_2$ sol–gel	Amperometric	65
Cyanide	GCE	HRP was immobilized into redox active [Zn–Cr–ABTS] layered double hydroxide	Amperometric	66
Nitric oxide	Pyrolytic graphite electrode	Embedded in a film of phosphatidylcholine (PC)	Amperometric	67
Total biogenic amine	Carbon-paste electrode	HRP was immobilized on graphite using bovine serum albumin (BSA), carbodiimide, and glutaraldehyde	Amperometric	68
Sulfides (HS$^-$, H$_2$S and S^{2-}).	Au electrode	HRP was immobilized on the surface of cysteamine SAM by cross-linking with glutaraldehyde	Amperometric	69
Hydrogen peroxide	Pt electrode	HRP was entrapped *in situ* by electropolymerization of pyrrole	Amperometric	70
Hydrogen peroxide	Optical fiber	HRP was immobilized by microencapsulation in sol–gel crystals derived from tetramethyl orthosilicate	Optical	71

product NADH can reduce Med to its reduction state Med_{red}. If Med is modified on an electrode, Med_{red} will be oxidized to Med_{ox}, and an electric signal is observed [76] (Figure 14.2a). Similar results can be achieved in the reaction of pyruvate to lactate as shown in Figure 14.2b.

Based on the above mechanism, amperometric biosensor for the detection of lactate (or NAD^+) can be formed by immobilizing NAD^+ (or lactate), LDH, and Med on electrodes. In contrast, amperometric biosensor for the detection of pyruvate (or NADH) can be prepared by immobilizing NADH (or pyruvate), LDH, and Med on electrodes. Some examples can be found in Table 14.7.

14.1.1.6 Pyruvate Oxidase

Pyruvate oxidase (PyOD, E.C. 1.2.3.3) was first found in *Escherichia coli* by Hager [81] in 1957. PyOD is a tetramer consisting of four similar subunits; each subunit combines a molecule of FAD tightly.

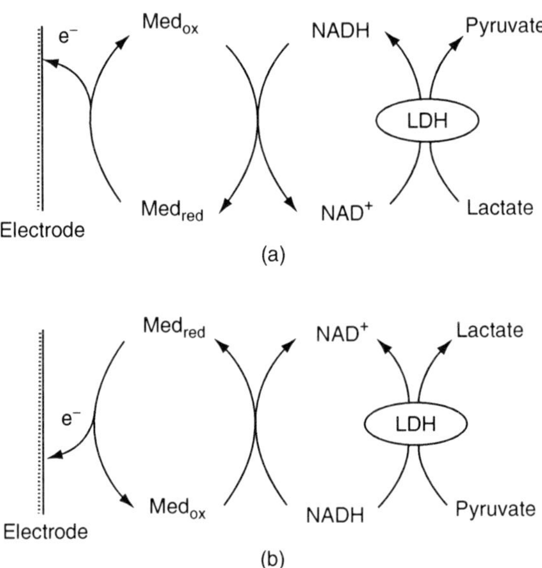

FIGURE 14.2 Induction of electron transferring during the reaction of lactate to pyruvate (a) and the reverse reaction of pyruvate to lactate (b) in the presence of Med. (Modified from Catherine, M., Simon, E., Toh, C.S., Bartlett, P.N., and Cass, A.E.G., *Anal. Chim. Acta.*, 453, 191, 2002. With permission.)

TABLE 14.7
Examples of Amperometric Biosensors Prepared by LDH

Substrates	Mediators	Signal Transducers	Immobilization Method of Enzyme	Ref.
Lactate	Toluidine blue O moiety	Carbon-paste electrode	LDH was immobilized with NAD⁺ on redox polymer and polyethylenimine	77
NAD⁺	Poly(3-ethylthiophene)/ poly(phenol red)	Pt electrode	LDH was immobilized with lactate on the poly(3-methylthiophene)/ poly(phenol red) membrane	78
Pyruvate	Electrochemically prepared PANI film	ITO glass plate electrode	LDH was immobilized with NADH on the PANI film	79
NADH	A thiol-terminated, sol–gel-derived, 3-D, silicate network	Polycrystalline Au electrode	LDH was immobilized on the Med with Au nanoparticles (NPs)	80

PyOD catalyzes the consumption of pyruvate and phosphate in the presence of oxygen, while hydrogen peroxide, carbon dioxide, and acetyl phosphate are generated. This reaction is shown below (14.17):

$$\text{Pyruvate} + \text{phosphate} + O_2 \xrightarrow{\text{PyOD}} \text{acetyl phosphate} + H_2O + CO_2 \qquad (14.17)$$

Based on Reaction 14.18, PyOD can be used to prepare biosensors for the direct detection of pyruvate [82] and phosphate [83]. PyOD is also involved in the biosensing detection of alanine with the assistance of other reactions including a dehydrogenation process catalyzed by alanine dehydrogenase (AlaDH, E.C. 1.4.1.1) (14.18) and a hydroxidation process catalyzed by salicylate hydroxylase (SHL, E.C.1.14.13.1) (14.19) [84].

$$\text{Alanine} + NAD^+ \xrightarrow{\text{ALaDH}} \text{pyruvate} + NADH \qquad (14.18)$$

$$\text{Salicylate} + NADH + O_2 \xrightarrow{\text{SHL}} \text{catechol} + NAD^+ + CO_2 \qquad (14.19)$$

14.1.1.7 Glutamate Oxidase

GLOD (E.C. 1.4.3.11) from *Streptomyces* is an extracellular heterotrimeric enzyme consisting of α, β, and γ subunits of molecular masses equal to 39, 19, and 16 kDa, respectively [85]. This enzyme specifically catalyzes the oxidative deamination of glutamate in the presence of water and oxygen with the formation of ketoglutarate, ammonia, and hydrogen peroxide as in Reaction 14.20. GLOD has excellent potential as the principal component in the biosensing determination of glutamate [86,87]:

$$\text{Glutamate} + O_2 + H_2O \xrightarrow{\text{GOLD}} \text{ketoglutarate} + H_2O_2 + NH_3 \qquad (14.20)$$

14.1.2 MICROORGANISMS

Microbial biosensors are an important category of biosensors, which use microorganisms as biological transducers. Based on the action mechanism, microbial biosensors can be divided into two kinds: electrochemical microbial biosensor and bioluminescent microbial biosensor. The electrochemical microbial biosensor is classified into respiratory activity detection biosensor and electrode activity detection biosensor. Biochemical oxygen demand (BOD) biosensor that belongs to the respiratory activity detection biosensor is a superior kind of biosensor. BOD is a commonly used environmental index showing the amount of oxygen that microbes require to decompose organic materials in a given wastewater sample.

In comparison with the enzymes used in biosensor, microorganisms can be easily manipulated and adapted to consume and degrade new substrate under certain cultivatable conditions [88–90]. Additionally, the progress in molecular biology or recombinant DNA technology has opened endless possibilities of tailoring microorganisms to improve the activity of an existing enzyme or express foreign enzyme or protein in host cell [91,92]. All these factors make microorganisms excellent biological transducers to construct biosensors [93].

Till date, there are mainly two categories of microorganisms used in the preparation of biosensors, bacterium (including *E. coli, Bacillus subtilis, Bacillus licheniformis,* and so on) and yeast (including *Trichosporon cutaneum, Saccharomyces cerevisiae, Arxula adeninivorans,* and so on). These microorganisms used in biosensors are introduced in detail as follows.

14.1.2.1 *Escherichia coli*

E. coli, which exists in the intestines of humans and animals, is a representative bacterium of the genus *Escherichia* and is chosen as a model organism in the biological research. Recently, *E. coli* was used to prepare microbial biosensors. Rainina et al. [94] utilized cryoimmobilized recombinant *E. coli* cells to develop a microbial biosensor for the direct detection of neurotoxins, which is capable of hydrolyzing a wide spectrum of OP pesticides and chemical warfare agents. The biological transducer was provided through the enzymatic hydrolysis of OP neurotoxins catalyzed by organophosphate hydrolase. In the reaction, protons are generated with P–O, P–F, P–S, or P–CN bonds cleaved, and the number of released protons corresponds with the quantity of organophosphate hydrolyzed and is measured by using a pH glass electrode as the physical transducer. The cryoimmobilized *E. coli* cells exhibited stable hydrolytic activity for over 2 months under storage in 50 mM potassium phosphate buffer at 4°C and, therefore, provide the potential for the development of a stable biotransducer for detecting various OP neurotoxins.

Biran et al. [95] used a cadmium-responsive promoter from *E. coli* fused to a promoterless *lacZ* gene to construct a biosensor. This whole-cell biosensor could detect nanomolar concentrations of cadmium in water and soil samples within minutes, and it can be used for continuous online and *in situ* monitoring.

14.1.2.2 *Bacillus subtilis*

B. subtilis is a species of the genus *Bacillus*, belonging to aerobic bacteria, which can catalyze the biochemical degradation of organic matter in wastewater and is used for the fabrication of BOD biosensor. Jia et al. [96] developed a novel type of BOD biosensor for water monitoring by coimmobilization *B. subtilis* and *T. cutaneum* in the sol–gel-derived composite material, which is composed of silica, the grafting copolymer of poly(vinyl alcohol) and 4-vinylpyridine (PVA-g-P(4-VP)).

B. subtilis still retains sufficient enzymatic viability and activity for biooxidation of organic materials even when it is killed by a short exposure to high temperature. Therefore, thermally killed *B. subtilis* can also be used to prepare BOD biosensor, and this biosensor can be stored in phosphate buffer solution at room conditions without BOD or nutrients even for extended periods of time, while most of the microbial BOD sensors would require BOD and addition of nutrients to sustain the living microorganisms [4]. Tan et al. [97] adopted a thermal method to kill *B. subtilis* and used it for sensing BOD of waters and wastewaters. The BOD sensor is fabricated by covering a dissolved oxygen probe with a biofilm containing the dead cells, and the measured BOD_5 data of industrial and synthetic wastewater samples matched well with the results obtained by the conventional American Public Health Association (APHA) method.

14.1.2.3 *Bacillus licheniformis*

B. licheniformis is another species of *Bacillus* that belongs to aerobic bacteria. Tan et al. [98] reported that *B. licheniformis* demonstrated a better ability to assimilate amino acids; therefore it was used to fabricate glutamate BOD biosensors. Suriyawattanakul et al. [99] coimmobilized *B. licheniformis* and *T. cutaneum* to achieve a great response to glucose on top of the Teflon membrane of a Clark oxygen electrode and to form a glucose or glutamate BOD biosensor with improved sensitivity and dynamic range. It is shown that a membrane loaded with *T. cutaneum* at 1.1×10^8 cells mL^{-1} cm^{-2} and *B. licheniformis* at 2.2×10^8 cells mL^{-1} cm^{-2} gave the optimum result.

Jiang et al. [100] immobilized *B. licheniformis* and two other kinds of microorganisms, *Dietzia maris* and *Marinobacter marinus*, on a PVA organically modified silicate (ORMOSIL) film embedded with an oxygen-sensitive Ru complex to form a glucose/glutamate BOD biosensor; the biosensor is applied for the BOD determination of seawater. This kind of BOD biosensor has a relatively long life, which could steadily perform up to 10 months.

14.1.2.4 *Gluconobacter oxydans*

G. oxydans cells contain membrane-bound aldose dehydrogenase, which catalyzes the oxidation of a wide range of sugars including all sugars present in lignocellulose hydrolysate [101]. Tkáč et al. [102] prepared a microbial biosensor by surface modification of a graphite electrode with *G. oxydans* cells and enhanced the sensitivity of amperometric detection by using hexacyanoferrate(III) as a mediator. The biosensor was used for the determination of total sugars during lignocellulose hydrolysate fermentation including D-glucose, D-galactose, D-xylose, D-mannose, and L-arabinose, and a good correlation was obtained between total sugars determined by the biosensor and by quantitative paper chromatography.

Reshetilov et al. [103] immobilized *G. oxydans* whole cells on a FET to detect xylose by monitoring extracellular pH changes resulting from xylose dehydrogenation. This FET-based biosensor could detect xylose at a lower limit of 0.5 mM and could keep a linear range of 5.0–30 mM. Reshetilov et al. [104] also immobilized whole cells of *G. oxydans* on chromatographic paper by simple physical adsorption and attached those cells to the surface of the Clark-type electrodes for xylose determinations. In contrast with the xylitol above-mentioned biosensor, the detection of xylose by this biosensor was not significantly affected by the presence of xylitol. It is suggested that this biosensor will be useful in monitoring conversions of the compounds of xylose and xylitol.

14.1.2.5 *Pseudomonas aeruginosa*

P. aeruginosa is a representative bacterium of the genus *Pseudomonas* and belongs to aerobic bacteria. It is reported that *P. aeruginosa* JI-104 can aerobically degrade trichloroethylene (TCE) as a sole carbon source [105]. The overall pathway of oxidative TCE degradation by *P. aeruginosa* JI-104 is predicted as follows: TCE is transformed to TCE oxide, which becomes dichloroacetic acid, glyoxylate, carbon monooxide, or formic acid successively, and finally carbon dioxide is produced. Han et al. [105] immobilized *P. aeruginosa* JI-104 isolated from the soil near a gasworks on a polytetrafluoroethylene (PTFE) filter and mounted onto chloride ion electrode to form a novel microbial TCE sensor. Dihaloelimination occurs during the biological transformation of TCE and chloride ion concentration is measured, and thus it is possible to predict the initial TCE concentration.

Elasriá et al. [106] fused the *P. aeruginosa* recA promoter to a promoterless *Vibrio fischeri* lux operon. This recA–lux fusion (pMOE15) was introduced into a wild-type *P. aeruginosa* strain FRD1, and recA expression was monitored by measuring 490 nm light production. The RM4440 strain responded to the increasing doses of ultraviolet radiation by an increase in its bioluminescence. RM4440 has the potential to be useful as a biosensor for the measurement of DNA-damaging agents in the environment.

P. aeruginosa can produce a kind of blue phenazine pigment, pyocyanin, which exists in the oxidized form and was reduced by the reaction between GOD and glucose. The reduced form was then converted back to the oxidized form by an oxidative reaction [107]. Kunihiko et al. [107] produced pyocyanin by immobilized *P. aeruginosa* cells in κ-carrageenan under a 0.01% PO_4^{3-}, 0.2% Mg^{2+}, 0.001% Fe^{2+}, 1% glycerin, 0.8% leucine, and 0.8% DL-alanine condition. Then pyocyanin purified by chloroform extraction and silica-gel column chromatography was used as a mediator fixed on a screen-printed electrode to prepare a biosensor for more accurate determination of glucose concentration.

14.1.2.6 *Pseudomonas fluorescens*

P. fluorescens HK44 harbors the pUTK21 plasmid (derived from the NAH7 plasmid), which codes for genes of the naphthalene degradation pathway and is divided into two operons. Both the operons are positively inducible by salicylate through the *nahR* gene product, therefore little of their activity is present constitutively, and a huge increase of activity is observed after induction. The *V. fischeri luxCDABE* gene cassette coding for bioluminescence was inserted into the *nahG* gene of the salicylate operon, thus gaining inducibility by salicylate or naphthalene [108,109], so it can be used for the determination of naphthalene and salicylate bioavailability.

Trögl et al. [110] immobilized cells of *P. fluorescens* HK44 to the thick silica films prepared from prepolymerized tetramethoxysilane. With these films, the concentration of salicylate can be detected to get a *P. fluorescens* HK44 biosensor. The kinetics and response of such biosensors were researched. It is concluded that there was a positive relationship between light emissions of immobilized *P. fluorescens* HK44 and salicylate as well as naphthalene concentration. It is also mentioned that alginate appeared to be a very good immobilization material for further biosensor development using *P. fluorescens* HK44 because of its good transport properties with respect to napthalene and salicylate.

Takayama et al. [111] constructed an electrochemical biosensor based on *P. fluorescens*. They immobilized whole cells of *P. fluorescens* TN5 on the surface of carbon-paste electrodes containing *p*-benzoquinone or its derivatives. The electrodes produced anodic currents for nicotinic acid because of the electrocatalytic action of the bacterial cells using the quinone compounds as an electron transfer mediator, and thus it could be used as a nicotinic acid biosensor.

14.1.2.7 *Pseudomonas putida*

Similar to *P. aeruginosa* and *P. fluorescens, P. putida* is also a kind of Gram-negative bacterium that is an obligate aerobe and is used to develop highly sensitive biosensors for BOD detection [112]. In addition, *P. putida* ML2 has a special property of aerobic catabolism to benzene, thus it can be used in the precise detection of benzene.

Lanyon et al. [113] have constructed a *P. putida* ML2 bacterial biosensor for the detection of benzene that is integrated within a flow injection analysis (FIA) system. *P. putida* ML2 cells were immobilized between two cellulose acetate membranes and fixed onto a Clark dissolved oxygen electrode. Biosensor responses were investigated with the FIA system, resulting in a linear detection range between 0.01 and 0.1 mM benzene. This investigation demonstrates that the *P. putida* ML2 biosensor has potential applications for the analysis of samples containing benzene. Josef et al. [114] developed another *P. putida* biosensor for the detection of whole benzene, toluene, ethylbenzene (BTE), and xylene ranges. In this biosensor, the bacterial strains of *P. putida* F1 were immobilized between two cellulose acetate membranes and fixed onto a Clark dissolved oxygen electrode. The *P. putida* F1 aerobically degrades benzene, toluene, and BTE. The BTE biosensor in kinetic mode FIA displayed a linear range of 0.02–0.14 mM benzene (response time, 5 min; baseline recovery time, 15 min), 0.05–0.2 mM toluene (response time, 8 min; baseline recovery time, 20 min), and 0.1–0.2 mM BTE (response time, 12 min; baseline recovery time, 30 min. Due to the differences in sensitivity, response, and baseline recovery times for BTE, it was possible to differentiate each compound in mixtures of these volatile organic compounds (VOCs). No response for xylenes could be obtained since they cannot be completely metabolized by this bacterial strain.

14.1.2.8 *Klebsiella oxytoca*

K. oxytoca can exhibit high hydrogen production activity and high oxygen tolerance [115]. Ohki et al. [116] used *K. oxytoca* AS1 to prepare a BOD biosensor. They mainly investigated the effect of cell properties, such as the number and growth phase of immobilized cells, on the sensor response. It is concluded that the response of such biosensor was almost independent of the cell number in the case of low BOD solutions, whereas the response increased with increasing cell number when high-BOD solutions were used. The growth phase of the cells immobilized in the membrane affected the sensor response, especially when the membrane was stored at 30°C for a long time. Cells immobilized at the beginning of the stationary growth phase were the most effective in terms of both sensitivity and preservability. The biosensor showed a higher resistance to some toxic substances such as phenol.

14.1.2.9 *Serratia marcescens*

Kim and Kwon [117] reported a microbial BOD biosensor consisting of *S. marcescens* LSY 4 and an oxygen electrode. The polymer of sodium styrene sulfonate was grafted on the surface of porous Teflon membrane to absorb the heavy metal ions permeating through the membrane. Tolerance against Zn^{2+} was induced for *S. marcescens* LSY 4 to make the cells less sensitive to the presence of heavy metal ions. The membrane modification and the Zn^{2+} tolerance induction showed some positive effects in such a way that they reduced the inhibitory effects of Zn^{2+} and Cd^{2+} on the sensitivity of the BOD sensor.

14.1.2.10 *Rhodococcus erythropolis*

R. erythropolis is a kind of aerobic, Gram-positive actinomycete. It has unique enzymatic capabilities for catalyzing the biotransformation and degradation of diverse xenobiotics. Due to its ability to catalyze oxidation and metabolism of diverse and unusual substrates including hydrocarbons and substituted phenols, *R. erythropolis* attracts interest in the area of bioremediation. The survival of *R. erythropolis* under adverse environmental conditions was higher than any other hydrocarbon-utilizing bacteria.

Elena et al. [118] employed the whole cells of *R. erythropolis* as receptor and used a Clark-type oxygen electrode as a transducer to form a microbial sensor for 2,4-dinitrophenol (2,4-DNP) determinations. The response of this biosensor to 2,4-DNP was shown to add up, and it was considered to originate from two components: the effect of 2,4-DNP as the respiratory substrate on the cells' respiration of receptor element and the stimulatory effect of 2,4-DNP as protonophore on the cells' respiration.

14.1.2.11 *Trichosporon cutaneum*

T. cutaneum is a kind of yeast that can oxidize organic compounds. Yang et al. [119] fabricated a miniature Clark-type oxygen electrode array and prepared a BOD biosensor based on *T. cutaneum*. Each oxygen electrode of this array comprised an Ag cathode and an Ag/AgCl anode. *T. cutaneum* was immobilized onto the cathode of an oxygen electrode using a photo-crosslinkable resin, and the sensor responded to the difference between the output of a yeast-immobilized electrode and that of a bare oxygen electrode. The miniature oxygen electrode arrays showed good characteristics for monitoring dissolved oxygen and could be mass-produced with assured quality.

Yano et al. [120] used *T. cutaneum* to develop a BOD microbial biosensor that applied to the determination of amino acids produced in meat during the aging process. The biosensor consisted of an oxygen sensor and a *T. cutaneum* membrane (Figure 14.3). The sensor signal corresponded to the increase of amino acid levels and to the viable count in the meat with the storage time in the course of the first aging stage. This increase is due to the fact that amino acids produced initially by enzymes in the meat serve as a source of nutrition for septic bacteria during the aging process, and as a result, the level of bacterial cells increases with increasing amounts of amino acids with the passage of time.

14.1.2.12 *Saccharomyces cerevisiae*

A new system is described for the amperometric detection of metal ions using recombinant *S. cerevisiae* strains as the biocomponent in the microbial sensor. For this purpose, plasmids were constructed with the Cu^{2+}-inducible promoter of the *CUP1*-gene from *S. cerevisiae* fused to the promoterless *lacZ*-gene of *E. coli*. The fusion construct is only transcribed and translated in the presence of Cu^{2+}. Subsequently, these plasmids were transformed into the yeast strains. Provided that Cu^{2+} is present, the selected transformed cells are capable of utilizing lactose as an energy source [121]. The Cu^{2+}-depending utilization of lactose leads to alterations in the oxygen consumption of the cells, which can be measured by amperometric detection with a Clark oxygen electrode (Figure 14.4).

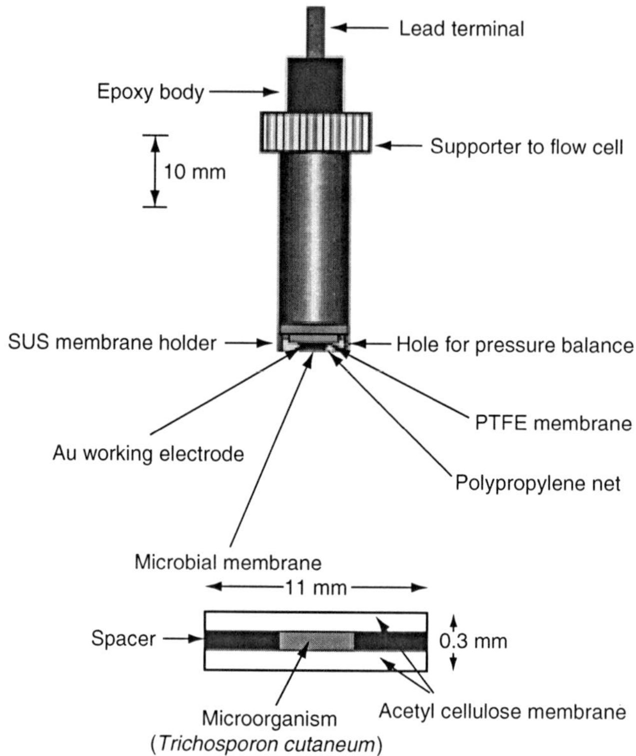

FIGURE 14.3 Microbial sensor for meat freshness. Microorganism: *Trichosporon cutaneum*. (From Yano, Y., Numata, M., Hachiya, H., Ito, S., Masadome, T., Ohkubo, S., Asano, Y., and Imato, T., *Talanta*, 54, 255, 2001. With permission.)

Lehmann et al. [121] prepared the first microbial biosensor to detect Cu^{2+} by this method. The sensor measured Cu^{2+} in a concentration range between 0.5 and 2 mM $CuSO_4$. In addition, they also developed an indirect amperometric measurement principle that allows the detection of samples containing Cu^{2+} and fast biodegradable substances.

Moreover, mutants of *S. cerevisiae* devoid of Cu, Zn-superoxide dismutase (SOD) are hypersensitive to a range of oxidants, hyperbaric oxygen, and hyperosmotic media; show lysine and methionine auxotrophy when grown under the atmosphere of air; and have a shortened replicative life span when compared with the wild-type strain. Ascorbate and other antioxidants can ameliorate these defects [122]. Zyracka et al. [122] employed the mutant of *S. cerevisiae* that lacked Cu, Zn-SOD as a tester to examine the possibility to use such yeasts for the detection of antioxidants. It is shown that a simple plate test based on the abolishment of leucine and methionine auxotrophy of SOD-deficient *S. cerevisiae* or restoration of growth on hypertonic medium can be used for the detection and semiquantitative estimation of concentrations of antioxidants.

14.1.2.13 *Arxula adeninivorans*

The yeast *A. adeninivorans* is found to have an amazingly broad substrate range: It assimilates all the sugars, polyalcohols, and organic acids except for ribose, lactose, and methanol [123]. As a result, an *A. adeninivorans*-based sensor should correlate with BOD_5 of most substrates and real samples [124]. Chan et al. [125] developed a microbial sensor for rapid measurement of the amount of biodegradable substances based on the salt-tolerant yeast *A. adeninivorans* LS3. They immobilized

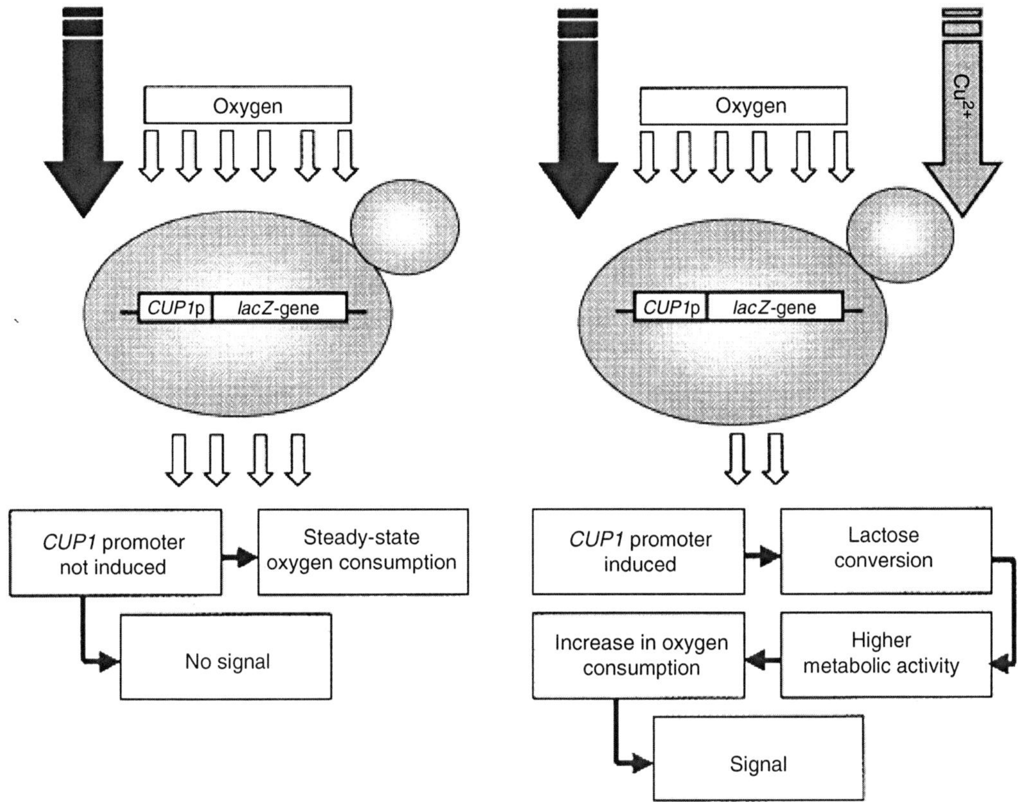

FIGURE 14.4 Principle of the Cu^{2+} measurement. (From Lehmann, M., Riedel, K., Adler, K., and Kunze, G., *Biosens. Bioelectron.*, 15, 211, 2000. With permission.)

A. adeninivorans in the hydrogel poly(carbamoyl)sulfonate (PCS), and the immobilized yeast membrane was placed in front of an oxygen electrode with -600 mV versus Ag/AgCl. The novel sensor makes it possible to monitor different types of wastewaters rapidly without pretreatment, and it can be used for an active process control of sewage treatment works [126].

14.1.2.14 *Torulopsis candida*

T. candida as a yeast can promote hydrocarbon to produce proteins. It is found that *T. candida* can assimilate a wide spectrum of organic compounds as an attractive alternative for *T. cutaneum* in BOD biosensor. Sugandhi et al. [127] employed *T. candida* to fabricate a BOD biosensor and evaluated it in the batch mode as well as under flow conditions.

14.1.2.15 *Pichia methanolica*

P. methanolica MN4 cells can be used to produce large amounts (up to 30% of the total protein of the cell) of highly active alcohol oxidase. Reshetilov et al. [128] developed such a biosensor by immobilizing *P. methanolica* on chromatographic paper and fixing on a Clark-type oxygen electrode. Of all substrates tested (ethanol, methanol, isopropanol, glucose, xylose, xylitol, arabinose, arabitol, glycerol, pyruvate, citrate, and acetate), the *P. methanolica*-based biosensor had a higher selectivity and was susceptible only to ethanol, methanol, and insignificantly to isopropanol.

14.1.3 DNA

DNA is the substance that makes up chromosomes and carries the genetic code in human beings and almost all other organisms. The information in DNA is stored as a code made up of four chemical bases: adenine (A), guanine (G), cytosine (C), and thymine (T). These DNA bases pair up with each other in the rule of A with T and C with G to form the basic units of DNA called base pairs. Each base is attached together to a sugar molecule and a phosphate molecule to construct the unit of nucleotide. Nucleotides are arranged in two long strands that form a spiral called double helix by the interaction of A–T and C–G [129].

DNA can also be used as molecular recognition element in biosensors. Based on the types of DNA used in biosensors and the mechanisms of action, there are in total two kinds of DNA biosensors, namely, single-strand DNA (ssDNA) biosensor and double-strand DNA (dsDNA) biosensor. The ssDNA biosensor uses an immobilized ssDNA as a probe to detect its own complementary ssDNA series by the interaction of DNA bases. The dsDNA biosensor is used to detect some molecules or ions that can interact with immobilized dsDNA based on the signals produced in the interaction.

Furthermore, based on the application of markers, DNA biosensors can be classified as marked DNA biosensor and unmarked DNA biosensor. In a marked biosensor, probe or target DNA is marked by fluorescent agents or electroactive agents, and the detection is fulfilled by the changes of fluorescent signals or redox signals. In contrast, no marks are used in an unmarked DNA biosensor, and the detection is realized by the changes of some physical or chemical information such as mass and the refractive indexes before and after the hybridization process of DNAs directly.

Similar to enzyme and microorganism biosensors, DNA biosensors can also be classified into electrochemical DNA biosensor, optical DNA biosensor, surface plasma DNA biosensor, etc. based on the difference of signal transducer.

Examples of DNA biosensors are listed in Table 14.8.

14.1.4 Antigens–Antibodies

Various substances act as antigens such as toxins, bacteria, foreign blood cells, and the cells of transplanted organs, which stimulate the production of antibodies when they are introduced into other bodies. Antibodies are protein substances produced in the blood or tissues in response to specific antigens. Antibodies can destroy or weaken bacteria and neutralize organic poisons, thus forming the basis of immunity. The binding of an antibody with its specific antigen that stimulated the formation of the antibody will result in agglutination, precipitation, complement fixation, greater susceptibility to ingestion, and destruction by phagocytes, or neutralization of an exotoxin.

Based on the special reaction of antigen with antibody, antigens (antibodies) can be used to prepare immunobiosensors for the qualitative or quantitative determination of corresponding antibodies (antigens) or even their accelerators and inhibitors by the changes of some physical or chemical signals such as optical, electrochemical, quality, and thermal signals during the reaction. Till now, lots of antigens (antibodies) have been used to construct immunobiosensors. Some of them are listed in Table 14.9.

14.2 INTERMEDIA MATERIALS

Intermedia materials are important components of biosensors. Up to now, various kinds of biosensors have been fabricated and their development depends on the application of new intermedia materials to a great extent. Because of their special characters, the intermedia materials are able to immobilize biorecognition molecules effectively or can function as excellent signal transducers. Usually more than one intermedia materials are needed in a biosensor to achieve the best stability and sensitivity. In this part, we review intermedia biomaterials widely used in biosensors. Some of them have been investigated for many years, while the others have been incorporated in biosensors only for a couple of years.

TABLE 14.8

Examples of DNA Biosensors

Immobilized DNA	Substrates	Signal Transducers	Immobilization Method of DNA	Type	Ref.
		Au disk electrode	The thiol-tagged probe DNA and 6-mercapto-1-hexanol were immobilized on the surface of electrode through thiol–Au binding	Electrochemical DNA biosensor	130
ssDNA	Complementary target oligonucleotide	Au substrates	DNA was immobilized by forming covalent amide bonds between carboxyl groups at the CNTs and amino groups at the ends of the DNA oligonucleotides	Electrochemical DNA biosensor	131
		Ag-plated surface	DNA was immobilized by the active coating of bovine serum albumin (BSA)	Acoustic wave DNA biosensor	133
		Au-covered quartz surface	DNA was immobilized on the gold quartz surface in NaCl solution	Quartz crystal microbalance (QCM) DNA biosensor	134
Biotinylated oligonucleotide (ssDNA)	Complementary target oligonucleotide	Resonant mirror	Biotinylated oligonucleotide was immobilized on the sensor surface by streptavidin	Optical DNA biosensor	132
dsDNA	Mitoxantrone	Glassy carbon electrode		Electrochemical DNA biosensor	135
	Toxic aromatic amines	Screen-printed electrodes	Electrodes were immersed in a stirred acetate buffer solution containing dsDNA for 120 s at a potential of +0.5 V versus SCE	Electrochemical DNA biosensor	136
	Benzo[a]pyrene (BaP)	Carbon paste electrode	dsDNA was immobilized on the electrode by applying a potential of +0.50 V for 5 min in 10 ppm dsDNA with 200 rpm stirring	Electrochemical DNA biosensor	137
	Organic analytes and metal	Flow cell fluidics	dsDNA was immobilized on a silica surface through avidin–biotin coupling	Waveguide DNA biosensor	138
Denatured DNA	Autoantibodies in blood serum	Stationary mercury film covered silver electrode	Denatured DNA was immobilized on cellulose nitrate film	Amperometric	139

14.2.1 CARBON NANOTUBES

Carbon nanotubes (CNTs) show intriguing performance when used as intermedia materials for biosensors. CNTs, which were discovered by Iijima in 1991 [151] and represent a new kind of carbon material. They are found in two distinct types of structures, namely, single-wall CNTs (SWCNTs) and multiwall CNTs (MWCNTs). SWCNTs comprise a cylindrical graphite sheet of nanoscale diameter

TABLE 14.9

Examples of Immunobiosensors Prepared by Antigens (Antibodies)

Target Substances	Substrates	Signal Transducers	Immobilization Method of Antigen (Antibody)	Type	Ref.
Atrazine antibodies	Atrazine	Au electrode of 10 MHz piezoelectric crystals	Atrazine antibodies were layered onto the gold electrode precoated with protein A	Piezoelectric crystal immunobiosensor	140
Protamine	Immunoglobulin M (IgM)	Piezoelectric crystal device	Protamine was immobilized by using either γ-aminopropyltriethoxy silane (γ-APTES) or 2.2.2-trifluoroethanesulfonyl chloride (tresyl chloride)	Piezoelectric crystal immunobiosensor	141
A-fetoprotein (AFP) antibody	AFP	MHz AT-cut quartz crystals with Au electrode	AFP antibody was immobilized onto the amine-coated surface by glutaraldehyde (GA) cross-linking	Piezoelectric crystal immunobiosensor	142
Antiestrogen antibody	Estrone	Pt electrode	Antibody was modified on the electrode by the direct electrochemical polymerization of pyrrole	Electrochemical immunobiosensor	143
Helicobacter pylori antigens	Immunoglobulin G (IgG) antibodies	GCE	*H. pylori* antigens were immobilized on the 3-aminopropyl-modified controlled pore glass	Electrochemical immunobiosensor	144
Carcinoembryonic antibody	Carcinoembryonic antigen	Screen-printed carbon electrode	Carcinoembryonic antigen was immobilized on the electrode with colloid Au and chitosan membrane	Electrochemical immunobiosensor	145
Sulfadiazine (SDZ)	SDZ antibody and SDZ residues sample	Dextran-coated silicon chip	SDZ was immobilized onto the surface of the dextran-coated silicon chip	Optical immunobiosensor	146
Antichloramphenicol (CAP) antibody	CAP	Solid support devised by installing a flow-through cell	Anti-CAP antibody was immobilized onto Biodyne B membrane pieces by a dipping procedure	Chemiluminescent immunobiosensor	147
Anti-2,4-dichlorophenoxyacetic acid (2,4-D) polyclonal antibodies	2,4-D	Chemiluminescent flow injection	Anti-2,4-D polyclonal antibodies are directly labeled with horseradish peroxidase	Chemiluminescent immunobiosensor	148
Protein A	Anti-BSA	Surface plasmon resonance	Protein A was immobilized on the Au surface by the heterobifunctional linker of N-succinimidyl-3-(2-pyridyldithio)propionate (SPDP)	Surface plasmon resonance immunobiosensor	149
Ivermectin-oxime	Ivermectin in bovine liver	Surface plasmon resonance	Ivermectin-oxime was immobilized onto the surface of a sensor chip by an amidating reaction by NHS/EDC	Surface plasmon resonance immunobiosensor	150

capped by hemispherical ends, while the MWCNTs comprise several to tens of incommensurate concentric cylinders of these graphitic shells with a layer spacing of 0.3–0.4 nm [151–153].

CNTs have excellent properties including high chemical and thermal stabilities, high elasticity, high tensile strength, ultrasmall size, and variable conductivity [151]. It was found that CNTs possess a high electrocatalytic effect and a fast electron transfer rate (ETR) [154–156]. MWCNTs are regarded as metallic conductors, a highly attractive property for an electrode, while SWCNTs can be metallic, semiconductors, or small band gap semiconductors depending on their diameter and chirality [157–159]. The CNTs can act as electrodes, generate electrochemiluminescence in aqueous solutions, and be derivatized with functional group that allows immobilization of biomolecules. The CNTs have high surface-to-weight ratio, which is accessible to both electrochemistry and immobilization of biomolecules. These properties, along with their favorable biocompatibility, make them excellent intermedia for the development of effective, low-cost environmental biosensors [160].

Purification of as-produced CNTs is essential to applications as intermedia biosensors. One of the most commonly used purification methods involves oxidative acid treatment, such as refluxing in dilute nitric acid or refluxing/sonication in a concentrated H_2SO_4/HNO_3 mixture [161]. The acid treatment is crucial for electrochemical properties of nanotubes, because it not only makes the nanotube stay dispersed in the solution but also leads to open-ended tubes containing either dangling bonds in organic solvents, which undergo further chemical reaction [162] or oxygenated functional groups such as quinones and carboxylic acids in polar solvents [161,163,164]. There are two critical problems to introduce CNTs to electrochemical biosensors, namely, how to incorporate CNTs onto the surface of electrodes and how to immobilize biological molecule to the electrode modified with CNTs. The techniques to assemble CNTs into biosensors are discussed in detail as follows.

14.2.1.1 Integration of Carbon Nanotubes [165]

14.2.1.1.1 Solution Casting Nanotubes onto Glass–Carbon Electrodes
As CNTs are insoluble in most aqueous solvents, they should be processed into a soluble product before casting onto GCEs. Homogeneous dispersions of CNTs can be achieved by oxidative acid treatments or with the aid of surfactants or polymers [166]. When the CNT-casting solutions are dropped directly onto the glassy carbon (GC) surface and allowed to dry, the electrode becomes ready for use [167,168]. The CNT-coated GCE, prepared by modifying GCE with CNTs dispersed in sulfuric acid [168], presented high sensitivity, low-potential, and stable amperometric sensing. CNTs have the ability to promote NADH electron-transfer reaction and suggest great promise for dehydrogenase-based amperometric biosensors.

SWCNTs treated with nitric acid during the purification process have been reported [169]; the carboxylic acid groups were introduced on the open ends of the SWCNTs. The nitric acid–purified SWCNT solution was cast on a GCE to form a CNT film. The film showed very stable electrochemical behavior and could be used to catalyze the electrochemical reaction of some biomolecules such as dopamine, epinephrine, and AA.

In Wu's work [170], with the aid of hydrophobic surfactant dihexadecyl hydrogen phosphate (DHP), MWCNTs were dispersed in water, achieving a MWCNT–DHP film-coated GCE, exhibiting remarkable electrocatalytic effects on the oxidation of dopamine (DA) and 5-hydroxytryptamine (5-HT), improving their oxidation peak currents and lowering their oxidation overpotential. On comparing with bare GCE, the modified electrode shows efficacy in detecting DA and 5-HT simultaneously and exhibits excellent stability and reproducibility. Other surfactants, such as *N*, *N*-dimethylformamide (DMF) [171] and cetyltrimethylammonium bromide (CTAB) [172], can be used to facilitate the dispersion of CNTs in aqueous solvents.

Comparing with common surfactants discussed above, polymers usually have more robust surface adsorption because of more involved interaction sites [173]. "Wrapping" of CNT in polymeric chains has been effective in improving their solubility without impairing their physical properties [174]. A variety of nonionic and ionic polymers were found capable of dispersing nanotubes [175–179]. For example, a widely used perfluorosulfonated polymer, Nafion polymer, with a polar side chain was found to solubilize CNTs in phosphate buffer solution or alcohol [180]. Wang et al. reported on the ability of Nafion to solubilize SWCNTs and MWCNTs and on the dramatically enhanced redox activity of hydrogen peroxide at CNT/Nafion-coated electrodes in connection with the preparation of oxidase-based amperometric biosensors [180]. Because of their unique properties such as ion exchange, discrimination, and biocompatibility, Nafion films have been used extensively for the modification of electrode surfaces and for the construction of amperometric biosensors [181,182].

14.2.1.1.2 Microfabrication of Nanoelectrode Ensembles and Arrays

Electrodes modified with nanotubes by drop-coating a random tangle of nanotubes onto the electrode surface take advantage of the bulk properties of CNTs. However, oriented CNT arrays possess advantage over the random tangle of CNTs. The open end of an MWCNT has a fast ETR similar to a graphite edge-plane electrode, while the SWCNT presents a very slow ETR and low specific capacitance, similar to the graphite basal plane [183]. The proper construction and orientation of the electrode is critical for its electrochemical properties. Several approaches to the production of aligned CNT arrays have been reported.

Liu et al. [184] used a bottom-up approach to fabricate a glucose biosensor based on CNT nanoelectrode ensembles. Low site density–aligned CNT arrays were grown from Ni nanoparticles (NPs) by plasma-enhanced chemical vapor deposition (CVD). A dielectric encapsulation was then applied, leaving half of the CNTs exposed to form inlaid nanoelectrode arrays (NEAs). Such an operation eliminates the need for permselective membrane barriers or artificial electron mediators, thus greatly simplifying the sensor design and fabrication (Figure 14.5).

Gooding et al. described a more versatile approach to the production of aligned CNT arrays by self-assembly [185] (Figure 14.6). The as-grown nanotubes were first chemically cut into short

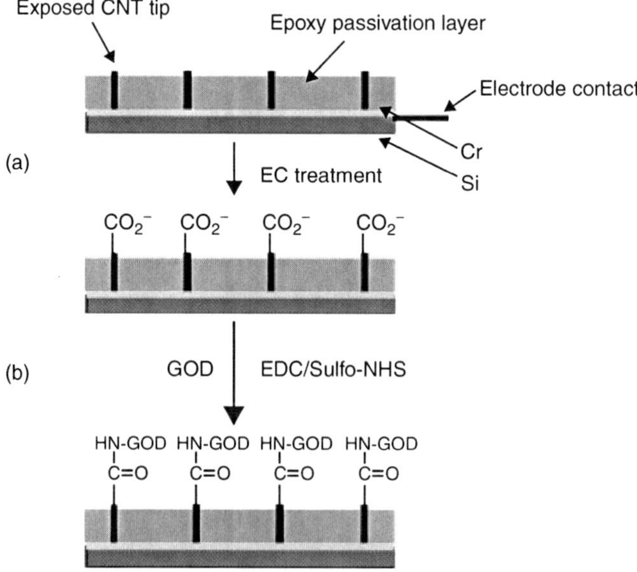

FIGURE 14.5 Fabrication of a glucose biosensor based on CNT nanoelectrode ensembles: (a) electrochemical treatment of the CNT NEEs for functionalization and (b) coupling of the enzyme (GOx) to the functionalized CNT NEEs. (From Lin, Y.H., Lu, F., Tu, Y., and Ren, Z.F., *Nano Lett.*, 4, 191, 2004. With permission.)

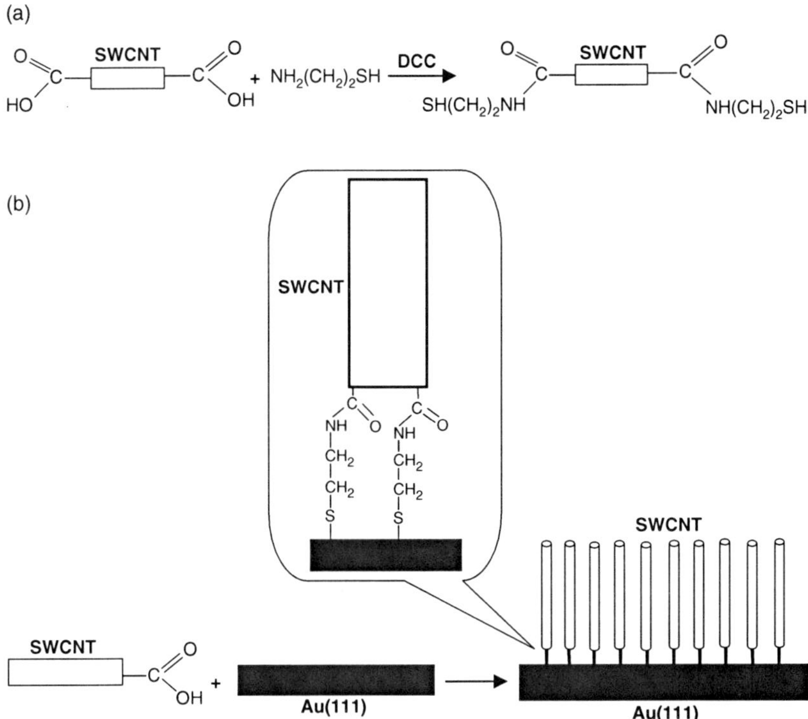

FIGURE 14.6 (a) Scheme for the thiolization reaction of carboxyl-terminated cysteamine (NH₂CH₂–CH₂SH) and (b) schematic diagram of the assembling structure of SW CNTs on gold. (From Liu, Z.F, Shen, Z.Y., Zhu, T., Hou, S.F., Ying, L.Z., Shi, Z.J., and Gu, Z.N., *Langmuir*, 16, 3569, 2000. With permission.)

pipes and thiol derivatized at the open ends. The ordered assembly of SWCNTs was made by spontaneous chemical adsorption to gold through Au–S bonds. Tapping mode atomic force microscopy (AFM) images clearly show that the nanotubes have been organized on gold, forming a self-assembled (SA) monolayer structure with a perpendicular orientation. This kind of chemical manipulation has great versatility and is not limited to the present system. One can design the terminal functionality of nanotubes and assemble them on various substrates by a predesigned bonding nature.

An alternative to self-assembling aligned nanotubes on an electrode surface is to grow aligned nanotubes directly on to an electrode surface. Sotiropoulou and Chaniotakis [186] performed it using the CVD method on a platinum electrode.

14.2.1.1.3 Attaching Individual or Microbundles of MWCNTs to the End of Wires

Nugent et al. [187] used arc-derived MWCNT microbundles to fabricate electrodes. The bundle that forms on the electrode during the electric arc discharge is broken open, and a microbundle of nanotubes is picked out and attached to the end of a copper electrode wire using a conductive silver paint. The electrodes show Nernstien behavior and fast electron-transfer kinetics for electrochemical reactions of $Fe(CN)_6^{3-/4-}$.

Boo et al. reported of an interesting needle-type nanobiosensor based on individual MWCNT [188]. The nanoneedles were fabricated by attaching a MWCNT to an etched tungsten tip using a nanomanipulator in a high-vacuum chamber. This attachment process was carried out in a field emission scanning electron microscope (JEOL, JSM-6700F) equipped with two piezoelectric nanomanipulator [189]. The nanoelectrodes can serve analytical functions as reliable as electrochemical nanosensors to detect electroactive species.

14.2.1.1.4 Mixing Nanotubes with a Binder and Packing Them as a Paste Electrode

Similar to carbon-paste electrodes, matrices with CNTs have recently been one of the focuses in the field of electrochemical sensors. In the electrochemical study employing CNT-modified electrodes by Britto et al. [190], nanotubes were dispersed in bromoform as a binder material and packed into a glass tube. The resultant electrode had randomly distributed tubes without any control over the alignment of the nanotubes. A variety of binders such as mineral oil [191], Teflon [192], and epoxy resins, [193] were explored to produce CNT pastes or composites.

14.2.1.2 Coupling with Biological Molecules

After the modification of electrodes with CNTs, the next key issue for the fabrication of biosensors is to immobilize biomolecules onto the modified electrodes. The simplest method is noncovalent immobilization of an enzyme by adsorbing the enzyme physically on the electrode surface modified with CNTs; one such example has been reported by Trojanowicz et al. for a screen-printed biosensor with OP hydrolase [194]. Streptavidin was found to adsorb on MWCNTs presumably by hydrophobic interactions between the nanotubes and hydrophobic domains of the proteins [195]. Chen et al. has also reported a simple and general approach to noncovalent functionalization of the sidewalls of SWCNTs, and subsequent immobilization of various biological molecules onto nanotubes with a high degree of control and specificity [196]. Noncovalent functionalization of CNTs has been reported for selective recognition and binding of target proteins and detection of clinically important biomolecules, such as antibodies associated with human autoimmune diseases [197].

Covalent immobilization of enzymes is another method by which enzymes and other redox proteins can be covalently immobilized to SWCNTs functionalized with carboxylic groups. The CNTs may be plugged into the enzymes in two ways [198]. In the first strategy, native GOD was covalently attached to the ends of the aligned tubes that allowed close approach to FAD, and direct electron transfer was observed with a rate constant of $0.3\ s^{-1}$. In the second strategy, FAD was attached to the ends of the tubes and the enzyme reconstituted around the surface-immobilized FAD. The latter approach allowed more efficient electron transfer to the FAD with a rate constant of $9\ s^{-1}$ (Figure 14.7).

Glucose is one of the most reported analytes detected through enzyme–CNT electrodes. CNT-modified gold electrodes described in Ref. 185 have been used to achieve a fast electron-transfer (i.e., in the case of GOD) between the redox active site of the enzyme, FAD, and the transducing electrode.

CNTs have also been utilized in the development of electrochemical DNA hybridization biosensors. The application of CNTs in electrochemical DNA biosensors includes two main aspects. On one hand, using CNTs as a novel substrate not only enables immobilization of DNA molecules but also serves as a powerful amplifier to amplify signal transduction event of DNA hybridization. On the other hand, CNTs can be employed as a powerful carrier to preconcentrate enzymes or electroactive molecules for electrochemical sensing of DNA hybridization as a novel indicator [199]. Various configurations of such biosensors have been described in recent years. DNA oligonucleotides can be strongly adsorbed onto the exterior surface of CNTs by nonspecific adsorption [200,201]. Covalent grafting of DNA oligonucleotides onto CNTs plays a more important role in sensitive and selective DNA biosensor. Aminated or carboxylated DNA oligonucleotides were covalently linked to carboxylated or aminated SWCNT-multilayer films through appropriate coupling chemistry, respectively [202].

14.2.2 POLYMER

14.2.2.1 Conducting Polymer Membrane

Since the discovery of high conductivity in doped polyacetylene in the 1970s [202,203], conducting polymers have attracted much interest and many of their applications including biosensors have

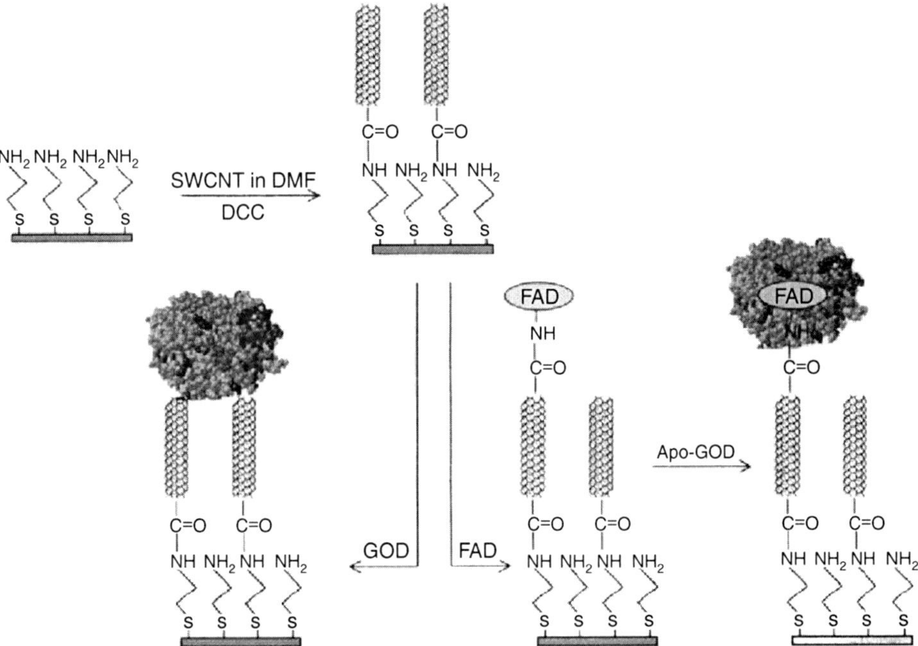

FIGURE 14.7 A schematic representation of the procedure for the modification of a SA monolayer modified Au electrode with aligned SW CNTs and their subsequent modification to allow direct electron transfer to GOD. (From Liu, J.Q., Chou, A., Rahmat, W., Paddon-Row, M.N., and Gooding, J.J., *Electroanalysis*, 17, 38, 2005. With permission.)

been explored. The electrical conducting polymers possess numerous features that allow them to act as excellent materials for immobilization of biomolecules and rapid electron transfer for efficient biosensors. Conducting polymers have conjugated backbone that can be oxidized or reduced by electron acceptors or donors, resulting in p-doping or n-doping materials, respectively. By adjusting the doping level, control of electronic property over the entire range from insulator to semiconductor and then to metal is feasible [204].

The conducting polymers can be produced by various techniques, for example, spin coating [205], SA monolayer [206], and Langmuir–Blodgett (LB) [204] methods. However, the most widely used technique is electrochemical synthesis because of its simplicity and reproducibility. Electrochemical polymerization occurs when suitable monomers are electrochemically oxidized to create active monomeric and dimeric species that react with each other to form a conjugated polymer backbone.

A number of favorable characteristics of conducting polymers for the application of biosensors are as follows: (1) direct and easy deposition on sensor electrode at room temperature by electrochemical oxidation of monomer, (2) control of thickness by varying either the potential or current with time, (3) modulation of the required electronic and mechanical properties by chemical modeling and synthesis, and (4) redox conductivity and polyelectrolyte characteristics of the polymer useful for sensor applications [207,208].

Conducting polymers are suitable matrix of enzymes because of their excellent electrical conductivity and favorable compatibility with biological molecules in neutral aqueous solutions. Organic conducting polymers as a convenient ingredient not only immobilize biomolecules, but also provide a microenvironment that can facilitate the direct electron transfer between biomolecules and the electrode. The majority of work has been carried out by redox or electronic conducting polymers, such as polypyrrole (PPy), polyaniline (PANI), and polythiophene.

The PPy polymer with low oxidation potential is easily formed from mild aqueous buffer solutions in which biomolecules are stable, so it has been widely used for the immobilization of enzymes, antibodies, and nucleic acids [209–211]. The polythiophene monomer is insoluble in water and requires higher potentials than PPy [212]. PANI polymers are formed from similar conditions as of PPy, but the formation of the most highly conducting form requires the presence of acid, which limits its use in biosensors because of the denaturization of biomolecules. Fortunately, the attachment of simple functional groups, such as sulfonates, to the monomer overcomes these problems [213].

There are several strategies for the immobilization of biomolecules using conducting polymers, namely, entrapment of biomolecules within electropolymerized films, electrosynthesis of biomolecules-functionalized monomers, and the attachment of the biomolecules to the underlying films.

14.2.2.1.1 Entrapment of Biomolecules within Electropolymerized Film

This one-step method is the most straightforward strategy of immobilization. When an appropriate potential is applied to an electrode soaked in an aqueous solution containing monomer and biomolecules, a polymer that incorporates biomolecules homogenously during its growth process is formed. It should be noted that such immobilization occurs under mild conditions without chemical reaction that could alter the activity of the biomolecule. The entrapment of enzymes in conducting polymers provides a facile means for ensuring proximity between the active site of the enzyme and the conducting surface of the electrode. This reagentless electrochemical approach is easily applicable to a wide variety of biological macromolecules.

This conventional electrochemical method of biomolecule entrapment was mainly focused on the immobilization of enzymes. GOD has been successfully entrapped in PPy films [214], PANI films [215], and in special copolymers [216]. Biosensors of other enzymes, such as peroxidase [217], COD [218], lactate oxidase [219], uricase [220], tyrosinase [212], and multienzyme that require sequential immobilization [221] or coimmobilization [222], have also been studied by the one-step strategy of immobilization. Although the immobilization of enzymes was widely studied by this method, few examples have been devoted to the immobilization of other biomolecule species such as antibodies and cells [223,224].

Theoretical models associated with the electrochemical entrapment of enzymes have also been studied along with the roles of polymer layer thickness, enzyme loading, and spatial location on the functioning of the biosensor [225–227].

14.2.2.1.2 Electrosynthesis of Biomolecules-Functionalized Monomers

For this procedure, monomers are first functionalized with biomolecules and then the combined monomers are electrosynthesized into copolymers. The first report was the covalent attachment of GOD to the PPy, terminal amine groups of the enzyme were chemically modified with pyrrole moieties, and the pyrrole-modified GOD was copolymerized with pyrrole to produce conducting polymer films containing covalently immobilized GOD. The resulting enzyme electrodes showed increased activity and thermal stability compared with PPy-immobilized GOD in which the enzyme was physically entrapped as a counteranion [228].

As an extension of the earlier work, a few reports of interaction of DNA with conducting polymers are available [229–231]. Livache et al. [232] used chemically modified DNA with a pyrrole moiety and proceeded to the polymerization of pyrrole to fabricate a DNA-based biosensor with a reliable DNA–PPy grafting. Korri-Youssoufi et al. [233] developed a synthetic route toward functionalized conjugated polymers and a copolymer of 3-acetic acid pyrrole and 3-*N*-hydroxyphthalimide (NHP) pyrrole with an aminooligonucleotide. The resulting modified copolymer was used for DNA recognition. Specific hybridization of the grafted oligonucleotide (ODN) with its complementary ODN target in solution induces a significant modification in the electrochemical response of PPy and enables a sensitive electrical reading of the recognition process.

14.2.2.1.3 The Attachment of Biomolecules to the Underlying Film

Being different from the above two strategies that can be proposed as "one-step procedure," this immobilization method could be called as a "two-step procedure" that involves electropolymerization of functionalized conducting polymers and then the attachment of biomolecules to the polymer surfaces.

For the two-step procedure, immobilization permits the selection of the optimum reaction conditions for each step. Since immobilization of biomolecules only takes place on the outer surface of the polymer, the access of polymer to biomolecules can be improved, and the attachment of the biomolecules to the functionalized polymer could be carried out in aqueous buffer solutions containing additives and stabilizers that could avoid damage to the biological entity.

There are three kinds of interactions between biomolecules and the underlying polymer for the attachment: adsorption, covalent bonding, and affinity interaction. The main binding forces of adsorption are static interactions between the polycationic matrix of the oxidated polymer and the total negative enzyme charge provided that the pH of the solution is higher than the isoelectric point (IEP) of the enzyme [234]. However, this technique suffers from desorption of enzyme from the immobilizing material into the sample solution during measurement. This procedure has been used for the preparation of cholesterol biosensors [235], urea sensors [236], and glucose biosensors [237,238].

Covalent linking is another interaction for biomolecules to be attached to the functionalized membrane. Apart from preventing the loss of biomolecules, this procedure improves the efficiency of the charge transfer process and increases the stability of the device [239]. Chemically reactive sites of a protein may be amino groups, carboxyl groups, phenol residues of tyrosine, sulfhydryl groups or the imidazole group of histidine, and in most cases amino and carboxyl groups of enzymes can be used for stable immobilizations by covalent bonding to polymer films functionalized by carboxyl or amino groups [240]. The covalent reaction conditions often partly denature the protein or lead to incomplete derivatization of the polymer surface. Therefore, effort has been focused on improving polymers for the grafting of biomolecules in terms of the performance of their chemically activated surfaces. An alternative method called postfunctionalization has been developed. The functional groups are attached onto the conducting polymer surface by electropolymerizing functioned thiophene, bithiophene, and pyrrole monomers with easy leaving groups such as *N*-hydroxysuccinimide (NHS) and NHP esters [241]. And the replaceable NHS or NHP groups can react easily by nucleophilic substitution with amines to form amide bonds. Thus, it is possible to anchor biomolecules with terminal amino functions onto the surface of conducting polymers functionalized with an activated ester. By this procedure, various biosensors have been prepared, such as enzymes [234] and oligonucleotides [242].

The affinity between biomolecules and films is another potent interaction for the surface modification of membranes. Compared with chemical modifications, it could improve the selectivity and orientation more effectively. One of the most important affinity interactions is the metal ion affinity, which originated from the "immobilized metal (ion) affinity chromatography" (IMAC) [243]. The technique is based on the differences in the affinity of proteins for metal ions bound to a metal-chelating substance, which is immobilized on a support membrane. Cooper et al. [244] further developed metal ion affinity binding for the immobilization of proteins onto the conducting polymers. In that procedure, Ni(II) was immobilized through its coordination to electrogenerated PPy films, *N*-substituted by carboxylate or imidazole groups, and then poly(histidine) and bacterial alkaline phosphatase bearing a chain of six histidines immobilized on the PPy-localized metal ions through specific interaction. Since proteins are now routinely engineered with terminal polyhistidine sequences, this immobilization procedure offers the great convenience of oriented immobilization of protein.

Electropolymerized PANI–poly(acrylate) and PANI–poly(vinyl sulfonate) films with electrochemically incorporated Ni(II) have been used to anchor the histidine-tagged enzyme [245,246].

Another attractive affinity interaction that has achieved wide acceptance for binding biological species to surfaces is avidin–biotin linkage, which presents a variety of specific advantages over other immobilization techniques. For example, the binding strength of biotin to streptavidin is nearly equal to that for a covalent bond ($K_D = 1 \times 10^{-15}$ M) [247]. This interaction is highly resistant to a wide range of organic solvents, pH range variations, and high temperatures, and it can be used to link any biomolecules possessing avidin or biotin labels. In addition, the biological activity of the biomolecule being immobilized by this interaction can also be preserved efficiently.

Biotins can be cooperated into the conducting polymers by oxidizing monomers labeled with biotin [246,248]. Subsequent avidins link to the functionalied polymers by the avidin–biotin affinity. A variety of biotinylated biomolecules have been fabricated, for example, GOD [248,249], nucleic acids [250], peptides, and bacteria [251].

14.2.2.2 Nanoconducting Polymer

The conducting polymers that are discussed in Section 14.2.2.1 function as a matrix of biomolecules in the form of bulk membrane. However, recently, nanoscaled forms of conducting polymers and their applications in the design of biosensors have attracted much interest because they have better properties compared with the bulk conducting polymers, such as larger surface area, better conductivity, and higher reaction ability. Several types of biosensors based on the nanoscaled conducting polymers have been reported.

Zhou et al. [252] fabricated an amperometric glucose biosensor based on platinum microparticles dispersed in nanofibrous PANI. The nanofibrous PANI film had been synthesized by pulse galvanostatic method. The single nanofibrous PANI has a diameter of 70–100 nm and a length of about 10 µm, and the nanofibrous PANI film exhibits a three-dimensional (3-D) structure with a large number of microgaps and micropores existing between the fibers. This structure results in a large specific surface area and good ionic and electronic conductivities of the film, which are beneficial for platinum dispersion and enzyme incorporation. So, it can be concluded that the nanofibrous PANI film can be used as a better supporting material for catalyst and enzyme.

There is another amusing approach for the immobilization of enzymes based on the nanoconducting polymers. Parthasarathy et al. [253,254] developed a template-based synthetic method to yield hollow PPy microcapsules of uniform diameter and length, and then they filled these microcapsules with high concentration of enzymes. This method is an ideal approach because it satisfies all the criteria that an ideal immobilization method requires, such as employing mild chemical conditions, allowing for large quantities of enzymes to be immobilized, providing a large surface area for enzyme–substrate contact with a small total volume, minimizing barriers to mass transport of substrate and product, and providing a chemically and mechanically robust system.

Since Martin et al. [255] explored the "template-synthesis" method, nano- or microtubes of many kinds of materials have been synthesized. It is feasible and facile to synthesize these microcontainers with various conducting polymers. Recently, Park et al. [256] reported a hollow microcylinder structure comprised of the conducting polymer, poly(3,4-ethylenedioxythiophene) (PEDOT); it worked as a container retaining water-soluble electroactive materials and played the role of a current collector for the electrochemical reaction of the species retained inside. The current collector exhibited a fine current response due to the redox reaction of $K_3Fe(CN)_6$, and the results show that guest materials can be stored in this capped cylinder structure without the problems associated with the use of organic solvents during the manufacturing processes.

As we have discussed above, the encapsulation method offers a number of important advantages such as general fabrication, chemically benign environment, and a large surface area for enzyme–substrate contact, so this biomolecule immobilization concept should find extensive applications in biosensors.

14.2.2.3 Nonconducting Polymer

Nonconducting polymers, which possess impressive advantages such as excellent permselectivity and high reproducibility, have also been emerging in biosensors as support matrices for the immobilization of biomolecules [257]. The property of the nonconducting polymers that are mainly discussed here is the permselectivity. As far as the permselectivity is concerned, the membrane synthesized by electropolymerization at about neutral pH showed excellent performance. The film growth is self-limited by its insulating and self-sealing character, and the resulting films are very thin (ca. 10–100 nm), so that the substrates and products can diffuse rapidly to and from the enzyme, and this diffusion will further increase the overall concentration of enzymes and may increase the current response. It has also shown that these films are continuous, hydrophobic, and "defect free," and they are able to reject interferents and hence can improve selectivity [258,259].

Work in this area involved enzyme entrapment in thin films that is electrochemically polymerized from phenol, phenylenediamine, or other monomers. Bartlett and Caruana [260] reported that the electropolymerization of phenol at a platinum electrode surface gave a thin-layer film with a thickness of 38 nm, and glucose biosensor was fabricated by repetitive potential cycling in an aqueous solution of phenol and GOD. Nakabayashi et al. [259] used poly(3-aminophenol) to immobilize ferrocene and HRP on a carbon-paste electrode for the development of H_2O_2 biosensor, and this biosensor is not easily influenced by oxidizable species such as L-AA and UA. Yang et al. [261] employed poly(m-phenylenediamine) (PMPD) for the fabrication of a needle-type glucose sensor with high selectivity. Since the permeability of PMPD film to interferents is lower than that of poly(o-phenylenediamine) and poly(p-phenylenediamine) films [262], the PMPD film is a promising material for fabricating glucose sensors.

As we have mentioned in Sections 14.2.2.1 and 14.2.2.2, PPy is one of the most extensively used conducting polymers in designing biosensors because of its high conductivity and stability as well as simplicity and flexibility of the immobilization procedure. Recently, a nonconducting PPy based on the overoxidation of pyrrole has emerged as a novel material for biosensor construction. Overoxidation of PPy (PPyox) appears to be attracted by the positive potentials in water- and oxygen-containing environment, and in this case it is moving toward partial destruction of polymeric backbone and generation of oxygen-containing (carboxyl, carbonyl, and hydroxyl) groups. The PPyox is a nonconducting, permselective polymer membrane with excellent interferential rejection properties and is often used as a discrimination membrane that significantly increases selectivity of electrochemical biosensors [263,264]. Many biosensors, such as glucose and cholesterol, have been investigated based on the enzymes immobilized on a PPyox-modified electrode [265–267].

14.2.3 Nanomaterials

Nanotechnology has recently become one of the most exciting forefront fields in analytical chemistry. Nanotechnology is defined as the creation of functional materials, devices, and systems through control of matter at the 1–100 nm scale. Owing to their small size, such nanomaterials have unique optical [268,269], electrical [270,271], magnetic [272,273], and catalytic [274] properties that differ from those of the bulk materials. Such properties, together with the diversity in composition (inorganic or organic and metals or semiconductors), the diversity of shapes (particles, rods, wires, tubes, cubes, tetrapods, or triangles), and the readiness for surface functionalization (physical, chemical, or biological), have enabled the fabrication of various functional nanoscale devices including biosensors [275–277].

Many interesting applications of nanomaterials in biosensors often incorporate biological components in the sensor transducer elements or separation phase or extraction materials [278]. Therefore, most literature reviewed herein focuses on nanomaterials conjugated with biological components. The review in this section divides nanomaterials into three sections, 1-D nanostructures, NPs, and nanoporous materials according to their shapes, followed by different types based on chemical composition. It is not a comprehensive coverage of these topics, but rather the most important advances relevant to novel developments in biosensor over the recent years are highlighted.

14.2.3.1 One-Dimensional Nanomaterials in Biosensor

One-dimensional nanostructures, such as CNTs, metal or metal oxide nanotubes, and conducting-polymer nanowires, are particularly attractive for biosensor application. Because of their high surface-to-volume ratio, high aspect ratio, and novel electron transport properties, their electronic conductance is hypersensitive to surface perturbations (such as those associated with the binding of macromolecules). Such 1-D materials thus offer the prospect of rapid (real-time) and sensitive label-free bioelectronic detection and massive redundancy in nanosensor arrays. The extreme smallness of these nanomaterials would allow the packing of a huge number of sensing elements onto a small footprint of an array device.

Since the applications of CNTs (Section 14.2.1), and conducting-polymer nanowires (Section 14.2.2.2) in biosensors have been reviewed in the previous sections, in this part, we mainly introduce several biosensor applications of metal and metal oxide 1-D nanostructures that have been reported recently.

It is known that gold electrodes have been increasingly used in designing electrochemical biosensors. However, enzyme immobilization on flat gold surfaces often suffers from low amounts of biomolecules and poor electrical contact to the transducer. Recently, Demoustier-Champagne and Delvaux reported on the fabrication of ensembles of gold nanotubes aligned parallel to each other and presenting uniform size and shape by electroless plating of gold into the pores of nanoporous polycarbonate track-etched membranes [279]. Then arrays of gold nanotubes were functionalized through the immobilization of enzymes using SA monolayers as anchor layers [280,281]. The resulting biosensors showed excellent properties, such as low cost, ease of fabrication, remarkable sensitivity, good reproducibility, and repeatability. Concerning the high sensitivity, there were two explanations [280]. First, it came from the higher roughness of the electroless Au surface of the electrode compared with flat gold film and from the tubular nature of the electrode, both leading to an increased surface area of the electrode for the same geometric area. Second, the amount of enzyme molecules keeping their activity is higher when they are immobilized within a porous system than on a flat surface, because the magnitude of analyte response is not only proportional to the enzyme loading but also to the enzyme activity on the electrode surface, and the Au nanoelectrode has better biocompatibility.

A disadvantage of metal nanomaterials that limits their applications in biosensors is the direct adsorption of redox proteins on unmodified metal surfaces, which usually leads to a dramatic change in the protein structures and significant loss of their bioactivity [282,283]. But for the metal oxides, the situation will change, because some metal oxides, such as zinc oxide semiconductors, have favorable biocompatibility.

Zinc oxide (ZnO) and its 1-D nanostructures have recently been investigated intensively due to their potential applications in optoelectronics [284,285]. The 1-D ZnO nanostructures have unique advantages including high specific surface area, nontoxicity, chemical stability, electrochemical activity, and high electron communication features, and more particularly, ZnO has a high IEP [286], which makes it suitable for the adsorption of low-IEP proteins or enzymes, and thus they may have great potential in the applications of biosensors.

Zhang et al. [287] reported a reagentless UA biosensor based on uricase immobilized on ZnO nanorods. The monodispersed ZnO nanorods were prepared by thermal evaporation approach [288] and dispersed in solution for the surface modification of GCE; the immobilization of uricase was done by casting 5 μL uricase on the ZnO membrane. This sensor showed high thermal stability and electrocatalytic activity to the oxidation of UA without the presence of an electron mediator. Glucose biosensor based on GOD immobilized on ZnO nanorod array has also been reported [289].

Similar to ZnO, nanostructured TiO_2 materials also show high biocompatibility and good retention of biological activity for protein binding [290,291]. TiO_2 nanotubes, fabricated by low-cost anodic oxidation of the pure titanium sheet, possess large surface areas and good uniformity and conformability over large areas, hence they are desirable for electrochemical biosensor design [291,292]. Liu et al. [293] investigated the coadsorption of protein with thionine on TiO_2 nanotubes for biosensor design. In the work, they first fabricated TiO_2 nanotubes by anodizing Ti sheets in a dilute HF solution and then coimmobilized HRP and thionine on the TiO_2 nanotube arrays by immersing the Ti/TiO_2 electrodes in a mixture of HRP and thionine solution. Electrochemical and spectroscopic measurements show that the TiO_2 nanotube arrays provide excellent matrices for the coadsorption of HRP and thionine and that the adsorbed HRP on these TiO_2 nanotube arrays not only effectively retains its bioactivity but also shows a high affinity for H_2O_2.

14.2.3.2 Nanoparticles in Biosensors

Inorganic NPs, such as metals, semiconductors, and magnetic particles, are clusters of a few hundred to a few thousand atoms that are only several nanometers long. Because of such small sizes, they have physical, electronic, and chemical properties different from those of bulk metals.

In noble metals, when the size of NPs decreases below the electron mean free path (the distance the electron travels between scattering collisions with the lattice centers), an intense absorption in the visible-near-UV that is absent in the spectrum of the bulk material appears, that leads to the surface plasmon band (SPB) observed near 530 nm for NPs. This extinction band arises when the incident photon frequency is resonant with the collective oscillation of the conduction electrons and is known as the localized surface plasmon resonance (LSPR) [268,294]. This LSPR gives these metallic NPs brilliant color in colloidal solution that intrigued scientists in the seventeenth century.

The LSPR spectrum depends on the NP itself (i.e., its size, material, and shape) and on the external properties such as the dielectric properties of the surrounding environment [295]; the induced wavelength shifts in the extinction maximum of NPs can be used to detect molecule-induced changes surrounding the NPs. The selectivity of the sensor is achieved by chemically modifying the NPs with SA monolayers that can be tailored to incorporate a wide variety of molecular recognition elements such as enzymes, antibodies, or DNA [296].

In LSPR techniques, a monolayer of noble metal NPs is adsorbed on an optically transparent, preactivated substrate (e.g., glass functionalized with amine or thiol groups) followed by an activation step of the particles themselves. Finally, a receptor is immobilized on the particle surface that binds to the target molecules of the sample under analysis. Spincasting polymers on top of the gold particles, leading to a refractive index change to which the metal particles respond optically, was found to increase the performance of this colorimetric biosensor [297,298].

Englebienne et al. first used the refractive index-dependent color change of spherical homogeneous 40 nm gold particles to develop a solution-phase immunoassay for monitoring the binding kinetics of antibody–antigen interactions in real time. After coating with monoclonal antibodies specific for human ferritin, human chorionic gonadotropin (hCG), and human heart fatty acid binding protein (hFABP), the NPs were incubated in a solution of their respective antigens [299,300]. This incubation caused a redshift in the LSPR extinction as well as an increase in the extinction at 600 nm (bathochromic and hyperchromic effects).

Several studies have been reported on gold NP-based UV–vis technique for the detection of DNA. This colorimetric detection method is based on the change in absorbance spectra (i.e., color) as particles are brought together by the hybridization of complementary DNA strands [301–304]. The limits of detection are reported in the range of tens of femtomoles of target oligonucleotide. These NP aggregation assays represent a 100-fold increase in sensitivity over conventional fluorescence-based assays [301].

Semiconductor quantum dots (QDs) have also been used to develop optical sensors based on fluorescence measurements [305,306]. QDs show size-tunable fluorescence emission and have a narrow and symmetric spectral line profile (the full width half maximum is typically 25–35 nm), making them ideal for simultaneous detection of multiple fluorophores by excitation of a single light source [307,308]. The photoluminescence has a long lifetime (~20–50 ns), which allows imaging of living cells without interference from background autofluorescence. QDs overcome several disadvantages of fluorescence dyes, which have intriguing stability against photobleaching [309], large molar extinction coefficients, high quantum yield [310], and large surface-to-volume ratios.

An application of QDs as sensors exploits the fluorescence resonance energy transfer (FRET). QDs are promising FRET donors or acceptors. Because of their continuously tunable adsorption and emission, and high FRET efficiency which has been well-documented with QDs connected to various acceptors [311,312], complexes are made by grafting complementary bioconjugates, such as antibody–antigen pairs.

Goldman et al. [313] used CdSe/ZnS core or shell QDs functionalized with antibodies to perform multiplexed fluoroimmunoassays for simultaneously detecting four toxins (Figure 14.8). This type of sensor could be used for environmental purposes for simultaneously identifying pathogens (like cholera toxin or ricin) in water.

Besides immunoassays, optical biosensors based on QDs can also be used to detect proteins (e.g., NADH or GOD) and organic molecules (e.g., AA and cholesterol) that are related to fundamental biological processes. As an example, specific binding of different proteins was observed through measurements of FRET between a CdSe–ZnS QD donor, attached to one of the proteins, and some organic acceptor dyes attached to the other protein under study. In the presence of specific interactions between both proteins, strong enhancement of the acceptor-dye fluorescence was observed [312]. In a more fundamental study, conjugation of BSA with luminescent CdTe NPs (capped with L-cysteine) resulted in a significant increase in the CdTe fluorescent emission, attributed to an efficient resonance energy transfer from the tryptophan moieties of the protein units to the CdTe NPs acting as acceptors [314].

Magnetic NPs have also been used in sensor applications. They can be prepared in the form of superparamagnetic magnetite (Fe_3O_4), greigite (Fe_3S_4), Maghemite (γ-Fe_2O_3), and various types of ferrites (MeO·Fe_2O_3, where Me = Ni, Co, Mg, Zn, Mn, etc.) [315]. Since the late 1990s, magnetoelectronics [316] has emerged as one of the several new platform technologies for biosensor and

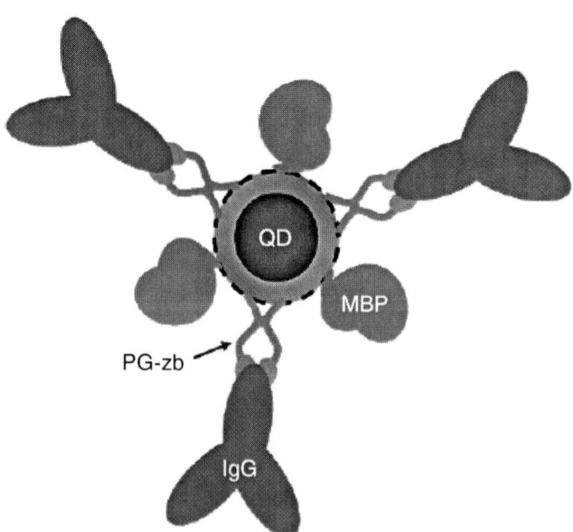

FIGURE 14.8 Cartoon of a mixed-surface QD conjugate. Both PG-zb adapter proteins binding antibodies through their Fc domain and MBPzb purification tool proteins are shown conjugated to the QD. (From Goldman, E.R., Clapp, A.R., Anderson, G.P., Uyeda, H.T., Mauro, J.M., Medintz, I.L., and Mattoussi, H., *Anal. Chem.*, 76, 684, 2004. With permission.)

biochip development. This technology is based on the detection of biologically functionalized micrometer- or nanometer-sized magnetic labels using high-sensitivity microfabricated magnetic field sensors. Although in its infancy, this technology offers high-sensitivity detection (to the level of a single molecular interaction, in principle), a stable labeling system, low-magnetic background, and cheap device components. Magnetic NPs have been widely used for the construction of biological assay systems, such as DNA hybridization [317] and ligand–receptor reactions [318,319].

Chemla et al. [320] developed a new technique for detecting biological targets using antibodies labeled with magnetic NPs. This technique uses a highly sensitive superconducting quantum interference device (SQUID) that only detected the antigen–antibody magnetic NPs. The NPs unlabeled to the antigen were not detected because they relax rapidly by Brownian rotation after pulses of magnetic fields were applied and do not contribute measurable signal. In this way, the ability to distinguish between bound and unbound labels enables homogeneous assays to be run without the need to separate and remove the unbounded particles.

Because of their unique physical (structural, electronic, magnetic, and optical) and chemical (catalytic) properties, NPs and their biosensor applications can be used in a variety of ways. NPs, including metals, semiconductors, and magnetic particles, have proved extremely useful in the preparation of optical sensors, electrochemical biosensors of DNA, enzymes, and proteins. Electrochemical biosensors based on nanoparticles have been widely investigated, as summarized in many elaborate reviews [321–324].

14.2.3.3 Nanoporous Materials in Biosensors

In addition to the nanotubes and NPs, novel materials such as porous silicon (PS) [325], porous carbon [326], and porous Al_2O_3 membranes [327] with pore size compatible with the dimension of the chemical–biological agents have been used for biosensor applications.

PS is a well-characterized and versatile inorganic material produced through a galvanostatic, chemical, or photochemical etching procedure in the presence of HF [328]. Depending upon the etching conditions, PS has a very complex, anisotropic, and nanocrystalline architecture of high surface area. Pore formation occurs in a unidirectional manner from the surface into the bulk, leading to aligned pores and columnar silicon structures. The PS surface is hydrophobic and the functionalization of the surface renders it as a biomaterial.

The immobilization of catalyst molecules within the pores involves the reaction of a silane-coupling agent (3-aminopropyl) triethoxysilane with the PS surface (partially oxidized), followed by the addition of a catalyst solution, forming the "microreactors." The porous enzyme microreactors show a ≤ 350-fold increase in GOD activity over those fabricated with planar silicon surfaces [329] with the specific activity showing dependence upon the doping of the porous layer, the anodization current, and the depth of the porous matrix.

Novel porous active carbon has shown to be a good matrix for the construction of highly stable biosensors [330]. The high conductivity of this carbon material is ideal for the electrochemical signal transduction; meanwhile, its high porosity allows the adsorption of large molecules, such as polyelectrolyte–enzyme complexes without adverse effects on the activity of the enzyme. And at the same time, the porous active carbon allows for high enzyme loading without the need for any chemical treatment of the enzyme. This material has been used with great success for the construction of highly stable and reproducible glucose and lactate biosensors [330–332].

Porous alumina membrane is well-known as a template for the preparation of nanotubes, nanofibrils, and nanowires of different materials. It can be also employed in the construction of biosensors providing an available relatively high surface area for the retention of enzymes or related bioactive compounds and allowing the development of biosensors that show a good operational stability [327–334].

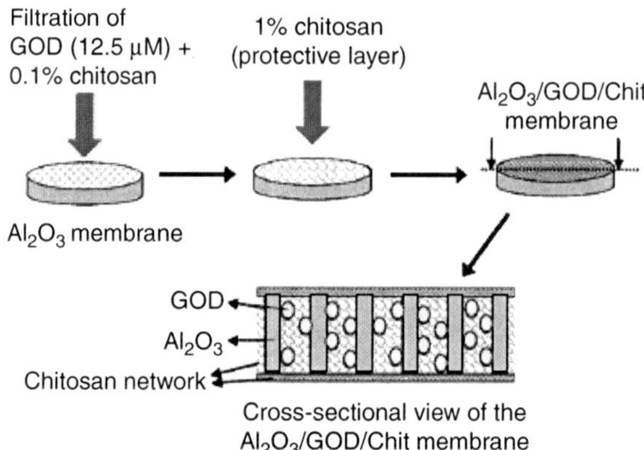

FIGURE 14.9 Immobilization of GOD in nanoporous alumina membranes. (From Darder, M., Aranda, P., Hernández-Vélez, M., Manova, E., and Ruiz-Hitzky, E., *Thin Solid Films*, 495, 321, 2006. With permission.)

Darder et al. [335] (Figure 14.9) reported a glucose biosensor employing porous alumina membrane as a matrix to immobilize GOD. In their work, nanoporous alumina membranes of different dimensions were made by electrochemical oxidation of aluminum in an acidic solution; these membranes were used to encapsulate GOD by procuring an external coverage with a thin layer of the biopolymer chitosan, which avoids enzyme leaching. The enzyme-modified membranes were then attached to the surface of a Pt electrode for the biosensor construction. The influence of membrane dimensions on the biosensor response was also studied.

14.2.4 FUNCTIONALIZED MONOLAYERS

Almost any surface can be modified by functionalized monolayers, which possess the desired specific electrical, optical, or chemical property. An ideal monolayer is described as perfectly aligned and closely packed alkane chains attached to a smooth surface. There are two kinds of functionalized monolayers, namely, LB membrane and SA monolayers. Such molecular assemblies have been demonstrated to be adapted for biosensor applications for the immobilization of biomolecules in a biomimetic environment.

14.2.4.1 Langmuir–Blodgett Membranes

The LB method is a powerful technique for transferring the Langmuir films at the air–water interface to a solid substrate. The Langmuir film is based on the particular properties of organic amphiphathic molecules such as lipids, phospholipids, or glycolipids. These organic molecules are composed of two distinct molecular regions: a hydrophilic ("water-loving") head group and a hydrophobic ("water-hating") tail group, which orient themselves at an air–water interface between the gaseous and the liquid phases, minimizing their free energy and forming an insoluble monolayer. For biological components, the tail groups are most often composed of one or two long alkyl chains.

The biosensors based on LB technology use an active film consisting of monolayers of an amphiphilic molecule in which the biomolecule is incorporated, and then the monolayer is transferred on a solid substrate to form one, two, or more mixed layers. The major interest in this technique is to create an organization of two components at the molecular scale; the very small thickness of such structures leads to biosensors with short response times.

The functionalization of LB films, conferring biospecificity, can be obtained by association (or insertion) of proteins, such as enzymes [336], antibodies [337], or specific ligands, presenting specific recognition properties. Insertion of enzyme molecules in LB films has been reported extensively

[338–340] and several bioactive proteins have been studied with regard to their potential applications in biosensing devices [341–343].

There are many advantages of LB films for making biosensors, such as orderly film on a molecular scale, short response time, one-step membrane fabrication, and biocompatible environment.

14.2.4.2 Self-Assembled Monolayers

As discussed in Section 14.2.1.1, on one hand, LB method is capable of transferring the monolayer from the air–water interface onto a solid support, and the multilayer could be formed by repetitive transfer, but those LB films are often thermodynamically unstable. On the other hand, self-assembled membrane (SAM) is not only thermodynamically stable but also capable of imprinting a desired function when assembling individual molecules into highly ordered architecture.

Molecular self-assembly is a key link among physics, chemistry, and biology, and it can be used to create novel nano- and microstructures, materials, and devices used in biosensors following the bottom-up procedure [344,345].

The term self-assembly involves the arrangement of atoms and molecules in an ordered form or even aggregation of functional entities without the intervention of humankind toward an energetically stable form [346]. Formation of an SAM is essentially an organization of molecules at solid–liquid interfaces induced by strong chemisorption between the substrate and the head group. The SAM offers several attractive features for its application of biosensors, such as molecular dimensions, high stability, good organization, and compatibility with metal substrates and biomolecules.

Many systems are capable of undergoing the process of self-assembly [347,348], for example, long chains of carboxylic acids ($C_nH_{2n+1}COOH$) at metal oxide substrates, organosilane species ($RSiX_3$, R_2SiX_2, or R_3SiX, where R is an alkyl chain and X a chloro- or alkoxygroup) at hydroxylated substrates such as glass, silicon, and aluminum oxide, and organosulfur-based species at noble metal surfaces. The last system has been most extensively used in biosensors because of its stability and physicochemical properties. Sulfur-containing compounds, for example, alkanethiols, dialkyl disulfides, and dialkyl sulfides, have a strong affinity for noble metal surfaces.

For Au electrodes, these films commonly consist of a methylene chain that has thiol functionality on one end that binds to the electrode and an organic functionality on the other end. SAM films have been used to immobilize proteins through covalent linkages [349], coordinative bonding [350], electrostatic attraction, [351] and hydrophobic interactions [352]. Electroactive end groups (for mediator or electron transfer function) of SAMs can be used as electrical wiring or for communication between the redox-active enzymes and the electrode surface.

The SAM films can also be used in the SPR sensors. Knoll et al. [353] used a variety of sulfur-containing compounds to create a wide range of biotinylated SA monolayers on Au surfaces, and the modified monolayers were then employed to bind streptavidin. Modification of biotin derivatives with long-chain hydroxythiols and dilution of the monolayer with short-chain alkanethiols are found to increase the effectiveness of binding to streptavidin.

14.2.5 Diamond

The biosensor development based on conductive diamond (sp^3-bonded) thin films is one of the frontiers of the integration of microelectronics technology and biotechnology in the very recent year [354,355]. Diamond possesses unparalleled properties including outstanding hardness, chemical robustness, and inertness with high thermal conductivity [356], as well as excellent electrical and optical properties [357]; moreover, diamond is also well-known for its biocompatibility and bioinertness [358,359]. These properties make it an ideal platform material for biointerfaces.

The diamond films on different substrates are obtained by CVD at reasonable cost, and the films can be made electrically conductive by selective incorporation of nitrogen or boron [360].

However, it is not possible to immobilize biomolecules directly because the deposited films are hydrophobic and chemically inert, so surface modification is necessary.

A variety of strategies have been developed for surface functionalization of the diamond thin films; one of them is the direct chemical or photochemical functionalization of the hydrogen-terminated surface [361–367]. In this approach, the hydrophobic hydrogen–terminated surfaces were functionalized either photochemically by UV excitation of halogen gases [362–364] or alkenes [361,367], thereby introducing chloro-, fluoro- or aminoalkyl groups, or chemically by reacting with the radical species generated from benzoyl peroxide [366]. Another commonly used approach is the application of pretreatment methods to introduce chemically reactive groups onto the films [368–372]. Some special techniques such as oxygen plasma treatment, anodic polarization, and the use of strong oxidizing acid are employed to introduce oxygen-containing functional groups onto the diamond film.

Tethering biomolecules is another important procedure for the whole biosensor fabrication. Yang et al. [361] described the attachment of DNA to nanocrystalline diamond (NCD) films using UV illumination (0.35 mW cm^{-2}, 254 nm). In their approach, vinyl groups of organic molecules were UV-linked to the hydrogen-terminated diamond surface. Applying a sulfosuccinimidyl 4-N-maleimidomethyl cyclohexane-1-carboxylate (SSMCC) cross-linker, thiol-modified DNA was subsequently tethered to hydrogen-terminated NCD films.

Enzymes such as GOD can also be immobilized onto conducting diamond films to form stable and sensitive biosensors. In the works of Wang et al. [373], GOD was attached to the ultrananocrystalline diamond (UNCD) surface by tethered aminophenyl functional moieties that were previously grafted to UNCD surface by electrochemical reduction of aryl diazonium salt. It causes less microstructure damage to diamond surface and has more stable C—C linkage at the interface compared with the surface oxidation approach in which the diamond surface is exposed to oxygen or other reactive gas plasmas.

Recent research shows that when diamond surfaces are covalently bonded to DNA or antibodies, the resulting biologically modified surfaces exhibit unusual chemical stability and perfect specificity in biomolecular recognition studies [374–376]. When bonded to enzymes such as redox enzymes, the whole system can exhibit excellent biocatalytic activity to analyte [373,377].

REFERENCES

1. Clark, L.C., Monitor and control of blood and tissue oxygen tensions, *Trans. Am. Soc. Artif. Intern. Organs*, 2, 41, 1956.
2. Stephen, A.W. and John, P.H., Chemically modified, carbon-based electrodes and their application as electrochemical sensors for the analysis of biologically important compounds: a review, *Analyst*, 117, 1215, 1992.
3. Updike, S.J. and Hicks, G.P., The enzyme electrode, *Nature*, 214, 986, 1967.
4. Swoboda, B.E.P. and Massey, V., Purification and properties of the glucose oxidase from *Aspergillus niger*, *J. Biol. Chem.*, 240, 2209, 1965.
5. Jones, M.N., Manley, P., and Wilkinson, A., The dissociation of glucose oxidase by sodium-n-dodecyl sulphate, *Biochem. J.*, 203, 285, 1982.
6. Leskovac, V. et al., Glucose oxidase from *Aspergillus niger*: the mechanism of action with molecular oxygen, quinones, and one-electron acceptors, *Int. J. Biochem. Cell. B.*, 37, 731, 2005.
7. Weibel, M. and Bright, H., The glucose oxidase mechanism, *J. Biol. Chem.*, 246, 2734, 1971.
8. Clark, L.C., The hydrogen peroxide sensing platinum anode as an analytical enzyme electrode, *Method. Enzymol.*, 56, 448, 1979.
9. Ianniello, R.M. and Yacynych, A.M., Immobilized enzyme chemically modified electrode as an amperometric sensor, *Anal. Chem.*, 53, 2090, 1981.
10. Marcos, S. et al., An optical glucose biosensor based on derived glucose oxidase immobilised onto a sol–gel matrix, *Sensor. Actuator. B Chem.*, 57, 227, 1999.
11. Fortier, G., Brassard, E., and Bélanger, D., Optimization of a polypyrrole glucose oxidase biosensor, *Biosens. Bioelectron.*, 5, 473, 1990.

12. Chen, Q. et al., β-Cyclodextrin cation exchange polymer membrane for improved second-generation glucose biosensors, *Anal. Chim. Acta*, 306, 201, 1995.

13. Yang, M.H. et al., Amperometric glucose biosensor based on chitosan with improved selectivity and stability, *Sensor. Actuator. B Chem.*, 101, 269, 2004.

14. Liu, G.D. and Lin, Y.H., Amperometric glucose biosensor based on self-assembling glucose oxidase on carbon nanotubes, *Electrochem. Commun.*, 8, 251, 2006.

15. Milardović, S. et al., Glucose determination in blood samples using flow injection analysis and an amperometric biosensor based on glucose oxidase immobilized on hexacyanoferrate modified nickel electrode, *Anal. Chim. Acta*, 350, 91, 1997.

16. Shankaran, D.R., Ueheara, N., and Kato, T., A metal dispersed sol–gel biocomposite amperometric glucose biosensor, *Biosens. Bioelectron.*, 18, 721, 2003.

17. Jorge, R.R., Enrique, L.C., and Beatriz, L.R., High stability amperometric biosensor based on enzyme entrapment in microgels, *Talanta*, 68, 99, 2005.

18. Chen, L.Q. et al., Genetic modification of glucose oxidase for improving performance of an amperometric glucose biosensor, *Biosens. Bioelectron.*, 17, 851, 2002.

19. Ferreira, M. et al., Enzyme-mediated amperometric biosensors prepared with the layer-by-layer (LbL) adsorption technique, *Biosens. Bioelectron.*, 19, 1611, 2004.

20. Yang, M.H. et al., Platinum nanowire nanoelectrode array for the fabrication of biosensors, *Biomater.*, 27, 5944, 2006.

21. Garjonyte, R. and Malinauskas, A., Amperometric glucose biosensor based on glucose oxidase immobilized in poly(*o*-phenylenediamine) layer, *Sensor. Actuator. B Chem.*, 56, 85, 1999.

22. Nagata, R. et al., Amperometric glucose biosensor manufactured by a printing technique, *Anal. Chim. Acta*, 304, 157, 1995.

23. Marek, T. and Hitchman, M.L., A potentiometric polypyrrole-based glucose biosensor, *Electroanalysis*, 8, 263, 1996.

24. Karyakin, A.A. et al., The improved potentiometric pH response of electrodes modified with processible polyaniline: application to glucose biosensor, *Anal. Commun.*, 36, 153, 1999.

25. Martin, M.F. et al., An optical glucose biosensor with eggshell membrane as an enzyme immobilisation platform, *Analyst*, 126, 1558, 2001.

26. Yang, X.F. et al., A fluorescent glucose biosensor based on immobilized glucose oxidase on bamboo inner shell membrane, *Biosens. Bioelectron.*, 21, 1613, 2006.

27. Tomasz, L. et al., Prussian blue-based optical glucose biosensor in flow-injection analysis, *Anal. Chim. Acta*, 447, 23, 2001.

28. Wu, X.J. and Choi, M.M.F., An optical glucose biosensor based on entrapped-glucose oxidase in silicate xerogel hybridised with hydroxyethyl carboxymethyl cellulose, *Anal. Chim. Acta*, 514, 219, 2004.

29. Göktuğ, T., Sezgintürk, M.K., and Dinçkaya, E., Glucose oxidase-β-galactosidase hybrid biosensor based on glassy carbon electrode modified with mercury for lactose determination, *Anal. Chim. Acta*, 551, 51, 2005.

30. Flegg, H.M., An investigation of the determination of serum cholesterol by an enzymatic method, *Ann. Clin. Biochem.*, 10, 79, 1973.

31. Richmond, W., The development of an enzymatic technique for the assay of cholesterol in biological fluids, *Scand. J. Clin. Lab. Inv.*, 29, 25, 1972.

32. Richmond, W., Preparation and properties of a bacterial cholesterol oxidase from *Nocardia* sp. and its application to enzyme assay of total cholesterol in serum, *Clin. Chem.*, 19, 1350, 1973.

33. Joseph, K., Lefebvre, G., and Germain, P., Membrane-bound cholesterol oxidase from *Rhodococcus* sp. cells: production and extraction, *J. Biotechnol.*, 33, 271, 1994.

34. Li, J.P., Peng, T.Z., and Peng, Y.Q., A cholesterol biosensor based on entrapment of cholesterol oxidase in a silicic sol–gel matrix at a Prussian blue modified electrode, *Electroanalysis*, 15, 1031, 2003.

35. Sean, B., Dyer, N., and Anthony, G.E., Amperometric determination of cholesterol in serum using a biosensor of cholesterol oxidase contained within a polypyrrole–hydrogel membrane, *Anal. Chim. Acta*, 448, 27, 2001.

36. Arya, S.K. et al., Application of octadecanethiol self-assembled monolayer to cholesterol biosensor based on surface plasmon resonance technique, *Talanta*, 69, 918, 2006.

37. Manoj, K.R. et al., Cholesterol biosensors prepared by layer-by-layer technique, *Biosens. Bioelectron.*, 16, 849, 2001.

38. Yan, Y.H., Xu, Y.H., and Li, S.P., Development of fiber optical biosensor of cholesterol based on fluorescence quenching, *Chin. J. Biomed. Eng.*, 23, 44, 2004.

39. Trettnak, W. and Wolfbeis, O.S., A fiberoptic cholesterol biosensor with an oxygen optrode as the transducer, *Anal. Biochem.*, 184, 124, 1990.

40. Motonaka, J. and Faulkner, L.R., Determination of cholesterol and cholesterol ester with novel enzyme microsensors, *Anal. Chem.*, 65, 3258, 1993.

41. Krug, A., Suleiman, A.A., and Guilbault, G.G., Enzyme-based fiber-optic device for the determination of total and free cholesterol, *Anal. Chim. Acta*, 256, 263, 1992.

42. Singh, S. et al., Covalent immobilization of cholesterol esterase and cholesterol oxidase on polyaniline films for application to cholesterol biosensor, *Anal. Chim. Acta*, 568, 126, 2006.

43. Karube, I. et al., Amperometric determination of total cholesterol in serum with use of immobilized cholesterol esterase and cholesterol oxidase, *Anal. Chim. Acta*, 139, 127, 1982.

44. Anon., Cholesterol oxidase and pollution, *Biofutur*, 138, 11, 1994.

45. Gómez, J.L. et al., Purification and properties of hydrophilic dimers of acetylcholinesterase from mouse erythrocytes, *Int. J. Biochem. Cell. B.*, 35, 1109, 2003.

46. Leuzinger, W., Goldberg, M., and Cauvin, E., Molecular properties of acetylcholinesterase, *J. Mol. Biol.*, 40, 217, 1969.

47. Yamada, H., Mori, N., and Tani, Y., Properties of choline oxidase of *Cylindrocarpon didymium* M-1. *Agr. Biol. Chem.*, 43, 2173, 1979.

48. Ohta-Fukuyama, M. et al., Identification and properties of the prosthetic group of choline oxidase from *Alcaligenes sp.*, *J. Biochem.-Tokyo*, 88, 197, 1980.

49. Ikuta, S. et al., Purification and characterization of choline oxidase from *Arthrobacter globiformis*, *J. Biochem.-Tokyo*, 82, 1741, 1977.

50. Cavener, D.R., GMC oxidoreductases: a newly defined family of homologous proteins with diverse catalytic activities, *J. Mol. Biol.*, 223, 811, 1992.

51. Fan, F., Ghanem, M., and Gadda, G., Cloning, sequence analysis, and purification of choline oxidase from *Arthrobacter globiformis*: a bacterial enzyme involved in osmotic stress tolerance, *Arch. Biochem. Biophys.*, 421, 149, 2004.

52. Vakurov, A. et al., Acetylcholinesterase-based biosensor electrodes for organophosphate pesticide detection, *Biosens. Bioelectron.*, 20, 1118, 2004.

53. Liu, G.D. and Lin, Y.H., Biosensor based on self-assembling acetylcholinesterase on carbon nanotubes for flow injection/amperometric detection of organophosphate pesticides and nerve agents, *Anal. Chem.*, 78, 835, 2006.

54. Francis, C.M. et al., An optical biosensor for dichlovos using stacked sol–gel films containing acetylcholinesterase and a lipophilic chromoionophore, *Talanta*, 69, 888, 2006.

55. Liu, B. et al., A potentiometric acetylcholinesterase biosensor based on plasma-polymerized film, *Sensor. Actuator. B Chem.*, 104, 186, 2005.

56. Kok, F.N. and Hasirci, V., Determination of binary pesticide mixtures by an acetylcholinesterase-choline oxidase biosensor, *Biosens. Bioelectron.*, 19, 661, 2004.

57. Doretti, L. et al., Acetylcholine biosensor involving entrapment of acetylcholinesterase and poly(ethylene glycol)-modified choline oxidase in a poly(vinyl alcohol) cryogel membrane, *Enzym. Microb. Tech.*, 27, 279, 2000.

58. Huang, Z.X. et al., Development of choline and acetylcholine pt microelectrodes, *Anal. Biochem.*, 215, 31, 1993.

59. Lin, Y.H., Lu, F., and Wang, J., Disposable carbon nanotube modified screen-printed biosensor for amperometric detection of organophosphorus pesticides and nerve agents, *Electroanalysis*, 16, 145, 2004.

60. Ciucu, A.A., Negulescu, C., and Baldwin, R.P., Detection of pesticides using an amperometric biosensor based on ferophthalocyanine chemically modified carbon paste electrode and immobilized bioenzymatic system, *Biosens. Bioelectron.*, 18, 303, 2003.

61. Veitch, N.C., Horseradish peroxidase: a modern view of a classic enzyme, *Phytochemistry*, 65, 249, 2004.

62. Hewson, W.D. and Hager, L.P., Peroxidase, catalases and chloroperoxidases. In Dolphin, D. (Ed.), *The Porphyrins*, Chap. 6, Academic Press, New York, 1979.

63. Yang, S.M. et al., Horseradish peroxidase biosensor based on layer-by-layer technique for the determination of phenolic compounds, *Sensor. Actuator. B Chem.*, 114, 774, 2006.

64. Yu, D.H. et al., Amperometric biosensor based on horseradish peroxidase-immobilised magnetic microparticles, *Sensor. Actuator. B Chem.*, 113, 749, 2006.

65. Chen, J. et al., Reagentless amperometric immunosensor for human chorionic gonadotropin based on direct electrochemistry of horseradish peroxidase, *Biosens. Bioelectron.*, 21, 330, 2005.

66. Shan, D., Cosnier, S., and Mousty, C., HRP/[Zn–Cr–ABTS] redox clay-based biosensor: design and optimization for cyanide detection, *Biosens. Bioelectron.*, 20, 390, 2004.

67. Liu, X.J. et al., Enhanced electron-transfer reactivity of horseradish peroxidase in phosphatidylcholine films and its catalysis to nitric oxide, *J. Biotechnol.*, 108, 145, 2004.

68. Castilho, T.J., Sotomayor, M.P.T., and Kubota, L.T., Amperometric biosensor based on horseradish peroxidase for biogenic amine determinations in biological samples, *J. Pharmaceut. Biomed.*, 37, 785, 2005.

69. Yang, Y.H. et al., An amperometric horseradish peroxidase inhibition biosensor based on a cysteamine self-assembled monolayer for the determination of sulfides, *Sensor. Actuator. B Chem.*, 102, 162, 2004.

70. Razola, S.S. et al., Hydrogen peroxide sensitive amperometric biosensor based on horseradish peroxidase entrapped in a polypyrrole electrode, *Biosens. Bioelectron.*, 17, 921, 2002.

71. Díaz, A.N., Peinado, M.C.R., and Minguez, M.C.T., Sol–gel horseradish peroxidase biosensor for hydrogen peroxide detection by chemiluminescence, *Anal. Chim. Acta*, 363, 221, 1998.

72. Shin, M.C., Yoon, H.C., and Kim, S., *In situ* biochemical reduction of interference in an amperometric biosensor with a novel heterobilayer configuration of polypyrrole/glucose oxidase/horseradish peroxidase, *Anal. Chim. Acta*, 329, 223, 1996.

73. Kumar, A. et al., Co-immobilization of cholesterol oxidase and horseradish peroxidase in a sol–gel film, *Anal. Chim. Acta*, 414, 43, 2000.

74. Li, H.Q. et al., An amperometric bienzyme biosensor for rapid measurement of alanine aminotransferase in whole blood, *Sensor. Actuator. B Chem.*, 119, 419, 2006.

75. Saha, A., Mandal, P.C., and Bhattacharyya, S.N., Radiation induced inactivation of enzymes—a review, *Radiat. Phys. Chem.*, 46, 123, 1995.

76. Catherine, M. et al., Immobilisation of lactate dehydrogenase on poly(aniline)–poly(acrylate) and poly(aniline)–poly-(vinyl sulphonate) films for use in a lactate biosensor, *Anal. Chim. Acta*, 453, 191, 2002.

77. Shu, H.C. and Wu, N.P., A chemically modified carbon paste electrode with D-lactate dehydrogenase and alanine aminotransferase enzyme sequences for D-lactic acid analysis, *Talanta*, 54, 361, 2001.

78. Warriner, K., Higson, S., and Vadgama, P., A lactate dehydrogenase amperometric pyruvate electrode exploiting direct detection of NAD^+ at a poly(3-methylthiophene): poly(phenol red) modified platinum surface, *Mater. Sci. Eng. C*, 5, 91, 1997.

79. Gerard, M. et al., Immobilization of lactate dehydrogenase on electrochemically prepared polyaniline films, *Electroanalysis*, 11, 450, 1999.

80. Jena, B.K. and Raj, C.R., Electrochemical biosensor based on integrated assembly of dehydrogenase enzymes and gold nanoparticles, *Anal. Chem.*, 78, 6332, 2006.

81. Gennis, R.B. and Hager, L.P., Pyruvate oxidase. In *The Enzymes of Biological Membranes*, Plennum Publishing Corp., New York, 1976.

82. Zapata, B.A.M., and Burstein, C., Enzyme electrode composed of the pyruvate oxidase from *Pediococcus* species coup led to an oxygen electrode for measurements of pyruvate in biological media, *Biosensors*, 3, 227, 1987.

83. Ngo, T.T., Single-enzyme-based amperometric assay for phosphate ion, *Appl. Biochem. Biotech.*, 13, 1272, 1986.

84. Kwan, R.C.H., Hon, P.Y.T., and Renneberg, R., Amperometric biosensor for rapid determination of alanine, *Anal. Chim. Acta*, 523, 81, 2004.

85. Arima, J. et al., Cloning of an L-glutamate oxidase gene from *Streptomyces* sp. X119-6 and its expression in *Escherichia coli*, In *Proceedings of The 18th Symposium on Trace Nutrients Research*, 2001.

86. Pan, S.T. and Arnold, M.A., Selectivity enhancement for glutamate with a naifon/glutamate oxidase biosensor, *Talanta*, 43, 1157, 1996.

87. Zhang, M.G., Mullens, C., and Gorski, W., Amperometric glutamate biosensor based on chitosan enzyme film, *Electrochim. Acta*, 51, 4528, 2006.

88. Jain, R.K., Dreisbach, J.H., and Spain, J.C., Biodegradation of *p*-nitrophenol via 1,2,4-benzenetriol by an *Arthrobacter* sp., *Appl. Environ. Microbiol.*, 60, 3030, 1994.

89. Leung, K.T. et al., Mineralization of *p*-nitrophenol by pentachlorophenol-degrading *Sphingomonas* spp., *FEMS Microbiol. Lett.*, 155, 107, 1997.

90. Spain, J.C. and Nishino, S.F., Degradation of 1,4-dichlorobenzene by a *Pseudomonas* sp., *Appl. Environ. Microbiol.*, 53, 1010, 1987.

91. Rensing, C. and Maier, R.M., Issues underlying use of biosensors to measure metal bioavailability, *Ecotoxicol. Environ. Saf.*, 56, 140, 2003.

92. Belkin, S., Microbial whole-cell sensing systems of environmental pollutants, *Curr. Opin. Microbiol.*, 6, 206, 2003.

93. Lei, Y., Chen, W., and Mulchandani, A., Microbial biosensors, *Anal. Chim. Acta*, 568, 200, 2006.

94. Rainina, E.I. et al., The development of a new biosensor based on recombinant *Escherichia coli* for the direct-detection of organophosphorus neurotoxins, *Biosens. Bioelectron.*, 11, 991, 1996.

95. Biran, I. et al., Online and *in situ* monitoring of environmental pollutants: electrochemical biosensing of cadmium, *Environ. Microbiol.*, 2, 285, 2000.

96. Jia, J.B. et al., Co-immobilized microbial biosensor for BOD estimation based on sol/gel derived composite material, *Biosens. Bioelectron.*, 18, 1023, 2003.

97. Tan, T.C. and Qian, Z.R., Dead *Bacillus subtilis* cells for sensing biochemical oxygen demand of waters and wastewaters, *Sensor. Actuator. B Chem.*, 40, 65, 1997.

98. Tan, T.C., Li, F., and Neoh, K.G., Microbial membrane modified dissolved oxygen probe for rapid biochemical oxygen demand measurement, *Sensor. Actuator. B Chem.*, 8, 167, 1992.

99. Suriyawattanakul, L. et al., The use of co-immobilization of *Trichosporon cutaneum* and *Bacillus licheniformis* for a BOD sensor, *Appl. Microbiol. Biotechnol.*, 59, 40, 2002.

100. Jiang, Y.Q. et al., Optical biosensor for the determination of BOD in seawater, *Talanta*, 70, 97, 2006.

101. Tkáč, J. et al., Determination of total sugars in lignocellulose hydrolysate by a mediated *Gluconobacter oxydans* biosensor, *Anal. Chim. Acta*, 420, 1, 2000.

102. Reshetilov, A.N. et al., FET-microbial sensor for xylose detection based on *Gluconobacter oxydans* cells, *Biosens. Bioelectron.*, 11, 401, 1996.

103. Reshetilov, A.N. et al., Evaluation of a *Gluconobacter oxydans* whole cell biosensor for amperometric detection of xylose, *Biosens. Bioelectron.*, 12, 241, 1997.

104. Han, T.S. et al., Microbial sensor for trichloroethylene determination, *Anal. Chim. Acta*, 431, 225, 2001.

105. Elasriá, M.O. and Miller, R.V., A *Pseudomonas aeruginosa* biosensor responds to exposure to ultraviolet radiation, *Appl. Microbiol. Biotechnol.*, 50, 455, 1998.

106. Ohfuji, K. et al., Construction of a glucose sensor based on a screen-printed electrode and a novel mediator pyocyanin from *Pseudomonas aeruginosa*, *Biosens. Bioelectron.*, 19, 1237, 2004.

107. King, J.M.H. et al., Rapid, sensitive bioluminescent reporter technology for naphthalene exposure and biodegradation, *Science*, 249, 778, 1990.

108. Burlage, R.S., Sayler, G.S., and Larimer, F., Monitoring of naphthalene catabolism by bioluminescence with *nah-lux* transcriptional fusions, *J. Bacteriol.*, 172, 4749, 1990.

109. Trögl, J. et al., Selectivity of whole cell optical biosensor with immobilized bioreporter *Pseudomonas fluorescens* HK44, *Sensor. Actuator. B Chem.*, 107, 98, 2005.

110. Webb, O.F. et al., Kinetics and response of a *Pseudomonas fluorescens* HK44 biosensor, *Biotechnol. Bioeng.*, 54, 491, 1997.

111. Takayama, K., Ikeda, T., and Nagasawa, T., Mediated amperometric biosensor for nicotinic acid based on whole cells of *Pseudomonas fluorescens*, *Electroanalysis*, 8, 765, 1996.

112. Chee, G.J., Nomura, Y., and Karube, I., Biosensor for the estimation of low biochemical oxygen demand, *Anal. Chim. Acta*, 379, 185, 1999.

113. Lanyon, Y.H. et al., Flow injection analysis of benzene using an amperometric bacterial biosensor, *Anal. Lett.*, 37, 1515, 2004.

114. Rasinger, J.D. et al., Evaluation of an FIA operated amperometric bacterial biosensor, based on *Pseudomonas putida* F1 for the detection of benzene, toluene, ethylbenzene, and xylenes (BTEX), *Anal. Lett.*, 10, 1531, 2005.

115. Minnan, L. et al., Isolation and characterization of a high H2-producing strain *klebsiella oxytoca* HP1 from a hot spring, *Res. Microbiol.*, 156, 76, 2005.

116. Ohki, A. et al., BOD sensor using *klebsiella oxytoca* AS1, *Int. J. Environ. Anal. Chem.*, 56, 261, 1994.

117. Kim, M.N. and Kwon, H.S., Biochemical oxygen demand sensor using *Serratia marcescens* LSY 4, *Biosens. Bioelectron.*, 14, 1, 1999.

118. Emelyanova, E.V. and Reshetilov, A.N., *Rhodococcus erythropolis* as the receptor of cell-based sensor for 2,4-dinitrophenol detection: effect of 'co-oxidation', *Process Biochem.*, 37, 683, 2002.

119. Yang, Z. et al., Fabrication of oxygen electrode arrays and their incorporation into sensors for measuring biochemical oxygen demand, *Anal. Chim. Acta*, 357, 41, 1997.

120. Yano, Y. et al., Application of a microbial sensor to the quality control of meat freshness, *Talanta*, 54, 255, 2001.

121. Lehmann, M. et al., Amperometric measurement of copper ions with a deputy substrate using a novel *Saccharomyces cerevisiae* sensor, *Biosens. Bioelectron.*, 15, 211, 2000.

122. Zyracka, E. et al., Yeast as a biosensor for antioxidants: simple growth tests employing a *Saccharomyces cerevisiae* mutant defective in superoxide dismutase, *Acta. Biochim. Pol.*, 52, 679, 2005.

123. Middelhoven, W.J., De Jong, I.M., and De Winter, M., *Arxula adeninivorans*, a yeast assimilating many nitrogenous and aromatic compounds, *Anton. Leeuw. Int. J. G.*, 59, 129, 1991.

124. Riedel, K. et al., *Arxula adeninivorans* based sensor for the estimation of BOD, *Anal. Lett.*, 31, 1, 1998.

125. Chan, C.Y. et al., Measurement of biodegradable substances using the salt-tolerant yeast *Arxula adeninivorans* for a microbial sensor immobilized with poly(carbamoyl) sulfonate (PCS) part I: construction and characterization of the microbial sensor, *Biosens. Bioelectron.*, 14, 131, 1999.

126. Lehmann, M. et al., Measurement of biodegradable substances using the salt-tolerant yeast *Arxula adeninivorans* for a microbial sensor immobilized with poly(carbamoyl)sulfonate (PCS)—part II: application of the novel biosensor to real samples from coastal and island regions, *Biosens. Bioelectron.*, 14, 295, 1999.

127. Sugandhi, G. et al., *Torulopsis candida* based sensor for the estimation of biochemical oxygen demand and its evaluation, *Electroanalysis*, 8, 698, 1996.

128. Reshetilov, A.N. et al., Characteristics of *Gluconobacter oxydans* B-1280 and *pichia methanolica* MN4 cell based biosensors for detection of ethanol, *Process Biochem.*, 36, 1015, 2001.

129. http://ghr.nlm.nih.gov/handbook/basics/dna

130. Liu, A.H. and Anzai, J.I., Use of polymeric indicator for electrochemical DNA sensors: poly(4-vinylpyridine) derivative bearing [Os(5,6-dimethyl-1,10-phenanthroline)2Cl]$^{2+}$, *Anal. Chem.*, 76, 2975, 2004.

131. Wang, S.G. et al., DNA biosensors based on self-assembled carbon nanotubes, *Biochem. Bioph. Res. Commun.*, 325, 1433, 2004.

132. Watts, H.J., Yeung, D., and Parkes, H., Real-time detection and quantification of DNA hybridization by an optical biosensor, *Anal. Chem.*, 67, 4283, 1995.

133. Zhang, H. et al., Bovine serum albumin as a means to immobilize DNA on a silver-plated bulk acoustic wave DNA biosensor, *Talanta*, 46, 171, 1998.

134. Lazerges, M. et al., *In situ* QCM DNA-biosensor probe modification, *Sensor. Actuator. B.Chem.*, 120, 329, 2006.

135. Brett, A.M.O. et al., Voltammetric behaviour of mitoxantrone at a DNA-biosensor, *Biosens. Bioelectron.*, 13, 861, 1998.

136. Chiti, G., Marrazza, G., and Mascini, M., Electrochemical DNA biosensor for environmental monitoring, *Anal. Chim. Acta*, 427, 155, 2001.

137. Kerman, K. et al., Electrochemical DNA biosensor for the determination of benzo[a] pyrene–DNA adducts, *Anal. Chim. Acta*, 450, 45, 2001.

138. Breimer, M.A., Gelfand, Y., and Sadik, O.A., Integrated capillary fluorescence DNA biosensor, *Biosens. Bioelectron.*, 18, 1135, 2003.

139. Babkina, S.S., Ulakhovich, N.A., and Zyavkina, Y.I., Amperometric DNA biosensor for the determination of auto-antibodies using DNA interaction with pt(II) complex, *Anal. Chim. Acta*, 502, 23, 2004.

140. Guilbault, G.G., Hock, B., and Schmid, R., A piezoelectric immunobiosensor for atrazine in drinking water, *Biosens. Bioelectron.*, 7, 411, 1992.

141. Suri, C.R., Rajem, M., and Mishra, G.C., Determination of immunoglobulin M concentration by piezoelectric crystal immunobiosensor coated with protamine, *Biosens. Bioelectron.*, 9, 535, 1994.

142. Tsai, W.C. and Lin, I.C., Development of a piezoelectric immunosensor for the detection of alpha-fetoprotein, *Sensor. Actuator. B Chem.*, 106, 455, 2005.

143. Gao, H. et al., Electrochemical immunoassay of estrone at an antibody-modified conducting polymer electrode towards immunobiosensors, *J. Electroanal. Chem.*, 592, 88, 2006.

144. Messina, G.A. et al., Continuous-flow/stopped-flow system using an immunobiosensor for quantification of human serum IgG antibodies to *Helicobacter pylori*, *Anal. Biochem.*, 337, 195, 2005.

145. Wu, J. et al., A disposable electrochemical immunosensor for flow injection immunoassay of carcinoembryonic antigen, *Biosens. Bioelectron.*, 22, 102, 2006.

146. Elliott, C.T. et al., The development of a rapid immunobiosensor screening method for the detection of residues of sulphadiazine, *Food Agr. Immunol.*, 11, 19, 1999.

147. Park, I.S. and Kim, N., Development of a chemiluminescent immunosensor for chloramphenicol, *Anal. Chim. Acta*, 578, 19, 2006.

148. Marquette, C.A. and Blum, L.J., Regenerable immunobiosensor for the chemiluminescent flow injection analysis of the herbicide 2,4-D, *Talanta*, 51, 395, 2000.

149. Lee, W. et al., Nanoscale fabrication of protein on self-assembled monolayer and its application to surface plasmon resonance immunosensor, *Enzym. Microb. Tech.*, 35, 678, 2004.

150. Samsonova, J.V., Determination of ivermectin in bovine liver by optical immunobiosensor, *Biosens. Bioelectron.*, 17, 523, 2002.

151. Iijima, S., Helical microtubules of graphitic carbon, *Nature*, 354, 56, 1991.

152. Ebbesen, T.W. et al., Electrical conductivity of individual carbon nanotubes, *Nature*, 382, 54, 1996.

153. Iijima, S. and Ichihashi, T., Single-shell carbon nanotubes of 1 nm diameter, *Nature*, 363, 603, 1993.

154. Chen, R.S. et al., Carbon fiber nanoelectrodes modified by single-walled carbon nanotubes, *Anal. Chem.*, 75, 6341, 2003.

155. Moore, R.R., Banks, C.E., and Compton, R.G., Basal plane pyrolytic graphite modified electrodes: comparison of carbon nanotubes and graphite powder as electrocatalysts, *Anal. Chem.*, 76, 2677, 2004.

156. Gong, K.P. et al., Sol–gel-derived ceramic-carbon nanotube nanocomposite electrodes: tunable electrode dimension and potential electrochemical applications, *Anal. Chem.*, 76, 6500, 2004.

157. Niyogi, S. et al., Chemistry of single-walled carbon nanotubes, *Acc. Chem. Res.*, 35, 1105, 2002.

158. Ajayan, P.M., Nanotubes from carbon, *Chem. Rev.*, 99, 1787, 1999.

159. Odom, T.W. et al., Structure and electronic properties of carbon nanotubes, *J. Phys. Chem. B*, 104, 2794, 2000.

160. Merkoçi, A. et al., New materials for electrochemical sensing VI: carbon nanotubes, *Trends Anal. Chem.*, 24, 826, 2005.

161. Liu, J. et al., Fullerene pipes, *Science*, 280, 1253, 1998.

162. Koshio, A. et al., A simple way to chemically react single-wall carbon nanotubes with organic materials using ultrasonication, *Nano Lett.*, 1, 361, 2001.

163. Hiura, H., Ebbesen, T.W., and Tanigaki, K., Opening and purification of carbon nanotubes in high yields, *Adv. Mater.*, 7, 275, 1995.

164. Kuznetsova, A. et al., Oxygen-containing functional groups on single-wall carbon nanotubes: NEXAFS and vibrational spectroscopic studies, *J. Am. Chem. Soc.*, 123, 10699, 2001.

165. Joshi, P.P. et al., Amperometric biosensors based on redox polymer-carbon nanotube-enzyme composites, *Anal. Chem.*, 77, 3183, 2005.

166. Lin, Y. et al., Advances toward bioapplications of carbon nanotubes, *J. Mater. Chem.*, 14, 527, 2004.

167. Musameh, M. et al., Low-potential stable NADH detection at carbon-nanotube-modified glassy carbon electrodes, *Electrochem. Commun.*, 4, 743, 2002.

168. Gan, Z.H. et al., Electrochemical studies of single-wall carbon nanotubes as nanometer-sized activators in enzyme-catalyzed reaction, *Anal. Chim. Acta*, 511, 239, 2004.

169. Luo, H.X. et al., Investigation of the electrochemical and electrocatalytic behavior of single-wall carbon nanotube film on a glassy carbon electrode, *Anal. Chem.*, 73, 915, 2001.

170. Wu, K.B., Fei, J.J., and Hu, S.S., Simultaneous determination of dopamine and serotonin on a glassy carbon electrode coated with a film of carbon nanotubes, *Anal. Biochem.*, 318, 100, 2003.

171. Wang, J.X. et al., Direct electrochemistry of cytochrome c at a glassy carbon electrode modified with single-wall carbon nanotubes, *Anal. Chem.*, 74, 1993, 2002.

172. Cai, C.X. and Chen, J., Direct electron transfer of glucose oxidase promoted by carbon nanotubes, *Anal. Biochem.*, 332, 75, 2004.

173. Duro, R. et al., Interfacial adsorption of polymers and surfactants: implications for the properties of disperse systems of pharmaceutical interest, *Drug Dev. Ind. Pharm.*, 1999, 25, 817.

174. O'Connell, M.J. et al., Reversible water-solubilization of single-walled carbon nanotubes by polymer wrapping, *Chem. Phys. Lett.*, 342, 265, 2001.

175. Lisunova, M.O. et al., Stability of the aqueous suspensions of nanotubes in the presence of nonionic surfactant, *J. Colloid Interface Sci.*, 299, 740, 2006.

176. Bandyopadhyaya, R. et al., Stabilization of individual carbon nanotubes in aqueous solutions, *Nano Lett.*, 2, 25, 2002.

177. Wang, H. et al., Shear-SANS study of single-walled carbon nanotube suspensions, *Chem. Phys. Lett.*, 416, 182, 2005.

178. Islam, M.F. et al., High weight fraction surfactant solubilization of single-wall carbon nanotubes in water, *Nano Lett.*, 3, 269, 2003.

179. Moore, V.C. et al., Individually suspended single-walled carbon nanotubes in various surfactants, *Nano Lett.*, 3, 1379, 2003.
180. Wang, J., Musameh, M., and Lin, Y.H., Solubilization of carbon nanotubes by nafion toward the preparation of amperometric biosensors, *J. Am. Chem. Soc.*, 125, 2408, 2003.
181. Fan, Z. and Harrison, D.J., Permeability of glucose and other neutral species through recast perfluorosulfonated ionomer films, *Anal. Chem.*, 64, 1304, 1992.
182. Fortier, G., Vaillancourt, M., and Belanger, D., Evaluation of nafion as media for glucose oxidase immobilization for the development of an amperometric glucose biosensor, *Electroanalysis*, 4, 275, 1992.
183. McCreery, L., In Bard, A.J. (Ed.), *Electroanalytical Chemistry*, vol. 17, 221, Marcel Dekker, New York, USA, 1991.
184. Lin, Y.H. et al., Glucose biosensors based on carbon nanotube nanoelectrode ensembles, *Nano Lett.*, 4, 191, 2004.
185. Liu, Z. et al., Organizing single-walled carbon nanotubes on gold using a wet chemical self-assembling technique, *Langmuir*, 16, 3569, 2000.
186. Sotiropoulou, S. and Chaniotakis, N.A., Carbon nanotube array-based biosensor, *Anal. Bioanal. Chem.*, 375, 103, 2003.
187. Nugent, J.M. et al., Fast electron transfer kinetics on multiwalled carbon nanotube microbundle electrodes, *Nano Lett.*, 1, 87, 2001.
188. Boo, H. et al., Electrochemical nanoneedle biosensor based on multiwall carbon nanotube, *Anal. Chem.*, 78, 617, 2006.
189. Kim, K.S. et al., *In situ* manipulation and characterization using nanomanipulator inside field emission-scanning electron microscope, *Rev. Sci. Instrum.*, 74, 4021, 2003.
190. Britto, P.J., Santhanam, K.S.V., and Ajayan, P.M., Carbon nanotube electrode for oxidation of dopamine, *Bioelectrochem. Bioenerg.*, 41, 121, 1996.
191. Valentini, F. et al., Carbon nanotube purification: preparation and characterization of carbon nanotube paste electrodes, *Anal. Chem.*, 75, 5413, 2003.
192. Wang, J. and Musameh, M., Carbon nanotube/teflon composite electrochemical sensors and biosensors, *Anal. Chem.*, 75, 2075, 2003.
193. Pumera, M., Merkoçi, A., and Alegret, S., Carbon nanotube-epoxy composites for electrochemical sensing, *Sensor. Actuator. B Chem.*, 113, 617, 2005.
194. Trojanowicz, M., Mulchandani, A., and Mascini, M., Carbon nanotubes-modified screen-printed electrodes for chemical sensors and biosensors, *Anal. Lett.*, 37, 3185, 2004.
195. Balavoine, F. et al., Helical crystallization of proteins on carbon nanotubes: a first step towards the development of new biosensors, *Angew. Chem. Int. Ed.*, 38, 1912, 1999.
196. Chen, R.J. et al., Noncovalent sidewall functionalization of single-walled carbon nanotubes for protein immobilization, *J. Am. Chem. Soc.*, 123, 3838, 2001.
197. Chen, R.J. et al., Noncovalent functionalization of carbon nanotubes for highly specific electronic biosensors, *Proc. Natl Acad. Sci.*, 100, 4984, 2003.
198. Liu, J. et al., Achieving direct electrical connection to glucose oxidase using aligned single walled carbon nanotube arrays, *Electroanalysis*, 17, 38, 2005.
199. He, P.G., Xu, Y., and Fang, Y.Z., Applications of carbon nanotubes in electrochemical DNA biosensors, *Mikrochim. Acta*, 152, 175, 2006.
200. Pedano, M.L. and Rivas, G.A., Adsorption and electrooxidation of nucleic acids at carbon nanotubes paste electrodes, *Electrochem. Commu.*, 6, 10, 2004.
201. Wu, K.B. et al., Direct electrochemistry of DNA, guanine and adenine at a nanostructured film-modified electrode, *Anal. Bioanal. Chem.*, 376, 205, 2003.
202. Jung, D.H. et al., Covalent attachment and hybridization of DNA oligonucleotides on patterned single-walled carbon nanotube films, *Langmuir*, 20, 8886, 2004.
203. Chiang, C.K. et al, Electrical conductivity in doped polyacetylene, *Phys. Rev. Lett.*, 39, 1098, 1977.
204. Malhotra, B.D. and Singhal, R., Conducting polymer based biomolecular electronic devices, *Pramana-J. Phys.*, 61, 331, 2003.
205. Jiang, L.S. et al., Sensing characteristics of polypyrrole–poly(vinyl alcohol) methanol sensors prepared by *in situ* vapor state polymerization, *Sensor. Actuator. B Chem.*, 105, 132, 2005.
206. Onoda, M., Tada, K., and Shinkuma, A., *In situ* polymerization process of polypyrrole ultrathin films, *Thin Solid Films*, 499, 61, 2006.
207. Gerard, M., Chaubey, A., and Malhotra, B.D., Application of conducting polymers to biosensors, *Biosens. Bioelectron.*, 17, 345, 2002.

208. Rajesh and Kaneto, K., A new tyrosinase biosensor based on covalent immobilization of enzyme on *N*-(3-aminopropyl) pyrrole polymer film, *Curr. Appl. Phys.*, 5, 178, 2005.

209. Serradilla R.S. et al., Hydrogen peroxide sensitive amperometric biosensor based on horseradish peroxidase entrapped in a polypyrrole electrode, *Biosens. Bioelectron.*, 17, 921, 2002.

210. Gooding, J.J. et al., Electrochemical modulation of antigen–antibody binding, *Biosens. Bioelectron.*, 20, 260, 2004.

211. Bidan, G. et al., Conducting polymers as a link between biomolecules and microelectronics, *Synthetic Met.*, 102, 1363, 1999.

212. Védrine, C., Fabiano, S., and Tran-Minh, C., Amperometric tyrosinase based biosensor using an electrogenerated polythiophene film as an entrapment support, *Talanta* 59, 535, 2003.

213. Wallace, G.G., Smyth M., and Zhao H., Conducting electroactive polymer-based biosensors, *TrAC-Trend. Anal. Chem.*, 18, 245, 1999.

214. Umana, M. and Waller, J., Protein modified electrodes: the glucose oxidase/polypyrrole system. *Anal. Chem.*, 58, 2979, 1986.

215. Skinner, N.G. and Hall, E.A.H.J., Investigation of the origin of the glucose response in a glucose oxidase & unknown; polyaniline system, *Electroanal. Chem.*, 420, 179, 1997.

216. Xue, H.G., Shen, Z.Q., and Li, Y.F., Polyaniline–polyisoprene composite film based glucose biosensor with high permselectivity, *Synthetic Met.*, 124, 345, 2001.

217. Razola, S.S. et al., Hydrogen peroxide sensitive amperometric biosensor based on horseradish peroxidase entrapped in a polypyrrole electrode, *Biosens. Bioelectron.*, 17, 921, 2002.

218. Trettnak, W., Lionti, I., and Mascini, M., Potentiometric discrimination between planar and octahedral anionic metal cyano complexes by liquid membrane electrodes based on lipophilic m-acrocyclic dioxopolyamines, *Electroanalysis*, 5, 753, 1993.

219. Palmisano, F., Centonze, D., and Zambonin, P.G., An *in situ* electrosynthesized amperometric biosensor based on lactate oxidase immobilized in a poly-o-phenylenediamine film: determination of lactate in serum by flow injection analysis, *Biosens. Bioelectron.*, 9, 471, 1994.

220. Dobay, R., Harsanyi, G., and Visy, C., Detection of uric acid with a new type of conducting polymer-based enzymatic sensor by bipotentiostatic technique, *Anal. Chim. Acta*, 385, 187, 1999.

221. Llaudet, E. et al., A three-enzyme microelectrode sensor for detecting purine release from central nervous system, *Biosens. Bioelectron.*, 18, 43, 2003.

222. Bongiovanni, C. et al., An electrochemical multienzymatic biosensor for determination of cholesterol, *Bioelectrochemistry*, 54, 17, 2001.

223. Campbell, T.E., Hodgson, A.J., and Wallace, G.G., Incorporation of erythrocytes into polypyrrole to form the basis of a biosensor to screen for rhesus (D) blood groups and rhesus (D) antibodies, *Electroanalysis*, 11, 215, 1999.

224. Deshpande, M.V. and Hall, E.A.H., An electrochemically grown polymer as an immobilisation matrix for whole cells: application in an amperometric dopamine sensor, *Biosens. Bioelectron.*, 5, 431, 1990.

225. Gooding, J.J., Hall, E.A.H., and Hibbert, D.B., Thick film to monolayer recognition layers in enzyme electrodes, *Electroanalysis*, 10, 1130, 1998.

226. Gros, P. and Bergel, A., Improved model of a polypyrrole glucose oxidase modified electrode, *J. Electroanal. Chem,.* 386, 65, 1995.

227. Bartlett, P.N., Archer, P.B.M., and Ling-Chung, S.K., Conducting polymer gas sensors part I: fabrication and characterization, *Sensor. Actuator.*, 19, 125, 1989.

228. Yon-Hin, B.F.Y. et al., Covalent electropolymerization of glucose oxidase in polypyrrole. Evaluation of methods of pyrrole attachment to glucose oxidase on the performance of electropolymerized glucose sensors, *Anal. Chem.*, 65, 2067, 1993.

229. Saoudi, B. et al., DNA adsorption onto conducting polypyrrole. *Synthetic Met.*, 87, 97, 1997.

230. Chehimi, M.M. et al., Adsorption of macromolecules onto conducting polymers, *Polymery*, 41, 75, 1996.

231. Bruno, F.F. et al., Enzyme mediated polymerization of phenol and aniline derivatives on a langmuir trough to form ordered 2-D polymer films, *J. Intel. Mat. Syst. Str.*, 5, 631, 1994.

232. Livache, T. et al., Biosensing effects in functionalized electroconducting conjugated polymer layers: addressable DNA matrix for the detection of gene mutations, *Synthetic Met.*, 71, 2143, 1995.

233. Korri-Youssoufi, H. et al., Toward bioelectronics: specific DNA recognition based on an oli-gonucleotide-functionalized polypyrrole, *J. Am. Chem. Soc.*, 119, 7388, 1997.

234. Geetha, S. et al, Biosensing and drug delivery by polypyrrole, *Anal. Chim. Acta*, 568, 119, 2006.

235. Kumar, A. et al, Immobilization of cholesterol oxidase and potassium ferricyanide on dodecylbenzene sulfonate ion-doped polypyrrole film, *J. Appl. Polym. Sci.*, 82, 3486, 2001.

236. Kuralay, F., Ö Zyörük, H., and Yıldız, A., Amperometric enzyme electrode for urea determination using immobilized urease in poly(vinylferrocene) film, *Sensor. Actuator. B Chem.*, 114, 500–506, 2006.

237. Dicks, J.M. et al., The application of ferrocene-modified n-type silicon in glucose biosensors, *Electroanalysis*, 5, 1, 1993.

238. Mu, S.L. and Xue, H.G., Bioelectrochemical characteristics of glucose oxidase immobilized in a polyaniline film, *Sensor. Actuator. B Chem.*, 31, 155, 1996.

239. Vidal, J.C. et al., Recent advances in electropolymerized conducting polymers in amperometric biosensors, *Mikrochim. Acta*, 143, 93, 2003.

240. Schuhmann, W. et al., Polypyrrole, a new possibility for covalent binding of oxidoreductases to electrode surfaces as a base for stable biosensors, *Sensor. Actuator. B Chem.*, 1, 537, 1990.

241. Calvo-Muñoz, M.L. et al., Electrochemical study by a redox probe of the chemical post-functionalization of N-substituted polypyrrole films: application of a new approach to immobilization of biotinylated molecules, *J. Electroanal. Chem.*, 578, 301, 2005.

242. Hiller, M. et al., Amperometric biosensors produced by immobilization of redox enzymes at polythiophene-modified electrode surfaces, *Adv. Mater.*, 8, 219, 1996.

243. Porath, J. et al., Metal chelate affinity chromatography, a new approach to protein fractionation, *Nature*, 258, 598, 1997.

244. Davis, J. et al., Spectroscopic evaluation of protein affinity binding at polymeric biosensor films, *J. Am. Chem. Soc.*, 121, 4302, 1999.

245. Halliwell, M.C. et al., Immobilisation of lactate dehydrogenase on poly (aniline)-poly (acrylate) and poly (aniline)-poly (vinyl sulphonate) films for use in a lactate biosensor, *Anal. Chim. Acta*, 453, 191, 2002.

246. Halliwell, M.C. et al., The design of dehydrogenase enzymes for use in a biofuel cell: the role of genetically introduced peptide tags in enzyme immobilization on electrodes, *Bioelectrochemistry*, 55, 21, 2002.

247. Pantano, P., Morton, T.H., and Kuhr, W.G., Enzyme-modified carbon-fiber microelectrodes with millisecond response times, *J. Am. Chem. Soc.*, 113, 1832, 1991.

248. Cosnier, S. et al., Electrogeneration of biotinylated functionalized polypyrroles for the simple immobilization of enzymes, *Electroanalysis*, 10, 808, 1998.

249. Cosnier, S. et al., A biotinylated conducting polypyrrole for the spatially controlled construction of an amperometric biosensor, *Anal. Chem.*, 71, 3692, 1999.

250. Livache, T. et al., Electroconducting polymers for the construction of DNA or peptide arrays on silicon chips, *Biosens. Bioelectron.*, 13, 629, 1998.

251. Da Silva, S. et al., Biotinylated polypyrrole films: an easy electrochemical approach for the reagentless immobilization of bacteria on electrode surfaces, *Bioelectrochemistry*, 63, 297, 2004.

252. Zhou, H.H. et al., Glucose biosensor based on platinum microparticles dispersed in nano-fibrous polyaniline, *Biosens. Bioelectron.*, 20, 1305, 2005.

253. Parthasarathy, R.V. and Martin, C.R., Enzyme and chemical encapsulation in polymeric microcapsules, *J. Appl. Polym. Sci.*, 62, 875, 1996.

254. Parthasarathy, R.V. and Martin, C.R., Synthesis of polymeric microcapsule arrays and their use for enzyme immobilization, *Nature*, 369, 298, 1994.

255. Martin, C.R., Nanomaterials: a membrane-based synthetic approach, *Science*, 266, 1961, 1994.

256. Jongseo, P., Jungsuk, K., and Yongkeun, S., Conducting polymer micro-tubules hosting electroactive species without guest modification, *Synthetic Met.*, 156, 714, 2006.

257. Miao, Y.Q., Chen, J.R., and Wu, X.H., Using electropolymerized non-conducting polymers to develop enzyme amperometric biosensors, *Trends Biotechnol.*, 22, 227, 2004.

258. Nakabayshi, Y. et al., Amperometric glucose sensors fabricated by electrochemical polymerization of phenols on carbon paste electrodes containing ferrocene as electron transfer mediator, *Anal. Sci.*, 14, 1069, 1997.

259. Nakabayashi, Y. and Yoshikawa, H., Amperometric biosensors for sensing of hydrogen peroxide based on electron transfer between horseradish peroxidase and ferrocene as a mediator, *Anal. Sci.*, 16, 609, 2000.

260. Bartlett, P.N. and Caruana, D.J., Electrochemical immobilization of enzymes. Part V. Microelectrodes for the detection of glucose based on glucose oxidase immobilized in a poly(phend) film, *Analyst*, 117, 1287, 1992.

261. Yang, Q.L., Atanasov, P., and Wilkins, E., Development of needle-type glucose sensor with high selectivity, *Sensor. Actuator. B Chem.*, 46, 249, 1992.

262. Murphy, L.J., Reduction of interference response at a hydrogen peroxide detecting electrode using electropolymerized films of substituted naphthalenes, *Anal. Chem.*, 70, 2928, 1998.

263. Ramanavičius, A., Electrochemical study of permeability and charge-transfer in polypyrrole films, *Biologija*, 2, 64, 2000.

264. Geise, R.J. et al., Electropolymerized films to prevent interferences and electrode fouling in biosensors, *Biosens. Bioelectron.*, 6, 151, 1991.

265. Guerrieri, A. et al., Electrosynthesized non-conducting polymers as permselective membranes in amperometric enzyme electrodes: a glucose biosensor based on a co-crosslinked glucose oxidase/over-oxidized polypyrrole bilayer, *Biosens. Bioelectron.*, 13, 103, 1998.

266. Vidal, J.C. et al., *In situ* preparation of a cholesterol biosensor: entrapment of cholesterol oxidase in an overoxidized polypyrrole film electrodeposited in a flow system; determination of total cholesterol in serum, *Anal. Chim. Acta*, 385, 213, 1999.

267. Vidal, J.C. et al., *In situ* preparation of overoxidized PPy/oPPD bilayer biosensors for the determination of glucose and cholesterol in serum, *Sensor. Actuator.*, 57, 219, 1999.

268. Daniel, M.C. and Astruc, D., Gold nanoparticles: assembly, supramolecular chemistry, quantum-size-related properties, and applications toward biology, catalysis, and nanotechnology, *Chem. Rev.*, 104, 293, 2004.

269. Alvarez, M.M. et al., Optical absorption spectra of nanocrystal gold molecules, *J. Phys. Chem. B*, 101, 3706, 1997.

270. Chen, S. and Murray, R.W., Electrochemical quantized capacitance charging of surface ensembles of gold nanoparticles, *J. Phys. Chem. B*, 103, 9996, 1999.

271. Hicks, J.F. et al., Dynamics of electron transfers between electrodes and monolayers of nanoparticles, *J. Phys. Chem. B*, 106, 7751, 2006.

272. Sun, Y. et al., Memory effects in an interacting magnetic nanoparticle system, *Phys. Rev. Lett.*, 91, 167206, 2003.

273. Mornet, S. et al., Magnetic nanoparticle design for medical applications, *Prog. Solid State Chem.*, 34, 237, 2006.

274. On, D.T. et al., Perspective in catalytic applications of mesostructured materials, *Appl. Catal. A*, 222, 299, 2001.

275. Zhao, J. et al., Direct electron transfer at horseradish peroxidase—colloidal gold modified electrodes, *J. Electroanal. Chem.*, 327, 109, 1992.

276. Wang, J., Liu, G., and Merkoci, A., Electrochemical coding technology for simultaneous detection of multiple DNA targets, *J. Am. Chem. Soc.*, 125, 3214, 2003.

277. Xiao, Y. et al., "Plugging into enzymes": nanowiring of redox enzymes by a gold nanoparticle, *Science*, 299, 1877, 2003.

278. Katz, E. and Willner, I., Integrated nanoparticle–biomolecule hybrid systems: synthesis, properties, and applications, *Angew. Chem. Int. Ed.*, 43, 6042, 2004.

279. Demoustier-Champagne, S. and Delvaux, M., Preparation of polymeric and metallic nanostructures using a template-based deposition method, *Mater. Sci. Eng. C*, 15, 269, 2001.

280. Delvaux, M. and Demoustier-Champagne, S., Immobilisation of glucose oxidase within metallic nanotubes arrays for application to enzyme biosensors, *Biosens. Bioelectron.*, 18, 943, 2003.

281. Delvaux, M., Walcarius, A., and Demoustier-Champagne, S., Electrocatalytic H_2O_2 amperometric detection using gold nanotube electrode ensembles, *Anal. Chim. Acta*, 525 , 221, 2004.

282. Yang, M., Chung, F.L., and Thompson, M., Acoustic network analysis as a novel technique for studying protein adsorption and denaturation at surfaces, *Anal. Chem.*, 65, 3713, 1993.

283. Jackson, D.R., Omanovic, S., and Roscoe, S.G., Electrochemical studies of the adsorption behavior of serum proteins on titanium, *Langmuir*, 16, 5449, 2000.

284. Xu, C.X. et al., Ultraviolet amplified spontaneous emission from self-organized network of zinc oxide nanofibers, *Appl. Phys. Lett.*, 86, 011118, 2005.

285. Roy, V.A.L. et al., Luminescent and structural properties of ZnO nanorods prepared under different conditions, *Appl. Phys. Lett.*, 83, 141, 2003.

286. Topoglidis, E. et al., Immobilisation and bioelectrochemistry of proteins on nanoporous TiO_2 and ZnO films, *J. Electroanal. Chem.*, 517, 20, 2001.

287. Zhang, F.F. et al., Immobilization of uricase on ZnO nanorods for a reagentless uric acid biosensor, *Anal. Chim. Acta*, 519, 155, 2004.

288. Yao, B.D., Chan, Y.F., and Wang, N., Formation of ZnO nanostructures by a simple way of thermal evaporation, *Appl. Phys. Lett.*, 81, 757, 2001.

289. Wei, A. et al., Enzymatic glucose biosensor based on ZnO nanorod array grown by hydrothermal decomposition, *Appl. Phys. Lett.*, 89, 123902, 2006.

290. Topoglidis, E. et al., Protein adsorption on nanocrystalline TiO2 films: an immobilization strategy for bioanalytical devices, *Anal. Chem.*, 70, 5111, 1998.

291. Zhang, J.K. and Cass, A.E.G., A study of his-tagged alkaline phosphatase immobilization on a nanoporous nickel–titanium dioxide film, *Anal. Biochem.*, 292, 307, 2001.

292. Gong, D. et al., Titanium oxide nanotube arrays prepared by anodic oxidation, *J. Mater. Res.*, 16, 2001, 3331.

293. Liu, S.Q. and Chen, A.C., Coadsorption of horseradish peroxidase with thionine on TiO2 nanotubes for biosensing, *Langmuir*, 21, 8409, 2005.

294. El-Sayed, M.A., Some interesting properties of metals confined in time and nanometer space of different shapes, *Acc. Chem. Res.*, 34, 257, 2001.

295. Kelly, K.L. et al., The optical properties of metal nanoparticles: the influence of size, shape, and dielectric environment, *J. Phys. Chem. B*, 107, 668, 2003.

296. Haes, A.J. and Van Duyne, R.P., A unified view of propagating and localized surface plasmon resonance biosensors, *Anal. Bioanal. Chem.*, 379, 920, 2004.

297. Okamoto, T., Yamaguchi, I., and Kobayashi, T., Local plasmon sensor with gold colloid monolayers deposited upon glass substrates, *Opt. Lett.*, 25, 372, 2000.

298. Nath, N. and Chilkoti, A., Label free colorimetric biosensing using nanoparticles, *J. Fluoresc.*, 14, 377, 2003.

299. Englebienne, P., Use of colloidal gold surface plasmon resonance peak shift to infer affinity constants from the interactions between protein antigens and antibodies specific for single or multiple epitopes, *Analyst*, 123, 1599, 1998.

300. Englebienne, P., van Hoonacker, A., and Valsamis, J., Rapid homogeneous immunoassay for human ferritin in the cobas mira using colloidal gold as the reporter reagent, *Clin. Chem.*, 46, 2000, 2000.

301. Taton, T.A., Mirkin, C.A., and Letsinger, R.L., Scanometric DNA array detection with nanoparticle probes, *Science*, 289, 1757, 2000.

302. Storhoff, J.J. et al., What controls the optical properties of DNA-linked gold nanoparticle assemblies?, *J. Am. Chem. Soc.*, 122, 4640, 2000.

303. Storhoff, J.J. et al., Sequence-dependent stability of DNA-modified gold nanoparticles, *Langmuir*, 18, 6666, 2002.

304. Storhoff, J.J. et al., One-pot colorimetric differentiation of polynucleotides with single base imperfections using gold nanoparticle probes, *J. Am. Chem. Soc.*, 120, 1959, 1998.

305. Smith, A.M. and Nie, S., Chemical analysis and cellular imaging with quantum dots, *Analyst*, 129, 672, 2004.

306. Wang, Y., Tang, Z.Y., and Kotov, A.N., Bioapplication of nanosemiconductors, *Mater. Today*, 8(5), 20, 2005.

307. Rosenthal, S.J. et al., Bar-coding biomolecules with fluorescent nanocrystals, *Nat. Biotechnol.*, 19, 621, 2001.

308. Tang, Z.Y. et al., Spontaneous organization of single CdTe nanoparticles into luminescent nanowires, *Science*, 297, 237, 2002.

309. Wu, X. et al., Immunofluorescent labeling of cancer marker Her2 and other cellular targets with semiconductor quantum dots, *Nat. Biotechnol.*, 21, 41, 2003.

310. Chan, W.C. and Nie, S., Quantum dot bioconjugates for ultrasensitive nonisotopic detection, *Science*, 281, 2016, 1998.

311. Clapp, A.R. et al., Fluorescence resonance energy transfer between quantum dot donors and dye-labeled protein acceptors, *J. Am. Chem. Soc.*, 126, 301, 2004.

312. Willard, D.M. et al., CdSe-ZnS quantum dots as resonance energy transfer donors in a model protein-protein binding assay, *Nano Lett.*, 1, 469, 2001.

313. Goldman, E.R. et al., Multiplexed toxin analysis using four colors of quantum dot fluororeagents, *Anal. Chem.*, 76, 684, 2004.

314. Mamedova, N.N. et al., Albumin-CdTe nanoparticle bioconjugates: preparation, structure, and interunit energy transfer with antenna effect, *Nano Lett.*, 1, 281, 2001.

315. Safarik, M.S., Magnetic nanoparticles and biosciences, *Monatsh. Chem.*, 133, 737, 2002.

316. Prinz, G.A., Device physics-magnetoelectronics, *Science*, 282, 1660, 1998.

317. Fan, Z.H. et al., Dynamic DNA hybridization on a chip using paramagnetic beads, *Anal. Chem.*, 71, 4845, 1999.

318. Guttenberg, Z. et al., Measuring ligand–receptor unbinding forces with magnetic beads: molecular leverage, *Langmuir*, 16, 8984, 2000.

319. Nishi, H. et al., A new method for histamine release from purified peripheral blood basophils using monoclonal antibody-coated magnetic beads, *J. Immunol. Meth.*, 240, 39, 2000.
320. Chemla, Y.R. et al., Ultrasensitive magnetic biosensor for homogeneous immunoassay PNAS, *Proc. Natl Acad. Sci.*, 97, 14268, 2000.
321. Katz, E., Willner, I., and Wang, J., Electroanalytical and bioelectroanalytical systems based on metal and semiconductor nanoparticles, *Electroanalysis*, 16, 19, 2004.
322. Hernández-Santos, D., González-García, M.B., and García, A.C., Metal-nanoparticles based electro-analysis, *Electroanalysis*, 14, 1225, 2002.
323. Wang, J., Nanomaterial-based electrochemical biosensors, *Analyst*, 130, 421, 2005.
324. MerkoÇi, A. et al., New materials for electrochemical sensing V. Nanoparticles for DNA labeling, *Trends Anal. Chem.*, 24, 341, 2005.
325. Stewart, M.P. and Buriak, J.M., Chemical and biological applications of porous silicon, *Technol. Adv. Mater.*, 12, 859, 2000.
326. Sotiropoulou, S. et al., Novel carbon materials in biosensor systems, *Biosens. Bioelectron.*, 18, 211, 2003.
327. Ballarin, B. et al., Chemical sensors based on ultrathin-film composite membranes—a new concept in sensor design, *Anal. Chem.*, 64, 2647, 1992.
328. Cullis, A.G., Canham, L.T., and Calcott, P.D.J., The structural and luminescence properties of porous silicon, *J. Appl. Phys.*, 82, 909, 1997.
329. Drott, J. et al., Pore morphology influence on catalytic turn-over for enzyme activated porous silicon matrices, *Thin Solid Films*, 161, 330, 1998.
330. Gavalas, V.G., Chaniotakis, N.A., and Gibson, T., Improved operational stability of biosensors based on enzyme-polyelectrolyte complex adsorbed into a porous carbon electrode, *Biosens. Bioelectron.*, 13, 1205, 1998.
331. Gavalas, V.G. and Chaniotakis, N.A., Polyelectrolyte stabilized oxidase based biosensors: effect of diethylaminoethyl-dextran on the stabilization of glucose and lactate oxidases into porous conductive carbon, *Anal. Chim. Acta*, 404, 67, 2000a.
332. Gavalas, V.G. and Chaniotakis, N.A., Lactate biosensor based on the adsorption of polyelectrolyte stabilized lactate oxidase into porous conductive carbon, *Microchim. Acta*, 136, 211, 2001.
333. Myler, S. et al., Ultra-thin-polysiloxane-film-composite membranes for the optimisation of amperometric oxidase enzyme electrodes, *Biosens. Bioelectron.*, 17, 35, 2002.
334. Heilmann, A. et al., Nanoporous aluminum oxide as a novel support material for enzyme biosensors, *J. Nanosci. Nanotechnol.*, 3, 375, 2003.
335. Darder, M. et al., Encapsulation of enzymes in alumina membranes of controlled pore size, *Thin Solid Films*, 495, 321, 2006.
336. Rosilio, V. et al., Penetration of glucose oxidase into organized phospholipid monolayers spread at the solution/air interface, *Langmuir*, 13, 4669, 1997.
337. Oh, B.K. et al., Fabrication of protein G LB film for immunoglobulin G immobilization, *Mater. Sci. Eng. C*, 24, 65, 2004.
338. Girard-Egrod, A.P., Morelis, R.M., and Coulet, P.R., Choline oxidase associated with behenic acid LB films. Reorganization of enzyme-lipid association under the conditions of activity detection, *Langmuir*, 13, 6540, 1997.
339. Wan, K., Chovelon, J.M., and Jaffrezic-Renault, N., Enzyme–octadecylamine Langmuir–Blodgett membranes for ENFET biosensors, *Talanta*, 52, 663, 2000.
340. Arisana, S. and Yamamoto, R., Quantitative characterization of enzymes adsorbed on to Langmuir-Blodgett films and the application to a urea sensor, *Thin Solid Films*, 210/211, 443, 1992.
341. Girard-Egrot, A.P., Godoy, S., and Blum, L.J., Enzyme association with lipidic Langmuir–Blodgett films: interests and applications in nanobioscience, *Adv. Colloid Interface Sci.*, 116, 205, 2005.
342. Yin, F., Shin, H.K., and Kwon, Y.S., A hydrogen peroxide biosensor based on Langmuir–Blodgett technique: direct electron transfer of hemoglobin in octadecylamine layer, *Talanta*, 67, 221, 2005.
343. Pal, P., Nandi, D., and Misra, T.N., Immobilization of alcohol dehydrogenase enzyme in a Langmuir–Blodgett film of stearic acid: its application as an ethanol sensor, *Thin Solid Films*, 239, 138, 1994.
344. Boozer, C., Yu, Q., Chen, S., Lee, C., Homola, J., Yee, S.S., and Jiang, S., Surface functionalization for self-referencing surface plasmon resonance (SPR) biosensors by multi-step self-assembly, *Sensor. Actuator. B Chem.*, 90, 22, 2003.
345. Jia, J.B. et al., A method to construct a third-generation horseradish peroxidase biosensor: self-assembling gold nanoparticles to three-dimensional sol–gel network, *Anal. Chem.*, 74, 2217, 2002.

346. Tecilla, P. et al., Hydrogen-bonding self-assembly of multichromophore structures, *J. Am. Chem. Soc.*, 112, 9408, 1990.

347. Ulman, A., *An introduction to ultrathin organic films*, Academic Press, Boston, MA, 1991.

348. Ulman, A., Formation and structure of self-assembled monolayers, *Chem. Rev.*, 96, 1533, 1996.

349. Collinson, M., Bowden, E.F., and Tarlow, M.J., Voltammetry of covalently immobilized cytochrome *c* on self-assembled monolayer electrodes, *Langmuir*, 8, 1247, 1992.

350. Trammell, S.A. et al., Orientated binding of photosynthetic reaction centers on gold using Ni-NTA self-assembled monolayers, *Biosens. Bioelectron.*, 19, 1649, 2004.

351. Clark, R.A. and Bowden, E.F., Voltammetric peak broadening for cytochrome *c*/alkanethiolate monolayer structures: dispersion of formal potentials, *Langmuir*, 13, 559, 1997.

352. Armstrong, F.A. et al., Fast, long-range electron-transfer reactions of a 'blue' copper protein coupled non-covalently to an electrode through a stilbene thiolate monolayer, *Chem. Commun.*, 3, 316, 2004.

353. Spinke, J. et al., Molecular recognition at a self-assembled monolayer: optimization of surface functionalization. *J. Chem. Phys.*, 99, 7012, 1993.

354. Swain, G.M., Anderson, A.B., and Angus, J.C., Applications of diamond thin films in electrochemistry, *MRS Bull.*, 23, 56, 1998.

355. Fujishima, A. and Rao, T.N., New directions in structuring and electrochemical applications of boron-doped diamond thin films, *Diam. Relat. Mater.*, 10, 1799, 2001.

356. Carlisle, J.A., Precious biosensors, *Nat. Mater.*, 3, 668, 2004.

357. May, P.W., Diamond thin films: a 21st-century material, *Phil. Trans. Roy. Soc. Lond.*, 358, 473, 2000.

358. Specht, C.G. et al., Ordered growth of neurons on diamond, *Biomaterials*, 25, 4073, 2004.

359. Garguilo, J.M. et al., Fibrinogen adsorption onto microwave plasma chemical vapor deposited diamond films, *Diam. Relat. Mater.*, 13, 595, 2004.

360. Amaratunga, G.A.J., A dawn for carbon electronics, *Science*, 297, 1657, 2002.

361. Yang, W.S. et al., DNA-modified nanocrystalline diamond thin-films as stable, biologically active substrates, *Nat. Mater.*, 1, 253, 2002.

362. Ando, T., Yamamoto, K., Suehara, S., Kamo, M., Sate, Y., Shimosaki, S., and Nishitanigamo, M., *J. Chin. Chem. Soc.*, 42, 285, 1995.

363. Ando, T. et al., Chemical modification of diamond surfaces using a chlorinated surface as an intermediate state, *Diam. Relat. Mater.*, 5, 1136, 1996.

364. Miller, J.B., Amines and thiols on diamond surfaces, *Surf. Sci.*, 439, 21, 1999.

365. Ohtani, B. et al., Surface functionalization of doped CVD diamond via covalent bond. An XPS study on the formation of surface-bound quaternary pyridinium salt, *Chem. Lett.*, 27, 953, 1998.

366. Tsubota, T. et al., Chemical modification of hydrogenated diamond surface using benzoyl peroxides, *Phys. Chem. Chem. Phys.*, 4, 806, 2002.

367. Strother, T. et al., Photochemical functionalization of diamond films, *Langmuir*, 18, 968, 2002.

368. Notsu, H. et al., Introduction of oxygen-containing functional groups onto diamond electrode surfaces by oxygen plasma and anodic polarization, *Electrochem. Solid State Lett.*, 2, 522, 1999.

369. Ando, T. et al., Vapour-phase oxidation of diamond surfaces in O_2 studied by diffuse reflectance Fourier-transform infrared and temperature-programmed desorption spectroscopy, *J. Chem. Soc. Faraday Trans.*, 89, 3635, 1993.

370. Granger, M.C. and Swain, G.M., The influence of surface interactions on the reversibility of ferri/ferrocyanide at boron-doped diamond thin-film electrodes, *J. Electrochem. Soc.*, 146, 4551, 1999.

371. Notsu, H. et al., Surface carbonyl groups on oxidized diamond electrodes, *J. Electroanal. Chem.*, 492, 31, 2000.

372. Notsu, H. et al., Hydroxyl groups on boron-doped diamond electrodes and their modification with a silane coupling agent, *Electrochem. Solid State Lett.*, 4, H1–H3, 2001.

373. Wang, J. and Carlisle, J.A., Covalent immobilization of glucose oxidase on conducting ultrananocrystalline diamond thin films, *Diam. Relat. Mater.*, 15, 279, 2006.

374. Yang, W.S., Butler, J.E., Russell, J.N. Jr., Hamers, R.J., Interfacial electrical properties of DNA-modified diamond thin films: intrinsic response and hybridization-induced field effects, *Langmuir*, 20, 6778, 2004.

375. Knickerbocker, T. et al., DNA-modified diamond surfaces, *Langmuir*, 19, 1938, 2003.

376. Lu, M.C. et al., Invasive cleavage reactions on DNA-modified diamond surfaces, *Biopolymers*, 73, 606, 2004.

377. Su, L. et al., Amperometric glucose sensor based on enzyme-modified boron-doped diamond electrode by cross-linking method, *Sensor. Actuator. B Chem.*, 99, 499, 2004.

Part IV

Other Biomaterials

15 Synthetic and Natural Degradable Polymeric Biomaterials

Sanjukta Deb

CONTENTS

15.1 INTRODUCTION

Polymers consist of molecules that have high molar masses and are composed of a large number of repeating units. Polymers occur in nature and can be found in living species such as proteins, collagen, and DNA. Synthetic polymers comprise of a large group of materials that have become an everyday commodity in life around us, ranging from the common carrier bag to heavy plastics. Due to the enormous range of synthetic polymers, they are often classified on the basis of their synthetic pedigree, such as condensation or addition polymers. Synthetic polymers have grown progressively to invade almost every commodity in our lives. A part of their growing popularity is due to the ability to produce them at high speed with controlled properties, at low cost, ease of fabrication, and with high resistance to aging. However, the abundance of synthetic polymers and their increasing use also generates a colossal amount of waste, making "recycling" an active part of our lives.

A huge amount of polymeric products are disposed worldwide daily, thus fabrication of recycled polymer waste is an important issue globally. However, not all polymers can be reprocessed or chemically degraded. There are various possible routes to eliminate polymeric wastes, but biodegradation and recycling are regarded as attractive solutions. There exists a group of polymers that can be made to degrade either through biodegradation or enzymatic processes, and such polymers are rapidly gaining importance and increasingly replacing nondegradable polymers.

Polymers considered "unstable" were deemed to be unsuitable for medical applications since materials were required to survive as long as possible within the body to be able to restore function. However, it became clear that polymers that were able to provide an appropriate function over a required period of time and degrade thereafter, could also prove to be beneficial in medicine. Polymers that were biodegradable were soon being exploited, and the development of a suture from poly(glycolic acid) (PGA) in the 1970s, triggered a spate of interest into degradable polymers and its application in medicine and dentistry. There are a variety of reasons to have a device that can be used as a temporary implant and will not require a second surgical intervention for removal. Besides eliminating the need for a second surgery, the biodegradation of implants presents other advantages. For example, a nonbiodegradable stainless implant used for fracture fixation tends to bear the maximum load during the healing phase, thus shielding the surrounding bone from body loads and making it resorb to an extent. Removal of implants from such sites can cause refracture whereas a degradable implant can be engineered to degrade at a rate that will allow for slow transfer of load during the healing process. Biodegradable polymers also offer tremendous potential as a drug delivery carrier, either as a drug delivery system alone or in addition to functioning as a medical device. Such polymers form a majority of the scaffolds desired for tissue engineering and regenerative medicine.

Polymers that can provide a temporary function are nevertheless required to fulfill a number of stringent criteria prior to their use in the human body. Parameters, such as their biocompatibility, resorbability, adequate mechanical support during the healing process, nontoxic response to degradation products, and their ability to be eliminated by natural pathways in the body, are features of importance. Easy processing, sterilizability, and adequate shelf life are other important considerations that have to be addressed.

Biomaterials intended for biomedical applications aim to develop artificial materials that can be used to restore or repair function of diseased or traumatized tissue in the human body, and thus improve the quality of life. In the last four decades, significant advances have been made in the development of biodegradable polymers for biomedical applications.

Polymers for biomedical applications are designed to be either biostable or bioabsorbable. Biologically stable polymers provide a permanent support over time and should ideally perform during the life-time of the patient, some examples being poly(methylmethacrylate) (PMMA), high-density poly(ethylene) (HDPE), and poly(tetrafluoroethylene) (PTFE) that are used for different applications. PMMA is mainly used as bone cements in hip and knee replacements and HDPE forms the articulating surfaces of hip and knee joints. However, bioabsorbable polymers are designed to provide temporary support and should absorb in the body over a period of time, some examples being poly(lactide) (PLA) and PGA used as degradable sutures, pins, and staples. A device that is able to provide a temporary support during the healing process is desirable for clinicians; and if its subsequent removal is not necessary, the device can greatly advantageous to the patient and the clinician, and reduce costs. Imagine an implant such as a bone screw or pin that is inserted to stabilize a fracture and performs its function during the stabilization process. It eventually degrades within the body and is eliminated by natural pathways.

This chapter provides an overview of degradable polymers in biomedical applications, including important aspects of the different polymers used, mechanism of degradation, and their applications. However, it will be prudent to mention that the degradable polymers discussed in this chapter are by no means exhaustive.

15.2 DEGRADABLE POLYMERS

Degradable polymers can be either of a natural origin or synthetically manufactured. Biodegradable polymers can be either natural or synthetic. In general, synthetic polymers offer greater advantages than natural materials in the way that they can be tailored to impart a wide range of predictable properties with a greater control on manipulation of physical, mechanical, and degradation properties. The synthesis of polymers in a laboratory or a manufacturing unit ensures the use of more reliable sources of raw materials, which eliminates the problems of immunogenicity that may be seen as a common occurrence in polymers from natural origins. Some examples of synthetic and naturally occurring polymers that have relevance in the field of biomaterials are presented in Table 15.1.

The essential component in a degradable polymer is the presence of a heteroatom within the backbone of the polymer. In general, a polymer with a $-C-C-$ backbone is stable and does not tend to degrade; however, the presence of anhydrides, esters, amide, etc. can confer biodegradable properties to the polymer. Biodegradability can therefore be engineered into polymers by the judicious introduction of chemical linkages such as anhydrides, esters and or amide bonds, among others polyesters, poly(ethylene oxide) (PEO), etc.

15.2.1 POLYESTERS

15.2.1.1 Poly(α-Hydroxyacids)

Biopolymers are of great interest in the field of biomaterials and their application in healthcare. However, there are some problems for practical applications such as their poor physical properties, poor processability, and high production costs. The polymers derived from α-hydroxy acids, namely, PLA and PGA, (Figure 15.1) have found the most extensive use, primarily as materials for sutures, dating back to the early 1960s due to their superior biocompatibility and acceptable degradation profiles.[1,2] These polymers remain popular for a variety of reasons including the fact that both of these materials have properties that allow hydrolytic degradation. Once degraded, natural pathways remove the degradation products, namely, the monomeric components of each polymer, glycolic acid that can be converted to other metabolites or eliminated by other mechanisms, and lactic acid that can be eliminated through the tricarboxylic acid (TCA) cycle.

The group of esters derived from α-hydroxy acids yield polymers such as PGA and PLA, which are hydrolytically unstable. Degradable polyesters derived from monomers such as lactide,

---

TABLE 15.1

Some Naturally Occurring and Synthetic Degradable Polymers

Natural Polymers	Synthetic Polymers
Albumin	Poly(lactic acid)
Alginates	Poly(L-lactic acid)
Collagen (proteins)	Poly(D,L-lactic acid)
Chitin, chitosan (polysaccharides)	Poly(glycolic acid)
Fibrin	Poly(ε-caprolactone)
	Poly(p-dioxanone)
	Trimethylene carbonate
	Polyanhydrides
	Polyorthoester
	Polyurethanes
	Poly(amino acids)
	Polyphosphazenes

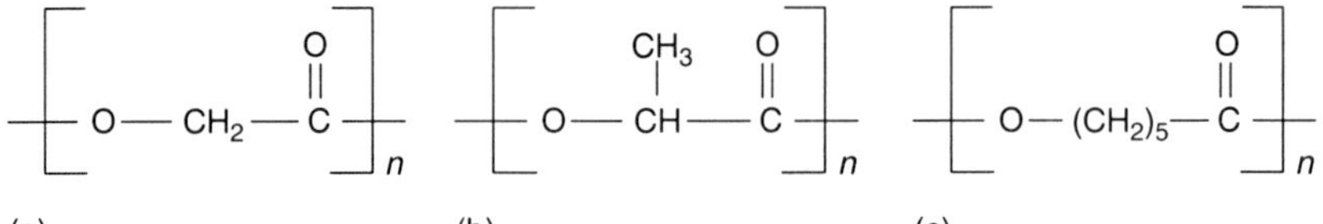

FIGURE 15.1 Structure of linear aliphatic polyesters (a) PGA, (b) PLA, and (c) PCL.

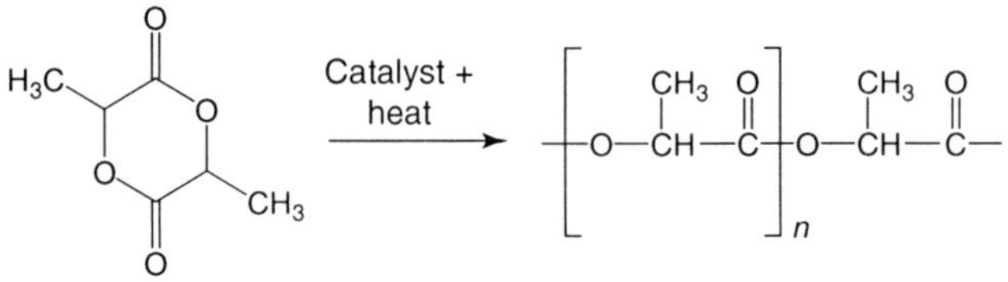

FIGURE 15.2 Ring opening polymerization of lactide in the presence of a catalyst and heat.

glycolide, and caprolactone are commonly used clinically. The degradation rates vary for each of the polymers; however, varying parameters such as molecular weight, crystallinity, copolymer, fabrication techniques, composite formation, etc. can vary the kinetics of degradation. Poly(lactic acid) (PLA) is one the most significant members of the degradable polymer family, which can be produced from abundant naturally occurring corns, sugars, or beetroot.

PGA belongs to the family of polyesters and is obtained through ring opening polymerization of glycolide, and it exhibits fairly rapid degradation rates. It is a crystalline polymer and the molecular weights can be varied by the method of synthesis. Poly(lactic) acid (PLA) is derived from lactic acid (Figure 15.2), which is a chiral molecule and can therefore exist as D and L isomers, the L-isomer being the biological metabolite. Hence, PLA is often referred to as PLLA, L-PLA (L-isomer), D-PLA (D-isomer), and PDLA/DL-PLA (mixture of D and L isomers), depending on the isomeric forms used.[3] The additional methyl group renders the polymer more hydrophobic than PGA and also exhibits slower degradation rates. PLLA is a thermoplastic material with a melting point (T_m) of about 180°C and a glass transition temperature (T_g) higher than room temperature.[4] Thus, PLLA can be processed into fibers, films, and blocks by techniques that are applicable for poly(ethyleneterephthalate) (PET) and various products with superior mechanical properties.

Polymer chains can be linear, branched, or cross-linked with other chains. Polymers can be amorphous or crystalline in nature and can typically comprise of both amorphous and crystalline domains. The greater the crystallinity, the more ordered the structure that results in a more "tightly bound" structure, restricting slippage between the adjacent polymer chains, which results in superior mechanical properties. These polymers are viscoelastic in nature. Increasing levels of amorphous domains within the polymer microstructure tend to enhance the rate of degradability and thus the absorption of the implant. Polymers in general are affected by temperature and exhibit a typical glass transition temperature. Polymers tend to undergo softening at a specific temperature and thus, polymers used for biomedical application should have a glass transition temperature well above the body temperature such that no distortion occurs as a result of polymer softening. Other factors that play an important role on the properties of polymers are the conformation, configuration, and orientation of the molecules. PGA and PLA undergo hydrolytic degradation and are totally degradable with water and carbon dioxide, its ultimate degradation products. The mechanical properties of PLA and PGA are diverse, and literature review suggests that comparisons are difficult because not only that the testing methods vary, the storage conditions, molecular weight, cyrstallinity, shape and form such as braided fibers, spun fibers, single and multifilament fibers, plates, films rods being different, they give rise to different mechanical properties. PGA fibers exhibit high strength and modulus, and are braided to form sutures due to its high stiffness. PGA sutures can lose 50% of their strength after 2 weeks and are generally totally absorbed within 4–6 months.[5] The biodegradation of the microspheres of PLA and PGA has been discussed in detailed by Anderson et al.[6] and they concluded that the rate of degradation is also dependent on the size of the microspheres in addition to molecular weight, sterilization, and processing parameters of the polymers.[6] Biodegradable polymers may be processed in a way similar to any engineering thermoplastic in that they can be melted and formed into fibers, rods, and molded parts. Final parts can be extruded, injection molded, compression molded, or solvent spun, or cast.[7] The molecular weight correlates with final properties of the implant such as the mechanical properties, stability, and absorption time. Most processing methods invariably influence the molecular weight, and factors such as residence time, temperature, shear, moisture, oligomeric units, and impurities, contribute to the given effect.[8] For example, the polymer poly(L-lactic acid) (PLLA) suffers chemical degradation at temperatures of 220°C and pre-drying of polymers before processing leads to minimal changes in molecular weight.

The degradation of aliphatic polyesters occurs mainly through the bulk degradation through hydrolysis. Hydrolytic degradation occurs as polymers (Figure 15.3) are in contact with tissue fluids or moisture and preferentially onsets at the amorphous regions of the polymeric network. Hydrolytic attack causes cleavage at the ester bonds, resulting in chain scission yielding low molecular weight species in the initial stages. Chain scission may also occur in presence of nonspecific esterases and carboxy peptidases, which can break down PGA into glycolic acid units. Both PLA and poly(ε-caprolactone) (PCL) can also be degraded enzymatically. As the bulk of the polymer substrate erodes, autocatalysis occurs within the core of the material due to the presence of the acidic degradation products that are contained within the matrix, as they are unable to diffuse out. The general trend observed in these semicrystalline polymers during the degradation is an increase in crystallinity as most of the amorphous regions degrade preferentially, followed by the loss of the crystalline phase. As this process continues, the polymer loses its mechanical strength and fragmentation occurs. Further hydrolysis yields smaller fragments that can be assimilated by phagocytes, while the soluble monomeric anions such as glycolate and lactate dissolve in the intercellular fluid. The glycolic acid is converted to glycine, then serine, and subsequently to pyruvic acid that enters the TCA cycle and is eliminated as carbon dioxide and water. PLA is broken down into lactic acid, which is converted to pyruvic acid and eliminated as carbon dioxide and water. PCL degrades to hydrohexanoic acid, a metabolizable metabolite.[9]

The degradation kinetics of poly(α-hydroxy acids) (PHA) is significantly affected by the molecular weight, morphology, and crystallinity. Properties such as crystallinity and morphology are strongly dependent on the thermal processing and sterilization techniques, which have a bearing on the rate of degradation, an important parameter in the designing of bioabsorbable devices. In general, higher molecular weight polymers possess superior mechanical properties and slower degradation rates in comparison with their lower counterparts. As the mechanism of degradation is autocatalytic in nature, and hydrolysis of PLA/PGA yields acids, higher molecular weight polymers have less acid-catalyzing groups present, and the longer chain length requires chain scission to occur more drastically until the oligomeric units are small enough to diffuse through the matrix, thus slowing the rate of degradation.[10] Morphology and crystallinity also play a major role in the degradation of the semicrystalline polymers, the amorphous regions being more prone to degradation than the crystalline domains. The processing parameters also strongly influence the mechanical properties, and increasing crystallinity through processing, annealing, and sterilization is reflected in the mechanical properties such as tensile strength and Young's modulus.[11] The mechanism of degradation in these polymers is via bulk and surface erosion, and the primary driving force is the relative hydrophilicity of the polymer that governs the ingress of aqueous solutions from the surface to within the bulk. As degradation begins, the accumulation of water-soluble degradation products causes an auto acceleration to occur, which causes more fluids to ingress within the bulk, further increasing the kinetics of the degradation process. The degradation process can be modulated by modification of the backbone of the polymer chain, and thus it provides the possibility of tailoring to regulate bulk degradation rates. Recently, it was hypothesized that surface erosion could be modified by tuning the hydrophobicity of a polymer backbone using a modular approach to polymer synthesis, wherein judiciously designed building blocks of varying lipophilicities are linked together using hydrophobic spacers. Based on this rationale, Xu et al. reported the synthesis of a library of polymers by designing macromonomer diols with differing lipophilicities, and then chemically reacting them with diacid spacers with thermal and physical properties distinct from pure PLLA and enhanced surface erosion behavior.[12]

The processing of PLA, PGA or copolymers, and subsequent sterilization techniques, has an impact on the molecular weight, crystallinity, and morphology of the resorbable implants. A systematic *in vivo* study by Chawla and Chang, with four different molecular weight PLA polymers implanted in rats, showed conclusively that the lower molecular weight polymers had a faster rate of degradation. This observation is associated with the difference in morphology and crystallinity.[13] Although, extrapolating *in vitro* degradation studies to *in vivo* models is not always linear, *in vitro* degradation studies confirm that degradation rates vary and thus the tailoring of copolymers to best justify a particular application is possible. The degradation of the suture Dexon based on PGA was reported to occur as a result of bulk degradation with selective attack on the amorphous regions.[14] Chu suggested that the diffusion of the oligomers was a significant component in the later stages of hydrolysis. The examination of the microstructure by scanning electron microscopy also supported the theory of the preferential attack and hydrolysis of the amorphous domains.[15] It was also reported that annealed specimens exhibited a faster rate of loss of mechanical properties than unannealed specimens when subjected to hydrolysis.[16,17] It is also important to note that a faster rate of the decrease in mechanical properties does not necessarily imply that it will exhibit a faster rate of degradation. Additionally, the degradation medium also influences the *in vitro* degradation rates. The degradation in both physiological and acidic media for Dexon and Vicryl were reported to not have a profound effect on the degradation, however, for the latter, maximum retention of tensile strength was obtained at a pH of 7.[18] In contrast, an alkaline buffer medium had a remarkable effect on the degradation and weight loss was reported to occur with increasing pH values.[19,20]

Surface chemistry and topography are important parameters for both biocompatibility and performance of biomedical devices. Any surface modifications that enhance cell adhesion, cell growth, and proliferation are advantageous for biomedical applications. Surface wettability is another important parameter since it has been established that moderately hydrophilic surfaces favor cellular adhesion and biocompatibility. Thus, covalent surface modification is generally favored over physical adsorption because of superior environmental stability. The molecular weight of PLLA and other aliphatic polyesters deteriorate through processing and sterilization, naturally influencing the overall degradation profile of the final processed polymer. Polymers generally tend to degrade as a result of processing and parameters such as temperature, residence time, presence of moisture, shearing action, and irradiation.[21]

The biocompatibility of PGA and PLA have been reviewed by Böstman and Pihlajamäki.[22] *In vitro* biocompatibility evaluation of these polymers is limited, however a large number of investigations report *in vivo* studies of particular devices.[23,24] The *in vitro* acute toxicity of two copolymers, namely, 70:30 poly (L,D, D,L-lactide) (PLDLA), and 90:10 poly(L-lactide-*co*-glycolide) (PLGA), were evaluated by the agar diffusion test and the filter test with L929 mouse fibroblasts.[25] The leachables from these copolymers obtained at temperatures of 37°C and 70°C, were assessed for mitochondrial succinate dehydrogenase activity by 3-(4,5-dimethylthiazol-2-yl)-2,5-diphenyltetrazolium bromide (MTT assay) and the incorporation of 5-bromo-2′-deoxyuridine (BrdU) into DNA of BALB 3T3 cells. Both materials revealed no signs of cytotoxicity during the agar diffusions and the MTT and BrdU assays PLDLA and PLGA showed similar results. The temperature at which the leachables were extracted was observed to exhibit an influence on the mitochondrial activity, with cells treated with extracts prepared at 37°C caused slight stimulation of mitochondrial activity and cells incubated with the 70°C media revealed a concentration-dependent decrease of mitochondrial activity. These *in vitro* results suggested that PLDLA and PLGA have satisfactory biocompatibility; however, high concentrations of the degradation products were reported to show a toxic influence on the cell culture systems used.[25] Adverse tissue response in PLA implants have been reported to be lower than PGA and foreign body response to PLLA would usually take longer *in vivo*. The crystalline debris yielded during degradation may be responsible for foreign body response and osteolysis, which are sometimes observed with PLLA.[26] Adverse inflammatory reactions in the long term have been known to occur with the use of slowly degrading bioabsorbable poly-L-lactide screws for bone fixation.[27] Complications from implants of lactide and glycolide occur typically at a rate of less than 10%. PCL is currently regarded as a nontoxic and tissue-compatible material[28] with good cell interaction in cell culture studies.[29] Thus, designing of devices for any biomedical application necessitates the tailoring of polymers to suit the physical, mechanical, and biological requirements.[10,30]

15.2.1.2 Poly(ε-Caprolactone)

PCL is derived by the ring opening polymerization of ε-caprolactone (Figure 15.4). It is a degradable polyester with a low melting point (~60°C) and a glass transition temperature (T_g) of −60°C. PCL is a hydrophobic, semicrystalline polymer, and has a relatively slow rate of degradation. PCL undergoes hydrolytic degradation and is assisted by enzymatic degradative processes. The molecular weight of the polymer influences especially the first stages of the degradation wherein random hydrolytic ester cleavage occurs autocatalyzed by the carboxyl end groups. The second stage of degradation sets in when the molecular weights are low and oligomers begin diffusing through the bulk matrix, at which point, fragmentation occurs.[31,32]

PCL has been studied for drug delivery applications and is especially compatible with hydrophobic drug entities, and high loading of the drug can be achieved. It has also been developed as a wound closure staples.[33]

15.2.1.3 Copolymers of PLA, PGA, and PCL

Copolymers based on PLA, PGA, PCL, and PEG confer a wide range of properties to polymers and thus open up new avenues for drug delivery, gene therapy, orthopedic implants, scaffolds for tissue engineering, and many other biomedical applications. The copolymers can be tailored to impart different crystallinity, morphology, molecular weight, thermal, and mechanical properties; thus the biodegradability can be controlled according to the clinical need. In order to alter, for example, the mechanical properties and degradation characteristics of polymers, copolymers can be fabricated. There is no linear relationship between the physical properties of the source homopolymers and the resulting copolymers.[34] The crystallinity of copolymers are lower than their related homopolymers, thus degrade more rapidly. For instance, the copolymer of PLLA and PGA with a ratio of 25:70 mol% of glycolide is largely amorphous and thus degrades more rapidly than PLLA itself. If PDLLA is a component of the PGA/PLA copolymer, the copolymer itself is amorphous in nature. The sequence of the component units in a copolymer linear chain also affects degradation rate. Thus block and random copolymers exhibit different degradation rates. Biodegradable polymers such as PLA and PGA are used extensively as scaffolds in tissue engineering for the regeneration of musculoskeletal tissues.[35,36] Copolymers and homopolymers can be fabricated into different sizes and shapes with differing molecular architecture and each of these parameters influence the degradation kinetics. Thus, *in vitro* degradation studies need to consider the effects of composition, porosity,[37] permeability, mechanical loading, and the effect of a dynamic flow medium experienced *in vivo*.[38]

The aliphatic polyesters are one of the most attractive groups of polymers that have been widely used in biomedical applications. The advent of the degradable suture using PLA, PGA, PCL, or

(a)

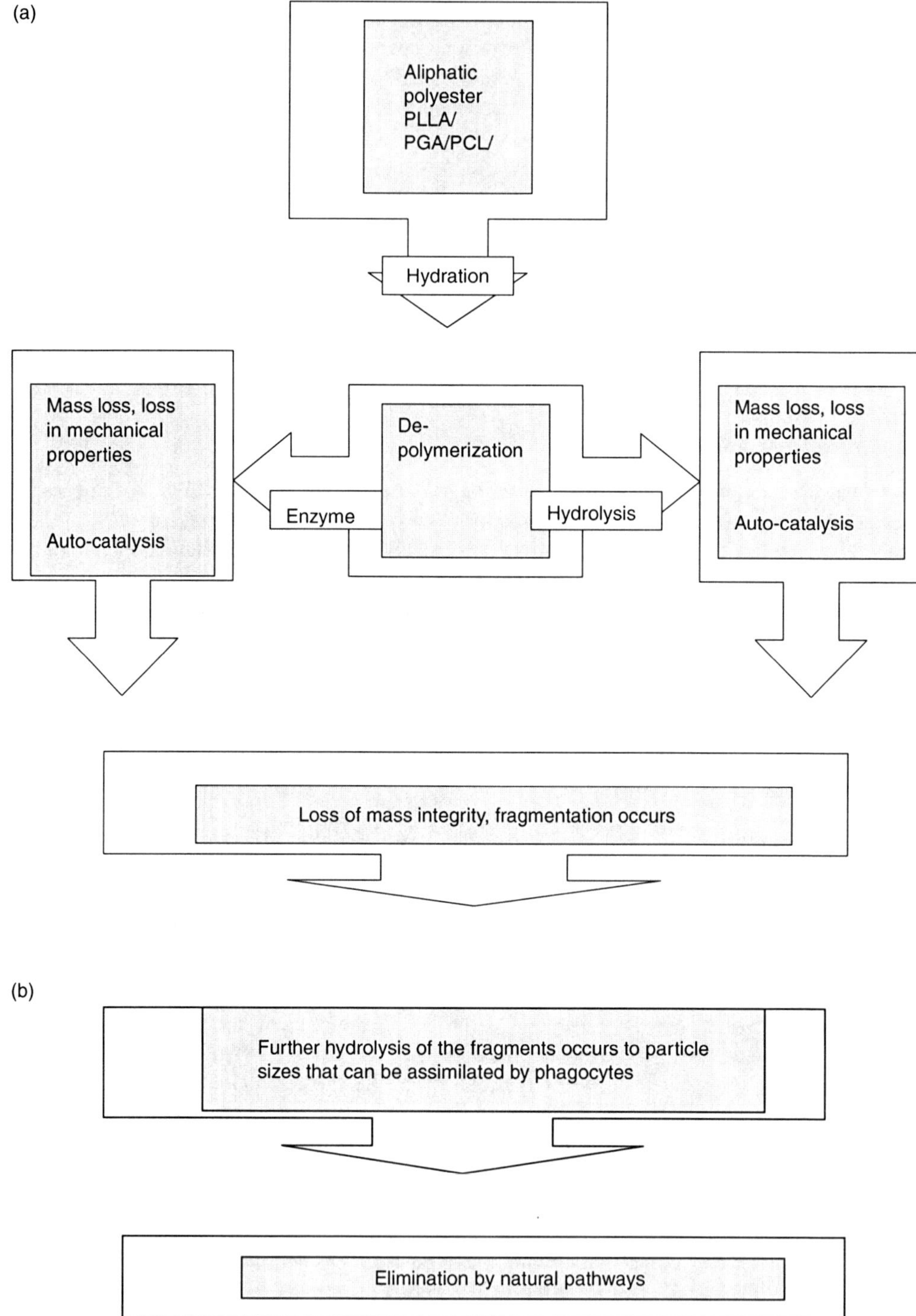

FIGURE 15.3 Sequence in the degradation of aliphatic polyesters.

PDS and its successful clinical use triggered a great deal of interest and thus a large number of biomedical applications have been researched. Biomedical applications range from orthopedic applications such as bone screws, pins and staples, to scaffolds used for tissue engineering in different applications such as the nerve, cardiovascular, ocular, and drug delivery applications. A few applications are discussed at the end of the chapter.

15.2.2 POLYDIOXANONE

Polydioxanone belongs to the poly(ether–ester) family, which is commonly used as a biodegradable suture material. Polydioxanones can be unsymmetrically substituted, yielding poly(1,4-dioxanone-2,5 diones), poly(1,3-dioxane-2-one), and poly(1,4-dioxane-2,3-dione). Poly(para-dioxanone), as shown in Figure 15.5, is primarily used as an absorbable suture material. It is a crystalline polymer that is obtained via the ring opening polymerization of p-dioxanone, in the presence of heat and organometallic catalysts.[39] Polydioxanone has a low glass transition temperature that ranges between 0°C and 10°C. The ether linkage within the polymeric backbone imparts flexibility to the polymer. The polymer has approximately 37–55% crystallinity and low-temperature processing is necessary to prevent depolymerization to the monomer. It is generally extruded into fibers to manufacture sutures.[39] Polydioxanone suture was first marketed by Ethicon and has been shown to be nontoxic. Monofilaments of PDS are absorbed within 6 months and mechanical strength decreases by 50% within 3 weeks; hence, it is advantageous for applications where rapid degradation is required.

Degradation of PDS proceeds through hydrolysis and changes in elastic modulus; pH and molecular weight, monitored over time, suggest that hydrolysis occurs at the ester bonds. The crystallinity is found to increase initially, suggesting that the amorphous regions undergo more rapid degradation followed by the crystalline regions. Elastic modulus decreases, as does the molecular weight with time. The surface morphological studies indicate that heterogeneous degradation does occur.[40] It is important to note that the geometry of the polymer, thickness, and shape govern the rate of degradation along with molecular weight and crystallinity, hence comparison between different studies is difficult. Copolymers of with p-dioxanone, lactides, and glycolides yield a family of polymers, which also find use in drug delivery systems. PDS has been investigated for arterial regeneration in rabbits for closure of abdominal wounds, for fixation of facial fractures, and for orbital floor reconstruction.[41]

15.2.3 POLYETHYLENE GLYCOL

Polyethylene oxide (PEO) is a polymer that has the repeat structural unit $-CH_2CH_2O-$ and finds application in drug delivery. The material known as poly(ethylene glycol) (PEG), possesses a similar

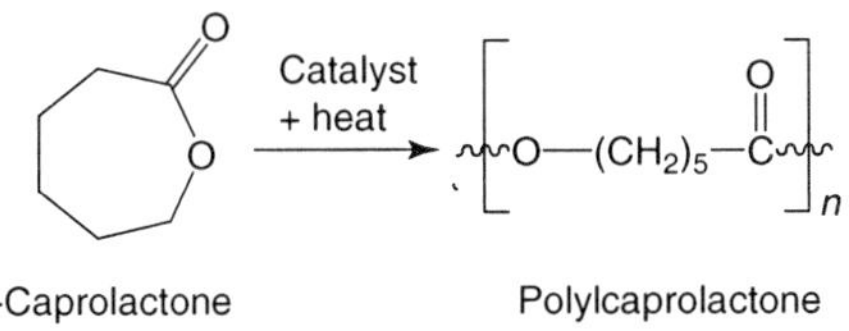

FIGURE 15.4	Synthesis of polycaprolactone from ε-caprolactone.

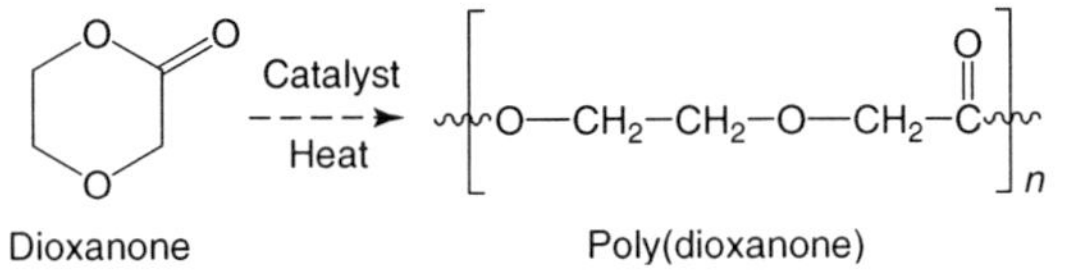

FIGURE 15.5	Synthesis of poly(dioxanone).

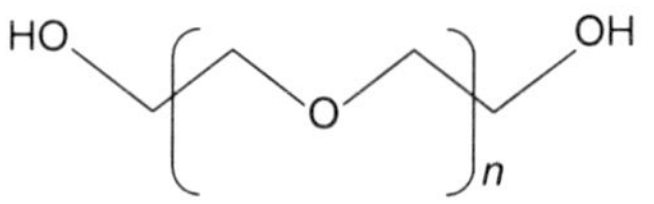

FIGURE 15.6   Polyethylene glycol.

repeating unit, however in addition, it has hydroxyl groups at each end of the molecule. Typically, high molecular weight polyethylene oxide polymers are used as biomaterials whereas PEG is frequently used with low degree of polymerization with "n" ranging from 12 to 400, although high molecular weight polymers are commercially available. PEO and PEG are highly biocompatible, which makes them attractive as biomaterials, and in addition, PEG with its hydroxyl end groups (Figure 15.6) can be synthetically linked with other polymeric units providing versatility in the properties of the modified polymers. PEG is soluble in water, methanol, dichloromethane, diethyl ether, and hexane. It can be covalently linked to hydrophobic molecules that yield surfactants.

PEG is a water-soluble and flexible polymer, the backbone similar to that of silicones. It has little specific interaction with biological molecules and is very useful in applying osmotic pressure. PEG[42,43] is nontoxic and used in a variety of medicinal and cosmetic products. Hydrogels of PEG are also good candidates for tissue engineering scaffolds because they are highly biocompatible and exhibit versatile physical characteristics based on their weight percent, molecular chain length, and crosslinking density.[44] It has been used in drug delivery and proteins attached covalently to PEG, enhances the efficacy of the drug due to improved dosing intervals and slow clearance from the blood. PEG is also a constituent in skin creams, laxatives, and toothpaste, etc.

PEGylation is a term that is increasingly being used to describe the ability to covalently link the PEG unit with other larger molecules, especially useful in the field of pharmaceutics. PEGylated proteins are commonly used, for example, PEGylated interferon as an injectable drug for Hepatitis C infection. PEG-fibrinogen hydrogels made up of protein fragments covalently bound to PEG-DA and crosslinked using UV photoinitiation have been reported, which allow the fibrinogen constituent to be covalently linked to functionalized PEG. A Michael-type addition reaction is used to form the ester bond between the free thiols in the fibrinogen cysteines and acrylate end groups on the PEG-DA (PEGylation).[45] PEG-fibrinogen hydrogels have also been synthesized using denatured fibrinogen fragments that are PEGylated with PEG-diacrylates, mixed with photoinitiator, and exposed to UV light to form a hydrogel material in the presence of a cell suspension. The advantage of this type of material lies in its mechanical properties while maintaining biological functionality. The elastic modulus of such PEG-fibrinogen hydrogel has been shown to be dependent on the molecular weight of the PEG constituent and proportional to the percent polymeric composition. These type of scaffolds can be very useful for cultivating cells in a 3D environment for tissue regeneration therapies.[46] Recent research has shown that it can aid in both peripheral and central nerve repair[47] and improve in spinal healing in animal models. Several groups have investigated PEO as an injectable polymeric device for chondral defects. The high degree of hydration in PEO gels acts as barrier to macromolecules involved in the immune response and it has an established biocompatibility. The potential for PEO in the repair of articular cartilage is high because of its ability to retain water and its crosslinking under facile conditions. PEG is currently under investigation for newer clinical applications such as colorectal cancer and paraplegia.

15.2.4   TRIMETHYLENE CARBONATE

A ring-opening polymerization of cyclic carbonate or lactones yields trimethylene carbonate. A variety of organocatalysts have been surveyed for the ring opening polymerization and excellent control on molecular weight and polydispersities can be obtained.[48] ABA-type triblock copolymers, poly(trimethylene carbonate)-poly(ethylene glycol)-poly(trimethylene carbonate), obtained via the ring-opening polymerization of trimethylene carbonate and initiated by dihydroxyl poly(ethylene glycol), have been reported and investigated for the release of anticancer drugs.[49] It is generally used as a plasticizer and has been incorporated in Maxon sutures.[50] More recently, nanoparticles of poly(trimethylene carbonate) (PTMC) and monomethoxy PEG-*block*-PTMC (mPEG-PTMC), with poly(vinyl alcohol) as a stabilizer, were synthesized with particles sizes in the range between 95 and 120 nm. The particles were reported to be stable over 20 weeks, and dexamethasone release studies conducted by using these nanoparticles showed that the release was diffusion controlled and, sustained release over 14 to 60 days was possible.[51]

15.2.5 POLY(α-AMINO ACIDS)

Poly(amino acids) widely occur in nature and synthetic analogs have been investigated for biomedical applications. Poly(α-amino acids) are synthesized from aspartic acid and glutamic acid, or can be fermented. Pure poly(α-amino acids) are highly crystalline, which results in slow rates of degradation and the antigenicity of these polymers can make *in vivo* use more challenging. Poly(esteramides) are the most commonly investigated of these group of polymers. Drug delivery applications have reported wherein covalent attachment of drugs to the polymer backbone has been achieved.[52]

15.2.6 POLY(ALKYL 2-CYANOACRYLATES)

Poly(alkyl 2-cyanoacrylates) are synthesized from cyanoacrylates. They have excellent adhesive properties as a result of the strong bonds that can form with polar substrates including living tissues and skin.[53–55] They are widely used as surgical adhesives.[56,57] Polycyanoacrylates are synthesized from cyanoacrylates as shown in Figure 15.7.

Polyalkylcyanoacrylates are used in several biomedical applications[58] and more recently with increasing interest in the field of nanotechnology, these polymers have also been prepared in nanoparticulate sizes and utilized in drug delivery.[59] These polymers have been investigated extensively for drug delivery. There have been three main generations of polyalkylcyanoacrylates drug delivery systems, the first being the conventional drug carriers where the molecules are rapidly eliminated from the blood stream by the macrophages, the second being stealth drug carriers in which the drug carriers avoid the macrophages due to the PEG chains on their surface;[60] thus, they are able to circulate for a longer time, however still do not target the tissue. The third generation drug carriers are called targeted drug delivery systems that can target a tissue or a cell due to the chemical grafting of PEG chains.[61] There is an increasing interest in this group of polymers for therapeutics, especially for cancer treatments, which involve highly toxic molecules in contact with healthy tissues.[62–64] Polymer colloidal drug delivery systems are considered promising for targeted drug delivery and compounds such as nucleic acids and peptides are being tethered to the poly(alkylcyanoacrylates), and it is one of the most promising group of polymers that are being investigated. This is due to the fact that cyanoacrylate monomers are able to form polymeric materials with biodegradable characteristics that may easily be controlled depending on the nature of the cyanoacrylic monomer used. Heparin-coated poly(isobutylcyanoacrylate) nanoparticles have

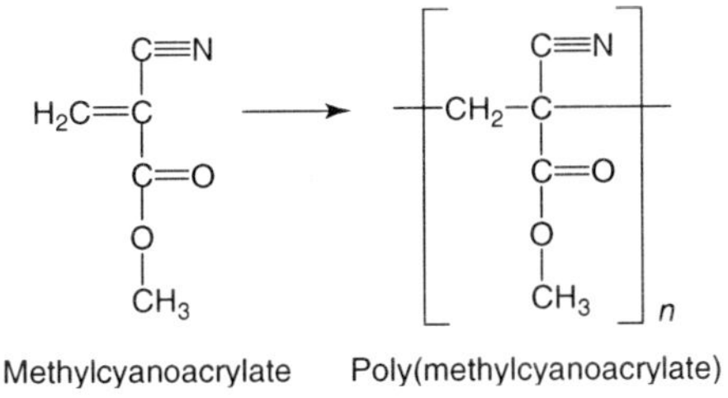

FIGURE 15.7 Polymerization of methylcyanoacrylate to poly(methylcyanoacrylate).

been recently developed to carry hemoglobin. These copolymers are able to form nanoparticles in water with a ciliated surface of heparin and are able to maintain the antithrombogenic properties of heparin and thus inhibit complement activation. Hence, these drug delivery systems are suitable tools in the treatment of thrombosis oxygen-deprived pathologies.[65] However, as stated above, many questions remain concerning the intracellular fate of nanoparticles, probably because the answers differ from one cell line to another and from one cyanoacrylic polymer to another. Whatever the answer, there is an urgent need to design nanoparticles which will be able to specifically deliver these molecules, either to the cytoplasm or to the nucleus, depending on the target.[66]

15.2.7 POLYURETHANES

Polyurethanes (PUs) consist of urethane linkages and the main backbone is produced by the reaction between a diisocyanate (aromatic or aliphatic) and polyol, typically polyethylene glycol or polyester glycol in presence of catalysts, as shown in Figure 15.8. Polyurethanes have extensive structure property diversity and are extremely favored for biomedical applications, especially for blood contacting devices. The properties of polyurethanes can be designed and are mainly governed by the choice of the polyol; however, the diisocyanate exerts some influence. Their popularity has been sustained as a direct result of their segmented block copolymeric character, which endows them

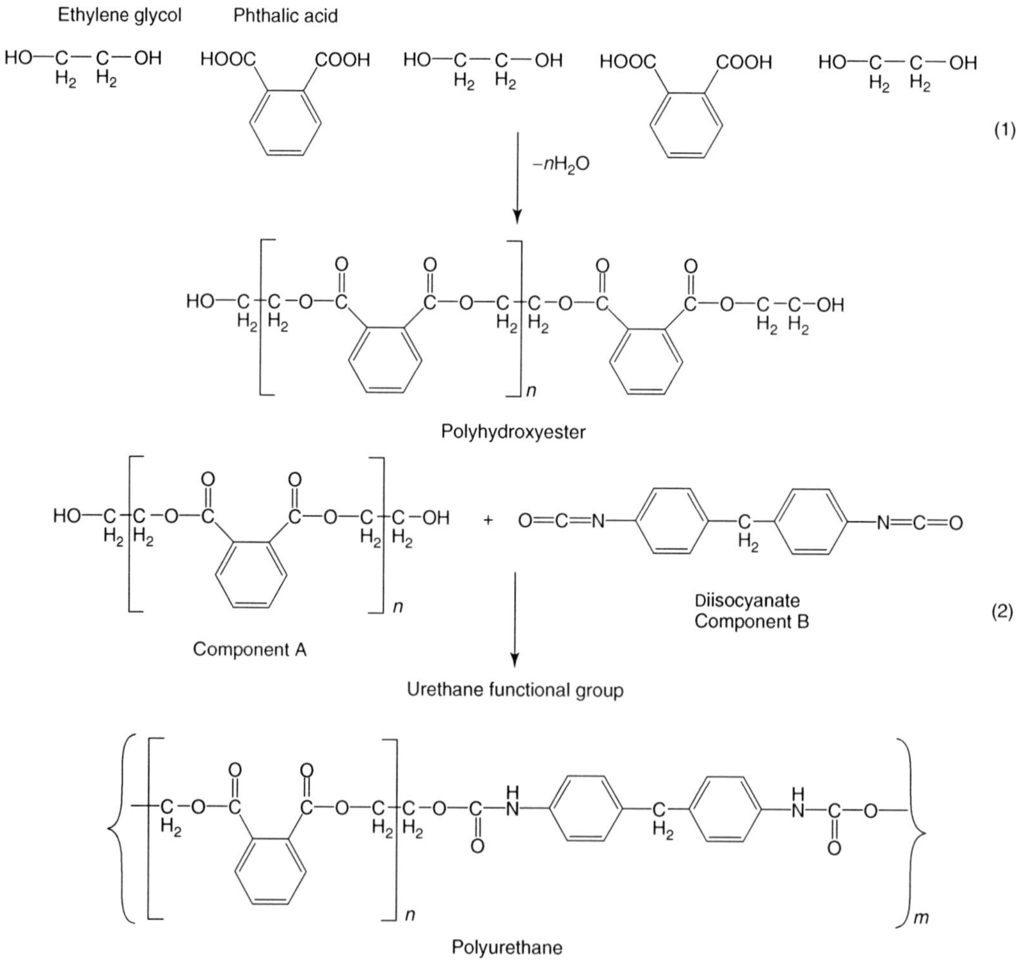

FIGURE 15.8 The formation of polyurethanes.

with a wide range of versatility in terms of tailoring their physical properties, blood and tissue compatibility, and more recently, their biodegradation character. Softer and more flexible polyurethanes result when linear difunctional polyethylene glycol segments, commonly called polyether polyols, are used to create the urethane links. This strategy is used to make elastomeric fibers and soft rubber parts, as well as foam rubber. More rigid products result if polyfunctional polyols are used, as these create a three-dimensional cross-linked structure, which again, can be in the form of low-density foams. The mechanical properties, density, hardness and other physical properties, can be modified by selection of appropriate monomers.

Poyurethanes have had a significant role in the development of medical devices ranging from catheters to artificial heart components. Biostable medical devices have been fabricated from polyurethanes due to their durability, elasticity, good fatigue resistance, and biotolerance. Furthermore, the propensity for bulk and surface modifications allow attachment of biologically active species such as anticoagulants and other biomolecules, which aid in the healing process. Segmented polyurethanes also show low bacterial adhesion and hemocompatibility in addition to good mechanical properties.[67,68] Polyester urethanes are hydrolytically unstable and hence are being increasingly modified with silicone containing moeities to restrict the chronic *in vivo* instability. Thus, devices such as breast implants and cardiovascular devices that require long-term biostability have caused concern. Polyurethanes have been the subject of extensive investigation in terms of biodegradation studies[69] and as a consequence, not only has there has been a move to develop more biostable implants but also to develop a new class of bioresorbable materials with all the versatility of PUs in terms of physical properties and biocompatibility. The designs of biodegradable PUs have incorporated comonomers such as lactide and glycolide, polycaprolactone units, and polyethylene oxide.

Polyurethane foam breast implants were first used in 1970s as a biostable implant.[70,71] In the late 1980s, it was reported that *in vitro* degradation of polyurethane could lead to formation of substances known to be carcinogenic in animals.[72] This information raised concerns on the potential carcinogenic effect of polyurethane breakdown products in humans; however, with the very low risk associated, this product was not banned by the The United States Food and Drug Administration (FDA). Subsequently, these implants were voluntarily withdrawn from the market in 1991. Polyurethane coatings have been used to decrease bacterial adhesion on implant surfaces[73,74] and enhanced blood compatibility has been achieved through different methods. There is a vast amount of literature on this subject and a detailed discussion is outside the scope of this chapter.

15.3 NATURAL DEGRADABLE POLYMERS

Polysaccharides form a group of polymers that have found extensive use in biomedical application. The nontoxicity of the polymers, their monomeric residues, facile chemical modifications to alter fluid uptake, their swellability, and a wide variety of chemical structures with excellent properties make them a versatile group of polymers for medical application.

15.3.1 ALGINATES

Alginic acid is an insoluble polysaccharide and the sodium, potassium, or ammonium salts are the alginates. Alginate is a water-soluble linear polysaccharide extracted from brown seaweed and is composed of alternating blocks of 1,4-linked α-L-guluronic (G) and β-D-mannuronic acid (M) residues. The structure is shown in Figure 15.9 and the binding between the two residues in the alginate molecule. Alginates are not random copolymers and the pattern of the two residues, D and M, differ according to the source of the algae, each of which have different conformational preferences and behavior, for example, the M/G ratio of alginate from *Macrocystis pyrifera* is about 1.6 whereas that from *Laminaria hyperborea* is about 0.45.

The β-D-mannuronic acid blocks and α-L-guluronic acid blocks can be arranged in different proportions and sequences along the polymer chain and the composition; sequences of the residues

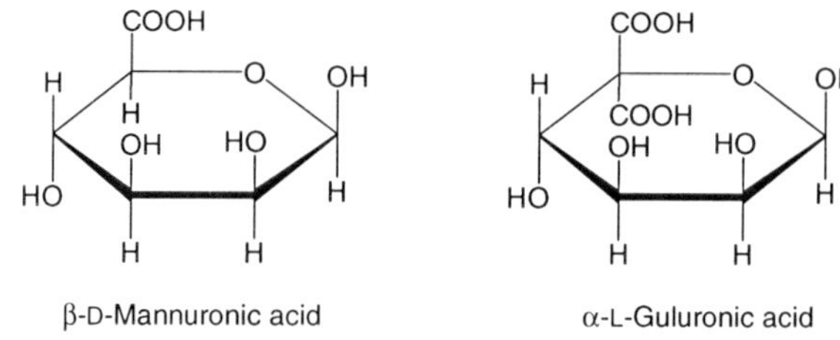

FIGURE 15.9 The M and G units of alginic acid.

and molecular weight determine the physical properties of the alginate.[75,76] The solubility of alginates and water retention capacity depends on the pH and precipitation occurs at about pH 3.5. The molecular weight also affects water holding capacity, and calcium alginates with low molecular weights or less than 500 residues exhibit higher water uptake and binding. Sodium alginate and most other alginates from monovalent metals are soluble in water, forming solutions of considerable viscosity. The rheological properties of alginate sols make them particularly useful as a thickening agent and have long been used in the pharmaceutical industry as thickening or gelling agents, as colloidal stabilizers and as blood expanders. Alginates are used to take impressions of the oral tissue due to their ability to undergo a transformation from the sol state to a gel state through ionotropic gelation in the presence of many multivalent ions such as Ca^{2+}. The crosslinking can be carried out under very mild conditions at low temperatures and high humidity. Alginates have been widely investigated for cartilage and bone regeneration, either as a scaffold or as carriers for biologically active molecules and drug delivery.[77–81]

15.3.2 CHITOSAN

Chitosan is a linear copolymer of glucosamine and *N*-acetyl glucosamine in a β-1-4 linkage, usually obtained from chitin. Chitin is the second most abundant natural polymer in the world after cellulose. Chitosan is produced by the deacetylation of chitin (Figure 15.10), which is the structural element of the shells of crustaceans such as crab and shrimps. The degree of deacetylation (%DA) and the molecular weight determine the properties of chitosan. The degree of deacetylation can be determined from nuclear magnetic resonance (NMR) data and ranges between 60% and 100% in commercial chitosan. Chitosan is positively charged and soluble in acidic to neutral solution with a charge density dependent on pH and the %DA-value.

The DA, which signifies the mole fraction of the N-acetylated units is a structural parameter and influences charge density, crystallinity, solubility and proneness to enzymatic degradation. Chitosan readily binds to negatively charged surfaces such as mucosal membranes and hence acts as a bioadhesive. It displays interesting properties such as biocompatibility, biodegradability, and its degradation products are nontoxic, nonimmunogenic and noncarcinogenic.[82] As a polysaccharide of natural origin, chitosan has many useful features such as nontoxicity, biocompatibility, biodegradability, and antimicrobial properties.[83] It exhibits excellent biological properties such as biodegradation in the human body, immunological, antibacterial, wound-healing activity, and is used as microcapsule implants for controlled release in drug delivery.[84] Chitosan is one of the most promising biopolymers for tissue engineering and possible orthopedic applications. In particular, the possibility to generate structures with predictable pore sizes and degradation rates makes it a suitable material as a bone graft alternative in orthopedic procedures.[85,86] It has been recently approved for use in bandages as it can cause rapid clotting. Chitosan has been found to be the material that supports gene delivery, cell culture, and tissue engineering.[87,88] It has also been proven to be safe for use as a pharmaceutical excipient and has properties that make it suitable for drug delivery applications. As chitosan shows great promise in controlled release, this material is being increasingly exploited for developing nano- and microparticles for drug delivery, gene therapy, and regenerative medicine.[89–91]

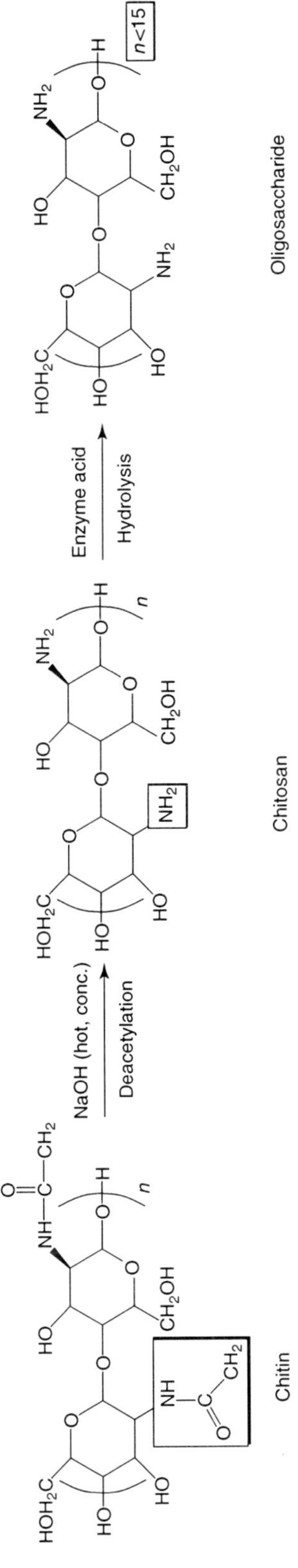

FIGURE 15.10 Chitin, chitosan, and the oligomeric saccharides.

15.3.3 ALBUMIN

Albumins are water-soluble proteins that also exhibit a degree of solubility in concentrated salt solutions. They are heat-sensitive and coagulate. Egg white contains albumin and the most commonly known albumin is serum albumin present in human blood. They are the most abundant blood plasma protein, which act as transport proteins for several steroid hormones and fatty acids. Being a naturally occurring protein in the human body, albumin has also been considered for biomedical applications. Surfaces of polymers have been modified by grafting albumin on their surfaces in order to enhance blood compatibility. Functionalized albumin has been covalently linked to polymers such as polyethylene, polycarbonates, and polypropylene, etc. The grafted albumin molecules are retained on the surface, even on exposure to blood for extended periods; they function as good oxygenators.[92] Laser welding technologies have also been used to join, repair, and create hemostasis on surfaces using human-serum-albumin based biodegradable biomaterials.

15.3.4 COLLAGEN

Collagen is another abundant protein, which is the main component of connective tissues in mammals. It has a long fibrous structure and is found as "collagen fibrils," which are tough bundles of fibrillar proteins. They possess good tensile strength and are a component of cartilage, tendons, ligaments, bone, and teeth. Collagen is also responsible for the elasticity and strength of the skin and its degradation leads to wrinkles and facilitate aging. Collagen has an amino acid composition, and interestingly, almost every third amino acid residue is a glycine unit and is known to contain large fractions of proline. There are at least 28 types of known collagens [from Wikipedia, the free encyclopedia]. Collagen Type I is the most abundant in human body, forms a structural component of bone and teeth, and is present in scar tissue and in tendons. Collagen has been known for its use as a "glue" since ancient times. More recently it has been widely used in soft tissue augmentation.[93] Collagen has been used to develop biologic patches and for purposes of tendon augmentation and is used in sports medicine,[94] namely Zimmer Collagen Repair and TissueMend (TEI Biosciences, Boston, MA, USA). Collagens on their own or in combination with silicones, glycosaminoglycans, fibroblasts, growth factors, and other substances are employed in the management of burns and act as artificial skin substitutes. Collagen-GAG scaffolds loaded with basic fibroblast growth factor have been reported to significantly enhance neovascularization and tissue remodeling in animal models.[95] Soft-tissue fillers, most commonly injectable collagen or fat, can help fill in these lines and creases, temporarily restoring a smoother, more youthful-looking appearance. When injected beneath the skin, these fillers plump up creased and sunken areas of the face. They can also add fullness to the lips and cheeks. Injectable fillers may be used alone or in conjunction with a resurfacing procedure, such as a laser treatment, or a recontouring procedure, such as a facelift.

15.3.5 HYALURONIC ACID

Hyaluron or hyaluronic acid (HA) is a non-sulfated glycosaminoglycan that is widely distributed throughout connective, epithelial and neural tissues. Hyaluronan is a polymer consisting of disaccharides with D-glucoronic acid and D-N-acetylglucosamine, linked via alternating beta-1,4 and beta-1,3 glycosidic bonds. It is one of the main components of the extracellular matrix, contributes significantly to cell proliferation and migration, and may also be involved in the progression of some malignant tumors. Polymers of hyaluronan can range in size from 10^2 to 10^4 kDa *in vivo*. Hyaluronan is a major component of the synovial fluid and is found to increase the viscosity of the fluid. It is also a main constituent of the articular cartilage, present as a coating on chondrocytes. The high molecular mass HA, which plays an important role in many biological processes such as tissue hydration, proteoglycan organization in the extracellular matrix, and tissue repair, has found application in several clinical treatments and cosmetic use. Degradation of HA is enzyme mediated and the responsible enzymes are hyaluronidases. The degradation products are oligosaccharides and low molecular weight hyaluron. HA was first developed as a biomedical product in the 1970s and used for eye surgery in the 1980s. Healon was used for corneal transplantation, cataract surgery, and retinal detachment.[96] It has been used in the treatment of osteoporosis and is generally administered as a course of injections.[97,98] This topic has been eloquently reviewed by Allison & Grande-Allen and further details are not within the scope of this chapter.[99]

15.4 APPLICATIONS

Degradable polymers have found widespread use as biomaterials for biomedical applications. Biomaterials have been used for skin, bone, cartilage, vascular, nerve, and drug delivery.[100]

15.4.1 ORTHOPEDICS

The use of bioabsorbable materials has become commonplace in orthopedic surgery. Screws, suture anchors, meniscal repair devices, bone plates, staples, and simple fracture fixation devices have expanded the armamentarium of the orthopedic surgeon, and are increasingly used for anterior cruciate ligament reconstruction, shoulder surgery, meniscal repair, and fracture care.[101–103] The three most commonly used polymers in clinical applications are PGA, PLA, and polydioxanone.[104] These polymers are α-polyesters or poly(α-hydroxy) acids and can be used for stabilization of fractures, osteotomies, bone grafts, and fusions, as well as for reattachment of ligaments, tendons, meniscal tears, and other soft tissue structures. The advantage of such devices is their resorbability, thus the need for a removal operation is overcome and long-term interference with tendons, nerves, and the growing skeleton is avoided. The polymeric devices also provide lower moduli, thus, problems associated with periprosthetic stress shielding and infections are reduced.[105] Poly-L-lactic bioabsorbable interference screws have been reported to provide clinical results, which are similar to metal interference screw for fixation of a central third bone-patellar tendon-bone graft in ACL reconstruction.

15.4.2 TISSUE ENGINEERING AND DEGRADABLE POLYMERS

The field of tissue engineering is a rapidly emerging field that aims to address a diverse range of clinical needs for the replacement of damaged or diseased tissues. Biomaterials, on its own, are able to address certain clinical needs through the development of prosthetic hearts, valves, blood vessels, and artificial breasts; however, only few perform adequately over the life span of a patient. Tissue engineering aims to create three-dimensional tissues and organs using autologous cells. The three main components of tissue engineering are namely the scaffold, appropriate cells, and the presence of appropriate growth factors. Thus, the scaffold is generally intended to provide the shape of the construct, which then is eliminated by the body, while the natural tissues regrow. Scaffolds thus form an integral part of the tissue-engineered construct and must be able to direct the arrangement of cells in an appropriate three-dimensional configuration and present molecular signals in appropriate spatial and temporal manner. Growth factors are increasingly employed to promote tissue regeneration with various biomaterial scaffolds. *In vitro* release kinetics of protein growth factors from tissue engineering scaffolds are often investigated in aqueous environment, which is significantly different from *in vivo* environment. Biodegradable polymers, thus form the basis of a large number of scaffolds that are used for tissue engineering; however, detailed discussion is outside the scope of this chapter. Nerve tissue engineering is expected to be one of the most promising methods for the restoration of central nerve system damages in health care. Spinal cord injury, particularly when it involves partial or complete transection of the cord, is devastating, as transected axons, in the absence of further intervention, do not regenerate. Research has been mainly focused on the development of regimes to overcome this lack of axon growth, and limited but significant strides have been made within the past decade. Three-dimensional distribution and growth of cells within porous scaffolds are thus of clinical significance. Surgical management of these injuries, especially where nerves have been severed so that apposing ends are separated by long gaps, usually involves grafting. Early literature shows evidence of the use of several materials such that inserting them in a tube bridges the cut ends of the nerve. Early literature shows evidence that both filled and unfilled experimental nerve chambers can assist in bridging the cut ends of a nerve. Degradable polymers such as copolymers of poly (lactic) acid-caprolactone and Type 1 collagen have been used in the construction of tubes that have been reported to significantly induce outgrowth of axons in comparison to ethylene–vinylacetate copolymers.[106] Polymeric porous nano fibers from poly-L-lactic acid have been reported to promote *in vitro* cell culture of nerve stem cells (NSC) while behaving as the extra cellular matrix. *In vitro* cell culture showed that the 3-D porous scaffold seeded with NSC, supported differentiation and neurite outgrowth. Thus nanostructured PLLA scaffold with NSCs can be used for repair while being able to deliver therapeutic macromolecules and growth factors in a controlled fashion.[107] One of the major challenges in fabricating three-dimensional scaffolds is the ability to maintain adequate diffusion of nutrients to cells. Small diameter blood vessels are important for vascular tissue engineering, and micropatterned porous polycaprolactone scaffolds using novel techniques of soft lithography that are able to transport nutrients adequately have been recently reported.[108] Polydioxanone suture has handling properties that are acceptable for use in vascular applications,[109] and it provides adequate mechanical support for sutured vessels to heal.

Cardiovascular devices: Biodegradable porous scaffolds for heart tissue engineering have also been reported. Not surprisingly, the porous structures have been created from well-established bioabsorbable polymers such as PLLA. A copolymer of 1,3 trimethylene carbonate and DL-lactide, prepared by compression molding using salt leaching techniques, has been reported by Pego et al;[110] this copolymer has been produced in a reproducible manner. These interconnected porous structures have been shown to exhibit adequate mechanical properties and cell material interactions to serve as scaffolds for cardiac cells. The copolymers were shown to be elastomeric in nature and allowed the adhesion and proliferation of cardiomyocytes and early signs of degradation were apparent at only 4 weeks. Electrospinning techniques have been recently applied for the fabrication of biomaterials. Electrospun PLGA scaffolds were also examined for attachment of cardiomyocytes. Electrospun nano- and microfibrous networks provided oriented scaffold structures that encouraged anisotropic cell growth. The cardiomyocytes were also reported to be sensitive to the composition of the construct, and functional studies of CMs on the scaffolds further confirmed the superior response on PLLA scaffolds compared to PLA10GA90 + PLLA and PLGA + PEG − PLA. Thus, electrospun scaffolds provide flexibility and guidance to growth and can be successfully applied for cardiac tissue constructs.[111,112] Biomaterials in the fabrication of stents have been largely restricted to metals because of the need for good mechanical properties, the ability to provide support in maintaining the lumen gain, nonthrombogenic abilities, and biocompatibility. The elastic moduli of most biomedical polymers are in the range of 1–5 GPa, which is one restricting factor for developing stents using polymers. Nevertheless, coating and stents as a whole have been carried out using biostable polymers and several biodegradable polymers. Biostable polymers made up of PET have been shown to possess adequate mechanical strength and the radial pressures exerted are similar to stainless steel meshes. However, *in vivo* testing indicates foreign body inflammatory response with some thickening of the neointimal wall.

Poly(L-lactide-*co*-glycolide) (PLGA) and PUs are the most widely investigated materials for coatings of coronary stents. The degradation behavior of the polymer is a critical factor in the controlled delivery of the drug in the stent system. For example, the rate of heparin release was reported to be slowest for PLLA, followed by PLGA (80/20), and finally PLGA (53/47) for coronary stent applications.[113] Thus the rate of drug release from PLGA stents, as has been indicated, is likely to depend on the copolymer ratio. Recently, Venkatraman et al.[114] imparted self-expanding capability to biodegradable PLLA stents (at 37°C) by adding PLGA (53/47). This effect was induced in the bilayered stents by fabricating them at 37°C. Poly(L-lactide-*co*-glycolide) (PLGA) stents have been investigated more in urological applications than in coronary applications. PUs have been extensively used for medical device applications because of their excellent biocompatibility. These polymers have been used as a coating material on stents to improve the antithrombogenic properties of Ta, corrosion resistance of Ni–Ti and biocompatibility of SS (stainless steel). It was also reported that PU coatings can improve endothelialization. Thus, while some studies advocated the use of PU for stents, others show contradictory evidence. Hence it is difficult to categorize PU as a good or poor stent material. Although PU has been used successfully in many cardiovascular devices (pacemaker lead wires, vascular grafts, artificial heart pumps, and inner surface coatings of artificial heart), it does not necessarily mean that the coating may be beneficial for stents. Fibrin, a natural biopolymer and an insoluble protein, is known to be biocompatible and biodegradable with viscoelastic properties. Fibrin has also been tested as a stent coating material with encouraging results in a porcine model.[112]

15.4.3 DRUG DELIVERY

Biodegradable polymers have been the subject of intense interest in the field of controlled drug delivery. The need for site-specific, targeted, and controlled release of drugs has been recognized because it can improve bioavailability, including longer circulation time, and slower clearance, which can decrease the systemic drug level in the body with the efficacy of the improved drug as breakdown of the drug is limited and patient compliance is not crucial. Controlled drug delivery is a challenging field as applications require drugs to be released either at one time, in days, weeks, or months, or sustained release in different tissues, such as tumor sites, diseased blood vessels, and others. Extensive research has been focused on improving and creating advanced drug delivery systems.[115–117] The fact that active proteins can now be synthetically prepared and drugs can be produced by molecular biology–based techniques has stimulated the research in the field of controlled drug delivery. Furthermore, improvements in the efficacy of the drug through the changes in the molecular structure of the active protein molecules and the possibility of sustained release have had a marked effect on patient health care.

Hydrogels based on drug delivery vehicles[118] are of current major interest with several products available commercially. Degradable hydrogel systems are of potential interest in drug delivery. West and Hubbell synthesized PLA-b-PEG-b-PLA hydrogels composed of PLA and PEGblock copolymers for protein release applications.[119] Metters et al. developed scaling laws to predict the degradation rates of PLA-b-PEG-b-PLA hydrogels based on macroscopic properties such as compressive modulus and volumetric swelling ratio.[120,121] Controlled delivery devices are generally diffusion-based release systems applicable to release of drugs intended for the systemic circulation, or for a localized site. The basic approach developed by Langer provided the foundation of a wide variety of implantable and injectable devices made primarily from degradable materials. Drug-eluting stents are now providing medical technology to decrease restenosis and are also able to treat more complex lesions in coronary heart disease. For example, TAXUS paclitaxel-eluting stent in a soft, hydrophobic, elastomeric triblock copolymer, poly(styrene-b-isobutylene-b-styrene), is an example of this new class of product.[122] Polyurethane has also been investigated in drug delivery systems. However, some studies have shown that PU coating can be accompanied by extensive inflammatory reactions.[123]

15.5 CONCLUSION

Polymers are versatile materials that allow tailoring of its final properties. The polymers discussed in this chapter are typically biocompatible and are able to perform adequately for a number of biomedical applications. Degradable polymers such as PLA, PGA, PCL, and PDS are able to offer excellent suture materials, however these and related polymers have been relatively less successful in providing adequate hard tissue replacement alternatives. Materials for bone reconstruction must not only be biocompatible but also provide mechanical support for tissue regeneration and thus polymeric scaffolds need to be further developed and assessed. Presently there are no real solutions for long-term replacements for some connective tissues, small diameter blood vessels, and nerve grafts. The clinical need for whole organs is high, and tissue engineering is one emerging field in regenerative medicine. There still exists need for three-dimensional tissue engineered matrices that are able to integrate with biological tissues, thereby necessitating the development of more intelligent scaffolds. Controlled and targeted drug delivery is becoming extremely important and there has been a certain amount of success with many of the technical hurdles to protein delivery being overcome, particularly as new drugs are developed in tune with delivery systems. The next challenge is gene delivery, which presents an entirely new set of scientific and technical issues, particularly when delivery is to be targeted to a single tissue or cell type in the body and long-term stable expression is desired. Current gene therapy approaches continue to face problems of immunological reaction to and low specificity of viral vectors; thus, synthetic polymer conjugates are exciting alternatives. Another important aspect is to establish the immune response to polymer debris. Although it has been speculated that biodegradable polymers induce inflammatory reactions because of an immune response to degradation products and nonreacted monomer compounds, basic mechanisms need to be further explored. In addition, the advent of the use of nanoparticulate materials and the effect of such particles from an immunological standpoint needs thorough investigation.

REFERENCES

1. Kulkarni R.K., Pani K.C. and Neuman C. et al., Polylactic acid for surgical implants, *Archives of Surgery*, 93, 839–843, 1966.
2. Kulkarni R.K., Moore G. and Hegyeli A.F. et al., Biodegradable poly(lactic acid) polymers, *Journal of Biomedical Materials Research*, 5, 169–181, 1971.
3. Vert M., Biomedical polymers from chiral lactides and functional lactones. Properties and applications, *Makromolekulare Chemie-Macromolecular Symposia*, 6, 109–122, 1986.
4. Vert M., Christel P., Chabot F. and Leray J., In: G.W. Hasting and P. Ducheyne, Editors, Degradable polymers, *Macromolecular Materials*, CRC Press, Boca Raton, FL (1984), pp. 119–142.
5. Shalaby S.W. and Johnson R.A., Synthetic absorbable polyesters, In: S.W. Shalaby, Editor, *Biomedical Polymers. Designed to Degrade Systems*, Hanser, New York (1994), pp. 1–34.
6. Anderson J.M. and Shive M.S., Biodegradation and biocompatibility of PLA and PLGA microspheres, *Advanced Drug Delivery Reviews*, 28, 5–24, 1997.
7. Middleton J.C. and Tipton A.J., Synthetic biodegradable polymers as orthopedic devices, *Biomaterials*, 21, 2335–2346, 2000.
8. von Oepen R. and Michaeli W., Injection moulding of biodegradable implants, *Clinical Materials*, 10, 21–28, 1992.
9. Pitt C.G., Chasalow F.I., Hibionada Y.M., Klimas D.M. and Schindler A., Aliphatic polyesters. I. The degradation of poly(e-caprolactone) *in vivo*, *Journal of Applied Polymer Science*, 26, 3779–3787, 1981.
10. Li S. and Vert M., Biodegradation of aliphatic polyesters, In: G. Scott and D. Gilead, Editors, *Degradable Polymers Principles and Applications*, Chapman & Hall, London (1995), pp. 43–87.
11. Callister W.D., *Materials Science and Engineering. An Introduction* (3rd ed.), Wiley, New York (1994) pp. 473–482.
12. Xiao-Jun X., Jay C.S. and Prasad S.V., Towards developing surface eroding poly(α-hydroxy acids), *Biomaterials*, 27, 3021–3030, 2006.
13. Chawla A.S. and Chang T.M.S., In-vivo degradation of poly(lactic acid) of different molecular weights, *Biomaterials, Medical Devices and Artificial Organs*, 13, 153–162, 1985–1986.
14. Chu C.C., Hydrolytic degradation of poly(glycolic acid): Tensile strength and crystallinity study, *Journal of Applied polymer Science*, 26, 1727–1734, 1981.
15. Chu C.C. and Campbell N.D., Scanning electron microscope study of the hydrolytic degradation of poly(glycolic acid) suture, *Journal of Biomedical Materials Research*, 16, 417–430, 1982.
16. Nakamura T., Hitomi S. and Watanabe S. et al., Bioabsorption of polylactides with different molecular properties, *Journal of Biomedical Materials Research*, 23, 1115–1130, 1989.

17. Li S.M., Garreau H. and Vert M., Structure property relationships in the degradation of massive poly (α hydroxy acids) in aqueous media. Part 3: Influence of the morphology of poly(L lactic acid), *Journal of Materials Science—Materials in Medicine*, 1, 198–206, 1990.

18. Chu C.C., A comparison of the the effect of pH on the biodegradation of two synthetic absorbable sutures, *Annals of Surgery*, 195, 55–59, 1982.

19. Makino K., Ohshima H. and Kondo T., Mechanism of hydrolytic degradation properties of poly(L-lactide) microcapsules: Effect of pH, ionic strength and buffer concentration, *Journal of Microencapsulation*, 3, 203–212, 1986.

20. Chu C.C. and Moncrief G., An *in vitro* evaluation of the stability of mechanical properties in various pH conditions, *Annals of Surgery*, 198, 223–228, 1983.

21. Weir N.A., Buchanan F.J., Orr J.F., Farrar D.F. and Boyd A., Processing, annealing and sterilisation of poly-L-lactide, *Biomaterials*, 25, 3939–3949, 2004.

22. Pihaljamaki H., Salminen S., Laitinen O., Tynninen O. and Bostman O., Tissue response to polyglycolide, polydioxanone, polylevolactide, and metallic pins in cancellous bone: An experimental study on rabbits, *Journal of Orthopaedic Research*, 24, 1597–1606, 2006.

23. An Y.H., Woolf S.K. and Friedman R.J., Pre-clinical *in vivo* evaluation of orthopaedic bioabsorbable devices, *Biomaterials*, 21, 2635–2652, 2000.

24. Ashammakhi N. and Rokkanen P., Review: Absorbable polyglycolide devices in trauma and bone surgery, *Biomaterials*, 18, 3–9, 1997.

25. Ignatius A.A. and Claes L.E., *In vitro* biocompatibility of bioresorbable polymers: Poly(L, DL lactide) and poly(L-lactide-*co*-glycolide), *Biomaterials*, 17, 831–839, 1996.

26. Hilkka H.P., Dorrit H., Terttu T., Pertti H. and Timo W., SR-PLLA and SR-PGA miniscrews: Biodegradation and tissue reactions in the calvarium and dura mater, *Journal of Cranio-Maxillofacial Surgery*, 27, 42–50, 1999.

27. Harri P., Ole B., Olli T. and Outi L., Long-term tissue response to bioabsorbable poly-L-lactide and metallic screws: An experimental study, *Bone*, 39, 932–937, 2006.

28. Corden T.J., Jones I.A., Rudd C.D., Christian P., Downes S. and. McDougall K.E., Physical and biocompatibility properties of poly-ε-caprolactone produced using *in situ* polymerisation: A novel manufacturing technique for long-fibre composite materials, *Biomaterials*, 21, 713–724, 2000.

29. Serrano M.C., Pagani R., Vallet-Regí M., Peña J., Rámila A., Izquierdo I. and Portolés M.T., *In vitro* biocompatibility assessment of poly(ε-caprolactone) films using L929 mouse fibroblasts, *Biomaterials*, 25, 5603–5611, 2004.

30. Li S., Garreau H. and Vert M., Structure–property relationships in the case of the degradation of massive poly(α-hydroxy acids) in aqueous media. Part 3: Influence of the morphology of poly(L-lactic acid), *Journal of Materials Science—Materials in Medicine*, 1, 198–206, 1990.

31. Jarret P., Benedict C. and Bell J.P. et al., Mechanism of the biodegradation of of polycaprolactone, *Polymer Preprints* (American Chemical Society, Division of Polymer Chemistry), 24, 32–33, 1983.

32. Pitt C.G., Chasalow F.I. and Hibionada Y.M. et al., Aliphatic polyesters. I. The degradation of poly(caprolactone) *in vivo*, *Journal of Applied polymer Science*, 26, 3779–3787, 1981.

33. Nobuto K., Kazunori Y., Harukazu T., Masanori Y. and Yoshie T., Primary stability of three posterior cruciate ligament reconstruction procedures: A biomechanical *in vitro* study arthroscopy, *The Journal of Arthroscopic and Related Surgery*, 21, 970–978, 2005.

34. Suggs L.J. and Mikos A.G., Synthetic biodegradable polymers for medical applications, In: J.E. Mark, Editor, *Physical Properties of Polymers Handbook*, Springer-Verlag, Berlin (1997), pp. 615–624.

35. Agrawal C.M., Best J., Heckman J.D. and Boyan B.D., Protein release kinetics of a biodegradable implant for fracture non-unions, *Biomaterials*, 16, 1255–1260, 1995.

36. Lo H., Kadiyala S., Guggino S.E. and Leong K.W., Poly(L-lactic acid) foams with cell seeding and controlled-release capacity, *Journal of Biomedical Materials Research*, 30, 475–484, 1996.

37. Athanasiou K.A., Schmitz J.P. and Agrawal C.M., The effects of porosity on degradation of PLA-PGA implants, *Tissue Engineering*, 4, 53–63, 1998.

38. Agrawal C.M., McKinney J.S., Lanctot D. and Athanasiou K.A., Effects of fluid flow on the *in vitro* degradation kinetics of biodegradable scaffolds for tissue engineering, *Biomaterials*, 21, 2443–2452, 2000.

39. Doddi N., Versfelt C.C. and Wasserman D., Synthetic absorbable devices of polydioxanone, U.S. Patent, 4, 052,988, 1976.

40. Sabino M.A., González S., Márquez L. and Feijoo J.L., Study of the hydrolytic degradation of polydioxanone PPDX, *Polymer Degradation and Stability*, 69, 209–216, 2000.

41. Lizuka T., Mikkonen P., Paukku P. and Lindqvist C., Reconstruction of orbital floor with polydioxanone plate, *International Journal of Oral and Maxillofacial Surgery*, 20, 83–87, 1991.

42. Sperinde J.J. and Griffith L.G., Synthesis and characterization of enzymatically-cross-linked poly(ethylene glycol) hydrogels, *Macromolecules*, 30, 5255–5264, 1997.

43. Hubbell J.A., Synthetic biodegradable polymers for tissue engineering and drug delivery, *Current Opinion in Solid State and Materials Science*, 3, 246–251, 1998.

44. Temenoff J.S., Athanasiou K.A., LeBaron R.G. and Mikos A.G., Effect of poly(ethylene glycol) molecular weight on tensile and swelling properties of oligo(poly(ethylene glycol) fumarate) hydrogels for cartilage tissue engineering, *Journal of Biomedical Materials Research*, 59, 429–437, 2002.

45. Lutolf M.P. and Hubbell J.A., Synthesis and physicochemical characterization of end-linked poly(ethylene glycol)-*co*-peptide hydrogels formed by Michael-type addition, *Biomacromolecules*, 4, 713–722, 2003.

46. Liora A. and Dror S., Biosynthetic hydrogel scaffolds made from fibrinogen and polyethylene glycol for 3D cell cultures, *Biomaterials*, 26, 2467–2477, 2005.

47. Krause T.L. and Bittner G.D., Rapid morphological fusion of severed myelinated axons by polyethylene glycol, *Proceedings of the National Academy of Sciences of the United States of America*, 87, 1471–1475, 1990.

48. King M.E and Kinney A.Y., Tissue adhesives: a new method of wound repair. *Nurse Pract.* 24, 64–73, 1999.

49. Zhang Y. and Zhuo R.X., Synthesis and drug release behavior of poly (trimethylene carbonate)-poly (ethylene glycol)-poly (trimethylene carbonate) nanoparticles, *Biomaterials*, 26, 2089–2094, 2005.

50. Hutmacher D., Hurzeler M.B. and Schliephake H., A review of material properties of biodegradable polymers and devices for GTR and GBR applications, *International Journal of Oral and Maxillofacial Implants*, 11, 667–678, 1996.

51. Zhang Z., Grijpma D.W. and Feijen J., Poly(trimethylene carbonate) and monomethoxy poly(ethylene glycol)-block-poly(trimethylene carbonate) nanoparticles for the controlled release of dexamethasone, *Journal of Controlled Release*, 111, 263–270, 2006.

52. Pisken E., Review, biodegradable polymers as biomaterials, *Journal of Biomaterials Science, Polymer Edition*, 6, 775–795, 1994.

53. Coover H.W., Dreifus D.W. and O'Connor J.T., Cyanoacrylate adhesives, In: I. Skeist, Editor, *Handbook of Adhesives* (3rd ed.), Van Nostrand Reinhold, New York (1990), pp. 463–477.

54. King M.E. and Kinney A.Y., Tissue adhesives: A new method of wound repair, *Nurse Practitioner*, 24, 66–73, 1999.

55. Oowaki H., Matsuda S., Sakai N., Ohta T., Iwata H., Sadato A., Taki W., Hashimoto N. and Ikada Y., Non-adhesive cyanoacrylate as an embolic material for endovascular neurosurgery, *Biomaterials*, 21, 1039–1046, 2000.

56. Reece T.B., Maxey T.S. and Kron I.L., A prospectus on tissue adhesives, *American Journal of Surgery*, 182, 40S–44S, 2001.

57. Pollak J.S. and White R.I., Jr., The use of cyanoacrylate adhesives in peripheral embolization, *Journal of Vascular and Interventional Radiology*, 12, 907–913, 2001.

58. Vauthier C., Dubernet C., Fattal E., Pinto-Alphandary H. and Couvreur P., Poly(alkylcyanoacrylates) as biodegradable materials for biomedical applications, *Advanced Drug Delivery Reviews*, 55, 519–548, 2003.

59. Barratt G., Couarraze G., Couvreur P., Dubernet C., Fattal E., Gref R., Labarre D., Legrand P., Ponchel G. and Vauthier C., Polymeric micro- and nanoparticles as drug carriers, In: S. Dumitriu, Editor, *Polymeric Biomaterials* (2nd ed.), Marcel Dekker, New York (2001), pp. 753–782.

60. Stella B., Arpicco S., Peracchia M.T., Desmaële D., Hoebeke J., Renoir M., D'Angelo J., Cattel L. and Couvreur P., Design of folic acid-conjugated nanoparticles for drug targeting, *Journal of Pharmaceutical Sciences*, 89, 1452–1464, 2000.

61. Calvo P., Gouritin B., Chacun H., Desmaële D., D'Angelo J., Noel J.P., Georgin D., Fattal E., Andreux J.P. and Couvreur P., Long-circulating PEGylated polycyanoacrylate nanoparticles as new drug carrier for brain delivery, *Pharmaceutical Research*, 18, 1157–1166, 2001.

62. Kattan J., Droz J.P., Couvreur P., Marino J.P., Boutan-Laroze A., Rougier P., Brault P., Vranckx H., Grognet J.M. and Morge X., Phase I clinical trial and pharmacokinetic evaluation of doxorubicin carried by polyisohexylcyanoacrylate nanoparticles, *Investigational New Drugs*, 10, 191–199, 1992.

63. Couvreur P., Kante B. and Roland M., Les vecteurs lysosomotropes, *Journal De Pharmacie De Belgique*, 35, 51–60, 1980.

64. Couvreur P., Kante B., Grislain L., Roland M. and Speiser P., Toxicity of polyalkylcyanoacrylate nanoparticles. II. Doxorubicin-loaded nanoparticles, *Journal of Pharmaceutical Sciences*, 71, 790–792, 1982.

65. Cedric C., Michael C.M., Christine V., Denis L., Patrick C. and Liliane L., Heparin coated poly(alkyl-cyanoacrylate) nanoparticles coupled to hemoglobin a new oxygen carrier, *Biomaterials*, 25, 3081–3086, 2004.

66. Kawasaki E.S. and Player A., Nanotechnology, nanomedicine, and the development of new, effective therapies for cancer: Review, *Nanomedicine: Nanotechnology, Biology and Medicine*, 1, 101–109, 2005.

67. Gustavo A.A., de Queiroz A.A.A. and Julio S.R., Immobilization of a nonsteroidal antiinflammatory drug onto commercial segmented polyurethane surface to improve haemocompatibility properties, *Biomaterials*, 23, 1625–1638, 2002.

68. Dong-an W., Jian J., Chang-you G., Guan-Hua Y. and Lin-xian F. Surface coating of stearyl poly(ethylene oxide) coupling-polymer on polyurethane guiding catheters with poly(ether urethane) film-building additive for biomedical applications, *Biomaterials*, 22, 1549–1562, 2001.

69. Santerre J.P., Woodhouse K., Laroche G. and Labow R.S., Understanding the biodegradation of poly-urethanes: From classical implants to tissue engineering materials, *Biomaterials*, 26, 7457–7470, 2005.

70. Ashley F.L., A new type of breast prosthesis: Preliminary report, *Plastic and Reconstructive Surgery*, 45, 421–424, 1970.

71. Ashley F.L., Further studies on the natural-Y breast prosthesis, *Plastic and Reconstructive Surgery*, 49, 414–419, 1972.

72. Batich C. and Williams J., Toxic hydrolysis product from biodegradable foam implant, *Journal of Biomedical Materials Research*, 23, 311–319, 1989.

73. Ignacio A.R., Jeffrey B.S. and David W.G., Polyurethane coatings release bioactive antibodies to reduce bacterial adhesion, *Journal of Controlled Release*, 63, 175–189, 2000.

74. Ji-Dong G., Microbial colonization of polymeric materials for space applications and mechanisms of biodeterioration: A review, *International Biodeterioration and Biodegradation*, Available online October 2006.

75. Kim J.H. and Kim S.C., PEO-grafting on PU/PS IPNs for enhanced blood compatibility—effect of pendant length and grafting density, *Biomaterials*, 23, 2015–2025, 2002.

76. Gombotz W.R. and Wee S.F., Protein release from alginate matrices, *Advanced Drug Delivery Reviews*, 31, 267–285, 1998.

77. Draget K.I., Skjak-Braek G. and Smidsrod O., Alginate based new materials, *International Journal of Biological Macromolecules*, 21, 47–55, 1997.

78. Yong-Dan T., Subbu S.V., Freddy Y.C.B. and Li-Wei W., Sustained release of hydrophobic and hydrophilic drugs from a floating dosage form, *International Journal of Pharmaceutics*, Available online 3 December 2006 (Science Direct).

79. Eiselt P., Yeh J., Latvala R.K., Shea L.D. and Mooney D.J., Porous carriers for biomedical applications based on alginate hydrogels, *Biomaterials*, 21, 1921–1927, 2000.

80. Alsberg V., Anderson K., Albeiruti A., Franceshi R.T. and Mooney D.J., Cell interactive alginate hydro-gels for bone tissue engineering, *Journal of Dental Research*, 80, 2025–2029, 2001.

81. Pornsak S. and Ross A.K., Development of polysaccharide gel-coated pellets for oral administration: 2. calcium alginate, *European Journal of Pharmaceutical Sciences*, 29, 139–147, 2006.

82. Ravi Kumar M.N.V., Muzzarelli R.A.A., Muzzarelli C., Sashiwa H. and Domb A.J., Chitosan chemistry and pharmaceutical perspectives, *Chemical Reviews*, 104, 6017–6084, 2004.

83. Marguerite R., Chitin and chitosan, properties and applications: Review, *Progress in Polymer Science*, 31, 603–632, 2006.

84. Meera G. and Emilia A.T., Polyionic hydrocolloids for the intestinal delivery of protein drugs: Alginate and chitosan—a review, *Journal of Controlled Release*, 114, 1–14, 2006.

85. Alberto D.M., Michael S. and Makarand V.R., Chitosan: A versatile biopolymer for orthopaedic tissue engineering: Review article, *Biomaterials*, 16, 5983–5990, 2005.

86. Barbosa M.A., Granja P.L., Barrias C.C. and Amaral I.F., Polysaccharides as scaffolds for bone regen-eration, *ITBM-RBM*, 26, 212–217, 2005.

87. Jayakumar R., Prabaharan M., Reis R.L. and Mano J.F., Graft copolymerized chitosan—present status and applications, *Carbohydrate Polymers*, 62, 142–158, 2005.

88. Thomas F., Rivelino M., Hui S.K. and Molly S.S., Chitin-based tubes for tissue engineering in the nerv-ous system, *Biomaterials*, 26, 4624–4632, 2005.

89. Sunil A.A., Nadagouda N.M. and Tejraj M.A., Recent advances on chitosan-based micro- and nanopar-ticles in drug delivery, *Journal of Controlled Release*, 100, 5–28, 2004.

90. Jiyoung M.D. and Kam W.L., Natural polymers for gene delivery tissue engineering, *Advanced Drug Delivery Reviews*, 58, 487–499, 2006.

91. Chunmeng S., Ying Z., Xinze R., Meng W., Yongping S. and Tianmin C., Therapeutic potential of chitosan and its derivatives in regenerative medicine, *Journal of Surgical Research*, 133, 185–192, 2006.

92. Kamath R. and Park K., Surface modification of polymeric biomaterials by albumin grafting using h-irradiation, *Journal of Applied Biomaterials*, 5, 162–173, 1994.

93. Hirsch R.J. and Cohen J.L., Soft tissue augmentation, *Cutis*, 78, 165–172, 2006.

94. Coons D.A. and Alan B.F., Tendon graft substitutes-rotator cuff patches, *Sports Medicine and Arthroscopy Review*, 14, 185–190, 2006.

95. Geutjes P.J., Daamen W.F., Buma P., Feitz W.F., Faraj K.A., and van Kuppevelt T.H., From molecules to matrix: Construction and evaluation of molecularly defined bioscaffolds, *Adamantiades-Behcet's Disease*, 585, 279–295, 2006.

96. Annick L., The use of mucoadhesive polymers in ocular drug delivery, *Advanced Drug Delivery Reviews*, 57, 1595–1639, 2005.

97. Fernandez L.J.C. and Ruano-Ravina A., Efficacy and safety of intraarticular hyaluronic acid in the treatment of hip osteoarthritis: A systematic review, *Osteoarthritis Cartilage*, 14, 1306–1311. E pub 2006.

98. Brockmeier S.F. and Shaffer B.S., Viscosupplementation therapy for osteoarthritis, *Sports Medicine and Arthroscopy Review*, 14, 155–162, 2006.

99. Allison D.D. and Grande-Allen K.J., Review. Hyaluronan: A powerful tissue engineering tool, *Tissue Engineering*, 12, 2131–2140, 2006.

100. Seal B.L., Otero T.C. and Panitch A., Polymeric biomaterials for tissue and organ regeneration review, *Materials Science and Engineering: R: Reports*, 34, 147–230, 2001.

101. Peter B., Maurus M.D. and Christopher C.K., Bioabsorbable implant material review, *Operative Techniques in Sports Medicine*, 12, 158–160, 2004.

102. Steven M., Raikin M.D., Alexander C., Ching M.D., Bioabsorbable fixation in foot and ankle, *Foot and Ankle Clinics of North America*, 10, 667–684, 2005.

103. Justin G., Recent innovations and future directions in external fixation of the foot and ankle, *Foot and Ankle Clinics of North America*, 9, 637–647, 2004.

104. Rezwan K., Chen Q.Z., Blaker J.J. and Aldo R.B., Biodegradable and bioactive porous polymer/inorganic composite scaffolds for bone tissue engineering, *Biomaterials*, 27, 3413–3431, 2006.

105. Warris E., Konttinen Y.T., Ashammakhi N., Suuronen R. and Santavirta S., Bioabsorbable fixation devices in trauma and bone surgery: Current clinical standing, *Expert Review of Medical Devices*, 1, 229–240, 2004.

106. Yannas I.V. and Hill B.J., Selection of biomaterials for peripheral nerve regeneration using data from the nerve chamber model, *Biomaterials*, 25, 1593–1600, 2004.

107. Yang F., Murugan R., Ramakrishna S., Wang X., Ma Y.-X. and Wang S., Fabrication of nano-structured porous PLLA scaffold intended for nerve tissue engineering, *Biomaterials*, 25, 1891–1900, 2004.

108. Sumona S., George Y.L., Joyce Y.W. and Tejal A.D., Development and characterization of a porous micro-patterned scaffold for vascular tissue engineering applications, *Biomaterials*, 27, 4775–4782, 2006.

109. Merrel S.W. and Lawrence P.F., Initial evaluation of absorbable polydioxanone suture for peripheral vascular surgery, *Journal of Vascular Surgery Oct*; 14452–7; 457–459, 1991.

110. Pêgo A.P., Siebum B., Van Luyn M.J.A., Gallego X.J., Van Seijen Y., Poot A.A., Grijpma D.W. and Feijen J., Preparation of degradable porous structures based on 1,3-trimethylene carbonate and D,L-lactide (co)polymers for heart tissue engineering, *Tissue Engineering*, 9, 981–994, 2003.

111. Xinhua Z., Harold B., Chiung-Yin C., Lihong Y., Dufei F., Benjamin S.H., Benjamin C. and Emilia E., Electrospun fine-textured scaffolds for heart tissue constructs, *Biomaterials*, 26, 5330–5338, 2005.

112. Gopinath M., Marc D.F., Devang P. and Mauli A.C., Biomaterials in the fabrication of stents coronary stents: A materials perspective review, *Biomaterials*, 28, 1689–1710, 2007.

113. Tan L.P., Venkatraman S.S., Sung P.F. and Wang X.T., Effect of plasticization on heparin release from biodegradable matrices, *International Journal of Pharmaceutics*, 283, 89–96, 2004.

114. Venkatraman S., Tan L., Joso J., Boey Y. and Wang X., Biodegradable stents with elastic memory, *Biomaterials*, 27, 1573–1578, 2006.

115. Peppas N.A., Intelligent therapeutics: Biomimetic systems and nanotechnology in drug delivery, *Advanced Drug Delivery Reviews*, 56, 1529–1531, 2004.

116. Langer R., Drug delivery and targeting, *Nature*, 392, 5–10, 1998.

117. Zachary H.J. and Nicholas A., Peppas Microfabricated drug delivery devices, *International Journal of Pharmaceutics*, 306, 15–23, 2005.

118. Chien-Chi L. and Andrew T.M., Hydrogels in controlled release formulations: Network design and mathematical modeling: Review, *Advanced Drug Delivery Reviews*, 58, 1379–1408, 2006.

119. West J.L. and Hubbell J.A., Photopolymerized hydrogel materials for drug-delivery applications, *Reactive Polymers*, 25, 139–147, 1995.
120. Metters A.T., Anseth K.S. and Bowman C.N., Fundamental studies of a novel, biodegradable PEG-b-PLA hydrogel, *Polymer*, 41, 3993–4004, 2000.
121. Metters A.T., Anseth K.S. and Bowman C.N., A statistical kinetic model for the bulk degradation of PLA-b-PEG-b-PLA hydrogel networks: Incorporating network non-idealities, *Journal of physical Chemistry B*, 105, 8069–8076, 2001.
122. Kalpana R.K., James J.B. and Kathleen M.M., The Taxus™ drug-eluting stent: A new paradigm in controlled drug delivery: Review, *Advanced Drug Delivery Reviews*, 58, 412–436, 2006.
123. Kondyurin A., Maitz M., Romanova V., Begishev V., Kondyurina I. and Guenzel R., Drug release from polyurethane coating modified by plasma immersion ion implantation, *Journal of Biomaterials Science, Polymer Edition*, 15, 145–159, 2004.

16 Electroactive Polymers as Smart Materials with Intrinsic Actuation Properties: New Functionalities for Biomaterials

Federico Carpi and Danilo De Rossi

CONTENTS

16.1 INTRODUCTION

The field of biomaterials is very broad. As largely discussed in this book, a biomaterial is typically conceived as a biocompatible and bioapplicable synthetic material, which is employed either to replace a part of a living tissue or to function in intimate contact with it. Accordingly, biomaterials are intended to interface with biological systems in order to evaluate, treat, augment, or replace biological functions of tissues or organs of the body. The rapidly growing basic science of biomaterials, along with continuous improvements on their fabrication and processing, provides fundamental benefits for medical devices that already use biomaterials in clinical practice, such as artificial hips, oral implants, vascular stents, drug delivery systems, etc.

The functional properties of each biomaterial are, of course, the key elements that determine its suitability for a specific application. As an example, both the structural support function and the interface properties with living bone offered by calcium hydroxylapatite coatings are vital for bone replacement implants. Likewise, surface functionalization (e.g., by plasma processing) is used to graft surface functional groups, so as to transform a bioinert material into a bioactive structure. Nowadays, such types of functional properties are largely studied and represent one of the biggest areas of investigation of the biomaterials science. On the contrary, another class of functional properties, the actuation properties that are potentially useful for several applications, are considerably less studied. Accordingly, this chapter intends to provide a brief survey on the classes of materials that could be employed for this purpose, along with the applications that could benefit from their use.

Actuation can be defined as a property shown by a material or a mechanism by which it is able to act upon its external environment by transducing a certain form of input energy into an external mechanical work. Electric motors, largely employed in many areas of technology, are examples of electromechanical actuators, that is, mechanisms that transduce electrical energy into work. Muscles, instead, are examples of biological materials acting as natural electrochemomechanical actuators; following a neural electrical command, they transform body's chemical energy (arising from ATP) into motion. So, a simple question may arise: Why should actuation properties be useful for certain biomaterials? This question can have several answers. One of them is directly provided by the latter example. In order to support or even replace injured muscular tissues, "artificial muscles" (also known as "pesudomuscular" actuators) would be necessary. They should ideally consist of biocompatible materials forming biomimetic actuation systems, which are capable of working with the typical performing features of natural muscles such as in terms of efficiency, compliance, lightweight, size, etc. In addition to prosthetic systems, further examples of medical devices requiring biomaterials with actuation properties could be mentioned as well: for instance, implantable drug delivery systems, implantable devices for analysis of body fluids, tools for minimally invasive surgery (e.g., active steerable catheters), etc.

The development of such different types of systems is not trivial and, in some cases, is very challenging. As an example, despite a large amount of efforts spent to develop prosthetic robotic arms driven by electric motors, no real "artificial muscles" (from a really biomimetic point of view, as mentioned above) are currently available. In fact, systems developed so far are at least stiff, heavy, cumbersome, and characterized by low efficiency. Figure 16.1 shows an example of prosthetic arms.

Similarly, nowadays the design of, for instance, either smart drug delivery systems, miniaturized and conformable to the human body, or steerable catheters endowed with actuation properties, enabling accurate, smoother, and safer endoscopic explorations, finds several challenging issues. In particular, they arise while attempting to simply adapt to such types of systems, conventional materials, and technologies of actuation. The inadequacy of this approach puts in evidence a strong need for new materials showing passive and active properties closer to their respective counterparts in biological tissues. New research avenues in this direction are currently being open by the so-called electroactive polymers (EAP), as described in the chapter.

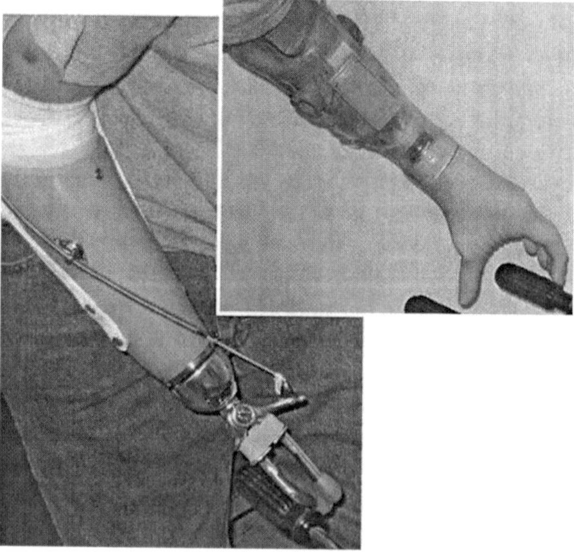

FIGURE 16.1　Examples of prosthetic arms. (Photo courtesy of U.S. Army.)

16.2 ELECTROACTIVE POLYMERS

The term "electroactive polymers" identifies a broad family of synthetic polymers sharing, as a common and fundamental feature, a capability of changing dimensions and/or shapes when a suitable electrical input is applied. Accordingly, they are studied as soft materials with intrinsic actuation properties. They are particularly attractive for their ability to show sizable active strains and/or stresses, large compliance, low density, low power consumption, ease of processing, and low costs. Due to such properties, EAP are currently considered the most promising class of materials for pseudomuscular actuators: their potential to implement a functional biomimesis of natural muscles is studied in the perspective development of future "artificial muscles" [1,2].

EAP can be classified according to a division into two main classes: ionic EAP and electronic EAP [1,2]. The first group comprehends materials whose actuation principles are based on diffusions of ions and solvents (as better clarified in the following paragraphs), while electronic EAP are activated (according to different mechanisms) by the direct application of an electric field. Both these groups can be further divided, depending on the specific actuation mechanism and the related types of materials. In particular, ionic EAP comprehend polymer gels, ionic polymer–metal composites (IPMC), conducting polymers and carbon nanotubes (which are conventionally classified as EAP, even though they are just nonpolymeric macromolecular materials). Electronic EAP include piezoelectric polymers, electrostrictive polymers, dielectric elastomers, and flexoelectric polymers. Table 16.1 summarizes this classification and reports, for each group, the most studied examples of polymers.

Although these materials have been known since many decades, they have found limited uses so far despite their potentialities. This should be mainly attributed to their scarce development toward mature technological levels. However, promising recent results in materials science, materials processing, and configuration design for such polymers are encouraging the concentration of efforts for a concrete exploitation of their performance, as briefly reported in the following discussion.

TABLE 16.1

Classification and Examples of EAP

EAP Class	EAP Subcategories	Examples of Materials
Ionic EAP	Polymer gels	Poly(acrylic acid) (PAAc)
		Poly(vinyl alcohol) (PVA)
		Modified Poly(acrylonitrile) (PAN)
	Ionic polymer–metal composites (IPMC)	Nafion/Pt
	Conducting polymers	Poly(pyrrole) (PPy)
		Poly(aniline) (PANi)
	Carbon nanotubes	Single-walled nanotubes
		Multiwalled nanotubes
Electronic EAP	Piezoelectric polymers	Poly(vinylidene fluoride) (PVDF)
	Electrostrictive polymers	PVDF-based copolymers, for example,
		Poly(vinylidene fluoride–trifluoroethylene) (P(VDF–TrFE)),
		Poly(vinylidene fluoride–hexafluoropropylene) (P(VDF–HFP))
	Dielectric elastomers	Silicone elastomers
		Acrylic elastomers
		Polyurethane elastomers
	Flexoelectric polymers	Liquid crystal elastomers

Regardless of the specific mechanisms of actuation (described in the following), it can be useful to underline as from now that ionic EAP require low driving voltages, while high fields are typically needed for electronic EAP. This means that electronic EAP are considerably less suitable for applications requiring implantable devices, which should work in strict contact with biological tissues. For this reason, this chapter will largely focus on ionic EAP (except for carbon nanotubes, which represent an actuation technology still far to be mature). Nevertheless, a glance at one of the most performing classes of electronic EAP, namely dielectric elastomers, will be provided as well by underlying their potential use for different types of biomedical applications.

16.3 POLYMER GELS

As early as the half of the last century, studies about water-swollen polymer gels converting chemical energy into mechanical work were reported [3–5]. These materials, consisting of soft elastic cross-linked polymer networks with fluid-filled interstitial spaces, are in fact capable of undergoing large deformations through swelling and deswelling. Reversible contractions and dilatations, due to reversible ionizations of suitable groups (e.g., polycarboxilic [—COOH] groups), can be obtained by alternating addition of alkalis and acids. Katchalsky denoted such transformations as mechanochemical reactions. According to such effects, these materials, which are generally amorphous without any particularly ordered molecular structure, can be easily deformed by external stimuli, to generate force or execute work upon their external environment. From a general point of view, reversible order–disorder transitions in gels can be induced by changes either in temperature, irradiation, electric fields, pH (by chemical or electrochemical activation) or solvent properties, as sketched in Figures 16.2 and 16.3.

When placed in contact with organic solvents, gels swell. Similarly, the presence of a polar solvent-like water can induce significant changes. As an example, spontaneous motions of gels placed in water have been reported [14,15]. In these types of systems, the driving force of the gel motion when it is placed in water originates from the spreading of the inner organic solvent out of the material, as represented in Figure 16.4 [15].

Electrical activations of water-swollen cross-linked polymer gels can be achieved by inserting the material between a couple of charged electrodes, causing anisotropic contractions with concomitant fluid exudations [16,17]. As an interpretation of such phenomena, the contraction response was

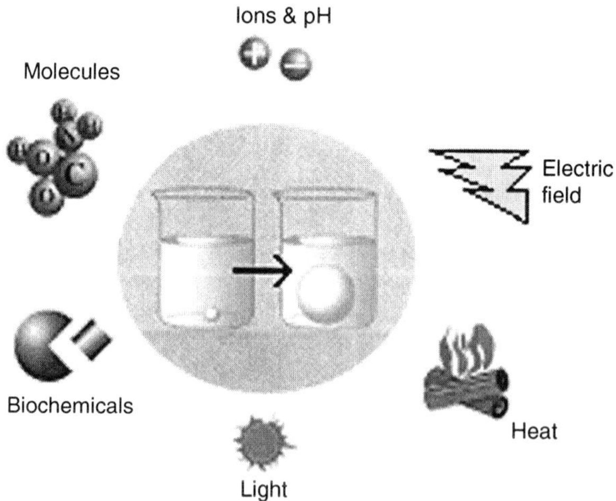

FIGURE 16.2 Different types of stimuli enabling a mechanical response of a polymer gel. Since many years, polymer gels are being studied for the development of low-voltage soft actuators [6–12]. As an example, they can be used to construct thermo-responsive diaphragms, capable of automatically opening and closing a valve [13]. They can show shape memory effects as well, as presented in the two frames of Figure 16.3.

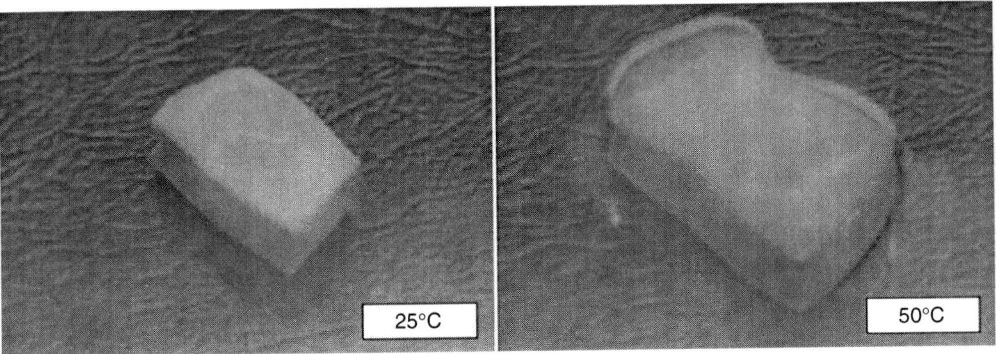

FIGURE 16.3   Thermal activation of a shape memory gel.

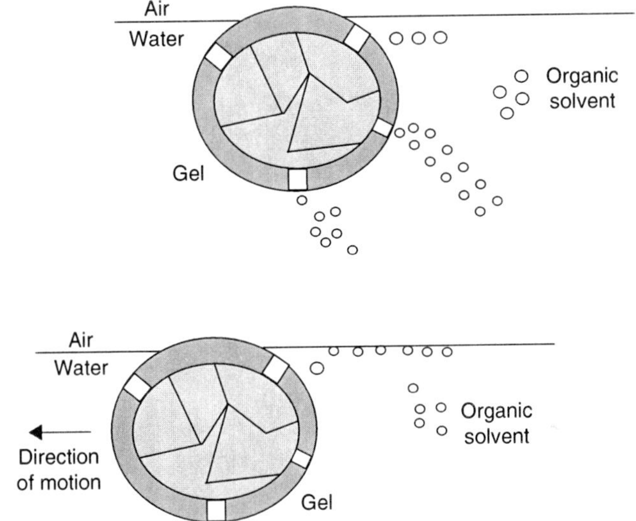

FIGURE 16.4   Spontaneous gel motion in water due to a spreading process of organic solvent.

ascribed to spatio temporal pH gradients generated by electrode reactions, which propagate inside the gel by electrodiffusion. In fact, this can cause mechanical rearrangements of the gel network by changes in the statistical length of the polymer chains [17].

Different types of devices have been proposed so far by exploiting such phenomena with different actuating configurations. Films, strips, membranes, and fibers are some examples of considered shapes. A significant example of application is represented by an electrically activated "chemical valve" membrane, capable of reversibly expanding and contracting its pore size in response to electrical stimuli [18]. In particular, by keeping the membrane dimensions constant, the contractile stress generated by the electrochemomechanical changes in the membrane expands its pore channels, permeable to solutes and solvent. Variable potential differences can therefore be used to electrically modulate the membrane permeability. Accordingly, such a type of system could be used as a permeation-selective membrane, continuously separating mixture of solutes with different molecular sizes.

One of the most important areas of biomedical application of polymer gels is represented by the controlled release of drugs. The purpose behind controlling a drug delivery is to achieve more effective therapies by eliminating the risk for under- or overdosing. In particular, controlled-delivery systems are intended to maintain drug levels within a desired range, with a delivery profile yielding a suitable blood level of the drug over long periods of time. In fact, with traditional administration of tablets or injections, the drug level in the blood rises after each administration of the drug and then decreases until the next one. In order to implement such controlled-delivery systems, polymer gels capable of releasing drugs when placed in appropriate biological environments are currently largely studied [19–23]. Hydrogels, in particular, offer very interesting properties [20]. When placed in the body, they are capable of swelling due to absorption of water or other body fluids (they can comprise 60–90% of fluid at equilibrium). The swelling process increases the aqueous solvent content within the polymer network, enabling the drug to diffuse through the swollen mesh into the external environment, as represented in Figure 16.5.

More generally, swelling can be achieved by means of different types of chemical–physical environmental stimuli (Figure 16.2), which are responsible of different mechanisms of activation. The most relevant examples are reported in Table 16.2.

A specific and largely studied application of such materials for controlled drug release consists of the therapy for diabetes. For this disease, the system should be able to deliver insulin upon

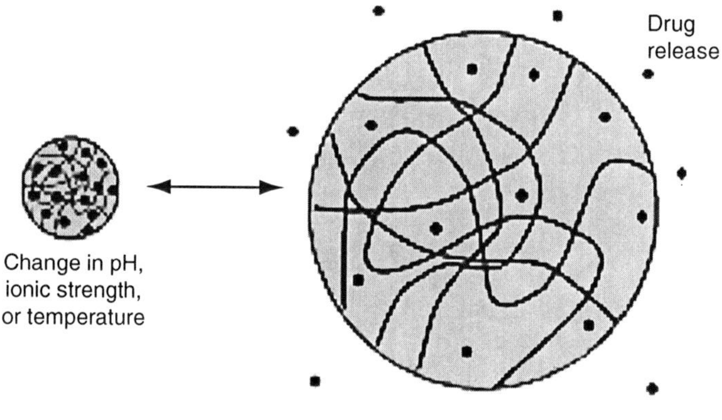

FIGURE 16.5   Schematic drawing of a drug delivery by swelling of an environmental-sensitive polymer gel. (Adapted from Brannon-Peppas, L., *Medical Plastics and Biomaterials Magazine*, November issue, 1997. With permission.)

TABLE 16.2
Polymer Gel Types and Activation Mechanisms for Drug Delivery

Environmental Stimulus	Polymer Gel Type	Mechanism of Activation for Drug Release
Change in pH	Acidic or basic hydrogel	Swelling
Change in ionic strength	Ionic hydrogel	Change in concentration of ions inside the gel, with related swelling
Change in chemical species	Hydrogel containing electron-accepting groups	Formation of charge/transfer complex, with related swelling
Change in enzyme–substrate	Hydrogel containing immobilized enzymes	Enzymatic conversion, with related swelling
Change in temperature	Thermo-responsive hydrogel poly(N-isopropylacrylamide)	Change in polymer–polymer and water–polymer interactions, with related swelling
Applied electric field	Polymer hydrogel	Electrophoresis of charged drug, with related swelling
Ultrasound irradiation	Ethylene–vinyl alcohol hydrogel	Ultrasound irradiation, with related temperature increase

Source: Brannon-Peppas, L., *Medical Plastics and Biomaterials Magazine*, November issue, 1997. With permission.

detection of glucose in the bloodstream. For this purpose, such systems are typically conceived according to the reaction of glucose in the blood with the enzyme glucose oxidase, which can be immobilized within the delivery polymer. In fact, this reaction causes a lowering of the pH, which induces a swelling of the polymer system with a related release of insulin. Examples of materials studied for such a purpose include copolymers containing N,N-dimethylaminoethyl methacrylate [24] or polyacrylamide [25]. Systems working on shrinking gels, rather than swelling, consisting of poly(methacrylic acid-g-poly(ethylene glycol)) copolymers, have been reported as well [26].

As shown by the examples mentioned above, the considerable promising results achieved so far are very encouraging. Nevertheless, it is necessary to stress here that further investigations and developments are still required in order to achieve reliable and safe clinical uses of such types of materials and systems.

16.4 IONIC POLYMER–METAL COMPOSITES

The IPMC are used to fabricate actuators capable of large deformations driven by low applied voltages [27,28]. They consist of polymer networks (such as Nafion, produced by Du Pont de Nemours, Wilmington, Delaware having in their molecular chain ionizable groups that can be dissociated in various polar solvents, showing a resulting net charge. These net charges of the network macromolecules are called polyions. They are electrically compensated by the presence of mobile counterions within the network. When equilibrated with aqueous solutions, the membranes are swollen and they contain a certain amount of water. Swelling equilibrium results from a balance between the elastic recovery force of the polymeric matrix and the water affinity to the fixed ion exchanging sites and the moving counterions. The water content depends not only on the hydrophilic properties of the ionic species inside the membranes, but also on the electrolyte concentration of the external solution. Such an ability of the membrane to swell in water can be controlled in an electric field due to the ionic nature of the membrane. For this purpose, two electrodes are placed in close proximity of the membrane and a low voltage (typically of the order of 1 V), below the threshold for electrolysis, is applied. As a result, electrophoretic migrations (due to the imposed electric field) of the mobile ions within the solution and through the macromolecular network can cause the network itself to be deformed accordingly [27–41]. In fact, the shifting of ions of the same polarity within the network results in both electrostatic interactions with the fixed charges of opposite polarity (contained in the side groups of the polymer chains) and transport of solvent molecules. Both these factors concur to produce a stress gradient between the opposite sides of the membrane. In particular, local expansions and collapses (swelling and deswelling) occur on the two sides of the membrane depending on the polarity of the nearby electrode. Accordingly, these phenomena determine a macroscopic bending of the structure. Figure 16.6 shows a schematic drawing of this electrochemomechanical activation.

The basic principle above described is exploited to use IPMC structures as actuators. The applied external voltage makes the structure bending toward the anode. By reversing the polarities of the electrodes, a bending toward the opposite direction is achieved. An increase of the voltage level causes a larger bending. When an alternate voltage is applied, the membrane undergoes movements like a swing. Of course, the displacement depends not only on the voltage magnitude, but also on the frequency (lower frequencies lead to higher displacements according to the device bandwidth) [27–41].

A typical material used to fabricate IPMC actuators consists of films of Nafion® (Du Pont de Nemours, Wilmington, Delaware an ion exchange membrane. Platinum electrodes are deposited on both sides of a film. The thickness of the actuator is typically around 0.2 mm. To maintain the actuation capability, the film needs to be kept moist. Structure and properties of Nafion membranes have been subjected to numerous investigations. One of the interesting properties of this material is its ability of absorbing large amounts of polar solvents, that is, water. Platinum ions, which are dispersed throughout the hydrophilic regions of the polymer, are subsequently reduced to the

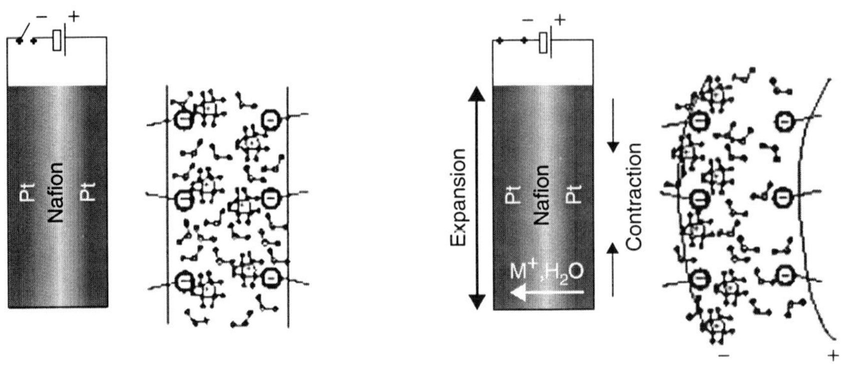

FIGURE 16.6   Working principle of IPMC rest condition (*left*); bending due to activation (*right*).

corresponding metal atoms. According to described mechanism of activation, IPMC actuators usually operate best in a humid environment, even though they can be made as encapsulated devices to operate in dry conditions.

Several applications of the bending function of IPMC actuators are currently being studied. Some of them concern the biomedical field in which the low-driving voltages required by this technology are particularly appealing. Within this ambit of application, a particular emphasis deserves to be given to the following examples [42]. A concept for a ventricular assist device has been proposed. It relies on the use of a few parallel IPMC bending units to be positioned around the heart ventricles, as shown in Figure 16.7. The benders are arranged so that to provide a compression of the ventricles, working as an assistance device.

A second type of concept under study consists of the development of a device proposed for surgical corrections of refractive errors in eyes. In particular, the idea relies on the use of IPMC bands to be positioned around the eyeball, as represented in Figure 16.8. The bands should be activated in order to modify the length of the eyeball in the direction of the optical axis; accordingly, the related corneal curvature should be exploited to induce refractive error corrections modulated by electrical signals. This type of system is conceived as equipped with a built-in coil, which is remotely energized by magnetic induction, so that it provides power for the activation (Figure 16.8).

Other types of applications of IPMC actuators are being studied as well, including artificial sphincters [42]. Nevertheless, for all these reported examples, it is worth stressing that from a technological point of view, one of the most challenging issues still open concerns the necessary improvement of the forces that an IPMC device can deliver. This is one of the main features that concur at present to limit the applicability of these materials for several fields .

16.5   CONDUCTING POLYMERS

Conducting polymers are chemically characterized by the bond conjugation, that is, carbon double bonds alternate with carbon single bonds along a polymer backbone. According to this feature, they are typically identified also as "conjugated polymers." When doped with ions, these materials can be characterized by high electrical conductivity values [43,44]. The conductivity of conjugated polymers can be reversibly changed by orders of magnitude, by changing the doping level. Unlike silicon, dopants can be easily inserted and removed from the spaces they occupy between the networks of the polymer chains. Moreover, in comparison with other semiconducting materials, the doping level can be very high: approximately one dopant counterion per three or four monomers.

Depending on the doping level, different electrical properties can be obtained, spanning from insulation, semiconduction, and conduction. Accordingly, conjugated polymers are being studied

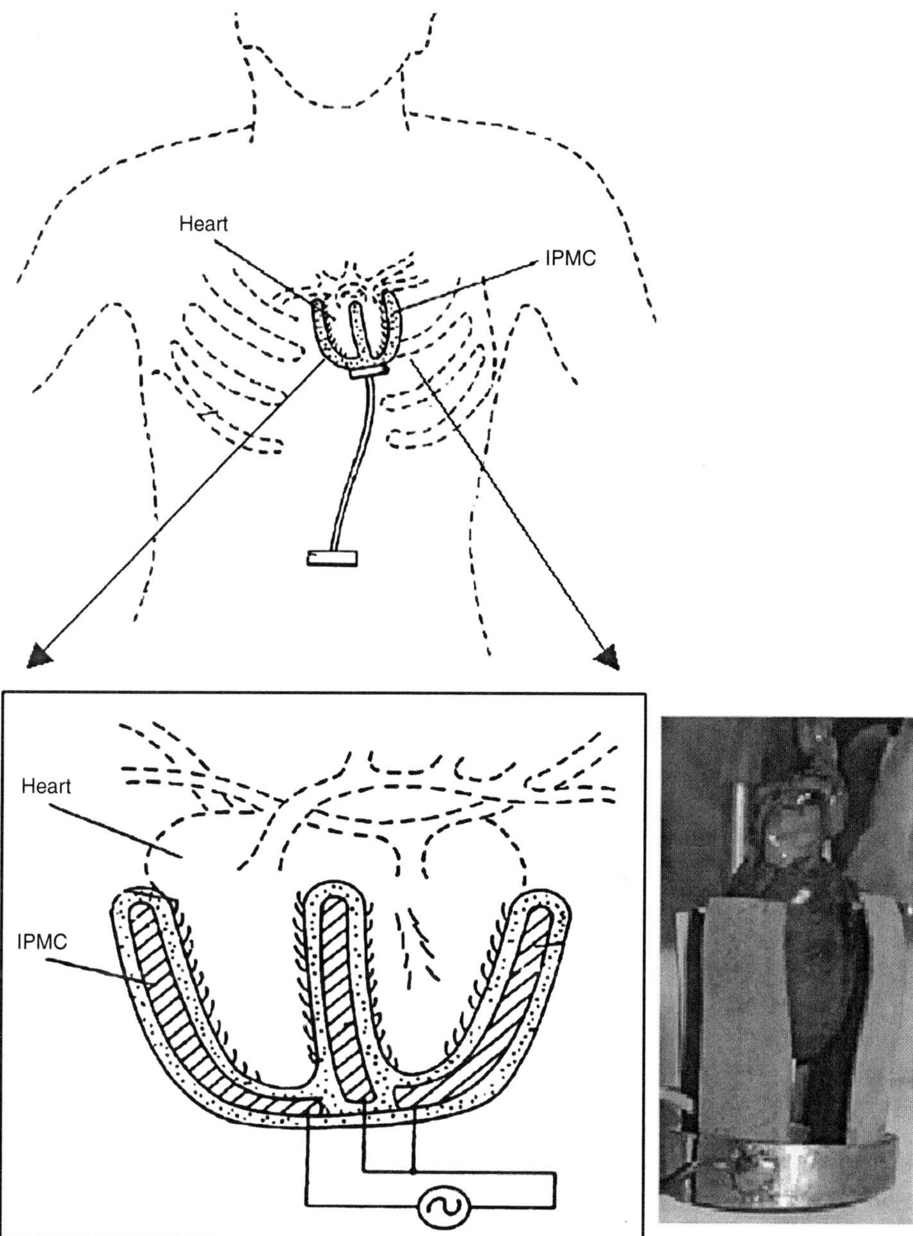

FIGURE 16.7   Concept and experimental prototype sample of a heart compression device made of IPMC benders. (Adapted from Shahinpoor, M., and Kim, K.J., *Smart Mater. Struct.*, 14, 197–214, 2005. With permission.)

for several fields of application by exploiting different types of physical effects [45]. Some examples deserve to be specifically mentioned. Since these materials are able to store a large amount of charge, they are of interest for batteries and supercapacitors. Another interesting property is their band-gap that allows electron–hole recombination, which has made these materials appealing for light-emitting diodes. Moreover, their optical properties (especially light absorption) can be voltage controlled so that conducting polymers have also been investigated for electrochromic devices.

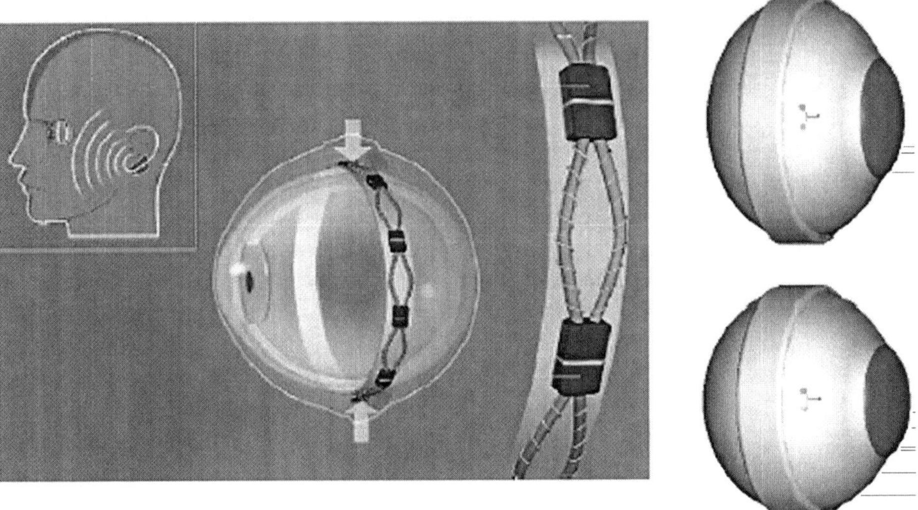

FIGURE 16.8 Scleral bands made of IPMC actuators conceived for corrections of ocular refractive errors. (Adapted from Shahinpoor, M., and Kim, K.J., *Smart Mater. Struct.*, 14, 197–214, 2005. With permission.)

Within the biomedical field, conjugated polymers present very interesting properties: biocompatibility, improvement of regeneration of tissues (e.g., uses in nerve guidance channels), neural communication, modulation of surface properties of neural recording electrodes, functionality as substrates for cell cultures, possibility of being produced in biodegradable/bioerodible forms, and possibility of being doped with biomolecules for controlled releases [46–50].

For the specific topic presented in this chapter, another property is, however, emphasized here: their actuation capabilities. For this purpose, conducting polymers are used as components of an electrochemical cell whose basic structure includes two electrodes immersed in an electrolyte. The conducting polymer material constitutes one or both the electrodes of the cell. By applying a potential difference between them, redox reactions cause strongly anisotropic and reversible volume variations of the material [51–53], which can be used for actuation [51–74]. In particular, three effects have been found to be responsible for dimensional and volume changes in conducting polymers: interactions between polymer chains, variation of the chain conformation, and insertion of counterions. The third effect is generally considered to be the most dominant. In fact, the commonly accepted explanation of the observed deformations attributes the dimensional changes to the input/output of ions (exchanged with the surrounding media) into/from the polymer sample, driven by an applied voltage. In particular, the voltage produces a variation of the polymer oxidation state, causing the necessary modification of the number of ions associated to each chain in order to maintain the global electroneutrality.

Several actuating configurations have been proposed in order to exploit the electromechanical properties of these materials. The most diffused structure is represented by the so-called unimorph bilayer bender. This kind of actuator consists of a film of active material coupled to a passive supporting layer. The structure is operated within an electrochemical cell, having a liquid electrolyte in which the device is immersed. The active polymeric layer of the actuator works as one electrode of the cell, while a counterelectrode and a third reference electrode are separately immersed in the electrolyte. One end of the bilayer is constrained, while the other end is free. The potential difference applied between the electrodes causes redox reactions of the conducting polymer. Since the conducting polymer and the passive layers are mechanically interlocked, when the polymer swells/shrinks, the passive layer that cannot modify its dimensions, transforms the conducting polymer displacement into a bending movement of the structure [70–74]. A different type of bender can be obtained by using the so-called bimorph structure. It consists of two layers of conducting polymer that work as electrodes and sandwich a solid polymer electrolyte. Following the application of a voltage difference between the polymer layers, one of them is oxidized and the other is reduced. Accordingly, they show an opposite variation of length. This causes a bending of the structure toward the shortening side [46,75]. The length variation of the electrodes and, therefore, the resulting bending can be reversed when the applied potential difference varies from a positive half-period to a negative one and vice versa.

As a different actuating configuration, fiber actuators made of conducting polymers have been proposed as well. They can consist of extruded fibers, covered by a thin layer of solid polymer electrolyte and a counterelectrode of conducting polymer [64]. Conducting polymer fibers have now become commercially available. For instance, Santa Fe Science and Technology Inc. produces polyaniline (PANi) fibers under the trademark of Panion. They have been used to fabricate linear actuators: a bundle of Panion fibers (operating as an actuating electrode) has been inserted into a Panion hollow fiber (counterelectrode) with a separator–electrolyte medium. This kind of actuator, tested with a [BMIM][BF4] ionic liquid electrolyte, has reported strains of about 0.3%, stresses of about 1.8 MPa, and redox cycle lifetimes in excess of 10^4 cycles [59].

State-of-the-art devices made of conducting polymers typically need driving voltages of the order of 1 V and are able to generate strains of the order of 1–10% for linear actuators and rotations up to $\pm 90°$ for benders, with large active stresses (up to tens of MPa). Nevertheless, such interesting performances usually correspond to several drawbacks, such as high response times and short lifetimes, whose relevance has to be evaluated in relation to the specific application of interest. Approaches to increase the achievable strains are currently the object of several studies. As a first method, since these materials are typically poor ion conductors, it can be useful to use thin polymer layers and to add water-filled pores or tunnels in order to allow fast diffusions of ions inside the polymer. As a second point, it can be useful to store the ions instead of transporting them. This can be done by using a solid polymer electrolyte (electrolyte storage configuration) or switching the ions between two different polymer layers through a solid polymer electrolyte (electrode storage configuration).

In order to fabricate conducting polymer structures having the main dimensions of the order of centimeters, different techniques have been proposed so far. They consist of classical procedures borrowed from many industrial sectors, where they are employed for different uses. Electrochemical deposition, casting, deep- and spin-coating are the most notable examples. They are briefly mentioned here. Electrochemical deposition or electropolymerization is performed by using an electrochemical cell whose liquid electrolyte contains the monomer under polymerization. The procedure consists of a growth of polymer layers typically via monomer oxidation. In particular, the polymer is deposited on the electrode where oxidation takes place (anode) [76,77]. This method can be used for direct fabrication of electrode/polymer bilayers. Alternatively, the active polymeric layer can successively be peeled off from the deposition electrode, so that it can be coupled to another type of passive substrate. Casting, deep- and spin-coating, and extrusion can be used for film and fiber fabrication if the material is available in solution phase. Following the material processing and shaping, the polymer solution is dried in an oven or by exposure to an infrared lamp. These techniques have been largely used for polyaniline [78,79] and certain forms of polypyrrole [80–83]. Bender actuators fabricated with such techniques can present, when fatigued, a separation of the film from the support (delamination) due to shear stresses generated at the layer interface by the bending movement during operation. Interface roughening, enriching the mechanical interlock between the two layers, has been demonstrated as being useful in order to reduce such a problem [84].

Different techniques have been used to microfabricate small-scale conducting polymer actuators, down to micron size. The most used microtechnologies consist of conventional procedures of surface and bulk micromachining derived from photolithography. They are implemented as sequential steps of layer depositions and etching removals [85,86]. With such methods, several examples of bending actuators have been reported, mainly related to Au/PPy bilayers fabricated onto silicon wafers with polymer thickness even down to 1 μm [85–89]. Many interesting applications of this kind of actuators have been described, including microgrippers [85,89], gates for "cell clinics" [85,89], self-assembling boxes [90,91], microrobots [85,89,92], and positioning microhinges [88]. Recently, different techniques such as ink-jet printing, soft lithography and deposition via controlled-volume or pneumatic microsyringes have been demonstrated as well. Ink-jet printing is a simple and fairly economical technique consisting of a drop-by-drop deposition of a polymer, previously dissolved in a volatile solvent, by using a printing head [93–95]. Soft lithography is a methodology derived from photolithography and includes microinjection molding in capillaries and microcontact printing [96–98]. Microinjection molding uses microfabricated stamps made of poly(dimethylsiloxane). The elastomeric stamps are filled up with a polymer solution and the excess of solvent is evaporated so that the polymer filling the microchannels assumes a specified geometry. The realized microstructure is then removed from the mold via lift-off [99]. The use of microsyringes as extruders mounted on micropositioning systems enables the deposition of polymers in two- and three-dimensional structures [100]. According to the principle of extrusion, two types of systems can be recognized: (1) those with pneumatic microsyringes, where the solution flow is enabled and regulated by compressed air and (2) those with volumetric microsyringes, driven by the controlled movement of a piston. All these systems have been used to fabricate benders. Some examples can be found in Refs. 101, 102.

The actuation technology based on conducting polymers has opened interesting perspectives and its important applications in the biomedical field are currently being studied [46]. Microfabricated benders to be used as gates for the so-called "cell clinics" represent an interesting example. They consist of a microcavity that can be closed with a lid activated by conducting polymer microbenders, working as active hinges, as shown in Figure 16.9. The microcavity can be equipped with sensors to study a single cell.

A second type of relevant area of application consists of controlled releases of biologically active agents by means of external electrical stimuli. As an example, very recently nanotubes of poly(3,4-ethylenedioxythiophene) (PEDOT) were fabricated and demonstrated to be useful for such a purpose (Figure 16.10) [103]. In particular, PEDOT nanotubular structures were fabricated by first producing, by electrospinning, nanofibers of biodegradable poly(L-lactide) (PLLA) or poly(lactide-co-glycolide) (PLGA); these fibers were used as templates for a following electrochemical deposition of the conducting polymers around the nanofibers. Then, the fiber templates were removed or allowed to degrade slowly.

As another example, a potential application of conducting polymer actuators deserves to be mentioned. It consists of the possible development of steerable catheters or endoscopes. They are

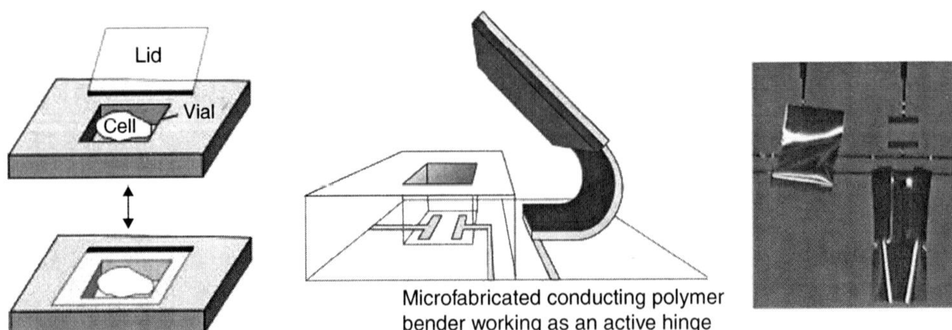

FIGURE 16.9   Cell clinic: Schematic drawings (*left* and *center*) and picture of a 100 μm × 100 μm sample (*right*). (Adapted from Smela, E., *Adv. Mater.*, 15, 481–494, 2003; Jager, E.W.H., Smela, E., Inganäs, O., *Science*, 290, 1540–1545, 2000. With permission.)

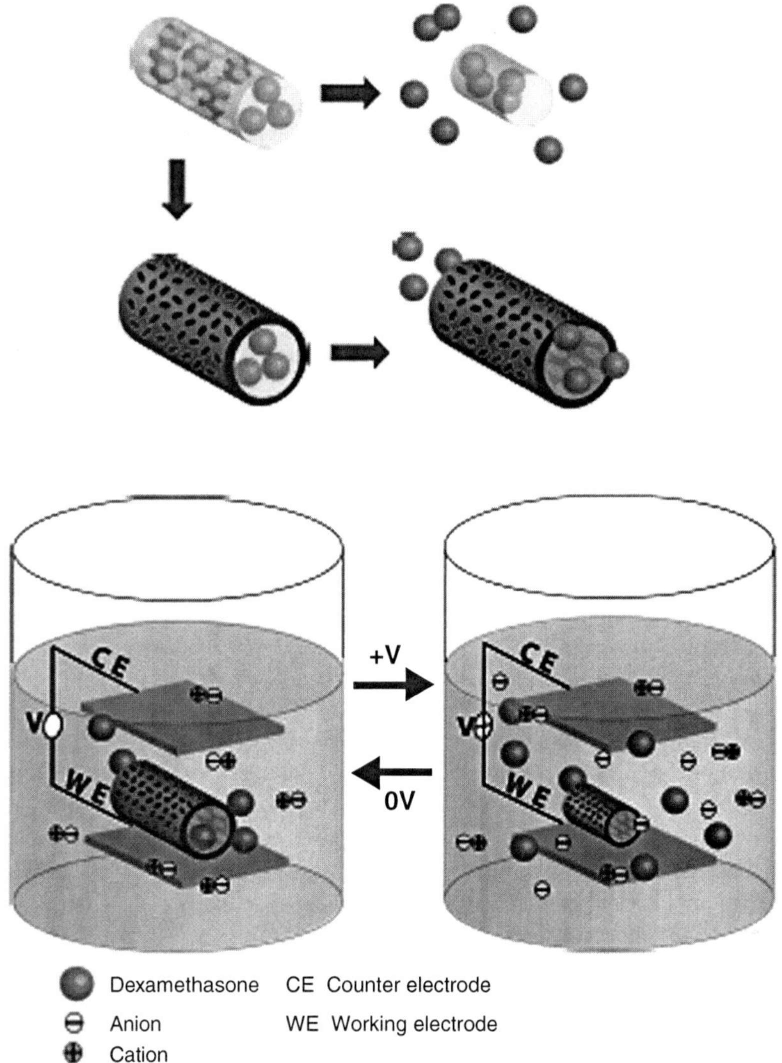

FIGURE 16.10 Conducting polymer nanotubes for controlled release of drugs (dexamethasone in the example). (Adapted from Abidian, M.R., Kim, D.H., Martin, D.C., *Adv. Mater.*, 18, 405–409, 2006. With permission.)

conceived as systems with intrinsic bending properties enabled by conducting polymer actuating elements embedded in the wall of the catheter itself [104]. They could contribute to make intra luminal interventions safer, easier, and more accurate. Figure 16.11 shows a schematic drawing of this concept.

In this respect, the Japanese company EAMEX has recently developed a hollow cylindrical tubing with multidirectional bending properties (Figure 16.12), which could provide interesting openings for this type of applications.

Although these examples are very promising, the actuation technology based on conducting polymers still requires basic improvements in order to achieve higher reliability, response speed, and lifetime.

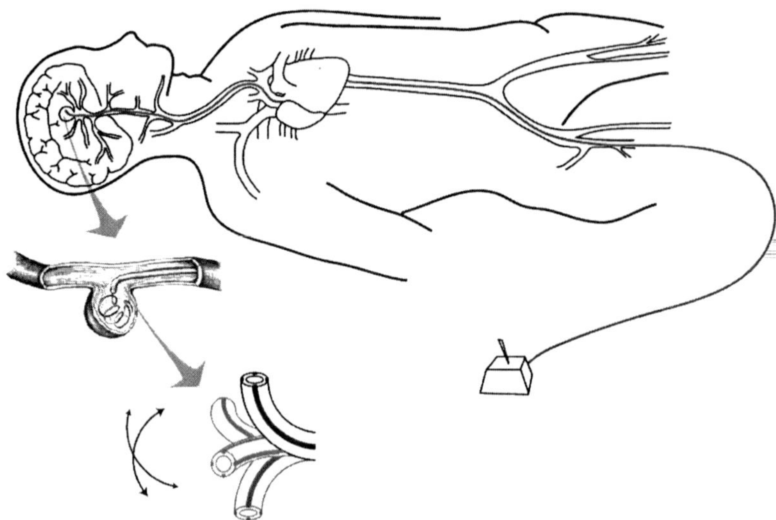

FIGURE 16.11 Concept of a steerable catheter equipped with conducting polymer actuators providing bending motions toward different directions. (Adapted from [105]).

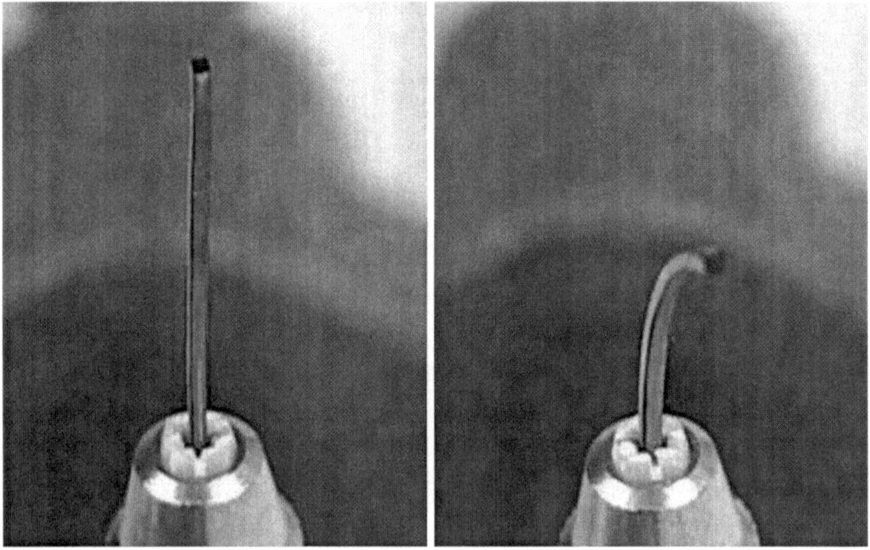

FIGURE 16.12 Prototype sample of a cylindrical tubing with multidirectional bending properties developed by EAMEX. (Adapted from [105].)

16.6 DIELECTRIC ELASTOMERS

The previous paragraphs have provided an overview on ionic EAP. As an example of electronic-type EAP, this paragraph briefly reports the main actuation features of dielectric elastomers. The interest for these materials arises from the fact that, within the overall EAP family, dielectric elastomers form at present one of the most performing subcategories in terms of output electromechanical properties. These materials consist of dielectric polymers with a low elastic modulus, which can present significant electrically induced strains. In particular, a dielectric elastomer actuator consists of a thin layer of an insulating rubber-like material sandwiched between two electrodes that must be compliant (deformable). The electrodes, which can be made for instance of carbon loaded elastomer or carbon grease, are electrically charged by the application of a high potential difference (typically of the order of kV). As a result, the activation of the material by the imposed electric field (usually of the order of 10–100 V/μm) causes a deformation at constant volume consisting of a squeezing of the dimension included between the electrodes and related expansions along the orthogonal directions [106–109]. Such a deformation is mainly due to the so-called Maxwell stress, arising from the electrostatic interactions among the free charges on electrodes. Although this kind of stress acts in any kind of dielectric material subjected to an applied electric field, for this technology the corresponding deformations are greatly emphasized by both the compliance of the electrodes and the softness of the dielectric polymer. These key features basically distinguish actuating devices made of dielectric elastomers from those based on different electric-field-driven dielectrics, such as a piezoelectric material [110] or an electrostrictive material [111]. In comparison with the latter, dielectric elastomers share a strain and stress dependence on the square of the electric field, but are capable of significantly larger deformations for comparable field strengths. This is due to a different activation mechanism and a lower elastic modulus. However, the latter feature reduces, as a counterpart, the achievable stresses.

Acrylic and silicone rubbers are the most significant types of dielectric elastomers used for actuation. Such kinds of polymers comprehend representative materials, which can be very compliant, being able of showing the highest actuating deformations among all EAP [107]. High-level actuation capabilities have been reported for certain types of acrylic polymers: thickness strains up to 60–70% at 400 V/μm, area strains up to 200% at 200 V/μm and corresponding stresses of some MPa [107]. Such performances are enabled by low elastic moduli and high dielectric strengths (dielectric breakdown can occur at electric fields up to about 500 V/μm). The highest active performances were achieved by prestretching the material: this operation was demonstrated to increase the dielectric strength, permitting the application of higher electric fields [107]. Besides acrylates, silicones (mainly polydimethylsiloxanes) offer attracting characteristics: they are easily processable (by spin-coating, casting, etc.) and permit the realization of rubber-like dielectrics with suitable elastic properties, arising from the flexibility of the material molecular chains. Certain silicone elastomers have been actuated with electric fields up to 100–350 V/μm, enabling thickness strains up to 40–50% and area strains up to 100%, with related stresses of 0.3–0.4 MPa [107].

The principle of electromechanical transduction in dielectric elastomers has been exploited by implementing devices with different types of geometries and structures. Examples include planar actuators [106–109], diaphragms [106], benders [106], linear extending devices, such as tubes [106,112] and rolls [106,113,114], linear contractile devices such as stacks [115], helical [116] and folded structures [117], etc.

Owing to the excellent figures of merit shown by several dielectric elastomers (very high actuation strains, considerable stresses, very fast response, high efficiency, stability, reliability, and durability), this class of EAP is nowadays considered as one of the most outstanding for polymer actuation. Nevertheless, a major drawback affects this performing technology: the high driving electric fields needed imply the use of the mentioned very high voltages (although at low currents). This is a significant disadvantage for several types of applications, especially in the biomedical area. In order to solve or at least reduce such a drawback, research efforts are today focused on the development of new elastomers with superior electromechanical properties, particularly by means of an increase of the dielectric permittivity [118]. However, the absence of significant contributions in this direction so far (due to both the challenging nature of the problem and the "youth" of this technology, launched at the end of the 1990s) prevents the adoption of dielectric elastomer actuation for devices that must work in contact with body tissues. Accordingly, different types of applications are emerging. Within the biomedical area, an example concerns the use of dielectric elastomer actuators for dynamic orthotic systems to be used for rehabilitation. In such a context, Figure 16.13 shows a prototype sample of a hand splint for rehabilitation of fingers, which is currently being developed in our laboratory.

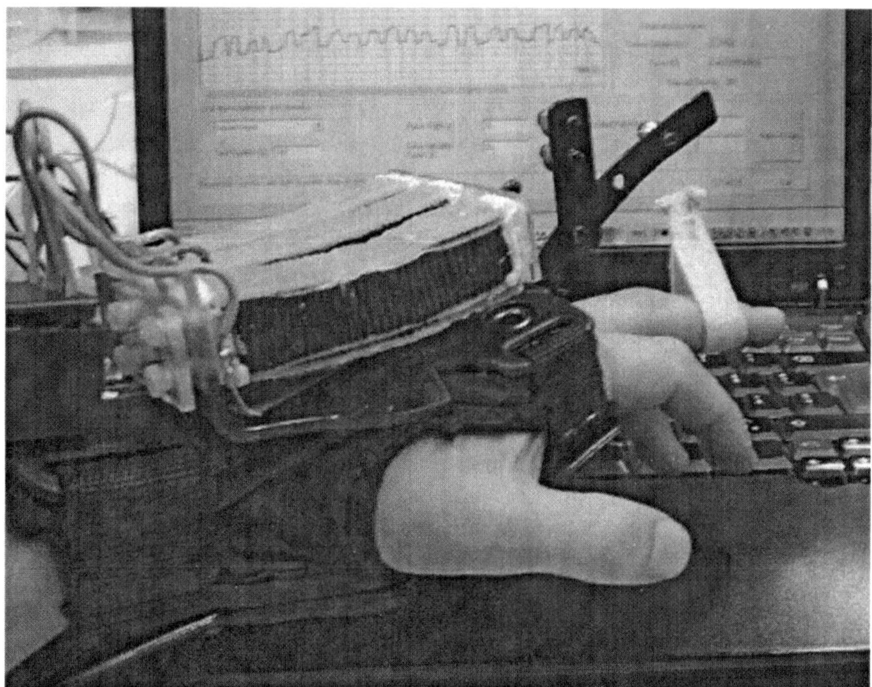

FIGURE 16.13   Prototype sample of a dynamic hand splint equipped with dielectric elastomer actuators.

16.7   CONCLUSIONS

This chapter has provided a brief survey about the most promising types of EAP, which are currently being studied for potential biomedical applications. They may find suitable uses for different kinds of tasks where materials with intrinsic actuation properties, controllable by external stimuli, are required. The main features of such materials, along with the state of the art of their related technology, have been presented. Although several interesting applications could be enabled by the use of these classes of polymers, basic challenging issues actually limit their applicability at present. In particular, polymer gels and IPMC typically offer high strains but low stresses, while an opposite behavior is shown by conducting polymers. These ionic EAP share low-driving voltages, particularly advantageous for a biological environment. Nevertheless, they also share low-response speeds, due to a diffusion-based control of their actuation mechanism, and poor efficiencies and durability, due to the electrochemical nature of the activation. On the contrary, dielectric elastomer actuators offer considerably superior electromechanical performances consisting of large, fast, and stable strains at moderate stresses. However, as a counterpart, they are characterized by the need of very high driving voltages, which discourage the use of this technology for intrabody applications. As a conclusion, it can be argued that an "optimal" EAP is not available at present and the selection of the most suitable material should be made according to the specific application of interest.

REFERENCES

1. Bar-Cohen Y. (Ed.), Electroactive polymer (EAP) actuators as artificial muscles. *Reality, Potential, and Challenges.* Second edition, Bellingham, WA: SPIE Press (2004).
2. Madden J. D. W. et al., Artificial muscle technology: physical principles and naval prospects, *IEEE J. Oceanic Eng.*, 29 (3), 706–728 (2004).

3. Kuhn W., Reversible dehnung und kontraktion bei änderung der ionisation eines netzwerks polyvalenter fadenmolekülionen, *Experimentia*, 5, 318–319 (1949).

4. Katchalsky A., Rapid swelling and deswelling of reversible gels of polymeric acids by ionization, *Experimentia*, 5, 319–320 (1949).

5. Kuhn W., Hargitay B., Katchalsky A., Eisenburg H., Reversible dilatation and contraction by changing the state of ionization of high-polymer acid networks, *Nature*, 165, 514–516 (1950).

6. Osada Y., *Advances in Polymer Sciences*, Berlin: Springer, 82, 1 (1987).

7. De Rossi D., Kajivira K., Osada Y., Yamauchi A. (Eds), *Polymer Gels*, New York: Plenum Press (1991).

8. Osada Y., Matsuda A., Shape-memory gel with order-disorder transition, *Nature*, 376, 219 (1995).

9. Osada Y., Murphy R. S., Intelligent gels, *Sci. Am.*, 268, 82–87 (1993).

10. Wasserman A., *Size and Shape Changes of Contractile Polymers*, New York: Pergamon Press (1960).

11. Okuzaki H., Osada Y., Electro-driven chemomechanical polymer gel as an intelligent soft material, *J. Biomater. Sci. Polym. Ed.*, 5 (5), 485–496 (1994).

12. Gong J. P., Osada Y., Gel actuators, in *Polymer Sensors and Actuators*, Osada Y. and De Rossi D. (Eds), Berlin: Springer, 272–294 (2000).

13. Tanaka T., Nishio I., Sun S.-T., Ueno-Nishio S., Collapse of gels in an electric field, *Science*, 218, 467–469 (1982).

14. Tanaka Y., Kagamo Y., Matsuda A., Osada Y., Thermoreversible transition of tensile modulus of hydrogel with ordered aggregates, *Macromolecules*, 28, 2574–257 (1995).

15. Gong J. P., Matsumoto S., Uchida M., Isogai N., Osada Y., Motion of polymer gels by spreading organic fluid on water, *J. Phys. Chem.*, 100 (26), 11092 (1996).

16. De Rossi D., Parrini P., Chiarelli P., Buzzigoli G., Electrically induced contractile phenomena in charged polymer networks: preliminary study on the feasibility of muscle-like structures, *Trans. Am. Soc. Artif. Intern. Organs*, 31, 60–65 (1985).

17. De Rossi D., Chiarelli P., Buzzigoli G., Domenici C., Lazzeri L., Contractile behaviour of electrically activated mechanochemical polymer actuators, *Trans. Am. Soc. Artif. Intern. Organs*, 32, 157–162 (1986).

18. Osada Y., Chemical valves and gel actuators, *Adv. Mater.*, 3, 107–108 (1991).

19. Zhang X.-Z., Chu C.-C., Temperature-sensitive poly(n-isopropylacrylamide)/poly(ethylene glycol) diacrylate hydrogel microspheres: formulation and controlled drug release, *Am. J. Drug. Deliv.*, 3 (1), 55–65 (2005).

20. Hoffman A., Hydrogels for biomedical applications, *Ann. NY Acad. Sci.*, 944, 62–73 (2001).

21. So Y. K., Young M. L., Drug release behavior of electrical responsive poly(vinyl alcohol)/poly(acrylic acid) IPN hydrogels under an electric stimulus, *J. Appl. Polym. Sci.*, 74, 1752–1761 (1999).

22. Brannon-Peppas L., *Polymers in Controlled Drug Delivery, Medical Plastics and Biomaterials Magazine*, November issue (1997).

23. Kwon I. C., Bae Y. H., Kim S. W., Electrically credible polymer gel for controlled release of drugs, *Nature*, 354, 291–293 (1991).

24. Kost J., Horbett T. A., Ratner B. D. et al., Glucose-sensitive membranes containing glucose oxidase: activity, welling, and permeability studies, *J. Biomed. Mater. Res.*, 19, 1117–1133 (1985).

25. Ishihara K., Kobayashi M., Shinohara I., Control of insulin permeation through a polymer membrane with responsive function for glucose, *Makromol. Chem. Rapid. Commun.*, 4, 327 (1983).

26. Dorski C. M., Doyle F. J., Peppas N. A., Preparation and characterization of glucose-sensitive P(MAA-g-EG) hydrogels, *Polym. Mater. Sci. Eng. Proc.*, 76, 281–282 (1997).

27. Oguro K., Asaka K., Takenaka H., Polymer film actuator driven by low voltage, *Proceedings of 4th International Symposium on Micro Machine and Human Science*, Nagoya, 39–40 (1993).

28. Asaka K., Oguro K., Nishimura Y., Mizuhata M., Takenaka H., Bending of polymer membrane-platinum composites by electric stimuli. Part I. Response characteristics to various waveforms, *Polymer J.*, 27, 436–440 (1995).

29. Asaka K., Oguro K., Bending of polymer membrane platinum composites by electric stimuli. Part II. Response kinetics, *J. Electroanal. Chem.*, 480 (1–2), 186–198 (2000).

30. Asaka K., Oguro K., Bending of polymer membrane-platinum composite by electric stimuli. Part III: self-oscillation, *Electrochimica. Acta.*, 45 (27) 4517–4523 (2000).

31. Abe Y., Mochizuki A., Kawashima T., Yamashita S., Asaka K., Oguro K., Effect on bending behavior of counter cation species in perfluorinated sulfonate membrane-platinum composite, *Polym. Advan. Technol.*, 9 (8), 520–526 (1998).

32. Onishi K., Shingo S., Asaka K., Fujiwara N., Oguro K., Morphology of electrodes and bending response of the polymer electrolyte actuator, *Electrochimica. Acta.*, 46 (5) 737–743 (2001).

33. Onishi K., Sewa S., Asaka K., Fujiwara N., Oguro K., Effects of counter ions on characterization and performance of a solid polymer electrolyte actuator, *Electrochimica. Acta.*, 46 (8) 1233–1241 (2001).

34. Shahinpoor M., Ion-exchange polymer-metal composites as biomimetic sensors and actuators, in *Polymer Sensors and Actuators*, Osada Y. and De Rossi D. (Eds), Berlin: Springer, 325–360 (2000).

35. Oguro K., Fujiwara N., Asaka K., Onishi K., Sewa S., Polymer electrolyte actuator with gold electrodes, *Proceedings of SPIE—The International Society for Optical Engineering*, 3669, 64–71 (1999).

36. Onishi K., Sewa S., Asaka K., Fujiwara N., Oguro K., Bending response of polymer electrolyte actuator, *Proceedings of SPIE—The International Society for Optical Engineering*, 3987, 121–128 (2000).

37. Tadokoro S., Yamagami S., Takamori T., Oguro K., Modeling of Nafion-Pt composite actuators (ICPF) by ionic motion, *Proceedings of SPIE - The International Society for Optical Engineering*, 3987, 92–102 (2000).

38. Bar-Cohen Y., Xue T., Joffe B., Lih S.-S., Shahinpoor M., Simpson J., Smith J., Willis P., Electroactive polymers (IPMC), low mass muscle actuators, *Proceedings of SPIE Smart Materials and Structure Conference*, San Diego, California, SPIE Publications, 3041–76 (1997).

39. Salehpoor K., Shahinpoor M., Razani A., Role of ion transport in dynamic sensing and actuation of ionic polymeric platinum composite artificial muscles, *Proceedings of SPIE Smart Materials and Structure Conference*, San Diego, California, SPIE Publications, 3330–09 (1998).

40. Shahinpoor M., Bar-Cohen Y., Simpson J. O., Smith J., Ionic polymer-metal composites (IPMCs) as biomimetic sensors, actuators and artificial muscles — a review, *Smart Mater. Struct.*, 7, R15–R30 (1998).

41. Nemat-Nasser S., Micromechanics of actuation of ionic polymer-metal composites, *J. Appl. Phys.*, 92 (5), 2899–2915 (2002).

42. Shahinpoor M., Kim K. J., Ionic polymer–metal composites: IV. Industrial and medical applications, *Smart Mater. Struct.*, 14, 197–214 (2005).

43. MacDiarmid A. G., Synthetic metals': a novel role for organic polymers, *Curr. Appl. Phys.*, 1, 269–279 (2001).

44. Heeger A. J., Semiconducting and metallic polymers: the fourth generation of polymeric materials, *J. Phys. Chem. B*, 105 (36), 8475–8491 (2001).

45. Carpi F., De Rossi D., Electroactive polymer based devices for e-textiles in biomedicine, *IEEE. T. Inf. Technol. B*, 9 (3), 295–318 (2005).

46. Smela E., Conjugated polymer actuators for biomedical applications, *Adv. Mater.*, 15 (6), 481–494 (2003).

47. Kim D.-H., Abidian M., Martin D. C., Conducting polymers grown in hydrogel scaffolds coated on neural prosthetic devices, *J. Biomed. Mater. Res. A*, 71A (4), 577–585 (2004).

48. Nyberg T., Inganäs O., Jerregård H., Polymer hydrogel microelectrodes for neural communication, *Biomedical Microdevices*, 4, 43–52 (2002).

49. Xinyan C., Lee V. A., Raphael Y., Wiler J. A., Hetke J. F., Anderson D. J., Martin D. C., Surface modification of neural recording electrodes with conducting polymer/biomolecule blends, *J. Biomed. Mater. Res.*, 56, 261–272 (2001).

50. Rivers T. J., Hudson T. W., Schmidt C. E., Synthesis of a novel, biodegradable electrically conducting polymer for biomedical applications, *Adv. Funct. Mater.*, 12, 33–37 (2002).

51. Baughman R. H., Shacklette L. V., in *Science and Application of Conducting Polymers*, Salaneck W. R., Clark D. T. and Samuelsen E. J. (Eds), New York: Adam Hilger (1990).

52. Baughman R. H., Conducting polymer artificial muscles, *Synthetic Met.*, 78, 339–353 (1996).

53. Smela E., Gadegaard N., Surprising volume change in PPY(DBS): an atomic force microscopy study, *Adv. Mater.*, 11 (11), 953–957 (1999).

54. Mazzoldi A., Carpi F., De Rossi D., 2004, Polymers responding to electrical or electrochemical stimuli for linear actuators, *Ann. Chim.-Sci. Mat.*, 29 (6), 55–64 (2004).

55. Ding J., Liu L., Spinks G. M., Zhou D., Wallace G. G., Gillespie J., High performance conducting polymer actuators utilising a tubular geometry and helical wire interconnects, *Synthetic. Met.*, 138, 391–398 (2003).

56. Ding J., Zhou D., Spinks G., Wallace G. G., Forsyth S., Forsyth M., MacFarlane D., Use of ionic liquids as electrolytes in electromechanical actuator systems based on inherently conducting polymers, *Chem. Mater.*, 15, 2392–2398 (2003).

57. Bay L., West K., Sommer-Larsen P., A conducting polymer artificial muscle with 12% linear strain, *Adv. Mater.*, 15 (4), 310–313 (2003).

58. Otero T. F., Cortes M. T., Artificial muscles with tactile sensitivity, *Adv. Mater.*, 15 (4), 279–282 (2003).
59. Lu W., Fadeev A. G., Qi B., Smela E., Mattes B. R., Ding J., Spinks G. M., Mazurkiewicz J., Zhou D., Wallace G. G., MacFarlane D. R., Forsyth S. A., Forsyth M., 2002, Use of ionic liquids for π-conjugated polymer electrochemical devices, *Science*, 297, 983–987 (2002).
60. Spinks G. M., Liu L., Wallace G. G., Zhou D., Strain response from polypyrrole actuators under load, *Adv. Funct. Mater.*, 12 (6–7), 437–440 (2002).
61. Bay L., Jacobsen T., Skaarup S., West K., Mechanism of actuation in conducting polymers: osmotic expansion, *J. Phys. Chem. B*, 105 (36), 8492–8497 (2001).
62. Lewis T. W., Spinks G. M., Wallace G. G., Mazzoldi A., De Rossi D., Investigation of the applied potential limits for polypyrrole when employed as the active components of a two-electrode device, *Synthetic Met.*, 122, 379–385 (2001).
63. Mazzoldi A., Della S. A., De Rossi D., Conducting polymer actuators: properties and modeling, in *Polymer Sensors and Actuators*, Osada Y. and De Rossi D. (Eds), Berlin: Springer, 207–244 (2000).
64. Mazzoldi A., Degl'Innocenti C., De Rossi D., Actuative properties of polyaniline fiber under electrochemical stimulation, *Mat. Sci. Tec. C*, 6, 65–72 (1998).
65. De Rossi D., Della S. A., Mazzold A., Performance and work capacity of a polypyrrole conducting polymer linear actuator, *Synthetic Met.*, 90, 93–100 (1997).
66. Della S. A., De Rossi D., Mazzoldi A., Characterization and modelling of a conducting polymer muscle-like linear actuator, *Smart. Mater. Struct.*, 6 (1), 23–34 (1997).
67. Gandhi M. R., Murray P., Spinks G. M., Wallace G. G., Mechanism of electromechanical actuation in polypyrrole, *Synthetic Met.*, 73, 247–256 (1995).
68. Chiarelli P., Della S. A., De Rossi D., Mazzoldi A., Actuation properties of electrochemical driven polypyrrole free-standing films, *J. Int. Mat. Syst. Struc.*, 6 (1), 32–37 (1995).
69. Kaneto K., Kaneko M., Min Y., MacDiarmid A. G., Artificial muscle: electromechanical actuators using polyaniline films, *Synthetic Met.*, 71, 2211–2212 (1995).
70. Otero T., Sansinena J. M., Soft and wet conducting polymers for artificial muscles, *Adv. Mater.*, 10 (6), 491–494 (1998).
71. Otero T. F. et al., Artificial muscles from bilayer structures, *Synthetic Met.*, 55–57, 3713–3717 (1993).
72. Pei Q., Inganäs O., Electrochemical muscles: bending strips built from conjugated polymers, *Synthetic Met.*, 57 (1), 3718–372 (1993).
73. Pei Q., Inganäs O., Lundström I., Bending bilayer strips built from polyaniline for artificial electrochemical muscles, *Smart Mater. Struct.*, 2, 1–6 (1993).
74. Smela E., Inganäs O., Lundström I., Conducting polymers as artificial muscles: challenges and possibilities, *J. Micromech. Microeng.* 3, 203–205 (1993).
75. Lewis T. W., Spinks G. M., Wallace G. G., De Rossi D., Pachetti M., Development of an all polymer electromechanical actuator, *Polymer Preprint*, 38 (2), 520–521 (1997).
76. Takashima W., Kaneko M., Kaneto K., MacDiarmid A. G., The electrochemical actuator using electrochemically-deposited poly-aniline film, *Synthetic Met.*, 71, 2265–2266 (1995).
77. Heinze J., Electrochemistry of conducting polymers, *Synthetic Met.*, 41–43, 2805–2823 (1991).
78. Wang H. L., Romero R. J., Mattes B. R., Zhu Y., Winokur M. J., Effect of processing conditions on the properties of high molecular weight conductive polyaniline fiber, *J. Pol. Sci. Part B*, 38 (1), 194–204 (2000).
79. Mattes B. R., Wang H. L., Yang D., Zhu Y. T., Blumenthal W. R., Hundley M. F., Formation of conductive polyaniline fibers derived from highly concentrated emeraldine base solutions, *Synthetic. Met.*, 84, 45–49 (1994).
80. Chinn D., Janata J., Spin-cast thin films of polyaniline, *Thin Solid Films*, 252, 145 (1994).
81. Lee J. Y., Kim D. Y., Kim C. Y., Synthesis of soluble polypyrrole of the doped state in organic solvents, *Synthetic Met.*, 74, 103 (1995).
82. Kim I. W., Lee J. Y., Lee H., Solution-cast polypyrrole film: the electrical and thermal properties, *Synthetic Met.*, 78, 177 (1996).
83. Miller E. K., Lee K., Heeger A. J., Lee J. Y., Kim D. Y., Kim C. Y., Reflectance studies of soluble polypyrrole doped with dodecylbenzene sulfonic acid, *Synthetic Met.*, 84, 821 (1997).
84. Pyo M., Bohn C. C., Smela E., Reynolds J. R., Brennan A. B., Direct strain measurement of polypyrrole actuators controlled by the polymer/gold interface, *Chem. Mater.*, 15 (4), 916–922 (2003).
85. Jager E. W. H., Smela E., Inganäs O., Microfabricating conjugated polymer actuators, *Science*, 290, 1540–1545 (2000).

86. Smela E., Microfabrication of PPy microactuators and other conjugated polymer devices, *J. Micromech. Microeng.*, 9, 1–18 (1998).

87. Smela E., Inganäs O., Pei Q., Lundström I., Electrochemical muscles: micromachining fingers and corkscrews, *Adv. Mater.*, 5, 630–632 (1993).

88. Smela E., Kallenbach M., Holdenried J., Electrochemically driven polypyrrole bilayers for moving and positioning bulk micromachined silicon plates, *J. Microelectrom. Syst.*, 8, 373–383 (1999).

89. Jager E. W. H., Smela E., Inganäs O., Lundström I., Application of polypyrrole microactuators. *Proceedings of SPIE—International Society of Optical Engineering*, 3669, 377–384 (1999).

90. Smela E., Inganäs O., Lundström I., Controlled folding of micrometer-size structures, *Science*, 268, 1735–1738 (1995).

91. Jager E. W. H., Inganäs O., Lundström I., Perpendicular actuation with individually controlled polymer microactuators, *Adv. Mater.*, 13 (1), 76–79 (2001).

92. Jager E. W. H., Inganäs O., Lundström I., Microrobots for micrometer-size objects in aqueous media potential tools for single-cell manipulation, *Science*, 288, 2335–2338 (2000).

93. Pede D., Serra G., De Rossi D., Microfabrication of conducting polymer devices by ink-jet stereolithography, *Mater. Sci. Eng. C*, 5, 289–291 (1998).

94. Chang S. C., Bharathan J., Yang Y., Helgeson R., Wudl F., Ramey M. B., Reynolds J. R., Dual-color polymer light-emitting pixels processed by hybrid inkjet printing, *Appl. Phys. Lett.*, 73, 2561–2563 (1998).

95. Hebner T., Wu C. C., Marcy D., Lu M. H., Sturm J. C., Ink-jet printing of doped polymers for organic light emitting devices, *Appl. Phys. Lett.*, 72, 519–521 (1998).

96. Whitesides G. M. et al., Soft lithography in biology and biochemistry, *Annu. Rev. Biomed. Eng.*, 3, 335–73 (2001).

97. Bao Z. N., Rogers J. A., Katz H. E., Printable organic and polymeric semiconducting materials and devices, *J. Mater. Chem.*, 9, 1895–1904 (1999).

98. Granlund T., Nyberg T., Roman L. S., Svensson M., Inganas O., Patterning of polymer light-emitting diodes with soft lithography, *Adv. Mater.*, 12, 269–273 (2000).

99. Vozzi G. et al., Microfabricated PLGA scaffolds: a comparative study for application to tissue engineering, *Mat. Sci. and Eng. C*, 20 (1–2), 43–47 (2002).

100. Vozzi G. et al., Microsyringe-based deposition of two-dimensional and three-dimensional polymer scaffolds with a well-defined geometry for application to tissue engineering, *Tissue Eng.*, 8 (6), 1089–1098 (2002).

101. Lewis T. W., Spinks G. M., Wallace G. G., De Rossi D., Pachetti M., Development of an all polymer electromechanical actuator, *Polymer Preprint*, 38 (2), 520–521 (1997).

102. Vozzi G., Carpi F., Mazzoldi A., Realization of conducting polymer actuators using a controlled volume microsyringe system, *Smart Mater. Struct.*, 15, 279–287, 2006.

103. Abidian M. R., Kim D.-H., Martin D. C., Conducting-polymer nanotubes for controlled drug release, *Adv. Mater.*, 18 (4), 405–409 (2006).

104. Della S. A., Mazzoldi A., De Rossi D., Steerable microcatheter actuated by embedded conducting polymer structures, *J. Intel. Mat. Syst. Str.*, 7 (3), 292–300 (1996).

105. EAMEX corporation, web site address: http://www.eamex.co.jp/index_e.html.

106. Pelrine R. E., Kornbluh R. D., Joseph J. P., Electrostriction of polymer dielectrics with compliant electrodes as a means of actuation, *Sensor. Actuat. A-Phys.*, 64, 77–85 (1998).

107. Pelrine R., Kornbluh R., Pei Q., Joseph J., High-speed electrically actuated elastomers with strain greater than 100%, *Science*, 287, 836–839 (2000).

108. Pelrine R., Kornbluh R., Kofod G., High-strain actuator materials based on dielectric elastomers, *Adv. Mater.*, 12 (16), 1223–1225 (2000).

109. Pelrine R., Kornbluh R., Joseph J., Heydt R., Pei Q., Chiba S. High-field deformation of elastomeric dielectrics for actuators, *Mater. Sci. Eng. C*, 11, 89–100 (2000).

110. Nalwa H. S., *Ferroelectric Polymers*, New York: Marcel Dekker, Inc. (1995).

111. Zhang Q. M., Bharti V., Zhao X., Giant electrostriction and relaxor ferroelectric behaviour in electron-irradiated poly(vinylidene fluoride-trifluoroethylene) copolymer, *Science*, 280, 2101–2103 (1998).

112. Carpi F., De Rossi D., Dielectric elastomer cylindrical actuators: electromechanical modelling and experimental evaluation, *Mater. Sci. Eng. C*, 24, 555–562 (2004).

113. Pei Q., Pelrine R., Stanford S., Kornbluh R., Rosenthal M., Electroelastomer rolls and their application for biomimetic walking robots, *Synthetic Met.*, 135–136, 129–131 (2003).

114. Pei Q., Rosenthal M., Stanford S., Prahlad H., Pelrine R., Multiple-degrees-of-freedom electroelastomer roll actuators, *Smart Mater. Struct.*, 13, N86–N92 (2004).
115. Schlaak H., Jungmann M., Matysek M., Lotz P., Novel multilayer electrostatic solid-state actuators with elastic dielectric, in *Smart Structures and Materials 2005: Electroactive Polymer Actuators and Devices*, Bar-Cohen Y. (Ed.), *Proceedings of SPIE* 5759 121–133 (2005).
116. Carpi F., Migliore A., Serra G., De Rossi D., Helical dielectric elastomer actuators, *Smart Mater. Struct.*, 14, 1210–1216 (2005).
117. Carpi F., Salaris C., De Rossi D., Folded dielectric elastomer actuators, *Smart Mater. Struct.*, 16, S300–S305 (2007).
118. Carpi F., De Rossi D., Improvement of electromechanical actuating performances of a silicone dielectric elastomer by dispers of titanium dioxide powder, *IEEE T. Dielect. El. In.*, 12 (4), 835–843 (2005).

17 Blood-Contacting Surfaces

Menno L.W. Knetsch

CONTENTS

17.1 INTRODUCTION

Upon implantation of a medical device, blood is the first tissue that comes into contact with the implant. This is caused by damage of tissue and blood vessels during the implantation procedure.

Lymphatic white cells, the B and T lymphocytes, are derived from lymphoid stem cells that are located in the lymphatic system, especially in the lymph nodes. These cell types represent the adaptive part of the immune system, catalyzing a specific response to each new invader, generating specific antibodies (B cells), and also priming cells to attack and remove the invader (T cells).

Furthermore, some additional white cells are present in the circulation like auxiliary cells, mast cells, and natural killer cells. These cells only represent a small fraction of the white blood cells and are not directly involved in the contact with synthetic surfaces.

17.2.3 PLATELETS

In the bone marrow, the megakaryocyte produces a large number of anuclear cellular fragments, called platelets that are important for blood coagulation and vessel wall repair.[3–6] These platelets have a half life of about 8–10 days, and inactive platelets will be removed in the spleen by macrophages. The platelets are mainly involved in the coagulation response, but also have a role in the attachment of leukocytes onto synthetic surfaces. The number of platelets in the blood can vary between 150 and 400×10^6/mL, but only a severe reduction of approximately 90% (below 20×10^6/mL) will result in serious bleeding complications, requiring transfusion to restore platelet levels.

17.2.4 PLASMA

Blood plasma is the liquid part of the blood in which all cells are suspended. A large array of ions, sugars, fatty acids, amino acids, proteins, and other soluble molecules are present in plasma.[7–9] The pH and osmolarity have to be kept constant to avoid damage to blood cells and tissues. The pH is kept constant at 7.4 by making use of the buffering capacity of carbonate ions. As a consequence, hyperventilation causes the pH of blood to drop as a result of an increased concentration of dissolved CO_2 and a shift in the balance of the carbonate ions. Eventually, this may result in fainting. Osmolarity is largely controlled by action of the kidneys that actively regulate the concentrations of ions. Increased levels of ions in the blood can lead to hypertension, which on the long run can damage the heart and vasculature. Blood sugar levels are also tightly controlled, with loss of control mechanisms resulting in diabetes. The effects of diabetes are both short-term (fainting, unconsciousness, and even coma) and long-term as for instance the diabetic foot that occurs as a result of impaired blood flow in the leg.[10–12] In this way an increased sugar level in the blood causes damage to the blood vessels, resulting in limb loss and in the worst case even death. Additionally, blood-contacting devices have a higher risk of failing in diabetic patients. The fatty acids and lipids in the blood are in general bound to transporter proteins. The low-density lipoproteins (LDL) and high-density lipoproteins (HDL) have long been used as an indicator for the risk of cardiovascular disease in humans. High LDL and low HDL have been associated with an increased risk in atherosclerosis, myocardial infarction, and stroke.[13–15]

An extensive array of different proteins is present in plasma.[7–9] The immune system (IgG, IgM, IgA), complement system (C3, C4, C5, C9, C1q), nutrient transport (apolipoproteins, transferrin), and coagulation (prothrombin, antithrombin (AT), factor XII, prekallikrein, plasminogen) are fully dependent on plasma proteins. Most of these proteins are released in the blood system by organs like the liver.

17.3 BLOOD VESSELS

Blood transports nutrients, waste products, gases, and (excess) heat throughout the body. Cells from the immune system can reach each tissue by moving through the blood vessels, and leaving the circulation when necessary. There are three major forms of blood vessels: (i) arteries, (ii) veins, and (iii) capillaries.[2] The anatomy of vessels is given in Figure 17.3. Capillaries and small postcapillary venules consist of only an endothelial layer with a basal lamina (tunica intima). The arteries and veins contain extra layers with smooth muscle cells (tunica media) and fibroblasts and collagen

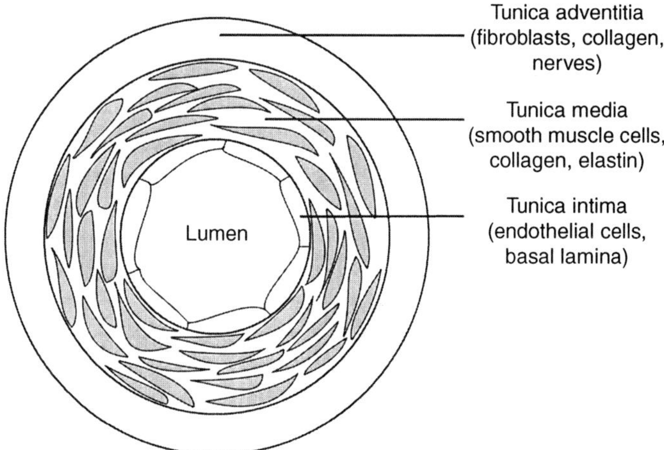

FIGURE 17.3 Blood vessels, except capillaries, are composed of three layers: the tunica intima, tunica media, and tunica adventitia. Capillaries lack the tunicae media and adventitia. The major components of each layer are given.

fibers (tunica adventitia). These layers give extra support and strength to large blood vessels, preventing rupture.

The arteries transport oxygen-rich blood from the heart to all tissues. The only exception is the pulmonary artery that comes from the heart and leads oxygen-poor blood to the lungs for oxygenation, and release of carbon dioxide. The blood pressure in the arteries is high, is reduced in the capillary bed, and is low in the veins. The veins transport the blood back to the heart. Veins contain valves to avoid retrograde flow. The surface area of the capillaries is large, especially in the lungs (efficient exchange of oxygen and CO_2) and the organs and tissues (nutrient and gas exchange). Because of this, capillaries only consist of one layer of endothelial cells on a thin basal lamina. This morphology enables efficient and easy exchange of gases and nutrients.

17.4 BLOOD-CONTACTING DEVICES

Blood-contacting devices are medical devices that are intended to function in direct contact with blood. These devices include vascular prosthesis, heart valves, intravenous catheters, blood bags, ventricular assist devise, guide wires, intravascular stents, hemodialysis filters, tubing for heart–lung machines, etc. To avoid loss of function, the surfaces of these devices should display no coagulation, inflammation, or hemolysis.[1,16–18]

The interaction of the synthetic surface with plasma proteins and the blood cells and platelets determines blood compatibility. The chemical composition and topography of the synthetic surface are of vital importance for blood compatibility. Additionally, some devices perform a mechanical task, like heart valves and blood-pumps. Hemolysis, or lysis of blood cells, by these devices is mostly dependent on the design of the moving parts.

The principal problem of all these devices is that they are more or less thrombogenic, meaning that they cause biomaterial-induced thrombus (blood clot) formation. To prevent failure of the device, often systemic anticoagulation drug therapy is used. The downside of this therapy is that it is chronic and increases the chance of hemorrhage for the patient. Therefore, biomedical engineers have designed a variety of surface modifications that aim to prevent thrombus formation on the surface. Some of these modification strategies will be discussed in this chapter. However, it should be kept in mind that in order to design successful blood-contacting surfaces, it is essential to understand the events that occur at the interface between blood and a synthetic surface.

17.5 INTERACTION OF BLOOD WITH SYNTHETIC SURFACES

17.5.1 Protein Adsorption

Upon first contact of blood with a synthetic surface, a rapid adsorption of plasma proteins will occur. This protein adsorption is not static and over time the composition of the adsorbed protein layer will change. This effect is called the Vroman effect, after Leo Vroman who first described this phenomenon in the late 1960s.[19–21] According to Vroman and coworkers, first the most abundant, and often small, proteins will adsorb, however with low affinity. These proteins will be replaced by, often larger, proteins with higher affinity for the surface, which are in general less prevalent in the blood. The mechanism of protein adsorption on synthetic surfaces still a much debated phenomenon. Protein adsorption is dependent on the physicochemical characteristics of the surface.[21–25] Some of these characteristics can be controlled during the synthesis of the surface, namely chemical composition, surface charge and hydrophilicity, surface topography, etc. In many cases adsorbed proteins will partly or completely denature, changing their structure and consequently their function.[21,25] Consequently, the nature of the surface can be radically changed by protein adsorption, like surface charge, and synthetic surface modifications that can become covered by adsorbed proteins. One can state that the surface of an implant rarely contacts cells and tissues. In fact it is the layer of adsorbed proteins that determines the behavior of cells and tissues in contact with synthetic surfaces.[26–28]

Given that the response of blood (coagulation, inflammation, complement activation) toward synthetic surfaces is governed by the nature of the adsorbed protein, directing protein adsorption is considered a valuable tool to control blood compatibility of surfaces. Many attempts have been made to either produce a completely protein-repellent surface or to manipulate protein adsorption in such a fashion that the desired cell–surface interaction is obtained. However of the protein-guiding surfaces none has been proven reliable and successful when in contact with flowing blood *in vivo*. Several blood compatibility strategies will be discussed in a later section (Section 17.6).

17.5.2 Coagulation

Blood coagulation is an essential part of the repair mechanism of the vascular system. The integrity of blood vessels has to be maintained, and therefore a complex mechanism of vessel repair has evolved.[1,29,30] Upon injury of a blood vessel, a primary plug is generated consisting mainly of platelets. This platelet plug primarily avoids further blood loss from the circulation.[31] This plug further activates a complex system of proteins, the coagulation system. Activation of coagulation leads to a stable blood clot, which avoids bleeding from the injury site.[5,17] In a second phase the damaged cell layers are repaired and the blood clot is removed in a process called fibrinolysis.[31,32]

The control of coagulation is of vital importance. The balance between coagulation and anticoagulation, called hemostasis, has to be controlled tightly. When the balance changes toward coagulation, thrombosis, and stroke or myocardial infarction may follow. In case of the balance shifting toward anticoagulation, excessive bleeding and hemorrhage, for example, in the joints or in the brain may follow. It is clear that the delicate balance of the coagulation system should not be disturbed by blood-contacting devices. Unfortunately, contact of synthetic surfaces with blood usually disturbs the balance and very often induces coagulation and consequently thrombus formation.[17]

Thrombus formation is triggered by two different pathways, the intrinsic and the extrinsic. Both pathways lead to the activation of the common pathway in which the central enzyme thrombin catalyzes the formation of fibrin from the plasma protein fibrinogen, resulting in a stable blood clot. All these systems will be discussed to generate a further understanding of the problems faced by biomedical engineers in trying to design blood-compatible surfaces.

17.5.2.1 Common Pathway

The central enzyme in blood coagulation is thrombin. This enzyme digests fibrinogen and thereby induces the formation of fibrin fibers and a fibrin network, stabilizing the thrombus or clot. The fibrin network is then cross-linked by factor XIIIa (FXIIIa) to the obtain an even more stable clot. During the formation of the clot, platelets, white blood cells and especially red blood cells get caught. This is the reason for the reddish appearance of blood clots. After the vessel damage or tissue damage has been repaired, the clot will be degraded by a process called fibrinolysis. The zymogen plasminogen is cleaved to form plasmin, which degrades the fibrin network.[31,33]

Thrombin is formed through cleavage of prothrombin by FXa with FVa (the prothrombinase complex). Both extrinsic and intrinsic pathways result in the activation of FXa and assembly of the prothrombinase complex. Because both pathways converge in this last stage of coagulation, it has been termed as the common pathway (Figure 17.4).

The activation of thrombin is dependent on Ca^{2+} and a negatively charged phospholipid surface.[30,34,35] The dependency of thrombin formation on calcium ions is exploited for anticoagulation of blood. Blood is often collected on citrate or ethylenediaminetetraacetic acid (EDTA), both chelators of calcium ions and thereby blocking coagulation of blood. In this way blood can be stored before it is used in the laboratory. Furthermore, the activity of prothrombinase relies on phospholipid (PL) surfaces that are enriched in the negatively charged phosphatidyl serine. For instance, these PLs can be the plasma membrane of (activated) platelets adhered to synthetic surfaces.

Thrombin can initiate the formation of additional thrombin by activating FVIII or FXI in a feedback upregulation of the intrinsic pathway.[17,30] In this way, traces of thrombin can be amplified to a burst of thrombin. The threshold thrombin concentration for the formation of a stable blood clot can be reached, and a full clotting response will follow.

Of course the inactivation of thrombin is as important as its activation. Active thrombin can be inactivated by binding it to AT, thereby forming an irreversible complex that is targeted for degradation (Figure 17.5). AT can also inactivate FXa by a very similar mechanism. The anticoagulant drug heparin, which mimics glycosaminoglycans present on the endothelial cells of the inner vessel wall,

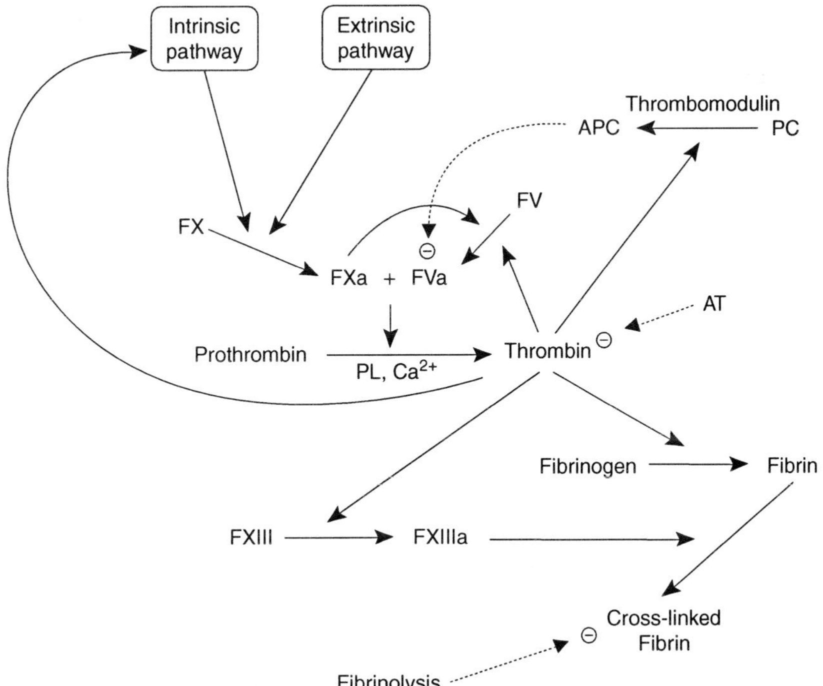

FIGURE 17.4 Common pathway of blood coagulation. AT, antithrombin; PC, protein C; APC, activated protein C; F, factor; PL, phospholipids.

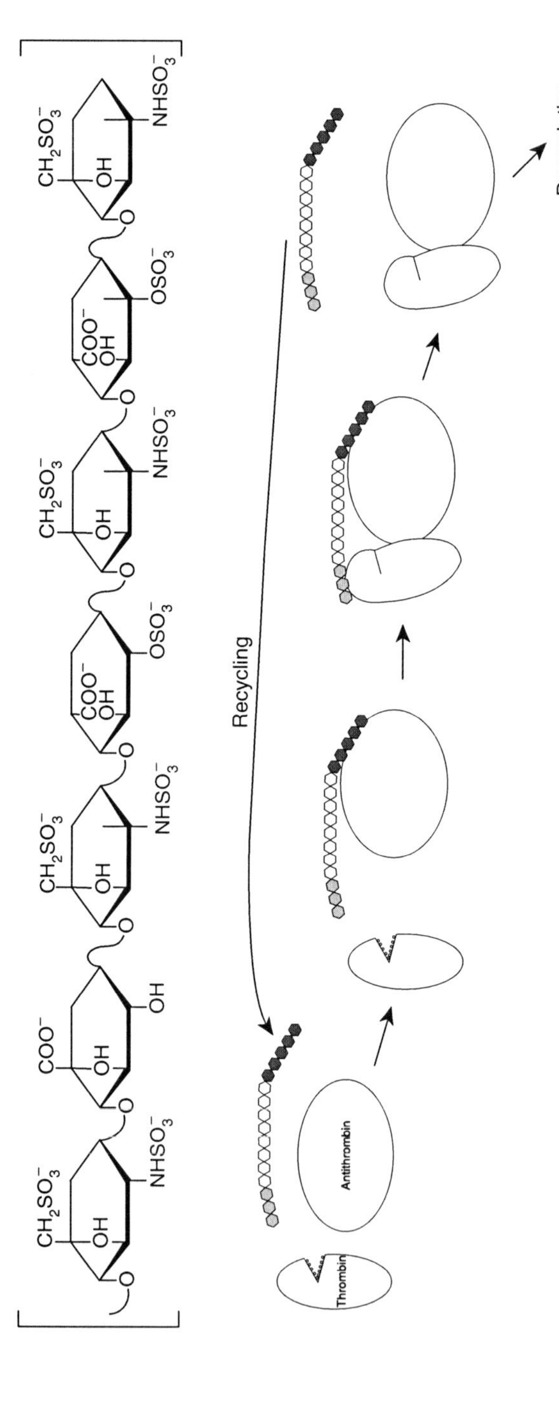

FIGURE 17.5 Structure of the anticoagulant heparin (upper) and inhibition of thrombin by heparin (lower). Note that heparin acts as a catalyst in inactivating thrombin.

makes use of this thrombin inactivation system. Heparin is a commonly used drug in the control of thrombosis and coagulation disorders.[35–37]

Heparin enhances the affinity of AT for thrombin or FXa, accelerating clearance of these enzymes from the blood. The heparin will release the thrombin–AT (or FXa-AT) complex, ready to interact with a following AT molecule. Because heparin works in a catalytic fashion, it is a favorite anticoagulant molecule for biomedical engineers. Other anticoagulant drugs like hirudin, which is derived from the medicinal leech *Hirudo medicinalis* targets the active site of thrombin.[38] These sorts of drugs can only inactivate one thrombin molecule while heparin can inactivate multiple thrombin molecules. Thrombin also induces its own inactivation, for instance by the activated protein C (APC) pathway.[39,40] The APC cleaves FVa, inhibiting prothrombinase, or FVIIIa, which is an essential component of the tenase complex, reducing FXa formation. A decrease in the ability of APC to inactivate thrombin is called APC resistance, and may result in deep vein thrombosis. This clotting disorder is often caused by mutations in the gene encoding FV, resulting in slower cleavage of FVa and thus a prolonged thrombin activity.[41] Also the use of oral contraceptives was shown to influence the inactivation of thrombin via this mechanism. The hormones present in oral contraceptives decrease the sensitivity of FVa for APC, prolonging the activity of thrombin and thus increasing the chance of deep vein thrombosis.[42] This shows that both coagulation and anticoagulation have to be kept in balance in order to prevent complications from the blood. As a consequence, many strategies for improved blood compatibility rely on synthetic surfaces that can induce inhibition of thrombin formation or activity.

17.5.2.2 Intrinsic Pathway

This pathway of blood coagulation is often referred to as the "contact activation" pathway. This is termed as contact activation because upon the contact of blood with a synthetic surface, a series of events is triggered that results in thrombus formation.[1,17,43] Negatively charged surfaces are especially good substrates for contact activation. For this reason the physiological importance of contact activation remains a matter of speculation since negatively charges surfaces *in vivo* are rare, especially in contact with blood.

In contact activation, first, adsorption of high-molecular-weight kininogen (HMWK), prekallikrein, and FXII to a surface occurs. The adsorbed HMWK will cleave prekallikrein and the formed kallikrein can in turn convert FXII to FXIIa. Together with HMWK, FXIIa activates FXI and the resulting FXIa will in turn convert FIX to FIXa. In fact the intrinsic pathway is a chain of zymogens that cleave and subsequently activate each other in a precise order. At the end of this pathway the formed FIXa together with FVIIIa will form the tenase complex that catalyzes the formation of FXa. This enzyme is a convergence point in coagulation and from here on the intrinsic pathway is activated, ultimately resulting in formation of a blood clot (Figure 17.6). The importance of the cofactor FVIIIa is known from the hemophilia-A patients who have a strongly increased bleeding tendency, especially in the joints. The most famous carriers of this bleeding disorder were some of the males in the Romanov, Russian tsar family. Hemophilia-B is caused by a deficiency in FIX, resulting in a much reduced thrombin response due to lack of positive feedback upregulation of the coagulation response.[44,45]

17.5.2.3 Extrinsic Pathway

The extrinsic pathway is driven by the generation of tissue factor (TF), also called thromboplastin.[1,17,46] This membrane protein is presented on the surface of cells after tissue damage, for instance, in the vessel wall. TF is not expressed by cells exposed to blood flow, but is present in cells of the subendothelium, the smooth muscle cells. Of course when a medical device is implanted into the patient, extensive tissue damage will occur and this pathway of coagulation will be triggered. For the wound healing response this is desirable, but for blood-contacting devices this response can be a complication.

TF will form a complex with FVII (TF.FVII), which can be activated to a TF.FVIIa complex by FIXa or by TF-FVIIa itself. Small amounts of activated FVIIa are constantly present in the circulation

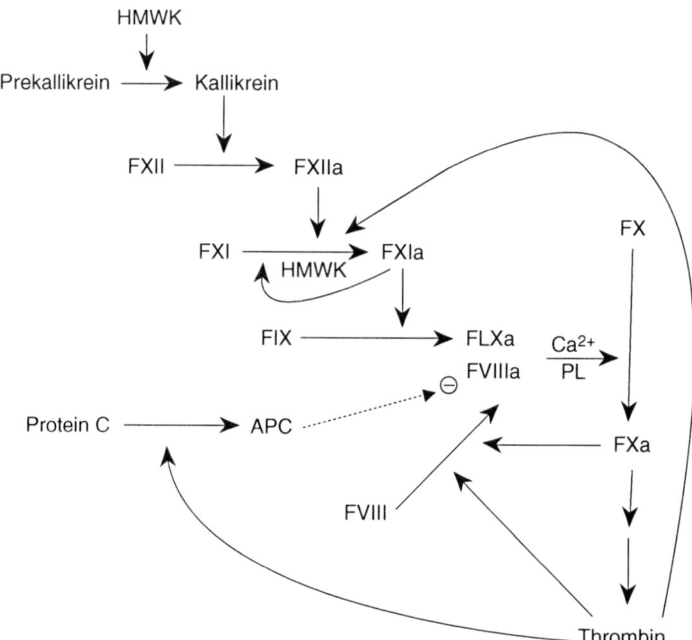

FIGURE 17.6 Intrinsic pathway of blood coagulation. HMWK, high-molecular-weight kininogen; F, factor; PC, protein C; APC, activated protein C.

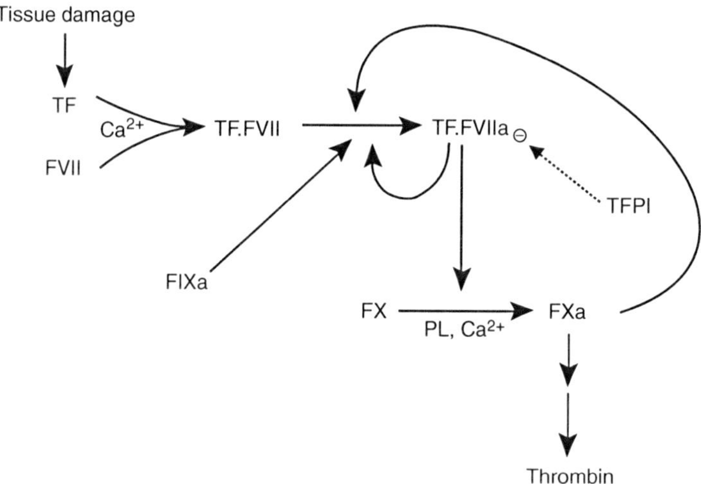

FIGURE 17.7 Extrinsic pathway of blood coagulation. TF, tissue factor; TFPI, tissue factor pathway inhibitor; PL, phospholipids.

and so the feedback upregulation is probably the most important mechanism of TF.FVII activation. The TF.FVIIa complex is also known as the extrinsic tenase complex. This means that the complex can activate FX to FXa. This will result eventually in the formation of thrombin and a blood clot, as described in the common pathway section (Figure 17.7). The TF.FVIIa complex is rapidly and efficiently inhibited by the tissue factor pathway inhibitor (TFPI).[47] Therefore, it is speculated that the extrinsic pathway is mainly involved in triggering of coagulation and that via feedback upregulation of the intrinsic pathway the burst of thrombin and thrombus formation are achieved.

17.5.3 Platelet Adhesion and Activation

Platelets are responsible for the formation of the initial plug in damaged vessels, subsequently cata-lyzing thrombus formation at that site.[5,17] Platelets normally flow along with the blood, until at a site of vessel damage the underlying extracellular matrix is exposed. Collagen and von Willebrand fac-tor (vWF) are exposed and the platelets contain receptors for these proteins on their surface. Revers-ible binding of vWF to the platelet membrane glycoprotein GP1b-V-IX or integrin-αIIbβ3 will slow down the platelets, causing them to roll over the damaged vessel wall. Now the platelets can bind to collagen via the collagen receptors GP-VI and integrin α2β1. GP-VI is the main receptor on platelets for collagen binding. Additionally, binding of collagen to integrin α2β1 has been demonstrated to result in activation of the platelets. The surface of activated platelets becomes enriched with nega-tive charge by the active translocation of phosphatidyl serine from the inner leaflet of the membrane to the outer leaflet, resulting in an increased negative charge on the outer surface.[5,48] This negatively charged surface is an excellent substratum for the propagation of the coagulation response. The for-mation and activity of the protein complexes that form FXa and thrombin are highly dependent on this negatively charged lipid surface for efficient activity. Furthermore, upon activation of platelets, these will excrete several chemical signals (adenosine diphosphate (ADP), thromboxane A2) that will induce further platelet adhesion (platelet aggregation) and activation. Activated integrin αIIbβ3 can bind to fibrinogen and act as a link between platelets, resulting in aggregation.[17,49]

Apart from binding to the subendothelial layers upon vessel damage, platelets also bind to synthetic surfaces. The binding and subsequent activation of platelets is accompanied by a marked change in morphology that can be easily monitored by electron microscopy (Figure 17.8).[50] The platelets have a round morphology directly after binding the surface. Then they form spike like extrusion from the main cell body, resulting in a dendritic cell shape. The platelets will start

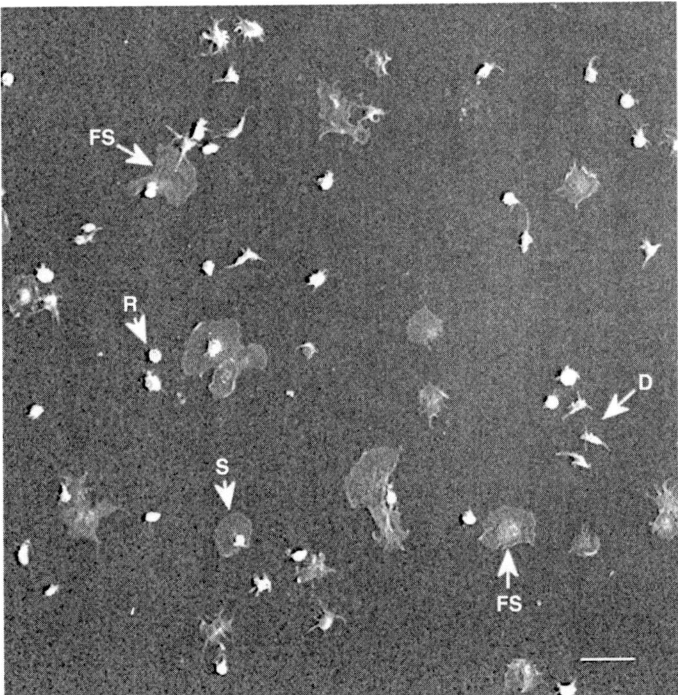

FIGURE 17.8   Adhered and activated platelets on a polyurethane sheet. Different stages of platelet activation can be observed. Round, freshly adhered (R), dendritic (D), spreading (S), and fully spread (FS). The scale bar represents 10 μm.

spreading, occupying more surface area until the fully spread morphology is reached, which is associated with full activation of the platelets. It has been shown that activated blood platelets shed small vesicular structures called microvesicles.[51–53] The microvesicles are highly thrombogenic and they have been proposed to play a role in coagulation and atherosclerosis, although some investigators doubt that these microvesicles actually occur *in vivo*. These investigators claim that the formation of microvesicles only occurs upon contact with foreign, synthetic surfaces. Fact is that in blood and blood products used for transfusion purposes these microvesicles are present.

Additionally, thrombin can activate platelets, increasing the amount of available negatively charged surface, resulting in rapid clot formation and clot propagation. This means that a combination of platelet adhesion and activation, and thrombin generation will induce blood clot formation on blood-contacting devices. In summary, platelets have an important role in coagulation and extensive adhesion and activation of platelets on synthetic surfaces should be avoided.

17.5.4 COMPLEMENT SYSTEM

The complement system is the first line of defense against pathogens invading in the blood.[4,17,54] It consists of a family of proteins that function or as proteases or as binding proteins. These proteins are also organized in a cascade (Figure 17.9) similar to the coagulation system (Figure 17.6). There are two pathways of complement activation. The classical pathway is mainly activated by antigen–antibody complexes. This will lead to the activation of the C1q,r,s complex that can proteolytically cleave C4 and C2. This results in the formation of the C3 convertase, C4b2a. The alternative pathway is triggered by the presence of foreign surfaces like bacteria or fungi or biomaterials. This pathway also results in a C3 convertase, namely C3bBb. In fact this pathway is always activated in

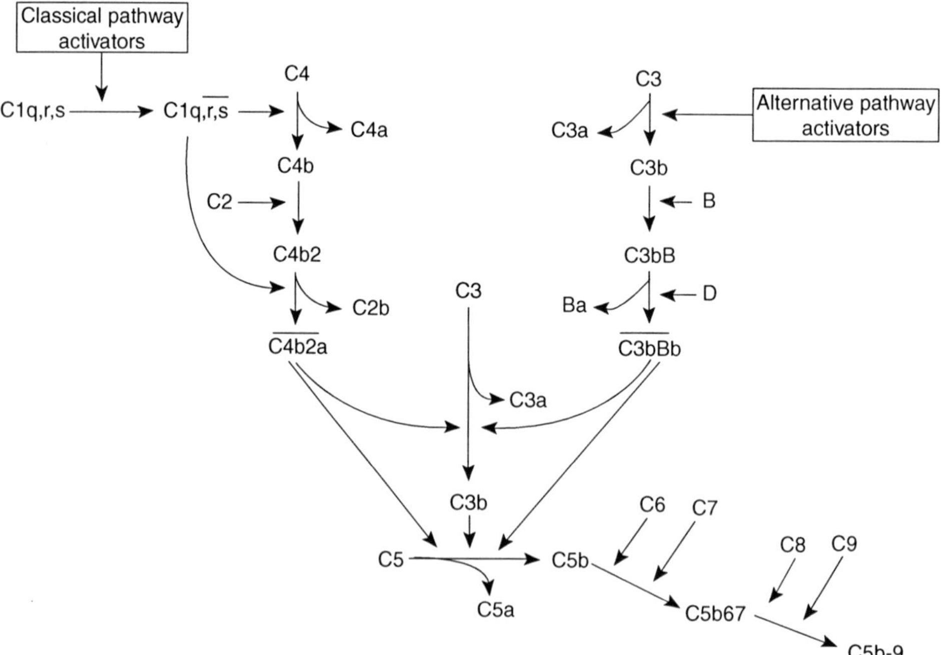

FIGURE 17.9 Complement system activation. The classical pathway is activated by antigen–antibody complexes, while the alternative pathway is being activated by the presence of cell walls of fungi or bacteria. Both pathways generate C3 convertase complexes (C4b2a and C3bBb), which results in cleavage of C3 into C3a and C3b. C3b can act as an opsonin or can induce the formation of the membrane attack complex (C5b-9), which can lyse cells or unicellular pathogens.

minute amounts, but upon the appearance of favorable conditions it triggers a full response. The C3 convertase complexes will cleave C3 in C3a and C3b. Especially C3b is an important component since it can act as an opsonin, making the surface it sticks to very attractive for the cellular components of the immune system (lymphocytes and leukocytes). It can also process C5 to C5b upon which sequential association with C6, C7, C8, and C9 will form the terminal complement complex (TCC). This complex is also known as the membrane attack complex since it can disturb membranes of cells and bacteria, resulting in cell lysis. In case of medical implants, the opsonization effect of C3b is especially worrying, since this may lead to a severe immune response in the blood that may result in failure of the device. Also some of the complement proteases have been implicated in activation of blood coagulation by activating some of the coagulation zymogens.[4,17]

17.5.5 LEUKOCYTES

Leukocytes directly interact with synthetic surfaces in the blood.[2,55] This interaction may be guided by proteins of the complement system (e.g., C3b). The normal function of leukocytes is to attack foreign bodies and if possible present (peptide-) parts on their surface (antigen-presenting cells). These so-called antigen-presenting cells will induce the production of antibodies by the B-cells. Monocytes will attempt to remove pathogens or foreign bodies from the circulation by simply ingesting them by phagocytosis. The neutrophiles will attack by producing peroxides and oxygen radicals, attacking the surface. The interaction of leukocytes with implanted materials will result in an inflammatory response.[55] This can be dangerous in case of a severe response (high fever, organ failure, and coma). Most materials however will elicit merely a moderate to mild inflammatory response that is however chronic. In solid tissues the inflammation results in the encapsulation of the implant into a fibrous capsule to minimize the interaction of the implant with the body. In fact the tissue is protected from further interaction by encapsulation. In the blood this response is of course not possible, but upon interaction of the surface with monocytes, TF will be presented on the membrane of these cells.[56,57] This TF will give rise to local coagulation and lead to the formation of a thrombus on the surface. Consequently, the function of the implant will be compromised, and in the worst case, distant embolization may occur when parts of the surface clot release. This can seriously compromise the health of the patient. The presence of a clot on the blood-contacting device almost always results in stenosis of a blood vessel and will therefore often lead to removal of the device from the patient.

17.6 SURFACES OF BLOOD-CONTACTING DEVICES

There is a large range of devices that are intended for direct contact with blood. In principle almost all implanted devices will contact blood, except the ones that are implanted into solid tissues, and the formation of a thrombus on the surface can be advantageous, since coagulation is a part of the wound healing and tissue regeneration response.

Biomedical devices that function in contact with blood are for instance, arterial stents, synthetic vessels, heart valves, catheters, guide-wires for percutaneous transluminal coronary angioplasty (PTCA), blood bags, hemodialysis filters, tubes of heart–lung machine, vena cava filters, etc. Since the effects of these implants can be systemic, the most vigorous testing of these devices is required. Toxic molecules as well as inflammatory molecules are easily spread throughout the whole body. Of course the biomedical industry has come up with a variety of strategies to minimize toxicity, inflammatory response, and biomaterial-induced coagulation to prevent premature failure of the device. There are roughly four major strategies that have been pursued over the last decades: (i) produce the blood-contacting device from inert materials or polymers; (ii) coat the implant with a polymer that contains favorable blood compatibility characteristics; (iii) generate a single endothelial cell layer on the blood contacting surface of an implant; and (iv) make the implant from living tissue *in vitro*, so called tissue engineering.

17.6.1 BIOINERT MATERIALS IN BLOOD-CONTACTING DEVICES

For a long period of time, the most accepted strategy to produce a successful blood-contacting device was to make use of materials to which no proteins would adsorb or no cells would interact with. This bioinert principle was based on the idea that when blood would not interact at all with the material, no adverse response could take place and therefore no complications of the device would occur.[58,59] It soon turned out that the favorite materials of the industry like poly(tetrafluoroethylene) (PTFE; Teflon) or poly(ethyleneterephthalate) (PET) were not as inert as they were thought to be (Figure 17.10). The manufacturers advertising for Teflon-coated frying pans claim that no substance would stick to it. This may be true at high temperatures, but when applied in a patient, proteins and cells will readily interact with Teflon surfaces. This does not mean that no successful implants consisting of PTFE or PET have been produced. Best known among them are the large diameter blood vessels (>5 mm inner diameter) made of PET or PTFE.[60,61] Especially prostheses that are intended to replace the aorta upon rupture, or in case of severe aortic aneurysms, have been very successful, saving many lives. Also the carotid or femoral arteries are frequently replaced by PTFE prosthesis.[62] The success rates depend on the health of the patient and the flow regime of the intended site of implantation. The higher the blood flows, the more chance of success since possible activators of coagulation are rapidly diluted under high blood flow.

Intravenous catheters are often made of polyvinylchloride (PVC) (Figure 17.10) and are vital for the application of drugs, fluids or nutrients to patients. The vast majority of these catheters remain in the vessel for only a couple of days, but some are inserted for several months into the large veins in the chest. The most common problems of these catheters are infection and coagulation. Therefore, these tubes are frequently flushed with the anticoagulant heparin. Infection can be treated with antibiotics, but in some severe cases the catheter has to be removed. So one can see that it is a challenge to design materials, which prevent coagulation and, at the same time, adhesion of bacteria. It has been shown that though inert materials perform reasonably well, eventually proteins and bacteria will adsorb and cause failure of the device.

Also polyurethanes are used or studied for blood-contact devices.[63] The advantage is that polyurethanes are a very versatile group of polymers. These materials are so-called block copolymers that contain soft and hard blocks. The easy chemical synthesis facilitates the design of materials with a variety of surface characteristics and mechanical properties. The disadvantage is that some of polyurethanes are degraded inside the body and that the degradation products often cause a severe inflammatory response.[64] The use of polyurethanes in blood contact devices is still under investigation and some positive studies have been reported for vascular prostheses.[63]

A new area of interest is the application of nanostructured surfaces of these materials. It has been shown that submicromolar or nanostructures can modulate the adhesion and viability of cells and bacteria. It remains to be determined how these surface topographies can be applied to manipulate the interaction of blood and cells with synthetic surfaces.

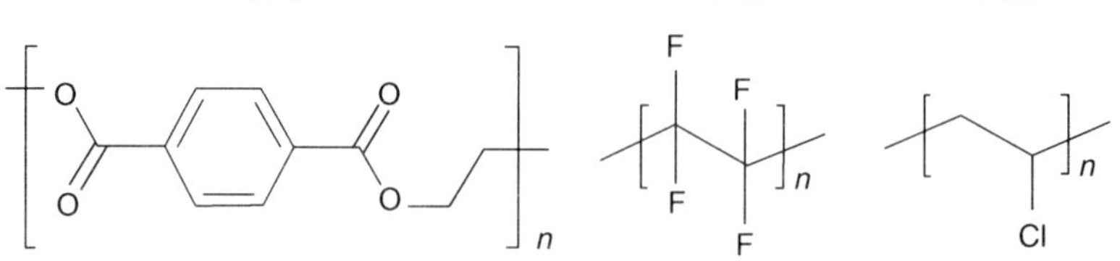

FIGURE 17.10   Structure of poly(ethyleneterephthalate) (PET), Teflon or poly(tetrafluoroethylene) (PTFE), and polyvinylchloride (PVC).

17.6.2 POLYMERIC COATINGS

For a number of implants, like for instance heart valves, the mechanical characteristics of the device direct the choice of material. It is not always possible to choose a material that combines both necessary mechanical characteristics and blood compatibility of the surface. Then often a polymeric coating is applied to the device. These coatings have several advantages since they can guide the surface characteristics of the device as well as act as a drug depot from which controlled, local release can take place.[65] In case of blood-contacting devices, a number of coatings have been designed. There are several groups of different coatings that aim to inhibit biomaterial-induced thrombus formation in a specific manner.

i. Coatings that present polymeric poly(ethylene oxide) (PEO) or poly(ethylene glycol) (PEG) on their surface have been extensively studied in the last years.[66–70] Actually, PEO and PEG are the same molecule as seen in Figure 17.11 and for the remainder of this chapter will be called PEG. These coatings aim to reduce the adhesion of proteins and cells. The chains of the hydrophilic PEG immobilize water molecules close to the surface, and this high water content is an unfavorable condition for the adhesion of plasma proteins, platelets, and cells like leukocytes. Therefore these PEG coatings are often referred to as protein-repellent surfaces.

These coatings have been applied on a wide variety of materials, but there are some drawbacks of PEG coatings. First of all, they are relatively difficult and thus expensive to produce on a large scale. It is not very difficult to attach PEG molecules to a surface on laboratory scale (square centimeters) but it is however quite a challenge to produce these coatings on a square meter scale, especially with a constant and high quality. Moreover these coatings are only useful when they can be handled without chance of damaging the coating. Even the smallest imperfection of the surface may open a possibility for proteins to adsorb and coagulation or inflammation to start. Although it is feasible to prepare perfect surfaces in the laboratory, industrial scale production of such surfaces is not trivial. Additionally, some recent *in vivo* studies have produced disappointing results of these coatings, with the gain in blood compatibility being modest at best.[71,72]

ii. Hydrogels and hydrophilic polymers are also being used to coat blood-contacting devices. The advantage of these coatings is that their relatively high hydrophilicity, and subsequently high water content, has been shown to decrease platelet adhesion and protein adsorption. These coatings can be used in combination with a large variety of materials but the solid attachment is not always straightforward. Since these hydrophilic coatings adsorb water, they have the tendency to expand and when not attached properly to the surface, they will detach from the device. The application of a base coating, which will anchor the main coating is often necessary. The fact is that the application of a hydrophilic coating on a medical device is not trivial and requires input from both chemists and engineers.[73]

The hydrophilic coatings can also be used as a drug depot since it is mostly straightforward in incorporating therapeutic drugs.[65,74,75] Upon contact with blood, the drug is slowly released, or in some cases exposed, at the surface. In this way drug release occurs at the site where it is most needed, namely at the surface of the device. Systemic application of drugs in the circulation has a disadvantage as limited

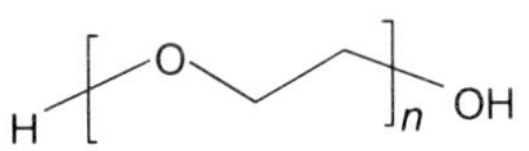

FIGURE 17.11 Chemical structure of poly(etheylene oxide), which is also known as poly(ethylene glycol).

diffusion to the wall of the vessels occurs, resulting in a low concentration of the drug close to the surface of the device. A well-known example of a coating that contains drugs is found on drug-eluting stents.[76,77] The bare metal is coated with a polymer from which paclitaxel or rapamycin are slowly released, inhibiting cell growth between the struts of the stent. In this way restenosis, or the reduction of the vessel lumen is avoided. Therefore the metal contributes to the mechanical properties of the device (expandibility and strength) while the coating influences the biological environment in such a way that restenosis is greatly reduced. The only downside of these drug-eluting stents is that they are more expensive, and are consequently often only used in more complicated situations. Therefore, some long-term clinical studies sometimes showed disappointing results.[78,79] But in straightforward stent placements, these drug-eluting stents could reduce restenosis from 15% to 20% to less than 2%. Also several coatings with heparin have been tested and are employed. This sulfated polysaccharide mimics heparan sulfate that normally appears on the endothelial surface.[75,80–84] Heparin can catalytically inhibit both factor X and thrombin (Figure 17.5), thus reducing the thrombin generation and thrombus formation near the coating surface. Because the heparin functions as a catalyst, it remains active for an extended period. This drug is also robust and can survive common sterilization protocols, like ethylene oxide gas, UV illumination, or gamma irradiation. There have been several additional attempts to cover the surface of blood-contacting devices with other drugs that influence coagulation of platelet adhesion and activation. Most of these coatings do show a significant effect on coagulation, but they are sensitive and will not be stable under sterilization conditions. Also the economics of some of these coatings is unfavorable, thus too expensive to use routinely.

    iii. Biomimetic and bioactive coatings are coatings that try to mimic the chemistry and topography of the endothelial layer that lines the vessels. In healthy individuals the endothelial cells that line the blood vessels, retain blood hemostasis.[85] This means that these cells counteract disturbances in the balance between coagulation and anticoagulation. To mimic this endothelial layer one can attempt to obtain a function endothelial cell layer on the implants. This will be discussed in the next session. Also attempts have been made to chemically synthesize a biomimetic coating, a coating that resembles the outside of endothelial cells. One example is the attachment of PLs to surfaces. This will result in a mono- or bilayer of PLs mimicking the cellular membrane. Also polymers containing the monomer 2-methacryloyloxyethyl phosphorylcholine (MPC), shown in Figure 17.12, are examples of biomimetic surfaces.[86,87]

MPC contains a side group that is identical to the head group of one of the major PLs of the cell membrane, phosphatidyl choline (PC). At present stents coated with polymers containing MPC are available. *In vitro* experiments showed reduced protein adsorption and platelet adhesion, resulting in improved blood compatibility.[86,87] These findings were confirmed in animal experiments, but long-term studies of the performance of MPC coatings in humans are not available at present. In this case the attempt is to mimic the cellular membrane, but the membranes that contact the circulating blood in humans have a much more complex structure containing many active proteins. Several attempts have been made to include some of these proteins in or couple these on polymeric coatings of blood-contacting devices. For instance, thrombomodulin, which plays an important role in thrombin inactivation, has been coupled with surfaces. *In vitro* experiments demonstrate decreased thrombus formation on such surfaces.[88] Attachment of tissue factor pathway inhibitor (TFPI) onto Dacron vascular grafts could counteract the excessive growth of cells, often the cause of stenosis of the graft.[89,90] Also urokinase, a stimulator of the fibrinolysis, the degradation of clots, was coupled with membranes, but only some *in vitro* experiments were performed, without much success.[91] Of course also other active components can be attached to surfaces, but there are certain major problems with these bioactive coatings. Firstly, they are laborious and expensive to produce, especially in large quantities, and the reproducibility is difficult to achieve. Secondly, the sterilization of such coatings is virtually impossible. Therefore the active component has to be included after sterilization, which

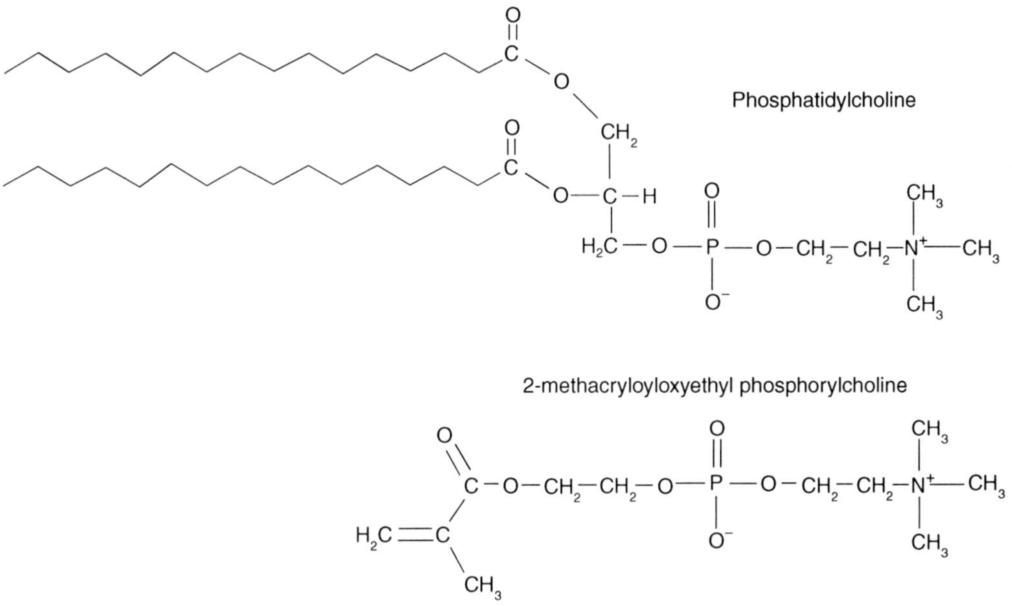

Phosphatidylcholine

2-methacryloyloxyethyl phosphorylcholine

FIGURE 17.12 Structure of di-palmitoyl phosphatidylcholine (PC) and 2-methacryloyloxyethyl phosphorylcholine (MPC).

means that there remains a risk of infection. Finally, these coatings are sensitive to storage conditions, which make them not very practical or economical.

17.6.3 LIVING CELL LAYER AS BOUNDARY LAYER

The most optimal contact layer for a blood-contacting device would be a functional layer of endothelial cells.[85] The endothelium is the inner layer of the blood vessels (Figure 17.3). The technique from which scientists attempt to produce a fully biological device or tissue is called tissue engineering and will be discussed later (Section 17.6.4). The control of hemostasis is one of the important functions of the endothelium. The endothelium secretes a number of molecules that play important roles in the regulation of coagulation, fibrinolysis, and inflammation. Heparan sulfate is exposed on the surface of endothelial cells and can catalyze the inhibition of thrombin and FXa by AT, a function that is mimicked by the anticoagulant drug heparin (Figure 17.5). Also activators of plasmin are secreted and these result in the degradation of formed thrombi. Formation of IL-10 and NO can reduce the inflammatory response and counteract the function of proinflammatory cytokines. As a result, the formation of an endothelial cell layer on blood-contacting devices has been a favorite subject of many biomedical engineers. Formation of an active and self-regenerating endothelial layer has been used to improve the performance of especially synthetic blood vessels.[92] One strategy attempts to make the endothelial cell layer form spontaneously after implantation of the device. The surface of the device is modified in such a way that it is an attractive substrate for endothelial cells.[28,93] Often extracellular matrix proteins like collagens, elastins, and fibronectin are used. Unfortunately, the proteins are not exclusively favorable for endothelial cells, but also accommodate other cell types like leukocytes and platelets, resulting in coagulation on such surfaces. In animal models, ingrowth of endothelial cells from the original vessel walls has been demonstrated to occur under optimal conditions. In human patients, however, the endothelial cells of the vessel walls demonstrate poor proliferation, indicating that no endothelialization occurs from the existing vessel walls.[94–97]

Endothelial progenitor cells (EPC) are not fully differentiated cells that are predestined to form endothelial cells. These cells are generated in the bone marrow and released in the circulation and are proposed to play a role in the repair of vessel walls.[98,99] The signals that trigger the release of these EPCs are being discovered (stromal cell-derived factor-1, SDF1), and this opens a new possibility to obtain an increased number of EPCs on the surface of the device, forming an endothelial layer. Devices that depend on spontaneous endothelialization are often referred to as off-the-shelf-implants. This means they can be employed instantaneously, are relatively cheap, and no specialized infrastructure is required for its use.

Another strategy involves the isolation of endothelial cells from a vessel biopsy conducted on the patient. The endothelial cells are isolated and multiplied in the laboratory. These cells are then seeded on the surface of the device, and subsequently the device is implanted. In some cases the endothelial cells are allowed to adhere and proliferate on the surface for several days in the laboratory before implantation is performed. A major disadvantage of such a strategy is that two operations are required, increasing the risk of infection and also increasing the total cost of the procedure. Though this endothelial cell-seeded vascular grafts performed well in animal models, the results in humans were disappointing.[100,101] One of the reasons for this difference in performance might be that in animal models, mostly young, healthy animals are used. In the clinic, the situation is very much different. The patients, who have to be treated, are frequently not in good condition. This means that harvesting of healthy endothelial cells from these patients is not easy, and in general yields are low. Additionally, these patients often have other diseases like diabetes that can dramatically influence the success rate of these synthetic vascular grafts. The step from the animal models toward the treatment of human patients has been a very difficult one and the simple strategy of seeding autologous endothelial cells has proven to be complicated and often unsuccessful. Because of the shortcomings of these cell-seeding experiments some scientists have reverted to tissue engineering, with which they attempt to construct fully biological and functional tissues *in vitro*. No doubt, in the future tissue engineering will produce functional tissues that can replace blood-contacting tissues, but at this moment success in this field seems distant.

17.6.4 Tissue Engineering

Since the purpose of this chapter is not to fully clarify tissue engineering, this topic will not be discussed in too much detail. However, there are many biomedical engineers trying to produce alternatives for blood-contacting devices using tissue engineering.

The *in vitro* production of functional tissues is a relatively new field within the science of biomedical engineering, called tissue engineering. The basic idea is that on a synthetic, porous scaffold cells are seeded and allowed to grow and differentiate, forming new functional tissue. These tissue-engineered products are then implanted into the patient, restoring the defect or replacing diseased tissues. The scaffold used is often biodegradable, so that no synthetic surfaces are left in the end. There are several tissue-engineered products that are pursued, which could act as an alternative for blood-contacting devices. Vascular prostheses, heart valves, pieces of heart muscle are all subjects of intense investigation. Almost a decade ago, the group of L'Heureux and coworkers has already succeeded in producing a complete tissue-engineered blood vessel.[102] Though the *in vivo* performance was not optimal, but the proof of principle was delivered. The biggest problem of all these tissue-engineering strategies is that the cells have to grow all the way through the scaffold, adopting the right differentiation at the right time. This has proven to be the hardest to achieve. The development of incubators that mimic the blood flow and conditions encountered by the native tissue (mechanic stress by beating heart, pulsatile shear stress by flowing blood) has greatly improved the survival of cells and formation of tissues.[103,104] The option to perform the incubation in the body has also been shown in mice, in case of vascular grafts.[105] But it does not seem very likely that such a strategy will be applied in large scale with patients very soon. Another problem is that the scaffold in which the cells are seeded has to be degraded at exactly the right time. Otherwise the consequences can be disastrous. Imagine the scaffold of a tissue-engineered coronary artery degrading prematurely.

17.7 BLOOD COMPATIBILITY TESTING

The testing of blood compatibility of medical implants has been laid down in the ISO standard 10993-part 4.[106,107] This norm describes standards, methods, and evaluation procedures that have to be followed in order to get approval for the use of a blood-contacting device. In general, blood-contacting devices have to be fully blood compatible, which means that no adverse effect of the device on blood can occur. Also the blood should not have adverse effects on the function and stability of the device. Overall, one can imagine that the safety requirements for permanent implants in contact with blood is quite strict, since the blood circulation can potentially spread a response initiated by an implant over the entire body.

For a blood-compatible material or surface to be called blood compatible, a number of requirements need to be fulfilled:

a. thrombus formation on the surface should be minimized or eliminated;
b. platelet adhesion and activation should be minimized or eliminated;
c. leukocyte adhesion and activation should be minimized or eliminated;
d. complement activation should be minimized or eliminated;
e. hemolysis, the damage to blood cells, should be minimized or eliminated; and
f. endothelial layer (endothelialization) formation should be promoted (in case of permanent implants).

Furthermore, the materials from which the blood-contacting device has been constructed should also not cause general or systemic toxicity (chemicals slowly leaching from the device). The extent of response that is acceptable depends very much on the time of contact and the place of implantation (on the skin or inside tissues).

The description of blood compatibility testing in the ISO 10993-4 standard gives guidelines for systematic testing of blood compatibility.[106] A major problem is that a large number of different assays and standard materials are being used. This results in many variables in testing of blood-contacting devices, making comparison of test results complicated and unreliable.

Blood compatibility tests can be performed *in vitro*, *ex vivo*, or *in vivo*. *In vitro* testing means that the device is tested in contact with blood from preferentially human donors outside the body. *Ex vivo* testing makes use of shunting blood from an animal or human directly to the test chamber. The blood can then be collected for analysis (single pass), or can be directed back into the circulation of the animal. For *in vivo* testing a suitable animal model is chosen, and the device is implanted in a tissue, that is representative for the intended use in humans. The choice of the animal model can strongly influence the outcome of the *in vivo* experiments, and therefore animal model and the procedure have to be chosen with care. The most preferred animal model would be nonhuman primates like chimpanzees or baboons. The use of such animals is bound to strict regulation and is also very expensive. Therefore, the most used animal models for implantation of blood-contacting devices are goats, sheep, pigs, and dogs. Extrapolation from the animal model to the human situation is not straightforward and should be done with extreme caution.

For different devices, different sets of experiments are required. This is determined by the intended use of the device, therefore if it will only contact the blood outside the body (canules, blood bags, collection tubes) implantation studies are not required. For short-term blood contact (catheters, hemodialysis equipment, guidewires, intravascular devices) or when the blood stays in the patient after contact, of course some *in vivo* testing is required, although long-term implantation studies are only required for implanted devices (like heart valves and vascular prostheses). *In vitro* testing is always performed in order to avoid complete failure in the more laborious and expensive *in vivo* experiments. In the remaining portion of this chapter some of the test procedures will be discussed in more detail, focusing on the ones most used.

17.7.1 THROMBIN GENERATION AND THROMBUS FORMATION

The activation of the coagulation cascade is one of the most common problems for blood-contacting devices. The adsorption of plasma proteins can lead, via the activation of the intrinsic pathway, to the generation of thrombin and subsequent thrombus formation. The formed blood clots can block blood vessels (thrombosis), and cause hypoxia and dysfunction of downstream tissues and organs. In the case of stents and synthetic blood vessels, this is the biggest concern. For other devices the release of small clot fragments (emboli) can result in distant embolization, leading to myocardial infarction, for instance.

Routinely coagulation disorders are determined *in vitro* measuring thrombin time (TT), activated partial thromboplastin time (APTT), or prothrombin time (PTT).[106,108–110] These assays depend on the fact that the formation of a blood clot is determined by the concentrations and activation state of the coagulation factors. In case of TT, the time in which a certain amount of thrombin results in a thrombus is determined. For the APTT the blood is challenged by an external stimulus that will activate the intrinsic pathway of the coagulation cascade. Finally, the PTT measures the clotting time upon addition of a combination of PL and TF so that the extrinsic pathway is triggered. The advantage of these methods is that they can be performed almost anywhere, they are very reproducible, and they are cheap. The disadvantage is that they are relatively insensitive and that they all depend on an external stimulus.[106,109,110] In fact, in the case of blood-contacting devices, one is not really interested in these parameters, but the biomaterial-induced thrombin generation is important. Also these clotting assays in general work with PPP.[110] The role of platelets, leukocytes, and even the erythrocytes is not taken into account, which is an oversimplification of the *in vivo* situation. Therefore, it is preferable to incubate the blood-contacting device with recalcified whole blood and measure the formation of thrombin and a clot.

The formation of blood clots is a very easy and effective way to estimate the performance of a blood-compatible surface (Figure 17.13). The device or material is incubated in whole blood, and the time it takes to form a clot on the surface is determined. This method is very effective in demonstrating the performance of good blood-compatible surfaces, since no clot will form on their surface when compared to a bad surface like bare steel, Teflon (PTFE), or glass.

The formation of a blood clot is preceded by the generation of thrombin, the central enzyme in coagulation (see Figure 17.4). For quantification, it is better to determine the time course of

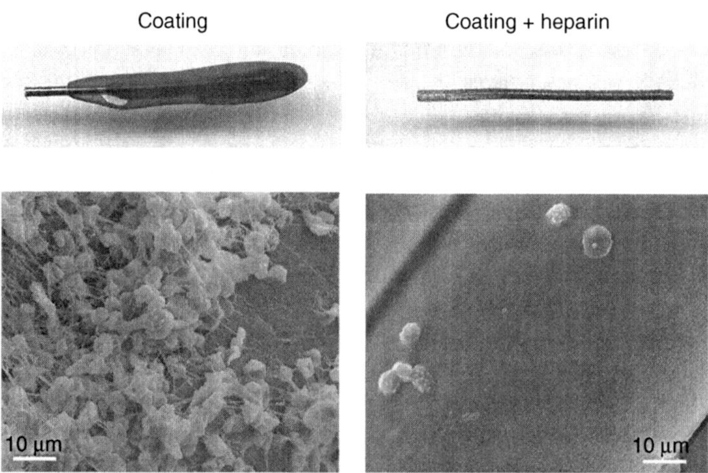

FIGURE 17.13 Clot formation on guidewires coated with a hydrophilic polymer. The inclusion of heparin in the coating inhibits blood clot formation. In the scanning electron micrographs, one can distinguish erythrocytes and fibrin. On the heparin containing coating, no thrombus was formed.

thrombin generation as well as the total amount of thrombin formation. Thrombin generation can be determined in several ways. The easiest way is to determine thrombin generation under static conditions. For this, preferably full blood is incubated with the blood-contacting surface and the concentration of thrombin is determined in samples taken over the period of the experiment.[74] The only problem is that when a clot has formed, the experiment has to be stopped since no homogenous samples can be drawn anymore. Since most thrombin generation occurs inside the clot, after clot formation, the time for thrombin generation is the only parameter that can be determined using this assay.[109,111] However, not only the lag time in thrombin generation is a parameter for blood compatibility, but also the so-called thrombin potential is important, which is an indicator for the total amount of thrombin formed.[109,112,113] This thrombin potential can be determined in PRP using a fluorescently labeled thrombin substrate. The blood-contacting material is incubated with PRP and fluorescent substrate, and fluorescence is constantly monitored. When the fluorescence is plotted against time, the slope of the curve is a direct measure for the concentration of active thrombin (Figure 17.14). This assay has recently been optimized and can now be seen as the golden standard to study hemostatic function of the blood. Since the method is very sensitive to a variety of parameters, it may be well suited to determine biomaterial-induced thrombin generation.

Dynamic incubations with blood mimic the *in vivo* situation better, although the choice of the flow rate, and consequently shear rates, are of critical importance. There are several methods for dynamic blood contact *in vitro*.[74] The first is to pump recalcified blood along the material or through a tube on which the surface coating of the device is deposited (Figure 17.15).

This blood can be analyzed for a number of coagulation parameters at the end of the conduit. The concentration of thrombin, thrombin–AT (TAT) complexes, fibrinogen degradation products, activation of the complement system, the consumption of platelets as a measure of platelet adhesion, can all be determined in the collected blood samples.[106] A second, regularly used, set-up is the closed-loop model, in which the inside of a tube is representative for the synthetic surface of an implant.[114] The blood can be left in the tube for any desired period of time, and samples can be taken at desired intervals although sampling means the system has to be stopped and opened, which is not an ideal condition in practice. Both these methods use only parts of the blood-contacting device and often also in another configuration, implying that these devices are not as used in the final device.

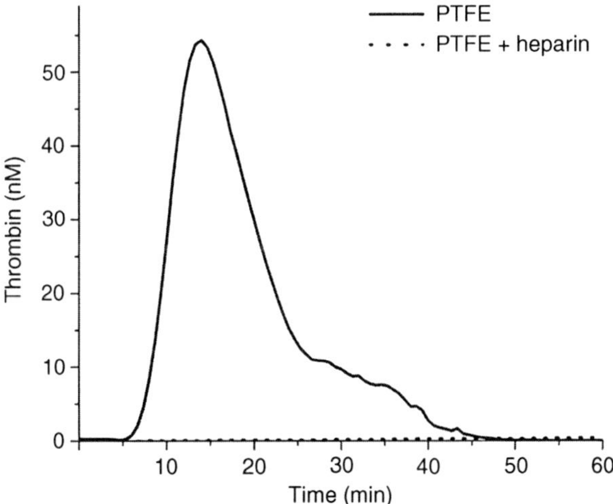

FIGURE 17.14 Thrombin generation using fluorescent substrate. The fluorescence over time is measured and the differential is plotted. The area under the curve represents the thrombin potential.

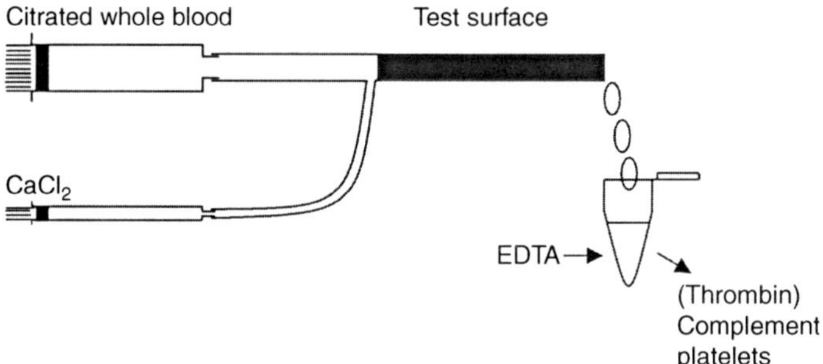

FIGURE 17.15 *In vitro* setup for dynamic testing of blood compatibility on a synthetic test surface. Anticoagulated blood (citrated) is recalcified and pumped over the test surface. Blood samples are analyzed for the desired parameters.

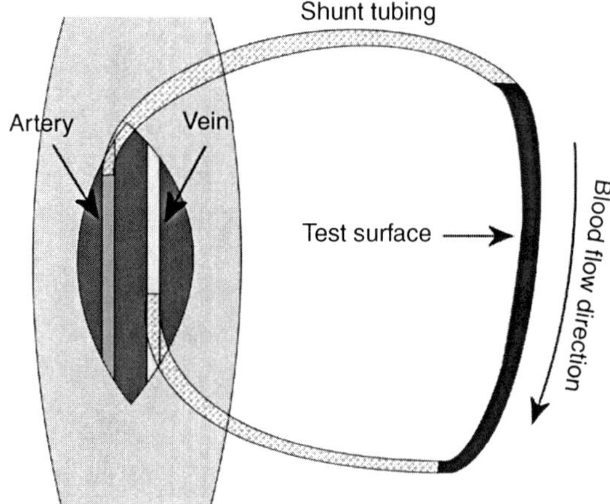

FIGURE 17.16 *Ex vivo* shunt model for blood compatibility testing.

Another way to test blood compatibility is to use an *ex-vivo* shunt model (Figure 17.16). This means that a bypass is connected to a major artery and vein of a test animal or a human volunteer, and the blood is guided over the test surface (which is at the inside of the tube).

In this way relevant flow regimes as well as possible variations in the blood are studied, for instance, as a result of medication. This sort of experiment is always prone to some form of risk, especially for embolization or severe clotting. Also the activation of the complement system can provoke unwanted reactions downstream the conduit in the body.

17.7.2 Platelet Adhesion and Activation

Platelets play a vital role in coagulation and therefore their interaction with blood-contacting devices is a valuable tool to study blood compatibility.[5,106] Upon adhesion of platelets, these become activated and subsequently a procoagulant surface is created. This means that the outer surface of the platelets will catalyze the generation of thrombin and thus result in thrombus formation on the device.[48] There are several ways to determine the interaction of platelets with synthetic surfaces.

17.7.2.1 Determination of Platelet Adhesion

Adhered platelets can be fixed on the surface of the device and subsequently studied by microscopy. Phase contrast microscopy can be used to count the amount of adhered platelets per area, but the determination of the morphology is rather difficult since the resolution of phase contrast microscopes is in general too low for determination of platelet morphology. Therefore either fluorescence microscopy or scanning electron microscopy is preferred. For fluorescence microscopy, the platelets are labeled with a fluorescent dye, which can be a nonspecific viability dye (like Calcein-AM or Cell Trace dyes). An easy method was discovered by accident.[115] When platelets are fixed with glutaraldehyde, they become fluorescent, and can be observed by fluorescence microscopy and counted. The most used method to observe adhered platelets is scanning electron microscopy. The platelets are fixed, and prepared for microscopy by dehydration and sputter coating with gold. It is a straightforward method for counting platelets per surface area. Additionally, different morphologies that occur upon activation of the adhered platelets can be analyzed through this method (Figure 17.8).[50] A disadvantage of such microscopy techniques is that they are relatively time-consuming, very laborious, and thus expensive. An alternative approach is to determine platelet adhesion by measuring of metabolic parameter like the enzyme lactate dehydrogenase (LDH).[115] The amount of LDH is a direct measure of the amount of adhered platelets.

17.7.2.2 Platelet Activation

An important parameter upon which the incubation of synthetic surfaces with platelets can be determined is platelet activation.[5,6,17] Adhered platelets that do not get activated will not contribute to coagulation. There are three ways to determine platelet activation: (i) platelet morphology, (ii) membrane markers, and (iii) secretion products (Figure 17.17).

Platelet morphology rapidly changes after initial adhesion and subsequent activation of platelets on synthetic surfaces.[50] The platelets are a round-shaped just after adhesion and before activation. Then pseudopods are extended from the central cell body after which the cells flatten and spread on the surface until the cell appears completely flat (like a pancake), covering a large surface. Upon activation, a number of specific markers get exposed on the outer surface of the platelet. One of these markers is P-selectin (also CD62p), a glycoprotein that has an important function in interaction with leukocytes. P-selectin can be demonstrated using specific antibodies coupled with fluorescent labels. Fluorescence microscopy or fluorescent-assisted cell sorting (FACS) analysis can be used to determine the amount of exposed P-selectin. Another frequently used marker is the PAC-1 antibody that binds to the activated integrin $\alpha_{IIb}\beta_3$. This integrin immobilizes fibrinogen on the surface of activated platelets. Use of a fluorescently labeled specific antibody enables the determination of activation.

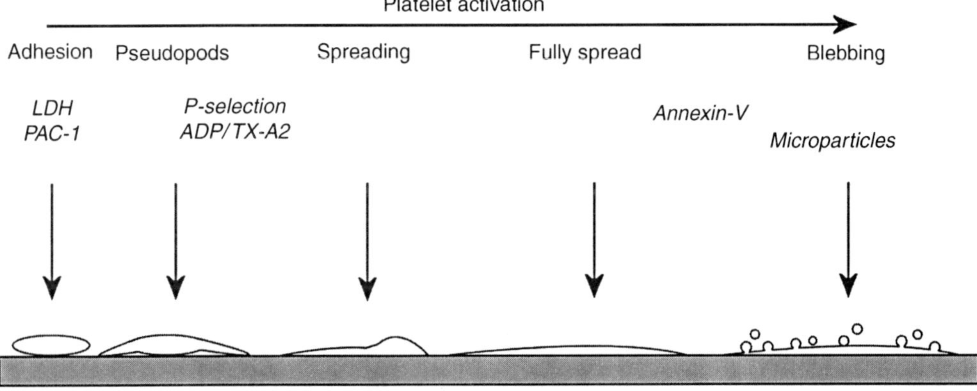

FIGURE 17.17 Schematic representation of platelet adhesion and activation on a synthetic surface. The markers that can be determined at different stages of platelet activation are given in italics. LDH, lactate dehydrogenase; PAC-1, antibody specific for activated integrin $\alpha_{IIb}\beta_3$; ADP, adenosine diphosphate; TX–A2, thromboxane-A2.

Upon platelet activation, the lipid composition of the platelet membrane is reshuffled in order to obtain a negatively charged surface on the outer membrane. To obtain this, negatively charged phosphatidyl serine (PSer) is actively transported from the inner leaflet of the plasma membrane to the outer leaflet, while uncharged PL (like phosphatidyl choline or PC) are transported in the opposite direction.[48] The negatively charged surface will catalyze the generation of thrombin and consequently the formation of thrombus. The protein annexin-A5 can specifically bind to PSer. Linking this protein to a fluorescent marker opens the possibility to determine platelet activation either by FACS analysis or by fluorescence microscopy.[116]

17.7.2.3 Secretion by Activated Platelets

Several molecules are secreted by activated platelets in order to obtain a full platelet response.[5,117,118] ADP, β-thromboglobulin, and thromboxane-A2 are major secretion products from activated platelets. These molecules can be determined by enzyme-linked immunosorbent assay (ELISA) or chromatography methods. However, the determination of these molecules is time-consuming and expensive. During activation the platelets shed microparticles, small vesicles originating from the platelet membrane.[51–53] These microparticles are efficient in catalyzing thrombin generation. Since these microparticles are much smaller than platelets, they can be determined by FACS analysis using backscattering of photons as a signal, and the number of these microparticles can be used as an indicator for platelet activation. The drawback of this method is that microparticles are easily formed, especially during collection of blood and preparation of PRP. The background level of microparticles can also be high, and thus sensitivity varies between assays.

17.7.3 Leukocyte Adhesion and Activation

The adhesion of leukocytes to blood-contacting devices has consequences for both the inflammatory response as well as coagulation on the surface of the devices.[17,18] The adhesion of neutrophils and monocytes to a synthetic surface will result in their activation. The natural response of these cells to foreign bodies can be exploited to study the interaction between leukocytes and implants. The adhesion of leukocytes can be determined in a variety of ways. First of all, phase contrast microscopy, fluorescence microscopy, and scanning electron microscopy can be used to visualize leukocytes adhered to synthetic surfaces. The adhesion is largely dependent on surface characteristics, as well as on the presence of platelets. So the incubation conditions are important for the outcome and interpretation of adhesion experiments. The best of course is to use whole blood, preferable in a dynamic setup. After incubation, cells adhered to the surface are fixed and prepared for microscopical examination. The number of adhered leukocytes and the morphology can be determined in this fashion. Also, viability assays can be applied to determine the amount of adhered leukocytes. These assays depend on the presence of certain metabolic enzymes that are present in every living cell. The MTT viability assay measures the level of a mitochondrial enzyme, succinate dehydrogenase, only present in live cells.[119] LDH is also frequently used to determine the number of live cells in a preparation.[116] The disadvantage of these viability assays is that platelets also carry these enzymes. Leukocytes are often associated with platelets, especially when adhered onto surfaces, so the viability assays have to be performed with caution using proper controls. The determination of DNA content in the cells adhered to a synthetic surface seems to be the best choice to quantify leukocyte adhesion.[120,121] Both platelets and erythrocytes do not posses a nucleus and consequently no significant amounts of DNA. There are a number of different DNA-binding dyes that can be used. Comparison to a standard curve allows for the exact quantification of the number of adhered cells.

The activation of leukocytes can be determined in whole blood using highly specific and sensitive ELISA protocols. The cytokines that are secreted by activated leukocytes, like IL-1b, IL-6, IL-8, and TNF-α, can be routinely determined in samples of blood.[2,17] Comparison with proper controls directly indicates the magnitude of the leukocyte response toward different materials. Isolated leukocytes can also be used in combination with synthetic surfaces. The morphology is an easy but subjective indicator for leukocyte activation. The production of cytokines is the best, most sensitive, and most precise indicator for leukocyte activation, which can be measured in whole blood samples.

17.7.4 COMPLEMENT ACTIVATION

Activation of the complement system is an important as well as a quick response of the blood upon contact with a biomedical implant (Figure 17.9).[2,17,18] All complement activation assays are based on the determination of one of the complement protein fragments. The complement system consists of a number of proteases and scaffold proteins. The appearance of cleaved fragments is a direct measure for the level of complement activation compared to a positive control lipopolysaccharides (LPS). One of these complement proteins is C3b that is at the convergence point between classical and alternative pathways. Another often determined component is the C5-9b, or also called the TCC or the membrane attack complex. This is the endpoint of the complement cascade. Both are determined using ELISA setups that are commercially available.

17.7.5 HEMOLYSIS

Hemolysis is defined as the lysis of blood cells. In order to determine blood compatibility, hemolysis is an important parameter that has to be determined.[106,122,123] Since over 99% of the blood's cells are erythrocytes, the increase of free hemoglobin in plasma is taken as a direct measure for hemolysis. Great care has to be taken in hemolysis measurements, since the basal level of free hemoglobin in blood preparations can vary significantly.

Hemolysis can be determined using a variety of different assays, but there is no generally accepted method. The different assays are based upon two major principles. A number of assays depend on direct optical measurement of hemoglobin. This means that the concentration of free hemoglobin in blood plasma is determined by spectrometry, making use of the unique adsorption spectrum of hemoglobin, with peaks at 415 nm, 541 nm, and 577 nm. The adsorption at these wavelengths can be used to directly determine the concentration of hemoglobin by quantifying the absorbance peak.

Several other hemoglobin assays are based on the use of chemical techniques and the addition of an agent that reacts with oxyhemoglobin. Especially benzidine chromogens are often used. The oxidation of benzidine derivates, like tetramethylbenzidine, by hydrogen peroxide is catalyzed by hemoglobin. The rate of the reaction is directly proportional to the concentration of hemoglobin. The drawback of these chemical methods is that they make use of highly toxic chemicals that are often expensive not only in purchase but also in disposal.

17.7.6 CELL COMPATIBILITY/ENDOTHELIALIZATION

For blood-contacting devices that have only limited exposure time to the blood, the interaction with cells is an unwanted phenomenon. However, for permanent implants that have to function for years inside the circulation, the formation of a functional endothelial cell layer on its surface will greatly improve the success rate of the device. For instance, for vascular prosthesis of heart valves, the endothelial cell layer on the surface is the best guarantee for long-term hemostasis. The endothelium will regulate coagulation and anticoagulation of the blood and the best part is that the layer can repair itself upon damage. Therefore many attempts have been made to seed endothelial cells on synthetic vascular grafts before implantation. Also the spontaneous endothelialization *in vivo* has been studied. The best and easiest methods are based on microscopy. The parts of the implant for scanning electron microscopy can be prepared in a straightforward way, but the pictures will only be seen if cells are present on the surface of the device (Figure 17.18). Fluorescence microscopy can be used to positively identify the cells as endothelial cells by making use of specific endothelial markers of which the CD31 or platelet-endothelial cell adhesion molecule-1 (PECAM-1) is most popular. There are more endothelial specific markers, which can be demonstrated using specific monoclonal antibodies. The cells can then be identified by microscopy or by FACS analysis after detaching them from the surface.

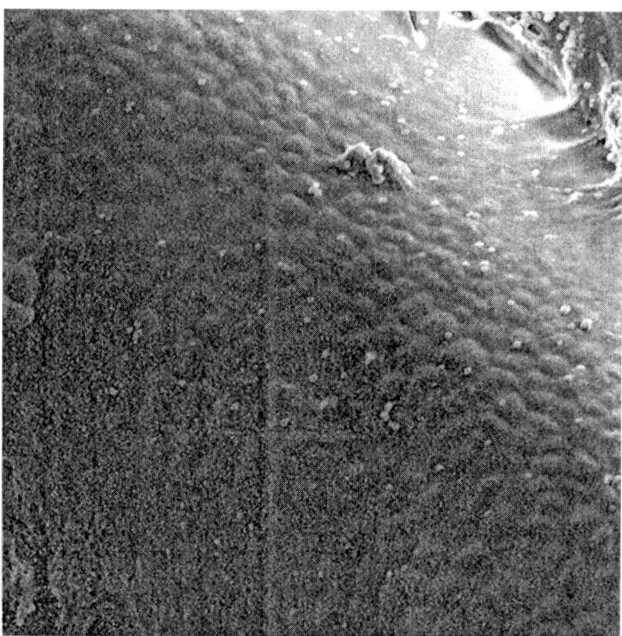

FIGURE 17.18 Luminal surface of a synthetic vascular graft lined with endothelial cells that formed spontaneously after 3-month implantation into the carotid artery of a goat.

17.8 CONCLUDING REMARKS

There are a wide variety of blood-contacting devices, ranging from blood bags to heart valves, from intravenous catheters to vascular prostheses. Although a number of these devices perform satisfactorily, some display poor blood compatibility, which means they provoke unacceptable responses upon contact with blood. The surfaces of such inadequate devices lead to coagulation, inflammation, hemolysis, or infection. For instance, devices that induce coagulation will only function properly when systemic anticoagulant therapy is applied simultaneously. This increases the risk of hemorrhage for the patient. Furthermore, the permanently implanted devices as well as the devices with large blood-contacting surfaces (hemodialysis filters, tubing of heart-lung machine and cardiac-assist devices) show significant activation of the immune system and consequently induce a moderate but chronic inflammatory response. The thrombogenicity of and inflammation on the surface compromise the function of blood-contacting devices, ultimately resulting in removal. In this chapter, several strategies have been discussed that aim to prevent coagulation and inflammation at synthetic surfaces. Currently most of these strategies are based on physicochemical manipulation of the surface. It is surprising that our increasing knowledge of blood and the immune response, together with an extensive understanding of polymer chemistry and its applications, has not culminated in the development of new materials that exhibit true blood compatibility. Of course, modifications of traditional materials like PTFE (Teflon), PET (Dacron), and polyurethanes have resulted in improved performance upon contact with blood, however, it is remarkable how few new biomaterials with excellent blood compatibility have been introduced over the last decades. Recently, increasing number of researchers use tissue engineering techniques to (i) construct surfaces with a functional self-regenerating endothelial cell layer or (ii) produce fully biological blood-contacting tissues in the laboratory. This is an exciting development that, without doubt, will lead in the formation of near perfect blood-contacting devices and tissues in future. Until then, the detailed study of blood-biomaterial interactions will require a multidisciplinary approach to solve the problems with current blood-contacting devices.

REFERENCES

1. Dee, K.C., Puleo, D.A., and Bizios, R., *Tissue Biomaterial Interaction*, 1st ed., John Wiley & Sons, Hoboken, NJ, 2002, chapter 4.
2. Bain, B.J., *Blood Cells: a Practical Guide*, 3rd ed., Blackwell, Oxford, U.K., 2002.
3. Alberts, B. et al., *Molecular Biology of the Cell*, 4th ed., John Wiley & Sons, New York, 2002.
4. Roitt, I., Brostoff, J., and Male, D., *Immunology*, 6th ed., Mosby, London, 2002.
5. Heemskerk, J.W.M., Bevers, E.M., and Lindhout, T., Platelet activation and blood coagulation, *Thromb. Haemost.*, 88, 186, 2002.
6. Bouchard, B.A. and Tracy, P.B., Platelets, leukocytes and coagulation, *Curr. Opin. Hematol.*, 8, 263, 2001.
7. Slack, S.M., Properties of biological fluids, in *Biomaterials Science*, Ratner, B.D. et al., Eds, Academic Press, San Diego, CA, 1996, 469.
8. Anderson, N.L. et al., The human plasma proteome, *Mol. Cell. Proteomics*, 3, 311, 2004.
9. Anderson, N.L. and Anderson, N.G., The human plasma proteome, *Mol. Cell. Proteomics*, 1, 845, 2002.
10. Guthrie, R.A. and Guthrie, D.W., Pathophysiology of diabetes mellitus, *Crit. Care Nurs.*, 27, 113, 2004.
11. Mush, B.E., Gagne, P., and Sheehan, P., Peripheral arterial disease: clinical assessment and indications for revascularization in the patient with diabetes, *Curr. Diab. Rep.*, 5, 25, 2005.
12. Ulbrecht, J.S., Cavanagh, P.R., and Caputo, G.M., Foot problems in diabetes: an overview, *Clin. Infect. Dis.*, 39, S73, 2004.
13. Huxley, R., Lewington, S., and Clarke, R., Cholesterol, coronary heart disease and stroke: a review of published evidence from observational studies and randomized controlled trials, *Semin. Vasc. Med.*, 2, 315, 2002.
14. McGovern, M.E., Taking aim at HDL-C. Raising levels to reduce cardiovascular risk, *Postgrad. Med.*, 117, 29, 2005.
15. Barter, P., HDL: a recipe for longevity, *Atherosclerosis Suppl.*, 5, 25, 2004.
16. Sefton, M.V., Gemmell, C.H., and Gorbet, M.B., What really is blood compatibility? *J. Biomater. Sci. Polymer Edn.*, 11, 1165, 2000.
17. Gorbet, M.B. and Sefton, M.V., Biomaterial-associated thrombosis: roles of coagulation factors, complement, platelets and leukocytes, *Biomaterials*, 25, 5681, 2004.
18. Anderson, J.M., Biological responses to materials, *Ann. Rev. Mater. Sci.*, 31, 81, 2001.
19. Vroman, L. and Adams, A.L., Identification of rapid changes at plasma-solid interfaces, *J. Biomed. Mater. Res.*, 3, 43, 1969.
20. Leonard, E.F. and Vroman, L., Is the Vroman effect of importance in the interaction of blood with artificial materials, *J. Biomater. Sci. Polymer Edn.*, 3, 95, 1991.
21. Krishnan, A., Siedlecki, C.A., and Vogler, E.A., Mixology of protein solutions and the Vroman effect, *Langmuir*, 20, 5071, 2004.
22. Gray, J.J., The interaction of proteins with solid surfaces, *Curr. Opin. Struct. Biol.*, 14, 110, 2004.
23. Malmsten, M., Formation of adsorbed protein layers, *J. Colloid Interface Sci.*, 207, 186, 1998.
24. Hlady, V. and Buijs, J., Protein adsorption on solid surfaces, *Curr. Opin. Biotech.*, 7, 72, 1996.
25. Nakanishi, K., Sakiyama, T., and Imamura, K., On the adsorption of proteins on solid surfaces, a common but very complicated phenomenon, *J. Biosci. Bioeng.*, 91, 233, 2001.
26. Knetsch, M.L.W., Aldenhoff, Y.B.J., and Koole, L.H., The effect of high-density-lipoprotein on thrombus formation on and endothelial cell attachment to biomaterial surfaces, *Biomaterials*, 27, 2813, 2006.
27. Allen, L.T. et al., Surface-induced changes in protein adsorption and implications for cellular phenotypic responses to surface interaction, *Biomaterials*, 27(16), 3096, 2006.
28. Wilson, C.J. et al., Mediation of biomaterial–cell interactions by adsorbed proteins: a review, *Tissue Eng.*, 11, 1, 2005.
29. Colman, R.W. et al., *Hemostasis and Thrombosis: Basic Principles and Clinical Practice*, 5th ed., Lippincott Williams & Wilkins, Philadelphia, PA, 2006.
30. Spronk, H.M.H., Govers-Riemslag, J.W.P., and ten Cate, H., The blood coagulation system as a molecular machine, *Bioessays*, 25, 1220, 2003.
31. Clemeston, K.J., Sticky fingers cement the relationship, *Curr. Biol.*, 9, R110, 1999.
32. Cesarman-Maus, G. and Hajjar, K.A., Molecular mechanisms of fibrinolysis, *Br. J. Haemotol.*, 129, 307, 2005.
33. Nesheim, M., Thrombin and fibrinolysis, *Chest*, 124, 33, 2003.

34. Zwaal, R.F.A., Comfurius, P., and Bevers, E.M., Lipid–protein interactions in blood coagulation, *Bioch. Biophys. Acta*, 1376, 433, 1998.
35. Dahlback, B., Blood coagulation, *Lancet*, 355, 1627, 2000.
36. Damus, P.S., Hicks, M., and Rosenberg, R.D., Anticoagulant action of heparin, *Nature*, 246, 355, 1973.
37. Petitou, M., Casu, B., and Lindahl, U., 1976–1983, a critical period in the history of heparin: the discovery of the antithrombin binding site, *Biochimie*, 85, 83, 2003.
38. Eldor, A., Orevi, M., and Rigbi, M., The role of the leech in medical therapeutics, *Haemostasis*, 10, 201, 1996.
39. Dahlback, B. and Villoutreix, B.O., The anticoagulant protein C pathway, *FEBS Lett.*, 579, 3310, 2005.
40. Dahlback, B. and Villoutreix, B.O., Regulation of blood coagulation by the protein C anticoagulant pathway: novel insights into structure–function relationships and molecular recognition, *Arterioscerl. Thromb. Vasc. Biol.*, 25, 1311, 2005.
41. Tans, G., Nicolaes, G.A., and Rosing, J., Regulation of thrombin formation by activated protein C: effect of the factor V Leiden mutation, *Semin. Hematol.*, 34, 244, 1997.
42. Rosing, J. et al., Low-dose oral contraceptives and acquired resistance to activated protein C: a randomized cross-over study, *Lancet*, 354, 2036, 1999.
43. Kaplan, A.P. and Silverberg, M., The coagulation-kinin pathway of human plasma, *Blood*, 70, 1, 1987.
44. Klinge J. et al., Hemophilia A: from basic science to clinical practice, *Semin. Thromb. Hemost.*, 28, 309, 2002.
45. Peyvandi, F. et al., Rare coagulation deficiencies, Haemophilia, 8, 308, 2002.
46. Steffel, J., Luscher, T.F., and Tanner, F.C., Tissue factor in cardiovascular diseases, *Circulation*, 113, 722, 2006.
47. Lwaleed, B.A. and Bass, P.S., Tissue factor pathway inhibitor: structure, biology and involvement in disease, *J. Pathol.*, 208, 327, 2006.
48. Zwaal, R.F.A., Comfurius, P., and Bevers, E.M., Surface exposure of phosphatidylserine in pathological cells, *Cell. Mol. Life Sci.*, 62, 971, 2005.
49. Rand, M.L., Leung, R., and Packham, M.A., Platelet function assays, *Transf. Apheresis Sci.*, 28, 307, 2003.
50. Ko, T., Lin, J., and Cooper, S.L., Surface characterization and platelet adhesion studies of plasma-sulphonated polyethylene, *Biomaterials*, 14, 657, 1993.
51. Heijnen, H.F.G. et al., Activated platelets release two types of membrane vesicles: microvesicles by surface shedding and exosomes derived from exocytosis of multivesicular bodies and alpha-granules, *Blood*, 94, 3791, 1999.
52. Nomura S., Function and clinical significance of platelet-derived microparticles, *Int. J. Hematol.*, 74, 397, 2001.
53. Tan, K.T. and Lip, G.Y.H., The potential role of platelet microparticles in atherosclerosis, *Thromb. Haemost.*, 94, 488, 2005.
54. Janatova, J., Activation and control of complement, inflammation, and infection associated with the use of biomedical polymers, *ASAIO J.*, 46, S53, 2000.
55. Anderson, J.M., Biological responses to materials, *Ann. Rev. Mater. Res.*, 31, 81, 2001.
56. Kappelmayer, J. et al., Tissue factor is expressed on monocytes during simulated extracorporal circulation, *Circ. Res.*, 72, 1075, 1993.
57. Tabuchi, N. et al., activated leukocytes adsorbed on the surface of an extracorporal circuit, *Artif. Organs*, 27, 591, 2003.
58. Xue, L. and Greisler, H.P., Biomaterials in the development and future of vascular grafts, *J. Vasc. Surg.*, 37, 472, 2003.
59. Ratner, B.D. and Bryant, S.J., Biomaterials: where we have been and where we are going, *Ann. Rev. Biomed. Eng.*, 6, 41, 2004.
60. Lau, H. and Cheng, S.W., Is the preferential use of ePTFE grafts in femorofemoral bypass justified? *Ann. Vasc. Surg.*, 15, 383, 2001.
61. Bordenave L. et al., *In vitro* endothelialized ePTFE prostheses: clinical update 20 years after the first realization, *Clin. Hemorheol. Microcirc.*, 33, 227, 2005.
62. Kannan, R.Y. et al., Current status of prosthetic bypass grafts: a review, *J. Biomed. Mater. Res.*, 74B, 570, 2005.
63. Tiwari, A. et al., New prostheses for use in bypass grafts with special emphasis of polyurethanes, *Cardiovasc. Surg.*, 10, 191, 2002.

64. Aldenhoff, Y.B.J. et al., performance of a polyurethane vascular prosthesis carrying dipyridamole coating on its luminal surface, *J. Biomed. Mater. Res.*, 54, 224, 2001.
65. Markou, C.P. et al., A novel method for efficient drug delivery, *Ann. Biomed. Eng.*, 26, 502, 1998.
66. Karrer, L. et al., PPS–PEG surface coating to reduce thrombogenicity of small diameter ePTFE vascular grafts, *Int. J. Artif. Organs*, 28, 993, 2005.
67. Xu, Z.K. et al., Tethering poly(ethylene glycol)s to improve the surface biocompatibility of poly(acrylonitrile-*co*-maleic acid) asymmetric membranes, *Biomaterials*, 26, 589, 2005.
68. Balakrishnan, B. et al., Chemical modification of poly(vinyl chloride) resin using poly(ethylene glycol) to improve blood compatibility, *Biomaterials*, 26, 3495, 2005.
69. Chung, C.W. et al., Poly(ethylene glycol)-grafted poly(3-hydroxyundecenoate) networks for enhanced blood compatibility, *Int. J. Biol. Macromol.*, 32, 17, 2003.
70. Unsworth, L.D., Sheardown, H., and Brash, J.L., Polyethylene oxide surfaces of variable chain density by chemosorption of PEO-thiol on gold: adsorption of proteins from plasma studied by radiolabelling and immunoblotting, *Biomaterials*, 26, 5927, 2005.
71. Park, K. et al., *In vitro* and *in vivo* studies of PEO-grafted blood-contacting cardiovascular prostheses, *J. Biomater. Sci. Polymer Edn.*, 11, 1121, 2000.
72. Hansson, K.M. et al., Whole blood coagulation on protein adsorption-resistant PEG and peptide functionalized PEG-coated titanium surfaces, *Biomaterials*, 26, 861, 2005.
73. Hanssen, H.H.L. et al., Metallic wires with an adherent lubricious and blood compatible polymeric coating and their use in the manufacture of novel slippery-when-wet guidewires: possible applications related to controlled local drug delivery, *J. Biomed. Mater. Res.*, 48, 820, 1999.
74. Aldenhoff, Y.B.J. et al., Coils and tubes releasing heparin. Studies on a new vascular graft prototype, *Biomaterials*, 25, 3125, 2004.
75. Peerlings, C.C.L. et al., Heparin release from slippery-when-wet guide wires for intravascular use, *J. Biomed. Mater. Res.*, 63, 692, 2002.
76. Lemos, P.A., Serruys, P.W., and Sousa, J.E., Drug-eluting stents, *Circulation*, 107, 3003, 2003.
77. Burt, H.M. and Hunter, W.L., Drug-eluting stents: a multidisciplinary success story, *Adv. Drug Deliv. Rev.*, 58, 350, 2006.
78. van der Hoeven, B.L. et al., Drug-eluting stents: results, promises and problems, *Int. J. Cardiol.*, 99, 9, 2005.
79. Tung, R. et al., Drug-eluting stents for the management of restenosis: a critical appraisal of the evidence, *Ann. Intern. Med.*, 144, 913, 2006.
80. Kocsis, J.F., Llanos, G., and Holmer, E., Heparin-coated stents, *J. Long Term Eff. Med. Implants*, 10, 19, 2000.
81. Nelson, S.R., deSouza, N.M., and Allison, D.J., Endovascular stents and stent-grafts: is heparin coating desirable? *Cardiovasc. Intervent. Radiol.*, 23, 252, 2000.
82. Shin, E.K. et al., efficacy of heparin coated stents in early setting of acute myocardial infarction, *Catheter Cardiovasc. Interv.*, 52, 306, 2001.
83. van der Giessen, W.J. et al., Heparin-coated coronary stents, *Curr. Interv. Cardiol. Rep.*, 1, 234, 1999.
84. Frank, R.D. et al., Anticoagulant-free Genius haemodialysis using low molecular weight heparin-coated circuits, *Nephrol. Dial. Transplant.*, 21, 1013, 2006.
85. Becker, B.F. et al., Endothelial function and hemostasis, *Z. Kardiol.*, 89, 160, 2000.
86. Nakabayashi, N. and Williams, D.F., Preparation of non-thrombogenic materials using 2-methacryloyloxyethyl phosphorylcholine, *Biomaterials*, 24, 2431, 2003.
87. Whelan, D.M. et al., Biocompatibility of phosphorylcholine coated stents in normal porcine coronary arteries, *Heart*, 83, 338, 2000.
88. Tseng, P.Y. et al., Membrane-mimetic films containing thrombomodulin and heparin inhibit tissue factor-induced thrombin generation in a flow model, *Biomaterials*, 27, 2637, 2006.
89. Sun, L.B. et al., Pretreatment of a Dacron graft with tissue factor pathway inhibitor decreases thrombogenicity and neointimal thickness: a preliminary animal study, *ASAIO J.*, 47, 325, 2001.
90. Sun, L.B. et al., Topically applied tissue factor pathway inhibitor reduced intimal thickness of small arterial autografts in rabbits, *J. Vasc. Surg.*, 34, 151, 2001.
91. Watanabe, S. et al., The *in vitro* and *in vivo* behavior of urokinase immobilized onto collagen-synthetic polymer composite material, *J. Biomed. Mater. Res.*, 15, 553, 1981.
92. Conte M.S., The ideal small arterial substitute: a search for the holy grail? *FASEB J.*, 12, 43, 1998.
93. Pawlowski, K.J. et al., Endothelial cell seeding of polymeric vascular grafts, *Front. Biosci.*, 9, 1412, 2004.

94. Tiwari, A. et al., Tissue engineering of vascular bypass grafts: role of endothelial cell extraction, *Eur. J. Vasc. Endovasc. Surg.*, 21, 193, 2001.

95. Dixit, P. et al., Vascular graft endothelialization: comparative analysis of canine and human endothelial cell migration on natural biomaterials, *J. Biomed. Mater. Res.*, 56, 545, 2001.

96. Seifalian, A.M. et al., Improving the clinical patency of prosthetic vascular and coronary bypass grafts: the role of seeding and tissue engineering, *Artif. Organs*, 26, 307, 2002.

97. Hoenig, M.R. et al., Tissue-engineered blood vessels, *Arterioscerl. Thromb. Vasc. Biol.*, 25, 1128, 2005.

98. Hunting, C.B., Noort, W.A., and Zwaginga, J.J., Circulating endothelial progenitor cells reflect the state of the endothelium: vascular injury, repair and neovascularisation, *Vox Sang.*, 88, 1, 2005.

99. Rotmans, J.I. et al., *In vivo* cell seeding with anti-CD34 antibodies successfully accelerates endothelialization but stimulates intimal hyperplasia in porcine arteriovenous expanded polytetrafluoroethylene grafts, *Circulation*, 112, 12, 2005.

100. Vara, D.S. et al., Cardiovascular tissue engineering: state of the art, *Pathologie Biologie*, 53, 599, 2005.

101. van der Zijpp, Y.J., Poot, A.A., and Feijen, J., Endothelialization of small-diameter vascular prostheses, *Arch. Physiol. Biochem.*, 111, 415, 2003.

102. L'Heureux, N. et al., A completely biological tissue-engineered human blood vessel, *FASEB J.*, 12, 47, 1998.

103. Engbers-Buijtenhuijs, P. et al., Biological characterisation of vascular grafts cultured in a bioreactor, *Biomaterials*, 27, 2390, 2006.

104. Niklason, L.E. et al., Functional arteries grown *in vitro, Science*, 284, 489, 1999.

105. Lepidi, S. et al., *In vivo* regeneration of small-diameter (2mm) arteries using a polymer scaffold, *FASEB J.*, 20, 103, 2006.

106. Part 4: Selection of tests for interactions with blood, *ISO standard 10993, Biological Evaluation of Medical Devices*, International organization for standardization, Geneva, 2006.

107. Seyfert, U.T., Biehl, V., and Schenk, J., *In vitro* hemocompatibility testing of biomaterials according to the ISO 10993-4, *Biomol. Eng.*, 19, 91, 2002.

108. van Oeveren, W. et al., Comparison of coagulation activity tests *in vitro* for selected biomaterials, *Artif. Organs*, 26, 506, 2002.

109. Hemker, H.C., Al Daeri, R., and Beguin, S., Thrombin generation assays: accruing clinical relevance, *Curr. Opin. Hematol.*, 11, 170, 2004.

110. Carr, M.E. and Martin, E.J., Evolving techniques for monitoring clotting in plasma and whole blood samples, *Clin. Lab.*, 50, 539, 2004.

111. Mann, K.G., Brummel, K., and Butenas, S., What is all the thrombin for? *J. Thromb. Haemost.*, 1, 1504, 2003.

112. Hemker, H.C. et al., The calibrated automated thrombogram (CAT): a universal routine test for hyper- and hypocoagulability, *Pathophysiol. Haemost. Thromb.*, 32, 249, 2002.

113. Hemker, H.C. and Beguin, S., Thrombin generation in plasma: its assessment via the endogenous thrombin potential, *Thromb. Haemost.*, 74, 134, 1995.

114. Hong, J. et al., A new *in vitro* model to study interaction between whole blood and biomaterials. Studies of platelet and coagulation activation and the effect of aspirin, *Biomaterials*, 20, 603, 1999.

115. Frank, R.D. et al., Glutaraldehyde induced fluorescence technique (GIFT): a new method for the imaging of platelet adhesion on biomaterials, *J. Biomed. Mater. Res.*, 52, 374, 2000.

116. Tamada, Y., Kulik, E.A., and Ikada, Y., Simple method for platelet counting, *Biomaterials*, 16, 259, 1995.

117. van England, M., et al., Annexin V-affinity assay: a review on an apoptosis detection system based on phosphatidylserine exposure, *Cytometry*, 31, 1, 1998.

118. Gurney, D., Lip, G.Y.H., and Blann, A.D., A reliable plasma marker of platelet activation: does it exist? *Am. J. Hematol.*, 70, 139, 2002.

119. Vistica, D.T. et al., Tetrazolium-based assays for cellular viability: a critical examination of selected parameters affecting formazan production, *Cancer Res.*, 51, 2515, 1991.

120. Lowik, C.W., et al., Quantification of adherent and nonadherent cells cultured in 96-well plates using the supravital stain neutral red, *Anal. Biochem.*, 213, 426, 1993.

121. Lui, S.M. and Cowan, J.A., A direct spectrophotometric method for monitoring the kinetics of T-cell cytolysis, *Biochimie*, 76, 452, 1994.

122. Cripps, C.M., Rapid method for the estimation of plasma haemoglobin levels, *J. Clin. Pathol.*, 21, 110, 1968.

123. Malinauskas, R.A., Plasma haemoglobin measurement techniques for the *in vitro* evaluation of blood damage caused by medical devices, *Artif. Organs*, 21, 1255, 1997.

18 Improving Blood Compatibility of Biomaterials Using a Novel Antithrombin–Heparin Covalent Complex

Leslie Roy Berry and Anthony Kam Chuen Chan

CONTENTS

18.1 INTRODUCTION

Use of biomaterials in clinical diagnosis and treatment is an increasingly prevalent application of chemical polymers.[1,2] Indeed, catheters,[3] stents,[4] heart valves,[5] bypass circuits,[6] dialysis devices,[7] and other devices constructed from biochemical polymers have enabled major advances in medical care. One persistent problem associated with the biomaterials involves biocompatibility of the polymer surfaces with blood. In particular, thrombotic complications induced by interactions between the biomaterials and the vascular system remain an obstacle to their functional utility.[8] This is a vexing issue especially in the pediatric population requiring catheters for blood sampling or treatment. Studies have clearly established that central venous catheters cause up to 90% of thromboses occurring in neonates[9] and approximately 60% of thromboses observed in children.[10] Clot formation in and around catheter lines not only prevents treatment from being received by the pediatric patient but leads to serious risk of thrombotic complications such as stroke.[11] Thus, obviation of clot induction by catheter surfaces would solve the major cause of thrombotic disease in children.

Evolution of a thrombus by biomaterial surfaces involves the activation of plasma coagulation proteins in a cascade pathway that leads to the production of thrombin. Systemic thrombin generation *in vivo* depends on a number of parameters. Parameters such as plasma levels of procoagulant or anticoagulant molecules and cell or extracellular matrix surfaces that initiate or inhibit the coagulation cascade control the hemostatic state within the individual.[12] Ultimately, activation of factors within the coagulation cascade determines the generation of thrombin from its precursor prothrombin.[13] Once generated, thrombin converts fibrinogen to fibrin monomer that polymerizes to form the fibrin clot.[14] Within the thrombotic process, thrombin is a key enzyme in the regulation of coagulation.[15] After the initial thrombin is formed, it can provide feedback to activate cascade factors such as FV,[16] FVIII,[17] and FXI[18] that are involved in its generation. Also, thrombin activates FXIII to FXIIIa, which can in turn cross-link fibrin to form a more stable clot.[19,20] Furthermore, thrombin activates platelets to bind with other cells or the fibrin within the clot[21] and converts thrombin-activatable fibrinolysis inhibitor into an active form that inhibits fibrinolysis.[22–24] In addition to these procoagulant features, thrombin can also act as an anticoagulant that limits its own formation. When bound to endothelial thrombomodulin, thrombin can activate protein C.[25] Activated protein C, along with cofactor protein S, converts FVa and FVIIIa into inactive forms incapable of accelerating thrombin generation.[26] Thus, thrombin has a multifunctional capability to affect the progress of coagulation. As a corollary, inhibition of thrombin would be a key step in the control of coagulation.

Antithrombin (AT) is a member of the family of serine protease inhibitors (serpins). AT acts mainly to irreversibly neutralize enzymes generated from activation of the coagulation cascade.[27] Thus, AT forms irreversible serpin–protease inhibitor complexes with FXIIa, FXIa, FIXa, FXa, and thrombin.[13,28,29] However, AT is most effective at thrombin inhibition, as evidenced by rate constant comparisons.[30] Further acceleration of thrombin reaction with AT can be affected by heparin and heparan sulfate glycosaminoglycans (GAGs). In the case of commercial unfractionated heparin (UFH), the rate of thrombin inhibition by AT is elevated at least 1000-fold.[31] This rate enhancement is due to two major factors. First, UFH molecules bind to AT through a unique oligosaccharide sequence[32] that induces a conformational chain in the serpin that makes it more reactive toward thrombin.[33] Second, UFH can act as a template that binds both thrombin and AT so that a tertiary complex is formed in which the UFH is a bridge that localizes the enzyme and inhibitor.[34] After thrombin and AT have reacted to produce an irreversible thrombin–AT (TAT) complex, massive structural changes in the AT moiety cause a decrease in affinity for the UFH so that the GAG can dissociate and catalyze another thrombin + AT reaction.[35] UFH's acceleration of thrombin inhibition allows for more effective neutralization by AT of the first thrombin formed after initiation of coagulation, so that propagation of thrombin generation from feedback activation is ablated.[17]

Although UFH, along with its low-molecular-weight derivatives, is the most common clinically used anticoagulant,[36,37] there are several major limitations associated with its application. One pharmacokinetic problem is that UFH has a short, dose-dependant intravenous half-life.[38] Rapid loss from the circulation results from nonspecific binding to positively charged plasma and cell surface proteins,[39] as well as passage through tissue layers because of its small size.[40] It is due to the variation in the UFH-binding proteins between individuals that UFH has such an unpredictable anticoagulant effect.[41] Other factors limiting UFH anticoagulation treatment and prophylaxis are biophysical in origin. The major issue relates to the resistance of UFH toward inhibition of coagulation factors adhering to surfaces. For example, noncovalent AT–UFH complexes are unable to neutralize FXa bound to phospholipid[42,43] and fibrin-bound thrombin.[44,45] Clinically, this is significant since evidence indicates major impacts from the lack of pacification of fibrin clot-associated procoagulant activity. Thus, the fact that there is an early recurrence of unstable coronary artery syndromes when UFH treatment is discontinued[46] gives credence to the concept that lack of neutralization of clot-bound thrombin by UFH influences clot propagation.[42–44] Although high doses of UFH might overcome resistance of surface-bound factors to inhibition, *in vivo* administration of such strong anticoagulation is not viable because of hemorrhagic complications.[47] Bleeding side effects of UFH have also hampered use of devices coated with heparin to prevent thrombosis. Leaching of surface-bound heparin from vascular devices has led to unwanted circulation of anticoagulant as well as loss of competency of surface coating.[48] Finally, since only about one-third of the starting UFH in commercial products have anticoagulant activity due to a lack of high affinity AT-activating binding sites,[49] much of the surface area coated with heparin is devoid of anticoagulant activity.

Given the issues surrounding heparin's clinical use, there has been an impetus to devise improved heparinoid derivatives to overcome these obstacles. One novel development is the creation of covalent complexes of AT and heparin (ATH). Rationales behind the conception of covalent ATH directly address UFH's major limitations. For example, if heparin is permanently linked to AT, the GAG moiety cannot dissociate to transverse tissue layers or form unfavorable interactions leading to loss from the circulation. Thus, covalent bonding to the serpin may result in an intravenous half-life that is closer to that of AT. In addition to increased retention in the circulation, activity of ATH will be maximal since the AT component will always be in its activated state because of ongoing effects from the conjugated heparin chain. Thus, thrombin inhibition rates will be increased relative to those of the dissociable noncovalent AT–UFH complexes. Since contacts between AT and heparin are maintained in ATH, a significant portion of the heparin will be shielded from interactions with plasma or cell surface proteins. This reduction in non-AT protein binding will engender a more predictable anticoagulant response since nonproductive interactions with nonanticoagulant proteins of varying concentrations are suppressed. A further consequence of reduced cell-receptor-protein binding of the ATH is that bleeding side effects may be lessened. In concert with the relief from many of UFH's sequelae with biological structures, the aforementioned properties and other aspects of ATH lend to even more improvement over heparin for coating of biomaterial polymers. Attachment of heparins to various commercial substrates on vascular devices is hampered by a lack of functional groups on the GAG that are easily linkable in a consistent fashion. In order to generate groups for immobilization, heparin is generally modified in ways that are somewhat destructive of its activity. Alternatively, ATH may be readily linked to surfaces of devices by utilizing the range of amino acid R'-groups on the AT. Moreover, linkage through the AT guarantees that the critical anticoagulant heparin chain will be directed away from the polymer surface to inhibit thrombin generation in the blood flow. Further, all ATH molecules coated on the surface will be permanently activated compared to surfaces with UFH in which only up to one-third of the molecules will be active. Thus, the overall potential of the projected characteristics of ATH to alleviate UFH's limitations encouraged the production of numerous covalent ATH complexes for study as a possible anticoagulant agent.

The purpose of this chapter is to give a thorough presentation of the development of ATH from its starting materials, with particular attention to its application as a biomaterial coating that improves biocompatibility. This approach is intended to introduce the reader to structural aspects and synthesis of AT, heparin, ATH, and ATH-containing surfaces, which will act as a reference guide for production of devices that are non- or antithrombotic when in contact with blood. AT structure–function will be described. Heparin structure and *in vivo* mechanisms will be outlined with respect to the long-established use of this anticoagulant in thrombosis prophylaxis and treatment. A general examination of ATH properties that directly address the major deficiencies of UFH derivatives will be made as a framework for the design of conjugates that should give the desired properties. Chemical and biological characteristics of ATH compounds that have been produced will be explored from a chronological perspective to give a flavor of the attempts toward optimization of this molecule. This perspective may be useful in providing insights for further improvements by future workers. Once development of the ATH conjugate has been discussed, the processes for coating surfaces with ATH will be described and the resultant performance *in vitro* and *in vivo* will be listed. Finally, the chapter ends with a synopsis of possible future paths for this new technology.

18.2 ANTITHROMBIN

18.2.1 CHEMICAL STRUCTURE OF ANTITHROMBIN

AT is a glycosylated polypeptide that belongs to a large family of serpins that have common structural and functional homology.[50–52] Over the entire group of these serpin proteins, the primary sequence homology is approximately 30%, and several tertiary structure characteristics are shared.[53] AT is synthesized in the liver and its transcript comes from a gene present on the long arm of chromosome 1.[54] In humans, the AT gene is spread over a continuous 19 kb stretch containing seven exons and six introns,[55,56] with an open reading frame of 1396 nucleotides that includes a 96-nucleotide-stretch coding for a 32-amino acid-signal peptide (which is removed from the N-terminal of AT prior to cellular secretion).[56] In the AT sequence, mammalians have sequence variation of 10–15% but high conservation around the reactive site.[57]

There are several important aspects of AT primary structure that create impact on its function and play a role in the more native covalent complexes prepared from heparin. This plasma serpin is a 60,000 Da single-chain polypeptide[58–60] that contains 432 amino acids and three pairs of disulfide bonds.[61] In particular, two of the disulfides link a somewhat unstructured length of 45 amino acid residues at the N-terminus with the third and fourth α-helices in AT. As will be seen later, the short N-terminal sequence beyond the last disulfide-bonded cysteine is an important feature involved in ATH formation from UFH. In terms of tertiary structure, AT from human plasma has 31% α-helix, 16% β-sheet, 9% β-turn, and 44% random coil.[62,63] Considering the type of the amino acid complement, AT has a net neutral pI because of the presence of significant amount of arginyl and lysyl residues that are the main contributors to the high-affinity UFH-binding regions.[53] A number of attempts have been made to get a full description of the AT three-dimensional structure to understand its functional activity. To this end, an x-ray crystal structure of the serpin with 3 Å resolution has been produced.[64] This analysis and studies by others have shown that AT can exist in either an active or an inactive (or latent) form[65] that occur together as a dimer during crystallization. Models of the active structure show a glycoprotein inhibitor with nine α-helices and three β-sheets.[64]

Posttranslational modification is restricted to complex type asparaginyl N-linked glycosylation that plays an important role in the functional activity of AT with regard to UFH catalysis of the inhibitor's reactions. *In vivo* AT glycosylation is carried out by a glycosyl-transferase at asparagines that are accompanied by specific neighboring sequences in areas of β-sheet structure. The initial step in this process involves placement onto the asparaginyl R-group of a tetraantennary, high-mannose glycan by transfer from a dolicol phosphate. These high-mannose glycans are then degraded by endoglycosidases to give a chitobiose-trimannose core, which acts as a base for the addition of monosaccharide residues to form the carbohydrate structures observed in the final glycoprotein that is excreted.[66] During this processing, variation can occur in the final type of glycan structures produced. For example, different degrees of branching are observed radiating out from the glycan core. Previous work has shown that glycosylation sites on AT can display mono-, bi-, tri- and tetraantennary-branched oligosaccharide chains.[67,68] In addition to heterogeneity in branching, the degree of substitution of terminal N-acetylneuraminic acid residues on AT glycans also varies.[69] Further variation is evident with the addition of fucosyl residues on glycans at Asn96 and Asn192.[67] In addition to alteration in the glycan structures themselves, subforms of AT have been described in which the number of oligosaccharides per polypeptide chain differs. AT molecules with three,[70] four,[71] and even five glycans have been discovered.[72] A number of factors have been muted as critical for influencing the degree of AT glycosylation. One general condition called carbohydrate-deficient glycoprotein syndrome leads to decreased glycosylation of AT by the golgi.[73] These under-glycosylated AT derivatives exhibit lower activity in anticoagulant functional tests. Overall, the main glycoforms of mammalian AT contain either four glycans (α-AT) or three glycans (β-AT) per molecule. Thus, in human plasma-derived AT, the fully glycosylated α-AT has N-amido glycosidically linked glycans on asparaginyl residues at positions 96, 135, 155, and 192.[74] The β-AT has the same carbohydrate as the α-isoform, except at asparagine 135 where no carbohydrate moiety is present.[75] Biosynthetic deficiency resulting in the three-glycan β product gives a subtype in which the heparin-binding affinity is increased,[76] which has significant implications for the likely population mixture that may result during some ATH syntheses. Thus, there is a wide range of variants within the AT family that have major differences in the key components of the molecule. These alterations in the overall molecular structure have important functional effects, as will be delineated in the following section (18.2.2).

18.2.2 FUNCTIONAL BIOCHEMISTRY OF ANTITHROMBIN

The AT anticoagulant has typical serpin structural features that control the action of the inhibitor toward its protease targets. A chronology of the developments leading to our present understanding of AT's mechanisms is illustrative in that it connects AT reactivity with its biological function *in vivo*. Consideration of the underpinnings of AT biochemical actions affecting the patient gives credence to the type of directions needed to construct covalent ATH complexes with advanced utility.

An early work on blood coagulation indicated that a circulating natural anticoagulant must be present since exogenous thrombin lost activity when mixed with plasma.[59,77] Initially, this "AT" molecule's activity in plasma was described as the "progressive AT activity." Early research by Robert Maclean in 1916 led to the discovery of an anticoagulant isolated from liver (i.e., UFH)[78] that effectively inhibited thrombin in the presence of an uncharacterized plasma protein. Since the plasma protein allowing heparin to exhibit its accelerating activity for thrombin inhibition had not been isolated, the molecule was designated as "heparin cofactor."[79] In an attempt to systematize classification of the AT and coagulant systems, nomenclature was suggested in the 1950s[80] whereby loss of thrombin activity due to fibrin-clot binding was called AT I, heparin cofactor activity was called AT II, and AT III was referred to progressive AT activity. In the 1960s and 1970s, purification and analysis of plasma proteins yielded data showing that a single protein possessed all the activities of the heparin cofactor and progressive AT.[59] Thus, ATs II and III were designated as AT III. Discussions evolving from the standardization subcommittee of the International Society of Thrombosis and Hemostasis finally led to the simple name of AT for this anticoagulant protein.

The mechanism of AT has been elucidated from a large wealth of investigations and it is now one of the best-understood protease inhibitors. AT reacts to neutralize activated coagulation factors by a stress-release mode in which initial cleavage of the inhibitor allows rapid relaxation from a high-energy state to a vastly altered form of AT in which the protease remains covalently linked and protected from hydrolytic release. As with many of the serpins, AT contains a reactive center loop near the C-terminus. As it approaches the reactive center, thrombin is attracted to a binding region close to the reactive center. Mutations discovered in AT such as Ala382 → Thr382[81] and Pro407 → Leu407[55] have established this thrombin-binding region to involve at least amino acid residues 382 and 407. In terms of the noncovalent AT-contact points on thrombin, a substitution of Gly226 to Val226 on the enzyme caused loss of the capacity for thrombin inhibition.[82] Molecular models have given indication that Gly226 extends into the specific recognition pocket on AT since the Val side chain was too large for the space required by the AT P_1 reactive center loop, the Arg393 R-group. Ultimately, specific binding of thrombin to AT allows for concomitant covalent bond formation. The peptide in the AT serpin that is targeted by thrombin or other proteases has been assigned the notation P_1-P_1', in which the P_1 Arg393 residue confers on AT its selectivity toward the coagulation factors.[52] Amino acids that are on the N-terminal side of P_1 add to the enzyme selectivity, such as Gly392 at position P_2 that selects for FXa and maintains covalent linkage with AT within the resultant FXa–AT complex.[27] Work is in progress to determine the significance of other residues, such as P_1 and Ser394 that are toward the C-terminus from P_1.

Reaction steps that ensue the first association of thrombin and AT are intricate. Initially, thrombin reacts with its AT substrate by acting on the inhibitor's Arg393 C-terminal amide bond using the protease-active serine. Thus, an ester between the thrombin serine hydroxyl oxygen and AT's

Arg393 carboxyl carbonyl group is formed. Prior to cleavage, AT has an active state called the "S-configuration" in which the reactive center P_1-P_1' bond is in the center of a stressed loop[83] that connects the β-sheet A strand 4 with β-sheet C strand 1 of the serpin.[84] This configuration is in a high-energy condition where the AT reactive center loop structure is contorted so that the reactive center is in a prominent position for protease reaction. After cleavage of the Arg393–Ser394 bond, but before the TAT ester bond can be hydrolyzed, a rapid release of the inherent tension of the now broken reactive center loop results in a massive rearrangement of the enzyme-linked inhibitor to its relaxed "R-configuration."[83] The extreme distortions imparted to thrombin within the enzyme-inhibitor complex disorders the structure so that the ester linking the thrombin to AT resists hydrolysis. Support for occurrence of these reaction steps has been derived from x-ray crystallographic structures and studies with antibodies that bind AT only when it is in enzyme–AT complexes or noncovalently bound to a P_{14}-P_1 tetradecapeptide, identical to that in the reactive center loop.[84–91] Findings showed that the thrombin-bound reactive center loop of AT is embedded within its β-sheet A and the serpin moiety has a highly modified overall structure that displays new epitopes that are not available to antibody recognition in the native, uncleaved AT. Indeed, additional x-ray and mutant AT variant investigations showed that the change in AT structure due to enzyme cleavage is so severe that the reactive center loop gets inserted into the β-sheet A up to the P_{12} residue and the C-terminus conformation is interpolated with thrombin.[92] In coincidence with this cleaved AT structure, the naturally occurring latent form of AT has a structure that also maintains the reactive center loop residues from P_{14} to P_3, inclusive, inserted within β-sheet A.[93] Thus, models of this reactive center loop–inserted AT structure show thrombin to be in the region of the β-sheet A pocket. This site keeps the thrombin isolated and permanently linked to AT in a pacified state.[94]

As stated earlier, UFH assists AT reaction with thrombin by accelerating its progress. One key component in this mechanism is that binding to UFH converts AT into a more reactive structure. Appearance of the AT-active state is evident from the increase in protein-intrinsic fluorescence, indicating the significant alteration in conformation as UFH continues its interaction. Loss of this UFH-associated fluorescence increase in Trp225 → Phe225 or Trp307 → Phe307 AT mutants indicates that these two Trp residues have altered environments because of the conformational change.[95] Further details of the UFH-induced AT-active conformation are evident. For example, the spectrum of Trp49 shifts toward the blue, indicating partial burial of this residue from UFH interaction. Alternatively, shift of the Trp225 to the red suggests that UFH may allow more solvent access for the R-group of this aromatic residue by retraction of Ser380. Studies with AT mutants have shown that the primary UFH-binding site is near the N-terminus,[96–99] with a second site between residues 107 and 156.[100] Experiments using alanine-scanning mutagenesis resulted in a large family of AT mutants, which could be tested for affinity to immobilized heparin. These studies determined that the key UFH-binding residues were as follows: Lys11, Arg14, Arg24, Arg47, Lys125, Arg129, and Arg145, which lay in a 5 nm trough on AT's surface.[101] In addition to these residues, a few other contact points on AT have been identified[93,94] where UFH binding may result in disruption of salt bridges of α-helix D with β-sheet B, allowing conversion to a serpin form that is more set for reactive center loop insertion into the β-sheet A.[101] Again, x-ray crystallography work showed that the high-affinity AT-binding site in UFH (pentasaccharide sequence) binds to particular AT-amino acid R-groups that, in turn, increases affinity between the two moieties and coincides with attaining the active AT conformation.[93] Further studies showing inhibition by P_{14}-P_3 peptide of the UFH induction of the AT-active conformation strongly confirmed the partial insertion effects of GAG binding.[102] In order to accelerate more thrombin + AT reactions, the UFH must be able to interact with other enzyme and serpin molecules once TAT inhibitor complex has formed. This is a logical consequence and simple tests have yielded proof. Consequently, AT bound to immobilized heparin was displaced by covalent reaction with thrombin to give free TAT complex and newly available heparin chains for fresh loads of AT.[35,103]

As exogenous UFH molecules can transform AT into an enhanced reactive state, the glycans on AT's polypeptide have a major influence on AT function. AT products made in baby hamster kidney (BHK) or chinese hamster ovary (CHO) cells have been shown to possess a 10 times lower UFH affinity[68,104] because of variable glycosylation on Asn155.[105] However, the major AT glycoforms that have been shown to have significant carbohydrate-related structure–function differences are the 4 glycan-containing α-AT and β-AT species that is missing a glycan at Asn135.[76,75] Of these human plasma-derived products, α-AT has reduced heparin affinity relative to β-AT,[76,106] which is not surprising since the Asn135 glycan is within the region of Lys125, Arg129, and Arg145 UFH-binding site residues. Therefore, it might be thought that covalent ATH preparations may tend to have a bias toward β-AT since there is no physical obstruction from the Asn135 glycan for heparin's approach during synthesis. However, steric issues between the Asn135-AT glycan and UFH with respect to AT binding to heparin are not the only factors. Rapid heparin-binding kinetic studies revealed that the glycan at Asn135 gives only a small reduction in initial weak binding.[106] It seems that the rate of conformational change to the final high-affinity complex with heparin is slower for α-AT, leading to an overall reduction in affinity relative to the β form.[106] Variation in heparin affinity between the two AT isoforms has extended to significant *in vivo* effects. Heparin-like GAGs such as heparan sulfate contain the pentasaccharide AT-binding sequence.[107] Research has shown that affinity to these heparinoids translates into regulation of AT pharmacodynamics since most β-AT is bound to heparan sulfate on vessel surfaces while the vast majority of α-AT remains in the circulation.[70] These data provide the potential for targeting heparin to areas of vascular damage by covalent linkage to a low glycan-containing AT that has increased vessel wall GAG affinity. Practical examples of such a design will be described later (Section 18.7).

18.3 HEPARIN

18.3.1 Chemical Structure of Heparin

UFH is derived from natural heparin in the mucosa of intestine and lung.[108] Heparin itself is part of the broad GAG classification of molecules[109] present in multi and single-celled organisms.[110] GAGs are polymers of uronic acid–hexosamine disaccharides that are synthesized in variable length straight chains.[111] Different subcategories of GAGs are defined by the type of uronic acid and/or the hexosamine makeup as well as type and degree of substituent groups present on the saccharide residues. For example, heparin and heparan sulfate have glucosamine, while chondroitin sulfates such as dermatan sulfate have galactosamine.[111] With respect to the uronic acid moiety, heparins and heparan sulfates are composed of mixtures of glucuronic and iduronic acids, but molecules of dermatan sulfate have only iduronic acid and other chondroitin species have molecules with only glucuronic acid residues.[111,112] Further refinement of structure is gained by groups present on the saccharide rings. Glucosamines in heparin and heparan sulfate are either N-acetylated or N-sulfated, while galactosamines of dermatan sulfate and chondroitin sulfates are mainly N-acetylated. Between heparin and heparan sulfate some statistical differences in hexosamine sulfation occur. Thus, >80% of heparin glucosamines are N-sulfated but roughly half of heparan sulfate glucosamines are sulfated.[113] Combined with the degree of O-sulfation in heparin (>2 O-sulfates/disaccharide)[114] relative to heparan sulfate (from 0.75 to 0.2 O-sulfates/disaccharide),[113] many features distinguish these GAGs as distinctly separate biosynthetic groups of molecules.

As stated, UFH is prepared from the native heparin in tissue. Heparin chains are built up as a posttranslational modification on a core protein within mast cells. Heparin GAGs, ranging from 60,000 to 100,000 Da, can number up to 10 per polypeptide and are attached to serine residues through O-glycosidic bonds.[115] Biosynthesis of heparin chains initiates by stepwise glycosyltransferase addition of monosaccharides to form a xylose–galactose–galactose–glucuronic acid linkage region sequence, the terminal xylose residue being glycosidically linked to a serine residue in the core polypeptide.[116] Chain growth continues to make a repeating disaccharide structure in which uronosyl-β-1 → 4 glycosaminosyl units are linked by α-1 → 4 bonds.[117] As indicated above, many functional group substituents are simultaneously added as the polysaccharide chain is synthesized. These modifications involve N-acetylases,[118] N-deacetylases,[118] O-sulfotransferases,[119] N-sulfotransferases,[120] glycosyltransferases,[121] and glucuronosyl-5-epimerases.[119] The order and degree of action for the various modifying enzymes is intricate and interrelated, which defines the final structures produced. Initially, as the nascent heparin chain grows, freshly synthesized regions are partially acetylated, sulfated, or unsubstituted on the glycosaminosyl nitrogen groups.[122] Both during and after this period,[122] the evolving chain is increased in N-sulfate by action of an N-deacetylase and an N-sulfotransferase.[118,122] Further modifications proceed following N-sulfation, with the O-sulfate- and uronic acid–type content within the final product being interdependent. Not long after the N-sulfotransferase reactions, a glucuronosyl-C5-epimerase converts glucuronosyl residues at the end of the chain into iduronosyls.[119] Although the epimerase drives the reaction toward the iduronosyl form, there is a significant reverse reaction that is only blocked if C6 of the glucosaminosyl residue or C2 of the iduronosyl residue becomes O-sulfated.[119] Within this O-sulfation pathway, interrelationships also exist whereby glucosaminosyl C6-O-sulfation can occur with or without 2-O-sulfate groups on the neighboring iduronosyl residue, but C2-O-sulfation of iduronosyls requires neighboring glucosaminosyl residues to be non-O-sulfated at the C6 position.[123] Furthermore, uronosyl residues are left nonsulfated, if glycosyl transfer of the next glucosamine occurs before the C2-O-sulfotransferase can act.[123] Apparently, O-sulfation is fairly effective during heparin GAG synthesis since ~78% of uronic acid residues in commercial heparins are iduronic[117] and ~75% of the iduronic acids are 2-O-sulfated.[117,124] By and large, both chain modification and length of heparins on the core protein are quite variable and partly controlled by conditions within the synthetic space like substrate availability and cell energetics.[125,126]

An important aspect for the type of UFH available for AT–heparin conjugation is the *in vivo* and *in vitro* processing that happens before and during commercial isolation. Heparin chains on proteoglycans produced by mastocytoma cells undergo partial depolymerization by an endoglucuronidase before storage in cytoplasmic granules.[127,128] This degradation within intestinal mucosa or lung mast cells is responsible for the reduced molecular weight range of 5000–30,000 observed in the free heparin chains of UFH prepared commercially. More recently, low–molecular weight heparin (LMWH) has been produced by partial depolymerization of UFH using HNO_2, base elimination after partial esterification of uronic acid carboxyls, heparinases, and heparitinases.[129,130] The reduced molecular weights of LMWHs (from 1800 to 12,000)[129] gives improved pharmacokinetics and biological characteristics relative to the starting UFH.

18.3.2 FUNCTIONAL BIOCHEMISTRY OF HEPARIN

In vivo, heparin and other GAGs mainly exist as proteoglycans that function as part of the structural architecture of the extracellular matrix and as a chemoattractant during processes in tissue.[131,132] In addition, heparin chains provide anticoagulant activity because of the ability to bind to AT or heparin cofactor II and catalyze their inhibition reactions with coagulation factors.[133] UFH catalysis of coagulation factor inhibition by AT *in vivo*[134] mostly involves the neutralization of thrombin and FXa.[135,136] Of these two coagulants, it has been shown that enhancement of thrombin's reaction with AT is the major mode of action for UFH clinical application.[137] In order to assist the *in vivo* inhibition of thrombin and FXa, heparin molecules must contain a specific pentasaccharide sequence that selectively binds with high affinity to AT.[138] In native rat skin mast cell proteoglycans, the pentasaccharide has been shown to occur variously[139] with most proteoglycans having chains without any pentasaccharides, while a minority of proteoglycans had GAG moieties with 1–5 pentasaccharides per chain.[140] Once final commercial production has been carried out, only one-third of UFH molecules on the average end up containing the high AT-affinity pentasaccharide.[141] However, very small subpopulations within the polydisperse commercial UFH preparations do exhibit two pentasaccharide sequences per molecule,[142] a fact that can have significant impact in some ATH synthetic designs. With regard to LMWH, however, the chain cleavages of UFH required to make these smaller molecules lead to a reduction of intact pentasaccharide.[136,143] In order to determine if there are better methodologies for retaining the active pentasaccharide in LMWHs, it would be instructive to know where this sequence resides are within UFH molecules. Previous work has demonstrated that although the AT-binding pentasaccharide is located fairly randomly in UFH chains,[144] there is a tendency for this active sequence to be expressed toward the aglycone or non-aldose half of the molecule.[145,146] The most recent work by our laboratory has taken advantage of this observation. Using thermal hydrolytic cleavage as a depolymerization method, UFH was heated at temperatures up to 115°C in aqueous 2-hydroxypyridine.[146,147] During this treatment, the 2-hydroxypyridine forms a protective sheath around UFH molecules, except at a somewhat central locus.[147] Thus, UFH undergoes minor degradation to yield a variable length inactive fragment containing the linkage region and an aldose-terminating product of uniform molecular weight that contains essentially all the original pentasaccharide activity. Isolation of the active material with an aldose gives the potential for a starting reagent with superior activity that may be covalently linked to AT through reaction chemistries involving the terminal aldehyde group.

The complete structural details and biosynthetic factors regarding the active pentasaccharide sequence have been established.[148] One feature observed to be a marker of the pentasaccharide was an unusual 3-O-sulfate group on the middle glucosamine residue.[149] It was later identified that 3-O-sulfation was mandatory for high AT affinity and anti-FXa activity.[150] Another critical component in the sequence is the occurrence of a nonsulfated glucuronic acid at the C4 position of the central 3-O-sulfated glucosamine residue.[148] Further work has elucidated the mode of pentasaccharide binding and activation of AT. Pentasaccharide interactions with AT occur through a two-stage mechanism that has been determined from studies of AT-binding to mono-, di-, tri-, and tetrasaccharide model derivatives.[151–153] In the first step, three residues at the nonaldose terminus of the pentasaccharide bind through charge attraction and hydrogen bonds to AT. This trisaccharide binding is weak in affinity but causes AT to undergo a conformational change to a form that is similar to that in the final activated state complex.[151] This conformational shift allows several amino acid R-groups, such as Arg47,[154] to come into contact with a charge cluster from the remaining two pentasaccharide residues and the 3-O-sulfate group on the central glucosamine,[153] all maintained in proper position by the skew boat conformation of the 2-O-sulfated iduronic residue four.[153] Binding of the final two saccharide units is responsible for locking heparin and AT into the final high-affinity complex state,[152,153] although no further conformational activation is induced in AT by association with residues four and five at the pentasaccharide aldose terminus.[154]

Although only the pentasaccharide sequence is required to accelerate AT inhibition of FXa, enhancement of thrombin neutralization necessitates a longer UFH chain since both protease and serpin need to bind for the maximal rate of thrombin inhibition to be achieved.[138] Experiments with distinct molecular weight heparin fractions have revealed that a minimum of 18–22 monosaccharide residues are required for the formation of heparin ternary complexes with AT and thrombin.[155] Thus, many LMWHs are unable to adequately accelerate thrombin inhibition when their chains are below this size limit. Interaction between thrombin and UFH occurs at an anion-binding exosite on thrombin[156] and negative charge groups on the GAG. Although no specific binding site for thrombin has been identified on UFH, increased charge density enhances affinity for the protease.[157] Due to the inability to bridge both AT and thrombin, LMWHs display reduced anti-thrombin to anti-FXa activity ratios versus UFH, which has been muted as the rationale behind lower antithrombotic activity of some LMWHs in vivo.[136] To emphasize this assertion, antithrombotic activity of the synthetic pentasaccharide has been reported as one of the lowest for LMWHs.[158] Alternatively, LMWH products have increased and more predictable intravenous half-lives compared to UFH.[159] Clearance of LMWH activity from the circulation occurs at a reduced rate because of decreased nonspecific protein binding,[160] and the fact that while UFH is removed by hepatic degradation and renal filtration, LMWH only disappears through the kidneys.[155] LMWH's two-compartment, single-phase elimination also leads to a simpler, more predictable treatment with reduced risk of hemorrhagic side effects.[161,162] Unfortunately, the multitude of depolymerization methods and isolation techniques makes for LMWH preparation with a range of inhibitory activities against thrombin.[163] Thus, treatment regimens must be determined for each LMWH product,[130] especially since (unlike UFH) overdosage cannot be fully reversed with protamine.[164] Development of a heparin derivative combining both high-AT-antithrombotic activities and a longer intravenous half-life would be a boon.

18.4 OVERVIEW OF COVALENT ANTITHROMBIN–HEPARIN COMPLEXES

18.4.1 LIMITATIONS OF CURRENT HEPARINS

Many clinical issues have evolved that have added increasing challenges to heparin use. These have given impetus for development of many new anticoagulant and antithrombotic drugs that are presently undergoing clinical trials. Limitations in heparin use arise from either pharmacokinetic problems or biophysical obstacles in pacifying prothrombotic activity on surfaces. Physical removal of UFH from the circulation involves binding to cell surfaces (such as hepatocytes) or passage through the kidneys.[155] These pharmacokinetic clearance mechanisms definitely involve free UFH separated from its noncovalent AT–UFH complex since AT and UFH in coinjected mixtures disappear from the circulation at different rates.[141] Due to variable protein interactions *in vivo*, UFH has an intravenous half-life in humans ranging from 18 min to 1 h.[155] To compensate for the rapid circulatory loss, UFH is administered by subcutaneous injection (which gives peak plasma levels at 4 h)[165] or given by slow intravenous infusion.[166] Although LMWHs have increased intravenous half-lives over UFH,[167] subcutaneous administration of LMWH gave peak plasma activity at 3 h that returned to background by 12 h.[161] Other interactions confound UFH application since heparin can bind to fluid-phase plasma protein,[168,169] platelets,[170] and endothelial surfaces.[171] Complexation of UFH and plasma proteins (other than AT and heparin cofactor II) occurs through nonselective charge attractions[172] and results in reduced activity.[168] UFH function is simply masked by its binding to basic plasma proteins since activity can be recovered by displacement with innocuous polyanions.[173] It is, in part, the variable association–dissociation of UFH from basic plasma and cell surface proteins that causes decreased regulation of heparin activity and reappearance of activity long after protamine neutralization (referred to as the heparin rebound effect).[173] Nonspecific plasma protein binding by UFH is somewhat molecular weight-dependent since LMWHs have reduced binding.[174,175] Biophysical limitations of heparin are seen in the lack of ability to inhibit fibrin-bound thrombin.[44,45] At prophylactic doses, UFH can even assist in accreting thrombin onto fibrin clots,[176] where thrombin in the resultant thrombin–UFH–fibrin–ternary complex[177] is resistant to reaction with AT·UFH.[178] This phenomenon results from an altered substrate reactivity by thrombin in the ternary complex[179] so that reaction against exogenous AT·UFH is reduced.[178] Studies show that LMWHs are also ineffective against clot-bound thrombin.[180] Further biophysical obstruction is evident in the reduced rate of UFH inactivation of FXa when bound to phospholipid surfaces within the prothrombinase complex.[181,182] Other UFH deficiencies involving adverse side effects have long been noted, the most significant of which is bleeding risk.[183]

Careful monitoring is required to maintain therapeutic levels of UFH activity without inducing hemorrhage[184] and regimens are designed to optimize the efficacy/bleeding ratio.[185] LMWH has a more predictable anticoagulant profile. Nevertheless, there is no clinical evidence that hemorrhagic complications are decreased for LMWH treatment compared with that for UFH.[186,187] Several other iatrogenic issues exist. Thrombocytopenia, arising from development of antibodies against epitopes from platelet-bound heparin,[188] precludes further UFH treatment. Although data from acute coronary syndrome patients has suggested that LMWH may have a lower risk of inducing thrombocytopenia,[183] LMWH is not recommended for the treatment of thrombocytopenia patients since LMWHs cross-react with about 80% of the antibodies from UFH-induced thrombocytopenia.[183] Finally, osteoporosis occurs in 17–36% of patients receiving chronic heparin treatment.[189,190]

To avert the shortcomings of heparin, several nonheparinoid anticoagulants have been investigated such as hirudin, hirulog, phe-pro-arg-chloromethyl ketone (PPACK), and ximelagatran.[191–195] Hirudin is a small-polypeptide (7000 MW) direct thrombin inhibitor that binds noncovalently with high affinity.[196] Hirolog is constructed from covalent linkage of an irreversible thrombin active site inhibitor to residues 53–65 of the hirudin C-terminal.[197] Studies have suggested that hirudin can inhibit clot-bound thrombin since no rebound of clot growth occurred after hirudin had been cleared.[198] Unfortunately, intravenous half-lives of hirudin[199] and hirolog[200] are not significantly longer than that of UFH, and coagulation does not appear to be terminated since markers of thrombin generation increase over time even after large hirudin doses.[201] PPACK is an irreversible, selective, direct thrombin inhibitor that can efficiently neutralize thrombin on fibrin clots.[202] Similar to the hirudin derivatives, PPACK is rapidly cleared[203] and has exhibited excessive bleeding risk associated with doses necessary to achieve plasma concentrations required for treatment.[204] Ximelagatran (which is metabolically converted to its active melagatran form *in vivo*) has shown promise since it had treatment outcomes rivaling heparins and could be taken orally.[195] Sadly, the compound has just been withdrawn by the manufacturer because of reports of serious hepatoxicity in a subpopulation of patients.[205] As this short survey illustrates, issues of efficaciousness, bioavailability, and hemorrhage in heparinoids have not been clearly overcome in newly developed agents. Thus, our laboratory and other researchers have attempted to address heparin's limitations by pursuing a more radical direction in heparinoid modification.

18.4.2 POTENTIAL ADVANTAGES OF COVALENT ANTITHROMBIN–HEPARIN COMPLEXES

Given that many of the deleterious effects of heparin occur when it is in the free state, dissociated from its target serpin, concepts were brought forward for permanently stabilizing AT complexes with heparin. A number of theoretical concepts that might logically ensue from the linkage of serpin to GAG incited the design of covalent ATH compounds. A discourse follows on this line of thought.

Many of the likely advantages of AT attachment to heparin revolve around the prevention of heparin dissociation from the inhibitor. Since AT in ATH cannot dissociate from the heparin chain, the serpin will always be in the activated state. Therefore, wherever the conjugated AT is located *in vivo*, it will always be in the most reactive form for inhibition of thrombin, FXa, etc. Furthermore, reaction with this highly activated anticoagulant will not depend on conditions within the fluid phase or tissue environment that might lead to disruption of the noncovalent AT–UFH complex. An added benefit associated with the lack of dissociation of heparin in ATH is that ATH should be readily able to inhibit fibrin clot-bound thrombin. Obviously, ATH heparin cannot detach to generate thrombin–heparin–fibrin complexes[177] that are resistant to inhibition by ATH.[178] Additionally, any attraction of thrombin–fibrin to heparin will necessarily also locate the activated AT moiety in the conjugate close to the bound thrombin for an inhibition reaction to take place. In conjunction with colocalization of ATH to the sites of coagulant insult, permanent complexation of AT with heparin should maintain the active heparin within the vascular space. Since heparin is fixed to AT in ATH, the heparin chains cannot be lost through glomerular filtration as the ATH is vastly increased in size.[141,206] Moreover, loss of activity from the circulation due to plasma or cell surface protein binding is likely to be curtailed because of masking of a significant proportion of the heparin chain that is forcibly associated with the AT polypeptide. Such perpetual interaction of a segment of the heparin will prevent other proteins to approach it because of steric hindrance. A primary advance in heparin application resultant from ATH preparation depends on the synthetic methodology employed. If AT is allowed to interact noncovalently prior to permanent bonding, selection could take place so that only heparin molecules with high-affinity pentasaccharide sequences appear in the ATH product. Thus, in adducts from such protocols, all serpins within the ATH molecules will be activated by a potent pentasaccharide, as opposed to the starting commercial UFH in which only one in three chains have the active sequence.[141,207] Once made, direct enhancement of heparin as an anticoagulant would be observed. Previous studies have indicated that binding of AT to heparin is the rate-determining step in heparin-catalyzed AT inhibition of thrombin.[208] Of course, linkage of heparin to AT eliminates this requirement. Other studies have revealed that a surfeit of heparin allows for simultaneous formation of AT-heparin and thrombin–heparin complexes, which are mutually repulsive.[30] ATH removes this roadblock by making simultaneous occurrence of heparin complexes with AT and thrombin impossible. Other features stemming from effective cloaking of AT surface areas may give ATH superior pharmacodynamics. Stable coverage of the AT polypeptide by heparin polysaccharide should sterically hinder proteases and some glycosidases. Reduction in degradation by this means elongates the circulatory half-life by preventing its conversion to products that are readily eliminated by the liver or spleen. In a similar manner, blockage of heparin–epitope recognition by the conjugated AT could make for a reduced immunological response. Therefore, if a smaller length of the heparin is available for external interactions, ATH may have a lowered induction of thrombocytopenic antibody generation akin to that of a LMWH.[183] In a similar sense, ATH heparin chains may mirror the LMWH's lack of capacity to trigger bone resorption in osteoporosis.[209] Finally, the major hemorrhagic side effects of heparin usage may be moderated if ATH remains in close contact. Platelet binding of ATH could be limited if the AT protein sufficiently interferes with adsorption to the PF4 receptor.[210,211] Alternatively, if ATH binds to PF4, factors responsible for aggregation may be muted by the presence of the AT protein. Overall, almost every category of heparin deficiency seems to be an object for improvement with a simple bonding to the GAG's natural serpin target. If these projections are true, ATH should lend itself to advancements in a number of clinical indications.

The limitations of heparins, to date, that have obstructed a number of its applications may be reachable with some of the enhanced structure and functions intrinsic in ATH. Increased rate of thrombin inhibition by ATH over UFH would significantly improve prophylactic treatment of prothrombotic conditions. If ATH more rapidly inhibits thrombin, then the ultralow concentrations of thrombin formed during the initiation stage of coagulation would not have the opportunity to cause the burst of coagulant activity from feedback activation of FV, FVIII, and FXI. In addition to the dampening of thrombin's activating function, a prolonged half-life of ATH over heparin means that prophylaxis by the conjugate may only require a single bolus injection. Thus, hospital and home care for ATH may be more facile and monitoring may be unnecessary if bleeding risk is lowered by a lack of platelet effects. The possibility that ATH can effectively inhibit clot-bound thrombin gives it a strong endorsement as an antithrombotic treatment agent. Thus, neutralization of fibrin clot-bound thrombin by ATH would be a major breakthrough, given that clot extension is believed to originate from fluid phase activation of coagulation by factors, such as thrombin, residing on the clot surface.[42–44] If the anticoagulant potency of ATH is as avid as suggested, the plasma concentrations required for successful treatment will be relatively low, which bodes well for reduction from the levels of drug that can induce bleeding. An increased half-life due to reduced renal loss adds to the lower estimate of ATH that should be necessary for proper medication and lowered hemorrhagic risk. The difficulty for ATH to pass through tissue because of size constraint leads to another option not available with heparin treatments. Size restriction of ATH could allow for sequestration within various vascular compartments. Therefore, ATH could be used to anticoagulate or pacify a region of interest without causing undesired anticoagulant effects in other spaces. One useful application of this property occurs in the respiratory distress syndrome (RDS) exhibited in premature infants. Underdevelopment of the lung in premature neonates, as well as acute or chronic lung damage in adults, causes permeability of plasma proteins into the airway.[212–214] Proteins of the coagulation cascade are eventually activated to deposit fibrin, a hallmark of RDS that complicates respiration,[215,216] increasing the occurrence and severity of long-term and chronic bronchopulmonary displasia.[217–223] Therefore, a pulmonary anticoagulant treatment could arrest much of the damage and fibrotic disease associated with prematurity. Previous work with UFH has shown that instead of being maintained within the lung, heparin is readily secreted from the alveoli into the systemic circulation.[40] Even if UFH could be retained in the airspace, it is unclear if sufficient amounts of AT are available for UFH to act. ATH may solve this problem. Migration of ATH complex across the lung membrane would be slow if at all, allowing the agent to inhibit coagulation in a concentrated state within the surfactant film on the epithelium. This application may be one of the more outstanding examples to encourage ATH development since it treats a disease state that can be predicted to occur in the premature population and cannot be properly addressed by other known agents. In this case, ATH may be an orphan drug.

18.5 DEVELOPMENT OF COVALENT ANTITHROMBIN–HEPARIN COMPLEXES

18.5.1 Concepts for Covalent Antithrombin–Heparin Synthesis

Forms of ATH incorporating structures with the inherent characteristics discussed above may represent the optimum heparinoid. To achieve this lofty goal, the type of conjugate structure devised will be crucial and dependent on the synthetic algorithm. Three paradigms can be envisaged to permanently link ATH. One option is for heparin molecules to be activated so that they can react with AT to covalently join the two macromolecules. This sequence of ATH preparation is one that may be more commonly followed. It is possible that some heparin derivatives may already possess reactive functional groups that can form a covalent bond with AT under appropriate conditions or with assistant reagents. Another alternative is that groups on AT can be activated so as to allow covalent bonding to heparin. Methodology of this type may define points on the AT polypeptide from which linkage to the heparin chain can be made. A third possibility is to allow AT and heparin to interact for noncovalent-binding associations to occur, followed by stabilization of the complex by using a bifunctional agent. Thus, one end of the bifunctional compound will covalently bond to AT, and the opposite end of the bifunctional compound will react with the heparin. In all the three reaction types, there is the theoretical possibility that, once activated, heparin molecules may become linked together or AT molecules may become bonded to themselves. To avoid these undesirable side products, careful designs must be employed using selective chemistries, particular stoichiometries, or special conditions that prevent their formation.

Consideration of conjugation by heparin activation involves awareness of the groups on GAGs that can be feasibly activated. Heparin functional groups that are candidates for activation (or are activated) include sulfonyl, carboxyl, amino, hydroxyl, and acetal. Both amino and acetal groups can potentially provide linkage through the heparin chain terminus, while sulfonyl and carboxyl groups would give bonds within the heparin molecule. Preference may tend toward heparin-chain terminus bonding to the AT polypeptide if structures similar to a core protein with glycosidically linked GAG chains found in heparin proteoglycans[116] are desirable. However, amino or acetal groups for end-point attachment of heparin to AT may be scarce, leaving the binding through internal functional groups on heparin potentially more practical. Some standard procedures can be applied for preactivation of heparin leading to ATH preparation. Carboxyl groups on heparins can be reacted with carbodiimide to produce an active intermediate that can then react with amino or hydroxyl groups from AT N-terminal, lysyl, seryl, or threonyl residues yielding amide or ester covalent linkages. ATH production using this protocol would directly join AT to the GAG. However, steric issues and optimum orientation of heparin with respect to the AT may preclude the development of useful complexes without first activating the internal heparin carboxyls with a spacer arm. Coupling through AT may have more options for chemically activatable groups but protocols may be more complicated. Amino acid R-groups include carboxyl, alkyl hydroxyl, phenyl hydroxyl, amino, imino, thiol, and thio ether, which provide a wide range of potential reactions to be exploited. However, the diversity of functional groups that could be activated for conjugation can, in themselves, interfere or overlap with each other leading to nonselectivity of linkage type and number or intramolecular AT linkage. Additionally, AT tertiary structure engenders a range of environments that alter reactivity of any one functional R-group type. Therefore, chemistries for activation and linkage must be more refined to get a consistent ATH yielded from initial activation of a small number of loci on AT. A potential example of ATH preparation by AT activation would be to react AT with N-hydroxysuccinimidyl-4-azidobenzoate. This reaction would give a photoactivatable benzoyl-amide on a lysyl amino. Incubation of this AT derivative with heparin, followed by treatment with light, gives bonding between the benzoyl linker and heparin. Some selectivity by AT activation protocols is possible by use of the AT glycans that are on the exterior of the protein and have some structures not observed in the polypeptide moiety. Thus, AT can be mildly treated with $NaIO_4$, which reacts with vicinal hydroxyls (at C8 and C9) on terminal N-acetylneuraminic acid residues of the glycans to give active aldehyde groups. The AT-aldehyde derivative can then be reacted with diamino-alkane + $NaBH_3CN$ to give an AT with a prominent alkyl-amine that will preferentially (relative to other AT R-groups) react with N-hydroxysuccin-imidyl-4-azidobenzoate to yield a photosensitive group for heparin coupling as above. The advantages of linkage through AT-glycan activation are that linkage location(s) is/are more controlled and the critical sites on the polypeptide, where enzyme reaction and heparin-binding reside, are unperturbed. Synthesis of ATH by simultaneous reaction with ATH by a bifunctional reagent or spacer is more complicated than initial activation of the serpin or the GAG alone. Since AT has R-groups with similar reactivity to functional groups on heparin, differentiation of heparin functional groups from those of AT is not practical. To somewhat control linkage points, it would be advisable to use hetero-bifunctional reagents that can select for AT R-groups not represented on heparin. Thus, at least one end of the bifunctional agent could be directed to a particular subset of locations on the AT as an anchor for positioning linkage on the heparin. To illustrate this concept, a reagent terminating with a vicinal dione would selectively react with the guanidinyl R-group of an AT arginyl residue. Linkage to heparin could then be completed at the opposite end of the reagent by a $-N(CH_3)_3^+$ group (attractive to polyanionic heparin) and a photoactivatable $-N_3$ function. The bifunctional linkage approach does allow for unmodified ATH to form a native complex prior to covalent stabilization. Unfortunately, even the most sophisticated approaches seem to lack selectivity on the placement of linkage points, and prevention of multilinkages that lead to reduced product activity is difficult.

As stated, formation of permanent linkage to AT through activated groups on the heparin species has been the main algorithm followed for ATH synthesis. The robust nature of heparin for performance of activation chemistries and minimal functional group types make for increased simplicity in method design.

18.5.2 CHEMICAL STRUCTURES AND *In Vitro* ACTIVITIES

Evolution of ATH design has followed a chronology that is illustrative of issues impacting product yield and anticoagulant functionality. Several reports have described isolation of noncovalent AT-UFH complexes.[224–227] However, without covalent bonds to hold the ATH together, even the most robust complexes are unlikely to be secure against dissociation by interaction with the vast array of molecules and cell surfaces *in vivo*.

Early endeavors toward permanently bonded AT–heparin utilized knowledge gained from investigations of chemical linkage of heparin to polymer surfaces and other macromolecules. Heparin coupling to albumin[228,229] and polysaccharides[230] gave insight into useful conjugation chemistries to build on. About 25 years ago Ceustermans et al. gave a broad survey of potential chemical routes attempting to realize ATH.[231] In one procedure, cyanogen bromide (CNBr) activated UFH (using the method of Cuatrecasas et al.)[232] was mixed with AT but no significant ATH was detected. Given that CNBr is most reactive with the few amino groups[231] of heparin molecules, attachment of active groups would be minimized. Consequently, many of the small number of CNBr activation points might also be distant from potential linkage groups on AT during noncovalent complexation. Other reaction schemes followed. Attempts were made to bind AT and UFH with the bifunctional 1,5-difluoro-2,4-dinitrobenzene,[231] according to the procedure of Zahn and Meienhofer[233,234] without success, again likely due to a paucity of heparin amino groups for nucleophilic substitution at the benzene ring. AT was modified with active groups by photochemical reaction with either 4-fluoro-3-nitrophenyl azide or 4-azido-phenacyl bromide and then mixed with heparin.[235–238] Negligible yields ensued, potentially arising from either intramolecular cross-linking reactions within AT or from lack of heparin–amino acceptor groups.

Finally, significant yields of AT–heparin conjugate were achieved by Ceustermans et al.[231] Preliminary attempts involved reaction of heparin with tolylene-2,4-diisocyanate according to the method of Clyne et al.[239–241] using basic conditions to increase amino (or hydroxyl) reactivity with the isocyanates. A very modest yield ($\leq$5%) was realized that was much reduced in ice-cold pH 9.5 borate because of accelerated hydrolysis of the isocyanates on the substituted heparin, prior to addition of AT. However, heparin modification with the more stable tolylene-2,4-diisothiocyanate (TDTC) according to Edman and Henschen,[242] prior to reaction with AT in pH 8.5 bicarbonate, gave a much improved 30% yield.[231] Further optimization of the process followed with the introduction of amino groups into the starting heparin. This was accomplished either by partial desulfation of glucosamine aminos or by the attachment of amino-terminating spacer arms to uronic acid carboxyls.[231] UFH was first chromatographed on immobilized AT to obtain the high-affinity fraction for modification. The pyridinium salt of high-affinity heparin, prepared by pyridine titration of the heparinic acid form, obtained by passage through Dowex 50, was partially N-desulfated by incubation in 95% dimethylsulfoxide at 23°C for 0.5 h.[243,244] Alternatively, high-affinity heparin was conjugated through the uronic carboxyl groups to 1,6-diamino-hexane using a carbodiimide.[231] Both amino-modified heparins were reacted with TDTC (in excess to the amino groups present) to give products with isothiocyanate functions for linkage with AT. Incorporation of isothiocyanate groups was improved 2-fold by partial N-desulfation and 2.9-fold by hexyl-amino modification.[231] However, ATH yield from either N-desulfated or hexyl-amino heparins remained at approximately 30% and up to 25% of the product molecules contained two ATs per heparin chain.[231] Table 18.1 gives activities from analyses of materials in such studies. N-desulfation decreased activated partial thromboplastin time (APTT), clotting time by 35% and anti-FXa activity (measuring ability to catalyze reaction of FXa with added AT) by 24%, compared to the starting high-affinity heparin (Table 18.1). Addition of hexyl-amino groups disrupted heparin function to an even greater degree causing 44% loss in APTT and 39% loss in anti-FXa (Table 18.1). Major functional reduction in both partially N-desulfated heparin and carboxyl-linked diamino-hexyl heparin would be expected since N-sulfates and carboxyls are key structures responsible for heparin anticoagulant activity.[245] Noncatalytic direct inhibition of FXa by hexyl-amino ATH was measured to have a second order rate constant of 2.1×10^6 M^{-1} s^{-1} (Table 18.1), one-third of that value was for noncovalent mixtures of high-affinity heparin and saturating amounts of AT.[231] It is possible that not all AT was being activated by the conjugated heparin since supplementation with additional heparin significantly increased the rate of FXa inhibition by the hexyl-amino ATH.[231] To eliminate inactive complexes (some of which may contain two AT per heparin chain), purification of hexyl-amino ATH product was performed on sepharose-conconavalin A,[246] in addition to chromatographic separations by ion exchange, gel filtration, and sepharose-AT.[231] Tests on the direct inhibition of thrombin by this highly purified hexyl-amino ATH gave a second order rate constant of 6.7×10^8 M^{-1} s^{-1} and a biomolecular rate constant of 2.5×10^8 M^{-1} s^{-1}, which was similar to the bimolecular thrombin inhibition rate of 2.2×10^8 M^{-1} s^{-1} for high-affinity heparin and saturating AT.[246] ATH was prepared by Hoylaerts et al. from high-AT-affinity hexyl-amino-derivatized molecular weight fractions (M_r = 4300 or 3200) of HNO$_2$-reacted UFH but complexes gave reduced second order rate constants for direct thrombin inhibition (2×10^7 M^{-1} s^{-1} and 3×10^5 M^{-1} s^{-1} for 4300 and 3200 M_r fractions, respectively) relative to ATH from full-length heparin.[246] This is consistent with a loss in the required heparin-binding of thrombin with short LMWH chains during inhibition by AT.[155]

Work by Björk et al., around the same time period as Ceustermans et al., resulted in ATH that was attached to the end groups of partially depolymerized heparin fragments.[247] High-AT-affinity fractions of HNO$_2$-treated UFH (having MW ranging from 3700[247] to 10,000[248] using this partial depolymerization protocol) were incubated with AT + NaBH$_3$CN.[247] In this system, the aldehydes on anhydromannose terminal residues of the heparin fragment form metastable Schiff bases with AT lysyl ε-amino groups, that are fixed by reduction.[247] ATH was separated from unreacted LMWH by gel filtration and finally isolated from unreacted AT on a heparin agarose column, to give an yield of 40% ATH from the starting AT. Since the coupling reaction occurs only at one active group

TABLE 18.1

Anticoagulant Activities of Heparins and Covalent Antithrombin–Heparin Complexes

			Activity							
			Antifactor Xa Catalytic Activity (U mg^{-1})			Antithrombin Catalytic Activity (U mg^{-1})			ATH + FXa Reaction Rate (M^{-1} s^{-1})	ATH + Thrombin Reaction Rate (M^{-1} s^{-1})
Methods	Start. Heparin	APTT of Mod. Heparin (% Start. Heparin)	Start. Heparin	Mod. Heparin	ATH	Start. Heparin	Mod. Heparin	ATH		
1	High-affinity UFH	65 ± 5	250	191 ± 28	—	—	—	—	—	—
2	High-affinity UFH	56 ± 7	250	153 ± 34	270	—	—	—	2.1 × 10^6	6.7 × 10^8
3	UFH modified to LMWH	—	~170 (UFH)	140 (LMWH)	5.2	~170 (UFH)	0 (LMWH)	0	—	—
4	UFH	—	168	—	Low	168	—	Low	—	6.7 × 10^7
5	UFH	100	209	209	861	198	198	754	3.8 × 10^6	3.1 × 10^9

Start. heparin, Initial source of heparin used for studies; APTT, activated partial thromboplastin time; Mod. heparin, activated heparin used for conjugation with antithrombin; ATH, covalent antithrombin–heparin complex; UFH, unfractionated heparin; LMWH, low molecular weight heparin. Methods: (1) ATH prepared by tolylene-2,4-diisothiocyanate linkage of N-desulfated high-affinity heparin to antithrombin;[231] (2) ATH prepared by tolylene-2,4-diisothiocyanate linkage of hexyl-amino substituted high-affinity heparin to antithrombin;[231,246,272] (3) ATH prepared by reduction by NaBH$_3$CN of Schiff base between aldehyde on high-affinity anhydromannose-terminating heparin and amino on antithrombin;[247,249] (4) ATH prepared by reaction of CNBr-activated heparin and antithrombin;[250,251] and (5) ATH prepared by Amadori rearrangement of Schiff base between aldehyde on aldose-terminating unfractionated heparin and amino on antithrombin.[141,261,264] on the terminus of each LMWH molecule, the chains are all connected to the AT moiety in the same way. The anti-FXa activity reported for the LMWH used was slightly lower than that of starting UFH (Table 18.1) and analyses showed that conjugates contain an average of 0.7 chains per AT.[247] Experiments with mixtures of Björk et al. ATH + FXa indicated that 98% of the complex was active and, unlike starting LMWH + AT, reactions with Björk et al. ATH were only mildly reduced by 1 M NaCl or polybrene (suggesting that the covalent linkage prevented disruption of AT activation by the LMWH).[247] Lack of polybrene neutralizability would prevent the capability of reversing anticoagulation by the agent if there were hemorrhagic complications. Assays of the LMWH used for Björk et al. ATH gave no detectable anti-thrombin catalytic activity (Table 18.1),[249] making the complex ineffective against thrombin. Thus, the Björk et al. complex could not address thrombin feedback of the coagulation cascade.

Mitra and Jordan, who were able to overcome previous failures employing CNBr as an activating reagent, have reported another active ATH product.[250] UFH + 57-fold molar excess of CNBr were reacted at pH 10.7 for 40 min at 23°C. After dialysis under basic conditions to remove unreacted CNBr, the activated heparin was reacted with AT (1 mol heparin per 0.02 mol AT) at pH 9.4 for 18 h at 5°C. During incubation, cyanate/iminocarbonate/N-nitrile active groups on the modified heparin reacted with lysyl amino groups on the AT to form amidine ester ($-O-CNH-NH-$), urethane ($-O-CO-NH-$), guanidine ($-NH-CNH-NH-$), or urea ($-NH-CO-NH-$) linkages. Removal of free heparin using immobilized Concanavalin A and removal of unreacted AT by heparin-sepharose chromatography gave a 40% yield of ATH with respect to starting AT.[250] Although no data was reported on the number of activated groups initially incorporated into the heparin by CNBr,[250] use of glycine to block excess active cyanate/iminocarbonate/N-nitrile groups after AT coupling[250,251] suggests that there was more than one reactive group per heparin and likely $\geq$ 1 GAG per AT in the final conjugate. Thrombin and FXa titrations of Mitra and Jordan ATH indicated that almost the entire product had potent inhibitory activity. Furthermore, the Mitra et al. ATH exhibited elevated fluorescence (relative to free AT) that was not enhanced further by addition of UFH, indicative of the fact that the AT moiety in all ATH molecules was fully activated by the covalently bonded heparin. Experiments studying inhibition of thrombin and FXa by Mitra and Jordan ATH in plasma suggested that inhibitory capacity was solely from direct reaction, with no extra catalytic activity evident.[250,251] Rate experiments were performed with Mitra and Jordan ATH + thrombin at equimolar concentrations, which allow for calculation of a biomolecular rate constant.[250] Results for the ATH gave a biomolecular rate of 6.7×10^7 M^{-1} s^{-1} (Table 18.1), while similar experiments with noncovalent AT + high-AT-affinity heparin gave a biomolecular thrombin inhibition rate of 2.0×10^7 M^{-1} s^{-1}, 3.3-fold slower than for Mitra and Jordan ATH. However, due to the fact that measurements were not made with inhibitor concentrations at 5 to 10 times greater than the enzyme (pseudofirst order conditions), comparison of the absolute reaction rates between covalent and noncovalent complexes is not possible.

Recent work by Chan et al.[141] has provided a new direction in ATH development. The fundamental difference in Chan et al.'s ATH construction is that no prior modification of either the AT or UFH reactants used to make the conjugate is required. Preparation of conjugate relies on novel observations on natural spontaneous reactions *in vivo* and the presence of a subpopulation of molecules within many commercial UFHs. Investigations in diabetic patients have established that hemoglobin and several plasma proteins undergo spontaneous glycation. Schiff base formation occurs between the C1 aldehyde of the open chain form of plasma glucose and the ε-amino of blood protein lysyl residues.[252] Bonding between sugar and polypeptide is stabilized by tautomeric Amadori rearrangement of protons on the glucosyl C1 and C2 to an ene-ol-amine and, eventually, a stable keto-amine.[252] The formation of these long-lived products in diabetics is significantly affected by glucose concentration, availability of amino groups, pH, and temperature. Nonenzymatic glycation of proteins has been shown to have measurable effects on the function of the molecule.[253] For example, brief increases in circulating glucose were shown to coincide with transient changes in AT activity,[254] while long-term exposure to high-glucose concentrations led to significant decreases in AT function,[255] a potential basis for development of thrombosis in severe diabetics.[256] Mechanistically, short-term interaction of glucose with AT may only produce temporary effects from the reversible Schiff base complex, while longer glucose incubation will lead to impact from the permanent Amadori product. Interestingly, it has been demonstrated that heparin's catalysis of AT reactivity can be inhibited by nonenzymatic AT glycation *in vitro*[257] and *in vivo*.[257] These data, combined with the observation that inhibitory effects of glycation on heparin activation of AT could be overcome by incubation with Na heparin before assay,[257] suggest that Schiff base/Amadori rearrangement products are formed at a particular residue that interacts closely with heparin. This selective glycation hypothesis was further strengthened by the fact that incubation of AT with 5 mM glucose for 10 days resulted in uptake of just 0.6 mol of glycose per mole of protein.[256] Other studies have shown that several residues on AT can form stable keto-amines.[258] However, even reactions with 0.5 M glucose lead to only one glucosyl modification per AT,[258] inferring that further glycation is unlikely if the protein is already glycated at one site. All these findings have given impetus to a novel potential mode for AT conjugation. Since heparin can affect and is affected by glycation of AT, aldose-containing heparin molecules may be capable of forming Schiff base or Amadori structures at particular sites in AT. As an adjunct to this concept, previous studies have revealed that a small portion of heparin molecules in fact terminate in aldose residues as opposed to a serine glycoside cap.[207] Thus, simple incubation of ATH under physiological conditions may yield covalent ATH. However, the prevailing thought in the field of nonenzymatic glycation has been that Schiff base–Amadori rearrangement of proteins with aldose-terminating polysaccharides is highly improbable. Although Amadori adducts have formed between insulin and maltose disaccharide,[259] it was considered that occurrence of Schiff bases between protein amino groups and polysaccharides is remote given that the aldose-end group represents a minor proportion of all residues in the polymer, approach of polysaccharide to the protein is much more sterically hindered, and the terminal aldose is much more likely to be in the hemiacetal (masked aldehyde) form.[260] As a consequence, spontaneous glycation between polypeptide amines and polysaccharide aldose-termini remained unexplored.

Chan et al. have conducted intensive experimentation to determine if practical preparation of ATH is feasible by either Schiff base and Amadori rearrangement or reduction of Schiff bases between AT and commercial UFH. Given that AT binds to and is activated by heparin through a high-affinity pentasaccharide, it would be important to develop a reaction setup, which allows for AT selection of heparin molecules where this active sequence is located close to the aldose terminus. Since only around 10% of molecules in commercial UFH contain a free aldose[207] and only about one-third of UFH chains have a pentasaccharide,[207] it was deemed that a 200 molar excess of UFH relative to AT may be necessary.[141] Trial experiments with various polypeptides and polysaccharides showed that glycation of protein by the polysaccharide aldose gave variable yields for a number of factors.[261] One critical issue was reaction temperature. Previous studies have shown that incubation of monosaccharide aldose with AT can increase the temperature at which thermal denaturation of the protein occurs.[262] As a corollary, it might be possible that increased temperature may be necessary to induce the conformation desired for linkage during aldose interaction with AT. Indeed, experiments revealed that while yields (in terms of AT) of ATH were ~5% at 37°C, production improved to 50% at 40°C.[261] An ATH synthetic method was standardized with heating of AT and UFH in phosphate-buffered saline (PBS) for 14 days, followed by removal of free heparin by hydrophobic chromatography and further purification by anion exchange to isolate conjugate from unreacted AT.[141] Analyses have verified that the resultant ATH contained one heparin per AT.[141,206] ATH product was partially digested with protease and heparin-containing peptides sequenced to determine the heparin linkage location within the AT polypeptide. Analyses determined that in the vast majority of ATH molecules (87%) the heparin aldose was bonded to the N-terminal amino group, followed by a minor subpopulation of complexes containing heparin chains linked to the ε-amino at Lys139.[263]

ATH prepared by Chan et al. displayed a rate for direct neutralization of FXa (Table 18.1) that was on par with the maximal value for noncovalent AT + high-affinity heparin.[264] With respect to thrombin, ATH prepared by Chan et al. possessed an extremely rapid second-order rate constant of 3.1×10^9 M^{-1} s^{-1} (Table 18.1),[141] one of the fastest ever reported. This potency may well have been derived from the fact that, unlike other ATH products, unmodified (undamaged) UFH is used in high molar excess to prepare the Chan et al. complex, which allows for selection by AT of the most active subpopulation of GAGs. Chan et al. ATH is also augmented during synthesis by the preferential coupling of heparin to the β-isoform of AT which, in combination with heparin, reacts at a two-fold faster rate than that for α-AT.[265] Further studies have established that Chan et al. ATH directly inhibits many of the activated coagulation factors at a much faster rate than noncovalent AT + UFH mixtures.[266] An unexpected finding was that the Chan et al. conjugate had potent activity for catalysis of exogenous AT inhibition of FXa and thrombin that was greater than the starting UFH or high-AT-affinity heparin (Table 18.1).[141] From in-depth studies, it has been discovered that heparin chains of ATH have at least one pentasaccharide and some 30–50% of the ATH heparin moieties have at least two high-AT-affinity sequences.[264] Other workers have reported that 1–3% of UFH molecules indeed have more than one high-affinity binding site for AT.[142,267] Given the vast surfeit of UFH over AT during reaction, the long incubation times during synthesis allowed for sampling of heparin molecules by AT until binding occurs by a pentasaccharide that is close to the aldose for covalent linkage to occur. In this sense, multipentasaccharide heparins would be preferred since dissociation by AT from one pentasaccharide would more likely lead to a short diffusion to the second pentasaccharide sequence on the same heparin chain (closer to the aldose terminus), as opposed to a longer distance of travel between heparin molecules. Further *in vitro* investigations have confirmed the anticoagulant utility of Chan et al. ATH. Comparisons between the conjugate and various heparinoids in activated plasma systems showed Chan et al. ATH to have superior efficacy in controlling thrombin generation. The covalent complex was more effective than either UFH or LMWH, at equivalent anti-FXa doses, in preventing contact phase-activated thrombin generation in adults, children, or newborn plasmas.[268] Experiments with a variety of activators further illustrated the increased avidity of Chan et al.'s ATH for inhibiting thrombin generation in hemophilic plasma relative to UFH and LMWH.[269] In all cases, the rapid neutralization by the Schiff base or Amadori ATH complex of the initial thrombin responsible for feedback activation of the cascade, coupled with the strong catalytic capacity to prevent further propagation of thrombin generation, would enhance its capability over other heparinoids.

18.5.3 EFFECTS *In Vivo*

In vivo testing of ATH complexes has been reported, with much of the data describing recent work with the Chan et al. compound. Primary investigations give information on pharmacokinetics, while some antithrombotic and hemorrhagic results are available from pathological animal models to assess functional potential in clinical disease states. A partial collection of pharmacokinetic data is given in Table 18.2.

ATH produced by Ceustermans et al. from N-desulfated, high-affinity heparin displayed biphasic disappearance from plasma in rabbits consisting of a short first phase or α-phase and slightly longer second or β-phase (Table 18.2).[231] In comparison, Ceustermans et al. ATH made from high-affinity hexyl-amino-modified heparin had a single α-phase elimination from plasma of slightly longer duration (Table 18.2).[231] Plasma half-lives for both these compounds were not more than three times longer than that for UFH in rabbits (single α-phase of 0.23 ± 0.03 h) and much shorter than the 11.0 ± 0.4 h determined for AT in the rabbit model.[231] Hastening of elimination for the hexyl-amino ATH complexes could well be expected through interaction with plasma and cell surface proteins, given the reports of binding by these ATH materials to histidine-rich glycoprotein.[172] ATH preparations of hexyl-amino derivatized LMWHs gave improved intravenous β-phase half-lives of 7–8 h (Table 18.2),[270,271] which was again about threefold longer than the corresponding

TABLE 18.2

Plasma Clearance of Heparins and Covalent Antithrombin–Heparin Complexes

	Intravenous Half-Life (h)		
Method	Heparin Precursor	ATH (α-Phase)	ATH (β-Phase)
1	0.23 ± 0.03	<0.5	0.65 ± 0.06
2	0.23 ± 0.03	0.89 ± 0.26	—
3	2.35 ± 0.17	1	7.85 ± 0.18
4	2.50 ± 0.18	1	7.63 ± 0.75
5	—	>UFH	—
6	—	<3	—
7	0.32	2.6	13

Methods: (1) ATH prepared by tolylene-2,4-diisothiocyanate linkage of N-desulfated high-affinity heparin to antithrombin;[231] (2) ATH prepared by tolylene-2,4-diisothiocyanate linkage of hexyl-amino substituted high-affinity heparin to antithrombin;[231,246,272] (3) ATH prepared by tolylene-2,4-diisothiocyanate linkage of hexyl-amino substituted high-affinity low–molecular weight heparin (MW = 3200) to antithrombin;[271,314] (4) ATH prepared by tolylene-2,4-diisothiocyanate linkage of hexyl-amino substituted high-affinity low–molecular weight heparin (MW = 4300) to antithrombin;[271,314] (5) ATH prepared by reduction by NaBH$_3$CN of Schiff base between aldehyde on anhydromannose-terminating heparin and amino on antithrombin;[247,249] (6) ATH prepared by reaction of CNBr-activated heparin and antithrombin;[250,251] and (7) ATH prepared by Amadori rearrangement of Schiff base between aldehyde on aldose-terminating unfractionated heparin and amino on antithrombin.[141,261,264]

free GAGs (half-lives of 3200 and 4300 LMWHs were 2.35 ± 0.17 h and 2.50 ± 0.18 h, respectively).[270] To test antithrombotic activity for hexyl-amino UFH- or LMWH-containing ATH, a Wessler rabbit thrombus prevention model was used, whereby, after systemic injection of different doses of test compounds, glass-activated plasma was incubated in a jugular vein segment for 10 min to semiquantitatively assess diminution of thrombus growth within the vessel.[272] When activated plasma was placed in the vessel segment up to 45–60 min after administration of anticoagulant, similar clot sizes were observed for all conjugates relative to equal mass doses of the corresponding noncovalent AT + heparinoid mixtures. When activated plasma was introduced from 60 to 120 min after anticoagulant injection, a reduction in size and number of thrombi was observed for the ATH products relative to noncovalent mixtures because of increased half-lives of the conjugates.[272] No data on bleeding side effects of Ceustermans et al. ATH is available. Regarding Björk et al. ATH, intravenous bolus injection of small amounts into 12-week-old mice gave successful antibody production against the human AT-containing complex,[249] although no pharmacokinetics was reported. Observations of low nonspecific binding to surface molecules of hybridoma cells[249] may indicate that the Björk et al. conjugate might have an increased intravenous half-life from reduced affinity for *in vivo* protein binding. However, a low 5.2 unit mg^{-1} anti-FXa activity measured for the conjugate in these studies makes for a dubious antithrombotic potential. More extensive study of *in vivo* efficacy of the Mitra and Jordan ATH has been done.[250,251] Blood samples were taken from rabbits after completion of intravenous infusion with 84 or 200 anti-FXa units kg^{-1} of ATH or UFH at 2 mL kg^{-1}. APTT tests of the samples showed functional activity for

ATH that was significantly longer than that for UFH and persisted up to 3 h after stoppage of perfusion.[250] The prolonged intravenous pharmacokinetics of Mitra and Jordan ATH over short half-life of UFH[273] would allow lower dosages to give successful prophylactic effects. Actual antithrombotic comparisons between the Mitra and Jordan product and other heparins *in vivo* may be warranted.

Extensive *in vivo* investigation of the Chan et al. keto-amine-linked ATH has been accomplished. Half-life studies in rabbits disclosed an intravenous α-phase (two-compartment model) half-life for both mass assay and anti-FXa activity of 2.5–2.6 h (Table 18.2), eightfold longer than UFH and fivefold shorter than the α-phase of AT.[141] The β-phase (three-compartment model) intravenous half-life for keto-amine ATH was measured to be 13 h (Table 18.2),[141] which was the longest disappearance value reported for ATH complexes to date. Investigation of nonselective plasma protein binding, a known mechanism for elimination of heparin activity, showed that Chan et al. complex had less binding than UFH, approaching that of LMWH.[274] Additional experiments indicated that uptake onto endothelial surfaces remarkably decreased for the keto-amine conjugate compared to UFH in noncovalent AT–UFH complexes,[274] which would allay loss of this ATH from the circulation by vessel wall binding. Given that Chan et al. ATH is prepared by simple incubation of unaltered commercial UFH with AT, an intriguing possibility exists that such a stable complex might already be generated from aldose-heparinoids *in vivo*. Attempts to isolate ATH after several bolus UFH injections were successful in obtaining a small quantity of identifiable product,[261] consistent with the potential for generation of conjugate from vascular AT and endogenous, nonprotein linked, heparin chains that are known to circulate in humans.[275–277] Subcutaneous administration of Chan et al. ATH resulted in very poor systemic adsorption but activities persisted up to 96 h after injection, with peak levels occurring at 24–30 h.[141] The much reduced capability, relative to UFH,[40] of the large keto-amine conjugate to pass through extravascular tissue suggested the ATH may be retained in sequestered spaces for applications such as anticoagulation treatment in the lung during RDS.[214,278–281] As a confirmation, intratracheal instillation of Chan et al. ATH into adult rabbits resulted in significant AT concentrations and anti-FXa activity in lavage fluids 48 h after treatment, without any of the human ATH antigen detected systemically.[141] Further experiments in full-term newborn rats demonstrated detectable anti-FXa activity in lavage fluid even 96 h after airway instillation of the complex. Moreover, even if lavaging did not retrieve the entire instilled activity and there was no evidence of ATH permeability into the circulation, anticoagulant or antithrombotic functioning of ATH on internal lung surfaces would still be the primary purpose for sequestration as premature newborn lungs develop. As evidence, experiments showed that Chan et al. ATH inhibited plasma-thrombin generation on fetal-distal-lung epithelium *in vitro* much more effectively than noncovalent AT and UFH,[282] or even covalent complexes of UFH or dermatan sulfate with heparin cofactor II[283] prepared by similar Schiff base or Amadori rearrangement chemistry.[284] Analysis of the data showed that the rapid rate of direct, noncatalytic inhibition of initial thrombin feedback activation of the cascade was a critical part of ATH's enhanced ability to inhibit expression of thrombin activity on epithelial surfaces.[282] Animal studies also validated keto-amine ATH as a superior systemic antithrombotic agent. Preformed thrombi in a rabbit jugular vein model had lower fibrin accretion and were reduced in size by a single ATH bolus injection, while clot size increased with similar mg kg^{-1} doses of AT + UFH noncovalent mixtures.[285] Other experiments showed that, at equivalent anti-FXa doses, Chan et al. ATH possessed significantly greater prophylactic capacity against thrombi formation than UFH in a rabbit arterial thrombosis prevention model.[286] Examination of interactions with fibrin–monomer proved that the covalent complex could prevent clot formation and extension by neutralizing fibrin-bound thrombin,[286,287] which can become protected from noncovalent AT-UFH by inclusion within thrombin–UFH–fibrin ternary complexes.[288] Hemorrhagic side effects were reduced for ATH versus infused equimolar mixtures of AT + UFH at similar plasma anti-FXa activities in rabbit bleeding ear experiments.[285] Indeed, bleeding risk to antithrombotic benefit analysis demonstrated a highly significant improvement over UFH for the ATH formed by Schiff base or Amadori rearrangement.[286]

18.6 SURFACE COATING WITH COVALENT ANTITHROMBIN–HEPARIN COMPLEXES

18.6.1 Chemistry and *In Vitro* Characterization

Pacification of blood-contacting biomaterial surfaces with ATH complexes has only been reported using the Chan et al. keto-amine adduct. In order to use ATH on devices used as blood conduits *ex vivo* or *in vivo*, chemistries had to be devised that took into consideration all the technical and biochemical issues that have caused serious impediments for biomaterial application.

As with the clinical application of heparin, biomaterials in contact with blood have a whole plethora of limitations from inappropriate activation of biomaterial surface-bound platelets and polymorphonucleocytes,[289,290] effects on flow from surface-bound plasma proteins that recruit increasing layers of cells, induction of blood or tissue cell inflammatory response,[291] complement activation,[292] and activation of coagulation. Historically, surface induction of coagulation has been the most problematic issue and various coatings have been applied to make surfaces less thrombogenic. Many coatings have inherent problems such as nonhomogeneous surface coverage, leaching of anticoagulant coating off the surface, or interactions with biological molecules that modify the coated surface, leaving it inactive or even procoagulant. Engineering design of chemistries to address the optimization of applying the desired agent onto the surface might be grouped into three broad methodology categories. Anticoagulant molecules might be coated by simple noncovalent adsorption, covalently bound to a polymer base coat that is itself not covalently linked to the device surface, or covalently bound (through an intervening linkage molecule) to the surface being coated. Noncovalent adsorption has the potential of maximal packing, which may more completely cover the surface, but loss of coating by mild interactions with macromolecules or by changing conditions *in vivo* would always remain a concern. As a consequence, noncovalent adsorption coating of anticoagulant molecules has been generally discounted as a viable option. Bonding of the anticoagulant molecule to a base polymer coating that is not covalently linked to the device surface can give good substitution, but strong abrasions may still be able to pull off large sections of the coverage. To optimize its prevention, careful selection must be made to use base coat monomers that have high affinity for the biomaterial, so as to get tight adhesion and dense covering before or at polymerization. Although covalent linkage of the agent being coated to the biomaterial surface itself would be the most secure, activation of the biomaterial for linkage can require harsh conditions that negatively alter its properties and complete coverage may be less likely. Potentially, either of the latter two coating methodologies may be more appropriate dependent on the biomaterial in question.

Coatings of covalent ATH may have theoretical aspects that might solve many problems associated with previous anticoagulant films on biomaterials. As with heparan sulfate in proteoglycans naturally found on the luminal side of vessels,[293] surface attachment of ATH would present the anticoagulant heparin chain in the proper orientation to interact with the blood coagulant system. Furthermore, the coating would already have an AT protein that may inhibit binding of further, unwanted, proteins from the circulation. Both AT[294] and heparin[295] have antiinflammatory properties and little immune response may be anticipated given that AT, heparin, and the Amadori rearrangement bonding are all natural products. In the case of Chan et al. ATH, the additional catalytic potency from ~1.5 pentasaccharides per heparin chain,[264] combined with the extremely rapid direct noncatalytic inhibition rate,[141] should be vastly superior to coatings of unprocessed commercial heparin or LMWH products. Thus, ATH combines the strengths of coatings of indirect (heparin) and direct (hirudin) thrombin inhibitors. Technical advantages are cogent for coating with ATH as opposed to many other anticoagulant agents. Unlike heparin alone, the AT in ATH affords many more functional groups for bonding to agents linking the anticoagulant to the device polymer surface. Apart from the numerous R-groups, human AT is endowed with many nucleophilic $-NH_2$ groups from its 37 lysyl ε-aminos,[61] whereas heparin amino groups are scarce.[231] Related to the preponderance of AT functional groups in ATH is the fact that multiple covalent bonds to the surface are easily foreseeable by attachment through the AT of ATH, as opposed to the difficulty of having multiple linkage points to heparin alone without potentially modifying groups within the pentasaccharide sequence. With multiple bonds to the ATH coating, leaching is less likely. In case of heparin coatings, it is precisely to avoid conjugation to the surface through the active sequences that end-point attachments have been developed, which indeed give better blood compatibility.

Several biomaterials composed of synthetic polymers used commercially *in vivo* have been coated with Chan et al. ATH using an array of chemical coating methods. Physical integrity, structural characteristics, and anticoagulant activities *in vitro* have been assessed. These are discussed with reference to the type of biomaterial and linkage chemistry used.

Attachment of keto-amine-linked ATH to an endoluminal graft, composed of polycarbonate with urethane extenders, has been achieved by direct covalent linkage.[296] The graft (Corethane) provided by Corvita Corporation was made from a finely woven material that was attached, through its weave to a stainless steel mesh that was flexible for elasticity during insertion within the blood vessel. Internal diameter of the graft was from 3 to 6 mm and wall thickness was <1 mm. Bonding was through urethane nitrogen atoms using chemistry based on the radical-initiated polymerization on poly(N-chloroamide) donor surfaces.[297] After modification of N-atoms using NaOCl, oligomeric chain growth of allyl glycidyl ether units was initiated by $-N\bullet$ radicals produced by concomitant reaction of the graft $-N-Cl$ groups with $Na_2S_2O_4$ or $Fe(NH_4)_2(SO_4)_2\cdot6H_2O$.[296] Previous work has ascertained that oligomers tend to contain 1–4.6 allyl glycidyl ether monomer units per point of attachment.[298,299] Once attachment of allyl glycidyl ethers was complete, endoluminal grafts were washed and incubated with ATH for reaction of AT amino groups with the surface epoxide groups.[296] Reviews indicate that surface-coating efficiency depends on a range of parameters including surface area and mode of drug linkage.[300] Previous work with polyurethane model surfaces by Chan et al. has confirmed high substitution of active allyl glycidyl ether by this method. Analysis of ATH coating on the polycarbonate urethane was by staining the surface for protein or GAG, followed by elution and quantification of the bound stain.[296] In addition, hirudin (used as a biomaterial coating clinically)[301,302] and heparin were coated by the same method for comparison. Graft densities were highest for ATH (~sixfold higher than heparin and 20-fold greater than hirudin) but leaching was similar for all three anticoagulants (a likely result of the direct covalent linkage modality).[296] As expected, the ability to directly inhibit thrombin *in vitro* was negligible for heparin alone while both ATH and hirudin surfaces neutralized significant amounts of thrombin. Binding of labeled AT (a measure of pentasaccharide content) was nine times greater for ATH relative to heparin-coated surfaces. Notable was the fact that the AT-affinity binding for ATH-coated surfaces was more enhanced over heparin coating than the ratio of surface-coating density for ATH versus heparin, consistent with ATH's greater pentasaccharide content.[264] Overall, ATH gives decidedly more effective degree of coverage and specific activity in this direct covalent attachment model.

Coating of Chan et al. ATH by covalent linkage to polymer base coats that were noncovalently adsorbed prior to polymerization on the biomaterial surface was investigated in a number of reports.[303–305] Polyurethane catheters, based on Carmeda technology (provided by Solomon Scientific), were used as the coating substrate. Catheters were from a combination of two types of polyurethane units[306] incorporated into polymer blocks and chain extenders prepared by 1:1 reaction of polyols and small diisocyanate monomers.[306,307] Heparin-coated catheters (i.e., CBAS) from Solomon were obtained for comparison in these studies. Polyurethane construction in the heparin-coated catheters was similar to that of the uncoated polyurethane and heparin was coated by end-point attachment by reduction of Schiff bases formed between anhydromannose aldehyde termini on partially HNO_2-depolymerized heparin and amine-rich polyurethane–urea dip coatings.[307,308] Application of ATH coatings to the polyurethane catheters was done by the following protocol.[305] Catheters were dip-coated in dichloromethane solutions of monomer mixtures (methyl methacrylate, ethylene glycol dimethacrylate, diurethane dimethacrylate, and polyethylene oxide (PEO) methacrylate) and a thermally labile initiator (azobisisobutyronitrile [AIBN]), followed by drying. ATH was premodified by reaction with NHS-PEO-acrylate to give ATH conjugates, a PEO spacer arm and polymerizable monomer group on the end. Catheters were heated in aqueous solutions of modified ATH and trace Triton X-114 surfactant so that radical-initiated polymerization of base coat and ATH spacer end groups could take place at the catheter surface. The resultant products had coatings of polymerized base coats with covalently incorporated PEO-linked ATH covering the polyurethane catheter support. A few experiments utilizing covalent link points to the catheter itself were achieved by first reacting N-atoms in urethane–urea groups on the catheter surfaces with isocyanate monomers at high temperature. Mainly, the vast majority of experiments omitted this direct covalent linkage to the catheter surface. Detailed physicochemical and activity measurements were performed on all surfaces. Fluorescence immunohistochemical analysis confirmed fairly uniform films of AT-containing product on the ATH-coated surfaces.[305] Surface tension calculated from contact angle measurements revealed that while both uncoated and heparin-coated polyurethane catheters were hydrophobic in nature, ATH-coated surfaces displayed a significant net hydrophilicity.[303] This hydrophilic character was considered more compatible with the aqueous systemic environment *in vivo*.[303] Determination of graft density in ATH coatings by use of radiolabeled ATH gave values in freshly prepared products of 26 pmol cm^{-2}.[304] Coating stability was examined by several consecutive saline washes using a roller pump. Under this shear stress, ATH surface density was rapidly reduced to a plateau level of 12 pmol cm^{-2}. However, a large proportion of the remaining ATH coating showed remarkable stability as roller pump washing with several treatments of a potent general protease only lowered ATH levels to around 7 pmol cm^{-2}.[304] Functional activity comparisons showed that ATH surfaces had 6.8 times the anti-FXa catalytic activity relative to commercial heparin-coated catheters[303] and uptake of AT from plasma was significantly greater (~twofold) for ATH than heparin coatings.[305] Finally, a survey of binding by various proteins after incubation of the catheters in plasma determined that, while both heparin and ATH (but not uncoated polyurethane) catheters bound significant amounts of AT, adsorption of other plasma proteins was much reduced for ATH.[305] In summary, many of the desirable *in vitro* characteristics for blood compatibility (high-coating density, stability, anticoagulant activity and low-protein binding) were embodied in surfaces with Chan et al. ATH covalently linked to a polymer base coat adherent to polyurethane catheters.

18.6.2   *In Vivo* Performance

Surfaces coated with Chan et al. ATH that had been extensively characterized *in vitro* were studied in a number of animal models. In particular, attention was given to the assessment of resistance to induction of clot formation as well as fibrin(ogen) accretion. The overall marker of effective value for coated devices within the vasculature was the ability to remain patent so that flow could continue to organ sites.

Endoluminal grafts covalently coated with Schiff base–Amadori ATH were compared to other direct thrombin inhibitors in a rabbit jugular vein model.[296] After coating, grafts (2 cm in length) were inserted within jugular vein segments and normal blood flow allowed to continue in the anesthetized animal for a 3 h period. At the end of this period, grafts were carefully explanted and rinsed. Weight of clot formed on the graft and accretion of labeled fibrin (from radiolabeled fibrinogen injected at onset of the experiment) were measured. This is considered a particularly harsh model for the coagulant system since rabbits do not take anesthesia well for prolonged periods.[296] Results from coating comparisons were dramatic. Surfaces coated with ATH showed significantly reduced clot masses than those on AT or hirudin-coated grafts.[296] Even more striking were the decreases in fibrin accreted on ATH explants compared to that of hirudin or nontreated controls. The possibility that surface activation and application of the active-linking agent to the graft may somehow have played a role in ATH biocompatibility was ruled out since similar experiments with grafts treated with the activator (NaOCl), initiator (Na$_2$S$_2$O$_4$), and linker (allyl glycidyl ether), but not ATH led to measurably increased clot formation relative to ATH surfaces.[296] Examination of plasma from samples taken over time gave further evidence of differences in large-scale activation of the coagulation cascade since there was a trend for increased TAT concentrations in experiments with uncoated or hirudin-coated endoluminal grafts relative to that with ATH.[296]

In vivo studies with polyurethane catheters having Chan et al. ATH-linked to polymerized base coats gave more detailed information about effects of ATH on surface pacification. Investigations involved either an acute protocol of accelerated coagulation stimulation[303] or chronic catheter survival.[304] In acute experiments, rabbits were injected with radiolabeled fibrinogen, immediately followed by insertion of catheters from the upper jugular vein down to the ventricle. Every 5 min, over a maximum of 4 h, blood would be taken up through the catheter, held in a syringe for 2 min to initiate activation and then be slowly reinjected, followed by saline flush. Time of occlusion was noted when blood could no longer be withdrawn. Experiments were terminated either at occlusion or after 4 h and the catheter removed, rinsed, and taken for determination of accreted radiolabeled fibrin(ogen) per hour of dwell time *in vivo*. While the average occlusion time for uncoated and commercially heparin-coated catheters, was less than 80 min, on no occasions did any of the ATH-coated catheters occlude during the experiment.[303] Correspondingly, rate of fibrin(ogen) accretion was significantly reduced for ATH relative to heparin-coated or uncoated catheters. Further studies were undertaken to determine mechanisms involved for ATH surface activity. Tests using catheters coated with base coat alone, base coat+ PEO-linking agent and catheters with base coats containing PEO-linked AT all showed greatly reduced occlusion times compared to results with ATH. Similarly, radioactive fibrin(ogen) accretion rates were increased with these catheters compared to ATH catheters. Thus, the full biocompatibility was exhibited only if AT coatings on the catheter surface also had a covalently linked heparin chain. Finally, the importance of the highly active heparin chains in ATH coatings was confirmed by treatment of ATH surfaces with $NaIO_4$ (to degrade the pentasaccharide), yielding occlusion times slightly less than that of uncoated controls and fibrin(ogen) accretion rates on par with heparin coatings.[303] Interestingly, $NaIO_4$ treatment of commercially coated heparin catheters had little effect on these coagulant parameters. Similar to *in vitro* tests for stability, the lack of occlusion by ATH catheter surfaces was retained even if the catheters were pretreated with a general protease.[303]

Chronic studies, employing a more clinical regimen, gave similar results to the acute experiments. After insertion of the catheter from the upper jugular vein to the ventricle in the rabbits, they were allowed to come out of anesthesia and were maintained in cages with free access to food and water. Twice daily, blood samples were taken through the catheter and then followed by saline flush. Occlusion was noted when fluid could neither be withdrawn or injected through the catheter. At occlusion, or after approximately 3 months, catheters were removed and examined. As with the acute studies, while uncoated and commercial heparin catheters occluded within 8 days, no ATH-coated catheters ever occluded over the entire experimental period.[304] This finding was remarkable since no anticoagulant was ever given to the rabbits systemically. Another point of note was that the average occlusion time for heparin-coated catheters (3.64 ± 0.78 days) was statistically shorter than even that for uncoated surfaces (7.84 ± 0.96 days). This initially curious result, on closer inspection, is not without some rationale. Although end-point attachment of heparin chains give better anticoagulant properties,[309] reports have shown it to be insufficient for good thrombin inhibition[35] without significant spacer arms (>2000 MW) added to the heparin-end terminus.[35] Even then, improved base coatings,[309] coimmobilization of heparin with AT,[310] and saturation of heparin-coated surfaces with free AT[311] have been tried to alleviate heparin-coating problems. Visual and electron microscopic observation of catheters in the Chan et al. study *ex vivo* revealed the expected high degree of thrombi associated with uncoated and heparin-coated surfaces. However, ATH coatings appeared essentially free of anything but a fine protein-like film. To understand topographic aspects of the three surfaces prior to *in vivo* implantation, atomic force microscopy was performed. Surprisingly, although ATH coatings resisted thrombosis, their surfaces were approximately seven times rougher than that of the other catheters.[304] Thus, it would seem that the activities of ATH coatings may be more relevant to their biocompatibility than any rheological effects of ATH surface geometry.

18.7 FUTURE DIRECTIONS

Thrombotic complications in the compatibility of biomaterials have been greatly addressed by application of anticoagulant coatings. Work over the last quarter century has led to a new class of "heparinoid" resulting from the natural marriage of AT with its clinical activator heparin by a covalent linkage of the two molecules. Recent work using nonenzymatic glycation has finally allowed a mechanism for selection of the optimum plasma AT and the most potent heparin for a linkage without obtrusive human chemical intervention. Vigorous structure–function and mechanistic studies have given a fairly well-defined product for progression to *in vivo* fluid-phase studies and, finally, investigation of a range of ATH surface coatings.

In order to launch ATH fluid phase and surface-bound biomaterials into clinical use, a number of issues stand out that must be addressed. One simple aspect is the production of pharmaceutical grade compound. This is theoretically straightforward. However, industrial scale-up under General Laboratory Practice (GLP) conditions requires careful technology transfer and proper selection criteria for the ATH starting materials. Recent work with some clinically approved AT products is instructive regarding new discoveries that might be gained during this process. Commercially obtained plasma-derived AT and a recombinant human AT produced in goats were each used to generate ATH complexes. Biodistribution studies showed that while plasma AT-containing ATH largely remained in the circulation during early time points, recombinant ATH rapidly became associated with arterial and venous walls, presumably due to altered N-linked glycosylation on the recombinant AT moiety.[312] Given that coagulation very commonly starts at the site of vessel wall damage,[313] selective targeting of ATH by the AT glycans may be an elegant mechanism for optimizing the conjugate's anticoagulant or antithrombotic function *in vivo*. Alternatively, presentation on biomaterial surfaces of ATH-containing AT with different N-linked glycosylation may selectively affect favorable interactions between the coated biomaterial and either fluid phase proteins or vascular tissue surfaces.

Finally, optimization of linkage technology for placing ATH complex onto biomaterials must be completed. Just as coating methods impact the effectiveness of other anticoagulant materials on blood-contacting device surfaces, ATH potency can best be exploited by the proper presentation upon biomaterials needing pacification within procoagulant environments. Given the progress made in the last 8 years, it seems feasible that coatings with covalent AT–heparin complexes can be rapidly developed for the initial phases of clinical trials.

REFERENCES

1. Pandit, H. et al., Total knee arthroplasty: The future, *J. Surg. Orthrop. Adv.*, 15, 79, 2006.
2. Nair, L.S. and Laurencin, C.T., Polymers as biomaterials for tissue engineering and controlled drug delivery, *Adv. Biochem. Eng. Biotechnol.*, 102, 47, 2006.
3. Bambauer, R. et al., Large bore catheters with surface treatments versus untreated catheters for vascular access in hemodialysis, *Artif. Organs*, 28, 604, 2004.
4. Commandeur, S., Van Beusekom, H.M., and Van der Giessen, W.J., Polymers, drug release, and drug-eluting stents, *J. Interv. Cardiol.*, 19, 500, 2006.
5. Sarraf, C.E., et al., Heart valve and arterial tissue engineering, *Cell Prolif.*, 36, 241, 2003.
6. Hsu, L.C., Heparin-coated cardiopulmonary bypass circuits: Current status, *Perfusion*, 16, 417, 2001.
7. Tobin, E.J. and Bambauer, R., Silver coating of dialysis catheters to reduce bacterial colonization and infection, *Ther. Apher. Dial.*, 7, 504, 2003.
8. Brash, J.L., Exploiting the current paradigm of blood-material interactions for the rational design of blood-compatible materials, *J. Biomater. Sci. Polym. Ed.*, 11, 1135, 2000.
9. Schmidt, B. and Andrew, M., Neonatal thrombosis: Report of a prospective Canadian and international registry, *Pediatrics*, 96, 939, 1995.
10. Male, C. et al., Central venous line-related thrombosis in children: Association with central venous line location and insertion technique, *Blood*, 101, 4273, 2003.
11. Chan, A.K. et al., Venous thrombosis in children, *J. Thromb. Haemost.*, 1, 1443, 2003.

12. Risberg, B., Andreasson, S., and Eriksson, E., Disseminated intravascular coagulation, *Acta Anaesthesiol. Scand.*, 95, 60, 1991.

13. Butenas, S., van't Veer, C., and Mann, K.G., "Normal" thrombin generation, *Blood*, 94, 2169, 1999.

14. Mosesson M.W., Fibrinogen and fibrin polymerization: Appraisal of the binding events that accompany fibrin generation and fibrin clot assembly, *Blood Coagul. Fibrinol.*, 8, 257, 1997.

15. Choay, J. et al., Structure–activity relationship in heparin: A synthetic pentasaccharide with high affinity for antithrombin III and eliciting high anti factor Xa activity, *Biochem. Biophys. Res. Comm.*, 116, 492, 1983.

16. Naito, K. and Fujikawa, K., Activation of human blood coagulation factor XI independent of factor XII: Factor XI is activated by thrombin and factor XIa in the presence of negatively charged surfaces, *J. Biol. Chem.*, 266, 7353, 1991.

17. Ofosu, F.A. et al., The inhibition of thrombin-dependent positive-feedback reactions is critical to the expression of the anticoagulant effect of heparin, *Biochem. J.*, 243, 579, 1987.

18. Ofosu, F.A., Liu, L., and Feedman, J., Control mechanisms in thrombin generation, *Semin. Thromb. Haemost.*, 22, 303, 1996.

19. Bereczky, Z., Katona, E., and Muszbek, L., Fibrin stabilization (factor XIII), fibrin structure and thrombosis, *Pathophysiol. Haemost. Thromb.*, 33, 430, 2003.

20. Muszbek, L., Adany, R., and Mikkola, H., Novel aspects of blood coagulation factor XIII. I. Structure, distribution, activation, and function, *Crit. Rev. Clin. Lab. Sci.*, 33, 357, 1996.

21. Devine, D.V. and Bishop, P.D., Platelet-associated factor XIII in platelet activation, adhesion, and clot stabilization, *Thromb. Haemost.*, 22, 409, 1996.

22. Bajzar, L. et al., Both cellular and soluble forms of thrombomodulin inhibit fibrinolysis by potentiating the activation of thrombin activable fibrinolysis inhibitor, *J. Biol. Chem.*, 273, 2792, 1998.

23. Boffa, M.B. et al., Plasma and recombinant thrombin activable fibrinolysis inhibitor (TAFI) and activated TAFI compared with respect to glycosylation, thrombin/thrombomodulin-dependent activation, thermal stability, and enzymatic properties, *J. Biol. Chem.*, 273, 2127, 1998.

24. Kokame, K., Zheng, X., and Sadler, J.E., Activation of thrombin activable fibrinolysis inhibitor requires epidermal growth factor-like domain 3 of thrombomodulin and is inhibited competitively by protein C, *J. Biol. Chem.*, 273, 12135, 1998.

25. Dahlback, B., The protein C anticoagulant system: Inherited defects as basis for venous thrombosis, *Thromb. Res.*, 77, 1, 1995.

26. Kisiel, W. et al., Anticoagulant properties of bovine plasma protein C following activation by thrombin, *J. Biol. Chem.*, 16, 5824, 1977.

27. Chuang, Y.J., Gettins, P.G., and Olson, S.T., Importance of the P2 glycine of antithrombin in target proteinase specificity, heparin activation, and the efficiency of proteinase trapping as revealed by a P2 gly→pro mutation, *J. Biol. Chem.*, 274, 28142, 1999.

28. Buller, H.R. and Ten Cate, T., Coagulation and platelet activation pathways. A review of the key components and the way in which these can be manipulated, *Eur. Heart J.*, 16, 8, 1995.

29. Nilson, I.M., Coagulation and fibrinolysis, *Scand. J. Gastroenterol.*, 137, 11, 1987.

30. Jordan, R.E. et al., The kinetics of hemostatic enzyme-antithrombin interactions in the presence of low molecular weight heparin, *J. Biol. Chem.*, 255, 10081, 1980.

31. Rezaie, A.R., Tryptophan 60-D in the B-insertion loop of thrombin modulates the thrombin-antithrombin reaction, *Biochemistry*, 35, 1918, 1996.

32. Mille, B. et al., Role of N- and C-terminal amino acids in antithrombin binding to pentasaccharide, *J. Biol. Chem.*, 269, 29435, 1994.

33. Olson, S.T. and Chuang, Y.J., Heparin activates antithrombin anticoagulant function by generating new interaction sites (exosites) for blood clotting proteinases, *Trends Cardiovasc. Med.*, 12, 331, 2002.

34. Danielsson, A.E. et al., Role of ternary complexes, in which heparin binds both antithrombin and proteinase, in the acceleration of the reactions between antithrombin and thrombin or factor Xa, *J. Biol. Chem.*, 261, 15467, 1986.

35. Byun, Y., Jacobs, H.A., and Kim, S.W., Mechanism of thrombin inactivation by immobilized heparin, *J. Biomed. Mater. Res.*, 30, 423, 1996.

36. Cundiff, D.K., Anticoagulation therapy thromboembolism, *Med. Gen. Med.*, 6, 5, 2004.

37. Vincentelli, A., Jude, B., and Belisle, S., Antithrombotic therapy in cardiac surgery, *Can. J. Anaesth.*, 53, S89, 2006.

38. Estes, J.W., Pelikan, E.W., and Kruger-Thiemer, E., A retrospective study of the pharmacokinetics of heparin, *Clin. Pharmacol. Ther.*, 10, 329, 1969.

39. Young, E. et al., Heparin binding to plasma proteins, an important mechanism for heparin resistance, *Thromb. Haemost.*, 67, 639, 1992.

40. Jaques, L.B., Mahadoo, J., and Kavanagh, L.W., Intrapulmonary heparin: A new procedure for anticoagulant therapy, *Lancet*, 7996, 1157, 1976.

41. Hirsh, J. et al., Heparin kinetics in venous thrombosis and pulmonary embolism, *Circulation*, 53, 691, 1976.

42. Eisenberg, P. et al., Importance of factor Xa in determining the procoagulant activity of whole-blood clots, *J. Clin. Invest.*, 91, 1877, 1993.

43. Prager, N.A. et al., Role of thrombin compared with factor Xa in the procoagulant activity of whole blood clots, *Circulation*, 92, 962, 1995.

44. Weitz, J.I. et al., Clot-bound thrombin is protected from inhibition by heparin-antithrombin III but is susceptible to inactivation by antithrombin III independent inhibitors, *J. Clin. Invest.*, 86, 385, 1990.

45. Hogg, P.J. and Jackson, C.M., Fibrin monomer protects thrombin from inactivation by heparin-antithrombin III: Implications for heparin efficacy, *Proc. Natl Acad. Sci. USA*, 86, 3619, 1989.

46. Theroux, P. et al., Reactivation of unstable angina after the discontinuation of heparin, *N. Engl. J. Med.*, 327, 192, 1992.

47. Palm, M. et al., Bleeding times in rats treated with heparin, heparin fragments of high and low anticoagulant activity and chemically modified heparin fragments of low anticoagulant activity, *Thromb. Haemost.*, 64, 127, 1990.

48. Kristensen, E.M. et al., Heparin coating durability on artificial heart valves studied by XPS and antithrombin binding capacity, *Colloids Surf. B. Biointerfaces*, 49, 1, 2006.

49. Hatton, M.W.C. et al., Tritiation of commercial heparins by reaction with NaB3H4: Chemical analysis and biological properties of the product, *Anal. Biochem.*, 106, 417, 1980.

50. Hunt, L.T. and Dayhoff, M.O., A surprising new protein superfamily containing ovalbumin, antithrombin-III, and alpha 1-protease inhibitor, *Biochem. Biophys. Res. Comm.*, 95, 864, 1980.

51. Carrell, R.W. et al., Active site of a1-antitrypsin: Homologous site in antithrombin-III, *Biochem. Biophys. Res. Comm.*, 93, 399, 1980.

52. Chandra, T. et al., Sequence homology between human alpha-1-antichymotrypsin, alpha-1-antitrypsin and antithrombin III, *Biochemistry*, 22, 5055, 1983.

53. Carrell, R.W., Christey, P.B., and Boswell, D.R., Serpins: Antithrombin and other inhibitors of coagulation and fibrinolysis: Evidence from amino acid sequences, in *Thrombosis and Haemostasis*, Verstraete, M., Vermylen, J., and Lijnen, R., Eds., Leuven University Press, Leuven, Belgium, 1987, chap. 1.

54. Takano, T. et al., Interstitial deletion of chromosome 1q [del(1)(q24q25.3)] identified by fluorescence in situ hybridization and gene dosage analysis of apolipoprotein A-II, coagulation factor V, and antithrombin III, *Am. J. Med. Genet.*, 68, 207, 1997.

55. Bock, S.C., Marrinan, J.A., and Radziejewska, E., Antithrombin III Utah: Proline-407 to leucine mutation in a highly conserved region near the inhibitor reactive site, *Biochemistry*, 27, 6171, 1988.

56. Prochownik, E.V., Bock, S.C., and Orkin, S.H., Intron structure of the human antithrombin III gene differs from that of other members of the serine protease inhibitor superfamily, *J. Biol. Chem.*, 260, 9608, 1985.

57. Niessen, R.W. et al., Sequence characterization of a sheep cDNA for antithrombin III, *Biochim. Biophys. Acta*, 1171, 207, 1992.

58. Abildgaard, U., Purification of two progressive antithrombins of human plasma, *Scand. J. Clin. Lab. Invest.*, 19, 190, 1967.

59. Rosenberg, R.D. and Damus, P.S., The purification and mechanism of action of human antithrombin-heparin cofactor, *J. Biol. Chem.*, 248, 6490, 1973.

60. Miller-Andersson, J., Borg, H., and Andersson, L.O., Purification of antithrombin III by affinity chromatography, *Thromb. Res.*, 5, 439, 1974.

61. Manson, H.E. et al., The molecular pathology of inherited human antithrombin III deficiency, *Transfus. Med. Rev.*, 3, 264, 1989.

62. Villaneuva, G.B., Predictions of the secondary structure of antithrombin III and the location of the heparin-binding site, *J. Biol. Chem.*, 259, 2531, 1984.

63. Petersen, T.E. et al., Primary structure of antithrombin III (heparin cofactor). Partial homology between a1-antitrypsin and antithrombin III, in *The Physiological Inhibitors of Coagulation and Fibrinolysis*, Collen, D., Wiman, B., and Verstraete, M., Eds., Elsevier, Amsterdam, The Netherlands, 1979, chap. 2.

64. Carrell, R.W. et al., Biological implications of a 3A structure of dimeric antithrombin, *Structure*, 2, 257, 1994.

65. Wardell, M.R. et al., Crystallization and preliminary X-ray diffraction analysis of two conformations of intact human antithrombin, *J. Mol. Biol.*, 234, 1253, 1993.

66. Fleischer, B., Mechanism of glycosylation in the golgi apparatus, *J. Histochem. Cytochem.*, 31, 1033, 1983.

67. Garone, L. et al., Antithrombin-heparin affinity reduced by fucosylation of carbohydrate at asparagine 155, *Biochemistry*, 35, 8881, 1996.

68. Bjork, I. et al., Decreased affinity of recombinant antithrombin for heparin due to increased glycosylation, *Biochem. J.*, 286, 793, 1992.

69. Borsodi, A. and Narasimhan, T.R., Microheterogeneity of human antithrombin III, *Br. J. Haematol.*, 39, 121, 1978.

70. Witmer, M.R. and Hatton, M.W., Antithrombin III-beta associates more readily than antithrombin III-alpha with uninjured and de-endothelialized aortic wall *in vitro* and *in vivo*, *Arterioscler. Thromb.*, 11, 530, 1991.

71. Carlson, T.H., Kolman, M.R., and Piepkorn, M., Activation of antithrombin III isoforms by heparan sulphate glycosaminoglycans and other sulphated polysaccharides, *Blood Coagul. Fibrinol.*, 6, 474, 1995.

72. Brennan, S.O. et al., New carbohydrate site in mutant antithrombin (7 Ile–Asn) with decreased heparin affinity, *FEBS Lett.*, 237, 118, 1988.

73. Stibler, H., Holzbach, U., and Kristiansson, B., Isoforms and levels of transferrin, antithrombin, alpha(1)-antitrypsin and thyroxine-binding globulin in 48 patients with carbohydrate-deficient glycoprotein syndrome type I, *Scand. J. Clin. Lab. Invest.*, 58, 55, 1998.

74. Picard, V., Ersdal-Badju, E., and Bock, S.C., Partial glycosylation of antithrombin III asparagine-135 is caused by the serine in the third position of its N-glycosylation consensus sequence and is responsible for production of the beta-antithrombin III isoform with enhanced heparin affinity, *Biochemistry*, 34, 8433, 1995.

75. Karlsson, G. and Winge, S., Separation between the alpha and beta forms of human antithrombin by hydroxyapatite high-performance liquid chromatography, *Protein Expr. Purif.*, 28, 196, 2003.

76. Turk, B. et al., The oligosaccharide side chain on Asn-135 of alpha-antithrombin, absent in beta-antithrombin, decreases the heparin affinity of the inhibitor by affecting the heparin-induced conformational change, *Biochemistry*, 36, 6682, 1997.

77. Howell, W.H., The coagulation of blood, in *The Harvey Lectures*, Lippincott, Philadelphia, 1918, chap. 7.

78. Marcum, J.A., Howell, W.H., and McLean, J., The experimental context for the discovery of heparin, *Perspect. Biol. Med.*, 33, 214, 1990.

79. Brinkhous, K. et al., The inhibition of blood clotting: An unidentified substance which acts in conjunction with heparin to prevent the conversion of prothrombin to thrombin, *Am. J. Physiol.*, 125, 683, 1939.

80. Seegers, W.H., Johnson, J.F., and Fall, C., An antithrombin reaction related to prothrombin activation, *Am. J. Physiol.*, 176, 97, 1954.

81. Devraj-Kizuk, R. et al., Antithrombin III-Hamilton: A gene with a point mutation (guanine to adenine) in codon 382 causing impaired serine protease reactivity, *Blood*, 72, 1518, 1988.

82. Whinna, H.C. and Church, F.C., Interaction of thrombin with antithrombin, heparin cofactor II, and protein C inhibitor, *J. Protein. Chem.*, 12, 677, 1993.

83. Carrell, R.W. and Owen, M.C., Plakalbumin, a2-antitrypsin, antithrombin and the mechanism of inflammatory thrombosis, *Nature*, 317, 730, 1985.

84. Schulze, A.J. et al., Structural aspects of serpin inhibition, *FEBS Lett.*, 344, 117, 1994.

85. Skriver, K. et al., Substrate properties of C1 inhibitor Ma (alanine 434—glutamic acid). Genetic and structural evidence suggesting that the P12-region contains critical determinants of serine protease inhibitor/substrate status, *J. Biol. Chem.*, 266, 9216, 1991.

86. Schulze, A.J. et al., Structural transition of alpha-1-antitrypsin by a peptide sequentially similar to beta-strand s4A, *Eur. J. Biochem.*, 194, 51, 1990.

87. Schulze, A.J. et al., Evidence for the extent of insertion of the active site loop of intact alpha 1 proteinase inhibitor in beta-sheet A, *Biochemistry*, 31, 7560, 1992.

88. Bjork, I. et al., Kinetic characterization of the substrate reaction between a complex of antithrombin with a synthetic reactive-bond loop tetradecapeptide and four target proteinases of the inhibitor, *J. Biol. Chem.*, 267, 19047, 1992.

89. Bjork, I. et al., Conversion of antithrombin from an inhibitor of thrombin to a substrate with reduced heparin affinity and enhanced conformational stability by binding of a tetradecapeptide corresponding to the P1 to P14 region of the putative reactive bond loop of the inhibitor, *J. Biol. Chem.*, 267, 1976, 1992.

90. Debrock, S. and Decleck, P.J., Characterization of common neoantigenic epitopes generated in plasminogen activator inhibitor-1 after cleavage of the reactive center loop or after complex formation with various serine proteinases, *FEBS Lett.*, 376, 243, 1995.

91. Nordling, K. and Bjork, I., Identification of an epitope in antithrombin appearing on insertion of the reactive-bond loop into the A beta-sheet, *Biochemistry*, 35, 10436, 1996.

92. Whisstock, J., Lesk, A.M., and Carrell, R., Modeling of serpin-protease complexes: Antithrombin-thrombin, alpha-1-antitrypsin (358Met−>Arg)-thrombin, alpha-1-antitrypsin (358Met→Arg)-trypsin, and antitrypsin-elastase, *Proteins*, 26, 288, 1996.

93. Skinner, R. et al., The 2.6 A structure of antithrombin indicates a conformational change at the heparin binding site, *J. Mol. Biol.*, 266, 601, 1997.

94. Jin, L. et al., The anticoagulant activation of antithrombin by heparin, *Proc. Natl Acad. Sci. USA*, 94, 14683, 1997.

95. Meagher, J.L. et al., Deconvolution of the fluorescence emission spectrum of human antithrombin and identification of the tryptophan residues that are responsive to heparin binding, *J. Biol. Chem.*, 273, 23283, 1998.

96. Koide, T. et al., Replacement of arginine-47 by cysteine in hereditary abnormal antithrombin III that lacks heparin-binding ability, *Proc. Natl Acad. Sci. USA*, 81, 289, 1984.

97. Owen, M.C. et al., Heparin binding defect in a new antithrombin III variant: Rouen, 47 Arg to His, *Blood*, 69, 1275, 1987.

98. Borg, J.Y. et al., Proposed heparin binding site in antithrombin based on arginine 47: A new variant Rouen-II, 47Arg to Ser, *J. Clin. Invest.*, 81, 1292, 1988.

99. Chang, J.Y. and Tran, T.H., Antithrombin III basel. Identification of a pro-leu substitution in a hereditary abnormal antithrombin with impaired heparin cofactor activity, *J. Biol. Chem.*, 261, 1174, 1986.

100. Smith, J.W. and Knauer, D.J., A heparin binding site in antithrombin III, *J. Biol. Chem.*, 262, 11964, 1987.

101. Ersdal-Badju, E. et al., Identification of the antithrombin III heparin binding site, *J. Biol. Chem.*, 272, 19393, 1997.

102. Skinner, R. et al., Implications for function and therapy of a 2.9 A structure of binary-complexed antithrombin, *J. Mol. Biol.*, 283, 9, 1998.

103. Hatton, M.W., Berry, L.R., and Regoeczi, E., Inhibition of thrombin by antithrombin III in the presence of certain glycosaminoglycans found in the mammalian aorta, *Thromb. Res.*, 13, 655, 1978.

104. Fan, B. et al., Heterogeneity of recombinant human antithrombin III expressed in baby hamster kidney cells. Effect of glycosylation differences on heparin binding and structure, *J. Biol. Chem.*, 268, 17588, 1993.

105. Olson, S.T. et al., Effect of individual carbohydrate chains of recombinant antithrombin on heparin affinity and on the generation of glycoforms differing in heparin affinity, *Arch. Biochem. Biophys.*, 341, 212, 1997.

106. Brieditis, T.B. et al., The oligosaccharide side chain on Asn-135 of alpha-antithrombin, absent in beta-antithrombin, decreases the heparin affinity of the inhibitor by affecting the heparin-induced conformational change, *Biochemistry*, 36, 6682, 1997.

107. Mertens, G. et al., Cell surface heparan sulfate proteoglycans from human vascular endothelial cells. Core protein characterization and antithrombin III binding properties, *J. Biol. Chem.*, 267, 20435, 1992.

108. Bianchini, P. et al., Heterogeneity of unfractionated heparins studied in connection with species, source, and production processes, *Semin. Thromb. Hemost.*, 23, 3, 1997.

109. Templeton, D.M., Proteoglycans in cell regulation, *Crit. Rev. Clin. Lab. Sci.*, 29, 141, 1992.

110. Lidholt, K., Biosynthesis of glycosaminoglycans in mammalian cells and in bacteria, *Biochem. Soc. Trans.*, 25, 866, 1997.

111. Ernst, S. et al., Enzymatic degradation of glycosaminoglycans, *Crit. Rev. Biochem. Mol. Biol.*, 30, 387, 1995.

112. Kobayashi, M. et al., Molecular cloning and characterization of a human uronyl-2-sulfotransferase that sulfates iduronyl and glucuronyl residues in dermatan/chondroitin sulfate, *J. Biol. Chem.*, 274, 10474, 1999.

113. Gallagher, J.T. and Walker, A., Molecular distinctions between heparin sulphate and heparin. Analysis of sulphation patterns indicates that heparin sulphate and heparin are separate families of N-sulphated polysaccharides, *Biochem. J.*, 230, 665, 1985.

114. Shively, J.E. and Conrad, H.E., Nearest neighbor analysis of heparin: Identification and quantitation of the products formed by selective depolymerization procedures, *Biochemistry*, 15, 3943, 1976.
115. Robinson, H.C. et al., A proteoglycan form of heparin and its degradation to single-chain molecules, *J. Biol. Chem.*, 253, 6687, 1978.
116. Iacomini, M. et al., "Linkage Region" sequences of heparins and heparan sulfates: Detection and quantification by nuclear magnetic resonance spectroscopy, *Anal. Biochem.*, 274, 50, 1999.
117. Lindahl, U. and Axelsson, O., Identification of iduronic acid as the major sulfated uronic acid of heparin, *J. Biol. Chem.*, 246, 74, 1971.
118. Riesenfeld, J., Hook, M., and Lindahl, U., Biosynthesis of heparin. Assay and properties of the microsomal N-acetyl-D-glucosaminyl-N-deacetylase, *J. Biol. Chem.*, 255, 922, 1980.
119. Jacobsson, I. et al., Biosynthesis of heparin. Substrate specificity of heparosan N-sulfate D-glucuronosyl 5-epimerase, *J. Biol. Chem.*, 259, 1056, 1984.
120. Miller, R.R. and Waechter, C.J., Partial purification and characterization of detergent-solubilized N-sulfotransferase activity associated with calf brain microsomes, *J. Neurochem.*, 51, 87, 1988.
121. Lind, T., Lindahl, U., and Lidholt, K., Biosynthesis of heparin/heparan sulfate. Identification of a 0-kDa protein catalyzing both the D-glucuronosyl- and the N-acetyl-D-glucosaminyltransferase reactions, *J. Biol. Chem.*, 268, 20705, 1993.
122. Lidholt, K. and Lindahl, U., Biosynthesis of heparin. The D-glucuronosyl- and N-acetyl-D-glucosaminyltransferase reactions and their relation to polymer modification, *Biochem. J.*, 287, 21, 1992.
123. Jacobsson, I. and Lindahl, U., Biosynthesis of heparin. Concerted action of late polymer-modification reactions, *J. Biol. Chem.*, 255, 5094, 1980.
124. Foster, A.B. et al., Amino-sugars and related compounds. Part IX. Periodate oxidation of heparin and some related substances, *J. Am. Chem. Soc.*, 85, 2279, 1963.
125. Lidholt, K., Kjellen, L., and Lindahl, U., Biosynthesis of heparin. Relationship between the polymerization and sulphation processes, *Biochem. J.*, 261, 999, 1989.
126. Toma, L., Berninsome, P., and Hirschberg, C.B., The putative heparin specific N-acetylglucosaminyl N-deacetylase/N-sulfotransferase also occurs in non-heparin-producing cells, *J. Biol. Chem.*, 273, 22458, 1998.
127. Ogren, S. and Lindahl, U., Cleavage of macromolecular heparin by an enzyme from mouse mastocytoma, *J. Biol. Chem.*, 250, 2690, 1975.
128. Ogren, S. and Lindahl, U., Metabolism of macromolecular heparin in mouse neoplastic mast cells, *Biochem. J.*, 154, 605, 1976.
129. Fareed, J. et al., Pharmacokinetics of low molecular weight heparins in animal models, *Semin. Thromb. Hemost.*, 25, 51, 1999.
130. Fareed, J., Haas, S., and Sasahar, A., Past, present and future considerations on low molecular weight heparin differentiation: An epilogue, *Semin. Thromb. Hemost.*, 25, 145, 1999.
131. Jaikaria, N.S. et al., Interaction of fibronectin with heparin in model extracellular matrices: Role of arginine residues and sulfate groups, *Biochemistry*, 30, 1538, 1991.
132. Zak-Nejmark, T. et al., Heparin modulates migration of human peripheral blood mononuclear cells and neutrophils, *Arch. Immunol. Ther. Exp. (Warsz)*, 47, 245, 1999.
133. Jeske, W. and Fareed, J., Antithrombin III-and heparin cofactor II-mediated anticoagulant and antiprotease actions of heparin and its synthetic analogues, *Semin. Thromb. Hemost.*, 19, 241, 1993.
134. Rosenfeld, R.D., Role of heparin and heparin-like molecules in thrombosis and athersclerosis, *Fed. Proc.*, 44, 404, 1985.
135. Frebelius, S., Hedin, U., and Swedenborg, J., Thrombogenecity of the injured vessel wall—role of antithrombin and heparin, *Thromb. Haemost.*, 71, 147, 1994.
136. Barrowcliffe, T.W. et al., The anticoagulant activity of heparin: Measurement and relationship to chemical structure, *J. Pharm. Biomed. Anal.*, 7, 217, 1989.
137. Liu, L. et al., Inhibition of thrombin by antithrombin III and heparin cofactor II *in vivo*, *Thromb. Haemost.*, 73, 405, 1995.
138. Wu, Y.I., Sheffield, W.P., and Blajchman, M., Defining the heparin-binding domain of antithrombin, *Blood Coag. Fibrinol.*, 5, 83, 1994.
139. Horner, A.A. and Young, E., Asymmetric distribution of sites with high affinity for antithrombin III in rat skin heparin proteoglycans, *J. Biol. Chem.*, 257, 8749, 1982.
140. Jacobsson, K.-G., Lindahl, U., and Horner, A.A., Location of antithrombin-binding regions in rat skin heparin proteoglycans, *Biochem. J.*, 240, 625, 1986.

141. Chan, A.K. et al., Covalent antithrombin-heparin complexes with high anticoagulant activity: Intravenous, subcutaneous and intratracheal administration, *J. Biol. Chem.*, 272, 22111, 1997.

142. Rosenberg, R.D. et al., Highly active heparin species with multiple binding sites for antithrombin, *Biochem. Biophys. Res. Comm.*, 86, 1319, 1979.

143. Thunberg, L. et al., On the molecular-weight-dependence of the anticoagulant activity of heparin, *Biochem. J.*, 181, 241, 1979.

144. Oscarsson, L.G., Pejler, G., and Lindahl, U., Location of the antithrombin-binding sequence in the heparin chain, *J. Biol. Chem.*, 264, 296, 1989.

145. Laurent, T.C. et al., The molecular-weight-dependence of the anti-coagulant activity of heparin, *Biochem. J.*, 175, 691, 1978.

146. Berry, L.R. and Hatton, M.W., Controlled depolymerization of heparin: Anticoagulant activity and molecular size of the products, *Biochem. Soc. Trans.*, 11, 101, 1983.

147. Berry, L.R. et al., Selective cleavage of heparin using aqueous 2-hydroxypyridine: Production of an aldose-terminating fragment with high anticoagulant activity, *Biochem. Biophys. Res. Comm.*, 346, 946, 2006.

148. Petitou, M. et al., Synthesis of heparin fragments. A chemical synthesis of the pentasaccharide O-(2-deoxy-2-sulfamido-6-O-sulfo-alpha-D-glucopyranosyl)-(1-4)-O-(beta-D-glucopyranosyluronic acid)-(1-4)-O-(2-deoxy-2-sulfamido-3,6-di-O-sulfo-alpha-D-glucopyranosyl)-(1-4)-O-(2-O-sulfo-alpha-L-idopyranosyluronic acid)-(1-4)-2-deoxy-2-sulfamido-6-O-sulfo-D-glucopyranose decasodium salt, a heparin fragment having high affinity for antithrombin III, *Carb. Res.*, 147, 221, 1986.

149. Kusche, M. et al., Biosynthesis of heparin. O-sulfation of the antithrombin-binding region, *J. Biol. Chem.*, 263, 15474, 1988.

150. Petitou, M. et al., Binding of heparin to antithrombin III: A chemical proof of the critical role played by a 3-sulfated 2-amino-2-deoxy-D-glucose residue, *Carb. Res.*, 179, 163, 1988.

151. Petitou, M. et al., A unique trisaccharide sequence in heparin mediates the early step of antithrombin III activation, *Glycobiology*, 7, 323, 1997.

152. Desai, U.R. et al., Mechanism of heparin activation of antithrombin. Role of individual residues of the pentasaccharide activating sequence in the recognition of native and activated states of antithrombin, *J. Biol. Chem.*, 273, 7478, 1998.

153. Desai, U.R. et al., Mechanism of heparin activation of antithrombin: Evidence for an induced-fit model of allosteric activation involving two interaction subsites, *Biochemistry*, 37, 13033, 1998.

154. Arocas, V. et al., The role of Arg46 and Arg47 of antithrombin in heparin binding, *Biochemistry*, 38, 10196, 1999.

155. Kandrotas, R.J., Heparin pharmacokinetics and pharmacodynamics, *Clin. Pharmacokinet.*, 22, 359, 1992.

156. e, J., Rezaie, A.R., and Esmon, C.T., Glycosaminoglycan contributions to both protein C activation and thrombin inhibition involve a common arginine-rich site in thrombin that includes residues arginine 93, 97, and 101, *J. Biol. Chem.*, 269, 17965, 1994.

157. Petersen, L.C. and Jorgensen, M., Electrostatic interactions in the heparin-enhanced reaction between human thrombin and antithrombin, *Biochem. J.*, 211, 91, 1983.

158. Lozano, M. et al., Suitability of low molecular weight heparin(oid)s and a pentasaccharide for an *in vitro* human thrombosis model, *Arterioscler. Thromb.*, 14, 1215, 1994.

159. Bergqvist, D., Low molecular weight heparins, *J. Intern. Med.*, 240, 63, 1996.

160. Young, E. et al., Ex-vivo and in-vitro evidence that low molecular weight heparins exhibit less binding to plasma proteins than unfractionated heparin, *Thromb. Haemost.*, 71, 300, 1994.

161. Bara, L. et al., Comparative pharmacokinetics (PK 10169) and unfractionated heparin after intravenous and subcutaneous administration, *Thromb. Res.*, 39, 631, 1985.

162. Hirsh, J. and Levine, M.N., Low molecular weight heparin, *Blood*, 79, 1, 1992.

163. Fareed, J. et al., Low molecular weight heparins: Are they different? *Can. J. Cardiol.*, 14, 28E, 1998.

164. Wolzt, M. et al., Studies on the neutralizing effects of protamine on unfractionated and low molecular weight heparin (Fragmin) at the site of activation of the coagulation system in man, *Thromb. Haemost.*, 73, 439, 1995.

165. Briant, L. et al., Unfractionated heparin and CY 216: Pharmacokinetics and bioavailabilities of the anti-factor Xa and IIa effects after intravenous and subcutaneous injection in the rabbit, *Thromb. Haemost.*, 61, 348, 1989.

166. Schran, H.F. et al., The pharmacokinetics and bioavailability of subcutaneously administered dihydro-ergotamine, heparin and the dihydroergotamine-heparin combination, *Thromb. Res.*, 31, 51, 1983.

167. Laforest, M.D. et al., Pharmacokinetics and biodistribution of technium 99m labelled standard heparin and a low molecular weight heparin (enoxaparin) after intravenous injection in normal volunteers, *Br. J. Haematol.*, 77, 201, 1991.
168. Manson, L. et al., The variable anticoagulant response to unfractionated heparin *in vivo* reflects binding to plasma proteins rather than clearance, *J. Lab. Clin. Med.*, 130, 649, 1997.
169. Young, E. et al., Induction of the acute-phase reaction increases heparin-binding proteins in plasma, *Arterioscler. Thromb. Vasc. Biol.*, 17, 1568, 1997.
170. Messmore, H.L. et al., *In vitro* studies of the interaction of heparin, low molecular weight heparin and heparinoids with platelets, *NY Acad. Sci.*, 556, 217, 1989.
171. Patton, W.A. 2nd. et al., Identification of a heparin-binding protein using monoclonal antibodies that block heparin binding to porcine aortic endothelial cells, *Biochem. J.*, 311, 461, 1995.
172. Lijnen, H.R., Hoylaerts, M., and Collen, D., Heparin binding properties of human histidine-rich glycoprotein: Mechanism and role in the neutralization of heparin in plasma, *J. Biol. Chem.*, 258, 3803, 1983.
173. Teoh, K.H. et al., Heparin binding proteins. Contribution to heparin rebound after cardiopulmonary bypass, *Circulation*, 88, 420, 1993.
174. Young, E. et al., *Ex-vivo* and *in-vitro* evidence that low molecular weight heparins exhibit less binding to plasma proteins than unfractionated heparin, *Thromb. Haemost.*, 71, 300, 1994.
175. Cosmi, B. et al., Effect of nonspecific binding to plasma proteins on the antithrombin activities of unfractionated heparin, low-molecular-weight heparin, and dermatan sulfate, *Circulation*, 95, 118, 1997.
176. Hogg, P.J. and Jackson, C.M., Heparin promotes the binding of thrombin to fibrin polymer. Quantitative characterization of a thrombin-fibrin polymer-heparin ternary complex, *J. Biol. Chem.*, 265, 241, 1990.
177. Hogg, P.J. et al., Binding of fibrin monomer and heparin to thrombin in a ternary complex alters the environment of the thrombin catalytic site, reduces affinity for hirudin and inhibits cleavage of fibrinogen, *J. Biol. Chem.*, 271, 26088, 1996.
178. Hogg, P.J. and Jackson, C.M., Fibrin monomer protects thrombin from inactivation by heparin-antithrombin III: Implications for heparin efficacy, *Proc. Natl Acad. Sci. USA*, 86, 3619, 1989.
179. Hogg, P.J. and Jackson, C.M., Formation of a ternary complex between thrombin, fibrin monomer, and heparin influences the action of thrombin on its substrates, *J. Biol. Chem.*, 265, 248, 1990.
180. Bendayan, P. et al., Dermatan sulphate is a more potent inhibitor of clot-bound thrombin than unfractionated and low molecular weight heparins, *Thromb. Haemost.*, 71, 576, 1994.
181. Rezaie, A.R., Prothrombin protects factor Xa in the prothrombinase complex from inhibition by the heparin-antithrombin complex, *Blood*, 97, 2308, 2001.
182. Brufatto, N. and Nesheim, M.E., The use of prothrombin(S525C) labeled with fluorescein to directly study the inhibition of prothrombinase by antithrombin during prothrombin activation, *J. Biol. Chem.*, 276, 17663, 2001.
183. Cohen, M., Heparin-induced thrombocytopenia and the clinical use of low molecular weight heparins in acute coronary syndromes, *Semin. Hematol.*, 36, 33, 1999.
184. Hull, R.D. et al., Optimal therapeutic level of heparin therapy in patients with venous thrombosis, *Arch. Intern. Med.*, 152, 1589, 1992.
185. Hirsh, J., Salzman, E.W., and Marder, V.J., Treatment of venous thromboembolism, in *Hemostasis and Thrombosis: Basic Principles and Clinical Practice*, Colman, R.W., Hirsh, J., Marder, V.J., and Salzman, E.W., Eds., J. P. Lippincott Company, New York, 1994, chap. 69.
186. Koopman, M.M. et al., Treatment of venous thrombosis with intravenous unfractionated heparin administered in the hospital as compared with subcutaneous low molecular weight heparin administered at home. The Tasman Study Group, *N. Engl. J. Med.*, 334, 682, 1996.
187. Levine, M. et al., A comparison of low molecular weight heparin administered primarily at home with unfractionated heparin administered in the hospital for proximal deep venous thrombosis, *N. Engl. J. Med.*, 334, 677, 1996.
188. Warkentin, T. et al., Heparin-induced thrombocytopenia in patients treated with low molecular weight heparins or unfractionated heparin, *N. Engl. J. Med.*, 332, 1330, 1995.
189. Dahlman, T., Lindvall, N., and Hellgren, M., Osteopenia in pregnancy during longterm heparin treatment: A radiological study *post partum*, *Br. J. Obstet. Gynaecol.*, 97, 221, 1990.
190. Barbour, L.A. et al., A prospective study of heparin-induced osteoporosis in pregnancy using bone densitometry, *Am. J. Obstet. Gynecol.*, 170, 862, 1994.

191. Hirsh, J. et al., Low molecular weight heparins (LMWH) in the treatment of patients with acute venous thromboembolism, *Thromb. Haemost.*, 74, 360, 1995.
192. GUSTO IIb investigators, A comparison of recombinant hirudin with heparin for the treatment of acute coronary syndromes. The global use of strategies to open occluded coronary arteries (GUSTO) IIb investigators, *N. Engl. J. Med.*, 335, 775, 1996.
193. Sarembock, I. et al., Effectiveness of hirulog in reducing restenosis after balloon angioplasty of atherosclerotic femoral arteries in rabbits, *J. Vasc. Res.*, 33, 308, 1996.
194. Verstraete, M., New developments in antiplatelet and antithrombotic therapy, *Eur. Heart J.*, 16, 16, 1995.
195. Corea, F. et al., Secondary prevention of cardioembolic stroke: Oldest and newest promises, *Clin. Exp. Hypertens.*, 28, 413, 2006.
196. Marki, W.E., The anticoagulant and antithrombotic properties of hirudins, *Thromb. Haemost.*, 64, 344, 1991.
197. Egner, U., Hoyer, G.A., and Schleuning, W.D., Rational design of hirulog-type inhibitors of thrombin, *J. Comput. Aided Mol. Des.*, 8, 479, 1994.
198. Agnelli, G. et al., Sustained antithrombotic activity of hirudin after its plasma clearance: Comparison with heparin, *Blood*, 80, 960, 1992.
199. Cardot, J.M., Lefevre, G.Y., and Godbillon, J.A., Pharmacokinetics of rec-hirudin in healthy volunteers after intravenous administration, *J. Pharmacokinet. Biopharm.*, 22, 147, 1994.
200. Fox, I. et al., Anticoagulant activity of Hirulog, a direct thrombin inhibitor, in humans, *Thromb. Haemost.*, 69, 157, 1993.
201. Zoldhelyi, P. et al., Persistent thrombin generation in humans during specific thrombin inhibition with hirudin, *Circulation*, 90, 2671, 1994.
202. Schumacher, W.A. et al., Effects of antithrombotic drugs in a rat model of aspirin-insensitive arterial thrombosis, *Thromb. Haemost.*, 69, 509, 1993.
203. Scott, N.A. et al., Local delivery of an antithrombin inhibits platelet-dependent thrombosis, *Circulation*, 90, 1951, 1994.
204. Hollenbach, S. et al., A comparative study of prothrombinase and thrombin inhibitors in a novel rabbit model of non-occlusive deep vein thrombosis, *Thromb. Haemost.*, 71, 357, 1994.
205. Schwienhorst, A., Direct thrombin inhibitors—a survey of recent developments, *Cell Mol. Life Sci.*, 63, 2773, 2006.
206. Paredes, N. et al., Mechanisms responsible for catalysis of the inhibition of factor Xa or thrombin by antithrombin using a covalent antithrombin-heparin complex, *J. Biol. Chem.*, 278, 23398, 2003.
207. Hatton, M.W.C. et al., Tritiation of commercial heparins by reaction of NaB3H4: Chemical analysis and biological properties of the product, *Anal. Biochem.*, 106, 417, 1980.
208. Pletcher, C.H. and Nelsestuen, G.L., The rate-determining step of the heparin-catalyzed antithrombin/thrombin reaction is independent of thrombin, *J. Biol. Chem.*, 257, 5342, 1982.
209. Muir, J.M. et al., A histomorphometric comparison of the effects of heparin and low molecular weight heparin on cancellous bone in rats, *Blood*, 89, 3236, 1997.
210. Amiral, J. et al., Platelet factor 4 complexed to heparin is the target for antibodies generated in heparin-induced thrombocytopenia, *Thromb. Haemost.*, 68, 95, 1992.
211. Lane, D.A. et al., Anticoagulant activities of heparin oligosaccharides and their neutralization by platelet factor 4, *Biochem. J.*, 218, 725, 1984.
212. Sprung, C.L. et al., Distribution of proteins in pulmonary edema, *Am. Rev. Respir. Dis.*, 136, 957, 1987.
213. Holter, J. et al., Protein permeability in the adult respiratory distress syndrome. Loss of size selectivity of the alveolar epithelium, *J. Clin. Invest.*, 78, 1513, 1986.
214. Brus, F. et al., Leakage of protein into lungs of preterm ventilated rabbits is correlated with activation of clotting, complement, and polymorphonuclear leukocytes in plasma, *Pediatr. Res.*, 39, 958, 1996.
215. Bachofen, M. and Weibel, E.R., Structural alterations of lung parenchyma in the adult respiratory distress syndrome, *Clin. Chest Med.*, 3, 35, 1982.
216. Gitlin, D. and Craig, J., The nature of the hyaline membrane in asphyxia of the newborn, *Pediatrics*, 17, 64, 1956.
217. Jobe, A.H., Pulmonary surfactant therapy, *N. Engl. J. Med.*, 328, 861, 1993.
218. Long, W., Thompson, T., and Sundell, H., Effects of two rescue doses of a synthetic surfactant on mortality rate and survival without bronchopulmonary dysplasia, *J. Pediatr.*, 118, 595, 1991.

219. The OSIRIS collaborative group, early versus delayed neonatal administration of a synthetic surfactant-the judgement of OSIRIS, *Lancet*, 340, 1363, 1992.
220. Liechty, E.A., Donovan, E., and Purohit, D., Reduction of neonatal mortality after multiple doses of bovine surfactant in low birth weight neonates with respiratory distress syndrome, *Pediatrics*, 88, 19, 1991.
221. Coalson, J.J. et al., Pathophysiologic, morphometric and biochemical studies of the premature baboon with bronchopulmonary dysplasia, *Am. Rev. Respir. Dis.*, 145, 872, 1992.
222. Saldeen, T., Fibrin-derived peptides and pulmonary injury, *Ann. NY Acad. Sci.*, 384, 319, 1982.
223. Fukuda, Y. et al., The role of intraalveolar fibrosis in the process of pulmonary structural remodelling in patients with diffuse alveolar damage, *Am. J. Pathol.*, 126, 171, 1987.
224. Jordan, R.E., Antithrombin-heparin complex and method for its production, U.S. Patent No. 4, 446, 126, 1984.
225. Eibl, J., Hetzl, E., and Linnau, Y., Method of producing an antithrombin III-heparin concentrate or antithrombin III-heparinoid concentrate, U.S. Patent No. 4, 510, 084, 1985.
226. Spannagl, M., Keller, R., and Schramm, W., A new AT III-Heparin-complex preparation: *In vitro* and *in vivo* characterisation, *Folia. Haematol.*, 116, 879, 1989.
227. Spannagl, M. et al., A purified antithrombin III-heparin complex as a potent inhibitor of thrombin in porcine endotoxin shock, *Thromb. Res.*, 61, 1, 1991.
228. Hennink, W.E. et al., Covalently bound conjugates of albumin and heparin: Synthesis, fractionation and characterization, *Thromb. Res.*, 29, 1, 1983.
229. Huhle, G. et al., Comparison of three heparin bovine serum albumin binding methods for production of antiheparin antibodies, *Semin. Thromb. Hemost.*, 20, 193, 1994.
230. Teien, A.N., Odegard, R., and Christensen, T.B., Heparin coupled to albumin, dextran and ficoll: Influence on blood coagulation and platelets, and *in vivo* duration, *Thromb. Res.*, 7, 273, 1975.
231. Ceustermans, R. et al., Preparation, characterization, and turnover properties of heparin-antithrombin III complexes stabilized by covalent bonds, *J. Biol. Chem.*, 257, 3401, 1982.
232. Cuatrecasas, P., Fuchs, S., and Anfinsen, C.B., Cross-linking of aminotyrosyl residues in the active site of staphylococcal nuclease, *J. Biol. Chem.*, 244, 406, 1969.
233. Zahn, H. and Meienhofer, J., Reaktionen von 1,5-difluor-2,4-dinitrobenzol mit insulin. 1. Mitt. synthèse von modellverbindungen, *Makromol. Chem.*, 26, 126, 1958.
234. Zahn, H. and Meienhofer, J., Reaktionen von 1,5-difluor-2,4-dinitrobenzol mit insulin. 2. Mitt. versuche mit insulin, *Makromol. Chem.*, 26, 153, 1958.
235. Fleet, G.W.J., Porter, R.R., and Knowles, J.R., Affinity labelling of antibodies with aryl nitrene as reactive group, *Nature*, 244, 511, 1969.
236. Staros, J.V. and Richards, F.M., Photochemical labeling of the surface proteins of human erythrocytes, *Biochemistry*, 13, 2720, 1974.
237. Bregman, M.D. and Levy, D., Labeling of glucagon binding components in hepatocyte plasma membranes, *Biochem. Biophys. Res. Comm.*, 78, 584, 1977.
238. Hixson, S.H. and Hixson, S.S., P-azidophenacyl bromide, a versatile photolabile bifunctional reagent. Reaction with glyceraldehyde-3-phosphate dehydrogenase, *Biochemistry*, 14, 4251, 1975.
239. Clyne, D.H. et al., The preparation of intermolecular conjugates of horseradish peroxidase and antibody and their use in immunohistology of renal cortex, *J. Histochem. Cytochem.*, 21, 233, 1973.
240. Schick, A.F. and Singer, S.J., On the formation of covalent linkages between two protein molecules, *J. Biol. Chem.*, 236, 2477, 1961.
241. Singer, S.J. and Schick, A.F., The properties of specific stains for electron microscopy prepared by the conjugation of antibody molecules with ferritin, *J. Biophys. Biochem. Cytol.*, 9, 519, 1961.
242. Edman, P. and Henschen, A., Sequence determination, in *Protein Sequence Determination: A Sourcebook of Methods and Techniques*, Needleman, S.B., Ed., Springer-Verlag, Berlin, Germany, 1975, page 232.
243. Inque, Y. and Nagasawa, K., Selective N-desulfation of heparin with dimethyl sulfoxide containing water or methanol, *Carb. Res.*, 46, 87, 1976.
244. Nagasawa, K. and Yoshidome, H., Solvent catalytic degradation of sulfamic acid and its N-substituted derivatives, *Chem. Pharm. Bull.*, 17, 1316, 1969.
245. Casu, B., Structure and biological activity of heparin and other glycosaminoglycans, *Pharmacol. Res. Comm.*, 11, 1, 1979.
246. Hoylaerts, M., Owen, W.G., and Collen, D., Involvement of heparin chain length in the heparin catalyzed inhibition of thrombin antithrombin III, *J. Biol. Chem.*, 259, 5670, 1984.

247. Bjork, I. et al., Permanent activation of antithrombin by covalent attachment of heparin oligosaccharides, *FEBS Lett.*, 143, 96, 1982.
248. Halluin, A.P., Protein heparin conjugates, U.S. Patent No. 5,308,617, 1994.
249. Dawes, J., James, K., and Lane, D.A., Conformational change in antithrombin induced by heparin probed with a monoclonal antibody against the heparin 1C/4B region, *Biochemistry*, 33, 4375, 1994.
250. Mitra, G. and Jordan, R.E., Covalently bound heparin-antithrombin III complex, U.S. Patent No. 4,689,323, 1987.
251. Mitra, G. and Jordan, R.E., Covalently bound heparin-antithrombin III complex, method for its preparation and its use for treating thromboembolism, European Patent No. 0-137-356, 1985.
252. Vlassara, H., Brownlee, M., and Cerami, A., Nonenzymatic glycosylation: Role in the pathogenesis of diabetic complications, *Clin. Chem.*, 32, B37, 1986.
253. Hall, P. et al., Functional activities and non-enzymatic glycosylation of plasma proteinase inhibitors in diabetes, *Clin. Chim. Acta*, 160, 55, 1986.
254. Ceriello, A. et al., Daily rapid blood glucose variations may condition antithrombin III biologic activity but not its plasma concentration in insulin-dependent diabetes. A possible role for labile non-enzymatic glycation, *Diabete. Metab.*, 13, 16, 1987.
255. Ceriello, A. et al., Decreased antithrombin III activity in diabetes may be due to non-enzymatic glycosylation—a preliminary report, *Thromb. Haemost.*, 50, 633, 1983.
256. Villanueva, G.B. and Allen, N., Demonstration of altered antithrombin III activity due to non-enzymatic glycosylation at glucose concentration expected to be encountered in severely diabetic patients, *Diabetes*, 37, 1103, 1988.
257. Brownlee, M., Vlassara, H., and Cerami, A., Inhibition of heparin-catalyzed human antithrombin III activity by non-enzymatic glycosylation. Possible role in fibrin deposition in diabetes, *Diabetes*, 33, 532, 1984.
258. Sakurai, T., Boissel, J.P., and Bunn, H.F., Non-enzymatic glycation of antithrombin III *in vitro*, *Biochim. Biophys. Acta*, 964, 340, 1988.
259. Brownlee, M. and Cerami, A., A glucose-controlled delivery system: Semi-synthetic insulin bound to lectin, *Science*, 206, 1190, 1979.
260. Hoffman, J., Larm, O., and Scholander, E., A new method for covalent coupling of heparin and other glycosaminoglycans to substances containing primary amino groups, *Carb. Res.*, 117, 328, 1983.
261. Berry, L., Chan, A.K.C., and Andrew, M., Polypeptide-polysaccharide conjugates produced by spontaneous non-enzymatic glycation, *Biochem. J.*, 124, 434, 1998.
262. Busby, T.F. and Ingham, K.C., Thermal stabilization of antithrombin III by sugars and sugar derivatives and the effects of non-enzymatic glycosylation, *Biochim. Biophys. Acta*, 799, 80, 1984.
263. Mewhort-Buist, T.A. et al., Structural effects of a covalent linkage between antithrombin and heparin: Covalent N-terminus attachment of heparin enhances the maintenance of antithrombin's activated state, *Biochem. J.*, 140, 175, 2006.
264. Berry, L. et al., Investigation of the anticoagulant mechanisms of a covalent antithrombin-heparin complex, *J. Biol. Chem.*, 273, 34730, 1998.
265. Chan, A.K.C. et al., Isoform composition of antithrombin in a covalent antithrombin-heparin complex, *Biochem. Biophys. Res. Comm.*, 309, 986, 2003.
266. Patel, S., Berry, L.R., and Chan, A.K.C., Analysis of inhibition rate enhancement by covalent linkage of heparin to antithrombin as a potential predictor of reaction mechanism, *Biochem. J.*, 141, 25, 2007.
267. Jordan, R.E. et al., Heparin with two binding sites for antithrombin or platelet factor 4, *J. Biol. Chem.*, 257, 400, 1982.
268. Chan, A.K.C. et al., Decreased concentrations of heparinoids are required to inhibit thrombin generation in plasma from newborns and children compared to plasma from adults due to reduced thrombin potential, *Thromb. Haemost.*, 87, 606, 2002.
269. Parmar, N. et al., Effect of heparins on thrombin generation in hemphilic plasma supplemented with FVIII, FVIIa, or FEIBA, *Clin. Lab.*, 51, 157, 2005.
270. Hoylaerts, M. et al., Covalent complexes between low molecular weight heparin fragments and antithrombin III—inhibition kinetics and turnover parameters, *Thromb. Haemost.*, 49, 109, 1983.
271. Collen, D.J., Novel composition of matter of antithrombin III bound to a heparin fragment, U.S. Patent No. 4,623,718, 1986.
272. Mattsson, C. et al., Antithrombotic properties in rabbits of heparin and heparin fragments covalently coupled to human antithrombin III, *J. Clin. Invest.*, 75, 1169, 1985.

273. Chan, A.K.C. et al., A novel antithrombin-heparin covalent complex: Antithrombotic and bleeding studies in rabbits, *Blood Coagul. Fibrinol.*, 9, 587, 1998.
274. Chan, A.K.C. et al., Binding of heparin to plasma proteins and endothelial surfaces is inhibited by covalent linkage to antithrombin, *Thromb. Haemost.*, 91, 1009, 2004.
275. Volpi, N., Cusmano, M., and Venturelli, T., Qualitative and quantitative studies of heparin and chondroitin sulfates in normal human plasma, *Biochim. Biophys. Acta*, 1243, 49, 1995.
276. Mitchell, L. et al., Circulating dermatan sulphate/heparin sulfate proteoglycan(s) in children undergoing liver transplantation, *Thromb. Haemost.*, 74, 859, 1995.
277. Andrew, M. et al., An anticoagulant dermatan sulfate proteoglycan circulates in the pregnant woman and her fetus, *J. Clin. Invest.*, 89, 321, 1992.
278. Singhal, K.K. and Parton, L.A., Plasminogen activator activity in preterm infants with respiratory distress syndrome: Relationship to the development of bronchopulmonary dysplasia, *Pediatr. Res.*, 39, 229, 1996.
279. Idell, S. et al., Pathways of fibrin turnover in lavage of premature baboons with hyperoxic lung injury, *Am. J. Respir. Crit. Care. Med.*, 149, 767, 1994.
280. Idell, S. et al., Local abnormalities in coagulation and fibrinolytic pathways predispose to alveolar fibrin deposition in the adult respiratory distress sydrome, *J. Clin. Invest.*, 84, 695, 1989.
281. Bertozzi, P. et al., Depressed bronchoalveolar urokinase activity in patients with adult respiratory distress syndrome, *N. Engl. J. Med.*, 322, 890, 1990.
282. Chan, A.K.C. et al., Effect of a novel covalent antithrombin-heparin complex on thrombin generation on fetal distal lung epithelium, *Am. J. Physiol.*, 274, L914, 1998.
283. Berry, L.R., Andrew, M., and Chan, A.K.C., Effect of covalent serpin-heparinoid complexes on plasma thrombin generation on fetal distal lung epithelium, *Am. J. Resp. Cell Mol. Biol.*, 28, 150, 2003.
284. Monagle, P. et al., Covalent heparin cofactor II-heparin and heparin cofactor II-dermatan sulfate complexes, *J. Biol. Chem.*, 273, 33566, 1998.
285. Chan, A.K.C. et al., A novel antithrombin-heparin covalent complex: Antithrombotic and bleeding studies in rabbits, *Blood Coagul. Fibrinolysis*, 9, 587, 1998.
286. Chan, A.K.C. et al., Antithrombin-heparin covalent complex: A possible alternative to heparin for arterial thrombosis prevention, *Circulation*, 106, 261, 2002.
287. Becker, D.L. et al., Exosites 1 and 2 are essential for protection of fibrin-bound thrombin from heparin-catalyzed inhibition by antithrombin and heparin cofactor II, *J. Biol. Chem.*, 274, 6226, 1999.
288. Berry, L.R., Becker, D.L., and Chan, A.K., Inhibition of fibrin-bound thrombin by a covalent antithrombin-heparin complex, *Biochem. J.*, 132, 167, 2002.
289. Bamford, C.H. and Al-Lamee, K.G., Chemical methods for improving the haemocompatibility of synthetic polymers, *Clin. Mater.*, 10, 243, 1992.
290. Karlsson, C., Nygren, H., and Braide, M., Exposure of blood to biomaterial surfaces liberates substances that activate polymorphonuclear granulocytes, *J. Lab. Clin. Med.*, 128, 496, 1996.
291. Tang, L. and Eaton, J.W., Inflammatory responses to biomaterials, *Am. J. Clin. Pathol.*, 103, 466, 1995.
292. Vanholder, R. and Lameire, N., Does biocompatibility of dialysis membranes affect recovery of renal function and survival? *Lancet*, 354, 1316, 1999.
293. Sanchez, J. and Olsson, P., On the control of the plasma contact activation system on human endothelium: Comparisons with heparin surface, *Thromb. Res.*, 93, 27, 1999.
294. Dickneite, G. and Leithauser, B., Influence of antithrombin III on coagulation and inflammation in porcine septic shock, *Arterioscler. Thromb. Vasc. Biol.*, 19, 1566, 1999.
295. Wendel, H.P. and Ziemer, G., Coating-techniques to improve the hemocompatibility of artificial devices used for extracorporeal circulation, *Eur. J. Cardiothorac. Surg.*, 16, 342, 1999.
296. Klement, P. et al., Blood-compatible biomaterials by surface coating with a novel antithrombin-heparin covalent complex, *Biomaterials*, 23, 527, 2002.
297. van Phung, K. and Schulz, R.C., Pfropfung von vinylverbindugen auf polyamide, *Macromol. Chem.*, 180, 1825, 1979.
298. Hoerl, H.H., Nussbaumer, D., and Wuenn, E., Surface grafting of microporous, nitrogen-containing polymer membranes and membranes obtained thereby, German Patent No. DE 3,929,648, 1990.
299. Heinrich, H.H., Nussbaumer, D., and Wuenn, E., Grafting of unsaturated monomers on polymers containing nitrogen, German Patent No. DE 4,028,326, 1991.
300. Raman, V.K. and Edelman, E.R., Coated stents: Local pharmacology, *Semin. Interv. Cardiol.*, 3, 133, 1998.

301. Phaneuf, M.D. et al., Covalent linkage of recombinant hirudin to poly(ethylene terephthalate) (Dacron): Creation of a novel antithrombin surface, *Biomaterials*, 18, 755, 1997.

302. Phaneuf, M.D. et al., Covalent linkage of recombinant hirudin to a novel ionic poly (carbonate) urethane polymer with protein binding sites: Determination of surface antithrombin activity, *Artificial Organs*, 22, 657, 1998.

303. Du, Y.J. et al., *In vivo* rabbit acute model tests of polyurethane catheters coated with a novel antithrombin-heparin covalent complex, *Thromb. Haemost.*, 94, 366, 2005.

304. Klement, P. et al., Chronic performance of polyurethane catheters covalently coated with ATH complex: A rabbit jugular vein model, *Biomaterials*, 27, 5107, 2006.

305. Du, Y.J. et al., Protein adsorption on polyurethane catheters modified with a novel antithrombin-heparin covalent complex, *J. Biomed. Mater. Res. A*, 80, 216, 2007.

306. Solomon, D.D. and Byron, M.P., Anti-infective and antithrombogenic medical articles and method for their preparation, U.S. Patent No. 4, 999, 210, 1991.

307. Solomon, D.D., McGary, C.W., and Pascarella, V.J., Permanently bonded antithrombogenic polyurethane surface, U.S. Patent No. 4, 642, 242, 1987.

308. Scholander, E., Process for preparing surface modification substances, Swedish Patent No. 6, 461, 665, 2002.

309. Gott, V.L. and Daggett, R.L., Serendipity and the development of heparin and carbon surfaces, *Ann. Thorac. Surg.*, 68, S19, 1999.

310. Miura, Y. et al., Anticoagulant acitivity of artificial biomedical materials with co-immobilized antithrombin III and heparin, *Biochimie*, 62, 595, 1980.

311. Cahalan, P. et al., Method for making improved heparinized biomaterials, U.S. Patent No. 5, 767, 108, 1998.

312. Chindemi, P.A. et al., Biodistribution of covalent antithrombin-heparin complexes, *Thromb. Haemost.*, 95, 629, 2006.

313. Egbrink, M.G. et al., Regulation of microvascular thromboembolism *in vivo*, *Microcirculation*, 12, 287, 2005.

314. Hoylaerts, M. et al., Covalent complexes between low molecular weight heparin fragments and antithrombin III—inhibition kinetics and turnover parameters, *Thromb. Haemost.*, 49, 109, 1983.

19 Surface Modification of Biomaterials Using Plasma Immersion Ion Implantation and Deposition

Xuanyong Liu, Ricky K.Y. Fu, and Paul K. Chu

CONTENTS

19.1 PLASMA SCIENCE AND TECHNOLOGY

Plasma is often called as the fourth state of matter. Generally, a solid substance melts into a liquid when the temperature is increased at a fixed pressure. The liquid then transforms into a gas as the temperature is further increased. Under high temperature, the molecules in the gas decompose to form atoms that move freely in random directions in space. If the temperature is further increased, the atoms decompose into freely moving charged particles, and the substance enters the plasma state. Thus, under certain conditions, a plasma can be thought of as a collection of electrons, single- and multiple-charged positive and negative ions along with neutral atoms, excited particles, electromagnetic radiation, molecules, and molecular fragments. In plasma, the densities of the excited particles, ions, and electrons as well as the intensity of the electromagnetic radiation far exceed those that are found in more mundane situations encountered elsewhere. An important feature of plasma is that the positive and negative particles are in a state of charge equilibrium, and the sum of the positive and negative charges in a sufficiently large volume is equal to zero. In fact, plasma technology is a dry, environmental-friendly, and cost-efficient process in a myriad of applications.

19.1.1 PLASMA SOURCES

To produce a plasma, electron separation from atoms or molecules in the gas state, or ionization, is required. Ionization occurs when an atom or a molecule gains enough energy from an outside excitation source or via interactions (collisions) with each other. In fact, to have a stable plasma discharge, the choice of heating mechanisms and geometric configurations for sustaining discharge is important. In most practical situations, the plasma is produced by an electrical discharge. Various forms of discharges such as radio frequency (RF), microwave, glow, and arc discharges have been developed. Generally, these discharges can be separated into two categories: gaseous and metallic plasma discharges. The RF, glow, and cathodic arc discharges are discussed in the following sections in detail.

19.1.1.1 Radio Frequency Discharge

RF discharges can be classified into two types according to the method of coupling the RF power with the load: capacitive coupling and inductive coupling. The setup typically consists of an RF generator, a matching network, and an antenna as shown in Figure 19.1. Commonly, the generator

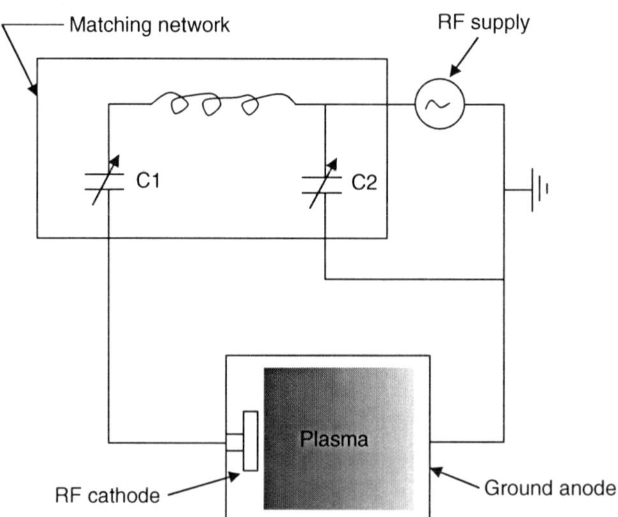

FIGURE 19.1 Schematic diagram of a capacitively-coupled plasma (CCP) plasma source with an equivalent electrical circuit.

operates at a frequency of 13.56 MHz, which is above the ion plasma frequency but below the electron plasma frequency. Therefore, electrons respond to the varying electric field, but ions experience only the average field. The pressure during discharge is between 10^{-3} and 100 Torr [1,2]. The plasma density in RF glow discharge in low pressure (10^{-3} to 1 Torr) varies from 10^9 to 10^{11}/cm^3, whereas that in medium pressure (1–100 Torr) can reach 10^{12}/cm^3 [3]. The low-pressure discharges have charge exchange mean free paths typically longer than the sheath dimensions at the substrate. Besides, the electron temperature of low-pressure discharge is usually in the range of 1–5 eV, and the electron energy distribution functions are close to Maxwellian. In addition, the ion temperature (0.1–0.5 eV) is somewhat higher than the gas temperature (0.03–0.1 eV) but much less than the electron temperature. The plasma potential of the RF discharge is typically in the range of 10–30 V above the wall potential and is proportional to the electron temperature [4].

19.1.1.2 Glow Discharge

A glow discharge is triggered by two common ways: thermionic filament glow discharge and pulsed high-voltage glow discharge. A simple thermionic discharge based on the electron emission from a hot cathode produces the desired plasma density by ionization of the background gas. Plasma generation requires a suitable selection of the cathode that is directly heated by a floating power supply that passes sufficient current through the filament to heat the cathode resistively to the emissive temperature. Usually, refractory metals are selected as the filament cathode as they are simple to fabricate and have sufficiently low evaporation rates and sputtering yields to provide a reasonable lifetime [5]. Thermionic discharges typically utilize electron currents that range from 1 A to several kilamperes depending on the types of gases used, plasma density, and plasma size. In addition, the voltage applied between the cathode and anode can be lower than the ionization energy and is commonly in the range of 25–100 V where the maximum of the ionization cross-section occurs for most gases.

In pulsed high-voltage glow discharge, the pulsed voltage serves the dual purpose of generating the plasma and accelerating the ions in the sheath to the substrate. The method is very versatile since it can be used practically for any electrode geometry and gases. The pulsed high voltage produces a sudden electric field between the substrate (cathode) and the surrounding system (anode). Free electrons that are emitted from the substrate are accelerated and collide with the gas molecules or the anode. Ions produced during the collisions continually strike the cathode to generate secondary electrons, which are accelerated back into the discharge volume. This discharge mechanism is described by the Paschen curves in gas discharge physics restricted by the minimum pressure of the process gas for a given geometry, voltage amplitude, and nature of the gas [6].

19.1.1.3 Cathodic Arc Discharge

In general, a cathodic arc plasma source is composed of two parts: plasma production unit and macroparticle filter. An arc discharge is characterized by a relatively high current (tens or hundreds of amperes) and a relatively low voltage (10–80 V) between the cathode and the anode. The vacuum arc is sustained by materials originating from the cathode. Before the arc is established, the atomic (molecular) density is not high enough to sustain the electrical discharge. When a feedback mechanism is established in which a very small area of the cathode surface is heated by electron emission, more particles are ejected as illustrated in Figure 19.2. The cathodic discharge is characterized by an ensemble of luminous cathode spots that move in a rapid and chaotic manner across the surface [7,8]. The plasma expands in all directions from the cathode spots toward the anode and vacuum chamber walls.

The cathode spot is small (10^{-8} to 10^{-4} m in diameter), but an intense plasma with a current density of 10^6–10^{12}/A^2 can be produced. The spot velocity is determined by factors that include the nature of the cathode, residual vacuum, and presence of the external magnetic field. The cathode erosion rate depends upon the state of the surface, and cathode spot characteristics change as the

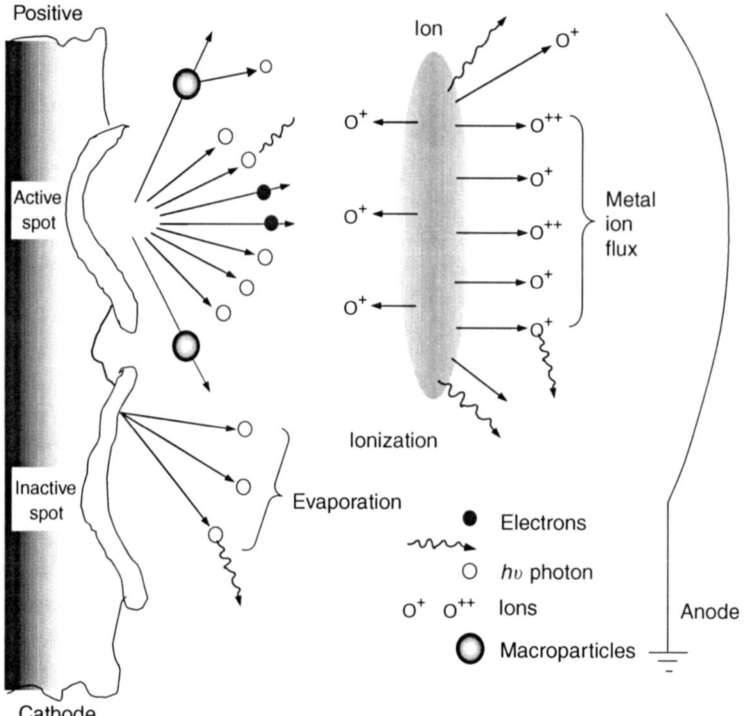

FIGURE 19.2 Particle emissions from the arc spots. (From Lafferty, J.M., *Vacuum Arcs—Theory and Applications*, Wiley, New York, 1980. With permission.)

surface is depleted of contamination and oxides during arcing. The materials ejected from the cathode spot are mainly ionized cathode materials together with microdroplets or macroparticles ranging from 0.1 to 100 μm in diameter. The electron density in the cathodic plasma can reach $10^{20}/cm^3$, and the expanding plasma produces a highly ionized jet with mean ion charge states greater than 1+ for many elements. Each cathode material has its own specific charge state distribution, which becomes constant for arc duration longer than about 200 s. Many attempts have been made to eliminate macroparticles. A curved duct filter with a magnetic field as shown in Figure 19.3 is commonly utilized to mitigate particle contamination from the arc. Another goal of the filter is to increase the plasma transport efficiency through the duct. An optimized 90° curved duct can achieve plasma transport efficiency of about 35% [9].

19.1.2 PLASMA PROPERTIES AND DIAGNOSTICS

The plasma is macroscopically neutral in an equilibrium state, that is, $n_e = n_i = n_o$, where n_e is electron density, n_i is ion density, and n_o is plasma density. However, at the edge of a bounded plasma, a potential exists to contain the more mobile-charged species. A nonneutral potential region formed between the plasma and the wall is referred to as a plasma sheath (Figure 19.4). In this situation, monoenergetic ions are accelerated by the sheath potential while the electron density decreases according to a Boltzmann factor.

The plasma medium is complicated in such a manner that the charged particles are affected by external electric and magnetic fields. Waves are important to carry energy from the surface of a plasma where the wave is excited into the bulk plasma, and the wave energy can be absorbed from the bulk plasma. Plasmas support both electromagnetic and electrostatic waves. Electromagnetic waves in plasmas are similar to those in dielectric materials and propagate due to the exchange of

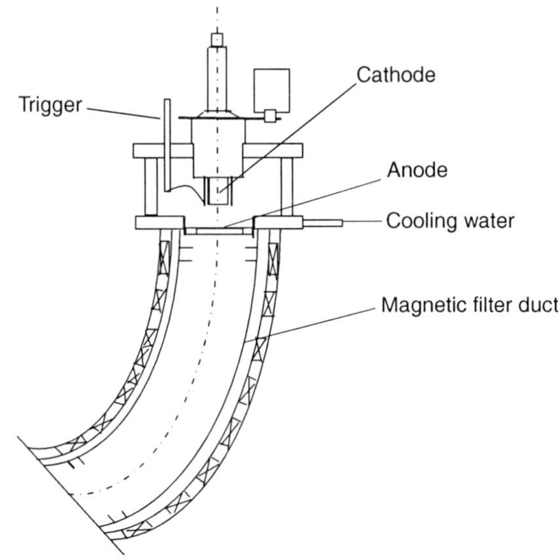

FIGURE 19.3 Schematic diagram of cathodic arc plasma source with a magnetic filter duct.

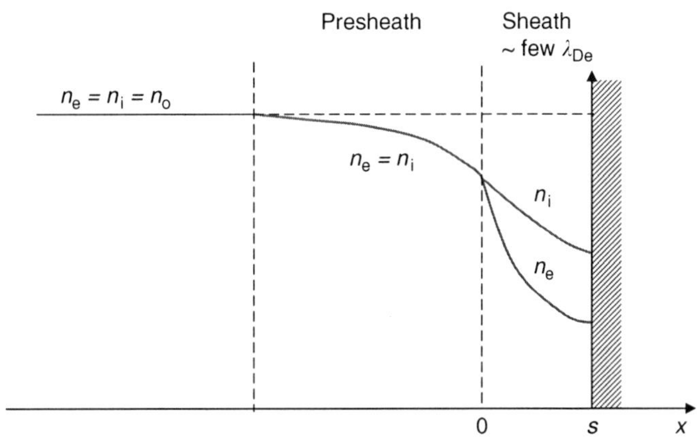

FIGURE 19.4 Qualitative behavior of plasma sheath and presheath in contact with a wall. (From Lieberman, M.A. and Lichtenberg, A.J., *Principles of Plasma Discharges and Materials Processing*, Wiley, New York, 1994. With permission.)

energy between electric and magnetic forms. In low-pressure cold plasma (electron temperature > ion temperature), the electron motion dominates the behavior of the waves as the mass of electron is much smaller than that of the ion. Thus, the plasma can be confined and enhanced by bounding the electron motions.

A metal probe inserted in a discharge and biased positively or negatively to draw electron or ion current is one of the most useful tools for diagnosing a plasma. A conducting probe smaller than the particle mean free path placed directly in the plasma is called a Langmuir probe [10]. The plasma electron density, electron temperature, and plasma potential can be measured from the current versus voltage characteristics of this probe. In this way, the energy of the ions striking the cathode can be inferred without the more difficult direct measurement.

Another technique to detect the plasma concentration is to use emission spectroscopy as most plasmas emit light in the infrared and ultraviolet ranges. A simple analytical technique is to measure the intensity of these emissions versus wavelength with the aid of a spectrophotometer. Using the observed spectral peaks, it is usually possible to determine the presence of neutral and ionic species. The relative concentrations of species can be obtained by correlating changes in the intensity with the plasma parameter changes.

19.2 PLASMA IMMERSION ION IMPLANTATION AND DEPOSITION

19.2.1 CONCEPTS AND FUNDAMENTALS OF PIII

Generally, a plasma immersion ion implantation (PIII) system consists of a vacuum chamber with a workpiece stage, plasma source, and high-voltage pulse modulator as shown in Figure 19.5. In the PIII process, a workpiece is immersed in plasma and pulsed to a high negative voltage with respect to the plasma potential, which is usually close to the ground potential of the chamber walls. The applied high voltage accelerates electrons away from the workpiece while accelerating the positive ions from the source plasma toward the workpiece, creating a plasma sheath around the workpiece and implanting the ions [11].

In the initial stage when the negative voltage is applied to the target, electrons are repelled on the time scale of the inverse electron plasma frequency to establish a positive space-charged region, and the potential profile can be described by the ion matrix sheath. Followed by ion collection or extraction and plasma sheath expansion, a quasistatic Child-Law sheath evolves. The evolution of the plasma sheath plays a very important role in PIII because it dictates the implantation process and can be used to predict process parameters and results including the implantation current, implantation dose, and impurities profile. Positive ions are accelerated by the electric field and implanted into the substrate with near-Gaussian depth distribution of which the projected range can be estimated by the TRIM simulation codes [12]. As implantation takes place on all exposed and biased surfaces, PIII can be a conformal treatment process for irregular targets, and the implantation time

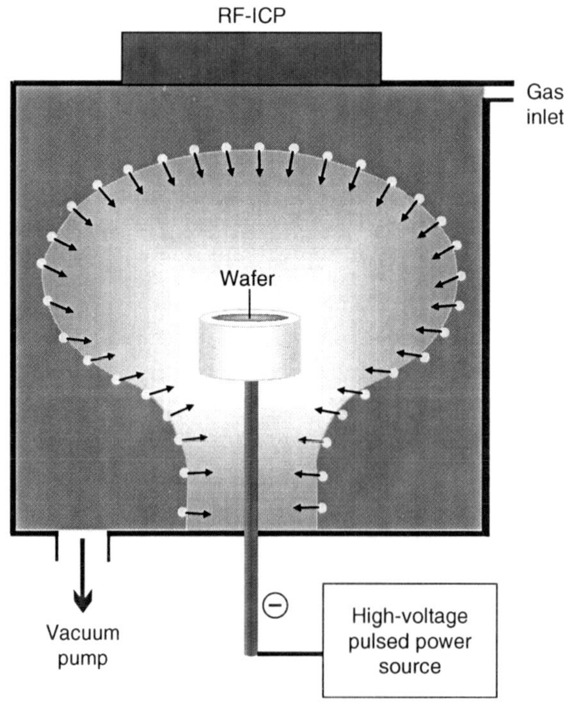

FIGURE 19.5 Schematic diagram of PIII system.

is independent of sample size with the proper control of the plasma sheath by varying the plasma density, bias potential, pulse duration, and configurations.

19.2.2 Ion–Solid Interactions Induced by Ion Implantation

The important considerations in any description of ion–solid interactions are the depth distribution of the implanted ions, ion irradiation damage and sputtering, novel synthesis and formation of materials by irradiation, as well as ion alloying [13–15]. An implanted ion penetrates a solid, slows down, and comes to rest. The total length of the ion trajectory in the solid is called the ion range R. As the incident ion makes many collisions with lattice atoms and displaces them from their lattice sites, these displaced atoms can in turn displace others, and the net result is the production of a highly disordered region along the path of the ion. At sufficiently high ion doses, these individual disordered regions may overlap, and an amorphous or metastable crystalline layer may form.

Ion irradiation is quite efficient in forming vacancy-interstitial pairs. The atomic displacements resulting from energetic recoiled atoms can be highly concentrated into small localized regions containing a large concentration of defects that are well in excess of the equilibrium value. If the defects are produced at temperatures at which they are mobile and can in part be annealed out, the balance between the rates of formation and annihilation leads to a steady state of excess concentration of defects. Since the atomic diffusivity is proportional to the defect concentration, an excess concentration of the defects leads to an enhancement in the diffusion process [16,17]. Thus, the final ion stopping range and the modified layer can be enhanced and extended by diffusion as shown in the right side of Figure 19.6. Experiments have shown that ordered alloys could become chemically disordered under irradiation. The effects of irradiation on the ordered alloy are described by the competing processes of chemical disordering, which is induced by atomic replacements resulting from displacement and cascade damage and chemical ordering, which is stimulated by radiation-enhanced diffusion [18,19]. When an ordered alloy is disordered by exposure to particle irradiation, thermodynamics will determine the strength of the driving force for the recovery of the chemical disorder. A driving force will always exist in alloys where the disordered state will not be in the equilibrium condition, and the primary limitation to reordering will be kinetic.

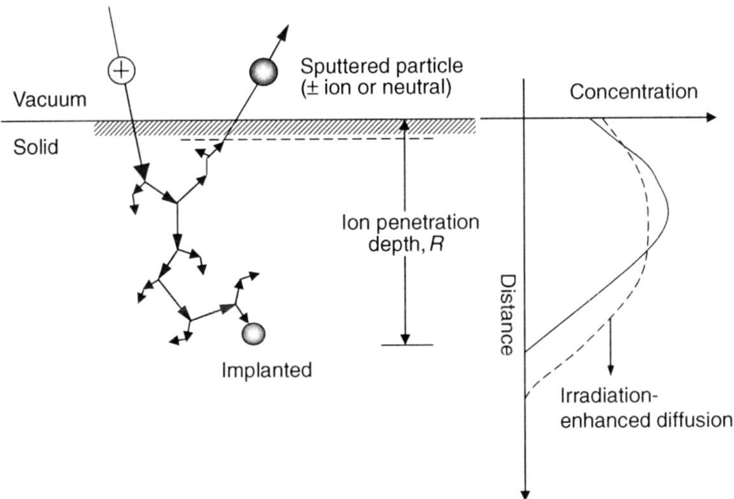

FIGURE 19.6   Schematic diagram of ion–solid interactions: the sputtering process and the irradiation-enhanced diffusion process. (From Borg, R.J. and Dienes, G.J., *An Introduction to Solid State Diffusion*, Academic Press, Boston, MA, 1988; Thompson, M.W., *Defects and Radiation Damage in Metals*, Cambridge University Press, Cambridge, MA, 1969. With permission.)

Ion implantation is a process in which virtually any element can be injected into the near-surface region of any solid. However, surface atoms will be removed by collisions between the incoming particles while atoms in the near-surface layers of a solid are removed by a process called sputtering, as shown in Figure 19.6. Sputtering sets the limit of the maximum concentration of implanted atoms that can be retained in a target material. The yield of sputtered atoms, that is, the number of sputtered atoms per incident ion, typically lies in the range of 0.5–20 depending upon ion species, ion energy, structure and composition of the target material, and experimental geometry [20,21]. Therefore, a high ion sputtering yield will result in a thin modified layer and a reduced retained dose.

Ion implantation has the ability to alloy any elemental species into the near-surface region of any substrate, irrespective of thermodynamic constraints such as solubility and diffusivity. These considerations coupled with the possibility of low-temperature processing have prompted exploration into applications where the limitations of dimensional changes and possible delamination associated with conventional coatings are the areas of concern. Interests in nonsemiconductor implantation have expanded from the initial friction and wear studies to other areas such as corrosion, oxidation, fatigue, conductivity, optical, and biomedical applications. In addition to metals, polymers and ceramics are receiving more attention from researchers with the principal objectives of increasing the conductivity, wettability, surface energy, and adhesion of polymers and investigating the fracture toughness and tribological properties of ceramics.

19.2.3 DEPOSITION PROCESS AND DYNAMICS

Plasmas used for deposition can be either single species or multiple species. Reactants in the plasma will diffuse to the substrate surface giving rise to chemical reactions and thin film deposition, and the details are illustrated in Figure 19.7. The parameters of the deposition process such as deposition rate and thin film structures can be varied by adjusting the working pressure and modes of substrate biasing [19,22–24]. RF, DC, and pulsed biases are the common modes of substrate biases. Typically, RF and DC biases are in the range of 0 V–1 kV while pulse biases can be varied from low-voltage thin film deposition to high-voltage ion bombardment. Bombardment with energetic particles has been observed to enhance a number of film characteristics and properties that are critical to the performance of thin films and coatings such as adhesion, densification of films grown at low substrate temperature, and modification of grain size and morphology, optical properties, and hardness and ductility.

Gaseous plasmas, such as hydrocarbons, methane, ethane, ethylene, acetylene, and benzene, are widely used in the synthesis of plasma-polymerized hydrogenated carbon films. In plasma

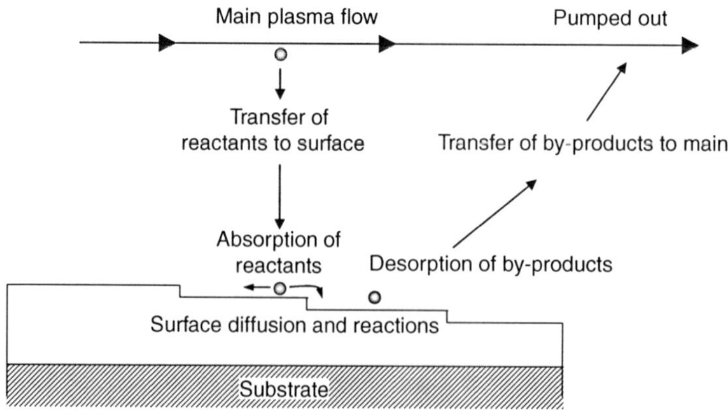

FIGURE 19.7 Schematic diagram of the sequential steps of deposition process.

polymerization, the transformation of low-molecular-weight molecules (monomers) into high-molecular-weight molecules (polymers) occurs with the assistance of energetic plasma species such as electrons, ions, and radicals. Polymer formation in plasma polymerization encompasses plasma activation of monomers to form radicals, recombination of the formed radicals, and reactivation of the recombined molecules. Plasma polymers do not comprise repeating monomer units but, instead, complicated units containing cross-linked, fragmented, and rearranged units from the monomers as well as a number of functional terminals.

Dual plasma deposition is a novel technology derived from PIII. In this process, gas and metal plasmas are simultaneously generated typically using a RF glow discharge source and a vacuum arc plasma source, respectively, or by direct introduction of the gas into the vicinity of the discharge area of the vacuum arc plasma source. Dual plasma deposition has many advantages as a thin-film technique. The obvious advantage is that a film composed of several elements (gaseous and metallic) with various compositions can be fabricated in the same instrument without breaking the vacuum. Several functional thin films with desirable properties can be synthesized by proper control of the plasma parameters and deposition modes. For instance, the technique can be used to fabricate optoelectronic materials such as ZnO, autocatalytic and biocompatible materials such as TiO_2, high dielectric constant materials such as ZrO_2 and TaO, apochromatic materials such as WO, electronic materials such as AlN, as well as hard-coating materials including TiN and metal-doped diamond-like carbon (DLC).

19.2.4 PIII VERSUS CONVENTIONAL BEAM-LINE ION IMPLANTATION

Conventional ion implantation is a line-of-sight process. During ion implantation, atoms or molecules are ionized and accelerated by an electrostatic field into a solid. In this way, a myriad of combinations of ions and substrates are possible, such as nitrogen into iron, boron into silicon, silicon into silicon, tellurium into gallium arsenide, and so on. The acceleration energy can be between a few hundred electron volts and several million electron volts. The ion penetration depth depends upon not only the energy, but also the mass of the ions and atomic mass of the solid [25]. Ions are extracted from the plasma by an extraction system, accelerated as a collimated beam to high energy, and then used to bombard the samples. In the semiconductor industry, a mass filter is added to obtain an ion beam consisting of a single ion species. The ion beam typically has a small cross-sectional area, and so either beam or sample rastering must be performed to achieve uniform implantation into a large sample. If the sample is nonplanar, sample rotation is required to implant all the surfaces. This manipulation adds complexity and in many cases casts a limit on the size of the workpieces that can be implanted in a cost-effective manner.

Since beam extraction optics, focusing optics, scanning, masking, and target manipulation are absent in PIII, the instrumentation is substantially cheaper and simpler than a conventional beam-line ion implanter. The smaller equipment footprint also bodes well for the space-conscious clean-room environment in the semiconductor industry. In PIII, the specimen is placed directly in the plasma and biased to high negative potential. Ions bombard normally to the entire surface of the sample with good conformality as long as the dimensions of the plasma sheath remain small compared with the sizes of the specimen features. The retained dose problem is also mitigated in PIII because ion acceleration occurs mostly perpendicular to the surface. Therefore, PIII circumvents the line-of-sight problem of conventional ion implantation and also alleviates the retained dose problem [26,27].

19.2.5 APPLICATIONS OF PIII

From the industrial viewpoint, PIII is attractive because of the simple instrumentation, low cost, and small footprint. The high throughput or efficiency of PIII is another big advantage because all surfaces are implanted simultaneously, and the implantation time is independent of the sample size [28]. A short processing time and high ion flux can be readily achieved. It is also relatively easy to adjust *in situ* instrumental parameters including the applied voltage, pulse width, pulsing frequency, working gas pressure, and discharging power to satisfy the processing requirements of different materials. Many significant applications have been developed since the mid-1980s in the semiconductor area. For instance, PIII has been used to form shallow junctions in submicrometer integrated circuits and to synthesize silicon-on-insulator (SOI) by implanting a high-dose oxygen or water vapor into a silicon wafer to form a continuous buried oxide layer (SPIMOX or separation by plasma implantation of oxygen) [29,30] or by implanting hydrogen or helium into a silicon wafer followed by wafer bonding and annealing in the commercial ion-cut process [31]. Other applications include surface modification of metals and alloys to enhance the corrosion resistance and tribological properties [32], thin film deposition [33], flat panel display fabrication [34], and so on.

Superficially, biomaterials are quite different from semiconductors. However, the knowledge acquired from plasma processing of semiconductors can be readily applied to that of biomaterials or vice versa. As an alternative to conventional ion implantation, there are advantages of using PIII and deposition (PIIID) to produce a functional surface on biomedical materials, and so it can also be used to enhance the surface properties of biomedical materials [35]. The surface composition, morphology, and microstructure of biomedical materials can directly impact the performance and lifetime of medical implants. In the area of biomaterials, the following two topics are being widely researched: (1) fundamental issues governing the bioactivity and tissue compatibility of biomaterials and medical implants and (2) mechanisms of biological responses such as anticoagulation of blood on artificial cardiovascular materials. Plasma immersion ion implantation is a novel technique in biomedical engineering offering omnidirectional processing capability and the possibility to introduce a myriad of different species at different energies into the materials to tailor the surface properties. Some of the bottlenecks and difficult problems that cannot be solved by conventional methods such as coatings can potentially be overcome by this technique, in addition to the extra benefits of PIII such as its excellent throughput and compatibility with medical implants with irregular geometries.

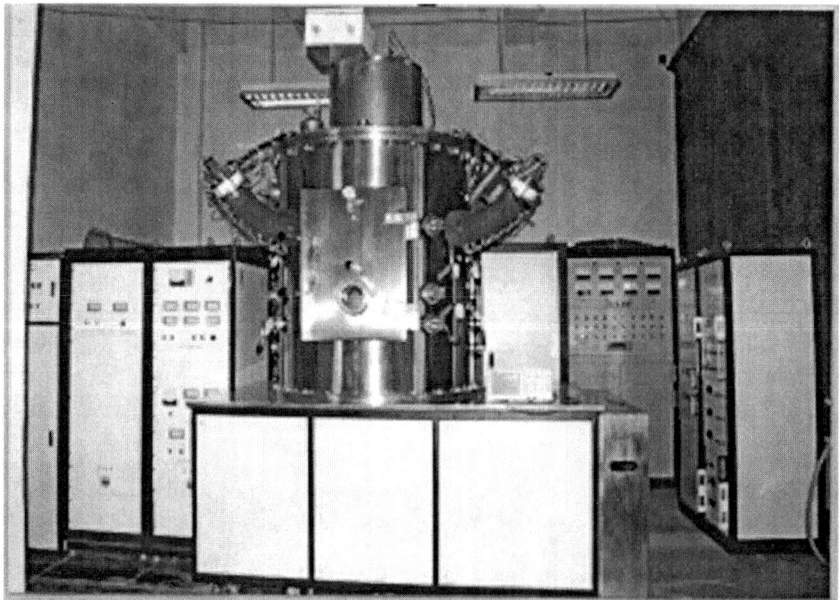

FIGURE 19.8 Photograph of the third-generation plasma immersion ion implanter. (From Chu, P.K., *Rev. Sci. Instrum.*, 72, 1660, 2001. With permission.)

When treating biomedical materials and components, hybrid processes incorporating gaseous and metal ion plasma implantation are sometimes more effective. In light of this and other requirements, researchers in Plasma Technology Limited and City University of Hong Kong designed and constructed a third-generation plasma immersion ion implanter for biomedical materials and engineering, and the design is flexible enough to enable other applications (Figure 19.8). In this chapter, we introduce the process and effects of PIIID to activate the surface of biomedical titanium alloys and silicon, mitigate Ni release of the biomedical NiTi alloys, improve the blood compatibility of blood-contacting materials, and improve the antibacterial property of biopolymers.

19.3 SURFACE ACTIVATION OF BIOMATERIALS

It is very important that biomaterials implanted into human bodies must have excellent bioactive surfaces. However, many biomaterials, such as titanium and its alloys, silicon, and some ceramics, are bioinert, thereby limiting their application in the clinical field. Therefore, it is a key issue in the field of biomaterials to improve the surface bioactivity of implanted materials. The bioactivity of titanium alloys, silicon, and titania coatings has been improved by plasma implantation of hydrogen, calcium, sodium, and other elements. The work on the surface activation of biomaterials by PIII conducted in City University of Hong Kong and Shanghai Institute of Ceramics are described here.

19.3.1 Hydrogen PIII

19.3.1.1 Improvement of Bioactivity on Silicon

In the past three decades, silicon has gradually been recognized as an essential trace element in the normal metabolism of higher animals, and the role of silicon in the human body has aroused interest in the biomedical community [37–41]. More silicon-containing materials are being investigated as potential materials in biomedical devices and medical implants. Both silicon-based microelectronics and biosensors have undergone tremendous technical development, but the bioactivity and biocompatibility of silicon are relatively not well understood. In fact, the surface biocompatibility of silicon is usually poor, and the interaction between silicon-based biosensors or micro electro mechanical system (MEMS) and the human body may not be desirable [42,43]. Long-term problems associated with the packaging and biocompatibility of Si chips have been identified to be major issues [44]. Therefore, it is necessary to improve the bioactivity and biocompatibility of silicon-based microelectronics and biosensors to meet the need of clinical applications.

Some attempts have been made to improve the bioactivity and biocompatibility of silicon wafers. For instance, Canham reported that apatite could be induced to form on the surface of microporous silicon films obtained by wet etching [45]. Dahmen et al. have shown that surface functionalization of amorphous hydrogenated silicon (a-Si:H) and amorphous silicon suboxide films (a-SiO$_x$:H) produced by a hydrosilylation reaction are largely biocompatible [46]. This feature suggests that Si "biochips" might be developed to bond directly with both living tissue and bone by surface modification. The ability to form apatite on materials soaked in a simulated body fluid (SBF) is commonly used by biomedical researchers to evaluate its bioactivity. The active Si—OH groups on the surface of silicon-based materials were thought to be effective to induce apatite precipitation on the surface of materials in SBF [47]. Our works have revealed that the bioactivity of silicon could indeed be enhanced by hydrogen PIII. An a-Si:H$_x$ layer can be formed on the surface of the hydrogen-implanted silicon wafer. After immersion in SBFs for a certain period, apatite could nucleate and grow on hydrogen plasma–implanted silicon wafers. The improvement of the bioactivity of silicon wafer was considered to result from the formation of the functional group, such as Si—H and Si—OH, on its surface.

Hydrogen was implanted into the polished silicon wafers using PIII in the plasma laboratory of the City University of Hong Kong. The chamber was evacuated to 0.6 Torr, and high-purity hydrogen gas was bled into the vacuum chamber to establish a working pressure of 0.5 mTorr. The instrumental parameters are listed in Table 19.1. Under these conditions, H_3^+ is the dominant ion species in the plasma [48]. Unlike beam-line ion implantation, the PIII hydrogen profile usually exhibits multiple peaks due to different implanted species such as H^+, H_2^+, and H_3^+. In addition, there exists certain amount of adsorbed hydrogen near the surface, and the hydrogen in-depth distribution is broader than that of a beam-line implant, also, as a result of a low-energy component.

The cross-sectional transmission electron microscopy (TEM) micrograph of the hydrogen-implanted silicon wafer in Figure 19.9 reveals the formation of defects. There exists a top amorphous zone (about 60 nm in thickness) and a dense dislocation zone (about 150 nm). The dense dislocation zone is located around the projected range of H_3^+. Figure 19.10 plots the atomic dislocation density versus depth derived from channeling-RBS (c-RBS) and the hydrogen elemental depth profile acquired by secondary ion mass spectrometry (SIMS). Hydrogen is mainly found on the near-surface to about 170 nm (~8 at.%), which is the projected range of H_3^+ obtained from the SRIM code. A total atomic displacement zone (amorphous silicon a-Si) is extended from the top surface to the depth of about 50 nm (slightly different from the TEM results due to calibration and instrumentation issues) followed by a dislocation zone located close to the projected range of H_3^+. Hence, the implanted sample consists of a highly hydrogen-doped surface with high crystalline disorder.

TABLE 19.1

Implantation Parameters

Implantation voltage (kV)	30
Pulse frequency (Hz)	50
Pulse duration (s)	500
RF discharge power (W)	1400
Implantation time (min)	20
Implantation dose/cm^2	~1.4 × 10^{17}

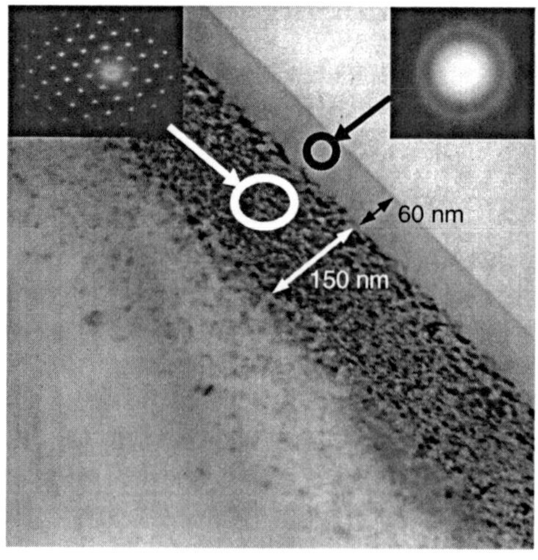

FIGURE 19.9 Cross-sectional views of hydrogen-implanted silicon wafer obtained from TEM analysis. (From Liu, X.Y. et al., *Biomaterials*, 25, 5575, 2004. With permission.)

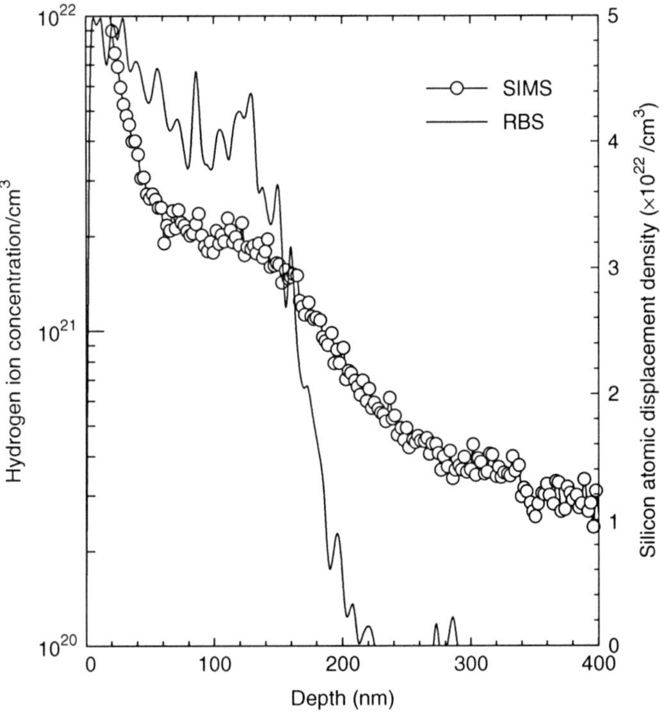

FIGURE 19.10 Depth profile of defects and hydrogen ion concentration in hydrogen-implanted silicon wafer obtained from RBS and SIMS. (From Liu, X.Y. et al., *Biomaterials*, 25, 5575, 2004. With permission.)

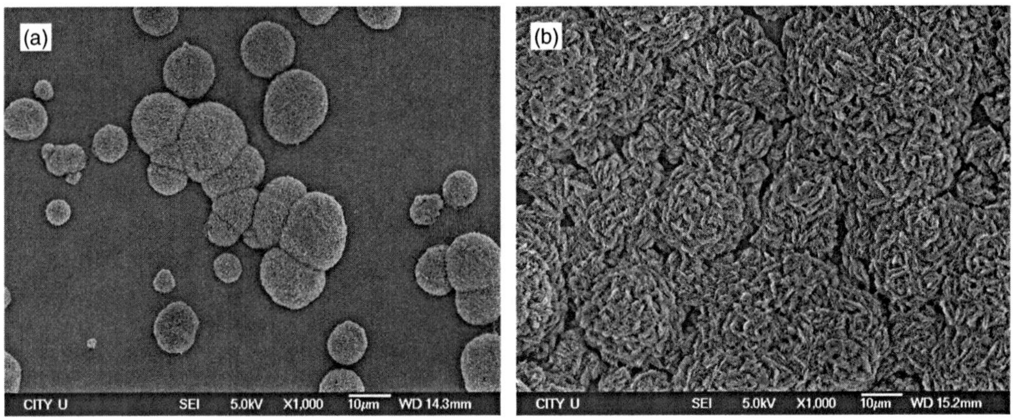

FIGURE 19.11 Surface views of hydrogen-implanted silicon wafer soaked in SBF for (a) 14 days and (b) 28 days. (From Liu, X.Y. et al., *Biomaterials*, 25, 5575, 2004. With permission.)

After immersion in the SBFs for 14 days, some single and clustered ball-shaped particles are observed on the surface of the hydrogen-implanted silicon surface (Figure 19.11a). The surface of the silicon wafer is, however, not covered completely. After an immersion time of 28 days, the surface is entirely covered by the newly formed layer (Figure 19.11b). The results obtained from x-ray diffraction (XRD) (Figure 19.12) and fourier transform infrared (FTIR) (Figure 19.13) show that carbonate-containing hydroxyapatite (HA) (bone-like apatite) is formed on the surface of the hydrogen-implanted silicon wafer soaked in SBF, and good bioactivity on the hydrogen-implanted silicon wafer can be inferred.

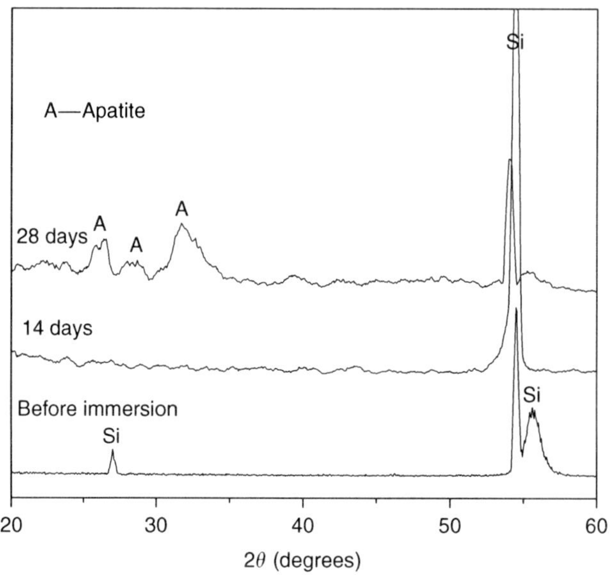

FIGURE 19.12   XRD patterns of hydrogen-implanted silicon wafer before and after being soaked in SBF for 14 and 28 days. (From Liu, X.Y. et al., *Biomaterials*, 25, 5575, 2004. With permission.)

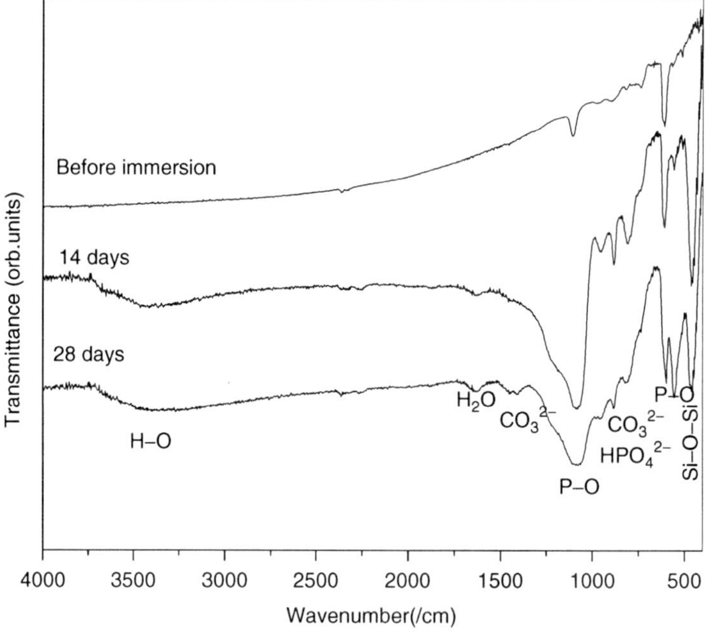

FIGURE 19.13   FTIR spectra of hydrogen-implanted silicon wafers before and after being immersed in SBF for 14 and 28 days. (From Liu, X.Y. et al., *Biomaterials*, 25, 5575, 2004. With permission.)

It is well known that the surface plays an important role in the response of the biological environment of the artificial biomedical device. Therefore, it is logical to believe that the improvement in the bioactivity on the implanted silicon wafer results from the surface modification through hydrogen implantation. The results from TEM, RBS, and SIMS reveal the presence of an amorphous hydrogenated silicon layer (a-Si:H$_x$) after hydrogen PIII. To clearly investigate the formation mechanism of bone-like apatite on the surface of the hydrogen-implanted silicon wafer, two comparative experiments have been conducted. One experiment is to investigate the bioactivity of hydrogenated silicon wafer with no surface damage, and the other one is to evaluate the bioactivity of argon-implanted silicon wafer, which possesses an amorphous surface but no hydrogen. After the hydrogenated silicon wafer and argon-implanted wafer are soaked in SBF for 28 days, no apatite particles can be found on either surface, indicating poor bioactivity on both the samples. The results suggest that only the formation of an amorphous hydrogenated silicon (a-Si:H$_x$) surface can improve the bioactivity of silicon wafer and can result in the formation of bone-like apatite on its surface after treatment in SBF. Experimental evidence has so far suggested that the formation of apatite requires the surface to be both amorphous and hydrogenated.

Hydrogen is known to interact with silicon in a wide variety of ways, including passivating the surface, deactivating dopants, and passivating shallow as well as deep levels [50]. In amorphous and polycrystalline silicon, hydrogen passivates dangling bonds by forming Si—H bonds. In our hydrogen PIII sample, many dangling bonds are produced [49], and the surface of the silicon wafer exhibits an amorphous network with disorders and defects [51]. In silicon, it is estimated that each H ion implanted at 30–100 keV produces approximately 10 Frenkel pairs. These defects provide many Si dangling bonds. The implantation-induced or preexisting dangling bonds can interact immediately with the implanted hydrogen to form Si—H bonds [52].

When the hydrogen-implanted silicon wafer is soaked in the SBF solution, the following reactions are believed to occur. The ≡Si—H structure is first hydrated to form silanol (≡Si—OH) by the following reactions:

$$\equiv\text{Si}-\text{H} + \text{H}_2\text{O} \rightarrow\ \equiv\text{Si}-\text{OH} + \text{H}_2 \qquad (19.1)$$

Afterward, the silanol (≡Si—OH) reacts with the hydroxyl ion to produce a negatively charged surface with the functional group (≡Si—O$^-$) as follows:

$$\equiv\text{Si}-\text{OH} + \text{OH}^- \rightarrow\ \equiv\text{Si}-\text{O}^- + \text{H}_2\text{O} \qquad (19.2)$$

At the same time, some water molecules may diffuse through the surface to react with the Si—H bonds or Si dangling bonds in the subsurface of the hydrogen-implanted silicon wafer to form an amorphous hydrated silicon layer. Therefore, after immersion in SBF, a negatively charged, amorphous, and hydrated silicon surface is formed.

The formation of a negatively charged surface on bioceramics and bioglasses is generally regarded to be important in the precipitation of apatite [53–55]. Due to the formation of the negatively charged surface, the calcium ions in the SBF solution are attracted to the negatively charged surface site of the silicon wafer. This action is followed by the arrival of HPO$_4^{2-}$ resulting in the formation of a hydrated precursor cluster consisting of calcium hydrogen phosphate. After the precursor clusters are formed, they spontaneously grow by consuming calcium and phosphate ions from the surrounding body fluid. The calcium phosphate phase that accumulates on the surface of the silicon wafer is initially amorphous. It later crystallizes to a carbonate-containing HA structure by incorporating carbonate anions from the solution within the amorphous calcium phosphate phase.

19.3.1.2 Improvement of Bioactivity on Nano-TiO$_2$ Coatings

Plasma-sprayed TiO$_2$ as bonding or composite coatings on Ti alloys has recently shown promising *in vivo* corrosion behavior as it acts as a chemical barrier against release of metal ions from the implants [56,57] in addition to its excellent biocompatibility [58], but its poor bioactivity has limited its application as the coating on hard tissue replacements. Nanosized surface topography may give biomedical implants special and favorable properties in a biological environments. Webster et al. [59–61] revealed that nanophase ceramics could promote osteointegration that is critical to the clinical success of orthopedic/dental implants. Osteoblast proliferation was observed to be significantly higher on nanophase alumina, titania, and HA in comparison with their conventional counterparts. Furthermore, compared with conventional ceramics, synthesis of alkaline phosphatase and deposition of calcium-containing minerals were significantly enhanced on osteoblasts cultured on nanophase ceramics. A nanostructured bioactive TiO_2 surface can be produced using a combination of nanoparticle plasma spraying and hydrogen PIII.

Commercially available nanosized TiO_2 powders were deposited onto titanium alloys using a atmospheric plasma spraying (APS) system under the modified spray parameters. Argon (40 slpm: standard liter per minute) and hydrogen (12 slpm) were used as the primary and auxiliary arc gases, respectively. The feeding rate of powders was about 10 g/min using argon (3.5 slpm) as the carrier gas. The arc current and voltage were 600 A and 70 V, respectively. The spraying distance was 100 mm. The thickness of the coatings was about 100 μm.

The high-magnification SEM view of the coating surface indicates that the surface of the nano-TiO_2 coating comprises particles less than 50 nm in size (Figure 19.14). The cross-sectional TEM views of the as-sprayed nano-TiO_2 coating also reveal that the outermost surface is composed of grains less than 50 nm (Figure 19.15a) and are consistent with the SEM results depicted in Figure 19.14. The thickness of this outer layer is about 500 nm. In the interior of the coating, most of the grains exhibit a columnar morphology with a diameter of about 100–200 nm, as shown in Figure 19.15b. The difference in the crystal growth between the surface and the interior of the coating depends mostly on the thermal history. During plasma spraying, the bulk of the coating tends to possess larger columnar grains due to the continuous heat provided by the plasma and subsequent melt, whereas the surface grains are subjected to less heating.

Hydrogen was implanted into the as-sprayed nano-TiO_2 coating using a multifunctional plasma immersion ion implanter [36,62,63]. The plasma chamber was evacuated to a background pressure of 0.6 Torr, and then high-purity hydrogen gas was bled into the vacuum chamber to establish a working pressure of 0.5 mTorr. The instrumental parameters were as follows: pulse voltage 30 kV, pulse frequency 200 Hz, pulse duration 30 μs, RF discharge power 1000 W, and implantation time 2 h.

After immersion in SBF for 2 weeks, the surface of the hydrogen PIII nano-TiO_2 coating was completely covered by an apatite layer, as shown in the surface views (Figure 19.16). The results obtained from our research indicate that only the hydrogen PIII nano-TiO_2 coating with

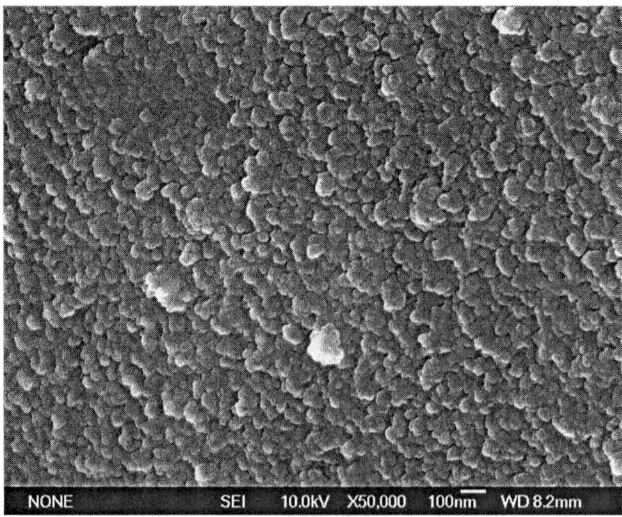

FIGURE 19.14 Higher magnification surface SEM views of the sprayed TiO_2 and nano-TiO_2 coating. (From Liu, X.Y. et al., *Biomaterials*, 26, 6143, 2005. With permission.)

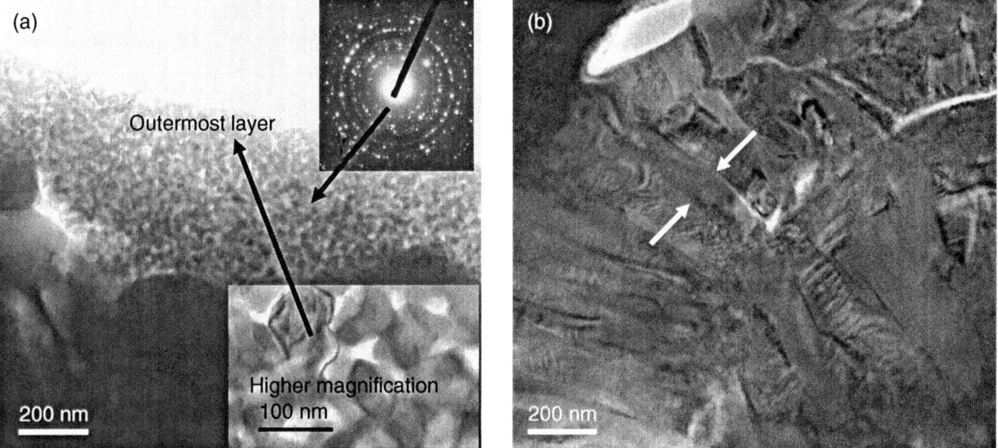

FIGURE 19.15   Cross-sectional TEM views of the as-sprayed nano-TiO_2 coating: (a) coating surface and (b) coating interior. (From Liu, X.Y. et al., *Biomaterials*, 26, 6143, 2005. With permission.)

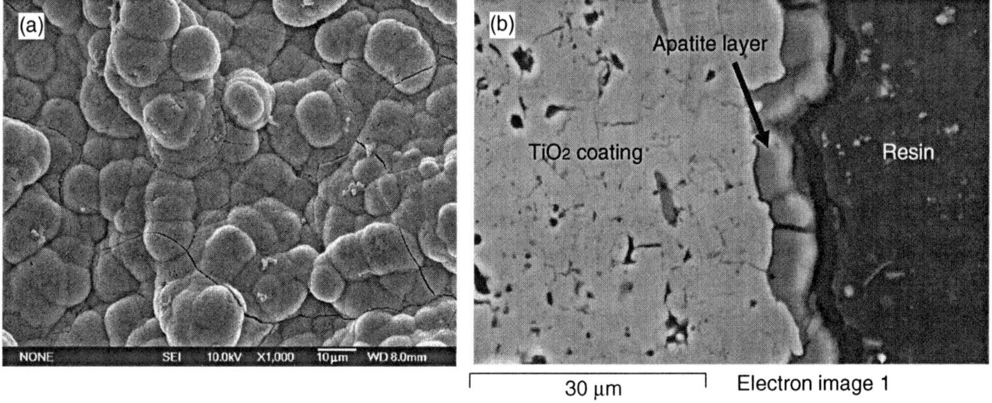

FIGURE 19.16   Surface (a) and cross-sectional (b) views of the hydrogen PIII nano-TiO_2 coating after soaking in SBF for 2 weeks. (From Liu, X.Y. et al., *Biomaterials*, 26, 6143, 2005. With permission.)

nanostructured surface possesses apatite formability. It can thus be inferred that the bioactivity of the plasma-sprayed TiO_2 coating depends on two factors: nanostructured surface composed of enough small particles and hydrogen incorporation.

It has been suggested that OH groups on ceramic surfaces are effective in inducing the formation of an apatite layer. For instance, gel-derived TiO_2 has been shown to induce surface apatite formation, but single crystal anatase and titania synthesized by hydrothermal methods cannot do so [65]. The difference is believed to be because of the Ti—OH functional groups forming a negatively charged surface on the titania gel. It is also believed to be one of the reasons for the surface bioactivity of the hydrogen PIII nano-TiO_2 and the lack of OH groups on the as-sprayed TiO_2 coatings.

The as-sprayed TiO_2 coating is highly oxygen-deficient. While the outermost surface of the as-sprayed TiO_2 coating can be immediately reoxidized via oxygen adsorption after it is exposed to air [66], the subsurface region in the coating is still oxygen-deficient. During hydrogen PIII, hydrogen ions react with the outermost bridge oxygen to form Ti—OH bonds because the reaction is energetically favorable, and two Ti(IV) are reduced to Ti(III) [67]. Eventually, a hydrogenated surface forms on the TiO_2. When the hydrogen PIII TiO_2 surface is soaked in SBF, Ti—OH reacts with the hydroxyl ion in the SBF to produce a negatively charged surface with the functional group Ti—O$^-$ as follows:

$$Ti\text{—}OH + OH^- \rightarrow Ti\text{—}O^- + H_2O \tag{19.3}$$

Adsorption of ions and molecules on the solid surface is a critical step in crystal growth. The deposition of calcium ions is the first and most crucial step of apatite nucleation in an ionic solution. This process is believed to initiate the growth of bone-like apatite on the surface of biocompatible implants [68]. The formation of a negatively charged surface gives rise to apatite precipitation because positive calcium ions are attracted from the solution [65]. On the hydrogen PIII nano-TiO_2 coating, in addition to hydrogen implantation that leads to a negatively charged surface, the formation of a nanostructured surface composed of enough small particles is required for the formation of apatite. It can be demonstrated by thermodynamic analysis that the surface or interfacial tension diminishes with decreasing particle size as a result of the increase in the potential energy of the bulk atoms of the particles [69]. Smaller particles with increased molar free energy are more likely to adsorb molecules or ions per unit area onto their surfaces in order to decrease the total free energy and to become more stable. The overall effect is a sufficiently high adsorption coefficient on the nano-TiO_2 surface so that the apatite can be formed.

19.3.2 Ca/Na PIIID of Titanium

Titanium and its alloys are generally the preferred materials for orthopedic and dental applications due to their relatively low modulus, excellent fatigue strength, excellent formability, good machinability, superior biocompatibility, and reasonable corrosion resistance. However, titanium also has relatively poor wear resistance and bioactivity [70]. Ion implantation has been used to harden the surface and reduce the friction coefficient of titanium in tribological applications, but the metal surface still requires further modification in order to achieve enhanced bioactivity or bone conductivity [71].

In protein-free solutions, it is possible to precipitate HA on an activated Ti surface with Ti—OH groups. The primary step is the formation of Ti—OH groups on the titanium surface. These Ti—OH groups are considered as nucleation points for calcium phosphate from supersaturated solutions [72,73], but this nucleation does not work in the presence of proteins [74]. The wet chemical method of Kokubo uses NaOH treatment of titanium for the induction of the Ti—OH groups and activation of the titanium surface, so that HA precipitates spontaneously from an SBF possessing an ion composition similar to blood plasma [75,76]. It has also been shown that HA precipitation after Na beam-line ion implantation follows the same chemistry as the Kokubo method. The Na-implanted Ti surface forms a sodium titanate layer when oxidized at 600°C in air and sodium titanate generates a Ti—OH hydrogel on the surface in an aqueous solution. The OH groups act as nucleation points for calcium phosphate precipitation from a supersaturated solution, among them is the HA [73,77]. Hanawa et al. investigated early bone formation on calcium ion–implanted titanium inserted into rat tibia. Their results reveal that Ca^{2+}-implanted titanium is superior to unimplanted titanium from the perspective of bone conduction [78].

As an alternative to conventional ion implantation, there are advantages of using PIIID to produce the functional titanium surface for better bone conduction. It is a nonline-of-sight process as opposed to conventional beam-line ion implantation. Therefore, under proper conditions, samples with a complicated shape can be treated with good conformality and uniformity without the need to resort to ion beam scanning and special target manipulation. In addition, since PIIID is usually conducted at low temperature and the target can be cooled, thermal deformation of the specimens can usually be minimized [62].

There are practical difficulties in the conduction of PIIID of sodium and calcium by the conventional cathodic arc technique because of their low melting point and high reactivity in air and with moisture. The low melting point makes stable and long implantation very difficult and the high reactivity imposes difficulty in handling as well as in the construction of a suitable cathode. The experiments used an evaporating ion source invented by the research staff in the City University of Hong Kong [79–81], as shown in Figure 19.17. In this source, instead of using electrical triggering to form the plasma, evaporation is used and on account of the high ionizing efficiency of Na and Ca, an intense Na and Ca plasma plume can be readily formed to conduct PIIID.

The implanted titanium samples possess a rough surface. Ball-like protuberances can be observed on the surface of the titanium sample implanted at 10 kV, as shown in Figure 19.18a. The titanium sample implanted at 20 kV is different from that implanted at 10 kV, and exhibits more salient features (Figure 19.18b). It can be observed that a new layer has formed on the surface of these

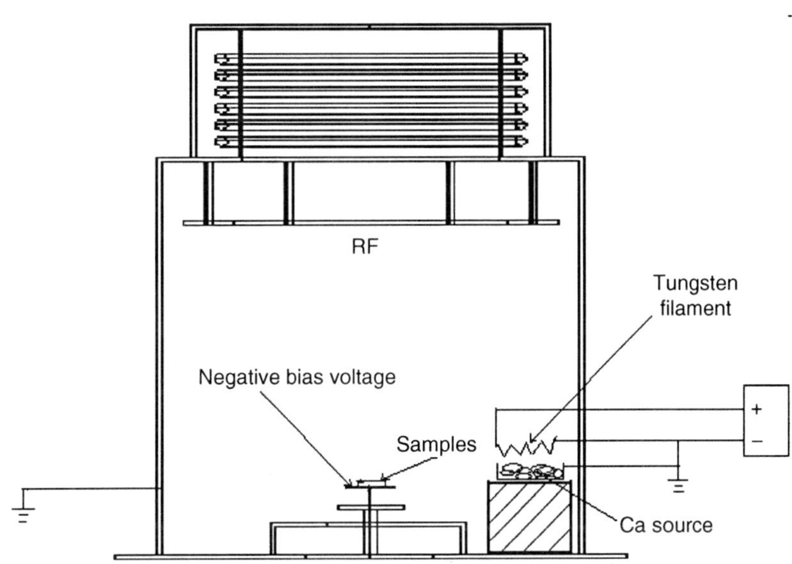

FIGURE 19.17   Schematic diagram of the Ca/Na PIIID system.

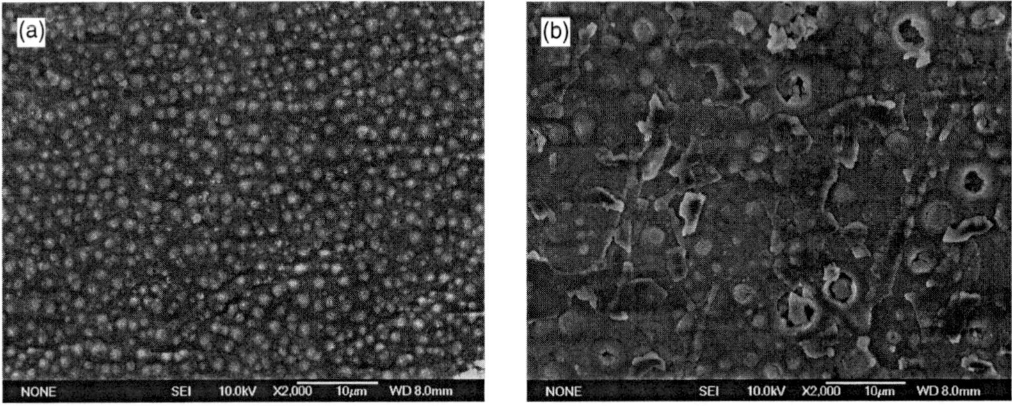

FIGURE 19.18   SEM micrographs of the Ca ion-implanted titanium: (a) 10 kV of bias voltage and (b) 20 kV of bias voltage. (From Liu, X.Y. et al., *Surf. Coating Tech.*, 191, 43, 2005. With permission.)

two implanted titanium samples and a higher bias (implantation) voltage creates more surface features possibly due to the higher amount of deposited energy and thicker calcium-containing layer.

The elemental depth profiles acquired by SIMS are plotted in Figure 19.19 as ion counts per second versus depth. Conversion to concentration is not done here due to the lack of a reference standard, but the qualitative information, particularly comparison among profiles, is reliable as they were acquired using the same analytical conditions. The SIMS profiles indicate that calcium has been successfully implanted into and deposited onto the sample and the implantation depth increases with higher bias voltages.

The XRD spectrum obtained from the implanted titanium indicates that the outermost layer is mainly composed of calcium hydroxide, as shown in Figure 19.20. Therefore, this layer is

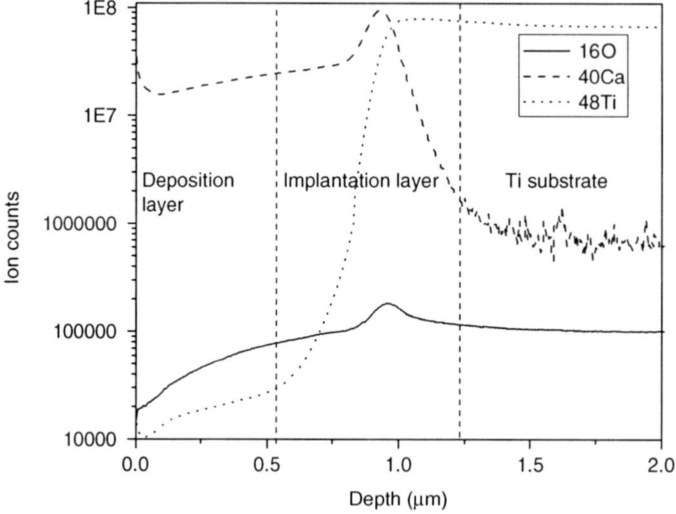

FIGURE 19.19 SIMS depth profiles: (a) 10 kV ion-implanted sample and (b) 20 kV Ca ion-implanted sample. (From Liu, X.Y. et al., *Surf. Coating Tech.*, 191, 43, 2005. With permission.)

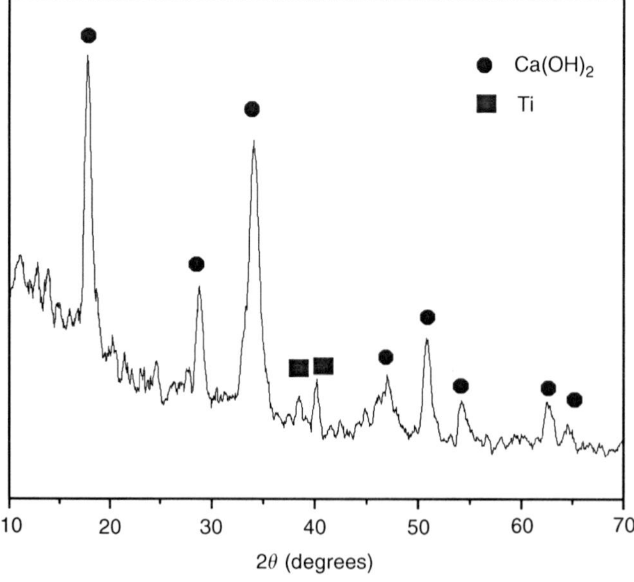

FIGURE 19.20 Thin-film XRD spectrum of Ca ion-implanted titanium at a bias voltage of 10 kV. (From Liu, X.Y. et al., *Surf. Coating Tech.*, 191, 43, 2005. With permission.)

composed of calcium hydroxide and calcium carbonate. This is because after calcium has been deposited onto the titanium surface, it reacts with ambient water and carbon dioxide upon exposure to air to form calcium hydroxide and calcium carbonate. Apatite can be observed on the surface of the Ca ion–implanted titanium at 10 kV of bias voltage after soaking in an SBF for 28 days, as shown in Figure 19.21.

Calcium is a very active metal that can be oxidized easily in air to form calcium oxide. In the experiments, a tungsten filament was employed to heat the calcium powders to produce the discharge current and calcium ions were plasma implanted by applying a pulsed high voltage to the titanium samples. During the off-cycle, calcium was deposited onto the sample surface. After the samples were taken out of the vacuum chamber, the surface calcium reacted immediately with oxygen in air to form calcium oxide (CaO), followed by adsorption of H_2O and CO_2 to form $Ca(OH)_2$ and $CaCO_3$. The process is schematically illustrated in Figure 19.22.

While in the SBF, calcium ions are released gradually from the sample surface into the SBF causing supersaturation of calcium ions in the body fluid in the vicinity of the surface. Hanawa has postulated that the calcium ion–implanted titanium surface is more positively charged due to the dissociation of hydroxyl radicals [83].

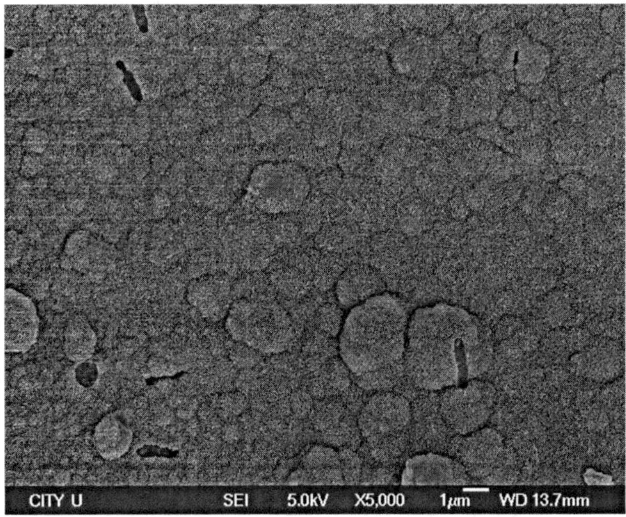

FIGURE 19.21 Surface views of the Ca ion–implanted titanium at a bias voltage of 10 kV soaked in a simulated body fluid for 28 days.

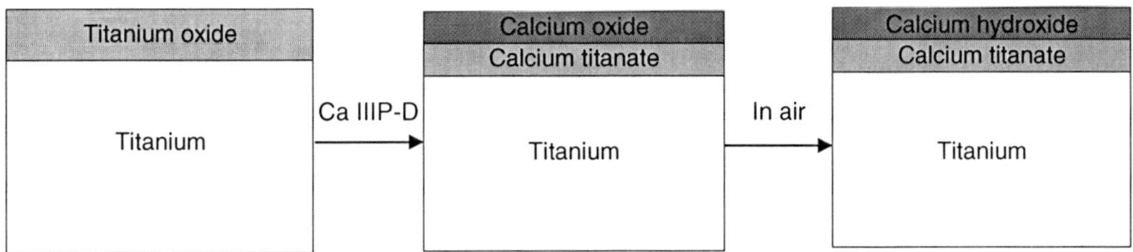

FIGURE 19.22 Schematic diagram of the surface reaction (cross-section of the Ca PIIID sample shown). (From Liu, X.Y. et al., *Surf. Coating Tech.*, 191, 43, 2005. With permission.)

The elemental depth profiles acquired from Na PIIID titanium prepared at chamber pressures of 4×10^{-2} Pa and 8×10^{-2} Pa are displayed in Figure 19.23 (left). It should be noted that PIIID is different from beam-line ion implantation in the sense that both deposition and implantation take place in the former process. The resulting depth profile thus consists of both high-surface concentration Na and an implanted component, as shown in Figure 19.23 (left). In high-temperature oxidation, sodium titanate is formed by releasing sodium into the solution during hydroxylation and leaving titanium hydroxide groups on the surface. The surface chemistry is the same as that on sodium ion beam-implanted titanium [73], except for a smaller projected range in the PIIID-treated samples. The process of oxidation, hydroxylation, and leaching of alkali metal is more complete in the more deeply ion-implanted sample 2 than the mainly deposited sample 1, as shown in Figure 19.24 (right). The surface composition of the NaOH-treated titanium has been analyzed in detail [75,76]. It consists of a porous, amorphous layer mainly composed of sodium titanate.

Precipitation of calcium phosphate was evaluated using SBF treatment and the results are shown in Figure 19.24. The beam line–implanted sample (Ti-II) exhibits very poor bioactivity, which is even worse than that of the untreated titanium (Ti). Nonetheless, it is very clear that the PIIID titanium sample (Ti PIII) induces significantly higher CaP precipitation and the efficacy is even better than that observed on the NaOH-treated sample. This phenomenon may be attributed to

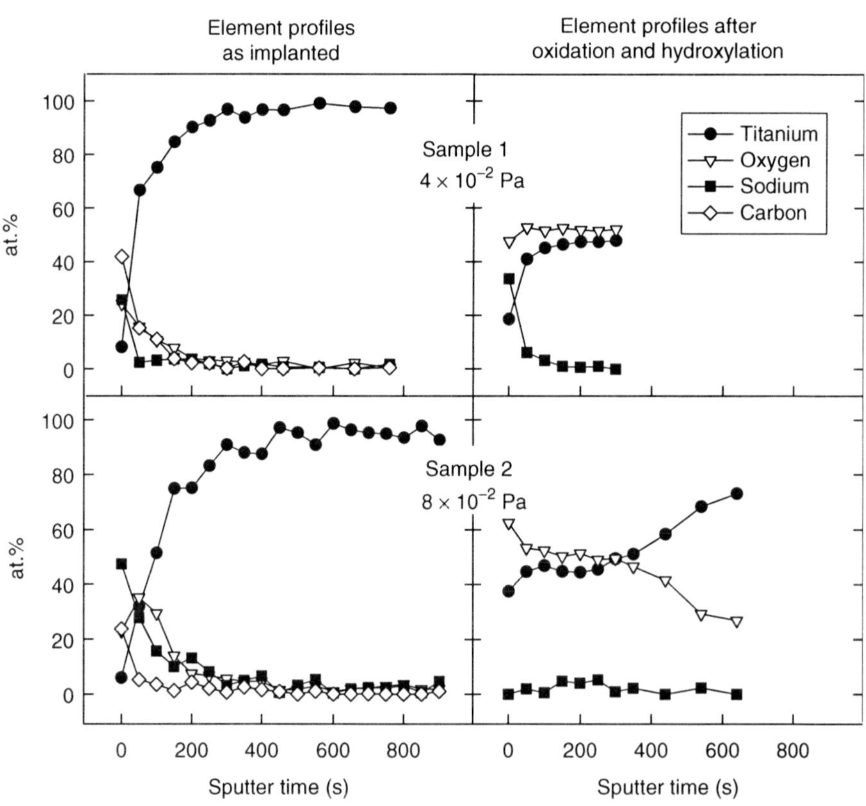

FIGURE 19.23 Depth profiles of the two samples implanted by Na PIIID at two pressure conditions as implanted and after oxidation and hydroxylation. (From Maitz, M.F. et al., *Biomaterials*, 26, 5465, 2005. With permission.)

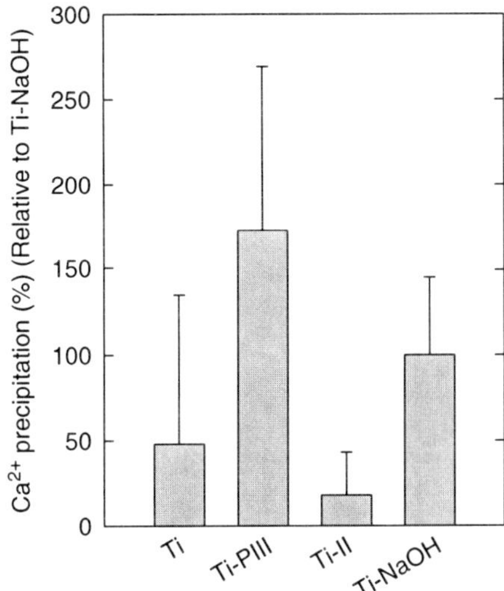

FIGURE 19.24 Bioactivity of the four samples as determined by the precipitation of calcium phosphate from a simulated body fluid after 24 h. The calcium phosphate precipitates are dissolved in HCl, and the calcium concentration in the solution is determined. The values are scaled to those of the NaOH-treated sample as 100%. Labels indicate Ti (untreated control), Ti PIII (Na plasma-implanted sample), Ti-II (beam-line implanted sample), and Ti-NaOH (NaOH-treated sample). (From Maitz, M.F. et al., *Biomaterials*, 26, 5465, 2005. With permission.)

the higher activity of the ion species in the plasma than in the solution, leading to a higher rate of titanate formation. However, more work is needed to verify this postulate.

19.4 SURFACE MODIFICATION OF NiTi ALLOY

Nickel titanium (NiTi) shape memory alloys are promising materials for surgical implants in orthopedics because of their unique shape memory effects (SME) and super elasticity (SE) that other common orthopedic materials such as stainless steels and titanium alloys do not possess. Their mechanical properties are also closer to those of cortical bones than stainless steels and titanium alloys. In terms of wear resistance, the materials are better than CoCrMo alloys used in bone trauma fixation [85]. Several other favorable properties of the materials have also been investigated [86–98] and good biocompatibility has been reported [85,89,99–109]. However, some negative effects have also been pointed out. For example, Berger-Gorbet et al. have found that the osteogenesis process and osteonectin synthesis activity in NiTi alloys are unfavorable compared to stainless steels and titanium alloys [110]. Jia et al. in their study revealed that the cell death rate was severe on NiTi alloys [111]. These problems are believed to stem from the poor corrosion resistance of the materials, thereby leading to an increase of the cytotoxicity. It is most likely that some toxic components released from the substrate cause cell death rather than apoptosis [112]. Shih et al. [113] reported that the supernatant and corrosive products from NiTi might result in the death of smooth muscle cells, especially when the amount of released nickel is higher than 9 ppm. A few other studies have reported that nickel ions [102,103] leached from the alloys cause allergic reactions in nickel hypersensitive patients [114–117]. While the homogeneity of the material microstructures and the surface morphology may alter the anticorrosion ability of NiTi alloys, there is no doubt that the corrosion resistance and antiwear properties of the materials must be enhanced before the materials can be widely used clinically, especially as orthopedic implants with couplings where fretting is expected.

It is known that titanium carbides and nitrides have excellent mechanical and chemical properties, for instance, good wear resistance, inactivity with a number of chemical substances, and outstanding hardness [118–124]. Titanium oxides are known to be fairly compatible with living tissues [125–128]. It is also inactive to many chemical reactions. In the surface coating industry, incorporation of C, O, and N into Ti alloys is quite common to improve both the mechanical and the corrosion properties of the substrates using various methods [129–134]. The use of PIII is more preferable for large samples, especially those with complex geometries, like orthopedic implants, because PIII is a conformal treatment process when conducted under proper conditions. PIII as a low-temperature process can enhance the mechanical properties of the specimens without altering the original dimension. In addition, PIII is not subjected to normal thermodynamic constraints such as impurity solubility. The implantation time is independent of the sample size. Using PIII, a gradual transition can be formed in the NiTi near-surface region, decreasing the possibility of delamination compared to the cases in which the coatings are put on. Here, the corrosion resistance and tribological properties as well as the cytocompatibility of the N, C, and O plasma-treated NiTi materials are illustrated. N_2, C_2H_2, and O_2 plasmas are used to introduce N, C, and O into NiTi substrates in the PIII system. The optimal implantation parameters of the N, C, and O PIII are listed in Table 19.2.

Figure 19.25a shows that a 100 nm thick titanium nitride surface layer is formed on the N PIII NiTi alloy. X-ray diffraction (XRD) and high-resolution x-ray photoelectron spectroscopy (XPS) analyses reveal that TiN is the only secondary phase present in the N-implanted layer. With regard to the acetylene-implanted layer, a titanium carbide layer with increasing Ti to C stoichiometric ratios is detected underneath the surface oxide layer. Figure 19.25b shows a 75 nm thick titanium carbide layer beneath a 25 nm surface oxide layer. The titanium chemical states are analyzed using high-resolution XPS and the oxides of Ti^{2+}, Ti^{3+}, and Ti^{4+} are found in the implanted layer. The results show that a titanium oxide layer about 120 nm thick beneath a 25 nm surface oxide layer is formed on the O PIII NiTi alloy (Figure 19.25c). It should be noted that in all cases, the nickel contents are suppressed to low levels in the near surface.

The hardness and the modulus profiles of the control sample, nitrogen-, acetylene-, and oxygen-implanted samples are shown in Figures 19.27a through 19.27d. The hardness of the control sample is 4.5 GPa and the Young's modulus is 57 GPa. All the surface-treated samples possess higher surface hardness and Young's modulus values compared to the control. In the nitrogen-implanted

TABLE 19.2

Implantation and Annealing Parameters

Sample	NiTi with Nitrogen Implantation	NiTi with Carbon Implantation	NiTi with Oxygen Implantation
Gas type	N_2	C_2H_2	O_2
RF (W)	1000	—	1000
High voltage (kV)	−40	−40	−40
Pulse width (μs)	50	30	50
Frequency (Hz)	200	200	200
Duration of implantation (min)	240	90	240
Base pressure (Torr)	7.0×10^{-6}	1×10^{-5}	7.0×10^{-6}
Working pressure (Torr)	6.4×10^{-4}	2.0×10^{-3}	6.4×10^{-4}
Dose/cm^2	9.6×10^{16}	5.5×10^{16}	1.0×10^{17}
Annealing pressure (Torr)	8.0×10^{-6}	1.0×10^{-5}	8.0×10^{-6}
Annealing temperature (°C)	450	600	600
Duration of annealing (h)	5	5	5

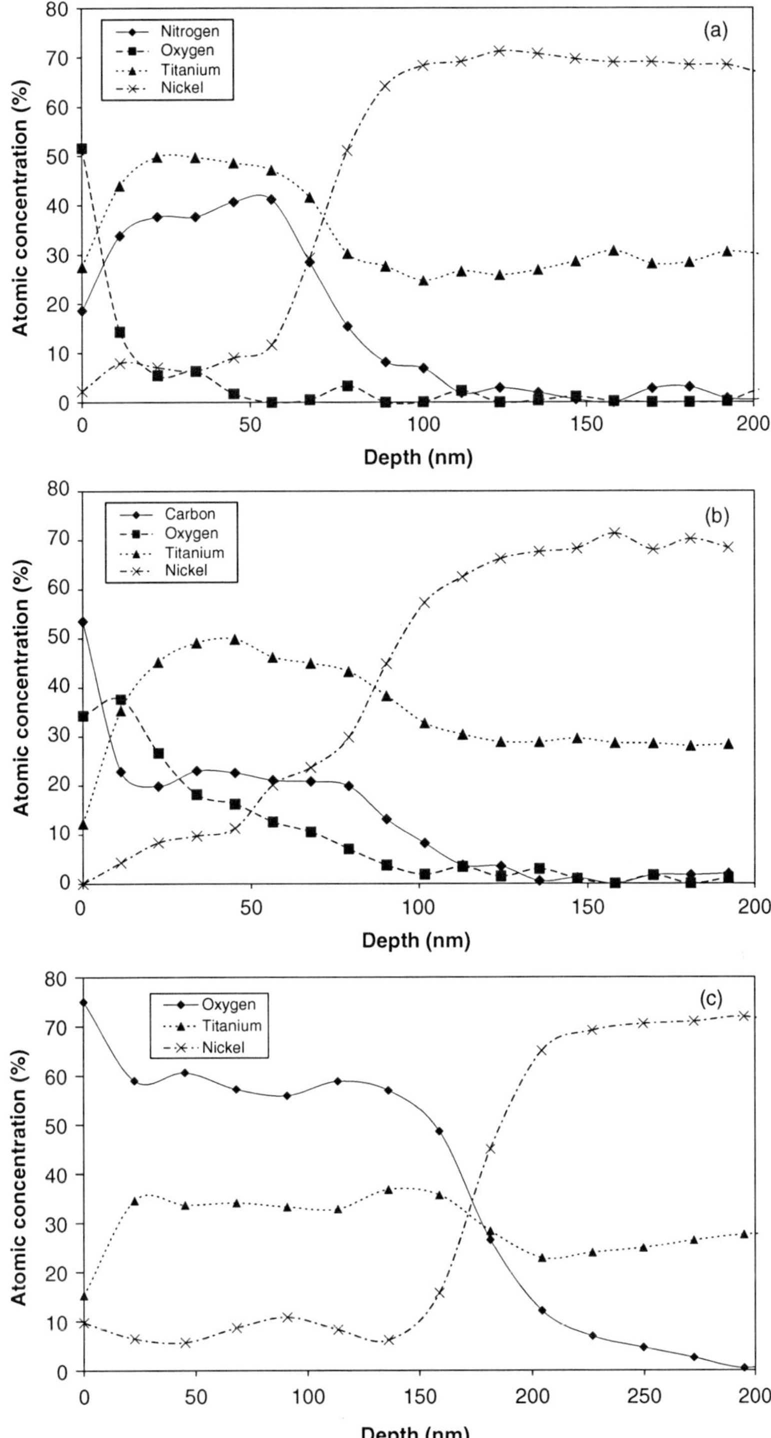

FIGURE 19.25   Depth profile of NiTi alloy after nitrogen (a), acetylene (b), and oxygen (c) PIII treatments. (From Yeung, K.W.K. et al., *J. Biomed. Mater. Res.*, 75A, 256, 2005. With permission.)

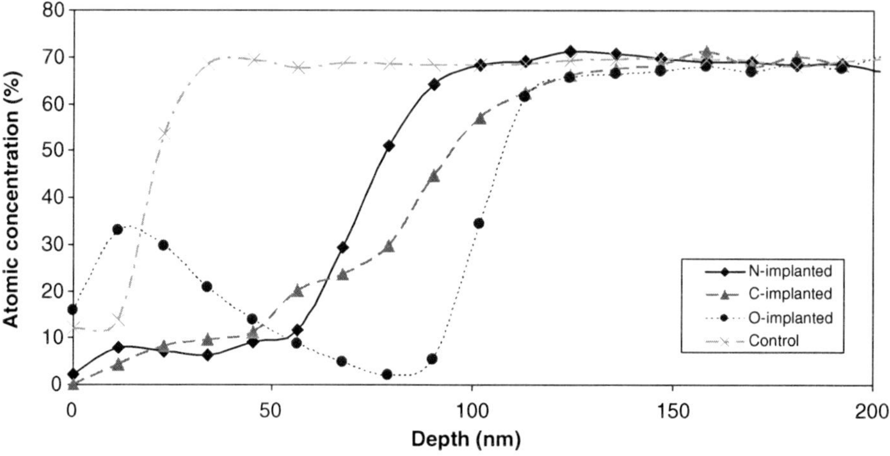

FIGURE 19.26 Ni depth profiles acquired from the three PIII samples and control.

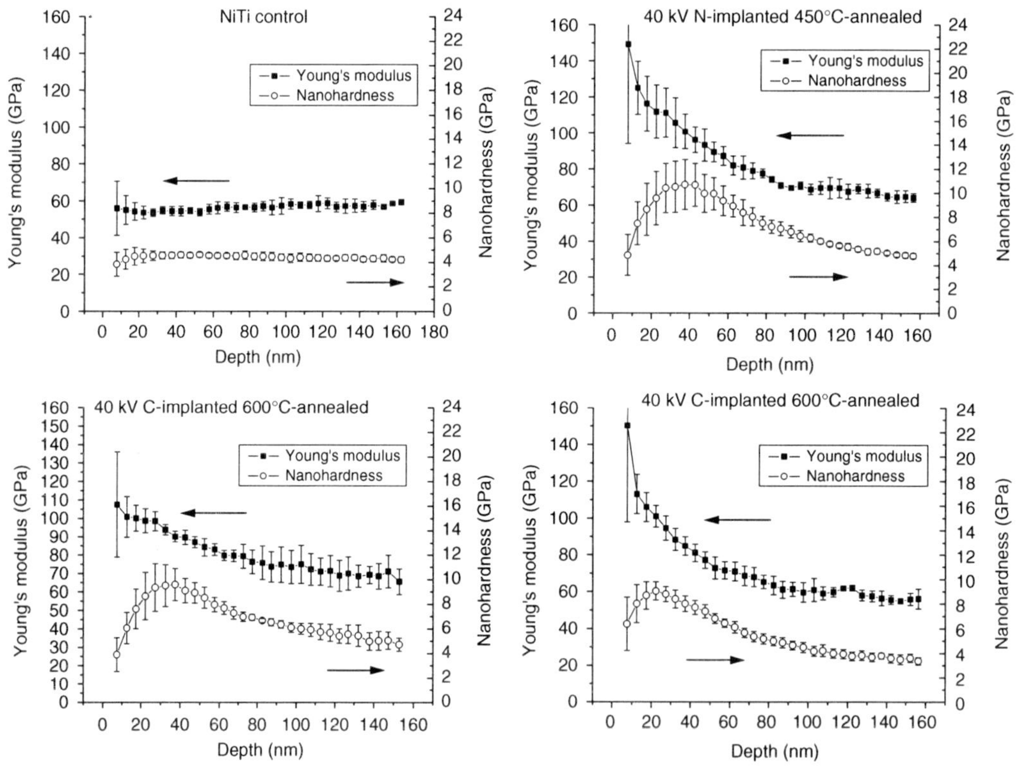

FIGURE 19.27 Hardness and modulus profiles of NiTi alloy before and after N, C, and O-PIII treatments. (From Yeung, K.W.K. et al., *J. Biomed. Mater. Res.*, 75A, 256, 2005. With permission.)

sample, the maximum hardness is 11 GPa at 40 nm from the surface. It gradually decreases to 5 GPa at 165 nm. The Young's modulus, being about 150 GPa at the topmost surface, decreases to 70 GPa gradually with depth. In the acetylene-implanted sample, the maximum hardness is 9.5 GPa at around 30 nm from the surface and gradually diminishes to 4.5 GPa at 150 nm. The Young's modulus exhibits the maximum value of 110 GPa at the topmost layer and then decreases gradually to a rather constant value of 70 GPa between 110 and 150 nm from the surface. The lower hardness value in the first 30 nm of this sample is probably due to surface moisture or oxide. In the oxygen-implanted sample, the modulus is found to be 150 GPa near the surface and progressively decreases to 55 GPa between 130 and 160 nm. The hardness is 9 GPa at 20 nm dropping to 3.5 GPa at 160 nm. It should be noted that these values are higher than that of the control sample of 57 GPa. The results suggest that the Young's modulus of the nitrogen-implanted sample is 163% or 14% higher than that of the substrate, whereas the hardness is 144% and 11% higher throughout the measurement. Hence, the nitrogen-implanted sample is mechanically stronger than the substrate. With regard to the acetylene-implanted sample, the hardness of the treated layer between 20 and 150 nm is 110% and 11% greater than that of the substrate, whilst the Young's modulus is 92% and 23% higher throughout the depth of the measurement. In the oxygen-implanted sample, the hardness at 20–70 nm is 100% and 11% higher and the modulus at 0–120 nm is 163% and 5% higher than that of the untreated substrate. Thus, the mechanical properties of all the treated layers are more superior to those of the untreated substrate [135,136].

Table 19.3 lists some of the essential readings from our electrochemical tests in lieu of the more complicated potentiodynamic curves. E_{corr} and E_b represent the corrosion and the breakdown potentials respectively. Higher E_{corr} and E_b values represent better corrosion resistance. The E_{corr} and E_b values of the control sample are −231 and 272 mV, respectively. The E_{corr} values measured from the nitrogen-, acetylene-, and oxygen-implanted samples are −163, −114, and −27 mV, respectively. The E_b values of the nitrogen-, acetylene-, and oxygen-implanted samples are 1120, 1170, and 867 mV, respectively. All the surface-treated samples exhibit higher E_{corr} and E_b values than the untreated sample. These results suggest that the corrosion resistance of the implanted samples is enhanced.

Table 19.4 displays the amounts of Ni leached from the surface-treated and untreated samples after the electrochemical tests, as determined by inductively coupled plasma mass spectrometry

TABLE 19.3

Essential Results from the Electrochemical Tests

Sample	Control	N-Treated	C-Treated	O-Treated
E_{corr} (mV)	−231	−163	−114	−27
E_b (mV)	272	1120	1170	867
Surface area (cm^2)	0.181	0.181	0.181	0.181

Source: Yeung, K.W.K. et al., *J. Biomed. Mater. Res.*, 75A, 256, 2005. With permission.

TABLE 19.4

Amounts of Ni and Ti Ions Detected in SBF by ICPMS after Electrochemical Tests

Sample	Ni Content (ppm)	Ti Content (ppm)
Control	30.2324	0.1575
N-treated	0.0117	0.0527
C-treated	0.0082	0.057
O-treated	0.0123	Not detectable

Source: Yeung, K.W.K. et al., *J. Biomed. Mater. Res.*, 75A, 256, 2005. With permission.

(ICPMS). The Ni and Ti concentrations released from the control sample are 30.2324 and 0.1575 ppm, respectively. The Ni concentrations from the nitrogen-, acetylene-, and oxygen-implanted samples are only 0.0117, 0.0082, and 0.0123 ppm, respectively. The Ti concentrations from the nitrogen- and acetylene-implanted samples are 0.0527 and 0.0057 ppm, respectively. The Ti concentration from the oxygen-implanted sample is undetectable. The results reveal that the amounts of Ni leached from all the treated samples are significantly reduced. The leached amount is only about 0.03–0.04% of that of the control sample.

All the plasma-implanted samples are well tolerated by the EGFP-expressing osteoblasts as shown in Figure 19.28. After culturing for 2 days, the cells start to attach to and proliferate on all the samples. After 4 days, cell proliferation on the untreated NiTi alloy samples was slightly higher than that of the nitrogen, oxygen, and acetylene PIII samples. However, the nitrogen PIII samples exhibit the highest degree of cell proliferation among the samples after 6 and 8 days of culturing. Cell proliferation on the acetylene- and oxygen-implanted samples was slightly lower than that on the NiTi control sample after 6 and 8 days, but the difference not significant.

Oxygen, nitrogen, or acetylene PIII can effectively suppress the leaching of nickel from the NiTi alloys. The enhancement phenomenon can be attributed to the high affinities of Ti toward N, C, and O as compared to Ni under high-temperature annealing. It provides a driving force to enrich the surface with the element forming a stronger chemical bond. The heat of formation of the lowest titanium oxide is −913 kJ/mole while that of NiO is −244 kJ/mole [137]. The heat of formation of TiN is −305.6 kJ/mole while nickel nitrides such as Ni_3N are unstable with respect to TiN [138]. The heat of formation of TiC is −773 kJ/mole [139] while that of NiC is not well established since the Ni−C phase diagram does not show stable carbides. The term nickel carbide may only stand for interstitial solid solutions of C in Ni, which possess the NaCl structure [140]. Therefore, the formation of titanium oxide, nitride, and carbide is energetically favored over the nickel counterparts and this is believed to account for the suppression of Ni in the implanted and annealed region. It should be noted that the degree of suppression does depend on the implantation parameters as reported by Tian et al. [137] in their study of the suppression of nickel in the stainless steel surface after nitrogen PIII.

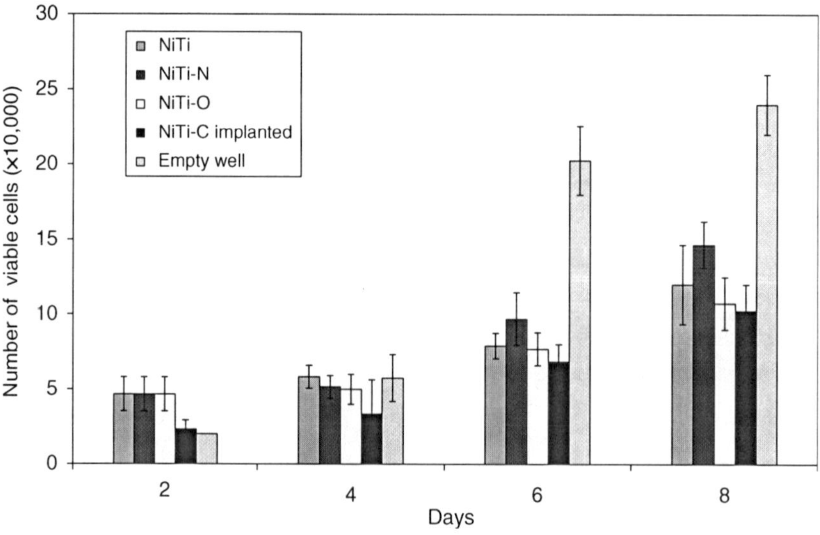

FIGURE 19.28 Cell proliferation on various NiTi alloys versus number of days. (From Yeung, K.W.K. et al., *J. Biomed. Mater. Res.*, 72A, 238, 2005. With permission.)

With regard to hardness and modulus enhancement, our nanoindentation results show that the treated surfaces possess higher Young's modulus and hardness than the untreated control surface. Hence, the surface mechanical properties of the treated samples are enhanced. The modified surfaces not only possess better corrosion resistance, but also are capable of resisting mechanical shocks. The efficacy of using PIII to strengthen the materials, surface mechanical properties such as hardness and elastic modulus [141] depends on the amorphous matrix composition and the size of precipitates [142]. Additionally, the corrosion resistance seems to be directly proportional to the surface conditions of metals. For instance, smooth surfaces usually give rise to higher corrosion resistance. A crack-free surface is always advantageous because of the reduced chance of localization of corrosive agent. Chemically inert materials such as metal oxides, nitride, or carbide can effectively reduce the permeability of the corrosive agent [143]. The wetting properties also govern the anticorrosion capability of a material.

Compared to the other treated and untreated NiTi alloys, the *in vitro* cell culture study indicates that the NiTi alloy after nitrogen implantation exhibits good biocompatibility. The cell proliferation rate on nitrogen-treated surfaces appears to be as good if not better than untreated NiTi alloy at the later time points [99,102,103,106,109]. This finding can be explained by Piscanec's study [144]. They reported the growth of the calcium phosphate phase on TiN-coated titanium implants, but no such activities were observed on the untreated titanium implants. The surface composition analysis revealed that this layer consisted of mixed precipitates of TiO_xN_y oxynitride. This layer promoted the deposition of Ca ions because of negative charges localized on the surface after the surface treatment. Therefore, this coating was favorable to the formation of bone-like materials under *in vivo* conditions. It was believed that the TiO_xN_y oxynitride layer also existed on the nitrogen-implanted NiTi alloy.

19.5 SURFACE MODIFICATION OF BLOOD-CONTACTING MATERIALS

19.5.1 DLC Thin Films

Diamond like carbon (DLC) thin films have been widely studied and used for many industrial purposes in the past 20 years due to their superior chemical, optical, electrical, and tribological properties. Their particularly favorable attributes include low friction coefficient, high hardness, and high wear resistance. They have been commercially used as the coating materials in many applications, for instance, shavers, cutting and drilling tools, protective coating for magnetic media and optical lenses. However, there has also been a lot of interest in DLC as biomedical coating materials since the materials not only possess excellent chemical and mechanical properties, but also are in general biocompatible [145–147]. Conventionally, metals or metal alloys are the dominant materials in medical implants, but relatively poor wear and corrosion resistance and inadequate biocompatibility are the drawbacks of some metallic materials. Therefore, DLC has been suggested to be a replacement in some applications. However, entire substitution of most medical devices with DLC is not practical. Hence, surface modification approach such as coating techniques is one of the potential solutions.

Initial studies of DLC in biomedical applications are mainly in the orthopedic field such as surface modification of artificial total hip and knee joints [148–151]. Most studies show that the DLC films are biocompatible, and the most important fact is that the tribological properties can be greatly improved by DLC films. However, in the cardiovascular field, there are fewer reports in the literature. Referring to the commercial products of cardiovascular devices such as artificial heart valves, rotary heart pumps, and stents, the crucial requirement of biocompatibility is the bioinertness to blood. In other words, the implants must avoid the occurrence of thrombogenesis. In practice, the hemocompatibility of the devices is not adequate and patients should continuously take anticoagulation medication after receiving implants. Hence, the development of a material with better blood compatibility is necessary. In this section, elemental-doped and undoped DLC films prepared by PIIID under different conditions are described.

The undoped and doped DLC films were fabricated by PIIID. Acetylene (C_2H_2) gas was used to produce carbon plasma for film deposition. The dopants were introduced into the vacuum chamber simultaneously via thermal- or electron-induced evaporation. Phosphorus- and calcium-doped DLC films were fabricated by using this method. C_2H_2 and Ar gases were bled into the chamber through two individual flow controls and inlets on top of the chamber. Figure 19.29 illustrates the schematic diagram of the basic experimental setup of PIIID for DLC films synthesis. By using the PIIID system with C_2H_2, amorphous hydrogenated carbon films can be produced. For elemental-doped DLC film fabrication, however, a dopant source is added to the system to provide additional ions for film deposition. In general, elemental powders are placed in a container and evaporated by means of heated filament and electron bombardment. The dopant vapor is created, mixed with the C_2H_2 gas, and eventually ignited into plasma by RF sources for film deposition as demonstrated in Figure 19.30.

19.5.1.1 Influence of Flow Ratio on Structure and Hemocompatibility

Using PIIID, DLC films are fabricated on silicon substrates at room temperature. By changing the C_2H_2 to Ar ($F_{C_2H_2}/F_{Ar}$) flow ratio during deposition, the effects of the reactive gas pressure and flow ratio on the characteristics of the DLC films are systematically examined to correlate to the blood compatibility. The Raman D-band to G-band intensity ratio is consistent with the adherent platelet quantity, both the ratio and platelets first increasing and then decreasing with higher $F_{C_2H_2}/F_{Ar}$ flow ratios. This implies that the blood compatibility of the DLC films is influenced by the ratio of sp^3 to sp^2, not by the absolute sp^3 or sp^2 content.

Using stylus profilometry, the film thicknesses are determined to be about 100, 130, 200, 240, and 300 nm at $F_{C_2H_2}/F_{Ar}$ flow ratios of 0.4, 0.6, 0.8, 1.0, and 1.2, respectively. As expected, the deposition rate is higher with increasing C_2H_2 flow rates. Figure 19.31 exhibits the 3D atomic force microscopy (AFM) morphology of the DLC films at $F_{C_2H_2}/F_{Ar}$ flow ratios of 0.6 and 1.2. The surfaces

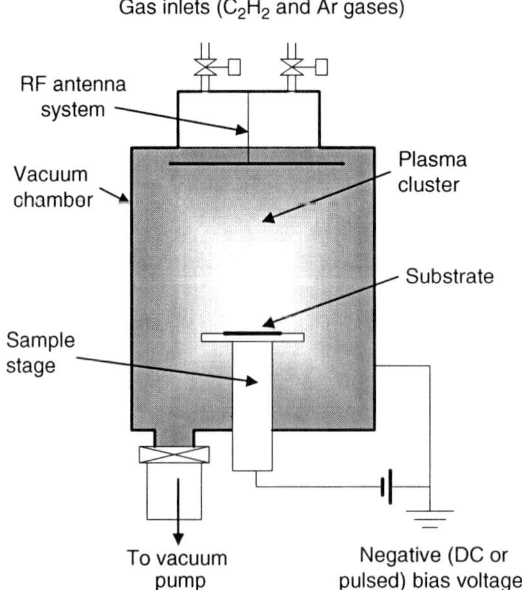

FIGURE 19.29 Schematic diagram of PIIID system for DLC synthesis.

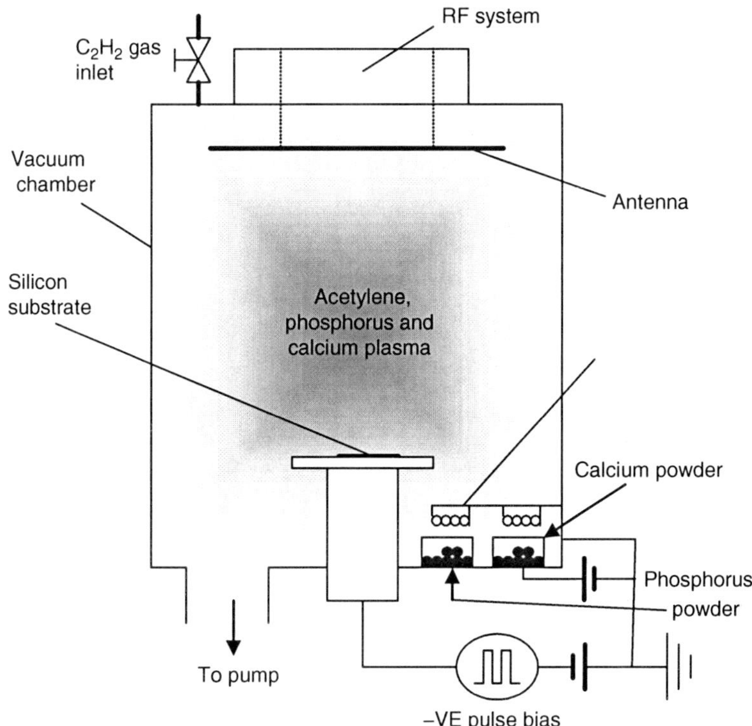

FIGURE 19.30   Schematic diagram of PIIID to deposit Ca, Ca and P, and P-doped DLC films.

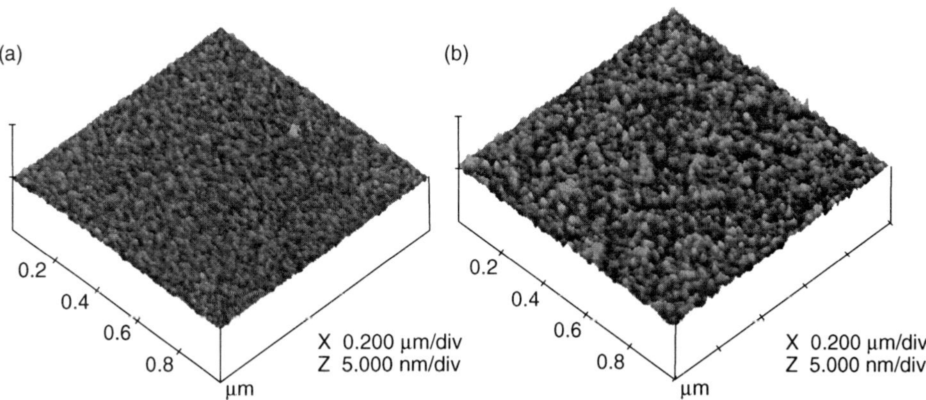

FIGURE 19.31   AFM micrographs of the DLC films prepared by PIIID at $F_{C_2H_2}/F_{Ar}$ ratios of (a) 0.6 and (b) 1.2. (From Chen, J.Y. et al., *Surf. Coating Tech.*, 156, 289, 2002. With permission.)

are relatively smooth, but a higher $F_{C_2H_2}/F_{Ar}$ flow ratio gives rise to a rougher surface, and it is due to the difference in the sp^3 content. The Raman spectra acquired from the DLC films prepared at different $F_{C_2H_2}/F_{Ar}$ flow ratios are shown in Figure 19.32. All the Raman spectra show a relatively sharp peak at around 1550/cm^{-1} and a shoulder at around 1345cm^{-1}, commonly referred to as the G-band and D-band, respectively. The latter becomes a shoulder of the former because the film is hydrogenated. It is found that the shifts of both the G- and D-peaks are the biggest and the G-peak width (full width half maximum [FWHM]) is the largest at a $F_{C_2H_2}/F_{Ar}$ flow ratio of 1.2. The changes in the Raman

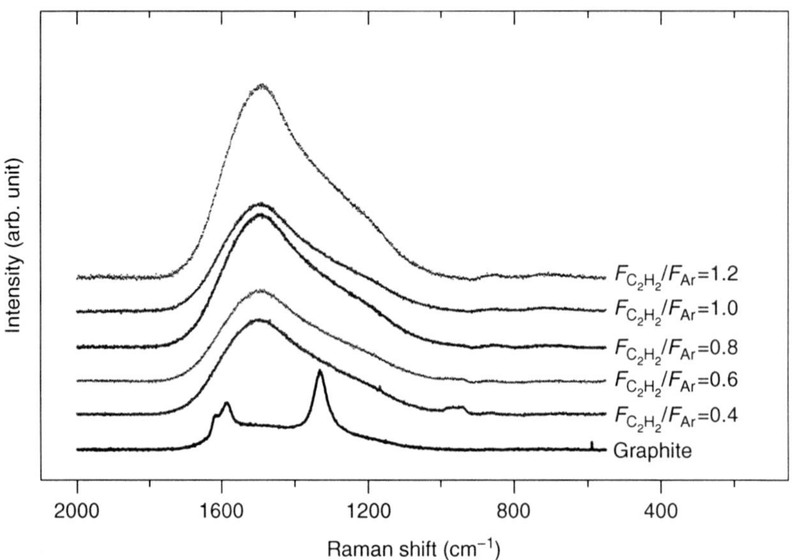

FIGURE 19.32 Raman spectra of DLC films fabricated at different $F_{C_2H_2}/F_{Ar}$ ratios. (From Chen, J.Y. et al., *Surf. Coating Tech.*, 156, 289, 2002. With permission.)

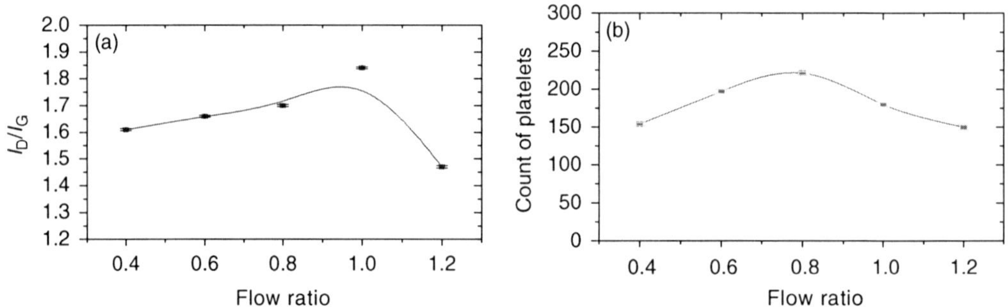

FIGURE 19.33 Effects of the $F_{C_2H_2}/F_{Ar}$ flow ratios on the intensity ratio of the D-band to G-band (a) and platelet counts (b). (From Chen, J.Y. et al., *Surf. Coating Tech.*, 156, 289, 2002. With permission.)

spectra indicate that smaller $F_{C_2H_2}/F_{Ar}$ flow ratios weaken the formation of DLC films with more fourfold coordinate bonds. That is, the sp^3 bond content is reduced at smaller $F_{C_2H_2}/F_{Ar}$ flow ratios. Both the peak width and I_D/I_G intensity ratio vary depending on the structure of the DLC films.

Platelet adhesion tests are conducted on the DLC film surface. After incubation in the platelet-rich plasma (PRP) for 20 min, the number of adherent platelets on the DLC film surface first increases, and then decreases with increasing $F_{C_2H_2}/F_{Ar}$ flow ratios. The platelet count is highest at a $F_{C_2H_2}/F_{Ar}$ flow ratio of about 0.8. After 3 h of incubation, the adherent platelets are too numerous to count. The amount of platelets on sample prepared under $F_{C_2H_2}/F_{Ar}$ flow ratio of 0.8 is the highest, and the accumulation of platelets is also most serious as manifested by several platelets interconnecting to form aggregation. In addition, serious pseudopodium of the adhered platelets is also observed serious on this sample.

Figure 19.33 displays the relationship between the Raman D-band to G-band intensity ratios and the platelet quantity for different $F_{C_2H_2}/F_{Ar}$ flow ratios. It can be readily observed that these two parameters agree well with each other. That is, both increase first and then decrease with increasing $F_{C_2H_2}/F_{Ar}$ flow ratios. The largest value is observed at a $F_{C_2H_2}/F_{Ar}$ flow ratio of 0.8–1.0. Taking into account the Raman results shown in Figure 19.6 which illustrates that the shift of both the G- and D-peaks is the biggest and the FWHM of the G-band peak is largest at a $F_{C_2H_2}/F_{Ar}$ flow ratio of 1.2, it can be inferred that the blood compatibility of the DLC film is influenced by the sp^3 to sp^2 ratio, not by the absolute sp^3 content or sp^2 content, and the hemocompatibility becomes worse when the sp^3 to sp^2 ratio increases.

19.5.1.2 Influence of Bias Voltage on Surface Property and Platelets Adhesion

Hydrogenated amorphous carbon films have been fabricated at room temperature. A mixture of acetylene (C_2H_2) and argon was introduced into the chamber and the plasma was triggered using RF. Film deposition was carried out at a constant RF power of 500 W. During the initial deposition of the base film, a higher negative DC bias voltage was applied to the sample holder to improve film adhesion by means of ion mixing. A series of DLC films were synthesized by adjusting the substrate bias voltage in subsequent deposition of the top films.

The Raman spectra acquired from the hydrogenated DLC (a-C–H) films prepared under different bias voltages are exhibited in Figure 19.34. A higher bias voltage (V_b) leads to the shift of the two peaks toward higher wave numbers and increasing I_D/I_G ratios. The positions of the G- and D-lines, G-full WHM and integrated intensity ratio (I_D/I_G) can be correlated with the sp^3/sp^2 bonding ratio [153], graphite cluster size [154,155], and disorder in these threefold coordinated islands [156]. Hence, the sp^3/sp^2 ratios in the a-C:H films cannot be derived directly from the Raman spectra, but nevertheless, some qualitative information can be extracted. Increases in the I_D/I_G ratio, shifting of the G-peak toward higher wave numbers, widening of the D-peak, and narrowing of the G-peak are caused by increase of the graphite-like component in the amorphous carbon films [157]. The results indicate that the film structure becomes more graphite-like with increasing substrate bias. One of the reasons is that the increase in substrate temperature induced by higher energetic ion

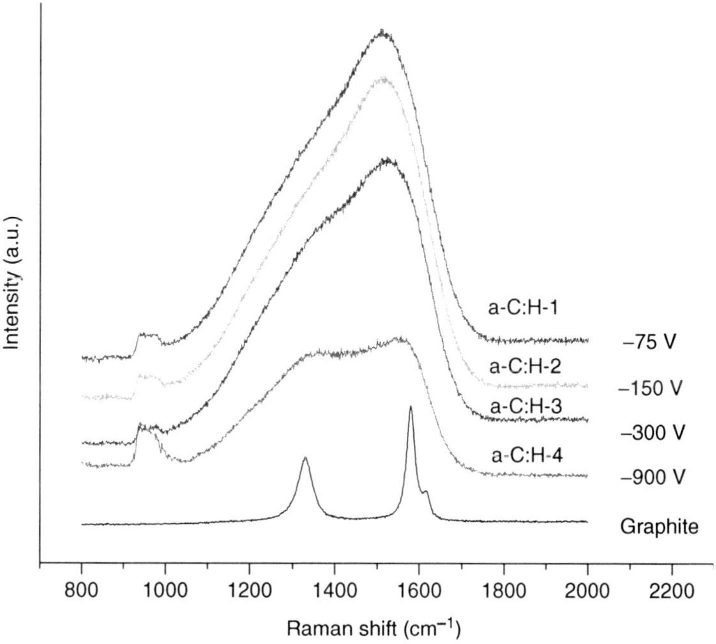

FIGURE 19.34 Raman spectra of the a-C:H films fabricated at different bias voltages. (From Yang, P. et al., *Biomaterials*, 24, 2821, 2003. With permission.)

bombardment promotes film graphitization, as it has been shown that such a graphitization process is thermally driven [158].

The surface energy (γ_s) and its polar and dispersive components $(\gamma_s^{p}$ and $\gamma_s^{d})$ are shown in Figure 19.35 together with the contact angle of water. The results show that all the surfaces have a hydrophobic nature with much higher γ_s^{d} than γ_s^{p}. As the absolute value of the bias voltage increases, the polar part of the surface energy decreases by nearly 60% from 6.4 to 3.8 mJ/m^2. The contact angle of water on the films is about 75°–85° and decreases with higher V_b. The trends are consistent with the change of the I_D/I_G ratio as displayed in Figure 19.36. The surface energy thus appears to be affected mainly by the sp^3 content in the films, and Pinzari's study on the wettability of diamond films in fact has shown similar effects [160].

Figure 19.37 exhibits the statistical results of the platelets adhered on the a-C:H film surfaces from PRP, and expresses as a percentage of platelets adhered on the stainless steel in the same test. After incubation in PRP for 15 min, the number of adherent platelets slightly decreases with increasing V_b (absolute value) and is less than that on the stainless steel surface. The percentage of unactivated platelets drops steeply from 30% to 8% when V_b is changed from −75 to −900 V. The percentage of unactivated platelets on stainless steel is in between.

Platelets are strongly surface activated by the a-C:H film deposited at high V_b (absolute value) compared to those at low V_b (absolute value). It is consistent with the variation of the polar component γ_s^{p} of the surface energy. The platelet attachment studies suggest that the adhesion behavior of the platelets is related to the surface energy of the film. The higher the absolute value of V_b, the lower is the value of γ_s^{p}, and accordingly, the higher is the activation of adherent platelets. Besides, the results show that when the bias V_b (absolute value) is increased, the interfacial energy of albumin and fibrinogen increases from 10.8 and 15.0 mJ/m^2 to 15.9 and 20.9 mJ/m^2, respectively. It is expected because protein molecules will undergo a conformational transformation when plasma protein adsorbs onto an artificial surface (higher interfacial energy) from its aqueous phase (lower interfacial energy). Thus, it suggests that the higher the interfacial energy γ_{sp}, the larger the conformation changes. Moreover, exacerbation of activation of the platelets adhered on the a-C:H film deposited at high V_b is probably due to the changes of fibrinogen conformation.

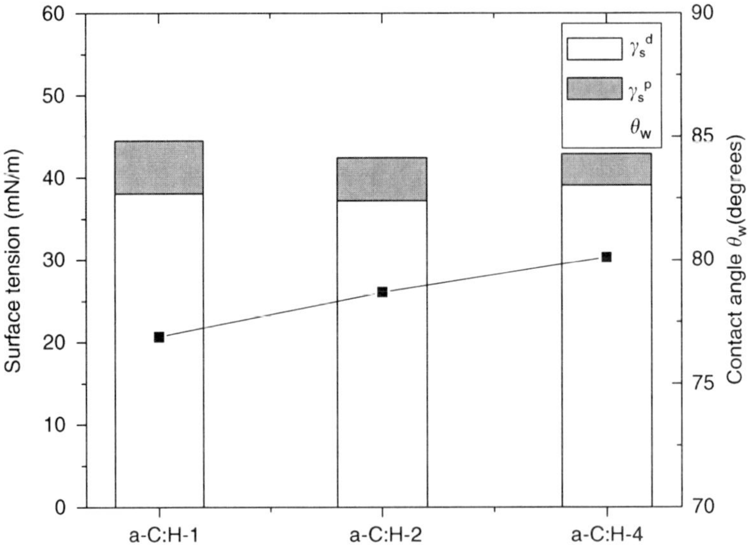

FIGURE 19.35 Surface energies (γ_s) and their polar and dispersive components $(\gamma_s^{p}$ and $\gamma_s^{d})$ of the a-C:H films. (From Yang, P. et al., *Biomaterials*, 24, 2821, 2003. With permission.)

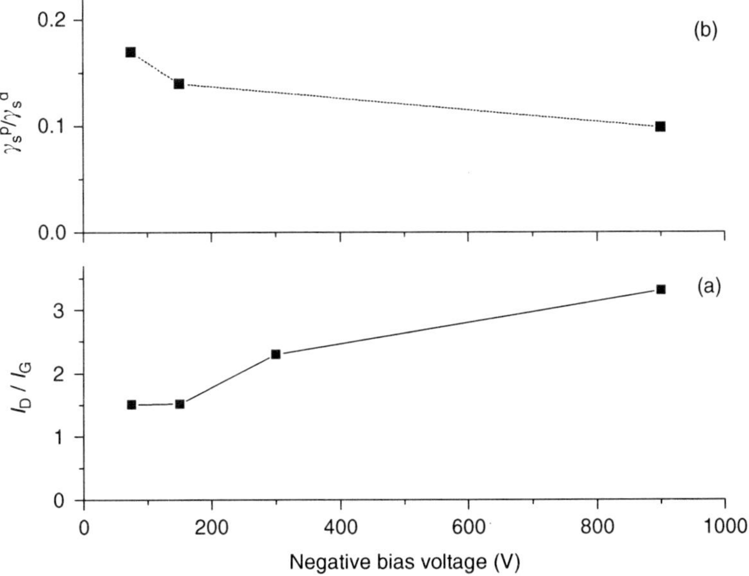

FIGURE 19.36 Effects of the bias voltage on (a) intensity ratio of the D-band to G-band and (b) ratio of polar/dispersive component of the surface energy. (From Yang, P. et al., *Biomaterials*, 24, 2821, 2003. With permission.)

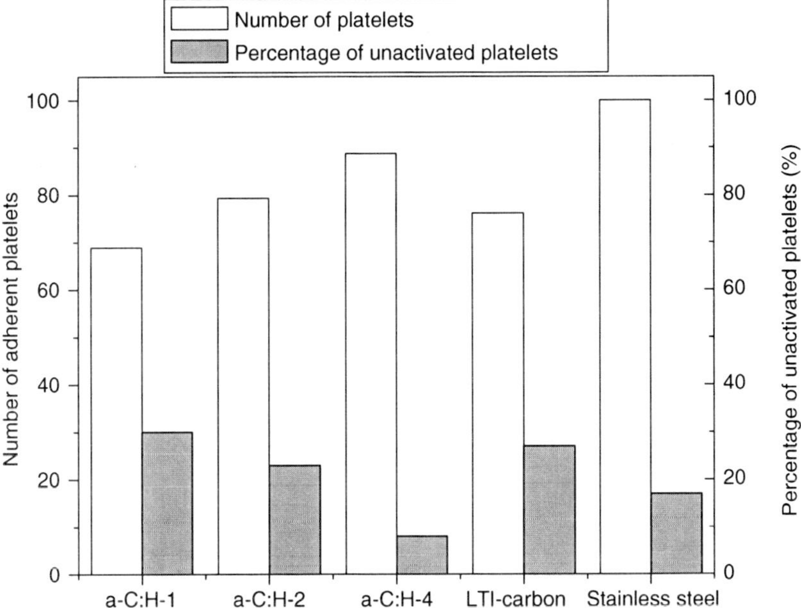

FIGURE 19.37 Quantity of platelets adhered on the surface of the a-C:H films synthesized at different bias voltages (15 min incubation in PRP) expressed as a percentage of platelets adhering to stainless steel in the same test. (From Yang, P. et al., *Biomaterials*, 24, 2821, 2003. With permission.)

All in all, the study of the surface energy of the films shows that the polar part of the surface energy decreases with increasing bias voltage, and the tendency is consistent with the change of the I_D/I_G ratios. It is believed that this trend is affected mainly by the reduction of the sp^3 content in the films. Activation and the quantity of adherent platelets on the surface of the a-C:H films are influenced by the substrate bias. The higher the bias V_b, the larger is the activation of the adherent platelets. This trend is consistent with the surface energy of the films. The effects can be attributed to the preference of albumin adsorption due to the higher W_a value of albumin that can be compared to that of fibrinogen and the changes of fibrinogen conformation, which has been caused by higher interfacial energy γ_{sp}. The blood compatibility of the a-C:H film deposited at −75 V is better than that exhibited by stainless steel and similar to that of LTI-carbon.

19.5.1.3 Influence of Annealing Temperature on Electrical Property and Blood Behaviors

Hydrogenated amorphous carbon films have been fabricated at room temperature using PIIID. After PIIID, annealing was carried out at 200–600°C for 30 min at reduced pressure ($<1 \times 10^{-3}$ Pa).

The position and width of the G-peak and I_D/I_G ratio as a function of the annealing temperature are shown in Figure 19.38. The shift in the G-band indicates the increase in size and number of the sp^2 carbons, and the increase in the observed I_D/I_G intensity ratio suggests that there is an increase in the number of ordered aromatic rings within the samples. The emergence of the D-band and the increase of the I_D/I_G ratio show that the materials have become nanocrystalline graphite [161]. The steep changes observed in the three curves at 300–400°C indicate that graphitization is promoted at higher annealing temperature arising from a diffusive mechanism. Ogwu has reported similar results [162].

The dependence of E_g, resistivity, and carrier concentration on annealing temperature is shown in Figure 19.39. As the band gap depends on the configuration of the sp^2 sites, the growth of the sp^2 cluster with increasing annealing temperature is the main reason for the observed band gap narrowing [164]. Both the resistivity and Hall mobility decrease with increasing annealing temperature and the trends are consistent with the Raman shift in the G-line. The steep changes at approximately 400°C in the two curves also agree with the Raman results. Thus, it appears that the increase of the electrical conductivity in the annealed a-C:H film is related to an increase in the sp^2 bonding carbon and ordered sp^2 cluster caused by graphitization.

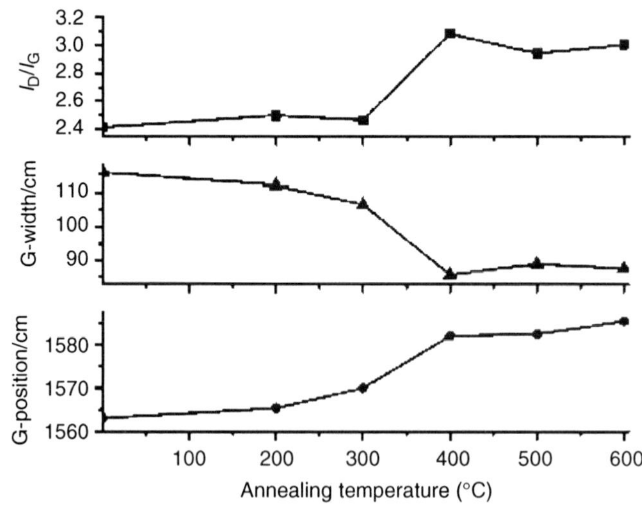

FIGURE 19.38 Intensity ratios of the D-band to G-band and width and position of G-band with annealing temperature derived from Raman spectra. (From Yang, P. et al., *Surf. Coating Tech.*, 177–178, 747, 2004. With permission.)

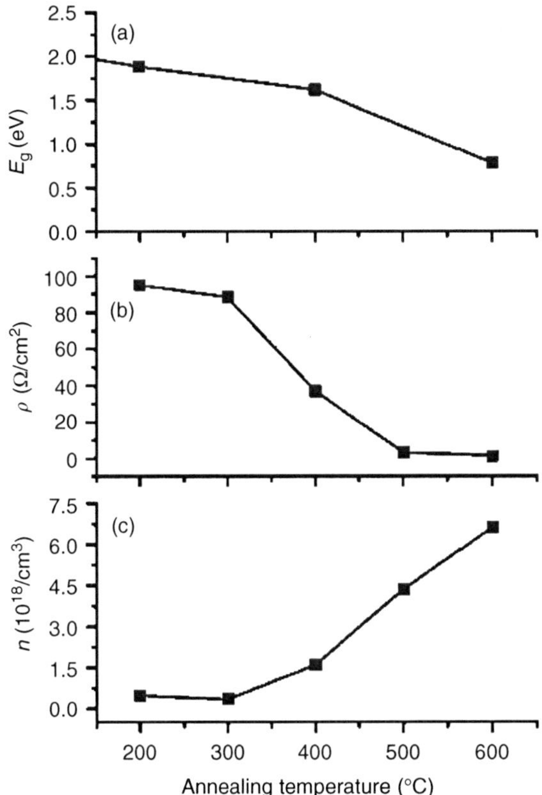

FIGURE 19.39   Band gap, resistivity, Hall mobility, and carrier concentration of a-C:H films as functions of annealing temperature. (From Yang, P. et al., *Surf. Coating Tech.*, 177–178, 747, 2004. With permission.)

Figure 19.40 exhibits the statistical results of the platelets adhered on the a-C:H films of different annealing temperatures from platelet rich plasma (PRP). In contrast with the results acquired from the as-deposited film, the numbering of adherent platelets on the annealed films decreases, fluctuates slightly from 200°C to 500°C, and increases slightly at 600°C. The unactivated platelet percentages of the annealed films are close to that of the as-deposited one when the annealing temperature is lower than 400°C, and the percentages decrease when the annealing temperature is higher than 500°C. The curve changes drastically at 400–500°C. It thus appears that annealing at a relatively low temperature cannot cause retrogression of blood compatibility of our a-C:H films, and the activation of platelets adhered on the a-C:H film surfaces is related to the change of the physical properties of the films.

When blood comes in contact with an artificial surface, the first event is protein adsorption. If the adsorbed protein such as fibrinogen is denatured, the coagulation factors or platelets will be activated, causing a series of cascade reaction of blood coagulation and then finally thrombosis. It has been shown that denaturing of fibrinogen and coagulation factors FV, FVIII, FIX depends on the transfer of its charges to the material, and this process is related to the electronic structure and properties of the material [165,166]. Fibrinogen has an electronic structure similar to that of a semiconductor. When a material possesses a wider band gap than fibrinogen, there are less local states in the band gap, lower carrier concentration and n-type structure, and consequently, fibrinogen denaturation is inhibited. Thus, it is reasonable that the as-deposited a-C:H film with a larger band gap and lower carrier concentration possesses lower surface activation of adherent platelets. It is probably the reason for the blood compatibility retrogression at a temperature higher than 400°C and the significant change in the electronic characteristics such as narrowing of the band gap (narrower than

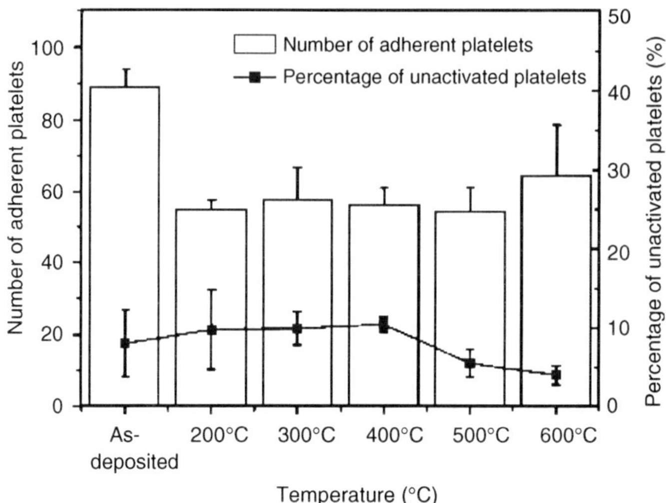

FIGURE 19.40 Quantity of platelets adhered on the surface of the a-C:H films annealed at different temperatures (15 min incubation in PRP). (From Yang, P. et al., *Surf. Coating Tech.*, 177–178, 747, 2004. With permission.)

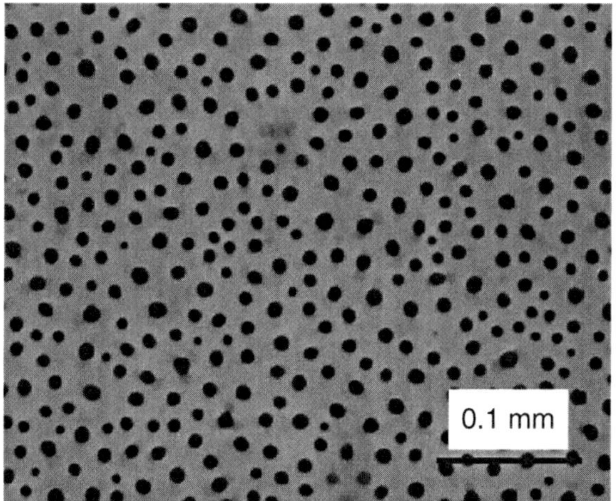

FIGURE 19.41 Optical micrograph of the surface of P-doped DLC. (From Kwok, S.C.H. et al., *Diam. Relat. Mater.*, 14, 78, 2005. With permission.)

the band gap of fibrinogen), order-of-magnitude increase of the carrier concentration, and of p-type conductivity. Hence, the blood compatibility of a-C:H films is affected by the electronic structure and improving the electronic structure is important for the abatement of platelet activation.

19.5.1.4 Influence of Elemental Doping on Film Characteristics

19.5.1.4.1 Phosphorus-doped DLC films (P-DLC)
Phosphorus, which is commonly found in inorganic phosphate rocks and in all living cells, is one of the essential elements in biological system. In this study, DLC films were firstly fabricated using acetylene gas in PIIID. Subsequent phosphorus implantation was conducted in the same vacuum chamber using high-voltage glow discharge so as to prepare P-doped DLC.

Dot-like features are observed in the P-doped DLC films as depicted in Figure 19.41. These microstructures with an average diameter of 8–18 mm and height of 30–50 nm are evenly distributed near the film surface. The total solid-surface free energy and its components were determined using double distilled water and diiodomethane. The surface free energy components of the different materials and biological substances are summarized in Table 19.5. The total surface free energy of the P-doped DLC increases from 42.9 to 72.4 mJ/m^2 and the polar component (γ_s^p) increases from 11.5 to 44.8 mJ/m^2. Moreover, the contact angle of water diminishes dramatically to 16.9°. These data indicate that the wettability is improved by phosphorus doping.

Figure 19.42 displays the statistical amount of adherent platelets on low-temperature isotropic pyrolitic carbon (LTIC), undoped-DLC, and P-doped DLC films after 20 min incubation. The number of adherent platelets on the P-doped DLC film is lower than that on LTIC, which is a common biomedical material. The morphology of adhered platelets is assessed and the platelets' shape

TABLE 19.5

Contact Angle and Surface Energy Components of Different Materials and Biological Substances

	Contact Angle (°)		Surface Energy (mJ/m^2)		
Substrate	Water	Diiodomethane	γ_s	γ_s^d	γ_s^p
LTIC	74.9	34.4	43.1	37.5	5.6
DLC	68.4	43.8	42.9	31.4	11.5
P-doped DLC	16.9	37.0	72.4	27.6	44.8
Blood	—	—	47.5	11.2	36.3
Fibrinogen	—	—	65.0	24.7	40.3
Albumin	—	—	65.0	31.38	33.62

Source: Kwok, S.C.H. et al., *Diam. Relat. Mater.*, 14, 78, 2005. With permission.

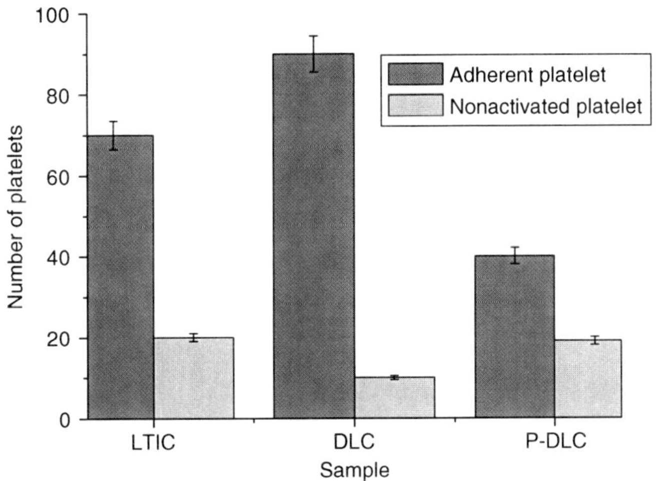

FIGURE 19.42 Quantity of platelets adhered on the surface of LTIC, DLC, and P-doped DLC. (From Kwok, S.C.H. et al., *Diam. Relat. Mater.*, 14, 78, 2005. With permission.)

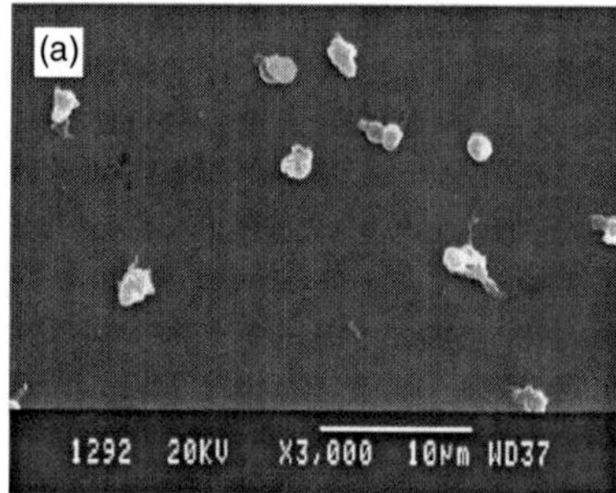
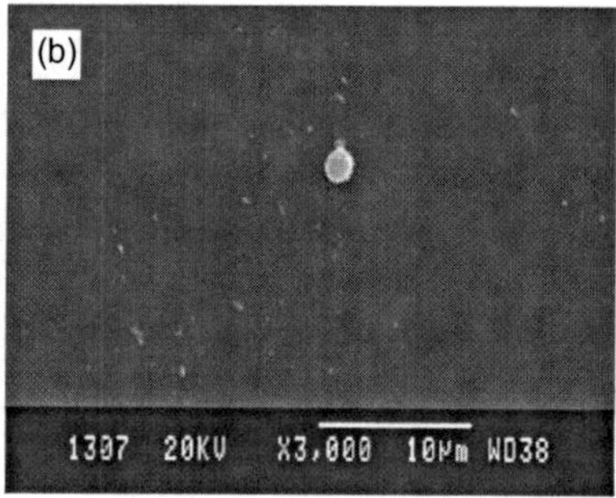

FIGURE 19.43 Morphology of adherent platelets observed by SEM on (a) LTIC (120 min incubation in PRP) and (b) P-doped DLC (120 min incubation in PRP). (From Kwok, S.C.H. et al., *Diam. Relat. Mater.*, 14, 78, 2005. With permission.)

changes on the different surfaces after 120 min incubation are compared. As shown in Figure 19.43, the adherent platelets on the P-doped DLC and LTIC are isolated and relatively round.

The interfacial tension is highest with albumin on the P-doped DLC film, but there are higher interfacial tensions between fibrinogen and LTIC or DLC. This suggests that albumin is preferentially adsorbed on P-doped DLC, whereas fibrinogen is preferentially adsorbed on LTIC and DLC. In particular, a high contribution of polar interaction between undoped DLC and albumin and an equal level of dispersive and polar interaction between undoped DLC and fibrinogen further prove the preferential adsorption of fibrinogen on the undoped DLC surface. Albumin preferential adsorption is known to passivate the surface of an implant and the preferential adsorption of fibrinogen or globulin will lead to favor coagulation and platelet activation. Furthermore, the interfacial tensions of three kinds of plasma proteins on the P-doped DLC surface are significantly lower than those on the undoped DLC and LTIC surfaces. Moreover, a mechanically stable blood–biomaterial interface is considered as another surface energetic criterion of biocompatibility of a foreign surface [168]. Because the cellular elements are compatible with blood and their interface with the medium is also mechanically stable, it is considered that a blood–biomaterial interfacial tension of about the same magnitude as the cell–medium interfacial tension ($\gamma_{SL} \approx 1$–3 dynes/cm) will provide a foreign surface with both long-term compatibility as well as mechanically stable interface with blood. It has been shown that the interfacial tension between the P-doped DLC film and medium (water) is 2.7 dynes/cm, which has the same magnitude as the cell–medium interfacial tension. Thus, the good hemocompatibility of the P-doped DLC coating is because it significantly minimizes the interactions with plasma protein giving rise to slight changes in the conformation of adsorbed plasma proteins and preferentially adsorbed albumin.

19.5.1.4.2 Calcium-Doped DLC Films (Ca-DLC)

Calcium (Ca), the fifth most abundant element in the earth's crust, is one of the essential elements in living organisms particularly pertaining to cell physiology. Moreover, calcium is a crucial constituent in bones and teeth formation and hence, it is an interesting dopant in DLC for biomedical applications. In this study, three doped DLC films, Ca-doped, Ca and P-doped, and P-doped DLC films, are produced.

The surface biocompatibility was assessed using *in vitro* platelet adhesion tests. Figure 19.44 displays the morphology and the quantity of the adhered platelets on the samples. The statistical results are presented in Figure 19.45. Both the P-DLC and Ca-DLC films show smaller numbers of adhered and unactivated platelets than LTIC. The results show that either Ca or P doping alone can enhance the hemocompatibility but not when acting together.

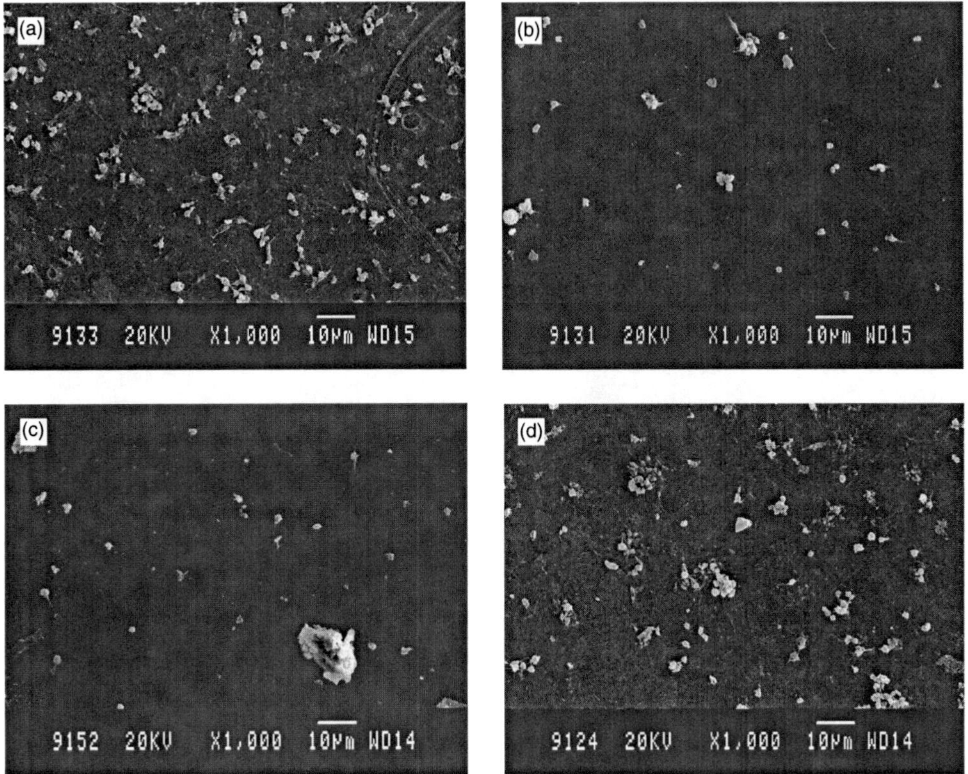

FIGURE 19.44 SEM photos showing adhered platelets on (a) CaP-DLC, (b) P-DLC, (c) Ca-DLC, and (d) LTIC control. (From Kwok, S.C.H. et al., *Diam. Relat. Mater.*, 15, 893, 2006. With permission.)

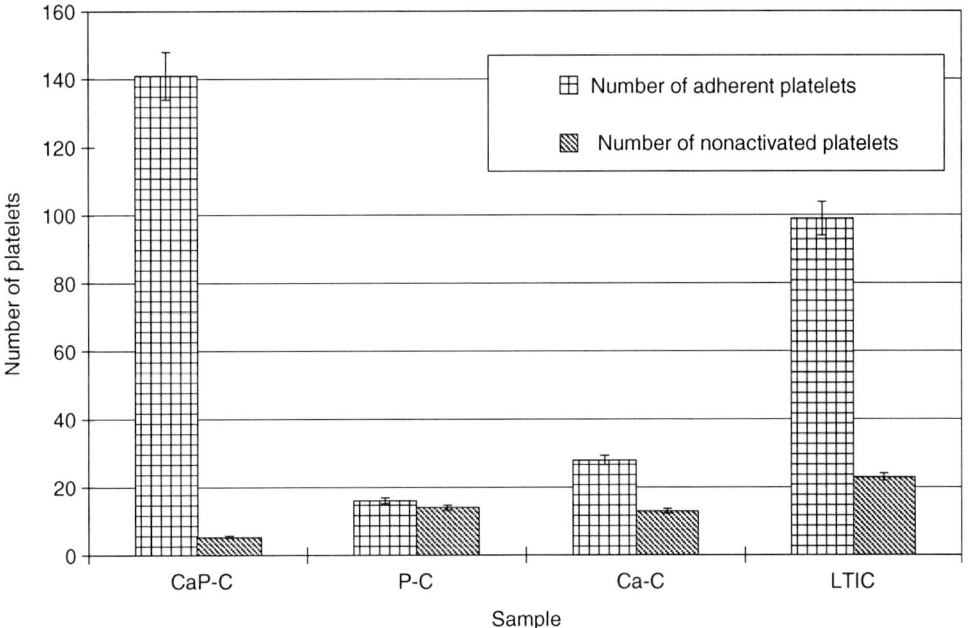

FIGURE 19.45 Quantity of platelets adhered on CaP-C, P-C, Ca-C; and LTIC. (From Kwok, S.C.H. et al., *Diam. Relat. Mater.*, 15, 893, 2006. With permission.)

TABLE 19.6

Interfacial Energies between Materials and Plasma Proteins

Biological Substances	Ca-DLC		CaP-DLC		P-DLC		LTIC	
	γ_{sp}	$\gamma_{sp}^{p}/\gamma_{sp}^{d}$	γ_{sp}	$\gamma_{sp}^{p}/\gamma_{sp}^{d}$	γ_{sp}	$\gamma_{sp}^{p}/\gamma_{sp}^{d}$	γ_{sp}	$\gamma_{sp}^{p}/\gamma_{sp}^{d}$
Fibrinogen	6.7	0.04	45.4	4.62	6.5	0.02	16.8	12.2
Albumin	11.2	0.11	35.8	6.31	10.7	0.08	11.8	46.6

Source: Kwok, S.C.H. et al., *Diam. Relat. Mater.*, 15, 893, 2006. With permission.

TABLE 19.7

Contact Angle (θ_w) and Interfacial Energy (γ_{sw}) between Different Materials (Samples) and Water

Materials	θ_w (°)	γ_{sw} (nJ/cm^2)
Ca-DLC	87.2	6.2
CaP-DLC	51	57.6
P-DLC	49	5.1
LTIC	74.9	24.2

Source: Kwok, S.C.H. et al., *Diam. Relat. Mater.*, 15, 893, 2006. With permission.

The interfacial energies (γ_{sp}) between plasma proteins and samples are shown in Table 19.6. Ca-DLC (0.11) and P-DLC (0.08) have lower values of $\gamma_{sp}^{p}/\gamma_{sp}^{d}$ for albumin (γ_{sp}^{p} and γ_{sp}^{d} represent the polar and dispersive components of the interfacial energy between proteins and materials) than CaP-DLC and LTIC, suggesting stronger adhesion of albumin. The $\gamma_{sp}^{p}/\gamma_{sp}^{d}$ ratio for fibrinogen is also small, but the total interfacial energy, γ_{sp}, is less than that of albumin, which means that less conformational changes occur. The results suggest that these surface energies are the primary factors for the good compatibility observed on Ca-DLC and P-DLC in the platelet adhesion test. Table 19.7 shows the results of the contact angles and calculated interfacial energies (γ_{sw}) between water and the films. Ca-DLC and P-DLC have the lowest values of interfacial energy (γ_{sw} = 6.2 and 5.1, respectively) with water (medium), indicating that both films have closer interfacial tension (1–3 nJ/cm^2) with the cell medium than CaP-DLC and LTIC. Hence, the platelet results are consistent with the calculated surface energy.

19.5.2 Ti–O Thin Film

Titanium oxide is widely used in optical and electrical applications because of its high refractive index and dielectric constant. It is also very attractive as a biocompatible protective coating on medical implants, where a protective surface layer of TiO$_2$ increases the wear resistance and hardness considerably. Dissolution of Ti metal ions from the rutile phase is one order of magnitude lower than that from anatase, and so rutile is the preferred phase with respect to biomedical applications

[170]. When a rutile titanium oxide layer is formed on the surface of a matrix, the blood compatibility can be improved significantly [166,170]. Several techniques to prepare titanium dioxide films have been reported, such as thermal oxidation [170], anodic oxidation [171], magnetron sputtering [172–175], cathodic vacuum arc deposition [176–178], and ion beam enhanced deposition (IBED) [166]. Titanium oxide films used in artificial heart valves have also been synthesized using PIIID technology in City University of Hong Kong and Southwest Jiaotong University, Chengdu, China [35,133,179].

The PIII system used in this work is schematically shown in Figure 19.46. A Ti cathode 14 mm in diameter was mounted on the metal vacuum arc plasma source. An oxygen plasma was sustained by RF in the vacuum chamber and at the same time, a titanium plasma was generated in the metal arc source and diffused into the vacuum chamber via a magnetic duct to eliminate deleterious macroparticles. The voltage on the sample was −50 V DC and the deposition time was 60 min. The deposition rate varied from 0.1 to 0.15 nm/s depending on the oxygen gas flow rate. To increase the adhesion between the film and silicon (100) substrate, a −3 kV pulse voltage (10 kHz, 5 μs) was applied to the sample during the first 10 min. Table 19.8 lists the instrumental

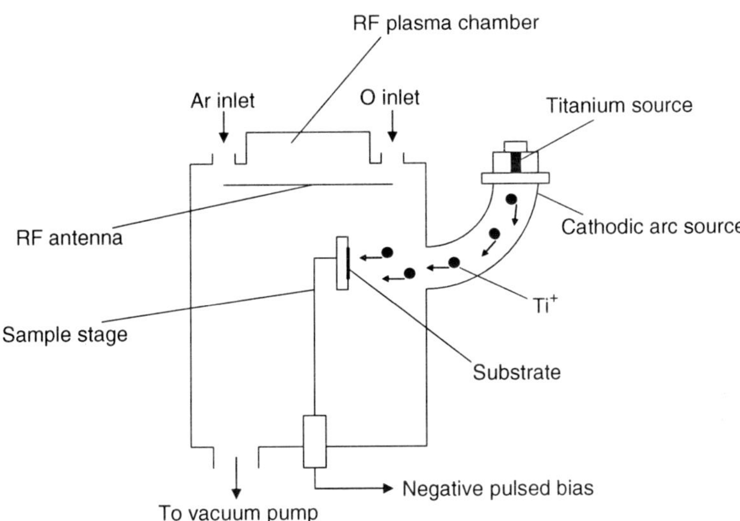

FIGURE 19.46 Schematic diagram of the PIII system applied to prepare the Ti–O thin film.

TABLE 19.8
Instrumental Parameters for Samples #1 to #5

Samples		#1	#2	#3	#4	#5
Vacuum arc	Pulse repetition rate (Hz)			65		
Metal plasma	Pulse width (ms)			1		
Source	Arc current (A)			180		
Oxygen gas flow (sccm)		3.1	5	7	10	15
Oxygen partial pressure ($\times 10^{-2}$ Pa)		0.63	0.93	1.2	1.7	2.7
RF power (W)				600		

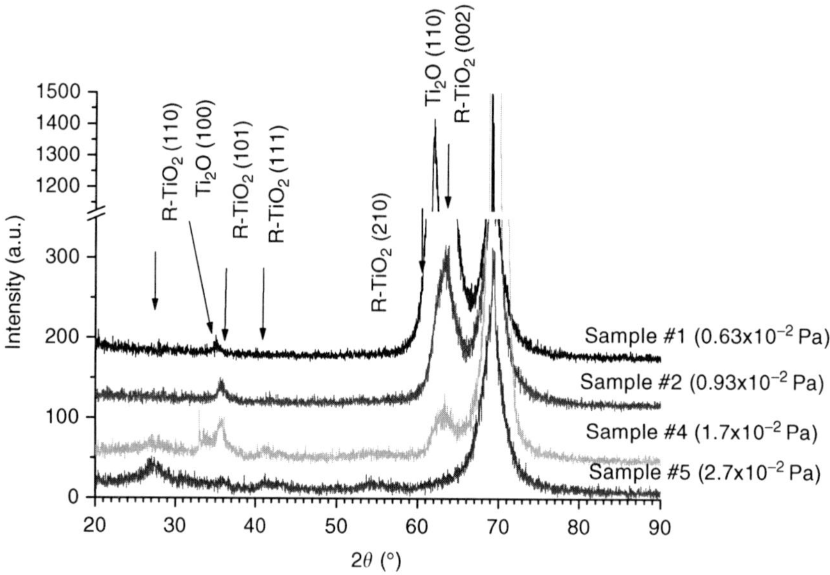

FIGURE 19.47   XRD patterns of the as-deposited titanium oxide films. (From Leng, Y.X. et al., *Surf. Coating Tech.*, 156, 295, 2002. With permission.)

parameters. The films were subsequently annealed *in situ* at 700°C for 60 min and then 750°C for 30 min at a base pressure of 1.5×10^{-3} Pa. The annealing apparatus comprised a resistively heated quartz tube.

The film is polycrystalline with coexisting Ti^{2+}, Ti^{3+}, and Ti^{4+}. The intensity of the (101) and (110) diffraction peaks goes up while that of the (002) diffraction peak diminishes with increasing oxygen partial pressure, as shown in Figure 19.47 [133]. Hence, Leng et al. [133] conclude that the growth on the (110) plane parallel to the surface becomes more dominant at higher oxygen partial pressure. The microhardness values obtained from TiO_2 shown in Figure 19.48 increase with oxygen partial pressure between 0 and 1.7×10^{-2} Pa. *In vitro* blood compatibility investigation indicates that the TiO_2 film has longer clotting time, lower hemolytic rate, less amounts of adherent platelets, less aggregation, and less pseudopodium of the adherent platelet [133]. *In vivo* tests also demonstrate that the TiO_2 film has much better hemocompatibility than LTIC [179], as shown in Figure 19.49.

To improve the mechanical properties, Leng et al. fabricate Ti—O/Ti—N duplex coatings on biomedical titanium alloys by metal PIII and reactive plasma nitriding/oxidation [180]. The presence of Ti—O improves the blood compatibility and the main effect of Ti—N is to improve the mechanical properties. Blood compatibility investigation reveals that the Ti—O/Ti—N duplex coatings are better than LTIC. In addition, tantalum nitride films with excellent mechanical and biomedical properties have been synthesized using a similar method [181]. Chen et al. prepared tantalum-doped Ti—O/Ti—N and obtained good mechanical property and blood compatibility results [182]. Studies have shown that TiO_2 has good blood compatibility due to the n-type semiconductivity with a wider band gap of 3.2 eV, low surface energy, and low critical surface force. The good surface physical properties preclude fibrinogen from denaturation and consequently prevent the blood coagulation process [166,170,183,184]. The blood–biomaterial interfacial tension $\gamma_{s \cdot blood}$ can influence the denaturing or distortion of fibrinogen. Furthermore, the activation of fibrinogen on the solid surface can be correlated with the electrochemical reaction between the protein and material

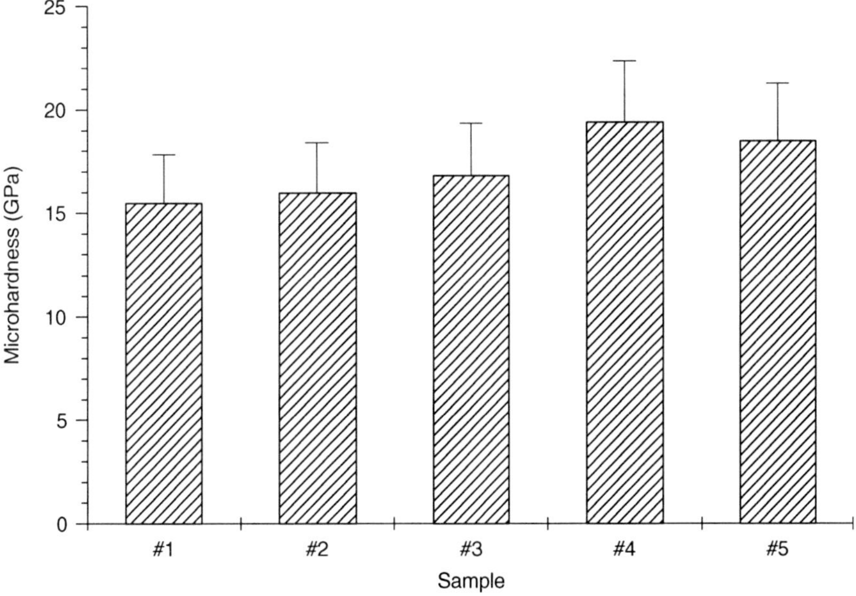

FIGURE 19.48 Microhardness of the TiO$_2$ films. (From Leng, Y.X. et al., *Surf. Coating Tech.*, 156, 295, 2002. With permission.)

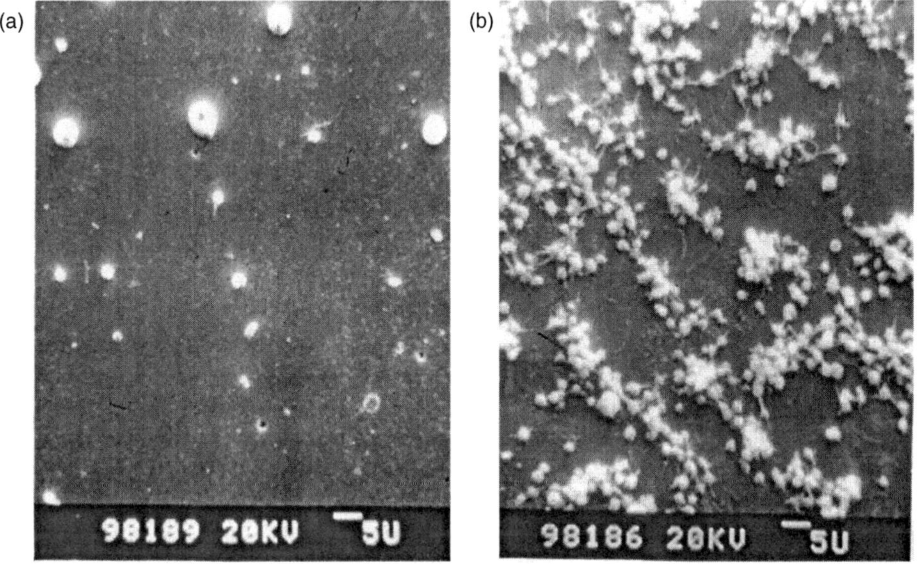

FIGURE 19.49 SEM (1000×) images showing less platelet adhesion on TiO$_2$ (a) than LTIC (b). (From Chu, P.K. et al., *Mater. Sci. Eng. R Rep.*, 36, 143, 2002. With permission.)

surface. It is postulated that the denaturing of fibrinogen is related to the charges of fibrinogen transferred to the material, as shown in Figure 19.50. During this process, fibrinogen decomposes and transforms into fibrin monomer and fibrin peptides, followed by cross-linking to form the irreversible thrombus [170].

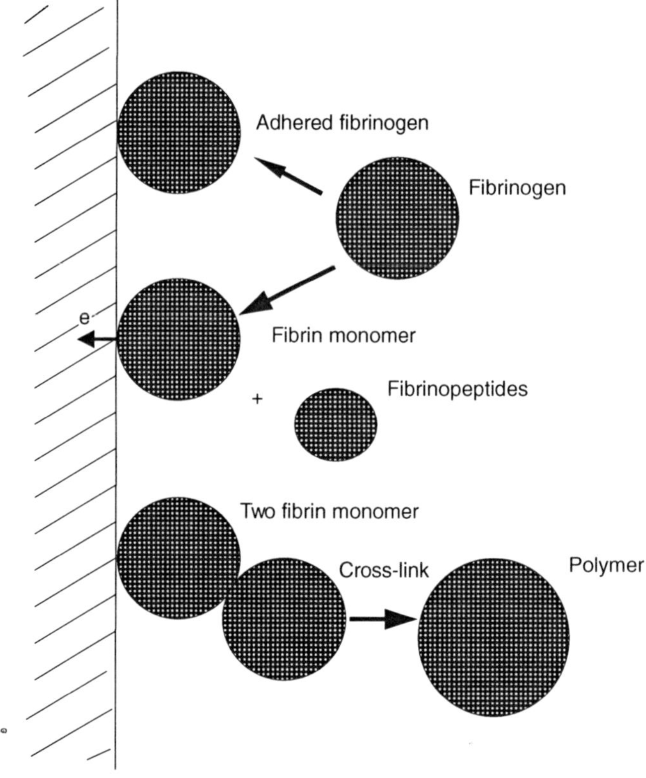

FIGURE 19.50 Interactions of fibrinogen with a solid via the charge transfer process. (From Chen, J.Y. et al., *Biomaterials*, 23, 2545, 2002. With permission.)

19.6 SURFACE MODIFICATION OF POLYMERS FOR ENHANCED ANTIBACTERIAL PROPERTIES

19.6.1 Cu-Implanted Polymers

Medical polymers are widely used in the treatment of diseases and biomedical implants because of their excellent mechanical properties and biological properties [185–187]. However, when medical polymers are implanted inside the human body, they can become places for microbes to adhere and breed, and thus infection of medical polymers is one of the major clinical complications [188–191]. Nowadays, there is an increasing interest in the development of anti-infective medical polymers by the biomedical industry. Antimicrobial properties on medical polymers can be achieved by two main approaches [192–196]. The first technique is the deposition of antibacterial reagents directly onto the surface of the polymers by means of vapor deposition, sputter coating, or ion beam–assisted surface modification and deposition. The second method is the direct incorporation of antibacterial reagents into the polymers.

Researchers in City University of Hong Kong found that Cu could be incorporated into the surface region of polyethylene (PE) by means of PIII to promote the antimicrobial properties [197]. Low-energy (several keVs) Cu PIII can introduce a large amount of Cu into the polymer without causing too much damage to the polymer surface [36,63,197–202]. Medical-grade PE specimens were implanted with Cu in a plasma immersion ion implanter equipped with a Cu cathodic arc plasma source and nitrogen PIII was performed to change the structure of the implanted region of the substrate. Compared to the single Cu PIII process, this dual plasma implantation process (Cu/N$_2$ PIII) can better regulate the copper release rate and improve the long-term antibacterial properties of the PE samples. This process thus creates a buried (stored) layer of the antimicrobial reagent with the ability to control the release of Cu by means of N$_2$ PIII. The antibacterial properties of the treated PE can thus be significantly enhanced particularly with respect to the long-term effects.

Medical-grade PE was inserted into the plasma immersion ion implanter equipped with a Cu cathodic arc plasma source. The arc was ignited using pulse duration of 300 μs, repetition rate of 30 Hz, and arc current of 1 A. The copper plasma was guided into the vacuum chamber by an electromagnetic field. The Cu PIII process was conducted by applying an in-phase bias voltage of −5 kV with a repetition rate of 30 Hz and a pulse width of 300 μs to the PE samples [36,63,197]. Another PE sample underwent N$_2$ plasma implantation at the same time. The nitrogen gas was bled into the vicinity of the copper arc discharge plume at a flow rate of 10 sccm (standard cubic centimeter) with the other processing conditions being similar to those of Cu PIII [200]. The working pressure in the vacuum chamber was $1 - 2 \times 10^{-4}$ Torr and the implantation time was 10 min.

Figure 19.51a shows that the implanted copper is located in the near-surface region as a result of the low implantation energy. The amount of implanted copper is about 11% at the peak (by comparing the ratio of copper to carbon), and the surface Cu concentration is about 3%, which stems from some surface deposition during PIII. Such surface Cu concentration offers immediate and direct killing of bacteria or inhibition of cells that are in contact with the materials surface [188,203]. Based on the metal ion antimicrobial mechanism [186,191], Cu ions are consumed during the antibacterial reactions, and so the effects of surface Cu can be short-lived. Furthermore, if the surface Cu concentration is too high, there are side effects on cells directly in contact with the material surface. Therefore, the sample, which has a relatively small amount of surface Cu and larger amount of embedded Cu, has many advantages. Most importantly, the buried Cu serves as a continuous supply of the antibacterial reagent to the surface to produce longer lasting antimicrobial effects. As shown in the result acquired from the Cu/N$_2$ PIII PE sample (Figure 19.51b), the in-depth copper profile is not affected significantly by N$_2$ plasma coimplantation. The nitrogen distribution is also similar to that of copper and so both chemical and physical interactions between the implanted N and Cu or polymer matrix in the implanted region can occur (to be discussed later in this chapter). The cross-sectional TEM image (Figure 19.52) of the Cu PIII PE sample reveals that the implanted Cu is segregated in the polymer matrix. In addition, no diffraction patterns can be obtained from the

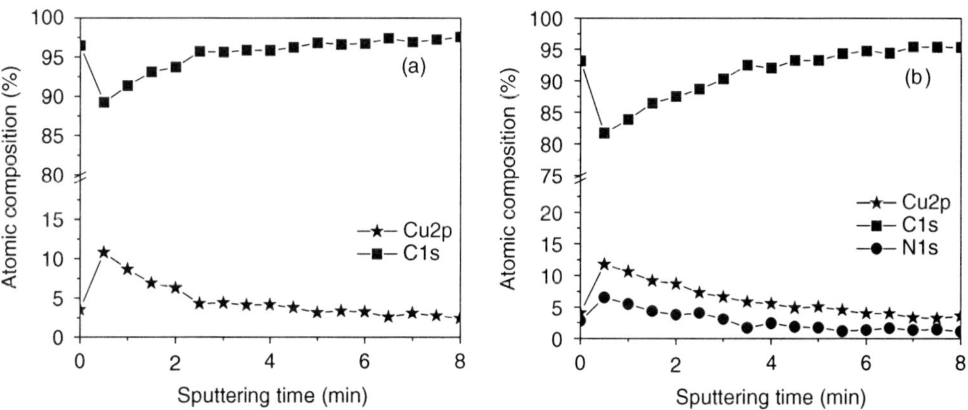

FIGURE 19.51 Elemental depth profiles acquired by XPS from (a) Cu PIII PE and (b) Cu/N$_2$ PIII PE. The argon ion-sputtering rate of 1 nm/min is approximated using that of silicon oxide under similar conditions. (From Zhang, W., Zhang, Y.H., Ji, J.H., Yan, Q., Huang, A.P., and Chu, P.K., *J. Biomed. Mater. Res.: Part A*, in press DOI.10.1002. With permission.)

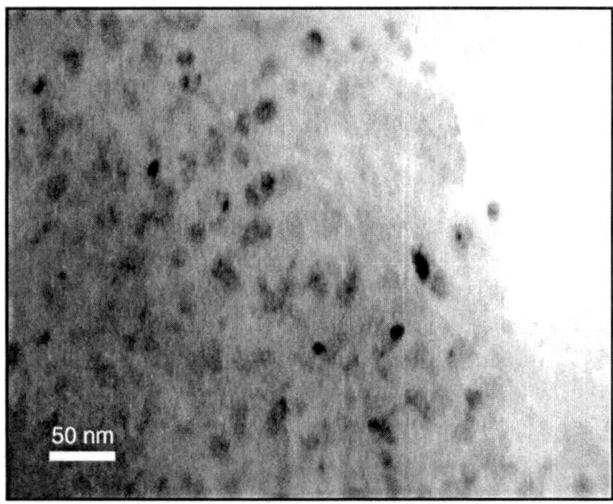

FIGURE 19.52   Cross-sectional TEM image of Cu PIII PE. (From Zhang, W., Zhang, Y.H., Ji, J.H., Yan, Q., Huang, A.P., and Chu, P.K., *J. Biomed. Mater. Res.: Part A*, in press DOI.10.1002. With permission.)

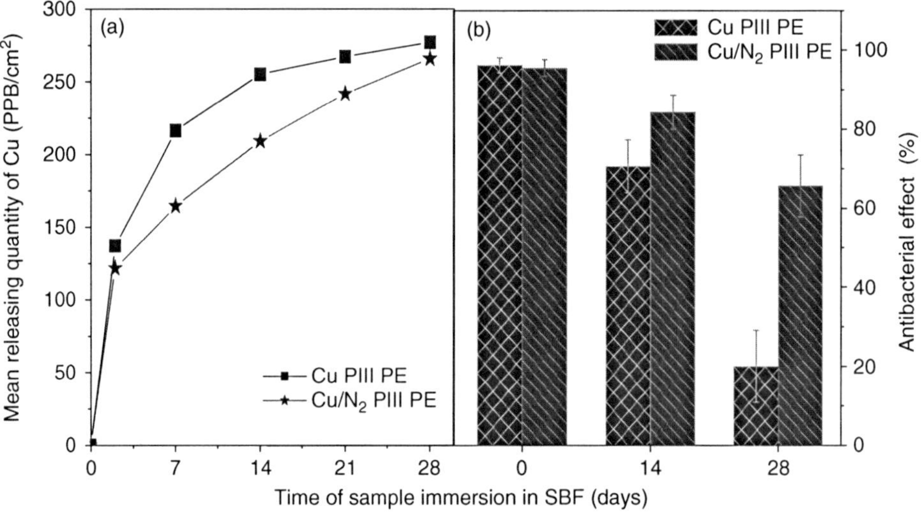

FIGURE 19.53   (a) Cumulative leached amounts of Cu from Cu PIII PE and Cu/N$_2$ PIII PE after various immersion times and (b) corresponding antimicrobial effects against *E. coli*. (From Zhang, W., Zhang, Y.H., Ji, J.H., Yan, Q., Huang, A.P., and Chu, P.K., *J. Biomed. Mater. Res.: Part A*, in press DOI.10.1002. With permission.)

sample further confirming that the implanted Cu is largely segregated in the polymer matrix. This segregated and unbonded Cu state is believed to facilitate effective out-diffusion.

The copper-leaching rate to the surface directly impacts the surface antibacterial effects. Therefore, ICPMS is conducted to evaluate the release rate of the implanted Cu from the substrates [205]. Figure 19.3a indicates high released quantities of Cu into the SBFs from the Cu PIII PE and Cu/N$_2$ PIII PE after 2 days. It has been reported that this amount of Cu does not raise health concerns [206]. Afterward, Cu out-diffusion from the Cu PIII PE sample diminishes. Figure 19.53a shows the cumulative amounts of leached Cu, and so a slower increase implies a lower degree of out-diffusion. In comparison, the Cu leaching rate from the Cu/N$_2$ PIII PE sample is steadier and approximately 10 ppb/day cm^2. This suggests that the N$_2$ plasma treatment is effective in regulating Cu out-diffusion and prolonging the surface antibacterial performance.

An *Escherichia coli* suspension with a concentration of 10^6 CFU/mL is employed to assess and compare the antimicrobial properties of the Cu PIII PE and Cu/N$_2$ PIII PE samples at immersion time periods of 0, 14, and 28 days (Figure 19.53b). Before they are immersed in SBF (i.e., day 0), both Cu PIII PE and Cu/N$_2$ PIII PE have excellent antibacterial effects against *E. coli*, that is, 96.2% and 95.5%, respectively. This mainly stems from the surface-deposited Cu that can deliver immediate antimicrobial effects. After immersion in SBF for 14 days, the Cu PIII PE and Cu/N$_2$ PIII PE still possess good antibacterial performances against such a high cell suspension in spite of the reduced Cu release rates. The antimicrobial effects against *E. coli* are 70.6% and 84.3%, respectively. It should be noted that the Cu/N$_2$ PIII PE sample exhibits better antibacterial effects. The difference is even more evident after immersion for 28 days. The results thus unequivocally demonstrate the excellent antibacterial effect of Cu/N$_2$ PIII. The process allows for the continuous release of buried Cu to retain the surface antibacterial ability for a longer period of time. In separate experiments, the prepared samples were stored under room temperature in air for 6 weeks and their antimicrobial effects were compared with those of freshly prepared samples. The antimicrobial effects against *E. coli* were found to hardly change, thus indicating excellent long-lasting effects during normal storage.

It is well known that the antimicrobial properties are primarily related to the release of the antibacterial reagent, Cu. In the absence of gettering effects, Cu out-diffusion from the substrate is believed to follow Fick's first law of diffusion [207,208]:

$$\frac{dN}{dt} = -DS\frac{dC}{dx}, \tag{19.4}$$

where N is the amount of copper, dC/dx is the Cu concentration gradient with distance, t is the time, S is the surface area of the samples, and D is the diffusion coefficient. Here, S is the same and dC/dx is more or less the same because the same Cu PIII conditions are used for both the samples. Consequently, the Cu diffusion rate, dN/dx, depends mainly on the diffusion coefficient, D. A diffusion process from the substrate consisting of two zones is being proposed, as schematically described in Figure 19.54. Diffusion in zone B is described by the above equation whereas that in zone A also depends on the chemistry and gettering effects between Cu, N, and the PE matrix.

Plasma immersion ion implantation is an effective method to introduce a large quantity of metal inorganic antimicrobials like Cu into organic medical polymers such as PE up to a depth of several hundred nanometers without causing appreciable damage to the polymer matrix. The use of N$_2$ PIII in concert with Cu PIII produces new polar unsaturated functional groups such as C=N and $-$C$\equiv$N in the near-surface of the polymer. They play an important role in regulating the out-diffusion rate of Cu and prolonging the antibacterial effects significantly. It demonstrates that an inorganic antimicrobial agent can be effectively incorporated into an organic biomedical polymer and by using a nitrogen plasma

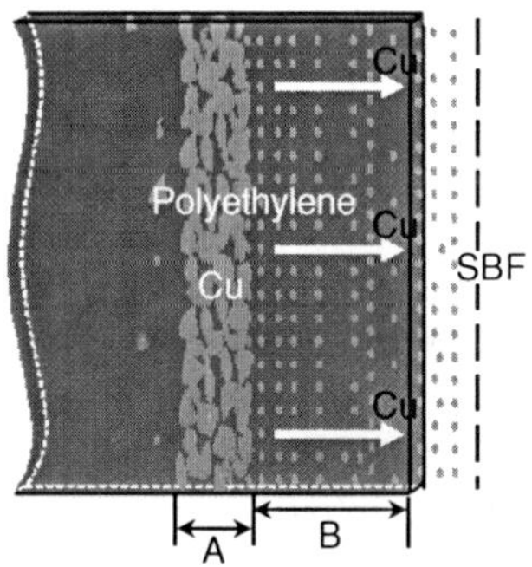

FIGURE 19.54 Schematic diagram illustrating two zones in the Cu-implanted polyethylene. (From Zhang, W., Zhang, Y.H., Ji, J.H., Yan, Q., Huang, A.P., and Chu, P.K., *J. Biomed. Mater. Res.: Part A*, in press DOI.10.2002. With permission.)

treatment, the release of Cu to the surface can be regulated. Consequently, the antimicrobial ability of the treated polymer can be prolonged significantly to increase its usefulness in medicine.

19.6.2 Grafting of Antimicrobial Reagents on Polymers

To obtain anti-infective properties, medical polymers are usually impregnated or compounded with some antibacterial or antimicrobial reagents [209,210]. These technologies require large quantities of the antimicrobial reagents, typically on the order of a few grams per square meter and the reagents are not immobilized on the surface. As a result, they are gradually released when these anti-infective polymers are embedded inside humans. They, therefore, pose great health hazards and it is necessary to develop alternative medical polymers or antibacterial surface treatments.

One of the ways to tackle this problem is to control the physicochemical interactions between the bacteria and medical polymer surface [211]. Surface modification of medical polymers or devices is a relatively simple and effective strategy to create a desirable surface and a number of surface modification techniques have been proposed to produce devices with antibacterial surfaces. Silver coatings, surface-immobilized PE oxide, surface thiocyanation, and surface modification by various gas plasmas (such as oxygen and argon) have been suggested [212–217]. PIII can be used to conduct surface modification for yielding superior surface with antibacterial properties. Polyvinyl chloride (PVC) is one of the common medical polymers [218–220]. Triclosan (2,4,4P-trichloro-2P-hydroxy-diphenylether) and bronopol (2-bromo-2-nitropropane-1,3-diol) are two types of compounds that exhibit immediate, persistent, broad-spectrum antimicrobial effectiveness as well as little toxicity in clinical use. They also deliver excellent biochemical and physical performances after plasma surface modification [221–223]. It is very significant and feasible to improve its antibacterial properties and decrease the degree of bacteria adhesion on medical-grade PVC using PIII technology.

The PVC was inserted into the plasma immersion ion implanter [36,63]. The O_2 plasma treatment was performed at the optimal conditions based on many trial experiments: Bias voltage -12 kV, voltage pulse width 20 µs, pulsing frequency 30 Hz, gas flow 35 sccm, RF power 1000 W, and treatment time 30 min. Under these conditions, sample charging was not serious and no arcing was observed during the experiments. After the initial plasma treatment, the samples were uniformly coated with the antibacterial reagent triclosan or bronopol in 20% alcohol. After the alcohol had volatilized, the samples were reloaded into the implanter and then underwent argon plasma ion bombardment to ensure that antibacterial reagent combined well with the PVC surface. The processing parameters were bias voltage -4 kV, RF power 1000 W, treatment time 30 min, and gas flow 35 sccm [224]. Again, these treatment conditions were based on trial experiments. Finally, the samples were washed three times using 70% ethanol to scour off loose triclosan or bronopol on the surface.

The surface of most medical-grade PVC is hydrophobic. On the other hand, triclosan and bronopol are hydrophilic and easily crystallized. In order to coat the PVC samples with these two antibacterial materials, the PVC surface must be modified. The PVC surface was firstly treated using oxygen plasma. The contact angles of distilled water in contact with the PVC surface before and after oxygen plasma modification were about 96° and 20°, respectively. This indicates that the O_2 PIII PVC surfaces are quite hydrophilic and the modified PVC can be coated effectively with the antibacterial reagents. The change in the surface hydrophilicity is because the C$-$C or C$-$H group on the surface of PVC is changed to C$-$O or C$=$O group by the oxygen plasma [36,63,225–227].

The antibacterial properties of samples treated with an oxygen plasma, coated with triclosan or bronopol, and then treated with an argon plasma are evaluated by plate-counting of *Staphylococcus aureus* and *E. coli*, which are the most representative bacteria, and the results are shown in Table 19.9. The antibacterial effects of the samples coated with triclosan against *S. aureus* and *E. coli* are 82.2% and 79.5%, respectively. This illustrates that after combining with the PVC surface, triclosan still possesses antibacterial properties. This phenomenon should be interpreted from the antibacterial mechanism of triclosan. Based on the results reported recently [221–223], triclosan acts as a nonspecific biocide by affecting the membrane structure and function of the bacteria. When it reacts with bacteria, triclosan

TABLE 19.9

Antibacterial Effects of Modified PVC at the Beginning and after 10 Days

Modified Conditions		Sample 1 (Treated with an Oxygen Plasma, Coated with Triclosan, and Then Treated with an Argon Plasma)		Sample 2 (Treated with an Oxygen Plasma, Coated with Bronopol, and Then Treated with an Argon Plasma)	
		0 day	10 days	0 day	10 days
Antibacterial effect	*S. aureus*	82.2	73.3	98.0	86.7
(modified/native)/%	*E. coli*	79.6	70.1	77.3	69.3

forms a stable ternary complex by interacting with amino acid residues of the enzyme active site. If the C—Cl bond is not destroyed during modification, it will still have antibacterial effects. However, when the molecule is fixed on PVC and its environment changes, its antibacterial effect degrades. From Table 19.9, the antibacterial performance of the sample coated with bronopol on *S. aureus* and *E. coli* is 98.0% and 77.3%, respectively, and the sample exhibits better antibacterial performance against *S. aureus* than against *E. coli*. The sample coated with triclosan has better antibacterial performance against *E. coli* than the sample coated with bronopol. Since plasma-treated surfaces tend to undergo changes with time, their antibacterial properties against *S. aureus* and *E. coli* degrade after 10 days.

19.7   SUMMARY

PIIID is a novel technique in biomedical engineering offering omnidirectional processing capability and the possibility to introduce a myriad of different species of different energies into the materials to tailor the surface properties. The surface microstructure, phase composition, and properties of many biomaterials, including metals, ceramics, and polymers, can be modified using PIIID. Excellent bioactivity can be introduced onto the surfaces of silicon and nano-TiO_2 coating using hydrogen PIII. This is because hydrogen PIII produces OH groups on the surface. The bioactivity of titanium can also be improved by Ca/Na PIIID. The PIII process can introduce energetic C, N, and O ions into the alloy surface so as to form a graded surface carbide, nitride, or oxide barrier layer. The stable Ti—C, Ti—N, and Ti—O bonds segregate the Ni, giving rise to a surface region depleted of nickel. Not only can Ni out-diffusion from the substrate be retarded by this method, but also the resulting mechanical properties are dramatically improved. Blood-compatible materials such as DLC and Ti–O thin film can be produced by PIIID. The characteristics of DLC films can be influenced by the flow rate, bias voltage, and annealing temperature during PIIID, and the blood compatibility of DLC films can be further improved by doping with elements such as Ca or P. Cu and antimicrobial reagents can be incorporated into the surface region of PE by means of PIII to promote the antimicrobial properties. Compared to the single Cu PIII process, a dual plasma implantation process (Cu/N_2 PIII) can better regulate the copper release rate and improve the long-term antibacterial properties of the PE samples. PIIID can also be used to conduct surface modification of medical polymers to yield superior surfaces with antibacterial properties.

ACKNOWLEDGMENTS

This work was jointly supported by Hong Kong Research Grants Council (RGC) Central Allocation Grant City U 1/04C, Hong Kong RGC Competitive Earmarked Research Grant (CERG) No. 112306, National Basic Research Fund under grant 2005CB623901, Shanghai Science and Technology R&D Fund under grant 07QH14016, and Foundation for the Author of National Excellent Doctoral Dissertation of PR China (FANEDD).

REFERENCES

1. Raizer, Y.P., Shneider, M.N., and Yatsenko, N.A., *Radio-Frequency Capacitive Discharges*, CRC Press, Boca Raton, FL, 1995.
2. Park, S.G. et al., Large area high density plasma source by helical resonator arrays, *Surf. Coating Tech.*, 133–134, 598, 2000.
3. Miyake, S. et al., Development of high-density RF plasma and application to PVD, *Surf. Coating Tech.*, 171, 131, 2000.
4. Lieberman, M.A. and Lichtenberg, A.J., *Principles of Plasma Discharges and Materials Processing*, Wiley, New York, 1994.
5. Ehlers, K.W. and. Leung, K.N., Some characteristics of tungsten filaments operated as cathodes in a gas discharge, *Rev. Sci. Instrum.*, 50, 356, 1979.
6. Brown, S.C., Basic data of plasma physics, the fundamental data on electrical discharges in gases, *Basic Data on Electrical Discharges in Gases*, American Institute of Physics, New York, 1993.
7. Lafferty, J.M., *Vacuum Arcs—Theory and Applications*, Wiley, New York, 1980.
8. Boxman, R.L., Sanders, D.M., and Martin, P.J., *Handbook of Vacuum Arc Science and Technology*, Noyes, Park Ridge, NJ, 1995.
9. Schulke, T., Anders, A., and Siemroth, P., Macroparticle filtering of high-current vacuum arc plasmas, *IEEE Trans. Plasma Sci.*, 25, 660, 1997.
10. Steinbruchel, C.H., Langmuir probe measurements on CHF_3 and CF_4 plasmas-the role of ions in the reactive sputter etching of SiO_2 and Si. *J. Electrochem. Soc.*, 130, 648, 1983.
11. Anders, A., *Handbook of Plasma Immersion Ion Implantation and Deposition*, John Wiley & Sons, Inc., Hoboken, NJ, 2, 2000.
12. Biersack, J.P. and Haggmark, L.G., A Monte Carlo computer program for the transport of energetic ions in amorphous targets, *Nucl. Instrum. Meth.*, 174, 257, 1980.
13. Rimini, E., *Ion Implantation: Basics to Device Fabrication*, Kluwer Academic, Boston, MA, 1995.
14. Mayer, J.W., Eriksson, L., and Davies, J.A., *Ion Implantation in Semiconductors*, Academic Press, New York, 1970.
15. Nastasi, M., Mayer, J.W., and Hirvonen, J.K., *Ion-Solid Interactions: Fundamentals and Applications*, Cambridge University Press, Cambridge, MA, 1996.
16. Adda, Y., Beyeler, M., and Brebec, G., Radiation effects on solid state diffusion, *Thin Solid Film*, 25, 107, 1975.
17. Borg, R.J. and Dienes, G.J., *An Introduction to Solid State Diffusion*, Academic Press, Boston, MA, 1988.
18. Thompson, M.W., *Defects and Radiation Damage in Metals*, Cambridge University Press, Cambridge, MA, 1969.
19. Auciello, O. and Kelly R., *Ion Bombardment Modification of Surfaces*, Elsevier, Amsterdam, 1984.
20. Andersen, H.H. and Bay, H.L., Sputtering yield measurements, in *Sputtering by Particle Bombardment I: Physical Sputtering of Single Element Solids, Topics Appl. Phys.* Behrisch, R., Ed., Vol. 47, Springer-Verlag, New York, 1981, 145.
21. Townsend, P.D., Kelly, J.C., and Hartley, N.E.W., *Ion Implantation, Sputtering and Their Applications*, Academic Press, New York, 1976.
22. Bunshah, R.F., *Handbook of Deposition Technologies for Films and Coatings: Science, Technology, and Applications*, Noyes Publications, Park Ridge, NJ, 1994.
23. Mattox, D.M., Particle bombardment effects on thin-film deposition: a review, *J. Vac. Sci. Tech. A*, 7, 1105, 1989.
24. Ensinger, W., Ion sources for ion beam assisted thin-film deposition, *Rev. Sci. Instrum.*, 63, 5217, 1992.
25. Ziegler, J.F., *Handbook of Ion Implantation Technology*, Elsevier Science Publishers, Amsterdam, North-Holland, 1992.
26. Smidt, F.A. and Sartwell, B.D., *Nucl. Instrum. Meth.*, B6, 70, 1985.
27. Grabowski, K.S. et al., Retention of ions implanted at non-normal incidence, in *Ion Implantation and Ion Beam Processing of Materials*, Hubler, G.K., Ed., Elsevier, New York, 1984, 615.
28. Chu, P.K. et al., Plasma immersion ion implantation—a fledgling technique for semiconductor processing, *Mat. Sci. Eng. R.*, R17, 207, 1996.
29. Min, J. et al., Buried oxide formation by plasma immersion ion implantation, *Mater. Chem. Phys.*, 40, 219, 1995.
30. Liu, J.B. et al., Formation of buried oxide in silicon using separation by plasma implantation of oxygen, *Appl. Phys. Lett.*, 67, 2361, 1995.

31. Lu, X., Plasma immersion ion implantation for SOI synthesis: SIMOX and ion-cut, *J. Electron. Mater.*, 27, 1059, 1998.

32. Zeng, Z.M. et al., Improvement of tribological properties of 9Cr18 bearing steel using metal and nitrogen plasma-immersion ion implantation, *Surf. Coating Tech.*, 115, 234, 1999.

33. Yu, C. and Cheung, N.W., Trench doping conformality by plasma immersion ion implantation (PIII), *IEEE Electron. Device. Lett.*, 15, 196,1994.

34. Bernstein, J.D. et al., Hydrogenation of polycrystalline silicon thin film transistors by plasma ion implantation, *IEEE Electron Device Lett.*, 16, 421, 1995.

35. Leng, Y.X., Properties of titanium oxide biomaterials synthesized by titanium plasma immersion ion implantation and reactive ion oxidation, *Thin Solid Films*, 377, 573, 2000.

36. Chu, P.K., Third-generation plasma immersion ion implanter for biomedical materials and research, *Rev. Sci. Instrum.*, 72, 1660, 2001.

37. Carlisle, E.M., Silicon as an essential trace element in animal nutrition, in *Silicon Biochemistry*, Evered, D. and O'Connor, M., Eds., John Wiley & Sons, New York, 1986, 123.

38. Hidebrand, M. et al., Silicon-responsive cDNA clones isolated from the marine diatom *Cylindrotheca fusiformis*, *Gene*, 132, 213, 1993.

39. Hench, L.L., Life and death: the ultimate phase transformation, *Thermochim. Acta*, 280/281, 1, 1996.

40. Xynos, D. et al., Bioglass (R) 45S5 stimulates osteoblast turnover and enhances bone formation *in vitro*: implications and applications for bone tissue engineering, *Calcif. Tissue Int.*, 67, 321, 2000.

41. Xynos, I.D. et al., Ionic products of bioactive glass dissolution increase proliferation of human osteoblasts and induce insulin-like growth factor II mRNA expression and protein synthesis, *Biochem. Biophys. Res. Comm.*, 276, 461, 2000.

42. Wise, K.D. and Najali, K., VLSI sensors in medicine, in *VLSI in Medicine*, Einspruch, N.G. and Gold, R.D., Eds., Academic Press, New York, 1989.

43. Madou, M. and Tierney, M.J., Required technology breakthroughs to assume widely accepted biosensors, *Appl. Biochem. Biotechnol.*, 41, 109, 1993.

44. Bowman, L. and Mendl, J.D., The packaging of implantable integrated sensors, *IEEE Trans. Biomed. Eng.*, 33, 248, 1986.

45. Canham, L.T., Bioactive silicon structure fabrication through nanoetching techniques, *Adv. Mater.*, 7, 1033, 1995.

46. Dahmen, C. et al., Surface functionalization of amorphous silicon and silicon suboxides for biological applications, *Thin Solid Films*, 427, 201, 2003.

47. Cho, S.B. et al., Dependence of apatite formation on silica gel on its structure: effect of heat treatment, *J. Am. Ceram. Soc.*, 78, 1769, 1995.

48. Fan, Z.N. et al., Surface hydrogen incorporation and profile broadening caused by sheath expansion in hydrogen plasma immersion ion implantation, *IEEE Trans. Plasma Sci.*, 28, 371, 2000.

49. Liu, X.Y. et al., Biomimetic growth of apatite on hydrogen-implanted silicon, *Biomaterials*, 25, 5575, 2004.

50. Pankove, J.I. and Johnson N.M., Hydrogen in semiconductors, *Semiconductors and Semimetals*, Academic Press, Boston, MA, 1991, 34.

51. Wang, L.W. et al., Damage in hydrogen plasma implanted silicon, *J. Appl. Phys.*, 90, 1735, 2001.

52. Tong, Q.Y. and Gösele, U.M., Wafer bonding and layer splitting for microsystems, *Adv. Mater.*, 11, 1409, 1999.

53. Li, P. and Zhang, F., The electrochemistry of glass surface and its application to bioactive glass in solution, *J. Non-Cryst. Solids*, 119, 112, 1990.

54. Li, P. et al., A role of hydrated silica, titania, and alumina in forming biologically active bone-like apatite on implant, *J. Biomed. Mater. Res.*, 28, 7, 1994.

55. Takadama, H. et al., Mechanism of biomineralization of apatite on a sodium silicate glass: TEM-EDX study *in vitro*, *Chem. Mater.*, 13, 1108, 2001.

56. Kurzweg, H. et al., Development of plasma-sprayed bioceramic coatings with bond coats based on titania and zirconia, *Biomaterials*, 19, 1507, 1998.

57. Nie, X. and Leyland, A., Deposition of layered bioceramic hydroxyapatite/TiO_2 coatings on titanium alloys using a hybrid technique of micro-arc oxidation and electrophoresis, *Surf. Coating Tech.*, 125, 407, 2000.

58. Ratner, B.D., A perspective on titanium biocompatibility, in *Titanium in Medicine*, Brunette, D.M. et al., Eds., Springer, Berlin, 2001, 1.

59. Webster, T.J., Siegel, R.W., and Bizios, R., Osteoblast adhesion on nanophase ceramics, *Biomaterials*, 20, 1221, 1999.

60. Webster, T.J. et al., Enhanced functions of osteoblasts on nanophase ceramics, *Biomaterials*, 21, 1803, 2000.
61. Webster, T.J. et al., Enhanced osteoclast-like cell functions on nanophase ceramics, *Biomaterials*, 22, 1327, 2001.
62. Chu, P.K. et al., Plasma surface modification of biomaterials, *Mater. Sci. Eng. R Rep.*, 36, 143, 2002.
63. Chu, P.K., Recent developments and applications of plasma immersion ion implantation (PIII), *J. Vac. Sci. Tech. B.*, 22, 289, 2004.
64. Liu, X.Y. et al., Plasma-treated nanostructured TiO_2 surface supporting biomimetic growth of apatite, *Biomaterials*, 26, 6143, 2005.
65. Li, P. et al., The role of hydrated silica, titania, and alumina in inducing apatite on implants, *J. Biomed. Mater. Res.*, 28, 7, 1994.
66. Pan, J.M. et al., Interaction of water, oxygen and hydrogen with TiO_2 (110) surfaces having different defect densities, *J. Vac. Sci. Tech. A*, 10, 2470, 1992.
67. Leconte, J. et al., Periodic ab initio study of the hydrogenated rutile TiO_2 (110) surface, *Surf. Sci.*, 497, 194, 2002.
68. Svetina, M. et al., Deposition of calcium ions on rutile (110): a first-principles investigation, *Acta Mater.*, 49, 2169, 2001.
69. Zhang, H. et al., Enhanced adsorption of molecules on surfaces of nanocrystalline particles, *J. Phys. Chem. B*, 103, 4656, 1999.
70. Long, M. and Rack H.J., Titanium alloys in total joint replacement—a materials science perspective, *Biomaterials*, 19, 1621, 1998.
71. Sioshansi, P. and Tobin, E.J., Surface treatment of biomaterials by ion beam processes, *Surf. Coating Tech.*, 83, 175, 1996.
72. Li, P. et al., The role of hydrated silica, titania and alumina in inducing apatite on implants, *J. Biomed. Mater. Res.*, 28, 7, 1994.
73. Pham, M.T. et al., Promoted hydroxyapatite nucleation on titanium ion implanted with sodium, *Thin Solid Films*, 379, 50, 2000.
74. Rzeszutek, K. et al., in 5th Asian Symposium, *Biomed. Mater.*, Hong Kong, 169, 2001.
75. Kokubo, T. et al., *In vivo* apatite formation induced on titanium metal and its alloys by chemical treatment, *Key Eng. Mater.*, 192–195, 3, 2001.
76. Kim, H.M. et al., Preparation of bioactive Ti and its alloys via simple chemical surface treatment, *J. Biomed. Mater. Res.*, 32, 409, 1996.
77. Pham, M.T. et al, Surface stimuli to precipitating hydroxyapatite on titanium, *J. Mater. Sci. Lett.*, 20, 295, 2001.
78. Hanawa, T. et al., Early bone formation around calcium-ion-implanted titanium inserted into rat tibia, *J. Biomed. Mater. Res.*, 36, 131, 1997.
79. Kwok, S.C.H., Wang, J., and Chu, P.K., Surface energy, wettability, and blood compatibility of phosphorus doped diamond-like carbon films. *Diam. Relat. Mater.*, 14, 78, 2005.
80. Li, L.H. et al., Hybrid evaporation-glow discharge source for plasma immersion ion implantation, *Rev. Sci. Instrum.*, 74, 4301, 2003.
81. Tian, X.B. et al., Flexible system for multiple plasma immersion ion implantation—deposition processes, *Rev. Sci. Instrum.*, 74, 5137, 2003.
82. Liu, X.Y. et al., Structure and properties of Ca plasma implanted titanium, *Surf. Coating Tech.*, 191, 43, 2005.
83. Hanawa, T., *In vivo* metallic biomaterials and surface modification, *Mater. Sci. Eng. A*, 267, 260, 1999.
84. Maitz, M.F. et al., Bioactivity of titanium following sodium plasma immersion ion implantation and deposition, *Biomaterials*, 26, 5465, 2005.
85. Ryhanen, J., *Biocompatibility Evaluation of NiTi Shape Memory Alloy*, University of Oulu, Finland, 1999.
86. Chen, M.F. et al., Bioactive NiTi shape memory alloy used as bone bonding implants, *Mater. Sci. Eng. C*, 24, 497, 2004.
87. Cragg, A.H. et al., Nitinol intravascular stent: results of preclinical evaluation, *Radiology*, 189, 775, 1993.
88. Dai, K. and Chu, Y., Studies and applications of NiTi shape memory alloys in the medical field in China, *Biomed. Mater. Eng.*, 6, 233, 1996.
89. Es-Souni, M. and Brandies, H.F., On the transformation behaviour, mechanical properties and biocompatibility of two NiTi-based shape memory alloys: NiTi42 and NiTi42Cu7, *Biomaterials*, 22, 2153, 2001.
90. Gil, F.X., Planell, J.A., and Manero, J.M., Relevant aspects in the clinical applications of NiTi shape memory alloys, *J. Mater. Sci. Mat. M.*, 7, 403, 1996.

91. Kong, X. et al., Effect of biologically active coating on biocompatibility of nitinol devices designed for the closure of intra-atrial communications, *Biomaterials*, 23, 1775, 2002.

92. Kujala, S. et al., Effect of porosity on the osteointegration and bone ingrowth of a weight-bearing nickel-titanium bone graft substitute, *Biomaterials*, 24, 4691, 2003.

93. Kujala, S. et al., Bone modeling controlled by a nickel-titanium shape memory alloy intramedullary nail, *Biomaterials*, 23, 2535, 2002.

94. Yang, P.J., Zhang, Y.F., and Ge, M.Z., Internal fixation with NiTi shape memory alloy compressive staples in orthopedic surgery, *Chinese Med. J.*, 100, 712, 1987.

95. Ryhanen, J. et al., Bone healing and mineralization, implant corrosion, and trace metals after nickel-titanium shape memory metal intramedullary fixation, *J. Biomed. Mater. Res.*, 47, 472, 1999.

96. Miyazaki, S., Medical and dental application of shape memory alloys, in *Shape Memory Materials*, Otsuka, K. and Wayman, C.M., Eds., Cambridge University Press, Cambridge, MA, 1998, 267.

97. Sanders, J.O. et al., A preliminary investigation of shape memory alloys in the surgical correction of scoliosis, *Spine*, 18, 1640, 1993.

98. Schmerling, M.A. et al., Using the shape recovery of nitinol in the Harrington rod treatment of scoliosis, *J. Biomed. Mater. Res.*, 10, 879, 1976.

99. Bogdanski, D. et al., Easy assessment of the biocompatibility of Ni-Ti alloys by *in vitro* cell culture experiments on a functionally graded Ni-NiTi-Ti material, *Biomaterials*, 23, 4549, 2002.

100. El Medawar, L. et al., Electrochemical and cytocompatibility assessment of NiTiNOL memory shape alloy for orthodontic use, *Biomol. Eng.*, 19, 153, 2002.

101. Putters, J. et al., Comparative cell culture effects of shape memory metal (nitinol), nickel and titanium: a biocompatibility estimation, *Eur. Surg. Res.*, 24, 378, 1992.

102. Kapanen, A. et al., Behaviour of nitinol in osteoblast-like ROS-17 cell cultures, *Biomaterials*, 23, 645, 2002.

103. Kapanen, A. et al., TGF-[beta]1 secretion of ROS-17/2.8 cultures on NiTi implant material, *Biomaterials*, 23, 3341, 2002.

104. Kapanen, A. et al., Effect of nickel-titanium shape memory metal alloy on bone formation, *Biomaterials*, 22, 2475, 2001.

105. Kujala, S. et al., Biocompatibility and strength properties of nitinol shape memory alloy suture in rabbit tendon, *Biomaterials*, 25, 353, 2004.

106. Rocher, P. et al., Biocorrosion and cytocompatibility assessment of NiTi shape memory alloys, *Scripta Mater.*, 50, 255, 2004.

107. Ryhanen, J. et al., *In vivo* biocompatibility evaluation of nickel-titanium shape memory metal alloy: muscle and perineural tissue responses and encapsule membrane thickness, *J. Biomed. Mater. Res.*, 41, 481, 1998.

108. Ryhanen, J. et al., Biocompatibility of nickel-titanium shape memory metal and its corrosion behavior in human cell cultures, *J. Biomed. Mater. Res.*, 35, 451, 1997.

109. Wever, D.J. et al., Cytotoxic, allergic and genotoxic activity of a nickel-titanium alloy, *Biomaterials*, 18, 1115, 1997.

110. Berger-Gorbet, M. et al., Biocompatibility testing of NiTi screws using immunohistochemistry on sections containing metallic implants, *J. Biomed. Mater. Res.*, 32, 243, 1996.

111. Jia, W. et al., Nickel release from orthodontic arch wires and cellular immune response to various nickel concentrations, *J. Biomed. Mater. Res.*, 48, 488, 1999.

112. Es-Souni, M. and Fischer-Brandies, H., On the properties of two binary NiTi shape memory alloys. Effects of surface finish on the corrosion behaviour and *in vitro* biocompatibility, *Biomaterials*, 23, 2887, 2002.

113. Shih, C.C. et al., The cytotoxicity of corrosion products of nitinol stent wire on cultured smooth muscle cells, *J. Biomed. Mater. Res.*, 52, 395, 2000.

114. Dalmau, L.B., Alberty, H.C., and Parra, J.S., A study of nickel allergy, *J. Prosthet. Dent.*, 52, 116, 1984.

115. Lamster, I.B. et al., Rapid loss of alveolar bone associated with nonprecious alloy crowns in two patients with nickel hypersensitivity, *J. Periodontol.*, 58, 486, 1987.

116. Espana, A. et al., Chronic urticaria after implantation of 2 nickel-containing dental prostheses in a nickel-allergic patient, *Contact Dermatitis*, 21, 204, 1989.

117. Sanford, W.E. and Niboer, E., Renal toxicity of nickel in humans, in *Nickel and Human Health Current Perspectives*, Nriagu, J.O., Ed., John Wiley & Sons, Inc., Canada, 1992, 123.

118. Mitura, E. et al., The properties of carbon layers deposited onto titanium substrates, *Diam. Relat. Mater.*, 5, 998, 1996.

119. Wu, S.K., Lee, C.Y., and Lin, H.C., A study of vacuum carburization of an equiatomic TiNi shape memory alloy, *Scripta Mater.*, 37, 837, 1997.

120. Huber, P. et al., Formation of TiN, TiC and TiCN by metal plasma immersion ion implantation and deposition, *Surf. Coating Tech.*, 174, 1243, 2003.

121. Liu, N. et al., Effect of nano-micro TiN addition on the microstructure and mechanical properties of TiC based cermets, *J. Eur. Ceram. Soc.*, 22, 2409, 2002.

122. Oliveira, M.M. and Bolton, J.D., High-speed steels: increasing wear resistance by adding ceramic particles, *J. Mater. Process. Tech.*, 92–93, 15, 1999.

123. Vaz, F. et al., Structural, optical and mechanical properties of coloured TiN_xO_y thin films, *Thin Solid Films*, 447–448, 449, 2004.

124. Kola, P.V. et al., Magnetron sputtering of tin protective coatings for medical applications, *J. Mater. Process. Tech.*, 56, 422, 1996.

125. Tan, L. and Crone, W.C., Surface characterization of NiTi modified by plasma source ion implantation, *Acta Mater.*, 50, 4449, 2002.

126. Mändl, S. et al., Investigation on plasma immersion ion implantation treated medical implants, *Biomol. Eng.*, 19, 129, 2002.

127. Nie, X., Leyland, A., and Matthews, A., Deposition of layered bioceramic hydroxyapatite/TiO_2 coatings on titanium alloys using a hybrid technique of micro-arc oxidation and electrophoresis, *Surf. Coating Tech.*, 125, 407, 2000.

128. Lackner, J.M. et al., Pulsed laser deposition of titanium oxide coatings at room temperature-structural, mechanical and tribological properties, *Surf. Coating Tech.*, 180–181, 585, 2004.

129. Li, M.C. et al., Corrosion behavior of TiN coated type 316 stainless steel in simulated PEMFC environments, *Corros. Sci.*, 46, 1369, 2004.

130. Wan, G.J. et al., TiN and Ti–O/TiN films fabricated by PIII-D for enhancement of corrosion and wear resistance of Ti—6Al—4V, *Surf. Coating Tech.*, 186, 136, 2004.

131. Pfohl, C. et al., Evaluation of the corrosion behaviour of wear-resistant PACVD coatings, *Surf. Coating Tech.*, 112, 114, 1999.

132. Maiya, P.S., Erck, R.A., and Moon, B.M., Failure and corrosion resistance of TiN and TiC coatings deposited on graphite by chemical vapor deposition, *Surf. Coating Tech.*, 102, 218, 1998.

133. Leng, Y.X. et al., Structure and properties of biomedical TiO_2 films synthesized by dual plasma deposition, *Surf. Coating Tech.*, 156, 295, 2002.

134. Liu, J.X. et al., Sol-gel deposited TiO_2 film on NiTi surgical alloy for biocompatibility improvement, *Thin Solid Films*, 429, 225, 2003.

135. Yeung, K.W.K. et al., Study of corrosion resistance, surface mechanical properties and cyto-compatibility of plasma immersion ion implantation treated NiTi shape memory alloys, *J. Biomed. Mater. Res.*, 75A, 256, 2005.

136. Yeung, K.W.K. et al., Investigation of nickel suppression and cyto-compatibility of surface treated NiTi shape memory alloy by using plasma immersion ion implantation, *J. Biomed. Mater. Res.*, 72A, 238, 2005.

137. Tian, X. et al., Oxygen-induced nickel segregation in nitrogen plasma implanted AISI 304 stainless steel, *Mater. Sci. Eng. A*, 316, 200, 2001.

138. Yokota, K. et al., Compositional structure of dual TiNO layers deposited on SUS 304 by an IBAD technique, *Surf. Coating Tech.*, 158–159, 568, 2002.

139. Huang, J.Y. et al., Microstructure investigations on explosive TiNi (or Ni)/TiC-composite-formation reaction during mechanical alloying, *Acta Mater.*, 44, 1781, 1996.

140. Badzian, A. and Badzian, T., Growth of diamond and nickel carbide crystals in the Ni—C—H system, *Diam. Relat. Mater.*, 5, 93, 1996.

141. Shi, W., Li, X.Y., and Dong, H., Improved wear resistance of ultra-high molecular weight polyethylene by plasma immersion ion implantation, *Wear*, 250, 544, 2001.

142. Girardeau, T. et al., Wear improvement and local structure in nickel-titanium coatings produced by reactive ion sputtering, *Thin Solid Films*, 283, 67, 1996.

143. Triantafyllidis, D., Li, L., and Stott, F.H., Surface properties of laser-treated ceramic materials, *Thin Solid Films*, 453–454, 76, 2004.

144. Piscanec, S. et al., Bioactivity of TiN-coated titanium implants, *Acta Mater.*, 52, 1237, 2004.

145. Hauert, R., A review of modified DLC coatings for biological applications, *Diam. Relat. Mater.*, 12, 583–589, 2003.

146. Grill, A., Diamond-like carbon coatings as biocompatible materials—an overview, *Diam. Relat. Mater.*, 12, 166, 2003.

147. Cui, F.Z. and Li, D.J., A review of investigations on biocompatibility of diamond-like carbon and carbon nitride films, *Surf. Coating Tech.*, 131, 481, 2000.
148. Allen, M., Myer, B., and Rushton, N., *In vitro* and *in vivo* investigations into the biocompatibility of diamond-like carbon (DLC) coatings for orthopedic applications, *J. Biomed. Mater. Res.*, 58, 319, 2001.
149. Dowling, D.P. et al., Evaluation of diamond-like carbon-coated orthopaedic implants, *Diam. Relat. Mater.*, 6, 390, 1997.
150. Ianno, N.J. et al., Deposition of diamond-like carbon on a titanium biomedical alloy, *Thin Solid Films*, 270, 275, 1995.
151. McLaughlin, J. et al., Properties of diamond like carbon thin film coatings on stainless steel medical guidewires, *Diam. Relat. Mater.*, 5, 486, 1996.
152. Chen, J.Y. et al., Blood compatibility and sp^3/sp^2 contents of diamond-like carbon (DLC) synthesized by plasma immersion ion implantation-deposition, *Surf. Coating Tech.*, 156, 289, 2002.
153. Robertson, J. and Reilly, E.P.O., Electronic and atomic structure of amorphous carbon, *Phys. Rev. B*, 35, 2946, 1987.
154. Lopinski, G.P., Semimetal to semiconductor transition in carbon nanoparticles, *Phys. Rev. Lett.*, 80, 4241, 1998.
155. Schwan, J. et al., Raman spectroscopy on amorphous carbon films, *J. Appl. Phys.*, 80, 440, 1994.
156. Beeman, D. et al., Modeling studies of amorphous carbon, *Phys. Rev. B*, 30, 870, 1984.
157. Valentini, L. et al., Ar-dilution effects on the elastic and structural properties of hydrogenated hard carbon films deposited by plasma-enhanced chemical vapor deposition, *Diam. Relat. Mater.*, 10, 1042, 2001.
158. Lai, K.H. et al., Mechanical properties of DLC films prepared in acetylene and methane plasmas using electron cyclotron resonance microwave plasma chemical vapor deposition, *Diam. Relat. Mater.*, 10, 1862, 2001.
159. Yang, P. et al., Activation of platelets adhered on amorphous hydrogenated carbon (a-C:H) films synthesized by plasma immersion ion implantation-deposition (PIII-D), *Biomaterials*, 24, 2821, 2003.
160. Pinzari, F. et al., Wettability of HF-CVD diamond films, *Diam. Relat. Mater.*, 10, 781, 2000.
161. Tang, Z. et al., Effect of mass-selected ion species on structure and properties of diamond-like carbon films, *J. Appl. Phys.*, 89, 1959, 2001.
162. Ogwu, A.A. et al., Characterisation of thermally annealed diamond like carbon (DLC) and silicon modified DLC films by Raman spectroscopy, *Physica B*, 269, 335, 1999.
163. Yang, P. et al., Structure and properties of annealed amorphous hydrogenated carbon (a-C:H) films for biomedical applications, *Surf. Coating Tech.*, 177–178, 747, 2004.
164. Robertson, J., Diamond-like amorphous carbon, *Mater. Sci. Eng. R Rep.*, 37, 129, 2002.
165. Feng, L. and Andrade, D.J., Protein adsorption on low-temperature isotropic carbon: II. Effects of surface charge of solids, *J. Colloid Interf. Sci.*, 166, 419, 1994.
166. Huang, N. et al., Blood compatibility of amorphous titanium oxide films synthesized by ion beam enhanced deposition, *Biomaterials*, 19, 771, 1998.
167. Kwok, S.C.H. et al., Surface energy, wettability, and blood compatibility phosphorus doped diamond-like carbon films, *Diam. Relat. Mater.*, 14, 78, 2005.
168. Ruckensten, E. and Gourisankar, S.V., A surface energetic criterion of blood compatibility of foreign surfaces, *J. Colloid Interf. Sci.*, 101, 436, 1984.
169. Kwok, S.C.H. et al., Biocompatibility of calcium and phosphorus doped diamond-like carbon thin films synthesized by plasma immersion ion implantation and deposition, *Diam. Relat. Mater.*, 15, 893, 2006.
170. Huang, N. et al., *In vitro* investigation of blood compatibility of Ti with oxide layers of rutile structure, *J. Biomater. Appl.*, 8, 404, 1994.
171. Pouilleau, J. et al., Structure and composition of passive titanium oxide films, *Mater. Sci. Eng. B*, 47, 235, 1997.
172. Amor, S.B. et al., Structural and optical properties of sputtered titania films, *Mat. Sci. Eng. B*, 47, 110, 1997.
173. Martin, N. et al., Characterizations of titanium oxide films prepared by radio frequency magnetron sputtering, *Thin Solid Films*, 287, 154, 1996.
174. Treichel, O. and Kirchhoff, V., The influence of pulsed magnetron sputtering on topography and crystallinity of TiO_2 films on glass, *Surf. Coating Tech.*, 123, 268, 2000.
175. Martin, N. et al., The effect of bias power on some properties of titanium and titanium oxide films prepared by R.F. magnetron sputtering, *Surf. Coating Tech.*, 107, 172, 1998.

176. Bendavid, A., Martin, P.J., and Takikawa, H., Deposition and modification of titanium dioxide thin films by filtered arc deposition, *Thin Solid Films*, 360, 2000, 241.
177. Takikawa, H. et al., Properties of titanium oxide film prepared by reactive cathodic vacuum arc deposition, *Thin Solid Films*, 348, 145, 1999.
178. Mändl, S. et al., Influence of ion energy on titanium oxide formation by vacuum arc deposition and implantation, *Nucl. Instrum. Meth. Phys. Res. B*, 178, 148, 2001.
179. Yang, P. et al., *In vivo* study of Ti—O thin film fabricated by PIII, *Surf. Coating Tech.*, 156, 284, 2002.
180. Leng, Y.X. et al., Fabrication of Ti—O/Ti—N duplex coatings on biomedical titanium alloys by metal plasma immersion ion implantation and reactive plasma nitriding/oxidation, *Surf. Coating Tech.*, 138, 296, 2001.
181. Leng, Y.X. et al., Biomedical properties of tantalum nitride films synthesized by reactive magnetron sputtering, *Thin Solid Films*, 398–399, 471, 2001.
182. Chen, J.Y. et al, The Second International Conference on Inorganic Materials, Santa Barbara, California, USA, P-99, Sept. 13–16, 2000.
183. Huang, N. et al., Investigation of blood compatibility of titanium oxide film doped with tantalum by sputtering deposition, in *Proceeding and Fabrication of Advanced Materials VIII*, Khor, K.A. et al., Eds., World Scientific Publishing Co. Pt. Ltd, Singapore, 2000, 341.
184. Chen, J.Y. et al., Antithrombogenic investigation of surface energy and optical bandgap and hemocompatibility mechanism of Ti(Ta^{+5})O$_2$ thin films, *Biomaterials*, 23, 2545, 2002.
185. Ramakrishna, S. et al., Biomedical applications of polymer-composite materials: a review, *Compos. Sci. Technol.*, 61, 1189, 2001.
186. Brocchini, S., Combinatorial chemistry and biomedical polymer development, *Adv. Drug. Deliver. Rev.*, 53, 123, 2001.
187. Rudnik, E., Resiak, I., and Wojciechowski, C., Thermoanalytical investigations of polyurethanes for medical purposes, *Thermochim. Acta.*, 320, 285, 1998.
188. An, Y.H. and Friedman, R.J., Concise review of mechanisms of bacterial adhesion to biomaterial surfaces, *J. Biomed. Mater. Res. A*, 43, 38, 1998.
189. Potera, C., Biofilms invade microbiology, *Science*, 273, 552, 1996.
190. Costerton, J.W., Stewart, P.S., and Greenberg, E.P., Bacterial biofilms: a common cause of persistent infections, *Science*, 284, 1318, 1999.
191. Nichols, R.L. and Raad, I.I., Management of bacterial complications in critically ill patients: surgical wound and catheter-related infections, *Diagn. Micr. Infec. Dis.*, 33, 121, 1999.
192. Favia, P. et al., Immobilization of heparin and highly-sulphated hyaluronic acid onto plasma-treated polyethylene, *Plasma process Polym.*, 3, 77, 1998.
193. Woo, G.L.Y., Mittelman, M.W., and Santerre, J.P., Synthesis and characterization of a novel biodegradable antimicrobial polymer, *Biomaterials*, 21, 1235, 2001.
194. Balazs, D.J. et al., Inhibition of bacterial adhesion on PVC endotracheal tubes by RF-oxygen glow discharge, sodium hydroxide and silver nitrate treatments, *Biomaterials*, 25, 2139, 2004.
195. Wang, J. et al., Bacterial repellence from polyethylene terephthalate surface modified by acetylene plasma immersion ion implantation–deposition, *Surf. Coating Tech.*, 186, 299, 2004.
196. Schierholz, J.M. and Pulverer, G., Investigation of a rifampin, fusidic-acid and mupirocin releasing silicone catheter, *Biomaterials*, 19, 2065, 1998.
197. Zhang, W. et al., Antimicrobial properties of copper plasma-modified polyethylene, *Polymer*, 47, 7441, 2006.
198. Fu, R.K.Y. et al., Surface composition and surface energy of teflon treated by metal plasma immersion ion implantation, *Surf. Sci.*, 573, 426, 2004.
199. Zhang, W. et al., Plasma surface modification of poly vinyl chloride for improvement of antibacterial properties, *Biomaterials*, 27, 44, 2006.
200. Zhang, W. et al., Effects of O$_2$ and H$_2$O plasma immersion ion implantation on surface chemical composition and surface energy of poly vinyl chloride, *Appl. Surf. Sci.*, 252, 7884, 2006.
201. Kostov, K.G. et al., Structural effect of nitrogen plasma-based ion implantation on ultra-high molecular weight polyethylene, *Surf. Coating Tech.*, 186, 287, 2004.
202. Boldyryeva, H. et al., High-fluence implantation of negative metal ions into polymers for surface modification and nanoparticle formation, *Surf. Coating Tech.*, 196, 373, 2005.
203. Cloete, T.E., Resistance mechanisms of bacteria to antimicrobial compounds, *Int. Biodeter. Biodegr.*, 51, 277, 2003.

204. Zhang, W., Zhang, Y.H., Ji, J.H., Yan, Q., Huang, A.P., and Chu, P.K, Antimicrobial polyethylene with controlled copper release, *J. Biomed. Mater. Res.: Part A* (in press). DOI.10.1002.
205. Poon, R.W.Y. et al., Formation of titanium nitride barrier layer in nickel–titanium shape memory alloys by nitrogen plasma immersion ion implantation for better corrosion resistance, *Thin Solid Films*, 488, 20, 2005.
206. Seth, R. et al., *In vitro* assessment of copper-induced toxicity in the human hepatoma line hep G2, *Toxicol. In Vitro*, 18, 501, 2004.
207. Ho, C.H. et al., Nanoseparated polymeric networks with multiple antimicrobial properties, *Adv. Mater.*, 16, 957, 2004.
208. Liu, Q. and Kee, D.D., Modeling of diffusion through nanocomposite membranes, *J. Non-Newton Fluid*, 131, 32, 2005.
209. Chen, K.S. et al., Immobilization of chitosan gel with cross-linking reagent on PNIPAAm gel/PP nonwoven composites surface, *Mat. Sci. Eng. C*, 26, 1, 2005.
210. Kalyon, B.D. and Olgun, U., Antibacterial efficacy of triclosan-incorporated polymers, *Am. J. Infect. Control*, 29, 124, 2001.
211. Speranza, G. et al., Role of chemical interactions in bacterial adhesion to polymer surfaces, *Biomaterials*, 25, 2029, 2004.
212. Mao, C., Qiu, Y.Z., and Sang, H.B., Various approaches to modify biomaterial surfaces for improving hemocompatibility, *Adv. Colloid Interf. Sci.*, 10, 5–17, 2004.
213. Yuan, Y.L., Ai, F., and Zang, X.P., Polyurethane vascular catheter surface grafted with zwitterionicsulfobetaine monomer activated by ozone, *Colloids Surf. B*, 35, 1–5, 2004.
214. Yang, M.R., Chen, K.S., and Tsai, J.C., The antibacterial activities of hydrophilic-modified nonwoven PET, *Mat. Sci. Eng. C*, 20, 167, 2002.
215. Kwok, C.S., Horbett, T.A., and Ratner, B.D., Design of infection-resistant antibiotic-releasing polymers II controlled release of antibiotics through a plasma-deposited thin film barrier, *J. Control. Release*, 62, 301, 1999.
216. Favia, P., Plasma treatment and plasma deposition of polymer for biomedical application, *Surf. Coating Tech.*, 98, 1102, 1998.
217. Balazs, D.J. et al., Inhibition of bacterial adhesion on PVC endotracheal tubes by RF-oxygen glow discharge, sodium hydroxide and silver nitrate treatments, *Biomaterials*, 25, 2139, 2004.
218. Kennedy, J.F., and Thorley, M., Polymers for the medical industry, *Carbohyd. Polym.*, 44, 175, 2001.
219. Akovali, G. et al., Mechanical properties and surface energies of low density polyethylene-poly (vinyl chloride) blends, *Polymer*, 39, 1363, 1998.
220. Gustin, B. and Wourm, P., Mechanical characterization of PVC dedicated to medical use, *RBM-News*, 18, 78, 1996.
221. Schweizer, H.P., Triclosan: a widely used biocide and its link to antibiotics, *FEMS Microbiol. Lett.*, 202, 1–7, 2001.
222. Braoudaki, M. and Hilton, A.C., Mechanisms of resistance in *Salmonella enterica* adapted to erythromycin, benzalkonium chloride and triclosan, *Int. J. Antimicrob. Ag.*, 25, 31, 2005.
223. Lian, H.Z. et al., A study on the stability of bronopol in bronopol lotion by ion-paired reversed-phase high performance liquid chromatography, *J. Pharm. Biomed. Anal.*, 5, 667, 1997.
224. Wang, J. et al., The effects of amorphous carbon films deposited on polyethylene terephthalate on bacterial adhesion, *Biomaterials*, 25, 3163, 2004.
225. Guruvenket, S. et al., Concise review of mechanism of bacteria adhesion to biomaterial surfaces, *Appl. Surf. Sci.*, 236, 278, 2004.
226. Triandafillu, K. et al., Adhesion of *Pseudomonas aeruginosa* strains to untreated and oxygen-plasma treated poly (vinyl chloride) (PVC) from endotracheal intubation devices, *Biomaterials*, 24, 1507, 2003.
227. Park, Y.W. and Inagaki, N., Surface modification of poly (vinylidene fluoride) film by remote Ar, H_2, and O_2 plasmas, *Polymer*, 44, 1569, 2003.

20 Biomaterials for Gastrointestinal Medicine, Repair, and Reconstruction

Richard M. Day

CONTENTS

20.1 INTRODUCTION

Biomaterials have been used for many years in the treatment of gastrointestinal conditions. Their applications range from biodegradable sutures and meshes to assist in the healing of laparotomy procedures, to the use of alginate-based raft-forming formulations, for the symptomatic treatment of heartburn and esophagitis. In addition to the continued use and development of traditional therapies, there is a growing interest in the design and fabrication of new biomaterials for a variety of other therapeutic applications associated with the gastrointestinal tract, such as nanotechnology-based drug delivery systems and tissue engineering. Before new therapies involving biomaterials can be successfully implemented, consideration needs to be given to the complexity of the gastrointestinal tract and the effect of this complexity on the delivery, longevity, and efficacy of the biomaterial.

The gastrointestinal tract in humans (also called the alimentary canal or gut) is a complex system of organs that carries out vital functions to maintain health. Its primary purpose is to extract energy, nutrients, and water from ingested food, which is achieved through a process called digestion before the remaining waste is expelled. In healthy adult humans, the gastrointestinal tract is approximately 7.5–9 m in length, extending from the mouth down to the anus. The gastrointestinal tract has various specialized regions within it that aid the different stages of the digestion process and help to maintain homeostasis. The upper gastrointestinal tract consists of the mouth, pharynx, esophagus, and stomach. The lower gastrointestinal tract consists of the small intestine (which is subcategorized into duodenum, jejunum, and ileum), the large intestine (which is subcategorized into cecum, colon, and rectum), and the anus. In addition to these regions, there are a number of related organs whose functions are integrated with those of the gastrointestinal tract. These organs include the liver, which secretes bile into the small intestine, and the pancreas, which secretes enzymes into the small intestine. Thus, both organs assist in the process of digestion. The wall of the gastrointestinal tract is made up of four concentric layers of tissue. The mucosa is the innermost layer facing the lumen of the gastrointestinal tract and is composed of the epithelium, lamina propria, and muscularis propria. Villi extending from the mucosal surface significantly increase the absorptive surface area of the intestine. The mucosa carries out highly specialized functions for each organ of the gastrointestinal tract, including the processes of absorption and secretion associated with digestion. It also maintains a barrier function against potentially harmful microorganisms that colonize the gut. The submucosa is composed of connective tissue and contains blood vessels, lymphatics, and nerves that extend into the mucosa and musclaris layers. The muscularis externa controls peristalsis and is composed of a circular inner muscle layer that contracts and prevents backwash of food in the lumen and a longitudinal outer muscle layer that contracts and shortens the tract. The outermost layer of the gastrointestinal tract is called the adventitia (or serosa) and is composed of several layers of connective tissue.

In addition to assisting nutrient absorption, the gastrointestinal tract is also a prominent part of the immune system, harboring abundant lymphoid tissues and immune cells. This system is particularly important since the gastrointestinal tract also plays host to a population of microflora, consisting predominantly of bacteria, whose density increases from the upper (almost sterile in the stomach) to the lower part (10^{12} bacteria per gram of colonic content) of the tract [1]. In healthy individuals, the immune system is programmed to distinguish resident commensal ("good") bacteria that colonize and coexist with the gut from harmful pathogenic bacteria that can cause illness. The immune system provides just one example of the potential problems faced when developing new devices for the gastrointestinal tract. Biomaterials need to avoid eliciting an immune response or become affected by other innate components associated with the gastrointestinal immune system, such as mucus and low pH (1–4) of the stomach, which might also interfere with biomaterials passing through the tract.

The recognition of biocompatibility as a fundamental requirement for the success of a biomaterial has led to the development of a variety of synthetic and modified natural polymers that offer not only optimal performance but also low toxicity and an ideal tissue response. In addition to considering the long-term biocompatibility of these materials, novel fabrication processes are frequently required that would provide a sufficient quantity of the biomaterial in a format that can be delivered to the site of delivery, which may not be easily accessible for the gastrointestinal tract.

This chapter discusses some of the old and new biomaterials that have been developed for use in therapeutic strategies to treat disorders associated with the gastrointestinal tract and describes the fabrication methods involved in their production.

20.2 BIOMATERIALS USED FOR GASTROESOPHAGEAL REFLUX DISEASE

20.2.1 Gastroesophageal Reflux Disease

Gastroesophageal reflux disease (GERD) is one of the most common disorders of the upper gastrointestinal tract, with epidemiological studies suggesting that almost 10% of adults in the United States experience heartburn daily. It is a chronic relapsing disease with 20–25% of patients receiving lifelong medical treatment [2,3]. GERD is most frequently caused by transient or permanent loss of the barrier function of the lower esophageal sphincter (also termed cardiac sphincter and gastroesophageal sphincter). Moderate to severe cases of GERD that are nonresponsive to medical therapy usually require antireflux surgery. To date, the mainstay of GERD antireflux therapy has been achieved with either open or laparoscopic fundoplication, a surgical procedure in which the upper part of the stomach is wrapped around the lower part of the esophagus. Due to the morbidity associated with general anesthesia, bleeding, organ injury, or infection, a move toward the development of minimally invasive endolumenal procedures for GERD has led to studies investigating the use of both biodegradable and nonbiodegradable materials delivered by endoscopic transoral approach.

20.2.2 Sphincter Augmentation Using Biomaterials

Several endolumenal procedures have been introduced into clinical practice, one of which is lower esophageal sphincter augmentation via endoscopic implantation of biomaterials. Early studies investigated the benefit of injecting bovine dermal collagen into the lower esophagus to bulk the submucosal tissue and augment the lower esophageal sphincter pressure, but the beneficial results were short-lived due to reabsorption of the collagen [4].

20.2.2.1 Ethylene Vinyl Alcohol Copolymer

Better clinical success has been reported with the biocompatible nonresorbable copolymer Enteryx (Boston Scientific Corp, Matick, Massachusetts), which is injected as a nonviscous liquid that rapidly forms a spongy solid *in situ*. Enteryx consists of an injectable solution of 8% ethylene vinyl alcohol copolymer dissolved in dimethyl sulfoxide. Ethylene vinyl alcohol copolymer (Figure 20.1) is a semicrystalline polymer derived from the hydrolysis of poly(ethylene-*co*-vinyl acetate) and is commercially available in a range of compositions, with a typical vinyl alcohol content of about 55–70 mol%. The vinyl alcohol content determines the melting point (T_m) of ethylene vinyl alcohol but is usually in the range of 170–190°C. The glass transition temperature (T_g) is 45–50°C and is independent of the vinyl alcohol content. Ethylene vinyl alcohol copolymers absorb large amounts

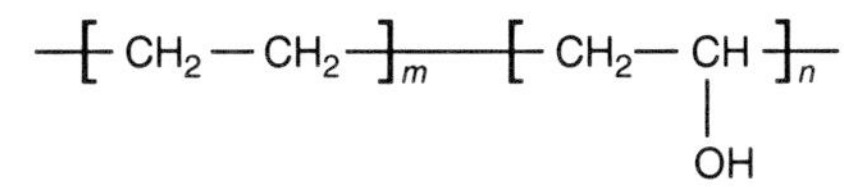

$$-\!\left[\text{CH}_2-\text{CH}_2\right]_m\!-\!\left[\text{CH}_2-\text{CH}\right]_n\!-$$
$$|$$
$$\text{OH}$$

FIGURE 20.1 Chemical structure of ethylene vinyl alcohol copolymer. It is a hydrolyzed copolymer of ethylene and vinyl acetate monomer.

of water, increasing as the ethylene content of ethylene vinyl alcohol decreases. The presence of water results in plasticization of the polymer, with T_g decreasing in more humid environments [5].

When mixed with polar physiological fluids, such as blood, the dimethyl sulfoxide in the Enteryx solution disperses, resulting in the hydrophobic copolymer becoming a solidified spongy mass. Enteryx can be injected through a 23–25 gauge needle due to its low viscosity before contact with physiological fluids, and the biocompatibility of its constituents is reported to be good [6]. The polymer becomes encapsulated in fibrous tissue after 3–6 months and has been shown to be durable for at least 3 years following implantation [6–8]. To enable visualization of the polymer under fluoroscopy, micronized tantalum powder (30% w/v) is added to the polymer/solvent mixture as a contrast agent.

20.3 BIOMATERIALS USED FOR GASTROINTESTINAL FISTULA REPAIR

20.3.1 Gastrointestinal Fistulas

Fistulas are a common complication of Crohn's disease, a chronic inflammatory disorder affecting any part of the gastrointestinal tract. Crohn's fistulas are most commonly present as a perianal manifestation in 14–38% of patients suffering from Crohn's disease in referral populations [9]. The pathogenesis of perianal fistulas remains unknown, but it is believed either they may begin as deep penetrating ulcers in the anus or rectum that extend over time due to feces being forced into the ulcer with the pressure of defecation [10], or they may arise due to an infection or abscess of the anal glands that exist at the base of the anal crypts [11–13]. Either way, fistulas are thought to form when there is no rapid compensatory fibrogenic response to fill up the defect [14]. Furthermore, fistulas might be perpetuated due to bacterial colonization by a variety of normal commensals of the lower gastrointestinal tract [15]. Although the options for treating fistulas in Crohn's disease continue to evolve, fistulas rarely heal. Medical therapies with proven efficacy for the treatment of Crohn's perianal fistulas include antibiotics, mercaptopurine and azathioprine, ciclosporin, tacrolimus, and infliximab [16]. Antibiotics are the most commonly used agents for Crohn's perianal fistulas, with clinical improvement usually seen after 6–8 weeks of metronidazole therapy, but fistulas frequently reoccur once metronidazole is discontinued [16]. The most successful treatment of perianal Crohn's disease is usually achieved when medical therapy is used in conjunction with surgery, but surgery carries the risk of causing incontinence [16].

20.3.2 Fistula Repair Using Biomaterials

20.3.2.1 Fibrin Glue

During the last decade, fibrin glue (also called fibrin sealant or fibrin tissue adhesive) has been proposed as an alternative to the cutting seton and mucosal advancement flap repair of complex fistulas. Due to its ease of application via injection, this procedure is considered safe and painless and without significant morbidity. Fibrin glue simulates physiological clot formation and was first used as a hemostatic agent at the beginning of the last century. Its use for surgical procedures progressed when a method was developed to combine highly concentrated fibrinogen with factor XIII (fibrin-stabilizing factor) and inhibitors of fibronolysis, such as aprotonin. Commercially available concentrated fibrinogen preparations became available during the 1970s, but the risk of viral transmission in pooled fibrinogen concentrates led to license revocation. Autologous human fibrinogen was used as an alternative, and despite subsequent development of viral elimination procedures and the relicensing of fibrin glue, autologous fibrin is still used for the closure of fistulas and in other surgical procedures [17].

Fabrication of fibrin glue is based on chemical reactions that occur during the physiological coagulation cascade. It is produced by mixing a fibrinogen solution containing factor XIII, fibronectin, and aprotonin with thrombin and calcium ions (Figure 20.2). Thrombin mediates the cleavage of fibrin monomers from fibrinogen, which spontaneously aggregate and form weak clot. Thrombin

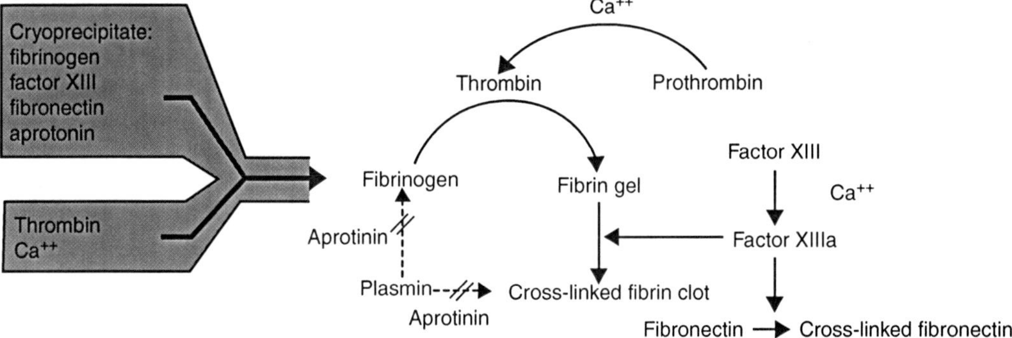

FIGURE 20.2 Schematic illustration of fibrin glue delivery and the chemical reactions that result in the production of cross-linked fibrin.

(and calcium ions) also activates factor XIII to XIIIa (also termed transglutamidase), which cross-links fibrin polymers solidifying the clot. The addition of aprotinin inhibits serine proteases, such as plasmin, which breakdown the fibrin clot via the process of fibrinolysis. Fibronectin present in the starting solution is also cross-linked by factor XIIIa. To prepare autologous fibrin, the patient donates approximately 400 ml of blood 3 weeks prior to surgery. The whole blood is centrifuged to separate the plasma, which is collected and stored at $-40°C$. The plasma is thawed at $4°C$ for 24 h, and the freeze–thaw process is repeated twice. The plasma is then centrifuged, and the autologous cryoprecipitate is collected, stored at $-40°C$, and thawed just prior to surgery [18]. The thawed cryoprecipitate is drawn into a syringe and connected via a Y-connector to a second syringe containing thrombin (1000 units/mL), calcium chloride, and aprotinin (Figure 20.2). Simultaneous delivery of the cryoprecipitate and thrombin via the Y-connector into the fistula tract creates the fibrin glue [18,19]. As the fibrin clots, it seals the fistula tract and thus provides a provisional matrix for the infiltration of fibroblasts and endothelial cells from the surrounding tissue, initiating tissue healing. Plasmin released from the surrounding tissue eventually causes lysis of the fibrin glue after 7–14 days. The rapid degradation of fibrin after a relatively short period of time may occur before complete tissue healing has taken place and possibly accounts for the disappointing published success rates, ranging from 10% to 85%, for fibrin glue injection of perianal fistulas [20]. Because of this low success rate a number of alternative materials that do not possess these inherent problems are being developed for use as filler materials that are likely to achieve higher success rates compared with the materials currently available. These alternative materials include collagen-based materials, such as Permacol (Tissue Science Laboratories Plc., Aldershot, Hampshire, U.K.) [21], and microspheres consisting of alginate/bioactive glass composites [22].

For any biomaterial developed for fistula repair, particular consideration should be given to countering bacterial infections, a problem frequently associated with medical implants that can require removal of the implant. This may be of particular significance in perianal fistulas since, unless thoroughly cleansed, the tracks that communicate with the gastrointestinal tract are likely to be colonized by gut bacteria [15].

20.4 BULKING BIOMATERIALS

20.4.1 FECAL INCONTINENCE

Fecal incontinence affects about 2% of the population and may be caused by defects or weakness of the internal anal sphincter [23]. Current treatment options include antidiarrheal drugs or sacral nerve stimulation, but these strategies are limited by expense and their short-term efficacy. Surgical reconstruction of the internal anal sphincter is usually unsuccessful in the majority of patients.

20.4.2 Injectable Bulking Materials

Injectable bulking agents constitute a feasible and attractive procedure to replace conventional surgery for a number of pathological conditions. Bulking agents have been used for many years to successfully treat patients with urinary incontinence [24]. As a result of this success, a small number of pilot studies have recently reported the use of bulking materials for the treatment of fecal incontinence in patients with weak but intact internal anal sphincter.

20.4.2.1 Polymer Microspheres

The first reported injectable bulking biomaterial used in the treatment of partial fecal incontinence was a paste of polytetrafluoroethylene (Teflon [Du Pont de Nemours & Company, Inc., Wilmington, Delaware] or Polytef), one of the most widely used biomaterials in medicine [25]. Polytef paste is a mixture of polytetrafluoroethylene, glycerin, and polysorbide fabricated as microspheres with sizes ranging from 4 to 100 μm, with 90% in the 4–40 μm range. Despite the reported therapeutic efficacy of Polytef, polytetrafluoroethylene-based materials have many drawbacks that limit their usefulness for sphincter augmentation. Moreover, polytetrafluoroethylene spheres have been found to migrate from the implantation site to distant organs and because they are nonbiodegradable are thought to have triggered granulomatous foreign body reactions, fever, and pneumonitis [26,27]. The problem of detecting transmigration of bulking biomaterials is exacerbated by materials, such as poly(methyl methacrylate), polytetrafluoroethylene, and silicone rubbers being radiolucent, that is, invisible with x-ray imaging. Because of the potentially serious clinical implications of this type of material, an ideal long-lasting injectable biomaterial is sought as a bulking agent for incontinence that is nonantigenic, volume-stable, and nonmigratory.

Microspheres remain an attractive choice for bulking materials due to their relative ease of delivery and ability to conform to the shape of the implantation site. A number of fabrication techniques for producing microspheres have been developed and reported to date, but the choice of the fabrication technique depends on the nature of the polymer, the intended use, and the duration of the therapy. Whichever technique is used, the following criteria should be achievable: (i) the yield of microspheres within the desired size range should be high, (ii) the quality of microspheres should be reproducible, and (iii) microspheres produced should be free flowing and should not aggregate or adhere to one another.

Emulsion solvent diffusion techniques are frequently used to produce microspheres and can be classified as either "in-water" methods or "in-oil" methods (Figure 20.3). The oil-in-water single

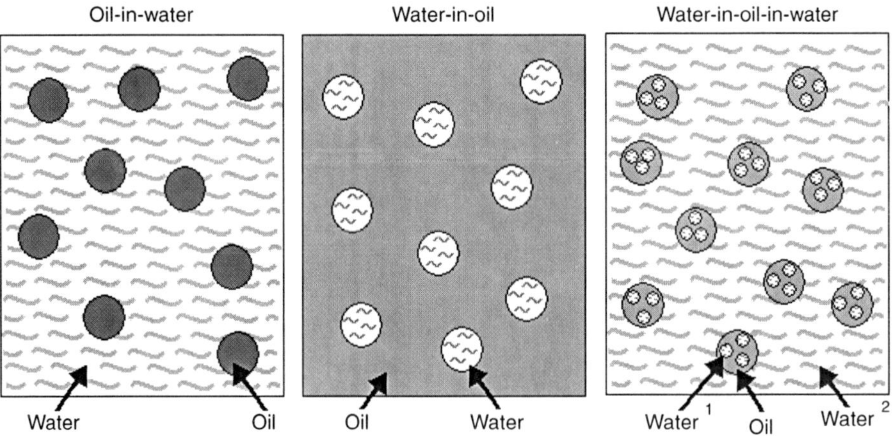

FIGURE 20.3 Schematic illustration of single and double emulsion processes for the fabrication of microspheres.

emulsion process involves dissolving a polymer, such as poly(lactic-*co*-glycolic acid), in a water-immiscible, volatile organic solvent, such as dichloromethane. The solution is then emulsified (with parameters of stirring rate and temperature optimized according to the polymer) in a large volume of water containing an emulsifier, such as poly(vinyl alcohol) (PVA), to yield an emulsion. To harden the oil droplets, the solvent is either evaporated by maintaining the emulsion at reduced pressure or at atmospheric pressure and the stir rate reduced, or extracted by transferring the emulsion to a large volume of quenching medium (with or without surfactant) into which the solvent diffuses out of the oil droplets [28–30]. The solid microspheres are then washed, collected by filtration, centrifugation, or sieving, and dried or freeze-dried to produce free-flowing microspheres.

A number of parameters can affect microsphere fabrication using the single emulsion process. The initial emulsification of the polymer is affected by the stirring rate and the temperature. The rate of solvent removal depends on the temperature of the quenching medium, atmospheric pressure, the ratio of emulsion volume to quench volume, and the solubility of the polymer and the solvent. The rapid removal of solvent by the extraction method can lead to more porous microspheres compared with those fabricated by the evaporation process. The oil-in-water single emulsion technique is widely used to encapsulate lipid-soluble drugs, such as steroids, but poor encapsulation efficiencies of water-soluble drugs has been reported because the drugs diffuse out or partition from the dispersed oil phase into the aqueous continuous phase. To increase the encapsulation efficiency of water-soluble drugs, water-in-oil (or oil-in-oil) single emulsion processes and double (multiple) emulsion processes (water-in-oil-in-water) processes have been developed (Figure 20.3) [28]. Water-in-oil emulsification involves dissolving the polymer and the drug in a water-miscible organic solvent, such as acetonitrile. An emulsion is produced by dispersing the polymer/drug solution into an oil, such as light mineral oil, in the presence of an oil-soluble surfactant such as Span. The organic solvent is evaporated or extracted and the oil removed from the microspheres using a solvent such as *n*-hexane. The water-in-oil-in-water method is useful for encapsulating water-soluble drugs, such as peptides and vaccines. An aqueous solution of drug is added to a vigorously stirred organic phase, consisting of polymer dissolved in a water-immiscible, volatile organic solvent, such as dichloromethane, to produce the first microfine water-in-oil emulsion. The first emulsion is then added to a larger volume of water containing an emulsifier, such as PVA, to form a water-in-oil-in-water emulsion. The solvent is subsequently removed by evaporation or extraction processes.

Poly(lactic-*co*-glycolic acid) microspheres have recently been evaluated as a potential bulking agent for the injection therapies, fabricated using a conventional oil/water emulsion and solvent extraction/evaporation technique, as outlined above [31]. Furthermore, radiopaque polymer microspheres that can be detected through x-ray fluoroscopy after injection have been developed, enabling direct monitoring of possible migration of the spheres *in vivo* or guidance for repeated treatment [32,33]. A copolymer of methyl methacrylate and 2-[2′,3′,5′-triiodobenzoyl]oxoethyl methacrylate was used to produce microspheres with intrinsic radiopacity due to the covalently bound iodine in the side chain [32]. The copolymer was prepared via a free-radical polymerization. To fabricate microspheres, the copolymer was dissolved in chloroform and added dropwise to a stirred solution of detergent (Dubro, Proctor & Gamble). This resulted in the drops of copolymer solution being split into smaller droplets by the turbulent aqueous medium. After continuous overnight stirring to allow evaporation of the solvent, the microspheres were thoroughly washed and freeze-dried. Experimental parameters found to influence the size and the distribution of the microspheres included the concentration of copolymer dissolved in chloroform, the speed of stirring, and the height from which the copolymer solution was dropped into the detergent solution, parameters that are generally applicable to all emulsification techniques used to produce microspheres. The authors of this study suggested that because the density of the microspheres (approximately 1.35 g/cm^3) closely matches that of surrounding soft tissue, the migration of microspheres might be reduced [32]. Moreover, if it was suspected that the microspheres were migrating to distant sites, they could be monitored relatively easily using x-ray fluoroscopy.

20.4.2.2 Collagen Bulking Materials

Collagen-based biomaterials have been evaluated for numerous medical applications. Contigen (CR Bard, Covington, Georgia), derived from bovine collagen, was the first approved injectable bulking agent on the U.S. market and has been extensively studied for urinary incontinence. Contigen is fabricated from dermal type I collagen that has been purified, cross-linked with glutaraldehyde solution, and dispersed in phosphate buffer saline. After injection, the collagen condenses into a fibrous network that is colonized by host connective tissue cells and vasculature, which gradually remodel and breakdown the implant. More recently collagen-based materials have been shown to be effective for use in the treatment of idiopathic fecal incontinence in which the beneficial effect appears to result from the mechanical effect of bulking the tissue with collagen, thus preventing fecal leakage [34].

Collagen-based biomaterials can be derived from bovine or porcine skin and porcine small intestinal submucosa or bladder. To prepare dermal-derived collagen-based materials, the fat and epidermis are first removed from the harvested hide, and then the dermis is soaked in detergent solutions. Povidone–iodine and hydrogen chloride solutions are used to remove microbial contaminants that may be present in the dermis, followed by hydroxide solutions to remove cellular debris and inactivate prions and any remaining viruses. Gamma irradiation is used to further sterilize the tissue [35].

Collagen used in biomaterials is usually cross-linked to improve the mechanical stability, immunogenic properties, and controlled biodegradability for long-term biomedical applications [36]. The predominant chemical treatment for collagen-based biomaterials has been cross-linking with glutaraldehyde, because it is inexpensive, readily available, and highly soluble in aqueous solution, resulting in a biomaterial that is less susceptible to biodegradation. The precise chemistry underlying the cross-linking of collagen by glutaraldehyde is not certain, but it is suggested that glutaraldehyde reacts with primary amines, cross-linking them in an inter- and intramolecular fashion via the formation of covalent bonds (Figure 20.4). This cross-linking occurs either by the formation of unstable Schiff base linkages through reaction of an aldehyde group with an amino group of lysine or hydroxylysine or by the formation of stable aldol condensation products between two adjacent aldehydes [37].

However, concerns have been raised regarding the use of glutaraldehyde cross-linked biomaterials since unstable glutaraldehyde polymers that can remain in the interstices of cross-linked bioprostheses may slowly leach out, causing prolonged local cytotoxicity [38]. Although the cytotoxic effects of glutaraldehyde cross-linked collagen can be decreased by extensive rinsing or by the addition of quenching reagents, such as propylhydroxybenzoate, methylhydroxybenzoate, and glycine [39], alternative cross-linking agents have been proposed. These include dicyclohexylmethane-4,4-diisocyanate (HMDI), which cross-links three amino acids in triple helix with hexamethylene diisocyanate. It is suggested that HMDI cross-linking produces fewer cytotoxic effects compared with those caused by glutaraldehyde cross-linking, where aldehyde leaching from the materials may cause an inflammatory response [35].

Although collagen is a naturally occurring biomaterial, the chemical processing it requires before it can be used as a long-term implant leads to a number of drawbacks. For example, although cross-linking slows down the rate of biodegradation of the collagen implant by cellular proteases, there is also a possibility that cross-linking may prevent cellular infiltration into the biomaterial from host tissue [35]. Furthermore, calcification of bioprostheses fabricated from tissue-derived

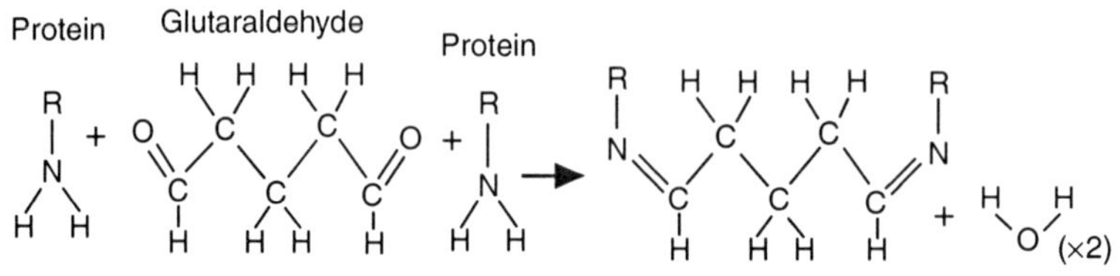

FIGURE 20.4 Cross-linking reaction of glutaraldehyde with primary amines on protein molecules.

biomaterials, such as collagen, represents a major clinical problem and appears to be encouraged by glutaraldehyde cross-linking. To overcome this problem, further chemical pretreatment of implants with biphosphonates has been proposed as a way of inhibiting calcification of the implants by interfering with crystal growth that prevents accumulation of calcium [40]. However, with each additional treatment stage, collagen becomes less like the original endogenous extracellular matrix material, which is its major attribute. Furthermore, as the collagen gradually degrades over time, the implant fails to conserve its volume, meaning repeat injections are usually necessary [41,42]. Besides leading to additional patient discomfort, this may also be clinically unsuitable for some patients as approximately 3% of patients treated with bovine collagen show allergic reactions preventing retreatment [43,44].

20.4.2.3 Zirconium Dioxide Microspheres

Durasphere (Carbon Medical Technologies, St. Paul, Minnesota) is another microsphere-type bulking agent that has been studied over short- and long-term periods in patients with an internal anal sphincter defect refractory to conservative management [45]. Durasphere consists of biocompatible and nonimmunogenic zirconium dioxide microspheres coated in pyrolytic carbon and suspended in a water-based carrier gel containing β-glucan. Although the size of microspheres ranges from 251 to 300 μm, which is considered to be approximately three times the migration threshold of 80 μm, microsphere migration has been reported to be visible on x-ray in some patients treated for stress urinary incontinence [46]. It has been suggested that the density of the bulk material (zirconium dioxide, 5.89 g/cm^3), which is much higher than the density of the surrounding soft tissue (approximately 1 g/cm^3), may account for the microsphere migration described [32].

20.5 BIOMATERIALS AND LAPAROTOMY PROCEDURES

20.5.1 INTRA-ABDOMINAL ADHESIONS

Adhesions are fibrous connections between tissues that occur as a result of tissue injury taking place during abdominal and pelvic surgery, radiation to abdominal or pelvic areas, or certain diseases, such as endometriosis. Postoperative intra-abdominal adhesions are a very common consequence of abdominal and pelvic surgery. Their formation is a major cause of morbidity, accounting for 60–70% of the all small bowel obstruction cases in the Western world [47]. Small bowel obstruction, as a result of adhesions, can cause abnormal orientation of the intestine, leading to strangulation and intestinal necrosis, with a high risk of morbidity and mortality. As a consequence of the common and serious nature of adhesions, there is an intensive area of biomaterials research devoted to developing materials that will prevent this condition. Therefore, the materials highlighted in this section do not form an exhaustive list, rather an indication of the type of materials that have been tested past and present.

20.5.2 BIOMATERIALS TO PREVENT INTRA-ABDOMINAL ADHESIONS

The most common objective in preventing adhesion formation using biomaterials has been to separate surgically traumatized internal tissue surfaces. Since the beginning of the twentieth century, many barrier materials, including silicones, polyvinyl pyrrolidine, oiled silk, and silver or gold foil, have been developed and tested in preclinical models, but most have been noneffective or have been found to exacerbate the problem [48].

20.5.2.1 Hyaluronic Acid–Based Biomaterials

The most effective barrier developed and tested in a prospective randomized clinical trial is a bioresorbable membrane called Seprafilm (Genzyme Corporation, Cambridge, Massachusetts), which is composed of chemically modified hyaluronic acid (sodium hyaluronate) and carboxymethylcellulose [49]. It is biocompatible and relatively easy to handle and apply. It readily adheres to tissues, turning into a hydrophilic gel after 24–48 h and provides a protective barrier over traumatized surfaces in the abdomen for up to 7 days during which time it is slowly reabsorbed from the abdominal cavity before being excreted from the body in 28 days [50].

Hyaluronic acid (also called hyaluronan or hyaluronate) is a glycosaminoglycan found abundantly in epithelial, connective, and neural tissues, where it is a chief component of the extracellular matrix. Because of its ubiquitous presence in the extracellular matrix of tissues and its biocompatibility, hyaluronic acid is an attractive biomaterial for biomedical applications. However, due to its poor biomechanical properties, it usually requires chemical modification, such as grafting onto natural or synthetic polymers, to produce mechanically robust materials. Fabrication of Seprafilm involves blending hyaluronic acid and carboxymethylcellulose, both of which are polyanionic polymers and contain carboxylic acid groups, followed by chemical modification with 1-(3-dimethylaminopropyl)-3-ethylcarbodiimide hydrochloride (carbodiimide) [51]. The carbodiimide modifies the negatively charged carboxylic acid groups and leaves a proportion of these groups cationic by the formation of *N*-acylurea. This creates an anionic–cationic cross-linked network that reduces the rate of *in vivo* degradation and absorption of both hyaluronic acid and carboxymethylcellulose polymers. This effect enables membranes prepared from this composite polymer to remain at the tissue surface longer to function as a barrier to separate the traumatized tissue surfaces [52].

However, the use of membranes and films such as Seprafilm is limited to surfaces easily accessible during surgery, and therefore alternative barrier approaches are being sought to prevent adhesion. One example is the use of an auto-cross-linked hyaluronic acid–derivative gel, which has been found to be effective in reducing adhesions after hemostasis [53,54]. Auto-cross-linked hyaluronic acid polymers, such as those produced by Fidia Advanced Biopolymers, Italy, are fabricated by an auto-cross-linking esterification reaction between the carboxyl groups and hydroxyl groups belonging to the same molecule and different molecules of hyaluronic acid, forming a mixture of lactones and intermolecular ester bonds [55]. By adjusting the reaction conditions, the level of cross-linking can be controlled. Because no additional bridging molecules are present between the cross-linked hyaluronic acid chains, only natural products are released during degradation of the hydrogel.

Further modifications to hyaluronic acid–based hydrogel barrier-type materials have included the incorporation of agents that inhibit cellular proliferation at the traumatized surface. Liu et al. recently reported on the *in vivo* efficacy of cross-linked hyaluronic acid films loaded with mitomycin C, an antitumour antibiotic that alkylates and cross-links DNA [56]. The use of an acrylamide derivative of mitomycin C enabled the incorporation of this agent into the films by conjugate addition chemistry [57].

20.5.2.2 Nanofibrous Sheets

Despite the reported success of these materials, there still remains a need to develop improved and inexpensive products that are effective in various surgical applications.

One example is the use of nanofibrous scaffolds, which are being considered for a number of different tissue engineering applications. They appear to offer a physical environment that more closely resembles that of native extracellular matrix, favoring cellular adhesion, proliferation, and differentiation compared with other human-made materials [58]. Zong and colleagues tested a novel nanostructured barrier fabricated by electrospinning poly(lactic-*co*-glycolic acid) copolymers designed to prevent postsurgery-induced abdominal adhesions [59]. The starting material is biocompatible and biodegradable and has previously been used in many FDA-approved implant devices, such as suture fibers. Electrospinning is a process that uses an electrostatic field to control the formation and the deposition of polymer fibers that can be submicron in diameter. The polymer solution at the tip of a nozzle is subjected to a large electric potential (typically 15–30 kV) and is separated by a distance from an oppositely charged target to create a static electric field. As the electric field potential increases,

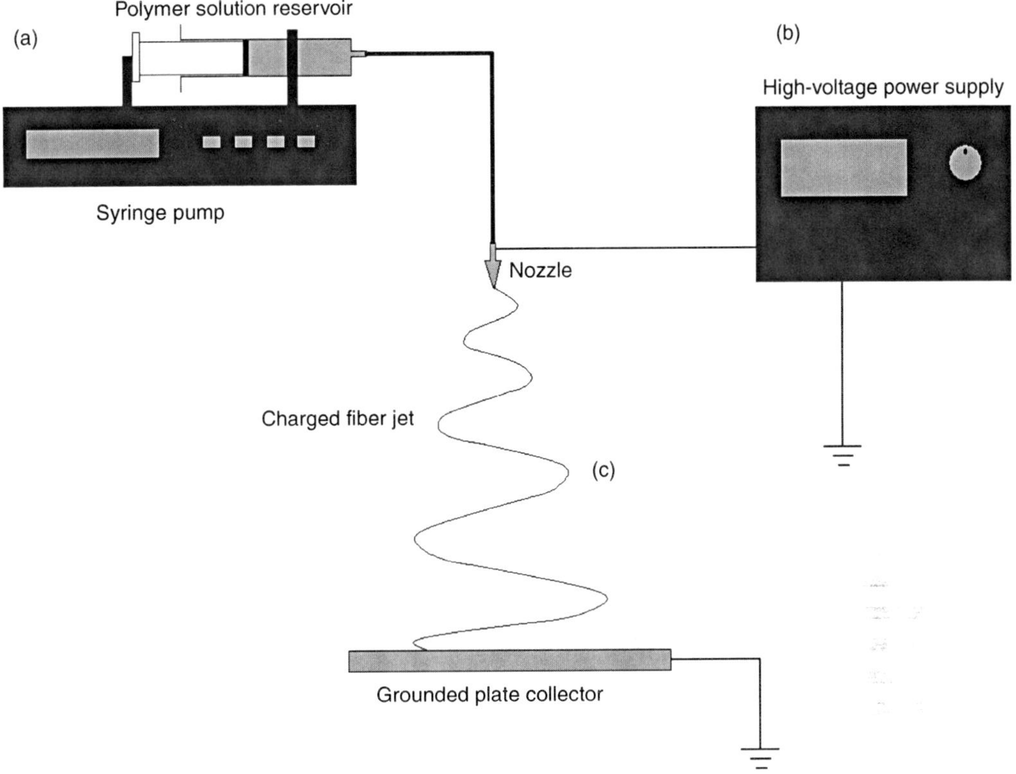

FIGURE 20.5   A schematic illustration of a typical electrospinning instrument. Parameters that affect the electrospinning process include (a) polymer concentration, viscosity, flow rate; (b) accelerating voltage; and (c) distance between nozzle and spinning atmosphere.

the electrostatic forces in the solution overcome the surface tension of the solution, and a thin jet of charged solution is ejected toward the oppositely charged target (Figure 20.5). The high surface area to volume ratio of the jet allows efficient solvent evaporation and further thinning of the jet. Processing parameters have a direct effect on the electrospun polymer fibers. These include solution concentration and viscosity, polymer flow/feed rate, spinning atmosphere, accelerating voltage, and tip-to-target distance [60].

Unmodified poly(lactic-*co*-glycolic acid) nonwoven nanofibrous membranes did not produce a significant reduction in adhesions compared with control groups. The ineffectiveness of the poly(lactic-*co*-glycolic acid) meshes was attributed to the substantial shrinkage of the nanofiber scaffold caused by the hydrophobic nature of poly(lactic-*co*-glycolic acid) when exposed to body fluids. The shrinkage reduced the tissue surface area effectively covered by the membrane, allowing an increased frequency of adhesions to form in the animal model studied. To overcome this problem, poly(ethylene glycol)/poly(D,L-lactide) was blended with poly(lactic-*co*-glycolic acid) to modify the hydrophobicity of the electrospun membrane. The hydrophilic PEG–PLA diblock copolymer maintained good membrane dimensional stability, resulting in effective coverage of the injured tissue surfaces and a significant reduction in the frequency of adhesions observed.

The barrier properties of the nonwoven nanofibrous membranes were further improved by incorporating antibiotics into the membranes. The antibiotic (cefoxitin sodium) was slowly mixed into the polymer solution before electrospinning. Although the role of antibiotics used in preventing adhesions remains uncertain, medicated barriers that locally delivered cefoxitin sodium exhibited excellent results for the prevention of adhesions [59].

20.6 TARGETED DRUG DELIVERY WITH BIOMATERIALS

20.6.1 Drug Delivery to the Colon

One of the most extensive areas of biomaterials research related to the gastrointestinal tract is the development of drug delivery devices. Biodegradable particulate carrier systems for oral drug delivery offer a number of potential benefits including enhancement of absorption, bioavailability, site-specific targeting, and a delivery system for oral immunization. This section will focus on the widely used oral administration route for drug delivery to the colon. The colon is an attractive site for drug delivery due to its less hostile environment compared with upper regions of the gastrointestinal tract, slower transit times allowing longer drug retention, and richness in gut-associated lymphoid tissue that facilitates efficient vaccine delivery. However, the bioavailability of peptide and protein drugs after oral administration can be low due to their instability in the gastrointestinal tract and low permeability through the intestinal mucosa. Therefore, a number of strategies have been developed to deliver intact molecules to the colon, including pH-sensitive coatings, timed-release systems, mucoadhesive systems, nanoparticles for site-specific accumulation, and polymers that are degraded by colonic bacteria. Many of these colon-targeted drug delivery systems are applied as coatings to conventional hard gelatin capsules [61].

Timed-release drug delivery systems are based on the principle of delivering drugs after a particular time, which is usually the time required to reach the colon after gastric emptying (3–4 h). However, this approach is limited since gastric emptying can vary considerably depending on the quantity and the type of food consumed and also the well-being of the patient.

The pH conditions of the gastrointestinal tract vary considerably along its length, increasing from acidic in the stomach (pH 1–4) to a neutral/slightly alkaline pH in the distal part of the small intestine and the colon. Colon targeting using polymer coatings that are pH-sensitive needs to withstand the acidic conditions of the stomach and proximal part of the small intestine before disintegrating in the neutral/alkaline pH of the colon. One of the most commonly used pH-dependent coatings is a copolymer of methacrylic acid and methyl methacrylate, such as Eudragit (Röhm Pharmaceuticals, Germany).

20.6.1.1 Chitosan-Based Drug Delivery Systems

Chitosan, a naturally occurring polymer, relies on different inherent properties to make it suitable for colonic specific delivery. These properties include (i) its sensitivity to biodegradation by lysozyme, an enzyme found highly concentrated in the colonic mucosa, and other colonic bacteria-derived enzymes and (ii) its mucoadhesive properties [62]. It is, therefore, a particularly attractive biomaterial because of its nontoxicity, biocompatibility, and biodegradability.

Chitosan is a copolymer of N-acetyl-D-glucosamine and D-glucosamine and is derived from chitin by alkaline deacetylation. Chitin is the second most abundant protein in nature, found in the exoskeleton of crustaceans, insects, and some fungi. To prepare chitosan, chitin is initially extracted from the shell of crustaceans by treatment for a few hours with 3–5% (w/v) NaOH aqueous solution at 80–90°C to remove proteins, followed by treatment with 3–5% (w/v) aqueous HCl to remove inorganic constituents of the shell. N-deacetylation of chitin to produce chitosan is achieved by treating the sample with 40–50% aqueous (w/v) NaOH solution at 90–120°C for 4–5 h. The crude precipitate of chitosan is washed in water and dissolved in 2% aqueous acetic acid. Any insoluble material is removed and the solution is neutralized with NaOH solution [63].

A hybrid colon-specific drug delivery system consisting of the pH-sensitive polymer Eudragit and chitosan has recently been developed [62]. Chitosan microspheres measuring 2–3 μm in diameter were prepared by spray-drying a solution of chitosan containing a model drug (sodium diclofenac), which was subsequently freeze-dried. The microspheres were encapsulated in Eudragit using an oil-in-oil solvent evaporation method. To do this, the microspheres were dispersed in a solution of

Eudragit (dissolved in a solvent consisting of acetone: ethanol) to produce an organic phase, which was then poured into liquid paraffin containing sorbitan trioleate (Span 85) and a foam suppressor (Antifoam A). The system was maintained under agitation for 3 h at room temperature to allow evaporation of the solvent. The encapsulated microspheres were collected, rinsed with *n*-hexane, and freeze-dried. Drug delivery from the microspheres was reported to occur after pH-dependent dissolution of the Eudagrit coating (the duration of which depended on the type of Eudagrit used), swelling of the chitosan microspheres, and dissolution of the model drug [62].

Mucoadhesive polymers offer increased drug bioavailability at target mucosal tissues without dilution or degradation in lumenal fluids. Prerequisites for a good mucoadhesive polymer include high flexibility of its polymer backbone structure and of its polar functional groups. Suggested mechanisms that may underlie the mucoadhesion between biomaterials and mucin include electrostatic adsorption (van der Waals, hydrogen bonds), wetting, diffusion, and fracture theories [64]. When hydrated, chitosan demonstrates good mucoadhesive properties through its interaction with mucin [65].

20.6.1.2 Alginate-Based Drug Delivery Systems

Another mucoadhesive polymer is alginate, a negatively charged polysaccharide derived from brown seaweed that is commonly used for the production of drug-loaded microparticles [66]. Because alginate beads are nontoxic orally and have high biocompatibility, they have been developed for use as controlled delivery devices to the colon for a number of different drugs [64,67,68]. Alginates undergo reversible gelation (coacervation) in the presence of divalent cations, such as Ca^{2+}, to form hydrogels [69]. Large beads (1–2 mm in diameter) can be readily produced by manually dropping an alginate solution from a syringe into a solution of calcium chloride. Fabrication of smaller beads down to about 200 μm in diameter can be achieved using a high electrostatic potential bead generator (Figure 20.6). This instrument uses an electrostatic potential to pull alginate droplets from a needle tip into a bath containing gelling ions, such as calcium chloride (Figure 20.7). Several parameters can be used to control the final size of the alginate beads produced and also the efficiency of drug entrapment. These parameters include the applied electrostatic potential, flow rate of polymer solution, needle diameter, gelling ion concentration, hardening times, and alginate composition, concentration, and viscosity [70,71].

Excellent mucoadhesive properties of alginate/chitosan beads to freshly excised pig intestine has been reported [64]. The beads, intended for colonic drug delivery, were prepared by complex coacervation using sodium alginate as a gel core. Sodium alginate (2% w/v) prepared in deionized water was dropped through a 0.45 mm syringe needle (1 mL/min) into a solution of calcium chloride (0.5–1.0% w/v) mixed with chitosan (0.5–1.5% w/v). The beads were allowed to harden for at least

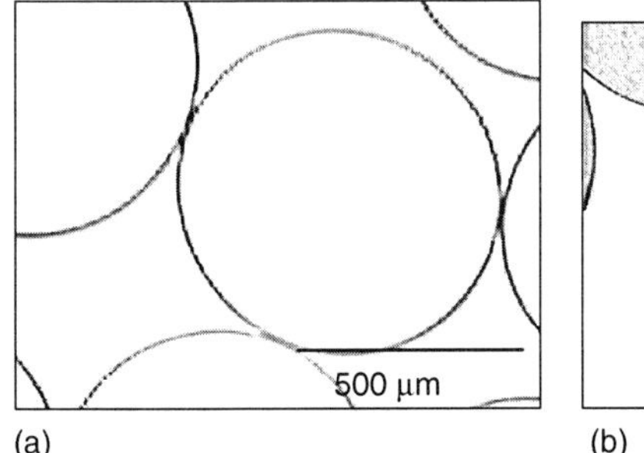

(a)

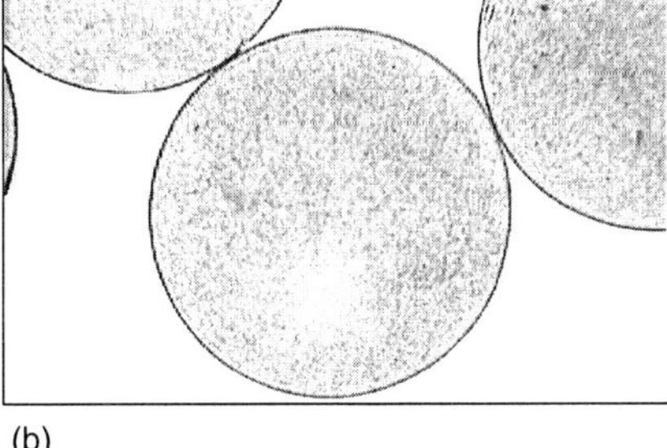

(b)

FIGURE 20.6 Alginate microspheres measuring approximately 600 μm in diameter containing (a) 0% or (b) 0.1% (w/v) 45S5 bioactive glass produced using an electrostatic bead generator. Alginate solution (1.5% w/v low viscosity) was delivered from a nozzle (outer diameter of 0.35 mm/inner diameter of 0.17 mm) at a flow rate of 9 mL/h and electrostatic potential of 3.6 kV into a gelling solution of 15 mM $CaCl_2$.

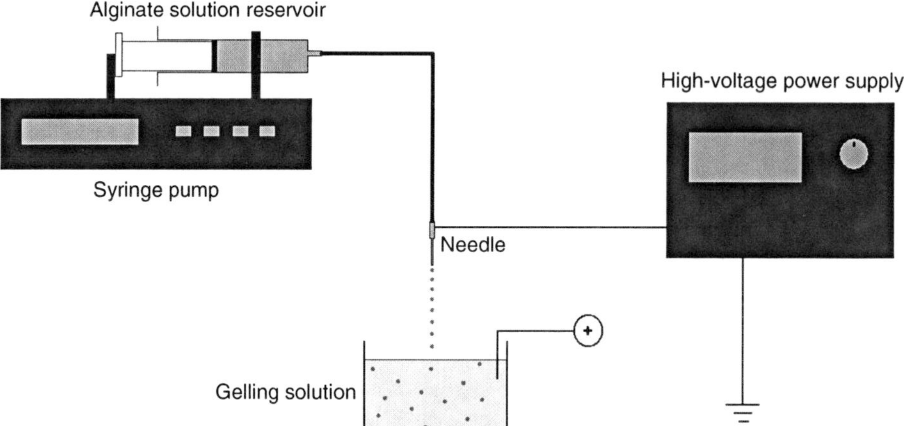

FIGURE 20.7 A schematic illustration of a typical electrostatic bead generator. The electrostatic potential between the needle delivering the alginate solution and the electroconductive gelling solution forces the droplets to fall from the needle tip before they grow to a point where they would fall due to their own weight.

2 h before washing in distilled water and drying at room temperature. Increasing the chitosan concentration was found to improve the number of beads attaching to the surface of the intestine after 1 h [64].

20.6.1.3 Nanoparticle Drug Delivery Systems

The efficiency of delivering drugs via oral routes to colon can be reduced in gastrointestinal diseases, such as inflammatory bowel disease, where symptoms may include diarrhea. This can lead to the accelerated elimination of microscopic drug delivery systems and a reduction of possible drug release at the target site. One suggested approach to overcome this problem is the reduction in size of the drug carrier down to nanoparticle-sized systems [72].

Nanoparticles are submicron colloidal carriers composed of natural or synthetic polymers. Various methods can be used to fabricate polymeric nanoparticles, but these processes can be broadly divided into two categories: those based on physiochemical properties such as phase separation and solvent evaporation (frequently used for hydrophobic or cross-linked water-insoluble hydrophilic polymers) and those based on chemical reactions such as emulsion polymerization and polycondensation (using, for example, hydrophobic vinyl monomers) [73]. Poly(lactic-*co*-glycolic acid) nanoparticles have been successfully prepared using an "in-water" emulsion solvent diffusion method [74]. Poly(lactic-*co*-glycolic acid) and a drug were dissolved in a solvent mix of acetone and ethanol, both of which dissolved in aqueous solution. When the polymer solution was poured into aqueous poly(vinyl alcohol) solution, the rapid diffusion of solvent into the aqueous phase (the Marangoni effect) resulted in the immediate formation of a submicron oil-in-water emulsion due to the immediate reduction of the interfacial tension and rapid diffusion of organic solvent into the aqueous phase. The nanosphere suspension was centrifuged and washed in distilled water to remove the aqueous phase containing solvent and freeze-dried to produce a free-flowing powder consisting of monodispersed nanoparticles approximately 250 nm in diameter [74]. Although this technique is relatively simple, its major drawback is the low entrapment efficiency when used with water-soluble drugs that leach from the nanoparticles during the solvent diffusion process. This problem was reduced by changing the dispersion medium from an aqueous solution ("in-water") to an oily medium ("in-oil") such as the medium chain triglyceride caprylate. Because the rapid diffusion of solvent into the oil medium did not occur, a surfactant, such as Span 80, was added to the polymer phase. The nanoparticles were collected and washed in *n*-haxane, suspended in a solution of PVA to prevent fusion and aggregation of the particles, and freeze-dried to produce a powder of nanoparticles approximately 700 nm in diameter [74]. Although the particles produced were still nanoscale, there was a substantial difference in the size of the particles produced using the two different techniques. When fabricating particulate carrier systems for oral drug delivery systems, particularly those intended for vaccine delivery, consideration should be given to the different particle sizes resulting from alternative fabrication techniques, as this may have implications for their efficacy in clinical applications. One example is the particle size-dependent exclusion phenomenon that exists in gastrointestinal mucosal tissue, where nanoparticles in the region of 100 nm show significantly greater uptake compared with larger nano/microparticles [75].

In addition to avoiding rapid elimination from the colon, nanoparticles also have the additional attribute of accumulating at sites of inflamed tissue, which could be used to facilitate the targeting of anti-inflammatory drugs to sites of colonic inflammation. This phenomenon is thought to occur through the uptake of nanoparticles by immune cells infiltrating the tissue and adhesion to the excessive amounts of mucus secreted in inflamed tissue, increasing the localization of drug delivery [76]. The selective delivery achievable with nanoparticle systems can therefore be applied to reduce the risk of severe adverse side effects associated with systemic administration of certain drugs and to achieve increased efficiency and tolerability [72].

Further selective drug delivery using nanoparticles has been achieved with pH-sensitive polymers developed for colonic drug delivery, whereby drug release is controlled by the sensitivity of the polymer to lumenal pH during intestinal passage [72]. The nanoparticles were prepared using an oil-in-water emulsification–solvent evaporation process. The pH-sensitive polymer (Eudragit P-4135F, Röhm Pharma Polymers, Japan) was dissolved in methylene chloride together with the immunosuppressant drug (tacrolimus). The solution was added to a 1% (w/w) solution of polyvinyl alcohol to form an oil-in-water emulsion using ultrasonication. The solvent was removed under reduced pressure, and the nanoparticles were washed in distilled water prior to freeze-drying in a 5% sucrose solution. The nanoparticles produced were approximately 450 nm in diameter and had high encapsulation efficiencies. Although the pH-sensitive nanoparticles and control (non-pH-sensitive) poly(lactic-*co*-glycolic acid) nanoparticles reduced the levels of adverse effects associated with systemic delivery of the drug, such as nephrotoxicity, in the mouse model of colitis used in the study, it is worth noting that the nanoparticle formulations were a less effective treatment for the control of the experimental colitis compared with subcutaneous delivery of the drug. This study illustrates the situation that frequently arises with the development of new "smart" materials. Although these new materials may solve one problem, they may give rise to additional problems that require further modification of the material.

20.7 BIOMATERIALS FOR INTESTINAL TISSUE ENGINEERING

20.7.1 INTESTINAL FAILURE AND TISSUE ENGINEERING

The intestine plays an essential role in maintaining the nutritional status of humans. A number of diseases can significantly disrupt the normal function of the intestine, resulting in a condition called intestinal failure. Children and adults with intestinal failure have a poor quality of life and suffer significant morbidity and mortality. This condition usually results in the patient receiving artificial feeding in the form of intravenous (parenteral) nutrition. In the United Kingdom, it is estimated that 20,000–25,000 adults and children are receiving long-term home parenteral nutrition at any point in time and that this figure is increasing by approximately 20% annually. Surgical options, such as transplantation, are reserved for patients with potential or actual life-threatening complications of parenteral nutrition due to the scarcity of donor organs, the side effects from immunosuppression, and much lower survival rates than from parenteral nutrition.

20.7.2 BIOMATERIALS USED FOR INTESTINAL TISSUE ENGINEERING

Although intestinal tissue engineering is currently not a viable therapeutic option for humans with intestinal failure, a number of research groups are developing biomaterials that can be used as scaffolds to support the engineering of intestinal constructs in small animal models. A variety of different scaffolds have been developed to date for intestinal tissue engineering, composed of both synthetic [77,78] and natural [79,80] polymers.

20.7.2.1 Fibrous Synthetic Polymer Scaffolds

To date, the most well-reported biomaterial used for intestinal tissue engineering has been a highly porous, synthetic, biodegradable polymer tube fabricated from nonwoven sheets of polyglycolic acid fibers [77]. Stabilized polyglycolic acid fibre–based tubes can be fabricated from polyglycolic acid meshes by physically bonding adjacent fibers using a spray-casting technique [81]. Rectangles of polyglycolic acid mesh composed of fibers with a diameter of approximately 12 μm were wrapped around a 3 mm diameter Teflon cylinder to form a tube, and the two opposing edges were interlocked to form a seam. The Teflon cylinder was rotated and solutions of poly(lactic-*co*-glycolic acid) and polylactic acid dissolved in chloroform were atomized and sprayed over the rotating polyglycolic acid mesh. Unlike poly(lactic-*co*-glycolic acid) and polylactic acid, polyglycolic acid is only weakly soluble in chloroform therefore the polyglycolic acid fibers were largely unaffected by the solvent-casting technique. The tubes were freeze-dried to remove residual solvent and removed from the Teflon cylinder.

The tubular scaffolds were capable of resisting relatively large compressive forces *in vitro* and maintained their tubular structure when implanted *in vivo*. The mechanical stability of the scaffolds was dictated by the extent of physical bonding, the polymer used to bond the polyglycolic acid fibers, and the processing conditions. Polylactic acid bonded tubes were more resistant to compressional forces compared with the poly(lactic-*co*-glycolic acid) bonded tubes, probably due to the crystalline nature of polylactic acid, making it stiffer compared with amorphous poly(lactic-*co*-glycolic acid). Simulated degradation of the tubes in an aqueous environment *in vitro* also markedly weakened the poly(lactic-*co*-glycolic acid) bonded tubes compared with the polylactic acid bonded devices. This effect was probably caused by the increased hydrophilic nature of poly(lactic-*co*-glycolic acid), leading to the adsorbed water acting as a plasticizer. Complete erosion of poly(lactic-*co*-glycolic acid) bonded fibers occurred within 11 weeks, whereas the polylactic acid bonded fibers degraded much more slowly [81].

The ability of this type of scaffolds to support tissue growth *in vivo* has been assessed by implanting them into a small animal model. Prior to implantation, the tubes were cold-gas sterilized with ethylene oxide and coated with a solution of collagen type I overnight to improve the biocompatibility of the polymer fibers. The collagen-coated tubes were subsequently washed with Hanks' balanced salt solution before cell seeding and implantation into the omenta of rats. In small animal models, such as rats, scaffolds fabricated using this approach have enabled small amounts of tissue-engineered intestine to be successfully grown and anastomosed to native small bowel, where it increased in size and became lined by well differentiated neomucosa, which could be maintained for up to 36 weeks [82].

20.7.2.2 Foam Synthetic Polymer Scaffolds

In addition to fibrous scaffolds, a number of alternative scaffolds for intestinal tissue engineering have also been developed. These include tubular scaffolds composed of PLGA foams fabricated by a thermally induced phase separation (TIPS) process [78]. TIPS has been used to fabricate a variety of micro- and macroporous foams. The technique involves the conversion of a single homogeneous polymer solution made at elevated temperature into two-phase separated domains via the removal of thermal energy. These domains are composed of a polymer-rich phase and a polymer-lean phase. The solvent crystallizes when the polymer solution temperature is lower than the solvent freezing temperature, which results in the polymer phase being expelled from the crystallization front.

Freeze-drying of the liquid–liquid phase-separated polymer solution removes the solvent, producing a foam structure with pores that have the geometry of the solvent crystals. Temperature gradients present along the direction of solidification may account for the pore anisotropy observed in foams fabricated using the TIPS process [83]. Various foam morphologies can be obtained by systematically changing parameters involved in the TIPS process, including polymer type and concentration, coarsening conditions, solvent or nonsolvent composition, and inclusion of an additive or particulates [84].

Tubular foam scaffolds fabricated using the TIPS process were prepared from poly(lactic-*co*-glycolic acid) dissolved in dimethylcarbonate under magnetic stirring to produce a 5% (w/v) polymer solution. The polymer solution was filtered through a 0.45 μm filter, cast onto a Petri dish and transferred into a lyophilization flask, which was subsequently frozen for 2 h in liquid nitrogen. The solvent in the cast polymer was then sublimated at −10°C for 48 h, and then at 0°C for an additional 48 h. Residual solvent was removed at room temperature. The polymer membranes were rolled into a tube and the opposing edges were joined by dissolving in chloroform and pressing them together. The resulting tube had a lumen approximately 3 mm in diameter and walls approximately 1.5–2 mm thick (Figure 20.8a). The porosity of the foam scaffolds was high (>93%) and the pore volume was calculated to be 11.5 cm^3/g. Two distinct pore sizes were present in the foam: macropores of ~100 μm average diameter and interconnected micropores of 10–50 μm diameter (Figure 20.8b) [78].

However, unlike the fibrous scaffolds previously described, scaffolds fabricated by the TIPS process failed to withstand compressive forces when implanted *in vivo* (Figure 20.9). Such loss of the lumenal structure would impede the use of these scaffolds for intestinal tissue engineering in which the ability to retain a tubular structure is crucial for the passage of nutrients through the gastrointestinal tract. Further modification of the processing parameters combined with improved polymer selection would probably increase the mechanical stability and prevent the scaffold collapsing.

The problem of good mechanical stability is not limited to tubular scaffolds produced by using the TIPS process. Without further modification, the ability of many of the different scaffolds developed to date, to resist compressive forces, is unlikely to be reproducible once the scaffold's lumenal dimension is increased to enable engineering of a construct with dimensions resembling that of native human intestine. Therefore, further modification of the biomaterials used to fabricate these scaffolds will be necessary to provide the additional mechanical strength required to prevent lumenal collapse.

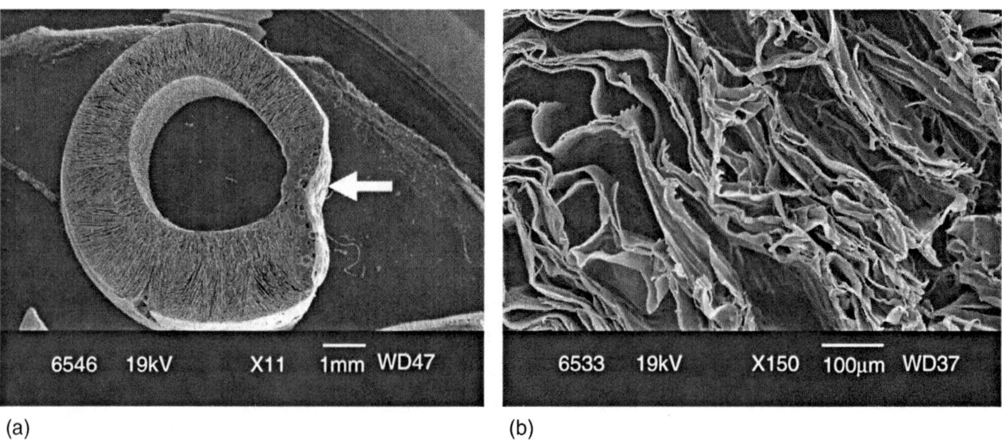

FIGURE 20.8 Scanning electron microscopy (SEM) of the microstructure of the tubular poly(lactic-*co*-glycolic acid) scaffolds fabricated using the TIPS process. (a) When the foams were rolled into tubes, the pores in the foam became highly oriented in radial direction. The arrow indicates the seam where the edge of the foam was dissolved with solvent to join the two edges. Loss of porosity occurs in these regions. (b) Higher magnification of the pore structure of the TIPS foams.

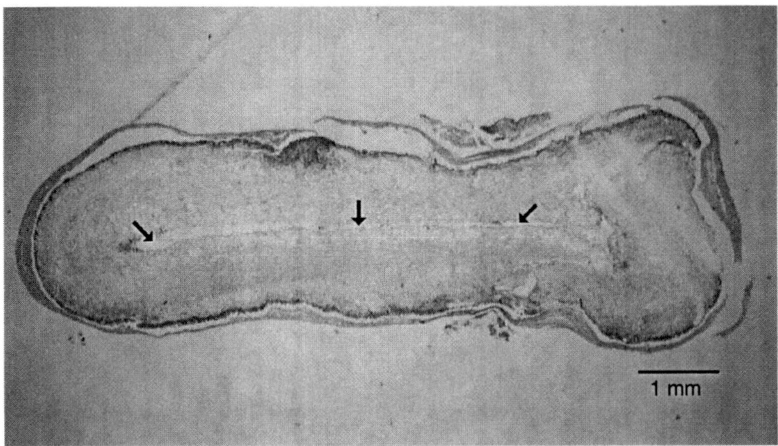

FIGURE 20.9 Tubes produced from poly(lactic-*co*-glycolic acid) foams fabricated using thermally induced phase separation techniques show poor mechanical stability when implanted *in vivo*, collapsing after 1 week of subcutaneous implantation. Arrows indicate the collapsed lumen in a histological cross-section of the implanted tube.

The problems associated with mechanical stability of the tubular scaffolds add to a list of obstacles arising from these early tissue engineering studies that have yet to be resolved before intestinal tissue engineering can be applied to humans, many of which can be attributed to the biomaterials currently being used to fabricate the scaffolds.

Other concerns raised include the ability to engineer sufficient lengths of intestine. Some of the tissue-engineered constructs produced to date have measured only approximately 1 cm in length. Even for a small animal model, such lengths of intestine are unlikely to produce a significant increase in the nutrient absorptive capacity of the intestine. Moreover, the production of a 1 cm length of engineered intestine has required all of the intestinal epithelial cells harvested from approximately one-and-a-half syngeneic donor intestines, a procedure that could not feasibly be translated to humans. The inefficient use of cells with this approach probably results from poor attachment and spreading of cells to the biomaterials used to fabricate the scaffolds. Future scaffolds might consist of biomaterials that have had key protein components of the intestine incorporated into them, which promote cell adhesion and spreading.

20.7.2.3 Collagen-Based Scaffolds

Naturally derived biomaterials, such as porcine small intestinal submucosa, have also been used for intestinal tissue engineering scaffolds [79,85]. Small intestinal submucosa is an obvious choice for intestinal tissue engineering since this biopolymer is derived from a tissue that in its native form provides support for the growth and differentiation of mucosal tissue while also functioning as a connective tissue structure that provides mechanical strength to the structure of the intestine [86]. Small intestinal submucosa biomaterials can be fabricated from freshly harvested porcine small intestine by inverting the tubular tissue and mechanically delaminating the outer muscular layers (tunica muscularis externa) and internal mucosal (tunica mucosa) layers from the submucosal tissue (tunica submucosa) [86]. The resulting submucosal tissue with basilar layers of the mucosa consists of a membrane about 80–100 μm thick. The membrane is rinsed in water, treated with an aqueous solution of 0.1% peracetic acid, and rinsed further in water and phosphate buffer saline to remove any remaining cells and to provide the small intestinal submucosa with a neutral pH. To increase the thickness of small intestinal submucosa, additional layers have been stacked on top before compressing and drying. Small intestinal submucosa is sterilized with 2.5 mRad gamma irradiation to produce a sterile, pyrogen-free biomaterial consisting of a complex mixture of extracellular matrix molecules including collagen type I, III, IV, V, VI; proteoglycans; glycoproteins; and glycosaminoglycans [79,87]. To make tubular scaffolds, the small intestinal submucosa has been soaked in saline to make it pliable and soft and wrapped around an appropriately sized glass tube before sewing the edges together with an absorbable suture [79].

The suitability of this type of material for intestinal tissue engineering remains uncertain. When pieces of tubular small intestinal submucosa scaffold measuring 6 cm long and 2 cm in diameter were anastomosed to the native intestine in a canine model, all recipients suffered significant morbidity. This was apparently caused by leakage from the site of anastomosis or stenosis caused by the tube collapsing [79]. Also, despite the large number of studies having reported successful use of small intestinal submucosa as an acellular xenograft material, concerns have been raised about the clinical safety and efficacy of small intestinal submucosa–derived biomaterials. Noninfectious edema and severe pain has been observed at sites of implantation in some patients, a response suggested to be caused by the possible retention of multiple layers of porcine cells and DNA material causing an inflammatory response [88].

20.7.2.4 Indirect Three-Dimensional Printed Scaffolds

Indirect three-dimensional printing is another approach that has been used to fabricate porous tissue engineering scaffolds that can be modified to include villi features, making them a suitable scaffold for intestinal tissue engineering [89]. Three-dimensional printing creates three-dimensional scaffold structures by ink-jet printing liquid solvent binder droplets to join loose particles of polymer. After the solvent has dissolved the polymer, it evaporates allowing the polymer to reprecipitate forming a solid structure. The remaining polymer particles are leached out to produce a porous scaffold. Porogens can also be mixed with the polymer to further increase porosity. The printing process is computer-aided, allowing parameters such as micro- and macrostructure, mechanical properties, porosity, and composition to be optimized. Indirect three-dimensional printing has been proposed as a way of overcoming limitations associated with direct printing, such as pore size, shape complexity associated with the use of organic solvent liquid binders, and the need for customized machines when using biodegradable polymers and solvents. Indirect three-dimensional printing involves printing a plaster mold and solvent-casting the polymer into the mold cavity. Molds to fabricate scaffolds with small villi (850 μm diameter, 150 μm apart) were designed by computer software. The water-based binder was printed onto layers of plaster powder (average particle size ~20 μm) to form a two-dimensional pattern. The process was repeated to form additional layers until the desired three-dimensional mold was completed. The molds were dried and infiltrated with polyethylene glycol to block surface pores in the mold and to increase its mechanical strength. For the solvent-casting process, sucrose particles (100–150 μm) were mixed into a solution of poly(lactic-co-glycolic acid) dissolved in chloroform and methanol and cast into the molds. After the scaffolds were freeze-dried, the molds and sucrose were leached simultaneously by immersing in deionized water. The outer surface of the scaffolds was further cleaned and modified by etching with ethanol and coated with fibronectin to increase adhesion, viability, and proliferation of rat intestinal epithelial cells seeded onto the surface. The epithelial cells were initially attached uniformly throughout the scaffold, but after longer periods of culturing, the cell density increased in the villi-shaped regions but remained low within the scaffold, possibly due to limited diffusion of oxygen and nutrients [89]. The use of such techniques to fabricate a scaffold containing villi is advantageous as it would increase the absorptive surface area of tissue-engineered intestinal construct.

20.7.2.5 Neovascularization of Intestinal Tissue Engineering Scaffolds

Sufficient neovascularization of tissue is essential to provide oxygen and nutrient delivery and removal of waste products to cells. Vascularization of tissue constructs is an important obstacle that is yet to be overcome satisfactorily in the engineering of any tissue larger than a few millimeters in volume. As with the majority of other organs tissue engineered to date, this problem affects intestinal tissue engineering [90]. A number of options have been suggested for modifying the biomaterials used to fabricate the scaffold to increase neovascularization. These include biodegradable polymers that provide localized and sustained growth factor release [91,92].

Incorporation of angiogenic growth factor proteins into polymeric devices is one way of stimulating neovascularization in the tissue-engineered construct that also enables the duration of growth factor release at the target site to be controlled. The duration of delivery can be influenced by protein loading, the type of polymer used to fabricate the device, and the processing conditions. Therefore, the type of growth factor, dosage, release kinetics, and duration of delivery are all parameters that require optimization. Growth factors can be incorporated into the scaffold either during or after scaffold fabrication. When biodegradable scaffolds are used, the growth factor is released as the scaffolds degrade, stimulating vascularization and tissue growth to replace the lost scaffold. The growth factors are released either via diffusion mechanisms, which are controlled by the porosity of the scaffold, or by erosion mechanisms.

A steady supply of growth factors, such as vascular endothelial growth factor (VEGF) and fibroblast growth factor-2 (FGF2) that show combined effects on angiogenesis and maturation of blood vessels is required to provide tissues with adequate exposure to the angiogenic stimulus. At the same time, because of the potent stimulatory effect of VEGF and other growth factors, systemic exposure is not desirable since it may enhance angiogenesis associated with pathological conditions, such as neoplasia or retinopathy. Therefore, scaffolds that provide sustained localized delivery of the growth factor are sought.

The most straightforward way to incorporate growth factors into tissue engineering scaffolds is to either soak the fabricated scaffold in a solution of the growth factor and rely on adsorption of the protein to the scaffold material or mix growth factors with the suspension of cells during the cell seeding process. Although both approaches are relatively easy to perform, the controlled release and duration of growth factor activity are usually not optimal.

A different approach relies on incorporating functional groups into the scaffold that will bind the growth factor and exert some control over the release of the protein. This has recently been demonstrated using acellular collagen–heparin scaffolds [93]. Porous collagen scaffolds were prepared by freeze-drying a solution of collagen dissolved in acetic acid. The scaffolds were cross-linked using 1-ethyl-3-dimethyl aminopropyl carbodiimide and N-hydroxysuccinimide in 2-morpholinoethane sulfonic acid in the presence of ethanol and heparin. After washing, the scaffolds were incubated in phosphate buffer saline containing either VEGF or bFGF. The covalently bound heparin in the collagen scaffold allowed coupling of the heparin-binding growth factors bFGF and VEGF. When implanted subcutaneously in an animal model, the dual growth factor–loaded scaffold led to the earlier establishment of a high-density vasculature that was well-developed when compared with the other acellular scaffolds tested [93].

Alternatively, an additional device, such as microspheres, capable of delivering growth factors can be incorporated into the scaffold to provide sustained and controlled localized delivery. Scaffolds containing polymer microspheres have been fabricated using a gas foaming or particulate leaching process that enables controlled release of VEGF [94]. The scaffolds were fabricated from either poly(lactic-co-glycolic acid) microspheres and VEGF or a mixture of poly(lactic-co-glycolic) microspheres, VEGF, and poly(lactic-co-glycolic) particulates ground to an average diameter of 125 µm. Poly(lactic-co-glycolic acid) microspheres were prepared using a double emulsion (water-in-oil-in-water) process incorporating VEGF. The first emulsion was prepared by dissolving the polymer in ethyl acetate into which an aqueous solution of the growth factor was mixed. Poly(vinyl alcohol) in ethyl acetate was mixed with the first emulsion and stirred into a solution of ethyl acetate, poly(vinyl alcohol) and water. The ethyl acetate was evaporated from the solution, allowing the microspheres to harden, which were then collected by filtration and freeze-dried. The polymer microspheres (with or without particles) were combined with NaCl particles (250–425 µm). Alginate was added to the mixture to increase incorporation and stabilization of the VEGF protein. The polymer or growth factor mixture was freeze-dried and pressed into a pellet using a Carver press. The pellets were equilibrated under high-pressure CO_2 before being rapidly returned to atmospheric pressure, causing thermodynamic instability that led to the polymer foaming and creating an interconnected structure around the NaCl particles. The NaCl particles were leached from the polymer structure scaffold to create a macroporous scaffold. The particulate polymer and microspheres fused to form a continuous homogeneous matrix with open pore structure. The different approaches used to incorporate VEGF into the scaffold led to different patterns of distribution of the growth factor in the scaffold and variations to the release kinetics. Directly incorporating VEGF led to it being located adjacent to scaffold pores and its rapid release, whereas pre-encapsulating the growth factor in microspheres prior to incorporation into the scaffold led to it being embedded deeply in the scaffold, which delayed its release [94]. The same approach was used to incorporate two different angiogenic growth factors (VEGF and platelet-derived growth factor) into a scaffold, creating a dual delivery system [95]. Here, one factor was mixed with the particulate polymer while the other was pre-encapsulated into the microspheres, resulting in the two growth factors being released at different rates.

Alginate microspheres containing fibroblasts and bioactive glass particles have also been used as angiogenic growth factor delivery devices [22]. Cells encapsulated in alginate microspheres are not exposed to the host's immune system and thus avoid rejection, but are able to receive oxygen and nutrients and release growth factors into the local host tissue. A solution of alginate-containing cells and bioactive glass particles was used to fabricate microspheres by coacervation in a solution of $CaCl_2$. The cells encapsulated in the microspheres were stimulated by the bioactive glass particles to secrete VEGF, which was released from the microspheres.

Since the process of neovascularization requires a number of different growth factors, the use of cells, provided with an appropriate stimulus such as bioactive glass, is likely to be advantageous over polymers providing single or dual growth factor delivery as it offers the ability to deliver several types of angiogenic growth factors at more physiologically relevant doses.

However, scaffold fabrication processes become limited when biological agents, such as growth factors, plasmid DNA, and viral vectors, are incorporated into the scaffold-processing techniques, which involve the use of high temperatures and solvents that would be detrimental to the biological activity of these agents. Composite polymers containing bioactive particles have been suggested to provide a solution to these problems. Third-generation biomaterials, such as bioactive glass, stimulate cell protein and gene expression [96]. The use of these nonbiological biomaterials can eliminate the need to incorporate biological factors into the scaffold fabrication process, avoiding the aforementioned problems while also potentially increasing the range of polymers/solvents/ temperatures that can be used to fabricate scaffolds and also increase the shelf life of prefabricated scaffolds. The use of bioactive glass particles in polymer scaffolds has recently been shown to stimulate angiogenesis. Polymer mesh scaffolds coated with a low concentration of bioactive glass and implanted subcutaneously *in vivo* were found to stimulate significantly greater infiltration of blood vessels into the polymer mesh compared with uncoated control scaffolds [97]. The mesh, consisting of woven poly(glycolic acid) fibers, was coated with 45S5 bioactive glass particles by immersing it into a stable slurry of glass particles in distilled water. After allowing the coated meshes to dry at room temperature, they were made porous again by flexing that left a thin coating of particles on the surface of the polymer fibers [97]. The angiogenic response observed has been suggested to result from the ability of certain bioactive glasses to stimulate cells infiltrating the scaffold to secrete angiogenic growth factors, such as VEGF, which stimulates angiogenesis and neovascularization [98,99].

20.8　SUMMARY

Biomaterials have been used for many centuries to assist therapeutic strategies associated with the gastrointestinal tract. Their usage continues to evolve with new applications, such as cavity filling materials combined with the use of key-hole surgery, nanotechnology-based drug delivery systems, and biologically active tissue engineering scaffolds, all of which are still in their infancies. With such a broad range of uses, there has been the parallel demand for new fabrication processes or the application of existing techniques to some of the new biomaterials.

Although many of the biomaterials used in the gastrointestinal tract have good safety profiles, issues have been raised about the long-term safety and efficacy of some of the newer materials, particularly relating to degradation products or migration of the implanted material. Further development of the materials will resolve many of the issues raised and improve their efficacies.

REFERENCES

1. O'Hara, A.M. and Shanahan, F. The gut flora as a forgotten organ. *EMBO Rep.*, 7, 688, 2006.
2. Pope, C.E. Acid-reflux disorders. *N. Eng. J. Med.*, 331, 656, 1994.
3. Locke, G.R. et al. Prevalence and clinical spectrum of gastroesophageal reflux: a population-based study in Olmsted County, Minnesota. *Gastroenterology*, 112, 1448, 1997.
4. O'Connor, K.W. and Lehman, G.A. Endoscopic placement of collagen at the lower esophageal sphincter to inhibit gastroesophageal reflux: a pilot study of 10 medically intractable patients. *Gastrointest. Endosc.*, 34, 106, 1988.
5. Aucejo, S., Marco, C., and Gavara, R. Water effect on the morphology of EVOH copolymers. *J. Appl. Polym. Sci.*, 74, 1201, 1999.
6. Louis, H. et al. Three years follow-up for initial GERD patients injected with EVOH polymer (abstr). *Gastroenterology*, 124, A419, 2003.
7. Peters, J.H., Silverman, D.E., and Stein, A. Lower esophageal sphincter injection of a biocompatible polymer: accuracy of implantation assessed by esophagectomy. *Surg. Endosc.*, 17, 547, 2003.
8. Mason, R.J. et al. Endoscopic augmentation of the cardia with a biocompatible injectable polymer (Enteryx) in a porcine model. *Surg. Endosc.*, 16, 386, 2002.
9. Sandborn, W.J. et al. AGA technical review on perianal Crohn's disease. *Gastroenterology*, 125, 1508, 2003.
10. Hughes, L. Surgical pathology and management of anorectal Crohn's disease. *J. R. Soc. Med.*, 71, 644, 1978.
11. Parks, A. Pathogenesis and treatment of fistuila-in-ano. *Br. Med. J.*, 1, 463, 1961.
12. Hawley, P.R. Anorectal fistula. *Clin. Gastroenterol.*, 4, 635, 1975.
13. Vasilevsky, C., Stein, B. In: Wexner S, Vernava A, eds. *Clinical Decision Making in Colorectal Surgery.* New York: Igaku-Shoin, 137, 1995.
14. Schuppan, D. and Freitag, T. Fistulising Crohn's disease: MMPs gone awry. *Gut*, 53, 622, 2004.
15. Seow-Choen, F. et al. Bacteriology of anal fistulae. *Br. J. Surg.*, 79, 27, 1992.
16. Schwartz, D.A. and Herdman, C.R. Review article: the medical treatment of Crohn's perianal fistulas. *Aliment. Pharmacol. Ther.*, 19, 953, 2004.
17. Hammond, T.M., Grahn, M.F., and Lunniss, P.J. Fibrin glue in the management of anal fistulae. *Colorectal Dis.*, 6, 308, 2004.
18. Mawatari, M. et al. Effectiveness of autologous fibrin tissue adhesive in reducing postoperative blood loss during total hip arthroplasty: a prospective randomised study of 100 cases. *J. Orthop. Surg.* (Hong Kong), 14, 117, 2006.
19. Sentovich, S.M. Fibrin glue for all anal fistulas. *J. Gastrointest. Surg.*, 5, 158, 2001.
20. Loungnarath, R. et al. Fibrin glue treatment of complex anal fistulas has low success rate. *Dis. Colon. Rectum.*, 47, 432, 2004.
21. Keshaw, H. et al. Development of a collagen-ceramic composite for fistula repair. *Gut*, 55, suppl II, A86, 2006.
22. Keshaw, H., Forbes, A., and Day, R.M. Release of angiogenic growth factors from cells encapsulated in alginate beads with bioactive glass. *Biomaterials*, 26, 4171, 2005.
23. Nelson, R. et al. Community-based prevalence of anal incontinence. *JAMA*, 274, 559, 1995.
24. Tsai, C.C., Lin, V., and Tang, L. Injectable biomaterials for incontinence and vesico-ureteral reflux: current status and future promise. *J. Biomed. Mater. Res. B Appl. Biomater.*, 77, 171, 2006.
25. Shafik, A. Polytetrafluoroethylene injection for the treatment of partial fecal incontinence. *Int. Surg.*, 78, 159, 1993.
26. Malizia, A.A. et al. Migration and granulomatous reaction after periurethral injection of polytef (Teflon). *JAMA*, 251, 3277, 1984.

27. Mittleman, R.E. and Marraccini, J.V. Pulmonary teflon granulomas following periurethral teflon injection for urinary incontinence. *Arch. Pathol. Lab. Med.*, 107, 611, 1983.
28. Jain, R.A. The manufacturing techniques of various drug loaded biodegradable poly(lactide-co-glycolide) (PLGA) devices. *Biomaterials*, 21, 2475, 2000.
29. Wu, X.S. Preparation, characterization, and drug delivery applications of mucrospheres based on biodegradable lactic/glycolic acid polymers. In: Wise et al., eds. *Encyclopedism Handbook of Biomaterials and Bioengineering.* New York: Marcel Dekker, 1151, 1995.
30. Arshady, R. Preparation of biodegradable microspheres and microcapsules: 2. Polylactides and related polyesters. *J. Control. Rel.*, 17, 1, 1991.
31. Cho, E.R., Kang, S.W., and Kim, B.S. Poly(lactic-*co*-glycolic acid) microspheres as a potential bulking agent for urological injection therapy: preliminary results. *J. Biomed. Mater. Res. B Appl. Biomater.*, 72, 166, 2005.
32. Saralidze, K. et al. Injectable polymeric microspheres with x-ray visibility. Preparation, properties, and potential utility as new traceable bulking agents. *Biomacromolecules*, 4, 793, 2003.
33. Aldenhof, Y.B. et al. Stability of radiopaque iodine-containing biomaterials. *Biomaterials*, 23, 881, 2002.
34. Kumar, D., Benson, M.J., and Bland, J.E. Glutaraldehyde cross-linked collagen in the treatment of faecal incontinence. *Br. J. Surg.*, 85, 978, 1998.
35. Winters, J.C. InteXen tissue processing and laboratory study. *Int. Urogynecol. J. Pelvic Floor Dysfunct.*, 17, S34, 2006.
36. Jorge-Herrero, E., Fernandez, P., and Turnay, J. Influence of different chemical crosslinking treatments on the properties of bovine pericardium and collagen. *Biomaterials*, 20, 539, 1999.
37. Jayakrishnan, A. and Jameela, S.R. Glutaraldehyde as a fixative in bioprostheses and drug delivery matrices. *Biomaterials*, 17, 471, 1996.
38. Huang-Lee, L.L.H., Cheung, D.T., and Nimni, M. Biochemical changes and cytotoxicity associated with the degradation of polymeric glutaraldehyde derived crosslinks. *J. Biomed. Mater. Res.*, 24, 1185, 1990.
39. Gendler, E., Gendler, S., and Nimni, M.E. Toxic reactions evoked by glutaraldehyde-fixed pericardium and cardiac valve tissue bioprostheses. *J. Biomed. Mater. Res.*, 18, 727, 1984.
40. Nimni, M.E. et al. Factors which affect the calcification of tissue-derived bioprostheses. *J. Biomed. Mater. Res.*, 35, 531, 1997.
41. Haferkamp, A. et al. Failure of subureteral bovine collagen injection for the endoscopic treatment of primary vesicoureteral reflux in long-term follow-up. *Urology*, 55, 759, 2000.
42. Block, C.A., Cooper, C.S., and Hawtrey, C.E. Long-term efficacy of periurethral collagen injection for the treatment of urinary incontinence secondary to myelomeningocele. *J. Urol.*, 169, 327, 2003.
43. DeLustro, F. et al. Reaction to injectable collagen: results in animal models and clinical use. *Plast. Reconstr. Surg.*, 79, 581, 1987.
44. Leonard, M.P. et al. Endoscopic subureteral collagen injection: are immunological concerns justified? *J. Urol.*, 160, 1012, 1998.
45. Davis, K., Kumar, D., and Poloniecki, J. Preliminary evaluation of an injectable anal sphincter bulking agent (durasphere) in the management of faecal incontinence. *Aliment. Pharmacol. Ther.*, 18, 237, 2003.
46. Pannek, J., Brands, F.H., and Senge, T. Particle migration after transurethral injection of carbon coated beads for stress urinary incontinence. *J. Urol.*, 166, 1350, 2001.
47. Ellis, H. The magnitude of adhesion related problems. *Ann. Chir. Gynaecol.*, 87, 9, 1998.
48. Ellis, H. Intraabdominal and postoperative peritoneal adhesions. *J. Am. Coll. Surg.*, 200, 643, 2005.
49. Becker, J.M. et al. Prevention of postoperative abdominal adhesions by a sodium hyaluronate-based bioresorbable membrane: a prospective, randomized, doubleblind multicenter study. *J. Am. Coll. Surg.*, 183, 297, 1996.
50. Beck, D.E. The role of Seprafilm™ bioresorbable membrane in adhesion prevention. *Eur. J. Surg.*, 577, 49, 1997.
51. Burns, J.W., Cox, S., and Walts, A.E., *Water Insoluble Derivatives of Hyaluronic Acid.* Cambridge, MA: Genzyme Corp, 1991.
52. Burns, J.W. et al. A hyaluronate based gel for the prevention of postsurgical adhesions: evaluation in two animal species. *Fertil. Steril.*, 66, 814, 1996.
53. De Iaco, P.A., et al. A novel hyaluronan-based gel in laparo-scopic adhesion prevention: preclinical evaluation in an animal model. *Fertil. Steril.*, 69, 318, 1998.

54. De Iaco, P.A. et al. Efficacy of a hyaluronan derivative gel in postsurgical adhesion prevention in the presence of inadequate hemostasis. *Surgery*, 130, 60, 2001.

55. Mensitieri, M. et al. Viscoelastic properties modulation of a novel autocrosslinked hyaluronic acid polymer. *J. Mater. Sci. Mater. Med.*, 7, 695, 1996.

56. Liu, Y. et al. Crosslinked hyaluronan hydrogels containing mitomycin C reduce postoperative abdominal adhesions. *Fertil. Steril.*, 83, 1275, 2005.

57. Li, H. et al. Synthesis and biological evaluation of a crosslinked mitomycin C-hyaluronan hydrogel. *Biomacromolecules*, 5, 895, 2004.

58. Ma, Z. et al. Potential of nanofiber matrix as tissue-engineering scaffolds. *Tissue Eng.*, 11, 101, 2005.

59. Zong, X. et al. Prevention of postsurgery-induced abdominal adhesions by electrospun bioabsorbable nanofibrous poly(lactide-*co*-glycolide)-based membranes. *Ann. Surg.*, 240, 910, 2004.

60. Deitzel, J. et al. The effect of processing variables on the morphology of electrospun nanofibers and textiles. *Polymer*, 42, 261, 2001.

61. Chourasia, M.K. and Jain, S.K. Pharmaceutical approaches to colon targeted drug delivery systems. *J. Pharm. Pharm. Sci.*, 6, 33, 2003.

62. Lorenzo-Lamosa, M.L. et al. Design of microencapsulated chitosan microspheres for colonic drug delivery. *J. Control. Release*, 52, 109, 1998.

63. Hejazi, R. and Amiji, M. Chitosan-based gastrointestinal delivery systems. *J. Control. Release*, 89, 151, 2003.

64. Wittaya-areekul, S., Kruenate, J., and Prahsarn, C. Preparation and *in vitro* evaluation of mucoadhesive properties of alginate/chitosan microparticles containing prednisolone. *Int. J. Pharm.*, 312, 113, 2006.

65. Fiebrig, I. et al. Transmission electron microscopy on pig gastric mucin and its interactions with chitosan. *Carbohydr. Polym.*, 28, 239, 1995.

66. Gomez, W.R. and Wee, S.F. Protein release from alginate matrices. *Adv. Drug Deliv. Rev.*, 31, 267, 1998.

67. Rahman, Z. et al. Characterization of 5-fluorouracil microspheres for colonic delivery. *AAPS Pharm. Sci. Tech.*, 7, E47, 1998.

68. Iruin, A. et al. Elaboration and "*in vitro*" characterization of 5-ASA beads. *Drug Dev. Ind. Pharm.*, 31, 231, 2005.

69. Smidsrod, O. and Skjak-Braek, G. Alginate as immobilization matrix for cells. *Trends Biotechnol.*, 8, 71, 1990.

70. Klokk, T.I. and Melvik, J.E. Controlling the size of alginate gel beads by use of a high electrostatic potential. *J. Microencapsul.*, 19, 415, 2002.

71. Sankalia, M.G. et al. Papain entrapment in alginate beads for stability improvement and site-specific delivery: physicochemical characterization and factorial optimization using neural network modeling. *AAPS Pharm. Sci. Tech.*, 6, E209, 2005.

72. Meissner, Y., Pellequer, Y., and Lamprecht, A. Nanoparticles in inflammatory bowel disease: particle targeting versus pH-sensitive delivery. *Int. J. Pharm.*, 316, 138, 2006.

73. Sakuma, S., Hayashi, M., and Akashi, M. Design of nanoparticles composed of graft copolymers for oral peptide delivery. *Adv. Drug Deliv. Rev.*, 47, 21, 2001.

74. Takeuchi, H., Yamamoto, H., and Kawashima, Y. Mucoadhesive nanoparticulate systems for peptide drug delivery. *Adv. Drug Deliv. Rev.*, 47, 39, 2001.

75. Desai, M.P. et al. Gastrointestinal uptake of biodegradable microparticles: effect of particle size. *Pharm. Res.*, 13, 1838, 1996.

76. Lamprecht, A. et al. Biodegradable nanoparticles for targeted drug delivery in treatment of inflammatory bowel disease. *J. Pharmacol. Exp. Ther.*, 299, 775, 2001.

77. Kaihara, S. et al. Regenerative signals for intestinal epithelial organoid units transplanted on biodegradable polymer scaffolds for tissue engineering of small intestine. *Transplantation*, 67, 227, 1999.

78. Day, R.M. et al. *In vivo* characterisation of a novel bioresorbable poly(lactide-*co*-glycolide) tubular foam scaffold for tissue engineering applications. *J. Mater. Sci. Mater. Med.*, 15, 729, 2004.

79. Chen, M.K. and Badylak, S.F. Small bowel tissue engineering using small intestinal submucosa as a scaffold. *J. Surg. Res.*, 99, 352, 2001.

80. Hori, Y. et al. Experimental study on tissue engineering of the small intestine by mesenchymal stem cell seeding. *J. Surg. Res.*, 102, 156, 2002.

81. Mooney, D.J. et al. Stabilized polyglycolic acid fibre-based tubes for tissue engineering. *Biomaterials*, 17, 115, 1996.

82. Kaihara, S. et al. Long-term follow-up of tissue-engineered intestine after anastomosis to native small bowel. *Transplantation*, 69, 1927, 2000.

83. Maquet, V. et al. Preparation, characterization, and *in vitro* degradation of bioresorbable and bioactive composites based on Bioglass-filled polylactide foams. *J. Biomed. Mater. Res. A*, 66, 335, 2003.

84. Nam, Y.S. and Park, T.G. Biodegradable polymeric microcellular foams by modified thermally induced phase separation method. *Biomaterials*, 20, 1783, 1999.

85. Ansaloni, L. et al. Experimental evaluation of Surgisis as scaffold for neointestine regeneration in a rat model. *Transplant Proc.*, 38, 1844, 2006.

86. Hodde, J. Naturally occurring scaffolds for soft tissue repair and regeneration. *Tissue Eng.*, 8, 295, 2002.

87. Badylak, S. et al. Resorbable bioscaffold for esophageal repair in a dog model. *Pediatr. Surg.*, 35, 1097, 2000.

88. Zheng, M.H. et al. Porcine small intestine submucosa (SIS) is not an acellular collagenous matrix and contains porcine DNA: possible implications in human implantation. *J. Biomed. Mater. Res. B, Appl. Biomater.*, 73, 61, 2005.

89. Lee, M., Dunn, J.C., and Wu, B.M. Scaffold fabrication by indirect three-dimensional printing. *Biomaterials*, 26, 4281, 2005.

90. Gardner-Thorpe, J. et al. Angiogenesis in tissue-engineered small intestine. *Tissue Eng.*, 9, 1255, 2003.

91. Babensee, J.E., McIntire, L.V., and Mikos, A.G. Growth factor delivery for tissue engineering. *Pharm. Res.*, 17, 497, 2002.

92. Nomi, M. et al. Principles of neovascularization for tissue engineering. *Mol. Aspects Med.*, 23, 463, 2002.

93. Nillesen, S.T. et al. Increased angiogenesis and blood vessel maturation in acellular collagen-heparin scaffolds containing both FGF2 and VEGF. *Biomaterials*, 28, 1123, 2007.

94. Ennett, A.B., Kaigler, D., and Mooney, D.J. Temporally regulated delivery of VEGF *in vitro* and *in vivo*. *J. Biomed. Mater. Res. A*, 79, 176, 2006.

95. Richardson, T.P. et al. Polymeric system for dual growth factor delivery. *Nat. Biotechnol.*, 19, 1029, 2001.

96. Hench, L.L. and Polak, J.M. Third-generation biomedical materials. *Science*, 295, 1014, 2002.

97. Day, R.M. Assessment of polyglycolic acid mesh and bioactive glass for soft-tissue engineering scaffolds. *Biomaterials*, 25, 5857, 2004.

98. Day, R.M. et al. *In vitro* and *in vivo* analysis of macroporous biodegradable poly(D,L-lactide-*co*-glycolide) scaffolds containing bioactive glass. *J. Biomed. Mater. Res. A*, 75, 778, 2005.

99. Day, R.M. Bioactive glass stimulates the secretion of angiogenic growth factors and angiogenesis *in vitro*. *Tissue Eng.*, 11, 768, 2005.

21 Biomaterials for Cartilage Reconstruction and Repair

Wojciech Swieszkowski, Miroslawa El Fray,
and Krzysztof J. Kurzydlowski

CONTENTS

21.1   ARTICULAR CARTILAGE BIOLOGY—STRUCTURE AND PROPERTIES

Cartilage is a type of dense connective tissue composed of collagenous or elastic fibers and chondrocytes embedded in a firm gel-like matrix of proteoglycans. It is an avascular tissue with extremely limited capacity for repair. It appears in three different forms in the human body (Figure 21.1):

1. *Elastic cartilage*—found in noses and ears (contains elastin, a collagen type II, scattered throughout the matrix);
2. *Fibrocartilage*—found in ligaments, tendons, intervertebral disks (composed primarily of collagen type I);
3. *Hyaline cartilage*—found in lining bones in the joints (called *articular cartilage* [AC]), such as the knee, the ankle, the hip, the shoulder, and in any other moving joint such as the fingers (made predominantly of type II collagen).

The hyaline cartilage, the most abundant type, is capable of withstanding repeated load-bearing activities (resistance to compression) and it evenly distributes this load to the underlying subchondral bone [1].

The main components of mature AC are chondrocyte cells, which make up to 10% of the volume of the extracellular matrix (containing interstitial fluid, several forms of collagen, proteoglycans, noncollagenous proteins, nonspecific lipids, glycoproteins, and trace amount of various growth factors). The collagen is present as woven fibrous network in a polysaccharide matrix containing hyaluronic acid (HA), chondroitin sulfate, keratin sulfates, and stabilizing proteins. The chondroitin and keratin sulfates have hydrophilic groups, which bind water helping to stabilize and strengthen the system. Collagen fibrils (mainly collagen type II) are responsible for the tensile and shear stiffness of cartilage, whereas proteoglycans are responsible for the biomechanical properties

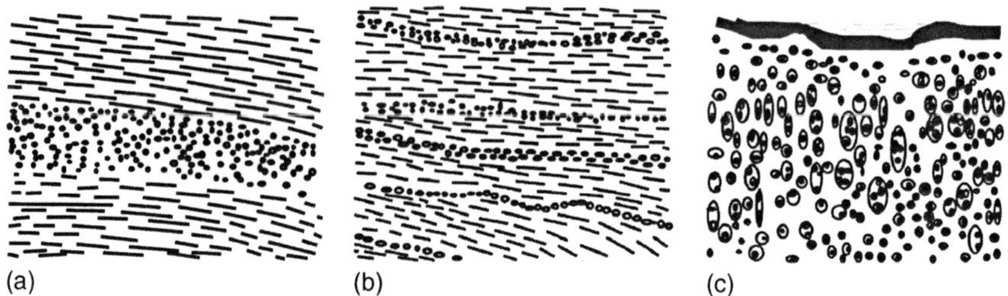

FIGURE 21.1 Schematic representation of three main types of cartilage: (a) elastic cartilage, (b) fibrocartilage, and (c) hyaline cartilage.

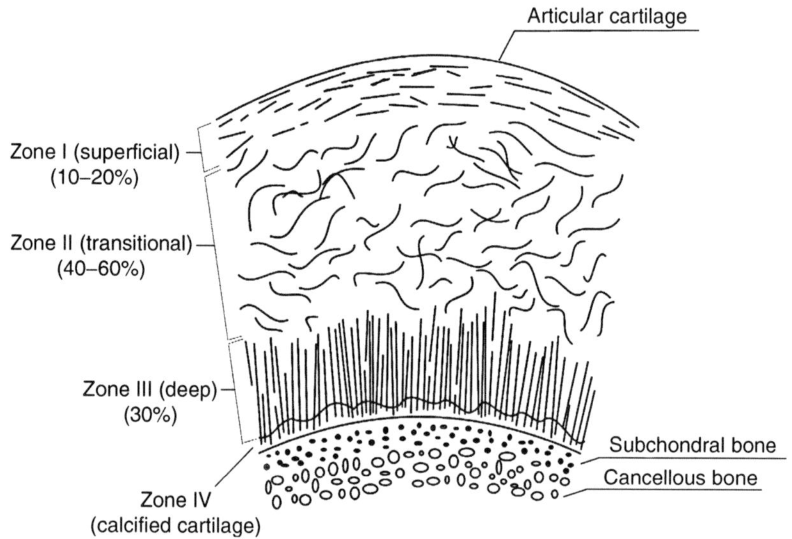

FIGURE 21.2 Articular cartilage (AC) architecture.

of cartilage in compression [2]. The liquid phase of the AC is mainly composed of water. Water makes up to 80% of the wet weight of AC [3]. Exudation and the movement of water through cartilage are dominant mechanisms controlling the compressibility of the tissue. When the cartilage is compressed, water moves aside, its thickness decreases, and the fluid leaks out of the matrix. Water keeps moving until an equilibrium pressure is obtained. When the loading is removed, water is drawn back into the cartilage. Working in a hydraulic fashion, the interstitial fluid can flow under compression within the cartilage and when the load is removed the fluid returns. Although AC lacks a network of capillaries to convey blood, it is instead nourished by the flow of synovial fluid.

From another point of view, AC is structurally graded, multilayered tissue with a fiber-reinforced composite structure. It is divided into four zones. Listing them from the articular surface (Figure 21.2), one can distinguish the (i) superficial zone, (ii) transitional (middle) zone, (iii) deep (radial) zone, and (iv) calcified cartilage zone. Each of them differs in chondrocytes arrangements, functions, and properties. Zone 1 is thin (10% of a total AC thickness) and contains flattened, horizontally distributed chondrocytes. Zone 2 is thicker (40–60% of a total thickness) and contains spherical chondrocytes. Collagen fibrils are horizontally arranged within zone 1, while in zone 2 they are randomly distributed. Zone 3 is characterized by columnar arrangement of spheroidal chondrocytes and vertical orientation of collagen fibrils (perpendicular to the joint surface). Zone 4 provides a direct fixation between the AC and the underlying subchondral bone. It contains smaller chondrocytes of lower level of metabolic activity (cells are surrounded by calcified extracellular matrix) [4].

Due to the complex gradient structure, AC shows anisotropic and nonlinear behavior in compression, tension, and shear. Moreover, the mechanical properties of cartilage depend on its height. The stiffness in axial direction increases with depth from the joint surface, especially in case of compressed cartilage [5]. A highly hydrated cartilage can be described as a poroviscoelastic material with a relatively low compressive stiffness (E = 0.1–2.0 MPa), Poisson's ratio (v = 0.2), and permeability (k = 5.0 × 10^{-15} m^4/N s) [6]. Despite the low stiffness, AC is able to transmit high loads (up to 10 times the body weight in the knee joint). Moreover, AC provides a low coefficient of friction of about 0.008 [5].

The functions of AC can be summarized as follows:

- Distributes high static and repetitive dynamic loads (up to 10 times the body weight)
- Protects cancellous bone from high stresses
- Provides a smooth, lubricated surface with a fluid film and a low coefficient of friction
- Reduces nominal contact pressure
- Guarantees joint conformity

21.2 REPAIR OF ARTICULAR CARTILAGE

Arthritis (*arth* = joint, *itis* = inflammation) is one of the oldest and most common diseases affecting human joints. It probably affects almost every person more than 60 years of age to some degree [7]. In general, arthritis affects approximately 15% of the total world population, and by the year 2020, this number is expected to increase to 18.2% due to increased aging. In arthritic joints, the cartilage is degraded, causing pain, loss of mobility, and joint stiffness. In addition to osteoarthritis, focal osteochondral injuries arising from sports are another cause for increasing applications of treatment methods. Due to limited potential for regeneration related to the absence of blood circulation, the treatment of cartilage defects is one of the most important problems in orthopedic surgery.

Unfortunately, in contrast to bone tissue, AC has a poor intrinsic capacity for repair. This limited cartilage regeneration is caused by (i) its avascular (and aneural) nature, (ii) relatively low cell density, (iii) low mitotic activity of the cells, and (iv) structural restriction to free migration of the cells.

The cartilage tissue response to injury or disease depends largely upon whether it involves only part of the tissue (partial-thickness defects) or extends to the subchondral bone (full-thickness defects).

Partial-thickness defects of AC resemble the clefts and fissures observed during the initial stages of osteoarthritis. Defects of this nature in mature tissue do not heal spontaneously. In such a tissue, a limited repair process takes place in response to the trauma within the tissue immediately adjacent to the site of the defect (a brief period of chondrocyte proliferation and matrix synthesis).

Full-thickness defects pass through the zone of calcified cartilage and penetrate the subchondral bone thereby gaining access to the cells that reside in the bone marrow space including the mesenchymal stem cells located therein. The repair response of this type of a defect results in the formation of a fibrocartilaginous tissue in the void. An immediate response to penetration of the subchondral bone by a full-thickness defect, in some cases, brings about the formation of hyaline-like AC. This repair tissue is a poor substitute for AC and, with time, there is marked degeneration of the repair tissue and continued degeneration of the native AC.

Restoring a damaged articular surface is quiet a challenge calling for a multidisciplinary approach that has to bring together research scientists, clinicians, and patients. Many new AC repair techniques have emerged in the past decades some of which appear to be very promising. The currently available treatments can be divided into four basic categories: (i) treatments that stimulate the bone marrow to form a repair tissue, (ii) transplantation of osteochondral autografts or allografts, (iii) implantation or transplantation of cultured autologous chondrocytes, and (iv) usage of resorbable scaffolding with or without cells.

Many of the arthroscopic repair strategies employed utilize the intrinsic repair response to induce the formation of a repair tissue within the defect [8].

Arthroscopic lavage and debridement are often used to alleviate joint pain. Lavage involves irrigation of the joint during arthroscopy. Debridement is the arthroscopic removal of damaged tissue from the joint, which has also been shown to alleviate pain and when used in conjunction with lavage, pain relief appears to last longer [9]. Both lavage and debridement, however, do not induce repair of AC in full-thickness defects.

Soft tissue grafts involving the transplantation of periosteum and perichondrium to full-thickness defects of AC have been used extensively in animal models and human clinical trials. It must be noted that periosteum has chondrogenic potential.

Osteochondral transplantation of autogenic and allogeneic tissues has been widely used to treat predominately large osteochondral defects. Though allogenic material derived from cadaveric donors has been used to treat osteochondral defects, an immune response is still a potential problem with this approach [10]. Autologous osteochondral grafts involve the removal of cylindrical plugs of osteochondral tissue from nonload-bearing regions of the AC, such as the femoral trochlear groove, and transplantation of the debrided full-depth defect. This procedure is limited by: 1) insufficient supply of donor tissue, 2) the difficulty of carving the host cartilage into the desired three-dimensional (3D) structure, 3) the chemical and mechanical instabilities of the graft, 4) mismatch of the articular surface of the donor and the host, and 5) an unfavorable immune response by synovial fluid [4].

Cell-based transplantation methods currently involve the transplantation of expanded autologous chondrocytes to the defects to form a repair tissue.

Autologous chondrocyte transplantation (ACT) in humans is a procedure involving the excision of a healthy biopsy by arthroscopy from a nonload-bearing region of the AC. The chondrocytes are then released by enzymatic digestion and expanded in culture. A second procedure is then performed by arthrotomy. The defect is debrided back to the healthy cartilage but not to the subchondral bone. A periosteal graft is taken from the medial tibia, sutured over the defect, and cultured autologous chondrocytes are then injected under the periosteal flap. Although, the ACT method is used very often, the repair tissue differs in structure from normal cartilage due to the lack of the preferential collagen arrangement, which could be found in the normal cartilage.

21.3   CARTILAGE RECONSTRUCTION—ARTIFICIAL CARTILAGE

Various materials, including biological and synthetic matrices with growth factors or chondrocytes, are used to restore, maintain, or improve tissue functions. Much attention is focused on the use of biocompatible synthetic matrices. Inorganic materials such as carbon fibers and hydroxyapatites, various polymers such as polytetrafluoroethylene, polyesters, poly(lactic acid) (PLA), and hydrogels such as poly(vinyl alcohol) (PVA) (Figure 21.3) have been used as artificial cartilage [11].

These materials are used very often as artificial osteochondral substitutes ("plugs") implanted in the cartilage defects to stop further fracture [12,13]. Meyer et al. [14] reported the clinical application of the plugs made of PVA hydrogel (SaluCartilage).

21.3.1   HYDROGELS

Hydrogels, both degradable and nondegradable, are widely studied for biomedical applications, including tissue engineering (TE), drug delivery, or cartilage repair. The network structure of polymeric hydrogels is made of cross-linked polar chains. This structure allows them to hold large amount of fluids (i.e., water) without dissolving. The hydrogels have a high permeability to small molecules and viscoelastic behaviors. These properties make hydrogels similar to biological tissues. These materials also show good biocompatibility. Cartilage reconstruction is generally based on polymeric hydrogels, which could form 3D porous scaffolds. Hydrogels for biomedical applications based on natural and synthetic polymers are hydrophilic polymer networks that may

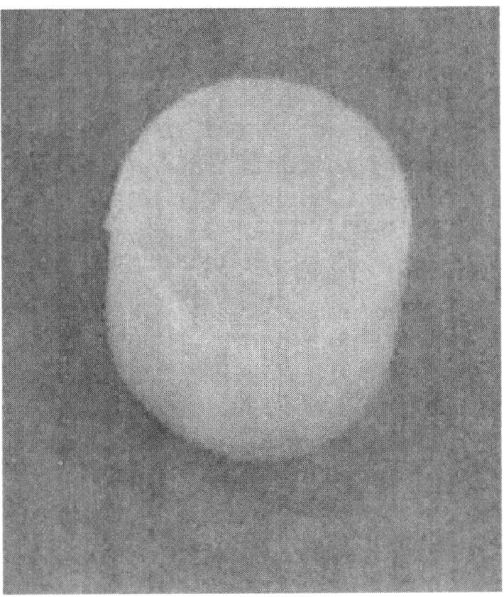

FIGURE 21.3   Poly(vinyl alcohol) (PVA) hydrogel.

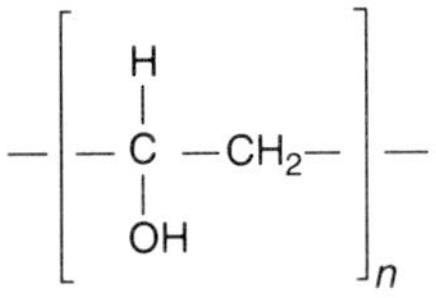

$$-\left[-\underset{\underset{\displaystyle OH}{|}}{\overset{\overset{\displaystyle H}{|}}{C}}-CH_2-\right]_n-$$

FIGURE 21.4   Chemical structure of poly(vinyl alcohol).

increase their weight in water by the amount varying from 10% to 20% up to 1000 times. Naturally derived hydrogel-forming polymers include collagen, chitosan, fibrin, gelatin, and HA. Synthetic polymers that may be used to form hydrogels are poly(ethylene oxide) (PEO), poly(acrylic acid) (PAA), poly(propylene fumarate-*co*-ethylene glycol) P(PF-*co*-EG), poly(hydroxy butyrate) (PHB), poly(vinyl pyrrolidone) (PVP), and PVA [15–17].

Hydrogels as materials for tissue replacement have many advantages, such as physical properties similar to natural cartilage, good transport of nutrients to the cells and products from the cells, biocompatibility, possibility of easy modification with cell adhesion ligands, etc. They can be injected *in vivo* as a liquid that gels at body temperature. However, one significant disadvantage of hydrogels is their low mechanical strength. For instance, Bray and Merrill [18] suggested, nearly 33 years ago, that PVA (Figure 21.4) might be a suitable material for synthetic AC applications. However, there was an 85% failure rate after 150 h from seven tests on a hip joint simulator.

One of the ways to improve the mechanical properties of PVA hydrogels is by the addition of a large amount of cross-linking agents. For hydrogels with hydroxyl or amino groups in the main chain, the most popular cross-linking agents are glutaraldehyde, acetaldehyde, and formaldehyde. Their reactions with polymer occur in the presence of sulfuric acid, acetic acid, or methanol [19–21]. For instance, the use of glutaraldehyde as cross-linking agent resulted in hydrogels of lower water contents (50%) with improved mechanical properties [22]. However, when the cross-linking density is altered, the swelling rates are reduced [23]. Because of the toxicity of these compounds that strongly influences the cell growth, some alternatives have been developed. Hydrogels were also obtained using gamma radiation in the presence of succinic or citric acid [24]. Other examples of nontoxic cross-linking agents are enzymes such as transglutaminase [25].

An alternative method of hydrogel preparation without using toxic additives is the freezing–thawing process in cycles repeated several times [26]. In this process, aqueous solution of PVA is frozen at $-20°C \pm 2$ and then thawed at room temperature, resulting in the formation of crystallites [27]. Such technological parameters as (i) number of freezing–thawing cycles, (ii) time of each operation, and also (iii) molecular weight and concentration of PVA determine the final properties of produced cryogels [28,29]. By cycling freezing–thawing process, the Young's modulus is significantly increased (up to 20 MPa) [30]. Moreover, after this process, the hydrogel is more thermally stable.

Ku et al. [31] described one of the methods of making the PVA cryogel in detail. In short, about 25% (by weight) aqueous solution of PVA (with M_n of above 70,000) was subjected to a series of freezing $(-20°C)$–thawing cycles, increasing the strength with each cycle. Then the samples were submerged in a deionized water bath and equilibrated at 37°C. Stammen et al. [32] and Swieszkowski et al. [33] investigated the mechanical properties of this type of hydrogel at 37°C. Cylindrical cryogel samples were compressed under displacement control at a rate of 508 mm/min until 35% strain was reached. Additionally, the material was tested in tension at a rate of 508 mm/min until failure. The failure strain of 226% was measured for such a material. Average tensile stress at failure was about 5 MPa. Unlike many other gels, the PVA cryogel did not soften or swell substantially at the body temperature.

To evaluate an elastic PVA implant for AC replacement, a numerical analysis was performed using finite element method (FEM) [33]. The objective of this study was to investigate the mechanical response of a PVA hydrogel as used for the articular surface of the glenoid component of a total shoulder arthroplasty. Based on numerical analyses, it was found that replacement of polyethylene with the hydrogel layer results in the significant reduction in the von Mises (Figure 21.5) and contact stresses together with the growth in contact area. The lower stresses in turn promote fluid film lubrication and reduce the wear and implant failure. This study showed a high potential of using PVA for articular surface in glenoid component.

Recently, Grant et al. [34] proposed an improvement of the PVA hydrogel biocompatibility by treating its surface with HA to mimic the viscous lubrication layer observed on AC. Such a treatment results in elastic modulus and friction coefficient similar to that reported for AC. Further improvement could be done by the addition of a lipid layer to the PVA hydrogel.

To improve the mechanical strength of hydrogels, multifunctional carboxylic acids taken from a large group of biologically active compounds present in metabolic pathway of chemical reactions

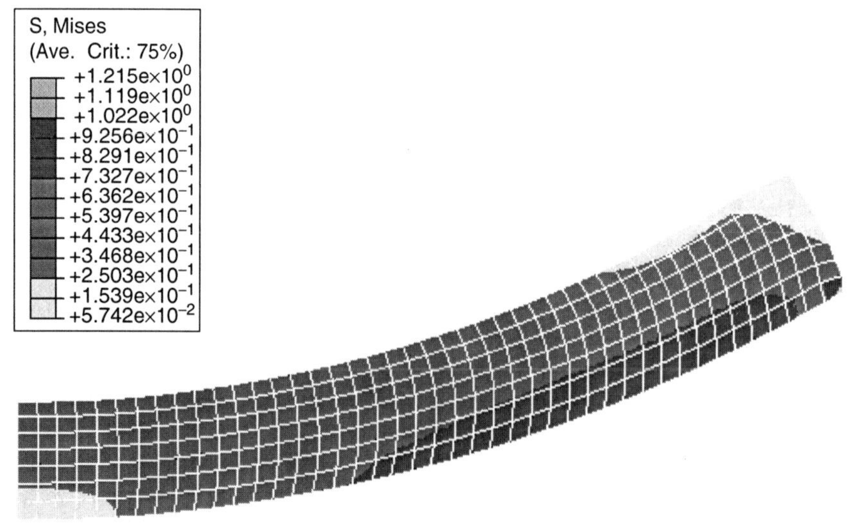

FIGURE 21.5 von Mises stresses for PVA-c layer with thickness of 2 mm.

occurring within the living organisms (including Krebs cycle) were applied by El Fray et al. as nontoxic cross-linking agents [35–37]. Due to the presence of two or more functional groups (carboxylic groups, hydroxyl groups), hydrogen bonds are additionally formed in the polymer network during freezing–thawing process, leading to cryogels with mechanical properties useful for cartilage repair. In applied freezing–thawing process, water acts as an expanding agent (porophor). When the PVA solution is subjected to freezing, the pure solvent crystallizes initially, while the solute stays in the liquid part of the specimen. Such a structure leads to stronger polymer–polymer and polymer–carboxylic acid interactions that result in stable 3D cryogel network [38]. The reactions proposed to occur between PVA and acids are presented in Figure 21.6.

The internal porosity of cryogels reveals significant correlation among number of freezing–thawing cycles, the chemical structure of additive, and the pore size and arrangement. PVA cryogel modified with succinic acid after nine freezing–thawing cycles shows highly porous structure with the pore size in the range of 1–2 µm (Figure 21.7a). The size of pores corresponds to the one

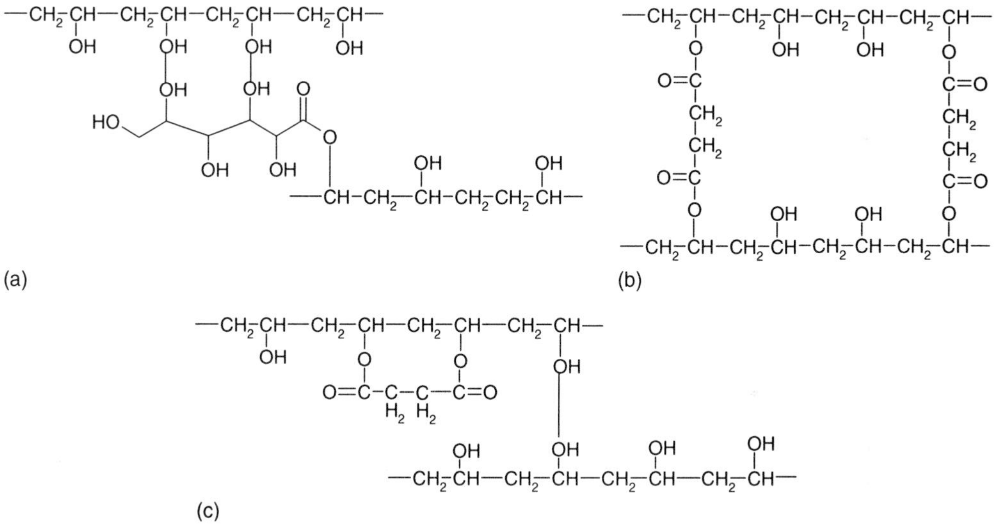

FIGURE 21.6 Scheme of possible reactions occurring between PVA chain and gluconic (a) and succinic acids (b and c).

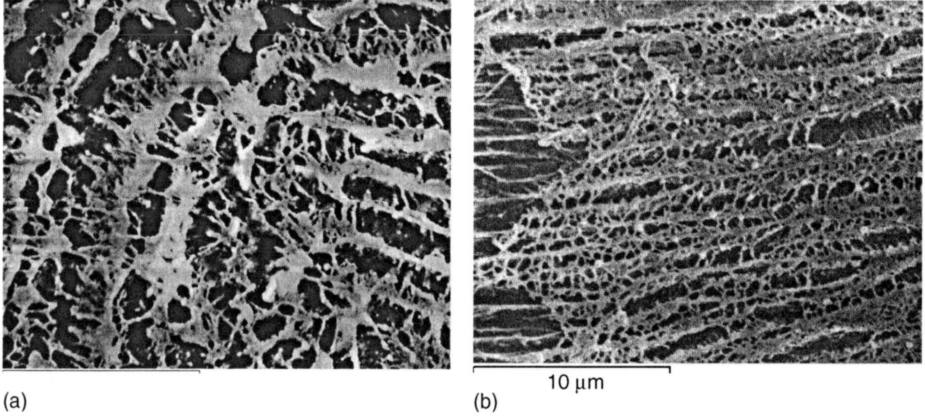

FIGURE 21.7 Internal porosity of PVA cryogel modified with (a) succinic acid and (b) gluconic acid.

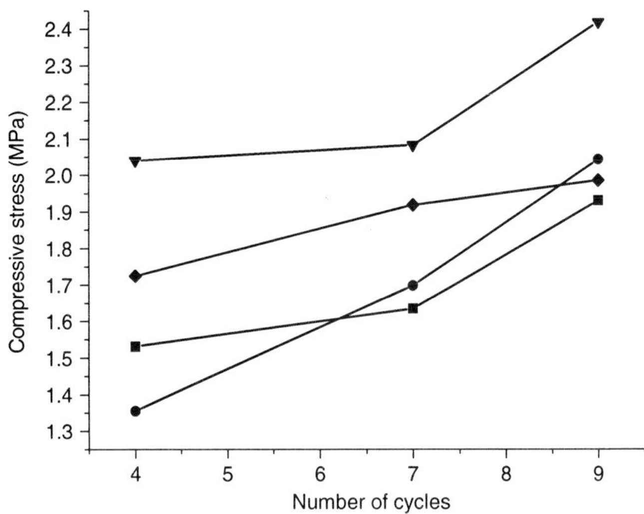

FIGURE 21.8   Compressive stress as function of freezing–thawing cycles: (■) 25% PVA, (●) 25% PVA 3% PVP, (♦) 25% PVA 3% succinic acid, and (▼) 25% PVA 3% gluconic acid.

observed by Watase et al. [39], but they differ in shape. PVA cryogels prepared using succinic acid are characterized by the ribbon-like and ordered structure than the honeycomb-like structure. After introducing multifunctional bioactive molecules of carboxylic acid (e.g., gluconic acid) (Figure 21.7b) as a cross-linking agent, long and parallel fibrils, bridged through thin lamella, form porous structure with a pore size less than 1 μm. In this case, pores of honeycomb-like structure are formed during subsequent freezing–thawing cycles.

High internal porosity strongly influences the mechanical properties of cryogels as illustrated in Figure 21.8. Materials with less ordered, mesh-like morphology obtained in a low number of freezing–thawing cycles and difunctional molecules exhibit lower compressive stress as compared to samples with multifunctional molecules subjected to higher number of freezing–thawing cycles. It has also been found that prepared blends were characterized by elastic modulus of $E_c = 7.2 - 14.1$ MPa at 60% strain, which is very well comparable to the properties of natural cartilage ($E_c = 1.9 - 14.4$ MPa by 30% of strain) [40].

Improvement in the characteristics of hydrogel could also be achieved by the addition of biological macromolecules. For this purpose, biopolymers such as collagen, found in the extracellular matrix, can be employed [40].

Another type of emerging polymeric biomaterial used for cartilage repair is poly(ethylene glycol) (PEG) hydrogel. PEG is widely used in many biomedical applications because of its combination of outstanding physicochemical and biological properties such as hydrophilicity, lack of toxicity, antigenocity, and immunogenocity [41]. PEG copolymers of ethylene oxide and propylene oxide can be used as injectable matrices for chondrocytes transplantation [41].

Microporous poly(2-hydroxyethyl methacrylate) (poly(HEMA)) gels were also investigated for use as replacement of AC [42]. The tensile strength of this material was almost 20 times lower than that for AC, which reduced the possibility of its use as artificial cartilage.

Another material that has potential in cartilage replacement is a semi-interpenetrating polymer (SIPN), which is synthesized from *N*-vinyl pyrrolidone-methyl methacrylate (copolymer) and reinforced with cellulose acetate butyrate (polymer) [43]. The tensile strength (10 MPa) and modulus (90 MPa) of this SIPN correspond with the mechanical properties of natural cartilage. Additionally, the elongation to break (120%) is greater than that of cartilage (80%). However, biocompatibility of such a polymer is still not fully tested (tests are still in progress).

21.3.2 Synthetic Segmented Polyesters and Polyurethanes

Synthetic segmented polyesters and polyurethanes are interesting materials for AC repair because of the versatility of the synthesis processes and useful intrinsic properties of a group of thermoplastic elastomers (TPE) by which these polymers are classified. The acronym TPE defines the polymers of specific properties being a consequence of a unique structure showing the lack of miscibility between discrete thermoplastic segments capable of forming rigid nanoscale domains or channels (hard segments) and covalently bonded to rubber-like segments (soft segments) (Figure 21.9). The hard domains render high mechanical strength. They also influence the processing conditions. The soft domains are responsible for elasticity and capacity to accumulate large strains—typical characteristic of elastomers [44].

Due to the covalent linkages between the chemically dissimilar segments, the rigid domains can form a 3D network of cross-linked domains, which are thermally reversible. The key property of TPE is their processability typical of the thermoplastics and the elasticity of vulcanized rubber. This is achieved by combining properties of the constituents—low glass transition of the soft, elastomeric component and high melting point of the glassy or semicrystalline thermoplastics.

The elastic properties and simultaneously thermoplastic character of TPE result from their molecular and submolecular structures, and morphology [45]. Due to the possibility of controlling the concentration of the hard and soft phases at the synthesis stage (polyester and polyurethane-type TPE are synthesized by step growth polymerization reactions), it is possible to produce TPE varying in their properties from hard thermoplastics to rubber-like materials [44].

Depending on the varying chemical nature of blocks, different combinations of semicrystalline and amorphous phases are possible. Hard blocks are crystallizable, as demonstrated by segmented (multiblock) copolymers of poly(butylene terephthalate) (PBT), with amorphous PEG forming soft blocks (Figure 21.10).

When the concentration of the soft segment is very low (30 wt.%), PBT-based poly(ester–ether) copolymers resemble cartilage material in terms of the mechanical properties [46–48]. Moreover, they are biodegradable and can be used as scaffolds for cartilaginous matrix formation [49].

Polyurethane TPE were intensively developed and applied for many years in such areas as biostable implantable devices (e.g., indwelling catheters, intra-aortic balloons, components of artificial heart or breast implants). Their chemical structure is presented in Figure 21.11.

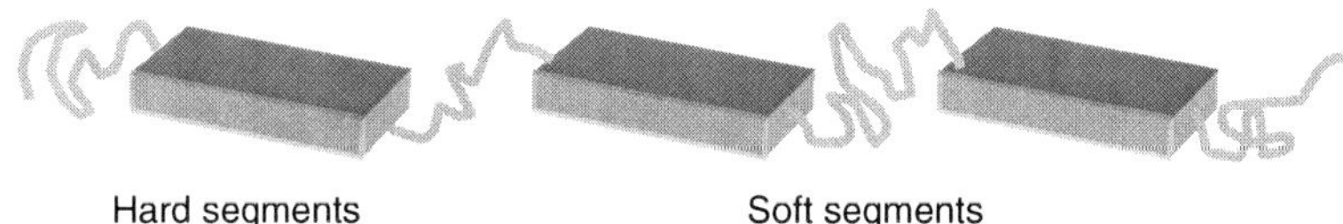

FIGURE 21.9 Schematic representation of segmented (multiblock) polyurethane.

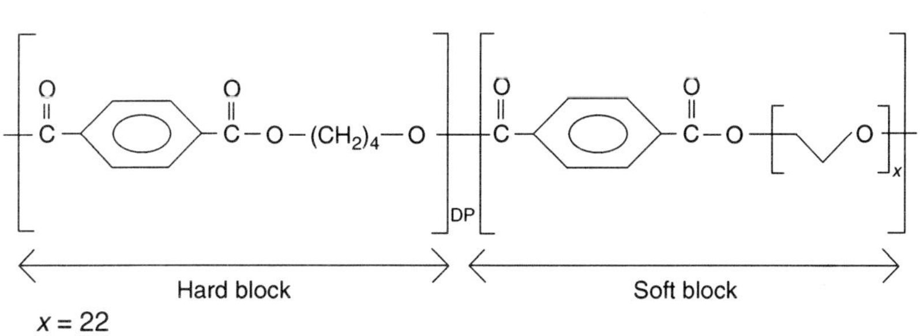

FIGURE 21.10 Schematic representation of multiblock poly(butylene terephthalate) (PBT).

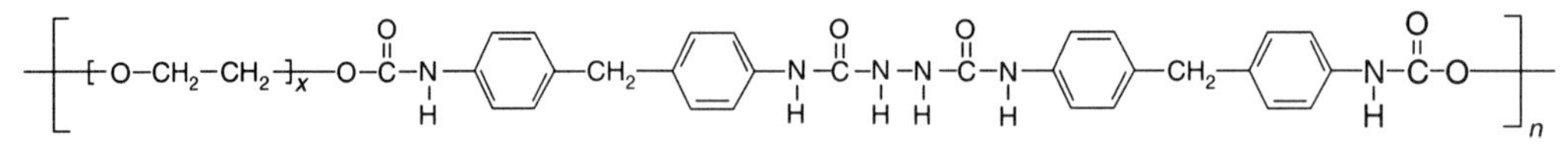

FIGURE 21.11 Schematic representation of TPE structure.

Due to the possibility of tailoring their structure and properties by careful selection of nontoxic monomers (or by using substrates leading to nontoxic by-products), designed biodegradable polyurethane systems are becoming interesting potential materials for cartilage reconstruction [50].

21.4 TISSUE ENGINEERING APPROACH

Current trends in AC regeneration involve the potential use of chondrocytes or chondroprogenitor cells (i.e., mesenchymal stem cells) as a source for TE. Combinations of cells with biodegradable scaffolds and growth factors are widely tested in the context of cartilage regeneration. One of the main issues in the cartilage TE is to design suitable scaffolds. In natural tissues, the extracellular matrix that surrounds cells in the body not only physically supports cells but also regulates their proliferation, differentiation, and morphogenesis. A scaffold, therefore, needs to provide the necessary support for cells to proliferate and maintain their differentiated functions. Ideally, a scaffold should have the following characteristics: (i) 3D and highly porous structure with an interconnected pore network for cell growth and transport of nutrients and metabolic wastes, (ii) biocompatible and bioresorbable with a controllable degradation and resorption rate to match cell or tissue growth *in vitro* and *in vivo*, (iii) suitable surface chemistry for cell attachment, proliferation, and differentiation, and (iv) mechanical properties to match those of the tissue at the site of implantation.

Three-dimensional scaffolds must support the loading of an appropriate cell source to allow successful infiltration and attachment in conjunction with appropriate bioactive molecules in order to promote cellular differentiation and maturation. Scaffolds could be modified with cell adhesion peptides, which show some promise of cell specificity. To make scaffolds more cell-friendly, the hydroxyl, carboxyl, and amine groups could be used on their surface to facilitate the attachment of peptides or biological molecules. Additionally, the presence of protein growth factors in the scaffold might stimulate differentiation and metabolism of the cells. Common growth factors are TGF-b and bone morphogenetic protein (BMP).

Two main types of polymeric materials used for scaffolds in AC regeneration—natural and synthetic biomaterials.

Collagen, fibrin, hyaluronan, alginate, starch, and chitosan-based matrices are among the most popular natural scaffold materials as they offer a substrate that would normally be found in the structure of native AC. Collagen (Figure 21.12) is a main component of the extracellular matrices of many tissues including skin, cartilage, bone, and ligaments. This fibrous polypeptide is mainly composed of glycine, proline, and hydroxyproline aminoacids. Fibrin can be produced from patient's own blood [51]. Alginate and chitosan are polysaccharides. Alginate can be obtained from brown algae while chitosan (Figure 21.13) from chitin by a deacetylation process. Chitin, however, is derived from the exoskeletons of crustaceans (shrimp, crab, and other shellfish).

With natural materials one may face problems of immunogenic compatibility, batch inconsistency, and low mechanical strength. Specifically engineered collagen-based scaffolds combined with unique peptide technology are currently offered to treat cartilage defects. However, the resulting materials are far away from the ideal cartilage.

Most of the mentioned natural polymers could be used in gel form. This is a significant advantage because the cell can be added to the scaffold made of gels and injected into the body before the material gelation. Then, the gel can be hardened by altering the pH of the solution [52] or by light agitation [53], allowing the scaffold to fill out the defect in the tissue. This TE approach does not require large incision to delivery cell with solid scaffolds into the body.

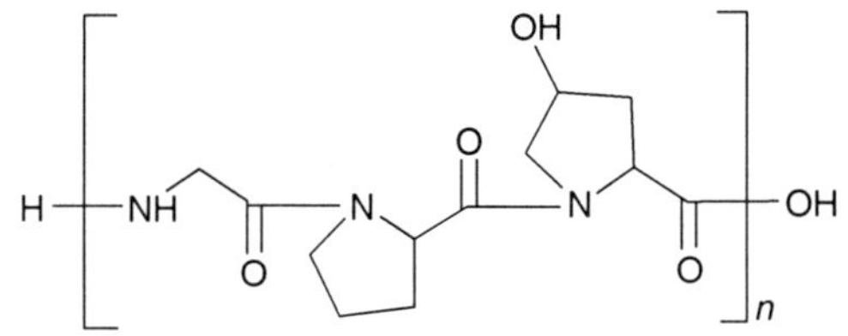

FIGURE 21.12   Chemical structure of collagen.

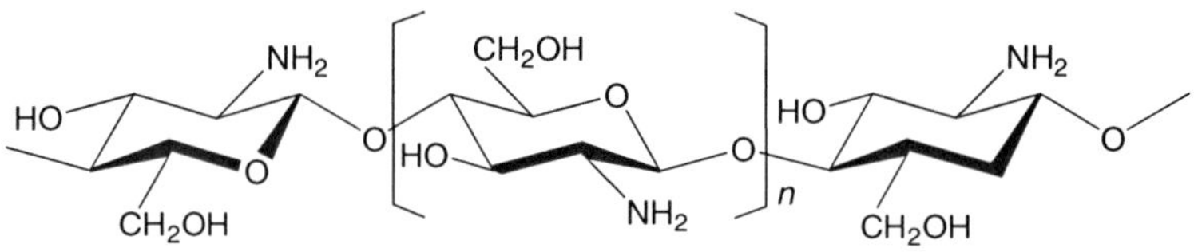

FIGURE 21.13   Chemical structure of chitosan.

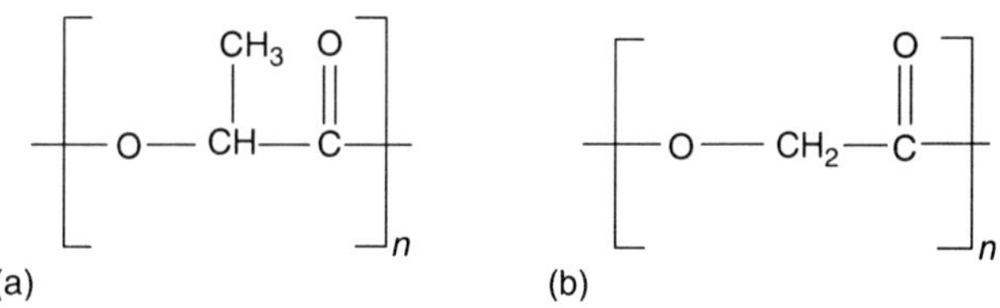

FIGURE 21.14   Chemical structure of (a) poly(lactic acid) and (b) poly(glycolic acid).

The most frequently used biodegradable and bioresorbable synthetic polymers are poly(glycolic acid) (PGA), PLA (Figure 21.14), and their copolymers, such as poly(lactic-*co*-glycolic acid) (PLGA). In addition, PLA can exist as two stereoisomers poly(L-lactic acid) (PLLA) and poly(D-lactide) (PDLA) or as a racemic mixture poly(DL-lactide) (PDLLA).

These biodegradable polymers offer the advantages such as good biocompatibility, biodegradability, bioresorbability, combined with required mechanical properties. Mechanical properties of these polymers, such as reaction to compression, are similar to normal beef cartilage. Moreover, they can be tailored to a wider range of properties and easily formed into the final products. The most important feature is that FDA has approved the use of these polymers in human body for medical and pharmaceutical purposes. The PLA, PGA, and their copolymers are biodegraded into lactic and glycolic acids and are then metabolized and excreted from the body as energy, carbon dioxide, and water. PLA is more water-repellent than PGA. This material is less crystalline and more slowly degrades. However, like cartilage, which is glassy, it is characterized by high crystallinity [54,55]. Synthetic poly-α-hydroxy ester substrates in the form of PGA- and PLLA-based scaffolds have shown to enhance the promotion of proteoglycans, chondrocyte proliferation, differentiation, and maturation in comparison to collagen-based scaffolds [56]. To improve the bioactivity of the synthetic materials, they are used very often in combination with natural HA or collagen [57].

TPE based on hydrophilic poly(ethylene glycol)-terephthalate (PEGT) and hydrophobic PBT block can also be used as carrier materials (scaffolds) for AC repair. The tensile modulus (E) and tensile strength for 300/55/45 (PEG/PEGT/PBT) copolymer are 187.5 and 15.3 MPa, respectively, while for 1000/70/30 they are about 34 and 5.3 MPa [46].

Synthetic scaffolds can be also produced from biodegradable elastomeric polyurethanes, which showed evidence as materials of high cell and tissue compatibility [58]. The biodegradable porous polyurethane scaffolds are characterized by high stimulation of seeded cells. These materials also stimulate the growth and biosynthetic activity of joint chondrocytes and maintain the varied

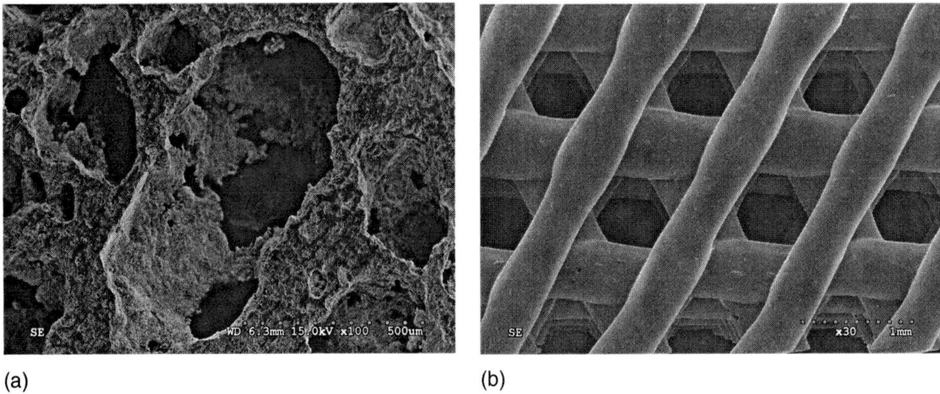

(a)   (b)

FIGURE 21.15   (a) Porous titanium scaffold made by powder sintering and (b) polymeric scaffold made using fusion deposition modeling (FDM) by group of D. Hutmacher (National University of Singapore).

phenotypes. This is due to profitable mechanical proprieties, durability, elasticity, and the controlled surface hydrophobicity of polyurethane scaffolds. In addition, the biodegradable polyurethanes show a relatively low *in vitro* degradation rate, which follows a low rate of changes within the chondral tissue [58]. Current research shows that 3D scaffolds prepared from linear, biodegradable polyurethanes can be used as chondrocytes carrier [59]; however, this is not an ideal scaffold.

In the majority of the TE approaches, the above-mentioned materials were used to produce 3D highly porous scaffolds for the cells. The high porosity is obtained by several methods, such as freezing–thawing, salt or ice leaching, casting, foaming, sintering (Figure 21.15a), solid freeform fabrication or rapid prototyping (Figure 21.15b), and fiber bonding.

When the cartilage defect is accompanied by subchondral bone, the regeneration of the so-called osteochondral defect requires the usage of a hybrid or biphasic scaffold, which has a specifically designed cartilage compartment and a bone compartment [60]. Swieszkowski et al. [61] analyzed two types of hybrid scaffolds: (i) the first biphasic scaffold consisting of fibrin (cartilage phase) and poly(ε-caprolactone) (PCL) (bone phase); (ii) the second type of scaffold using PCL as a cartilage phase and PCL–TCP as a bone phase. The fusion deposition modeling (FDM) was used for scaffolds fabrication (Figure 21.15b). The results of *in vivo* animal studies demonstrated that the porous PCL and PCL–TCP scaffolds promoted bone healing. Integration of a regenerated cartilage with native one was problematic. A better cartilage regeneration was obtained when the PCL scaffold has been used.

Application of PLGA microspheres in TE was also reported [62]. The characteristics of cartilage-like tissue as a result of PLGA microspheres–chondrocyte arrangement showed to be very similar *in vitro* to properties of natural tissue, and they can find applications in TE [62].

21.5   TOTAL JOINT REPLACEMENT

When AC is severely damaged because of a trauma or diseases such as osteoarthritis or rheumatoid arthritis, the total joint replacement (TJR) is the most widely used treatment method.

TJRs are designed to mimic the anatomical joint structure and function as much as possible using available engineering techniques and materials. The affected and painful joint surfaces are removed and replaced by two components, which restore the concave and convex geometry of articulating surface of natural joint. The concave component material consists mainly of the ultra high–molecular weight polyethylene (UHMWPE).

UHMWPE was classified as a form of high-density polyethylene (HDPE) in the early 1960s [63]. It has been fabricated using the Ziegler process [64]. UHMWPE has a molecular weight ranging between 3.1 and 5.67 g/mol million. For comparison, the molecular weight of HDPE is lower than

200,000 g/mol. The high molecular weight results in a high resistance to deformation and significantly higher abrasion and wear resistance compared with HDPE (Table 21.1). The volumetric wear rate for HDPE might be four times higher than UHMWPE [65].

UHMWPE, after approval by FDA in the year 2000, can be replaced by a highly cross-linked and thermally stabilized UHMWPE that has recently become the most widely used alternative to conventional UHMWPE for hip arthroplasty. Cross-linking is a process in which polyethylene molecules are bonded together to form a stronger material (Table 21.2) [66], with substantially improved wear resistance. Such materials are processed by irradiation with a total dose ranging from 50 to 105 kGy. Radiation cross-linking has been performed using gamma and electron beam radiations with the polymer in the solid or molten state. Recently, a postirradiation thermal treatment of irradiated UHMWPE is strongly recommended to improve polymer resistance to long-term oxidative degradation. The ionizing radiation reduces the concentration of free radicals in the polymer, which are responsible for the polymer oxidation.

TABLE 21.1

Physical Properties of High-Density Polyethylene (HDPE) and Ultra High–Molecular Weight Polyethylene (UHMWPE)

Property	HDPE	UHMWPE
Molecular weight (10^6 g/mol)	0.05–0.25	2–6
Melting temperature (°C)	130–137	125–138
Poisson's ratio	0.40	0.46
Specific gravity	0.952–0.965	0.932–0.945
Tensile modulus of elasticity* (GPa)	0.4–4.0	0.8–1.6
Tensile yield strength* (MPa)	26–33	21–28
Tensile ultimate strength* (MPa)	22–31	39–48
Tensile ultimate elongation* (%)	10–1200	350–525
Impact strength, Izod* (J/m of notch; 3.175 mm thick specimen)	21–214	>1070 (no break)
Degree of crystallinity (%)	60–80	39–75

Source: Adapted from Kurtz, S.M., in *Total Joint Replacement*, Elsevier Science & Technology, San Diego, CA, 2004. With permission.

TABLE 21.2

Physical Properties of Cross-Linked Ultra High–Molecular Weight Polyethylene

Property	Cross-Linked UHMWPE
Melting temperature (°C)	135.8 ± 5.6
Tensile modulus of elasticity* (MPa)	860 ± 206
Tensile yield strength* (MPa)	321.1 ± 2.5
Tensile ultimate strength* (MPa)	29.3 ± 7.7
Tensile elongation at fracture (%)	212 ± 61
Degree of crystallinity (%)	245.3 ± 5.3

Source: Adapted from Lewis, G., *Biomaterials*, 22, 371–401, 2001. With permission.

For convex side of the artificial joint, metals (titanium or CoCr alloys) or ceramic (aluminum ceramic) components are used. These components are equipped with short or long stems, which can be fixed to the trabecular bone by means of bone ingrowth to a porous surface with or without porous hydroxyapatite (HA) coating or by means of poly(methyl methacrylate) (PMMA) cement [67]. To fixate the prosthetic components, a surgeon has to remove not only affected and painful joint surfaces but also much of the healthy bone [68].

Although millions of TJRs are performed annually to improve quality of life of the patients, despite the early and mid-range follow-up good results of the human load–bearing joint replacement, the complications of artificial joint are inevitable, with an incidence of approximately 14% in 12–15 years after shoulder replacement and up to 70% of the total hip replacements (THR) after 10 years or less. The complications result in pain, reduction of the range of joint movements, loosening of components, and finally in a revision operation [33].

One of the main reasons of these complications is the failure or degradation of the implant biomaterials. The biomaterials such as metals and polymers (synthetic or natural), ceramics and their composites degrade and lose their original properties due to exposure to *in vivo* conditions [67]. The implant biomaterials subjected to highly demanding conditions such as high stresses and high cyclic loadings, coupled with aggressive body environment, degrade in time, losing their properties such as strength and wear or corrosion resistance. The undesirable degradation takes place in the form of wear, corrosion, deformation, creep, fatigue, fractures, and oxidation of the biomaterials. Despite all the progresses made in regenerative medicine, these phenomena are recognized as major factors limiting the success of the TJR.

Abrasion, burnishing, pitting, erosion, and delamination were found to be the most predominant modes of *in vivo* degradation (wear and cold flow) of polyethylene in TJR. From the scanning electron micrographs of the exposed surfaces of the retrievals, it was found that fine multidirectional scratches were dominant (Figure 21.16a). In addition to the scratches, flakes and rim erosion are also observed. Two implants revealed pitting areas and surface microcracks, which most likely resulted from subsurface fatigue. Polyethylene delamination was observed for metal-backed component. Some of the implants were completely worn out, in some places, to the metal backing.

In vivo degradation products such as particulate and ionic wear and corrosion debris cause aggressive biologic response that can lead to synovitis, periprosthetic bone loss, and aseptic loosening of the implants [67]. The polyethylene wear particles migrate into the periprosthetic spaces and stimulate the activity of the macrophages by the release of cytokines, which activate the osteoclasts,

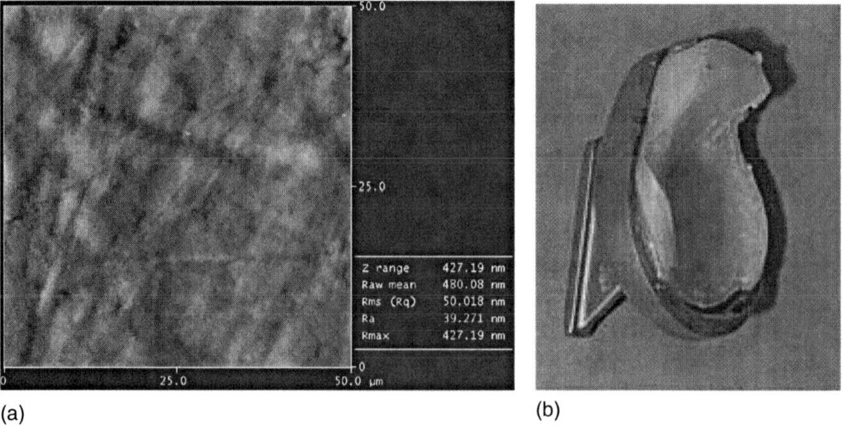

(a)   (b)

FIGURE 21.16 Atomic force microscope (AFM) image of (a) the polyethylene surface with multidirectional scratches and (b) degradation and wear of the glenoid component.

and these osteoclasts lead, in the long term, to the bone resorption around the prosthesis [68]. Increased concentrations of circulating metal-degradation products of fretting corrosion of the metallic implants may also induce the bone resorption and have deleterious biological effects over the long term [69]. Additionally to these negative biological effects, deformation and damage of the implant materials disturb the stabilizing function of the implant. It was found, for instance, that glenohumeral instability after arthroplasty was associated with the wear of the glenoid component [70] (Figure 21.16b).

There are many factors that influence the material wear and degradation in TJRs (Figure 21.17). Design and manufacturing process takes into account geometry of the prostheses, surface roughness, loading characteristics, and lubrication condition. By comparing anatomical and artificial joints, it can be concluded that while healthy human joints are lubricated by fluid film, all current artificial joints with relatively hard-bearing surfaces are lubricated by the boundary and mixed lubrication, which results in wear, and consequently wear debris from articulating surfaces [71]. Among the material factors, the material properties are crucial. However, details of manufacturing process, sterilization, and handling may profoundly alter these properties. Design of the artificial joints is of paramount importance. Insufficient thickness of the polyethylene component influences wear of the TJRs.

Bartel et al. [72] indicated that in order to minimize wear, a minimum thickness of 8–10 mm should be chosen for tibia component and 6–8 mm for acetabular components. Contact surface geometry described by radial clearance (or degree of conformity) between the radii of curvature of the articulating surfaces of components is another geometrical factor affecting the wear of implants. Low joint conformity might result in high contact stresses and could contribute to faster implant wear and failure. Swieszkowski et al. [73] reported that the peak stress generated in nonconforming glenoid components under conditions of normal living can be as high as 25 MPa; since this exceeds the polyethylene yield strength deformation, wear of the components can be expected.

The major factor responsible for the failure of polyethylene implants is oxidative degradation of polymer induced by sterilization with γ-irradiation. The irradiation results in the generation of free radicals in polyethylene. These free radicals may react with oxygen that could diffuse into polyethylene during shelf storage or *in vivo*, causing the polymeric chain scission, which in turn, will lower the molecular weight of PE, increase the density, stiffness, and brittleness, and reduce the fracture strength and elongation to failure. Any of these changes could dramatically affect the wear resistance [63].

Material fatigue could be the reason of the subsurface cracking in the polyethylene components of the knee implants. These cracks very often propagate to the surface of the implants, causing the fracture of the polymeric components. The fatigue and structure defects of the biomaterials may

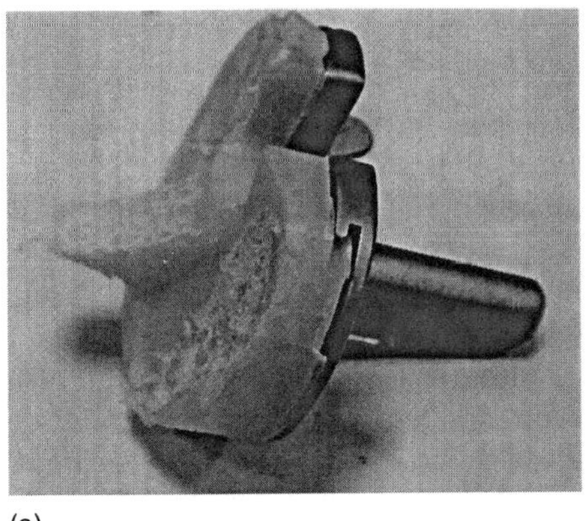

(a)

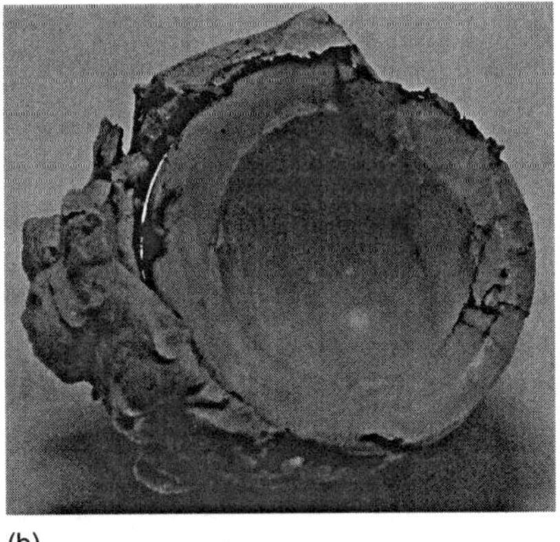

(b)

FIGURE 21.17 Wear, oxidation, and fracture of the (a) tibia and (b) acetabular components.

result in the fracture of the metallic stem in the THR. Aggressive fatigue loading of cemented artificial joints is responsible for the formation of microcracks in bone cement and stem/bone micromotions [67].

Another issue is related to the fact that after insertion of prosthesis–a bone, prosthesis structure is a composite one. It consists of bonded elements with different elastic and geometrical properties. These differences result in an altered load distribution in the artificial joint, as compared to the natural one [67]. In natural joints, the loads are distributed over the entire cross-section of the proximal part of the bone (i.e., femur). In the case of an artificial joint, the load is partially transformed by shear forces across the bone–cement–prosthesis interfaces. This altered load transfer leads to increased stresses at the cement–prosthesis interface and unloading of the bone away from prosthesis. The interface shear stresses are further increased due to the stiffness ratio between the prosthesis and the bone, typically at the order of 10:1 and higher. In addition, the bending displacements in the bone surrounding the stem are reduced because of relatively high flexural stiffness of the prosthesis. The change in load distribution increases the stress in some regions and reduces it in other regions. Areas with higher loads may experience an increase in bone mass, while areas with reduced load may experience a decrease. Moreover, for an inadequate proximal fit of the stem, either initially as an effect of bone preparation, or gradually postoperatively as the effect of stem subsidence, the proximal load transfer is bypassed in favor of distal one. This bypass mechanism as well as stress shielding causes failure of the arthroplasty [67].

To improve joint replacement in terms of long-term component fixation and wear properties, future work should also be concentrated on the design of advanced prosthetic materials, which will better mimic AC properties [33], such as water content, stiffness, shock absorption, promoting fluid film lubrication, and low coefficient of friction.

One of the biomaterial design conflicts is between mechanical and biological compatibilities. Many load-bearing implants require materials with a strength and durability stronger than bone, because the implant lacks the ability of living bone to repair localized damage due to fatigue or overloading. Strong materials should

- distribute high static and repetitive dynamic loads (up to 2500 N);
- protect the cancellous bone from high stresses; and
- allow to obtain a firm attachment to the underlying bones, leading to a long-term fixation.

On the other hand, soft material for bearing is needed to

- improve wear properties of bearing surfaces in TJR;
- provide a smooth, lubricated surface with fluid film and low coefficient of frictions;
- reduce nominal contact pressure; and
- increase joint congruence.

The soft material and its elastic deformation have been found to be the most significant factor in the prediction of the film fluid and low friction capability in artificial joints [71]. Cushion articulating surfaces consisting of low elastic modulus materials, which can articulate with full fluid film lubrication, are needed to mimic the natural lubrication of the joint where synovial fluid lubricates the bone cartilage interface [74]. Moreover, when the fluid film breaks down, such as during periods of heavy loading with little movement or at the start of movement, this biomaterial must give low friction and a low wear rate in these conditions of mixed or boundary lubrication. Recent studies have shown that polyurethane as a soft bearing material, which is articulated against a highly polished metallic surface, provides a lower coefficient of friction as compared with standard polyethylene versus metal bearings [75]. When polyurethane was replaced with water-swollen hydrogel, the friction was considerably reduced [76].

It can be concluded that the most appropriate design for load-bearing artificial joints would be an advanced material, which will be soft as well as strong enough. In comparison with homogeneous materials, composites offer a variety of advantages, which can be useful during the design of the advanced material. These include the possibility for engineers to exercise considerable control over material properties. By varying the type and distribution of the reinforcing phase in the composite, it is possible to obtain a wide range of elastic properties to enable better mechanical compatibility with bone and the other tissue while maintaining high strength and durability.

21.6 SUMMARY

The human body is generally adoptive to the articular joints; however, these joints must satisfy a long list of requirements that can be met with the application of several materials formed into composite structures. By gradually changing the material combinations, volume fractions and anisotropy at different locations, very effective and efficient structures can be produced. Articular cartilage can be modeled as a fiber-reinforced, porous, permeable composite material. Fluid-filled, porous engineering materials can be used to reconstruct the subchondral bone properties. Presently, it is not possible to replace these structures with the same effectiveness by engineering materials and designs. When the AC and subchondral bone layers are resected in human joint arthroplasty, the biomaterials (i.e., metal and polyethylene) used to replace and mimic them do not fulfill properties and functions of natural composite structures. Existing differences between natural and artificial materials can be the reason for unsatisfactory results of TJRs. Complications occur over several years, as a result of the introduction of interfaces, decreased lubrication properties, and changed load distribution. Structure and properties of the cartilage and subchondral bone should be restored in prosthesis design.

Currently, most of the repair strategies meet the aim to regenerate defected AC, although, many fail to prevent future degeneration of the repaired surrounding host tissues. The repair tissue is often of a fibrocartilaginous nature without the zonal organization of AC. Where hyaline cartilage is produced, it is often of an immature nature and does not have a true articular surface.

Future research may need to focus on the combination of biodegradable scaffolds and autologous cells to produce a mechanically functional hyaline repair tissue. The advanced materials (i.e., fiber-reinforced composites or other hybrid materials) fabricated using modern, rapid manufacturing techniques and nanotechnologies may offer new opportunities. These materials should better mimic the functional, physical, and mechanical behavior of tissues in anatomical joints.

ACKNOWLEDGMENTS

We would like to thank Prof D. Hutmacher for his inspiration and sharing his knowledge in tissue engineering with us.

REFERENCES

1. Reis R.L., *Biodegradable Materials in Tissue Engineering and Regenerative Medicine*, John Andrews, New York, 2004.
2. Temenoff J.S., Mikos A.G., Review: tissue engineering for regeneration of articular cartilage, *Biomaterials*, 2000 (21), 431–440.
3. Zdebiak P., El Fray M., The perspectives of polymeric hydrogels and thermoplastic elastomers as cartilage–like materials, *Inżynieria Biomateriałów*, 2006 (54–55), 27–35.
4. Mow V.C., Ratcliffe A., Structure and function of articular cartilage and meniscus. In: Mow V.C., Hayes W.C., eds. *Basic Orthopaedic Biomechanics*, Lippincott-Raven Publisher, Philadelphia, PA, 1997, 113–177.
5. Chen A.C., Bae W.C., Schinagl R.M., Sah R.L., Depth- and strain-dependent mechanical and electromechanical properties of full-thickness bovine articular cartilage in confined compression, *J. Biomech.*, 2001 (34), 1–12.

6. Mow V.C., Ateshian G.A., Lubrication and wear of diarthrodial joints. In: Van C.M., Wilson C.H., eds. *Basic Orthopaedic Biomechanics*, 2nd ed., Lippincott-Raven Publisher, Philadelphia, PA, 1997, 275–317.

7. Redman S.N., Oldfield S.F., Archer C.W., Current strategies for articular cartilage repair, *Eur. Cell. Mater.*, 2005 (9), 23–32.

8. Jin Z.M., Dowson D., Fisher J., Ohtsuki N., Murakami T., Higaki H., Moriyama S., Prediction of transient lubricating film thickness in knee prostheses with compliant layers, *Proc. Inst. Mech. Eng.* [H], 1998 (212), 157–164.

9. Chang R.W., Falconer J., Stulberg S.D., Arnold W.J., Manheim L.M., Dyer A.R., A randomized, controlled trial of arthroscopic surgery versus closed-needle joint lavage for patients with osteoarthritis of the knee, *Arthritis Rheum.*, 1993 (36), 289–296.

10. Langer F., Gross A.E., West M., Urovitz E.P., The immunogenicity of allograft knee joint transplants, *Clin. Orthop.*, 1978 (132), 155–162.

11. Hasegawa M., Sudo A., Shikinami Y., Uchida A., Biological performance of a three-dimensional fabric as artificial cartilage in the repair of large osteochondral defects in rabbit, *Biomaterials*, 1999 (20), 1969–1975.

12. Noguchi T., Yamamuro T., Oka M., Kamur P., Kotoura Y., Hyon S., Ikada Y., Poly(vinyl alcohol) hydrogel as an artificial articular cartilage: evaluation of biocompatibility, *J. Appl. Biomat.*, 1991, 2(2), 101–107.

13. Oka M., Chang Y.-S., Nakamura T., Ushio K., Toguchida J., Gu H.-O., Synthetic osteochondral replacement of the femoral articular surface, *J. Bone Join. Surg. B*, 1997, 79(6), 1003–1007.

14. Meyer C., Horas U., Horbelt R., Schnettler R., Dislocation of artificial cartilage (SaluCartialge), *Unfallchirurg*, 2005, 108(2), 163–166.

15. Drury J.L., Mooney D.J., Hydrogels for tissue engineering: scaffold design variables and applications, *Biomaterials*, 2003 (24), 4337–4351.

16. Hoffman A.S., Hydrogels for biomedical application, *Adv. Drug Deliv. Rev.*, 2002 (43), 3–12.

17. Thomas J., Lowman A., Marcolongo M., Novel associated hydrogels for nucleus pulposus replacement, *J. Biomed. Res.*, 2003 (67A), 1329–1337.

18. Bray J.C., Merrill E.W., Poly(vinyl alcohol) hydrogels for synthetic articular cartilage material, *J. Biomed. Mater. Res.*, 1973 (7), 431–443.

19. Hennink W.E., Van Nostrum C.F., Novel crosslinking methods to design hydrogels, *Adv. Drug Deliv. Rev.*, 2002 (54), 13–36.

20. Osada Y., Kajiwara K., *Gels Handbook*, Academic Press, San Diego, CA, 2001.

21. Hassan Ch.M., Peppas N.A., Structure and application of poly(vinyl alcohol) hydrogels produced by conventional crosslinking or by freezing/thawing methods, *Adv. Polym. Sci.*, 2000 (153), 37–65.

22. Cauich-Rodriguez J.V., Deb S., Smith R., Effect of cross-linking agents on the dynamic mechanical properties of hydrogel blends of poly(acrylic acid)-poly(vinyl alcohol-vinyl acetate), *Biomaterials*, 1996 (17), 2259–2264.

23. Anseth K.S., Bowman C.N., Brannon-Peppas L., Mechanical properties of hydrogels and their experimental determination, *Biomaterials*, 1996 (17), 1647–1657.

24. Ajji Z., Preparation of poly(vinyl alcohol) hydrogels containing citric or succinic acid using gamma radiation, *Radiat. Phys. Chem.*, 2005 (74), 36–41.

25. Sperinde J.J., Griffith L.G., Synthesis and characterization of enzymatically-cross-linked poly(ethylene glycol) Hydrogels, *Macromolecules*, 1997 (30), 5255–5264.

26. Stauffer S.R., Peppas N.A., Poly(vinyl alcohol) hydrogels prepared by freezing-thawing cyclic processing, *Polymer*, 1992 (33), 3932.

27. Peppas N.A., Turbidimetric studies of aqueous PVA solutions, *Makromol. Chem.*, 1975 (176), 3433.

28. Hickey A.S., Peppas N.A., Mesh size and diffusive characteristics of semicrystalline poly(vinyl alcohol) membranes prepared by freezing/thawing techniques, *J. Membr. Sci.*, 1995 (107), 229.

29. Lozinsky V.I., Solodova E.V., Zubov A.L., Simenel I.A., Study of cryostructuration of polymer systems XI. The formation of PVA cryogels by freezing-thawing the polymer aqueous solutions containing additives of some polyols, *J. App. Polym. Sci.*, 1995 (58), 171.

30. Ariga O., Kato M., Sano T., Nakazawa Y., Sano Y., Mechanical and kinetic properties of PVA hydrogel immobilizing–galactosidase, *J. Ferment. Bioeng.*, 1993, 76(3), 203–206.

31. Ku D.N., Braddon L.G., Wootton D.M., Poly(vinyl alcohol) cryogel, US Patent No. 5,981,826, 1999.

32. Stammen J.A., Williams S., Ku D.N., Guldberg R.E., Mechanical properties of a novel PVA hydrogel in shear and unconfined compression, *Biomaterials* 2001 (22), 799–806.

33. Swieszkowski W., Ku D., Bersee H., Kurzydlowski K.J., An elastic material for cartilage replacement in arthritic shoulder joint, *Biomaterials*, 2006 (27), 1534–1541.

34. Grant C., Twigg P., Egan A., Moody A., Smith A., Eagland D., Crowther N., Britland S., Poly(vinyl alcohol) hydrogel as a biocompatible viscoelastic mimetic for articular cartilage, *Biotechnol. Prog.*, 2006, 22(5), 1400–1406.

35. El Fray M., Pilaszkiewicz A., Swieszkowski W., Kurzydlowski K.J., Polymer hydrogel and method of preparation thereof. Polish Patent Pending P 378849 (2006) 1–10.

36. Pilaszkiewicz A., El Fray M., Święszkowski W., Kurzydłowski K.J., Chemically and physically cross-linked poly(vinyl alcohol) hydrogels for cartilage repair, *E Polymer.*, 2005, P_013, 1–6.

37. El Fray M., Pilaszkiewicz A., Swieszkowski W., Kurzydlowski K.J., Morphology assessment of chemically modified and cryostructured poly(vinyl alcohol) hydrogel, *Eur. Polym. J.*, submitted.

38. Lozinsky V.I., Cryotropic gelation of poly(vinyl alcohol) solutions, *Russ. Chem. Rev.*, 1998 (67), 573–586.

39. Watase M., Nishhinari K., Thermal and rheological properties of poly(vinyl alcohol) hydrogels prepared by repeated cycles of freezing and thawing, *Makromol. Chem.*, 1988 (189), 871–880.

40. Giusti P., Lazzeri L., Barbani N., Narducci P., Bonaretii A., Palla M., Lelli L., Hydrogels of poly(vinyl alcohol) and collagen as new bioartificial materials, *J. Mater. Sci. Mat. Med.*, 1993 (4), 538–542.

41. Minchewa R., Manalova N., Sabov R., Kjurkchiev G., Rashkov I., Hydrogels from chitosan crosslinked with poly(ethylene glycol) diacid as bone regeneration materials, *E Polymer*, 058 2004.

42. Filmon R., Basle M.F., Barbier A., Chappard D., Poly(2-hydroxy ethyl methacrylate)-alkaline phosphatase: a composite biomaterial allowing *in vitro* studies of bisphosphonates on the mineralization process, *J. Biomater. Sci. Polym. Ed.*, 2000 (11), 849–868.

43. Corkhill P.H., Trevett A.S., Tighe B.J., The potential of hydrogels as synthetic articular cartilage, *Proc. Instn. Mech. Eng. Part H, Eng. Med.*, 1990 (204), 147–155.

44. El Fray M., Nanostructured elastomeric biomaterials for soft tissue reconstruction, *Oficyna Wydawnicza Politechniki Warszawskiej, Warszawa* (2003) 1–144.

45. Fakirov S., *Handbook of Condensation Thermoplastic Elastomers*, Wiley-VCH, Verlag GmbH & C., New York, 2005.

46. Van Blitterswijk C.A., van den Brink J., Leenders H., Bakker D., The effect of PEO ratio on degradation, calcification and bone-bonding of PEO/PBT copolymer (polyactive), *Cells Mater.*, 1993 (3), 23–36.

47. Kellomäki M., Paasimaa S., Grijpma D.W., Kolppo K., Törmälä P., *In vitro* degradation of polyactive 1000PEOT70PBT30 devices, *Biomaterials*, 2002 (23), 283–295.

48. Deschamps A.A., Grijpma D.W., Feijen J., Poly(ethylene oxide)/poly(butylene terephthalate) segmented block copolymers: the effect of copolymer composition on physical properties and degradation behavior, *Polymer*, 2001 (42), 9335–9345.

49. Malda J., Woodfeild T.B.F., van der Vloodt F., Kooy F.K., Martens D.E., Tramper J., van Blitterswijk C.A., Rielse J., The effect of PEGT/PBT architecture on oxygen gradients in tissue engineered cartilaginous constructs, *Biomaterials*, 2004 (25), 5773–5780.

50. Chia S.L., Gorna K., Gogolewski S., Alini M., Biodegradable elastomeric polyurethane membranes as chondrocyte carriers for cartilage repair, *Tissue Eng.* (epub 2006 Jun 1).

51. Lee K.Y., Mooney D.J., Review. Hydrogels for tissue engineering, *Chem. Rev.*, 2001, 101(7), 1869–1879.

52. Gentleman E., Nauman E.A., Livesay G.A., Dee K.C., Collagen composite biomaterials resist contraction while allowing development of adipocytic soft tissue *in vitro*, *Tissue Eng.*, 2006, 12(6), 1639–1649.

53. Mann B.K., Gobin A.S., Tsai A.T., Schmedlen R.H., West J.L., Smooth muscle cell growth in photopolymerized hydrogels with cell adhesive and proteolytically degradable domains: synthetic ECM analogs for tissue engineering, *Biomaterials*, 2001, 22(22), 3045–3051.

54. Moran J.M., Pazzano D., Bonassar L.J., Characterization of polylactic acid-polyglycolic acid composites for cartilage tissue engineering, *Tissue Eng.*, 2003 (9), 63–70.

55. Lee C.T., Huang C.-P., Lee Y.-D., Biomimetic porous scaffolds made from poly(L-lactide)-g-chondroitin sulfate blend with poly(L-lactide) for cartilage tissue engineering, *Biomacromolecules*, 2006 (7), 2200–2209.

56. Grande D.A., Halberstadt C., Naughton G., Schwartz R., Manji R., Evaluation of matrix scaffolds for tissue engineering of articular cartilage grafts, *J. Biomed. Mater. Res.*, 1997 (34), 211–220.

57. Yoo H.S., Lee E.A., Yoon J.J., Park T.G., Hyaluronic acid modified biodegradable scaffolds for cartilage tissue engineering, *Biomaterials*, 2005 (26), 1925–1933.

58. Grad S., Kupsik L., Gorna K., Gogolewski S., Alini M., The use of biodegradable polyurethane scaffolds for cartilage tissue engineering: potential and limitations, *Biomaterials*, 2003 (24), 5163–5171.

59. Gorna K., Gogolewski S., Biodegradable porous polyurethane scaffolds for tissue repair and regeneration, *J. Biomed. Mater. Res. Part B*, 2006 (79), 128–138.

60. Gao, T.J., Tuominen T.K., Lindholm T.S., Kommonen B., Lindholm T.C., Morphological and biochemical difference in healing in segmental tibial defects implanted with biocoral or tricalcium phosphate cylinders, *Biomaterials*, 1997 (18), 219–223.

61. Swieszkowski W., Ho S.T.B., Kurzydlowski K.J., Hutmacher D.W., Repair and regeneration of osteochondral defects in the articular joints, *Biomol. Eng.*, 2006 (in press).

62. Mercier N.R., Costantino H.R., Tracy M.A., Bonassar L.J., Poly(lactide–*co*–glycolide) microspheres as a moldable scaffold for cartilage tissue engineering, *Biomaterials*, 2005 (26), 1945–1952.

63. Kurtz S.M., (eds.). *The UHMWPE Handbook. ULTRA-High Molecular Weight Polyethylene in Total Joint Replacement*, Elsevier Science & Technology, San Diego, CA, 2004.

64. Birnkraut H.W., Synthesis of UHMWPE. In *Ultra-High Molecular Weight Polyethylene as a Biomaterial in Orthopedic Surgery*, Eds. Hogrefe & Huber Publishers, 1991.

65. Edidin A.A., Kurtz S.M., The influence of mechanical behavior on the wear of four clinically relevant polymeric biomaterials in a hip simulator, *J. Arthroplasty*, 2000 (15), 321–331.

66. Lewis G., Properties of crosslinked ultra-high molecular weight polyethylene, *Biomaterials*, 2001 (22), 371–401.

67. Huiskes R., Verdondchot N., Biomechanics of the artificial joints: the hip. In: Mow C., Hayes W., eds. *Basic Orthopaedic Biomechanics* 2nd ed., Lippincott-Raven Publisher, Philadelphia, PA, 1997, 395–460.

68. Swieszkowski W., Figurska M., Bersee H.E.N., Kurzydlowski K.J., *In vivo* degradation and wear of biomaterials in total joint replacement, In: Lekszycki T., Maldyk P., eds. *Biomaterials in Orthopaedic Practice*, 2005, 97–115.

69. Shahgaldi B.F., Heatley F.W., Dewar A., Corrin B., *In vivo* corrosion of cobalt-chromium and titanium wear particles, *J. Bone Joint Surg. Br.*, 1995, 77(6), 962–966.

70. Weldon 3rd E.J., Scarlat M.M., Lee S.B., Matsen 3rd F.A., Intrinsic stability of unused and retrieved polyethylene glenoid components, *J. Shoulder Elbow Surg.*, 2001, 10(5), 474–481.

71. Dowson D., Fisher J., Jin Z.M., Auger D.D., Jobbins B., Design considerations for cushion form bearings in artificial hip joints, *Proc. Inst. Mech. Eng.* [H], 1991, 205(2), 59–68.

72. Bartel D.L., Bicknell V.L., Wright T.M., The effect of conformity, thickness, and material on stresses in ultra-high molecular weight components for total joint replacement, *J. Bone Joint Surg. Am.*, 1986, 68(7), 1041–1051.

73. Święszkowski W., Bednarz P., Prendergast P., *Proc. Inst. Mech. Eng., Part H, J. Eng. Med.*, 2003 (217), 49–57.

74. Auger D.D., Dowson D., Fisher J., Cushion form bearings for total knee joint replacement. Part 1: design, friction and lubrication, *Proc. Inst. Mech. Eng.* [H], 1995, 209(2), 73–81.

75. Quigley F.P., Buggy M., Birkinshaw C., Selection of elastomeric materials for compliant-layered total hip arthroplasty, *Proc. Inst. Mech. Eng.* [H], 2002, 216(1), 77–83.

76. Caravia L., Dowson D., Fisher J., Corkhill P.H., Tighe B.J., Friction of hydrogel and polyurethane elastic layers when sliding against each other under a mixed lubrication regime, *Wear*, 1995 (181–183), 236–240.

Index

A

O

Q

R

S